CONTRACEPTIVE TECHNOLOGY

ON

Patty Cason, Carrie Cwiak, Alison Edelman, Deborah Kowal,
Jeanne M. Marrazzo, Anita L. Nelson, Michael S. Policar,
Founding Author: Robert A. Hatcher

JONES & BARTLETT
LEARNING

World Headquarters
Jones & Bartlett Learning
25 Mall Road
Burlington, MA 01803
978-443-5000
info@jblearning.com
www.jblearning.com

Jones & Bartlett Learning books and products are available through most bookstores and online booksellers. To contact Jones & Bartlett Learning directly, call 800-832-0034, fax 978-443-8000, or visit our website, www.jblearning.com.

Substantial discounts on bulk quantities of Jones & Bartlett Learning publications are available to corporations, professional associations, and other qualified organizations. For details and specific discount information, contact the special sales department at Jones & Bartlett Learning via the above contact information or send an email to specialsales@jblearning.com.

ISBN 978-1-284-25503-4 (paperback with Navigate eBook)

ISBN 978-1-284-25506-5 (eBook)

25505-8

Production Credits
Vice President, Product Management: Marisa R. Urbano
Vice President, Content Strategy and Implementation: Christine Emerton
Director, Product Management: Matthew Kane
Product Manager: Tina Chen
Director, Content Management: Donna Gridley
Content Strategist: Carol Brewer Guerrero
Director, Project Management and Content Services: Karen Scott
Manager, Program Management: Kristen Rogers
Program Manager: Dan Stone
Senior Digital Project Specialist: Angela Dooley
Senior Product Marketing Manager: Lindsay White
Content Services Manager: Colleen Lamy
Senior Director of Supply Chain: Ed Schneider
Product Fulfillment Manager: Wendy Kilborn
Composition: S4Carlisle Publishing Services
Cover Design: Briana Yates
Text Design: Kristin E. Parker
Senior Media Development Editor: Troy Liston
Rights & Permissions Manager: John Rusk
Rights Specialist: Maria Leon Maimone
Cover Image (Title Page, Part Opener, Chapter Opener): © Yuri Hoyda/Shutterstock
Printing and Binding: Sheridan Saline

Library of Congress Cataloging-in-Publication Data
Library of Congress Cataloging-in-Publication Data unavailable at time of printing.

LCCN: 2023031587

6048

Printed in the United States of America
27 26 25 24 23 10 9 8 7 6 5 4 3 2 1

Dedication

The editors dedicate this book to its readers, who have continued to provide quality care to their patients in the face of the recent harrowing events—from the pandemic to the June 2022 Supreme Court *Dobbs* ruling. Many of these crises are still rippling through our lives and the lives of those we serve. In spite of this, you are committed to enhancing the health and well-being of those you serve by trying to learn the most current and accurate information about reproductive health. We applaud your dedication.

The editors would also like to acknowledge the profound debt we owe to our authors, who wrote their chapters while juggling extremely busy schedules, teaching, seeing patients, and conducting research. Some wrote chapters while leading the charge in their own states to protect reproductive rights. These hardworking authors prioritized the time to contribute to this book because, at their core, they are committed teachers. They stayed true to the tradition established by those who contributed to earlier editions.

One of these contributors, our late colleague Felicia Hance Stewart (1943–2006), noted at the beginning of the 21st century that we are all "engaged in a critically important and deeply moral undertaking. Reproductive health care enables individuals and couples to make and implement some of the most important decisions that shape their lives, and that also shape society... In sum, reproductive health care makes an essential contribution to the human infrastructure we count on for our society's well-being, opportunity, security, and freedom."[1] We hope that this book will help guide your practice to continue your work as ethically driven, dedicated teachers, clinicians, and champions of reproductive health and freedom.

Respectfully yours,

The Editors of *Contraceptive Technology, Twenty- Second Edition*

---

1 Stewart FH. Preface. In: Hatcher RA, Trussell J Stewart FH, Nelson AL, Cates, Jr. W, Guest F, Kowal D [eds]. Contraceptive technology. Eighteenth revised edition. New York, NY: Ardent Media, Inc., 2004.

Note to Readers:

Words Matter

Words we use have power, and their use can affect our thoughts and actions toward someone else. The authors of *Contraceptive Technology* endeavor to use words that encourage a collaborative and nonlabeling person-centered partnership between provider and client. Within the limitations of the English language and currently accepted grammar, we endeavor to use words of inclusion that respect those we serve, equitably regardless of their gender identity, sexual orientation, ability, racial identity, ethnicity, religion, or income. (Words that label gender identity, sexual orientation, racial identity, ethnicity, or other characteristics have been maintained when citing published studies and documents that report those specific participant characteristics.)

Contents

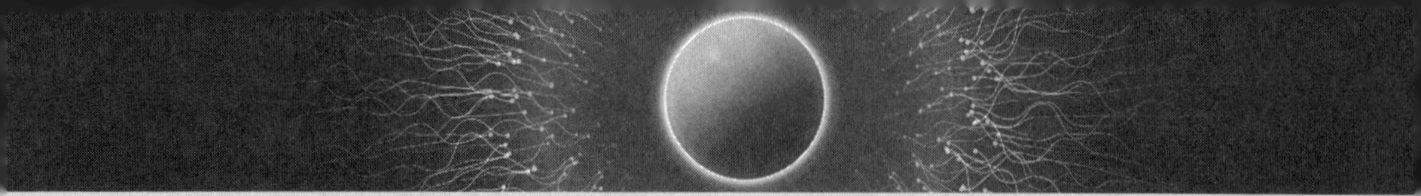

List of Tables

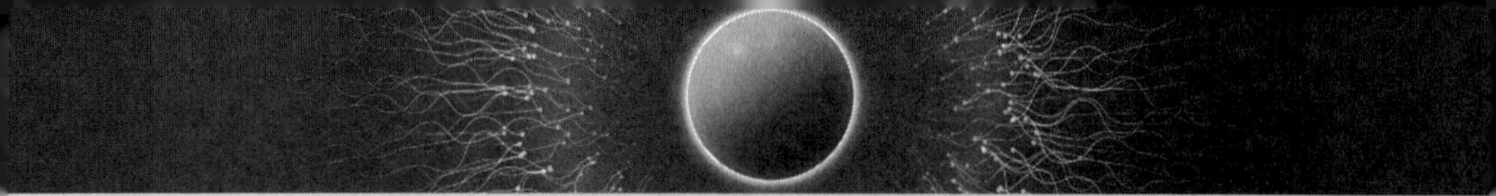

List of Figures

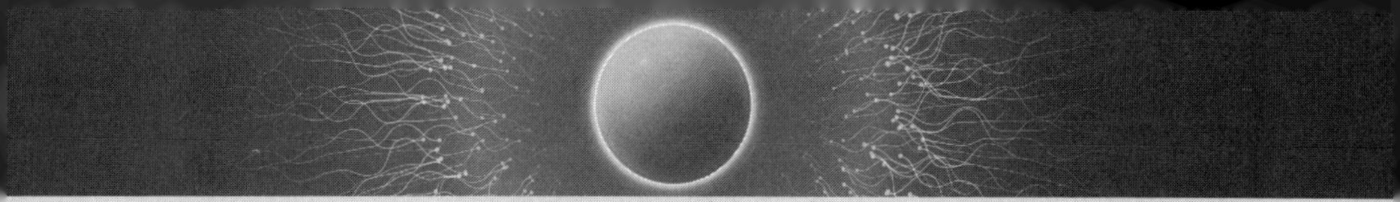

List of Boxes

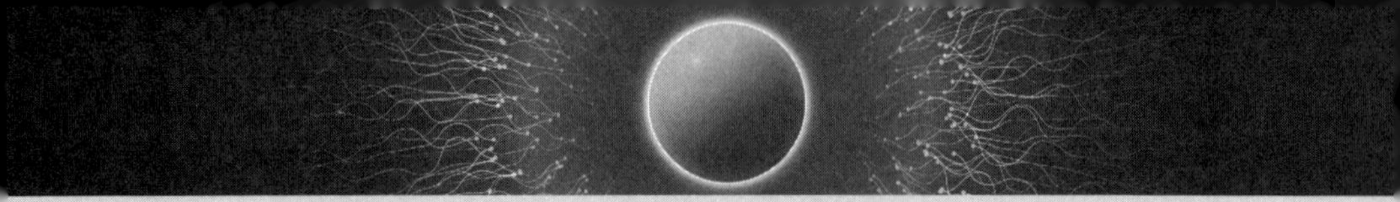

Preface

It's a New Day

Readers of the Twenty-Second Edition of *Contraceptive Technology* are facing a new reality. Family planning changed overnight when the Supreme Court overturned *Roe v. Wade* in the *Dobbs* decision on June 24, 2022. We are now living in a world where many of our clients have lost autonomy with respect to their own bodies, as half of the states in our nation have restricted or criminalized abortion care. As a human right, abortion is an essential option for health care in a world where gender-based inequities in power and violence continue. We recognize that even before this reversal of federal protections, many individuals already faced extreme barriers in accessing the full spectrum of reproductive health care services. As this book goes to press, opponents of abortion continue to use state and federal courts as a means to curtail access to safe, cost-effective medications for abortion care, creating uncertainty and potential danger for pregnant persons and their health care providers.

As we confront restricted options in providing reproductive health care, many family planning providers have grown discouraged. We borrow the optimism of our founding author and senior editor, Robert A. Hatcher, MD, MPH. He says that a sailor once taught him a lesson about the power of resilience in the face of change: "In a gale, I can't change the direction of the wind, but I can adjust my sails." Dr. Hatcher tells us, "We may not be able to change the antiabortion gale winds in the immediate future, but we can adjust a number of things we are doing to increase access to the reproductive care our clients seek."

We cannot know the future, but so far we have seen providers and advocates create networks across state lines to get people the services they want and need. We have heard the voices of millions rise up to object to the human rights violations and harms imposed by the criminalization of reproductive health care.

How can we help individuals for whom a current pregnancy is unacceptable to them—a threat to life, health, and well-being—yet are not able to obtain an abortion? We can enhance some of the things we are doing already: Person-centered counseling helps providers effectively communicate with their clients about fertility, contraception, and being prepared for pregnancy. We can also link clients to safe sources of information. People who have this essential information can make informed choices for themselves.

For those not immediately facing the need for abortion, contraception is our primary tool to prevent pregnancy. Over the years, new contraceptive technologies have been developed that improve effectiveness, convenience, and noncontraceptive benefits. But a wide variety of barriers still persist that limit the potential for individuals to control their own fertility. Full contraceptive access is by no means universal, and people do not always know about all their contraceptive options.

For those seeking to use permanent contraception, implants, and IUDs—the most convenient and effective methods—many barriers persist. Access is paramount. Avoid imposing delays; some ways to streamline contraceptive access include:

- Update consent forms and create policies that do not require that a patient be screened for cervical cancer or STIs prior to placement.
- Ensure all necessary instruments and supplies are available and the schedule is flexible enough to allow same-day placements when that is the patient's preference.
- Create policies and a practice culture that do not discourage uptake.

Individuals must be able to trust that they have control over how they choose to use a given method, and that implants and IUDs can be removed immediately upon request. Reports of side effects deserve serious and prompt attention.

- For injectable contraceptives, expand the use of self-injection of the DMPA Sub-Q version and Quick Start protocols.
- For those seeking pills, patches, or rings:
    - Use Quick Start protocols.
    - Dispense as many cycles as possible—ideally a full year (13 cycles) of supplies.
    - Maintain multiple ways for clients to access prescriptions, refills, and supplies—in office, online, from pharmacists, and soon, over the counter.
- For those using barrier and behavioral methods:
    - Ensure adequate supplies of condoms that fit.
    - Identify apps that are accurate and confidential.
    - Support techniques to improve the effectiveness of coitus interruptus.
    - Expand the availability of over-the-counter methods to enable users of those methods to maximize their contraceptive success.

Consider routinely prescribing and dispensing emergency contraceptive pills (ECPs) in advance of need. This enables the client to have ECPs on hand for immediate use if there are barriers to securing them, and it may lift the burden of out-of-pocket cost off the user's shoulders. Report unprofessional practices if an individual is prevented from obtaining their prescription.

Under restricted and criminalized access to abortion, even those using an effective method may choose to use a second method of contraception, particularly condoms, if they want additional protection against sexually transmitted infections. The stakes for some clients have shifted dramatically.

Early in this publication's life, Dr. Hatcher led the way by distributing free copies of textbooks to legislators, schools, and key opinion leaders; testifying before lawmakers; and ensuring that the voices of his clients were heard in the press. In 1973, Dr. Hatcher served as a co-plaintiff in the lawsuit challenging the Georgia law creating barriers to abortion for women whose life or health was threatened by a pregnancy; the favorable ruling prevailed in appeal to the US Supreme Court (*Doe v. Bolton* 410 U.S. 179 [1973]). In the tradition that Robert Hatcher established 50 years ago with his mimeographed, stapled booklet and through all the editions that followed, this twenty-second edition of *Contraceptive Technology* combines the latest evidence-based information, practice tips, person-centered counseling skills, and client education—with a strong thread of advocacy. As today's authors, editors, and readers carry that torch forward, we reflect on Bob Hatcher's remembrance of William Shakespeare's quote, "What's past is prologue," and his conclusion that the past sets the stage, but we determine what happens next. We remember his promise: "We haven't seen anything yet." There are many more steps we can take to defend reproductive rights, to learn more about and from our clients, to provide the best possible care to all, and to model evidence-based, ethical, morally driven, compassionate, and inclusive care. We hope this book will help readers and their clients achieve these goals.

Patty Cason
Carrie Cwiak
Alison Edelman
Deborah Kowal
Jeanne Marrazzo
Anita Nelson
Michael Policar

With gratitude to Dr. Hatcher for his leadership in the field.

Contributors

Editors

Patty Cason, MS, FNP-BC
Assistant Clinical Professor
UCLA School of Nursing
Envision Sexual and Reproductive Health
Los Angeles, California

Carrie Cwiak, MD, MPH
Professor
Director, Complex Family Planning Division and Fellowship
Department of Gynecology and Obstetrics
Emory University School of Medicine
Atlanta, Georgia

Alison Edelman, MD, MPH
Professor
Director, Complex Family Planning Fellowship
Director, Division of Complex Family Planning
Editor, Cochrane Fertility Regulation Review Group
Oregon Health & Science University
Portland, Oregon

Deborah Kowal, PA, MA
Executive Editor
Contraceptive Technology
Atlanta, Georgia

Jeanne M. Marrazzo, MD, MPH
Director, Division of Infectious Diseases
C. Glenn Cobbs, M.D., Endowed Chair in Infectious Diseases
Executive Vice Chair, Department of Medicine
University of Alabama at Birmingham School of Medicine
Birmingham, Alabama

Anita L. Nelson, MD
Professor, Obstetrics and Gynecology
Western University of Health Sciences Professor
Professor Emeritus, Obstetrics and Gynecology
David Geffen School of Medicine at UCLA
Los Angeles, California

Michael S. Policar, MD, MPH
Professor Emeritus
Obstetrics, Gynecology, and Reproductive Sciences
University of California, San Francisco, School of Medicine
Senior Medical Advisor, California Office of Family Planning
San Francisco, California

Founding Author/Editor: Robert A. Hatcher, MD, MPH
Professor Emeritus
Department of Gynecology and Obstetrics
Emory University School of Medicine
Atlanta, Georgia

Authors

Rebecca H. Allen, MD, MPH
Professor
Department of Obstetrics and Gynecology and Medical Science (Section of Medical Education)
Warren Alpert Medical School of Brown University
Providence, Rhode Island

Maureen K. Baldwin, MD, MPH
Associate Professor
Division of Complex Family Planning
Obstetrics and Gynecology
Oregon Health & Science University
Portland, Oregon

Amanda Y. Black, MD, MPH
Professor
Obstetrics and Gynecology
Dr. Elaine Jolly Chair in Women's Health Research
University of Ottawa
Ottawa, Canada

Sarah E.K. Bradley, PhD, MHS
Public Health Demographer
Washington, DC

Jewel A. Brown, MD
Complex Family Planning Fellow
Department of Obstetrics and Gynecology
University of California Davis
Sacramento, California

Anne E. Burke, MD, MPH
Fellowship Director, CFP
Division Director, Family Planning
Associate Professor, Gynecology and Obstetrics
Johns Hopkins University School of Medicine and Bloomberg School of Public Health
Baltimore, Maryland

Patty Cason, MS, FNP-BC
Assistant Clinical Professor
UCLA School of Nursing
Envision Sexual and Reproductive Health
Los Angeles, California

Beatrice A. Chen, MD, MPH
Associate Professor
Department of Obstetrics, Gynecology, and Reproductive Sciences
University of Pittsburgh
Pittsburgh, Pennsylvania

Melissa J. Chen, MD, MPH
Associate Professor
Division of Complex Family Planning
Department of Obstetrics and Gynecology
University of California, Davis
Sacramento, California

Kelly Cleland, MPA, MPH
Executive Director
American Society for Emergency Contraception
Lawrenceville, New Jersey

Kelly Culwell, MD, MPH
Assistant Clinical Professor
Division of Complex Family Planning
Department of Obstetrics, Gynecology, and Reproductive Services
University of California, San Diego
Head of Research and Development
Sebela Women's Health
San Diego, California

Carrie Cwiak, MD, MPH
Professor
Director, Complex Family Planning Division and Fellowship
Department of Gynecology and Obstetrics
Emory University School of Medicine
Atlanta, Georgia

Nicole Economou, MD, MPH
Assistant Clinical Professor
Division of Complex Family Planning
Department of Obstetrics and Gynecology
University of California, Davis
Sacramento, California

Alison Edelman, MD, MPH
Professor
Director, Complex Family Planning Fellowship
Director, Division of Complex Family Planning
Editor, Cochrane Fertility Regulation Review Group
Oregon Health & Science University
Portland, Oregon

Crystal Goldsmith, MD, MS
Director of Family Planning
Department of Obstetrics and Gynecology
Kaiser Permanente Northern California
Oakland, California

Frances Grimstad, MD, MS
Division of Gynecology
Department of Surgery
Boston Children's Hospital
Assistant Professor of Obstetrics, Gynecology, and Reproductive Biology
Harvard Medical School
Boston, Massachusetts

Leo Han, MD, MPH
Assistant Professor
Division of Family Planning
Department of Obstetrics and Gynecology
Oregon Health & Science University
Portland, Oregon

Miles S. Harris, BSN, MSN, FNP-BC, AAHIVS
Director of Gender-Affirming Care, University of California Davis Health
Health Sciences Assistant Clinical Professor
Betty Irene Moore School of Nursing at UC Davis
Sacramento, California

Jenny A. Higgins, PhD, MPH
Bissel Professor of Reproductive Health, Rights, and Justice
Director, UW Collaborative for Reproductive Equity
Professor of Obstetrics and Gynecology
University of Wisconsin-Madison
Madison, Wisconsin

Melody Y. Hou, MD, MPH
Professor
Clinical Obstetrics and Gynecology
Division of Family Planning
Department of Obstetrics and Gynecology
University of California, Davis School of Medicine
Sacramento, California

Rachel K. Jones, PhD
Principal Research Scientist
Guttmacher Institute
New York, New York

Zoë Julian, MD, MPH, FACOG
Core Faculty Physician
Department of Obstetrics and Gynecology
Wellstar Kennestone Regional Medical Center
Marietta, Georgia

Melissa Kottke, MD, MPH, MBA
Professor
Department of Gynecology and Obstetrics
Director, Jane Fonda Center
Emory University School of Medicine
Atlanta, Georgia

Chance Krempasky, BSN, MSN, WHNP-BC, FNP-BC, AAHIVS
Associate Director of Medicine—Education
Callen-Lorde Community Health Center
Clinical Professor of Nursing
Columbia University School of Nursing
New York, New York

Megan Lawley, MD, MPH
Assistant Professor
Director of Undergraduate Medical Education for GYN/OB
Associate Director, Complex Family Planning Fellowship
Department of Gynecology and Obstetrics
Emory University School of Medicine
Atlanta, Georgia

Jeanne M. Marrazzo, MD, MPH
Director, Division of Infectious Diseases
C. Glenn Cobbs, M.D., Endowed Chair in Infectious Diseases
Executive Vice Chair, Department of Medicine
University of Alabama at Birmingham School of Medicine
Birmingham, Alabama

Samuel Master, DO
Assistant Professor
Department of Pediatrics
Division of Child and Adolescent Health
Columbia University Irving Medical Center
New York, New York

Melissa C. Matulich, MD, MAS
Assistant Professor
Division of Complex Family Planning
Department of Obstetrics and Gynecology
University of California, Davis
Sacramento, California

Biftu Mengesha, MD, MAS
Associate Professor
University of California, San Francisco
Department of Obstetrics, Gynecology, and Reproductive Sciences
San Francisco, California

Elizabeth A. Micks, MD, MPH
Affiliate Associate Professor
Department of Obstetrics and Gynecology
University of Washington
Seattle, Washington

Taniqua A. Miller, MD, MSCP
Menopause Health Expert
Boundless Midlife Health
Atlanta, Georgia

Anita L. Nelson, MD
Professor and Chair
Obstetrics and Gynecology
Western University of Health Sciences Professor
Pomona, California
Emeritus, Obstetrics and Gynecology
David Geffen School of Medicine at UCLA
Los Angeles, California

Brian T. Nguyen, MD, MSc
Program Director, Fellowship in Complex Family Planning
Associate Professor, Department of Obstetrics and Gynecology
Keck School of Medicine, University of Southern California
https://www.theemergelab.com · https://www.malecontraception.center
Los Angeles, California

Siripanth Nippita, MD, MS
Clinical Associate Professor
Director, Division of Family Planning
Department of Obstetrics and Gynecology
NYU Grossman School of Medicine
New York, New York

Talita Oseguera, CNM, WHNP-BC, MSN
Certified Nurse Midwife
CHOICES: Center for Reproductive Health
Memphis, Tennessee

Ina U. Park, MD, MS
Professor
Department of Family and Community Medicine, and
Department of Obstetrics, Gynecology, and Reproductive Sciences
UCSF School of Medicine
San Francisco, California
Medical Consultant, Division of STD Prevention
Centers for Disease Control and Prevention
Atlanta, Georgia

Maureen Paul, MD, MPH
Affiliate staff physician
Department of Obstetrics and Gynecology
Beth Israel Deaconess Medical Center
Boston, Massachusetts

Lola Pellegrino, BSN, MSN, ANP-BE, WHNP-BC
Clinical Director, Women's Health
Callen-Lorde Community Health Center
New York, New York

Michael S. Policar, MD, MPH
Professor Emeritus
Obstetrics, Gynecology, and Reproductive Sciences
University of California, San Francisco, School of Medicine
San Francisco, California
Senior Medical Advisor, California Office of Family Planning
Sacramento, California

Chelsea B. Polis, PhD
Senior Scientist, Epidemiology
Center for Biomedical Research
Population Council
New York, New York

Joely Pritzker, MS, FNP-C
Family Nurse Practitioner
Vista Community Clinic
National Trainer for Envision SRH
Encinitas, California

Shaalini Ramanadhan, MD, MCR
Assistant Professor
Division of Complex Family Planning
Department of Obstetrics and Gynecology
Oregon Health & Science University
Portland, Oregon

Charita L. Roque, MD, MPH
Assistant Professor
Western Michigan University Homer Stryker M.D. School of Medicine
Department of Obstetrics and Gynecology
Kalamazoo, Michigan

Jessica N. Sanders, PhD, MSPH
Family Planning Research Director
Assistant Professor
Obstetrics & Gynecology
Health Sciences Center, University of Utah
Salt Lake City, Utah

John S. Santelli, MD, MPH
Professor
Population and Family Health and Pediatrics
Columbia University
New York, New York

George F. Sawaya, MD
Professor
Obstetrics, Gynecology and Reproductive Sciences
University of California, San Francisco School of Medicine
Director, Colposcopy Clinic
Zuckerberg San Francisco General Hospital
Director, Cervical Dysplasia Clinic
University of California, San Francisco
San Francisco, California

Eleanor Bimla Schwarz, MD, MS
Professor of Medicine
University of California, San Francisco
Chief, Division of General Internal Medicine
San Francisco General Hospital
San Francisco, California

Alexandra Sherman, WHNP-BC, MSCP
Nurse Practitioner
Department of Obstetrics and Gynecology
Emory Healthcare
Atlanta, Georgia

Markus J. Steiner, PhD, MSPH
Senior Epidemiologist
Product Development and Introduction Department
FHI 360
Durham, North Carolina

Riley J. Steiner, PhD, MPH
Senior Director, Research and Evaluation
Power to Decide
Washington, DC

Shivika Trivedi, MD, MSc
Assistant Professor
Department of Obstetrics and Gynecology
University of Chicago School of Medicine
Chicago, Illinois

David Turok, MD, MPH
Professor, Director, ASCENT Center for Reproductive and Sexual Health
Chief, Division of Family Planning
Department of Obstetrics and Gynecology
University of Utah School of Medicine
Salt Lake City, Utah

Rachel Peragallo Urrutia, MD, MS
Associate Professor
Division of General Obstetrics and Gynecology
Department of Obstetrics and Gynecology
University of North Carolina Chapel Hill
Chapel Hill, North Carolina

Jennifer Villavicencio, MD, MPP
Obstetrician-Gynecologist and Complex Family Planning Specialist
Public Policy, Communications & Equity Expert
Washington, DC

Lee Warner, PhD, MPH
Chief, Women's Health and Fertility Branch
Division of Reproductive Health
Centers for Disease Control and Prevention
Atlanta, Georgia

Reviewers

Lauren Abern, MD
Assistant Professor
Department of Gynecology and Obstetrics
Emory University
Atlanta, Georgia

Jessica M. Atrio, MD, MSc
Associate Professor
Director, Complex Family Planning Fellowship
Department of Obstetrics and Gynecology
Albert Einstein College of Medicine
New York, New York

Deborah Bartz, MD, MPH
Associate Professor
Harvard Medical School
Department of Obstetrics and Gynecology
Brigham and Women's Hospital
Boston, Massachusetts

Jewel A. Brown, MD
Complex Family Planning Fellow
Department of Obstetrics and Gynecology
University of California Davis
Sacramento, California

Megan Cohen, MD, MPH
Assistant Professor
Division of Complex Family Planning
Department of Obstetrics and Gynecology
Oregon Health & Science University
Portland, Oregon

Alyssa Colwill, MD, MPH
Assistant Professor
Department of Obstetrics and Gynecology
Oregon Health & Science University
Portland, Oregon

Blair G. Darney, PhD, MPH
Associate Professor
Division of Family Planning
Department of Obstetrics and Gynecology
Oregon Health & Science University
Health Systems & Policy, OHSU/Portland State Univ. School of Public Health
Portland, Oregon

Cristen Dalessandro, PhD
Adjunct Assistant Professor
University of Utah Health
Department of Obstetrics and Gynecology
Division of Family Planning
Salt Lake City, Utah

Christine Dehlendorf, MD, MAS
Professor and Vice Chair for Research, Family and Community Medicine
Director, Person-Centered Reproductive Health Program
Departments of Family and Community Medicine,
Obstetrics, Gynecology and Reproductive Sciences,
and Epidemiology and Biostatistics
University of California, San Francisco
San Francisco, California

Jodie Dionne, MD
Associate Professor of Medicine
Division of Infectious Diseases
University of Alabama at Birmingham Heersink School of Medicine
Birmingham, Alabama

Kathryn Dirks, CNM, FNP
Grady Health Systems
Atlanta, Georgia

David L. Eisenberg, MD, MPH, FACOG
Professor
Interim Chief, Division of Family Planning
Director, Complex Family Planning Fellowship
Department of Obstetrics and Gynecology
Washington University in St. Louis School of Medicine
St. Louis, Missouri

Anne N. Flynn, MD, MSHP
Assistant Clinical Professor
Department of Obstetrics and Gynecology
University of California Davis
Sacramento, California

J. Dennis Fortenberry, MD, MS
Donald Orr Professor of Adolescent Medicine
Professor of Pediatrics
Indiana University School of Medicine
Department of Pediatrics
Indianapolis, Indiana

Maria F. Gallo, PhD
Professor and Associate Dean of Research
College of Public Health
The Ohio State University
Columbus, Ohio

Katherine Glaser, MD, MPH
Assistant Clinical Professor
University of Arizona
Chief of Obstetrics and Gynecology
Tuba City Regional Health Care Corporation
Tuba City, Arizona

Laura Greenberg, MD
Reproductive Endocrinology, Retired
Portland, Oregon

Sadia Haider MD, MPH
Associate Professor
Vice Chair for Research and Faculty Affairs
Director, Division of Family Planning
Department of Obstetrics and Gynecology
Rush University
Chicago, Illinois

Tiffany Hailstorks, MD, MPH
Assistant Professor
Division of Family Planning
Department of Gynecology and Obstetrics
Emory University School of Medicine
Atlanta, Georgia

Mitzi Hawkins, MD
Assistant Professor
Chief, Division of Gynecology
San Francisco Veteran Affairs Medical Center
University of California-San Francisco
San Francisco, California

Victoria H. Jennings, PhD
Professor Emerita
Georgetown University
Washington, DC

Rebecca A. Jackson, MD
Robert B. Domush, MD, Chair in Obstetrics and Gynecology Education
Professor of Obstetrics, Gynecology and Reproductive Sciences and Epidemiology and Biostatistics
Division Chief Zuckerberg San Francisco General Hospital & Bixby Reproductive Global Health Center
University of California, San Francisco
San Francisco, California

Jeffrey T. Jensen, MD
Professor of Obstetrics and Gynecology, School of Medicine
Professor, Oregon National Primate Research Center
Vice-Chair of Research, Obstetrics and Gynecology, School of Medicine
Director of the Women's Health Research Unit, Center for Women's Health, School of Medicine
Portland, Oregon

Kelly A. Johnson, MD, MPH
Assistant Professor of Medicine, Division of Infectious Diseases
University of California San Francisco
San Francisco, California
Public Health Medical Officer, STD Control Branch
California Department of Public Health
Sacramento, California

Andrew Kaunitz, MD, FACOG, NCMP
Tenured Professor & Associate Chair
Department of Obstetrics and Gynecology
University of Florida College of Medicine
Jacksonville, Florida

Jessica K. Lee, MD
Assistant Professor, Obstetrics and Gynecology
University of Maryland School of Medicine
Baltimore, Maryland

Abigail Liberty, MD, MSPH
Clinical Fellow
Division of Complex Family Planning
Department of Obstetrics and Gynecology
Oregon Health & Science University
Portland, Oregon

Laura D. Lindberg, PhD
Professor
Department of Urban-Global Public Health
Rutgers School of Public Health
Newark, New Jersey

Meredith Manze, MPH, PhD
Assistant Professor
Department of Community Health and Social Sciences
CUNY Graduate School of Public Health and Health Policy
New York, New York

Alice Mark, MD, MSc
Independent consultant
Boston, Massachusetts

Raegan McDonald-Mosley, MD, MPH
Chief Executive Officer for Power to Decide
https://powertodecide.org/

Hillary McLaren, MD
Assistant Professor
Section of Complex Family Planning
Department of Obstetrics and Gynecology
University of Chicago School of Medicine
Chicago, Illinois

Rachel Rapkin, MD, MPH
Ryan Program Director
Associate Professor
Department of Obstetrics and Gynecology
University of South Florida
Tampa, Florida

Liz Romer, DNP, FNP
Assistant Professor
Department of Pediatrics
Section of Adolescent Medicine
University of Colorado School of Medicine
Aurora, Colorado

Dawn Russell, MD, NCMP
Assistant Professor
Medical Director of Women's Services, Emory Johns Creek Hospital
Department of Gynecology and Obstetrics
Emory University School of Medicine
Atlanta, Georgia

Jennefer Russo, MD, MPH
Chief Medical Advisor
DuPont Clinic
Los Angeles, California

Robyn Schickler, MD, MSc
Chief Medical Officer
Planned Parenthood of Southwest and Central Florida
Tampa, Florida

Rebecca G. Simmons, MPH, PhD
Assistant Professor
Division of Family Planning
Department of Obstetrics/Gynecology
University of Utah
Salt Lake City, Utah

Neetu Khurana Sodhi, DO, MPH
Assistant Clinical Professor of Obstetrics and Gynecology
Western University of Health Sciences
Physician and Owner
Bloom Obstetrics and Gynecology
Tarzana, California

Andrea Swartzendruber, PhD, MPH
Epidemiology and Biostatistics Department
College of Public Health
University of Georgia
Athens, Georgia

Julia Thompson, MS
Data Analyst, Department of Biostatistics
Columbia University Irving Medical Center
New York, New York

Suji Uhm, MD, MPH
Assistant Professor
Dept of Obstetrics, Gynecology, and Reproductive Sciences
University of Pittsburgh
Pittsburgh, Pennsylvania

Nisha Verma, MD, MPH, FACOG
Assistant Professor
Department of Gynecology and Obstetrics
Emory University School of Medicine
Atlanta, Georgia

Stephen Weiss, MD, MPH
Assistant Professor
Division GYN Surgical Specialties
Department of Gynecology and Obstetrics
Emory University School of Medicine
Atlanta, Georgia

Pamela Xandre
Associate Professor
CSULB Nursing School
Nurse Practitioner, Obstetrics and Gynecology
Providence St. Joseph's Hospital
Orange, California

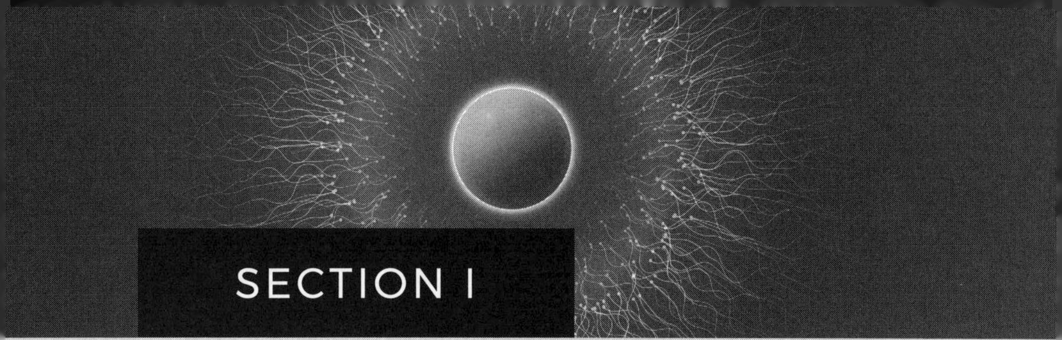

SECTION I

Foundations

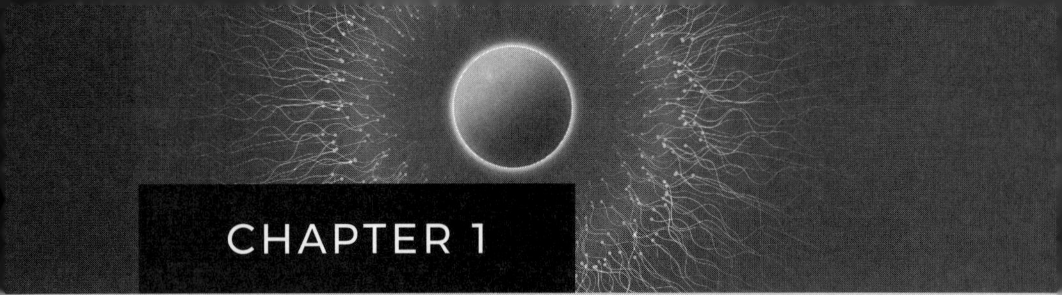

CHAPTER 1

Reproductive Justice within Reproductive Health Care

Talita Oseguera, CNM, WHNP-BC, MSN
Zoë Julian, MD, MPH, FACOG

True contraceptive equity and reproductive freedom will not be realized without investment in reproductive justice–aligned frameworks for care provision.

The criminalization of gender-affirming care for queer, transgender, nonbinary, and gender expansive communities; the Supreme Court decisions in *Dobbs v. Jackson Women's Health Organization;* and state-level abortion bans and restrictions have led to some of the most violent attacks on bodily autonomy and reproductive freedom in recent times. People will continue to lose critical access to evidence-based, life-saving care, with minoritized communities most heavily affected. As front-line health care providers in sexual and reproductive health care, pregnancy care, primary care, and contraceptive and/or abortion care, many of us are already fatigued from the ongoing COVID-19 pandemic, especially while the long-term public health, social, and economic effects continue to impact the well-being of individuals and communities living in the United States. With limited resources and support, health care providers have attempted to provide compassionate, comprehensive care in a health care system that fails too many, too often. We are simply doing our best to provide high-quality services in what feels like persistent "unprecedented times." In these times, pregnancy options are severely limited, and people may be forced to continue pregnancies and parent children without the option of safe abortion. Threats to contraception access flood the news while social programs designed to assist people in providing for and parenting their existing children in their homes continue to lose funding.

The current climate is not unique in our country's history. To understand a new way forward, it is essential that we contextualize these events within a long legacy of reproductive coercion and control in the United States. From the arrival of the first colonizers violating the human rights and land sovereignty of Indigenous peoples to the advent of chattel slavery, our country's birth is indivisible from white supremacy, misogyny, ableism, and transphobia. These interlocking, intersecting systems of oppression[1] manifest as sexual and reproductive harm in the form of medical experimentation, inadequate health care, forced sterilization, as well as deliberate misinformation directed toward Black and Indigenous communities—all contributing to sexual, reproductive, and perinatal health inequities and injustice.

The advent of the field of obstetrics and gynecology occurred in parallel to growth of chattel slavery, as enslavers sought out white, male medical doctors to ensure the reproductive capability and sustainability of their enslaved Black workforce.[2] Some Black enslaved people were subjected to prolonged medical experimentation without any anesthesia, while others were forced to assist these white male physicians in their surgical experimentation.[2] The legitimacy of this growing field also required widespread misinformation in the form of government-funded smear campaigns rooted in racism and misogyny to denigrate the sacred, esteemed work of Black and Indigenous midwives.[3] In more modern times, these same interlocking, intersecting oppressions are illustrated by obstetric racism.[4] Obstetric racism[4] is a specific oppressive experience that sits at the intersection of misogyny, anti-Black racism, and obstetric violence uniquely experienced by Black birthing people in the United States. In similar ways, minoritized communities are uniquely burdened at the intersections of racism, transphobia, and reproductive coercion, impacting equity in all aspects of reproductive health care.

Modern examples that threaten contraceptive equity and reproductive freedom include a legacy of forced sterilization, including coercive sterilization under federally funded programs.[5,6] Incarcerated pregnant people are specifically targeted, a function of reproductive policing.[5,6] Coercive eugenics and sterilization practices include those endured by Mexican people at a Los Angeles County hospital,[7] unwanted sterilizations performed on people in California prisons,[7] and in North Carolina, where 30% of forced sterilizations were inflicted on young girls under the age of 18.[7] Discriminatory contraceptive counseling and long-acting reversible contraception provision targeted at the Black community,[8] as well as drafted legislation requiring contraception for access to social services, posed additional threats.[5] In some states, pregnancy became a tool of leverage in which prosecutors offered reduced sentences in exchange for women agreeing to being sterilized.[5]

With the introduction of the contraceptive implant in the 1990s, many states legislated policies that either required or gave more benefits to women who relied on government aid if they agreed to long-term implantation of this provider-controlled, highly effective contraception method.[5] These examples illustrate how structural and obstetric racism compromise opportunities for historically marginalized communities and Black people with capacity for pregnancy to obtain or use pregnancy-related health services free from the fear or experience of harm and coercion.[4]

Unsurprisingly, evidence shows Black people feel more distrust and less comfort with clinician-controlled contraceptive methods compared to their white counterparts, affecting equitable contraceptive use.[8-10] In one study, participants across races spontaneously voiced the perception that their health care providers attributed unintended pregnancy to a failure to use contraception effectively, of which abortion is a symbol.[8] When people's preferences for features of contraceptive methods were considered among racial and ethnic differences, no single contraceptive method matched all desired features of any racial or ethnic group.[8] However, there is discrepancy between the preferences of people of color and the features of currently available highly effective methods.[8] Provider-centered health care delivery perpetuates inequities, and therefore care delivery systems need to be reorganized and centered on patient needs and values.

The overexposure of interlocking oppressions, from trans-Atlantic slavery through the post-Civil Rights era, contribute to present-day epidemiology of sexual and reproductive health inequities.[11] Instead, marginalized communities deserve sexual and reproductive freedom. The reproductive policing occurring throughout the United States is about attempting to control the reproductive health of individuals and is also a part of a continual ideology of white supremacy and patriarchy that manipulates and controls populations.[11] The United States fails its women, girls, and gender expansive communities on multiple health matrices; it leads the industrialized world in infant and maternal mortality as well as sexually transmitted infections, all while promoting fetal protection laws and personhood clauses as well as interventions that harm reproductive health. Perinatal health outcomes continue to worsen, with the most significant burden of inequity falling on Black birthing communities.[12]

Addressing sexual and reproductive health through a historical lens and ensuring the implementation of structurally tailored, culturally congruent programs, research, and health care delivery efforts rooted in Reproductive Justice (RJ) principles is foundational for moving beyond health equity to achieve reproductive freedom. There is no choice when there is inadequate access. "Our society will not be free until the most vulnerable people are able to access the resources and full human rights to live self-determined lives without fear, discrimination, or retaliation."[11]

Coined by 12 Black women scholars and activists in 1994, RJ encompasses Black feminist ideology, reproductive rights, and social justice to contextualize reproductive health within an intersectional human rights framework.[11] Here, we offer rearticulation of the principles of Reproductive Justice as they apply to reproductive health care provision, including contraception:[12]

1. *Every person has the right to decide if and when to become pregnant and to determine the optimal conditions under which they will birth*, with equitable access and utilization of culturally relevant options and opportunities for contraception, abortion, pregnancy, labor, birth, and postpartum.
2. *Every person has the right to prevent or end a pregnancy* and can do so via options that are accessible, approachable, acceptable, available and accommodating, affordable, and appropriate.
3. *Individuals have the right to parent children they already have with dignity and with the necessary social supports in safe, affordable, and sustainable environments* and healthy, thriving communities without fear or threat of violence, intimidation, coercion, or control from individuals or the government.
4. *Individuals have the right to disassociate sex from reproduction, including through the use of contraception and abortion*, and that healthy sexuality and pleasure are essential components to whole and full human life.

This RJ-aligned reproductive health praxis provides a blueprint for models of reproductive health care that bring us closer to a more free, liberated future, where a whole-person approach is required past that of human rights and abortion discourse.[12] RJ framework takes into account that policing, coercing, limited information, and restricting decision-making ability do not happen in isolation from historical, political, personal, structural, cultural, and economic institutions. Providing full-spectrum contraceptive options and granting time for decision making improves self-efficacy and promotes autonomous decisions.[10] Employing community-based, Reproductive Justice–aligned models of care, where people and their communities actively participate in decision making, build upon individuals' inherent strengths and assets, ensure individuals keep their power to lead fully self-determined lives, and can improve health and equitable quality of life.[11] Person-centered contraceptive counseling emphasizing patient values, shared decision making, and both informed consent and informed refusal can minimize coercion while still addressing unintended pregnancy.[10] Maintaining the human right to full bodily autonomy is a minimum.

Additonal resource: https://www.sciencedirect.com/science/article/pii/S0146000520300483?via=ihub

References

1. Taylor K-Y. How we get free: Black feminism and the Combahee River Collective. Chicago, IL: Haymarket Books; 2017.
2. Owens DC. Medical bondage: race, gender, and origins of modern gynecology. Athens, GA: University of Georgia Press; 2015.
3. Muigai W. "Something wasn't clean": Black midwifery, birth, and postwar medical education in All My Babies. Bull Hist Med. 2019;93(1):82-113.
4. Davis D-A. Reproductive injustice: Racism, pregnancy, and premature birth. New York, NY: New York University Press; 2019.
5. Roberts DE. Killing the Black body: race, reproduction, and the meaning of liberty. New York, NY: Vintage Books, 1999.
6. Goodwin M. Policing the womb: invisible women and criminalization of motherhood. New York, NY: Cambridge University Press, 2020.
7. Tajima-Pena R. No Mas Bebes. United States: Moon Canyon Films; 2016.
8. Jackson AV, Karasek D, Dehlendorf C, Foster DG. Racial and ethnic differences in women's preferences for features of contraceptive methods. Contraception. 2016;93(5):406-11.
9. Thorburn S, Bogart LM. Conspiracy beliefs about birth control: barriers to pregnancy prevention among African Americans of reproductive age. Health Educ Behav. 2005;32(4):474-87.
10. Brandi K, Woodhams E, White KO, Mehta PK. An exploration of perceived contraceptive coercion at the time of abortion. Contraception. 2018;97(4):329-34.
11. Ross L, Derkas E, Peoples W, Roberts L, Bridgewater P, eds. Radical reproductive justice: Foundation, theory, practice, critique. New York, NY: Feminist Press at CUNY; 2017.
12. Julian Z, Robles D, Whetstone S, et al. Community-informed models of perinatal and reproductive health services provision: a justice-centered paradigm toward equity among Black birthing communities. Semin Perinatol. 2020;44(5):151267.

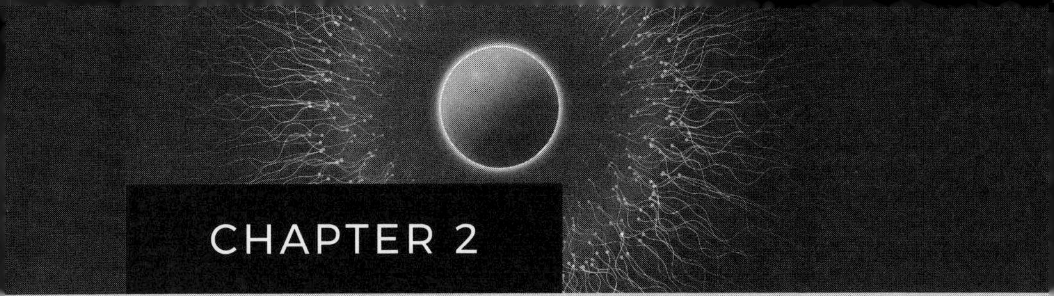

CHAPTER 2

Understanding the Physiology of the Menstrual Cycle

Anita L. Nelson, MD

KEY POINTS

- The menstrual cycle is key to understanding fertility, infertility, fertility control, and of course, cycling disorders.
- The purpose of the menstrual cycle is to establish pregnancy.
- The menstrual cycle relies on highly organized coordination of the hypothalamic–pituitary–ovarian axis and the ovarian–endometrial compartment.
- New information about cycle control centers in the hypothalamus provides new targets for treatment of vasomotor symptoms and an array of other reproductive problems.
- Menstruation is rare in other species, even among those who form placentas. Menstruation in humans is needed because of the reproductive advantages provided by spontaneous decidualization.

Mastering the physiology of the menstrual cycle is key to understanding most reproductive health topics that affect those born with a uterus, including contraception, pregnancy, endometrial cancer, infertility, menopause, and of course, menstrual irregularities. In this chapter, we update the classical understanding of the physiology of the menstrual cycle to include new insights that have greatly expanded our understanding. We also highlight impacts of key steps of the cycle and see how they can be applied to clinical situations. Chapter 3 details how to approach and characterize normal cycling compared to menstrual disorders; this chapter provides the foundational understandings of the underlying causes of menstrual disorders and explains why the recommended therapies work. Other chapters in this book discuss various contraceptive options; this chapter helps the reader understand how those methods work and why they may offer certain health benefits and, potentially, could cause certain side effects.

Overview

The purpose of the menstrual cycle is to establish pregnancy. The menstrual cycle is controlled by a multitiered system, which involves both the hypothalamic–pituitary–ovarian (HPO) axis and the ovarian-endometrial compartment (**Figure 2-1**). The HPO axis is responsible for hormonal cycling—producing the right amount of sex steroids at the right times in the cycle to heal the uterus, mature the oocyte for ovulation, create the right conditions for fertilization to take place, facilitate successful implantation of the conceptus (establishment of pregnancy), and support that pregnancy. Ovarian hormones are important not only for such reproductive success but are also vital to the healthy functioning of many other organ systems, such as the skeletal, metabolic, and cardiovascular systems. The ovarian–endometrial compartment is responsible for the repeated sequence of endometrial cell proliferation and the remarkable cellular differentiation, shedding, and regeneration that can occur up to 400 times in a reproductive lifespan. While these are by themselves complex, highly coordinated systems, other factors, both intrinsic and extrinsic, can affect the function of each of these compartments, each of which can lead to menstrual irregularities and/or compromised fertility.

The HPO Axis (The Ovarian Cycle)

The HPO axis relies on both negative and positive feedback to produce ovulatory cycling. The signals that flow in a hierarchal, top-down system from the hypothalamus to the pituitary, and then from the pituitary to the ovary, are all stimulatory. The hypothalamus uses pulses of the decapeptide gonadotropin-releasing hormone (GnRH) to control the pituitary's production and release of two different gonadotropins—follicle stimulating hormone (FSH) and luteinizing hormone (LH)—in different amounts at different times in the cycle to regulate the activities of the ovary, including ovarian hormone production. Ovarian hormones stimulate endometrial activity. In the absence of stimulation from the higher centers, no activity in the ovaries or endometrium is possible. On the other hand, the signals from the ovary to the higher centers can be either inhibitory (negative feedback) or stimulatory (positive feedback). Both the hypothalamus and the pituitary can assess various aspects of ovarian activity by monitoring circulating levels of sex steroids (estrogens and progesterone) and other hormones (inhibins and activin) produced by the ovary (**Figure 2-2**).

A successful ovulatory cycle requires that mature receptors on the neurons above the GnRH pulse generator in the ventral hypothalamus obtain information about the circulating levels of ovarian hormones and even of the gonadotropins to determine how much stimulation should be applied to the pulse generator to produce the right signals to send to the anterior pituitary. The gonadotroph cells in the anterior pituitary interpret the pattern of signals coming from the hypothalamus in the context of the levels of the ovarian hormones (estrogen, progesterone, inhibin) that they detect in the circulation to determine the appropriate amounts of gonadotropins they should release. These gonadotropins are carried in the bloodstream to the ovaries, where they stimulate the production of sex steroids and other hormonal proteins needed to enable ovulation and to prepare the uterus for pregnancy. This complexity helps explain why most cycles immediately

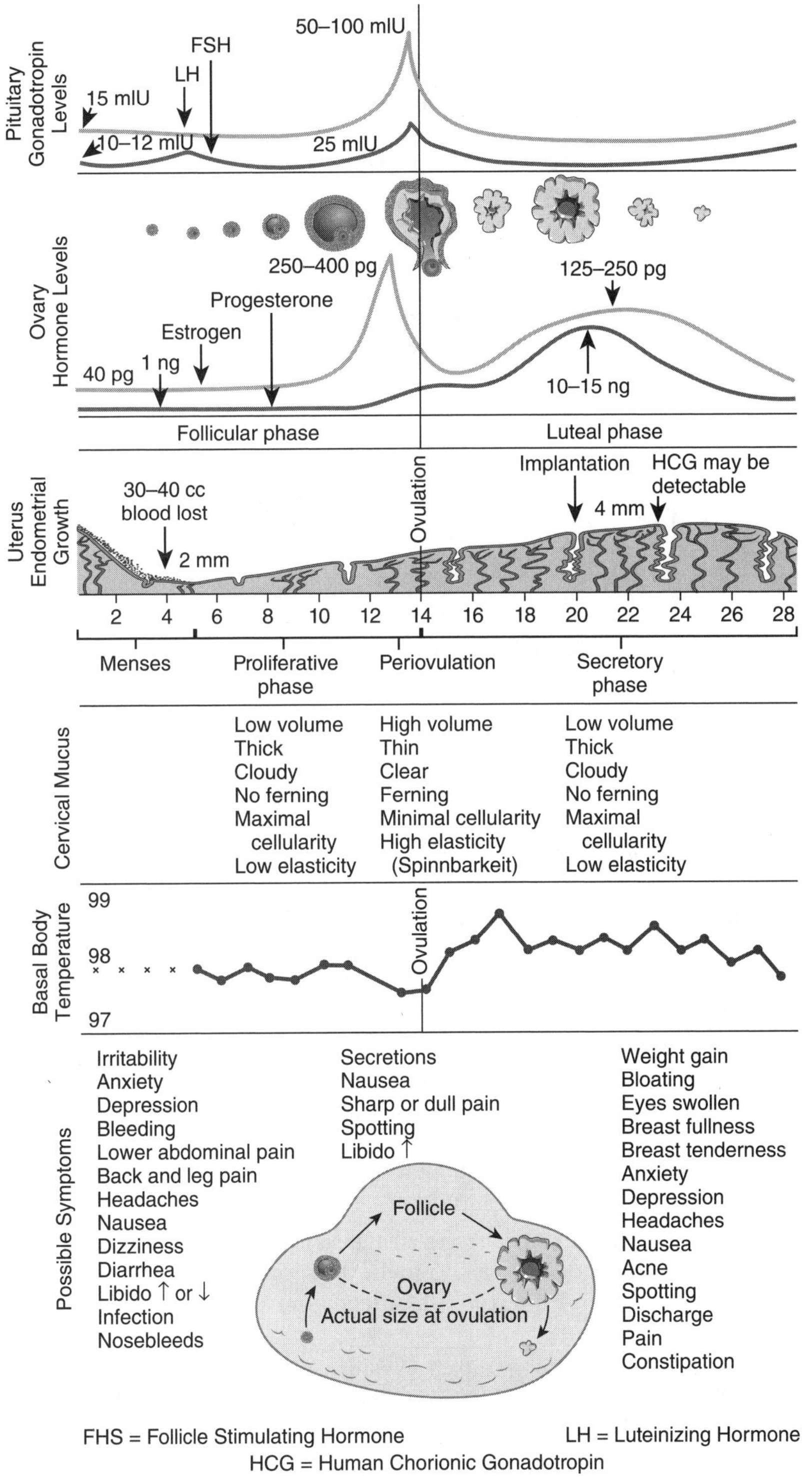

Figure 2-1 Comprehensive summary of menstrual cycle events.

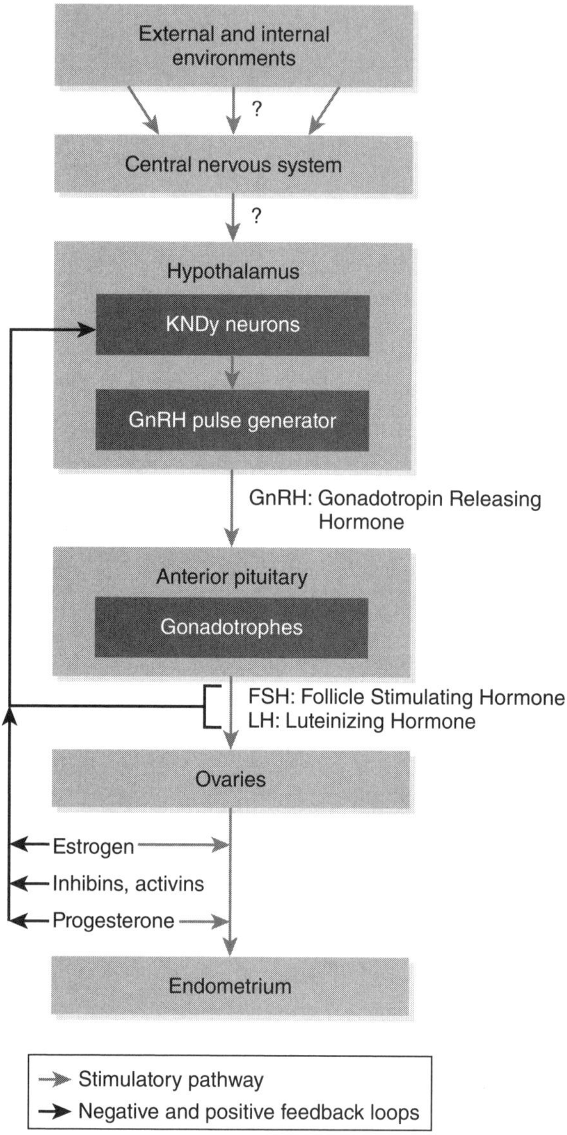

Figure 2-2 Regulation of the menstrual cycle.

following menarche do not quite get all the steps right and are not ovulatory. During the 30 years between ages 15 to 45 years, monthly cycling can produce around 400 mature ova for possible fertilization from the millions of primordial follicles formed in utero.

To understand how this all works in detail, let us start with a clean slate. Assume that the corpus luteum in the ovary from the prior cycle has involuted (collapsed) and is no longer producing hormones. The half-lifes of estradiol, estrone, and progesterone are short to allow for timely and accurate feedback to the brain. Because of this, once the corpus luteum involutes, circulating levels of estrogen and progesterone rapidly fall. The hypothalamus will detect a hormonal deficit in the circulation (the absence of negative feedback) and take action to start to replenish those hormones, which starts a new cycle.

Clinical Application

- *Because naturally produced estrogens and progesterone have short half-lives, they have not been used for once-daily dosing for contraception; longer-acting, synthetic versions of those hormones are generally needed to provide both contraceptive protection and good cycle control.*

Hypothalamic–Pituitary Overview

The hypothalamus contains a GnRH pulse generator that controls the stimulation of the entire system.[1] This pulse generator seems to be controlled by neurons that produce key neurotransmitters collectively called KNDy [for kisspeptin (K), neurokinin B (NKB), and dynorphin (D)]. These neurons (especially those that produce neurokinin B) assess the need for more stimulation from GnRH by monitoring circulating levels of ovarian hormones and pituitary gonadotropins.[2–6]

Clinical Applications

Without stimulation from the hypothalamus, the entire HPO system shuts down. All downstream activity stops; levels of FSH, LH, and E2 are all low. This is what is seen with functional hypothalamic amenorrhea[7] (see the discussion on secondary amenorrhea in Chapter 3, Menstrual Disorders).[4]

The recognition of the role that the KNDy neurons have in controlling GnRH release provides new targets for both contraceptive development and for treatment of postmenopausal vasomotor symptoms. Stopping the release of neurotransmitters that trigger GnRH pulses from the hypothalamus keeps the adjacent thermoregulatory areas in the hypothalamus quiescent and blocks the development of hot flashes.[5] These agents may also treat precocious puberty or help during transition for pubertal transgender patients.

Hypothalamus

The hypothalamus stimulates the production and release of varying amounts of glycoproteins FSH (follicle stimulating hormone) and LH (luteinizing hormone) by the anterior pituitary using only GnRH pulses. GnRH cannot be measured in a routine clinical setting, but its presence can be seen in its impacts on FSH and LH levels. The hypothalamus sends GnRH in *pulses* through the hypophyseal portal circulation to the gonadotropic cells in the anterior pituitary. Pulsatile secretion is very efficient compared to constant release. It uses less energy, and it does not desensitize the target cells in the anterior pituitary. Importantly, pulsatility enables coding of the signals from the hypothalamus. By varying the *amount* of GnRH in each pulse and *how often* GnRH pulses are sent to the anterior pituitary (the *intensity* and *frequency* of the GnRH pulses), the hypothalamus can cause the gonadotrophs in the pituitary to vary the ratios and amounts of FSH and LH they produce and release at any one time. As mentioned above, the situation is a little more complicated than that. The gonadotrophs in the pituitary must integrate the pulsatile GnRH signals they receive from the hypothalamus with the information they receive from the circulation about ovarian hormonal production to release with appropriate amounts of FSH and LH needed at that time in the cycle.

Clinical Applications

- *Constant levels of GnRH in place of pulsatile release cause an inevitable, reversible downregulation of GnRH receptors in the pituitary.*[6,9] *GnRH agonists such as leuprolide and goserelin, provide constant high levels of GnRH. This means that even though GnRH pulses continue to be delivered to the pituitary from the hypothalamus, they are not perceived by the gonadotrophs. Only very little FSH or LH is released, which shuts down ovarian activity and causes amenorrhea. This is how GnRH agonists suppress the HPO axis and create a "pseudomenopause" that is used to treat precocious puberty as well as estrogen-sensitive neoplasms, such as endometriosis. However, because estrogen production is suppressed by this therapy, women experience hot flashes and are at risk for osteoporosis. The impacts generally limit the duraction of use for these agents.*
- *Using a slightly different mechanism, the new GnRH antagonists, such as elagolix and relugolix, directly and immediately block the pituitary receptors for GnRH, so GnRH pulses from the hypothalamus cannot be detected by the pituitary.*[10] *This suppresses the HPO axis and has the same impacts as the agonist analogs. These agents are currently used on label to treat estrogen-related problems like pain from endometriosis and heavy menstrual bleeding due to uterine fibroids.*[7]

Ovarian Overview

The patterns of release of FSH and LH from the pituitary stimulate the ovary through an elaborate, orchestrated series of steps to prepare for pregnancy. These include:

- The rescue and growth of a cohort of ovarian preantral follicles in each ovary
- Stimulation of the theca and granulosa cells in those dozens of follicles in each ovary to produce androgens, estrogens, inhibins, and activin
- Selection of one dominant follicle for ovulation, while inducing atresia of all of the other competing follicles

Very high levels of estradiol are produced and released from the dominant follicle just prior to ovulation to facilitate many vital aspects of fertilization, such as:

- Changes in cervical mucus that permit sperm to enter the upper track through the cervix
- Reversal of the uterine contraction patterns to help carry the sperm into upper tract
- Production of low levels of progesterone to create a concentration gradient to guide the sperm to the egg for fertilization
- Preparation of the egg (oocyte) for fertilization (completion of meiosis and, with sperm penetration of the oocyte, creation of a haploid gamete)

Following rupture of the dominant follicle at ovulation, the remnants of the dominant follicle collapse to form a corpus luteum cyst, which will produce high levels of progesterone, estrogen, and other factors in the luteal phase. These hormones prepare the endometrium for successful implantation and to support the needs of the pregnancy for the first 10–12 weeks of its existence. If there is no successful implantation of a blastocyst, the corpus lluteum stops functioning and undergoes atresia (involution), and all hormonal production stops.

It should be noted that, as opposed to the follicles that are recruited, the number of preantral and small (≤ 8 mm) antral follicles is fairly constant throughout the menstrual cycle. The granulosa cells in these follicles produce anti-Müllerian hormone (AMH). AMH levels measured at any time in the cycle can reflect ovarian reserve, which may be useful to predict fertility potential.

Breaking this down into more detail, the actions in the HPO axis are best divided into three phases: the follicular phase (preparation for ovulation), the preovulatory LH surge, and the luteal phase (preparation for implantation and support of the pregnancy). It is easy to remember these because the first phase is about development of the dominant follicle and the last is about the yellowed-colored corpus luteum (luteum means yellow).

Follicular Phase of the HPO Axis

The follicular phase starts with the first day of menses and ends on the day of the LH surge. The length of the follicular phase depends upon the rate of maturation of the follicles, which can be quite variable. The primary objective of the follicular phase is the development of both a dominant follicle and the preparation of a secondary oocyte ready for ovulation. Although at birth there are nearly a million oocytes distributed in the stroma of the ovaries, only about half of them survive to puberty. A continuous supply of developing follicles (each with an oocyte) emerges in the ovaries in waves throughout each cycle.[8,11] Several hundred follicles start to grow each cycle. Most of the smaller follicles are doomed; they do not have receptors for gonadotropins, so they do not produce significant levels of sex steroids. They rapidly degenerate and disappear. As a result, the number of remaining oocytes (and the quality of those oocytes) decreases with increasing age. AMH levels decline, reflecting reduced ovarian reserve.

At the beginning of the follicular phase of the cycle, GnRH pulses have high frequency and low amplitude. The resulting FSH and LH released from the pituitary rescue cohorts of about 30 early antral ovarian follicles that have matured enough to have receptors for FSH and LH. Each such follicle is composed of granulosa cells surrounding a central core that contains the diploid oocyte frozen in the first meiotic prophase (see **Box 2-1**). A second layer of theca cells develops around the granulosa cells surrounding the edge of the follicle. Receptors for LH are found on the outer (superficial) layer of theca cells; the granulosa cells in the inner layer have receptors primarily for FSH but have also limited numbers of LH receptors.

These layers of specialized cells proliferate and work cooperatively to synthesize and secrete estradiol (**Figure 2-3**). Under the stimulation of LH, each theca cell transports low-density lipoprotein cholesterol (LDL-C) through the cell membrane and converts it to cholesterol. Cholesterol is then converted in that cell through a series of steps (that mirrors reactions in the adrenal gland) to pregnenolone, progesterone, 17-α-OH progesterone, and finally into two different androgens: androstenedione and testosterone. When those androgens exit the theca cells, some go into the general circulation and some enter the granulosa cells that directly surround the follicle. In the granulosa cells, under the stimulation of FSH, these androgens are aromatized into estradiol (E2). Androstenedione can be first aromatized into estrone (E1) and then converted to estradiol (E2), or it can be converted into testosterone and then aromatized into estradiol.

Box 2-1 Oocyte to Zygote in Detail

The number of germ cells maximizes at about 7 months gestational age, when there are about 7 million primordial germ cells (oogonia) in the fetal ovary. Those cells begin meiotic division and become primary oocytes. Their losses are high; just prior to birth, there are only 1 or 2 million remaining primary oocytes. These oocytes are frozen in the diplotene stage of the first meiotic prophase and are encased in surrounding granulosa cells as primordial follicles. Follicles can stay in this arrested stage for up to 50 years. Individual follicles often progress to primary (preantral follicles) without FSH or LH stimulation prior to puberty, but they are all are doomed to have unsuccessful development. These failures account for the drop in number of follicles (to 500,000 follicles) that are available at the time of puberty. Only about 400 of those mature during the reproductive life.

Clinical Applications

- *The long period of meiotic arrest exposes the primary oocyte to potentially adverse influences that may contribute to errors in subsequent division, like the nondisjunction errors that are seen in trisomy. This helps explain why advanced maternal age is a risk factor for trisomy.*

At the time of puberty, the process of regular recruitment of primordial follicles into a pool of growing follicles begins. Primordial follicles are recruited at a regulated rate to avoid premature exhaustion of that pool. Anti-Müllerian hormone levels may play a role in controlling that rate. Most primordial and primary follicles undergo rapid atresia. However, if a follicle is rescued in the early follicular phase by FSH and LH, it will continue to grow and to differentiate. Once activated, primordial follicles enter the preantral phase and can be identified as an enlarged oocyte surrounded by increasing layers of cuboidal granulosa cells. Theca cells collect around the periphery. For 77 to 85 days, this primary oocyte synthesizes large amounts of RNA that will later be needed for its own maturation and fertilization. Some of those proteins are assembled into an extracellular coat between the oocyte and the adjacent follicular cells called the zona pellucida. As the granulosa cells continue to proliferate, viscous fluids containing hormones start to collect in the center. This marks the start of the antral phase. As noted below, the ratio of estrogens to androgens within the follicular field is crucial to determining the survival of the follicle. Only those follicles with high levels of estrogen in the fluid can continue to grow.

Within hours of the beginning of the LH surge, the chromosomes in the oocyte reactivate and progress through the remaining steps of the first meiotic division. After duplicating the chromosomes, however, the follicle divides very unevenly. Half of the chromosomes and almost all of the enriched cytoplasm go into one cell (the secondary oocyte). The other set of chromosomes is combined into a small bag of cytoplasm, is cast off as the first polar body, and then dies. The chromosomes in the secondary oocyte enter the second meiotic division, line up on the second metaphase spindle, and freeze. Protein synthesis continues, but the new proteins that are made at this time prepare the oocyte for fertilization.

The oocyte is ovulated in this arrested second meiotic metaphase state. Ova are usually fertilized within 12 hours of ovulation. Many sperm bind to the zona pellucida but only one penetrates through that layer using its activated acrosomal enzymes from the sperm cap. The remaining portion of the sperm head fuses with the oocyte membrane. The sperm nucleus is incorporated into the ooplasm. After the sperm nucleus joins the ooplasm, the oocyte releases cortical granules that change the oocyte membranes and the zona pellucida. Also following this penetration, under the influence of waves of calcium, the oocyte completes the second meiotic division and sends one set of chromosomes into a second small polar body, which is extruded. This leaves haploid sets of chromosomes from maternal and paternal sources to unite to create a euploid zygote. All remaining sperm binding sites are removed; the zona pellucida around the egg becomes impenetrable by other sperm. The fertilization process is complete. Implantation in the endometrium to establish a pregnancy will not occur for at least 5 to 7 days, if it happens at all. About 60% of fertilized ova never implant; they are lost and resorbed. During the transit time to the endometrium, considerable differentiation of the conceptus occurs but there is no growth in size. The conceptus has no external source of energy; it relies on the proteins synthesized by the ova earlier.

Clinical Implications

- *The copper ions released from copper IUDs can interfere with sperm capacitation and thus block the sperm's ability to produce the acrosomal reaction needed to penetrate through the zona pellucida into the oocyte for fertilization.*
- *Interference with calcium wave generation potentially could block oocyte maturation and the sperm's ability to fertilize a haploid egg. This could be a novel target for new contraceptive methods.*

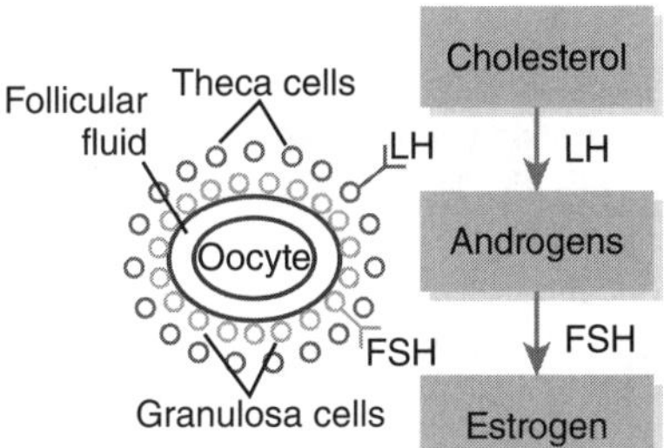

Figure 2-3 The two-cell hypothesis of ovarian follicle development and function.

Anita L Nelson, MD, PCOS generic 2019.

In the follicular phase, FSH also stimulates the granulosa cells to make other important hormone peptides, including inhibin B and activin. Inhibin B amplifies the impact estradiol has providing negative feedback at the level of the pituitary. Activin opposes that negative feedback and stimulates FSH secretion. More importantly, under the stimulation of FSH, activin also triggers the formation of more receptors for LH and FSH on the granulosa cells. Both estradiol and androgens, in combination with FSH, stimulate the formation of more granulosa cells surrounding the follicle. LH also stimulates the production of prostaglandins that may be important later for ovulation.

Both androgens and estradiol diffuse into the follicular fluid that bathes the oocyte as that fluid compartment expands in size. The ratio of estrogen to androgen in the follicular fluid is central in determining survival of the follicle. High levels of estrogen are needed for the follicle to continue to grow. Excessive androgen can induce follicular atresia. Significant amounts of the estradiol, testosterone, and inhibin B produced by the ovaries enter into the general systemic circulation, where those hormones have profound impacts on a wide variety of organ systems. Those circulating hormone levels are also critical to closing the feedback loop to the pituitary and the hypothalamus to ensure subsequent appropriate levels of FSH and LH are released to foster further development of the follicles.

Clinical Applications

- *Very high systemic levels of androgens can suppress follicular development and prevent production of estrogen. Danazol, a weak androgen, can help treat estrogen-dependent endometriosis for this reason. Similarly, androgens used by trans-men can dampen ovarian function.*
- *However, lower levels of androgens (but still with a high androgen to estrogen ratio in the follicular fluid) can protect the follicle from undergoing apoptosis for months—during which time the follicles do not grow but continue to produce excessive amounts of testosterone. In this situation, excess testosterone enters the general circulation and promotes the development of acne, hirsutism, and even male pattern balding—all characteristics seen in polycystic ovary syndrome (PCOS). Chapter 3 explains the reasons for this response.*
- *Following menopause, ovarian production of estrogen, progesterone, activin, and inhibins drops. In the absence of negative feedback, levels of FSH and LH increase markedly. These changes are why measuring gonadotropins and estradiol levels can help make the diagnosis of premature ovarian insufficiency.*
- *However, because the negative feedback loop from the ovary to the upper centers depends on more than just estradiol, we cannot follow FSH levels to titrate the dosing of postmenopausal hormonal therapy for vasomotor symptoms the way TSH levels are used to monitor thyroxin treatment. Instead, we must follow symptoms.*

Selection of a Dominant Follicle

Early in the follicular phase, dozens of small ovarian follicles are stimulated by FSH and LH to produce estradiol, inhibin B, and activin and to make many more FSH receptors and more granulosa cells. However, even collectively, all these small follicles are able to release only relatively low levels of hormones into the circulation. Because the levels of circulating hormones still are low, they provide little negative feedback to the upper elements of the HPO axis. The hypothalamus continues to send out GnRH pulses and the pituitary continues to respond to those pulses by releasing measurable amounts of FSH and LH. The ovarian follicles respond more robustly to each subsequent round of FSH and LH release; both the numbers of cells on each follicle and the numbers receptors on each cell increase dramatically over time.

It is important to note that some follicles start the cycle with many more receptors than other follicles. The follicles that start with more receptors are more likely to bind more of the available gonadotropins, produce more hormones, and make even more receptors. Greater production of hormones is linked to the growth of the follicle. As a result, generally one follicle begins to grow faster than all the others. The fluid surrounding the oocyte in this growing follicle expands more rapidly. Estrogens accumulate in the follicular fluid and reach a level that makes the follicle far less dependent on FSH for its continued growth and development. Such a dominant follicle is generally established by cycle day seven. At this stage, FSH and estrogen act together to stimulate the development of LH receptors on the granulosa cells, which is necessary for the follicle to enter into the preovulatory phase of follicular growth. Growth factors such as insulin, insulin-like growth factor (IGF), fibroblast growth factor (FGF), and epidermal growth factor (EGF) also influence the growth of the follicles and their production of androgens and estrogens.

Clinical Applications

- *Excessive amounts of insulin and IGF in the ovary can induce excessive production of androgens, which can contribute to the development of PCOS. That is why insulin-sensitizing agents, such as metformin, that reduce circulating insulin levels can help treat PCOS, particularly in patients with prediabetes.*
- *By providing pharmacologic levels of hormones early in the cycle, many of the high-dose hormonal contraceptive methods, such as depot medroxyprogesterone acetate (DMPA), can suppress early follicular development. This means that systemic levels of estrogen will be lower than normal, which may be the basis for the problems some women have with dry vaginas and bone loss with prolonged use of those methods.*
- *Most hormonal contraceptive methods do not significantly suppress follicular development but do suppress development of a dominant follicle. This explains why women using combined hormonal methods are likely to have polycystic-appearing ovaries and adequate levels of estrogen to protect bone.*

Atresia of Nondominant Follicles

If only one follicle ovulates each cycle, what happens to all those other follicles in the cohort? Without the necessary hormonal stimulation, these follicles undergo atresia. With every round of FSH and LH release, the ovarian follicles collectively produce increasing levels of estradiol and inhibin B, which are released into the circulation. Both the hypothalamus and the pituitary detect those high levels, and, in classic negative feedback fashion, they reduce their stimulation; the release of FSH and LH drops. Only the follicle with the greatest numbers of granulosa and theca cells that have the highest concentrations of LH and FSH receptors will be able to continue to grow in this bleak environment. The smaller follicles with fewer receptors are not able to capture adequate amounts of FSH or LH to survive. As a result of this and other local factors, including cytokines and change in the ratio of inhibin A and B, these smaller follicles stop functioning altogether and undergo atresia.

Estrogen Rise Prior to the LH Surge

As the smaller follicles stop functioning, fewer and fewer follicles remain to contribute estradiol and inhibin to the circulation. Circulating levels of estradiol and inhibin B drop so low that negative feedback to the pituitary and hypothalamus is reduced significantly. In the absence of significant negative feedback, the hypothalamus and pituitary respond. FSH and LH levels rise again. This time, though, the dominant follicle is primed with many granulosa and theca cells with many receptors for LH and FSH. So, when the FSH and LH levels rise, this follicle releases large amounts of estradiol. By this point in the cycle, the dominant follicle also has granulosa cells with LH receptors that can produce small amounts of progesterone. Prolonged periods (over 48 hours) of high levels of estradiol (200% to 400% above early follicular levels) combined with the very modest levels of progesterone released by this dominant follicle induce a switch in the hypothalamus and pituitary from negative feedback to positive feedback.[12] In positive feedback, the high levels of estrogen from the ovaries will prompt the hypothalamus and pituitary to secrete *more* FSH and LH to induce ovarian production of even *more* estrogen. Androgen production rises and progesterone levels (while still low) increase mildly to 0.5 ng/mL.[9] Inhibin A production replaces inhibin B. All this results in the outpouring pituitary gonadotropins, particularly LH—which we call the "LH surge"—that precedes ovulation.

As noted earlier, the high levels of estrogen in the preovulatory period are critical for other aspects of fertilization.

- High levels of estrogen change cervical mucus. For most of the cycle, cervical mucus is thick, tenacious, and impenetrable; it blocks entry of the sperm (and the pathogens they carry) into the upper genital track. However, in the face of high levels of estrogen, hydrophilic mucins in the cervical mucus increase dramatically. The viscosity of the mucus drops. Profuse, watery mucus protrudes from the cervix into the vagina forming the classic spinnbarkeit sign (increased elasticity or "egg-white" texture). This mucus has channels that are slightly wider than a sperm head to provide the sperm safe harbor from the acidity of the vagina and an entry pathway for the sperm to be carried into upper tract. A characteristic ferning pattern can be seen microscopically on slides after this estrogenized mucus has dried.
- This abundant cervical mucus also provides a source of vaginal lubrication, which contributes to mid-cycle increase in sexual arousal and the observed increase in frequency of coitus around the time of ovulation.
- High levels of estrogen also reverse the direction of uterine contractions. During most of the cycle, the uterus spontaneously contracts from the fundus toward the cervix, to expel its contents. During the LH surge, the contractions start from the cervix and propagate upward to the fundus, creating a current to help the sperm propel through the cervix into the endometrium and toward the ostia of the fallopian tubes.
- Estrogen is necessary for the cilia in the fallopian tubes to maintain their secretory activity and to increase the spontaneous muscle contractions along the tubes. Both of these changes are needed to support the sperm and to push them toward the egg for fertilization and later to move the zygote toward the endometrial cavity for implantation.

Clinical Applications

- **Fertility Awareness Methods for Contraception and for Conception.** *Many fertility awareness methods (like the Billings Method and the Two-Day Method) rely on these estrogen-induced changes in cervical mucus to identify at-risk days for* *conception. Many couples seeking pregnancy may use these methods to enhance their success by timing coitus more accurately.*

- **Hormonal Contraception.** *By providing high levels of progestin throughout the cycle, hormonal contraceptives (with or without estrogen) can interfere with conception in several ways and can have other impacts on users.*
  - *Progestins block the changes that estrogen has on cervical mucus mid-cycle. Consequently, the cervical mucus remains thick and impenetrable to the sperm at all times in the cycle, even if an LH surge occurs.*
  - *Progestins keep the uterine contractions moving from the fundus to the cervix, which reduces the number of sperm that enter the upper track.*
  - *Progestins thin the tubal epithelium and slow the ciliary action needed for fertilization and timely implantation. If conception does occur, this slowing of the cilia can increase the risk for ectopic implantation of conceptus.*
  - *Progestins reduce vaginal lubrication due to lack of cervical mucus, which may cause complaints of vaginal dryness.*
- **Infertility.** *In conditions of chronic estrogen production, as seen with obesity or PCOS, there is no surge in estrogen production to trigger positive feedback. Drugs like clomiphene can be used to block the negative feedback from that peripheral production of estrogens by binding to the estrogen receptors in the hypothalamus and pituitary so that those estrogens cannot bind. The upper elements of the HPO axis then perceive that there has been a large drop in circulating systemic estrogen levels. In the absence of negative feedback, there is an increase the release of FSH and LH to potentially jump-start an ovulatory cycle. Similarly, aromatase inhibitors, such as letrozole, halt production of estrogen and decrease the negative feedback and promote an increase in the production and release of FSH and LH.*

Preovulation/Ovulation Phase

The surge in LH induces major changes in both the oocyte and its surrounding follicular cells. In the first two hours of the LH surge, the output of both estrogens and androgens rises, but that output rapidly decreases later. The outer layers of the granulosa cells cease all proliferation, stop converting androgens to estrogen, and start to synthesize progesterone instead. They also develop receptors to bind progesterone, which will itself fuel positive feedback. Thus, just before ovulation, the unruptured dominant follicle begins to produce increasing amounts of progesterone.[12] At this point in the cycle, progesterone serves several important functions for fertility:

- Progesterone is essential for ovulation itself—it helps trigger the LH surge.
- The gradient of progesterone from the ovarian dominant follicle along the fallopian tube helps guide the sperm to the tube on the side on which ovulation occurred (chemotaxis).
- Progesterone promotes transition to the luteal phase.

Clinical Applications

- **Fertility Awareness Methods.** *The progesterone-induced temperature drops and subsequent temperature rises around the time of the ovulation are used in fertility awareness methods that rely on basal body temperatures to help identify ovulation.*

- **Emergency Contraception.** *Pharmacologic levels of progestin, such as levonorgestrel in Plan B or in high-dose oral contraceptives when given prior to the onset of the LH surge, provide strong negative feedback to the hypothalamus and pituitary, which blocks the LH surge and prevents ovulation. Similarly, high levels of estrogen (such as diethylstilbestrol [DES]) can do the same, although the risk of VTE generally precludes its use for this indication these days.*

  Anti-progestins (such as ulipristal acetate in ella) given either before the LH surge or as the LH levels are rising can block the actions of progesterone, stop the LH surge, and thus block or significantly delay ovulation to prevent fertilization.

Ovulation

At the end of the preovulatory phase, the size of the dominant follicle increases rapidly in diameter (up to 18–25 mm) due to rapid increase in follicular fluid. This fluid dramatically expands the follicle until its perimeter is stretched out into a thin rim of granulosa cells, basement, and theca cells. The intracellular matrix between the granulosa cells breaks down and the blood flow to the follicle increases. The oocyte migrates to one edge of the follicle attached by only a thin stalk of granulosa cells. The follicular wall thins more, and blood flow to the area stops. A stigma (bulge) forms on the surface of the ovary. The overlying ovarian cortex breaks down under the influence of progesterone-induced proteolytic enzymes, like matrix metalloproteinases and serum proteases. These agents further decrease the tensile strength of the follicle. Prostaglandins induce the smooth muscle fibers in the outer layer of the follicle to contract and expel the oocyte. Ovulation occurs approximately 30 to 36 hours after the start of the LH surge and about 10 to 12 hours after the LH peak. The follicular fluid flows out of the follicle into the peritoneal cavity, carrying the oocyte with it. At this point, the oocyte is surrounded by a cumulus of granulosa cells (cumulus oophorous) and by a clear zona pellucida. The oocyte generally adheres to the surface of the ovary until the muscular contractions and ciliary movement of the fallopian tube facilitate its entry into the fallopian tube.

Ovulation changes the entire endocrinology of the follicle, converting it into a corpus luteum, which produces large amounts of progesterone, estrogen, and inhibin A. The residual parts of the follicle collapse into the space formally filled by the fluid and a clot forms. At this point in time, the collapsed follicle is composed of a fibrin core surrounded by several layers of granulosa cells wrapped within a fibrous outer thecal capsule. This becomes the corpus luteum.

Clinical Applications

- **Contraception.** *Compounds that block the action of proteolytic enzymes could help prevent breakdown of the follicle wall and prevent the extrusion of the oocyte. This would result in a luteinized unruptured follicle that could not be fertilized. Meloxicam has been shown to increase the efficacy of LNG-EC, presumably via this mechanism.*
- **Mittelschmerz.** *The muscular cramping of the fallopian tube as well as the rupture of the follicle can cause midcycle ovulation pain a person can feel on one side of the pelvis for 12–24 hours.*

- **Ovulatory Hemoperitoneum.** *Women who are anticoagulated or have other bleeding diatheses can have significant intraperitoneal hemorrhage when the oocyte is extruded from the vascularized follicle. Timely clot formation may not be possible for them.*

Luteal Phase

The luteal phase starts with ovulation and ends with the first day of menses. Its length is determined by the lifespan of the corpus luteum, and is generally fixed at around 14 days. As noted, an LH surge is necessary to extrude the oocyte from the dominant follicle and allow for the formation of the corpus luteum from the remaining elements of that follicle. Under the stimulation of LH, the granulosa cells undergo luteinization and differentiate into granulosa luteal cells. Theca cells differentiate into the theca luteal cells. Both join capillaries and connective tissue to form the corpus luteum.

GnRH pulses in the luteal phase are high-amplitude, low-frequency pulses. The pituitary responds to those pulses by releasing FSH and LH to stimulate the granulosa luteal and theca luteal cells to produce androgens, progesterone, estradiol, and inhibins. Progesterone enhances the negative feedback effects of estradiol, so FSH and LH levels remain relatively low. Importantly, high levels of progesterone block positive feedback effects of estradiol, preventing another LH surge and ovulation. Both estradiol and progesterone rise to their maximum levels 5 to 7 days after ovulation, around the time the morula should arrive in the endometrial cavity. If there is no implantation, the corpus luteum starts to undergo programmed cell death (apoptosis) 9 or 10 days after its formation and circulating hormones return to baseline levels, which then triggers the hypothalamus and pituitary to stimulate the beginning of the next cycle. With time, that old corpus luteum is replaced by an avascular scar called the corpus albicans (**Figure 2-4**). However, if implantation does occur, the human chorionic gonadotropin (hCG) made by the syncytiotrophoblast cells of the invading blastocyst sustain the function of the corpus luteum until the placenta can support the pregnancy by itself.

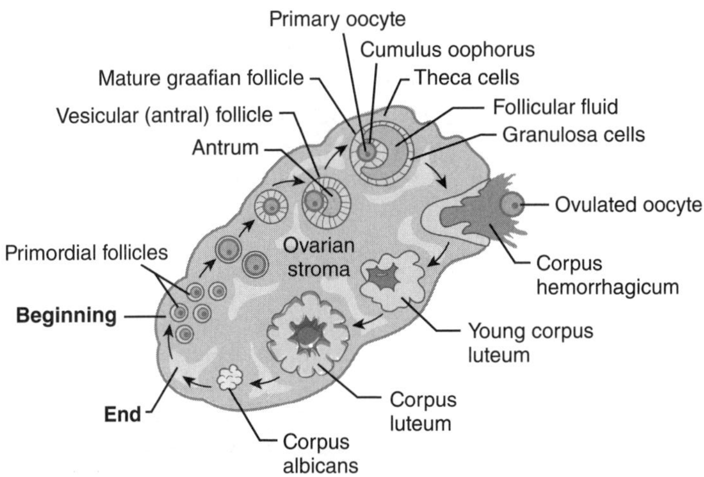

Figure 2-4 Picture of ovary with different cysts.

Box 2-2 **Timing of the Different Ovarian and Endometrial Phases**

Ovarian Phases	Endometrial Phases
Follicular (E_2 dominance)	Menstrual
Preovulatory/LH surge	Proliferative (E_2 dominance)
Luteal (P_4 dominance—atresia)	Secretory (P_4 dominance)

Ovarian–Endometrial Component (The Endometrial Cycle)

The endometrium undergoes remarkable cyclic changes in response to ovarian hormonal stimulation delivered by the systemic circulation (**Box 2-2**). As a result, the classic phases of this compartment rather closely match those of the HPO phases but are named after changes that occur in the endometrium: the menstrual phase, the proliferative phase, and the secretory phase.

Functionally, the endometrium is organized into two layers (**Figure 2-5**). The outer one-third of the endometrium, called the functional layer (the functionalis), is further away from the myometrium. It undergoes dramatic cyclic changes in morphology and function during the menstrual cycle and is sloughed off during menstruation when pregnancy is not successfully established. The inner portion of the endometrium, called the basal layer (the basalis), remains constant throughout the cycle. It is the source for the cyclic regeneration of the functional layer. The vascular supply to the endometrium is somewhat complicated. The basal layer is perfused by straight branches from the vessels running along its base in the myometrium. As these straight branches ascend through the basal layer, they start to coil and become the foundation of the spiral arteries that feed the upper portion of the basal layer and the base of the functional layer. These spiral arteries give off coiled blood vessels that undergo significant changes throughout the cycle to perfuse the growing functional layer. Contraction of the spiral arteries at the end of the cycle is the first uterine response to the failed ovarian corpus luteum and thus is the first step in menstruation.

Menstrual Phase

The first day of menstruation marks the beginning of a new cycle. The first four to five days of the cycle are defined as the menstrual phase. In response to the drop in circulating levels of progesterone (and estrogen) that comes with involution of the corpus luteum, prostaglandin-mediated vasoconstriction of the spiral arteries at the junction between the endometrial layers causes coordinated ischemic injury to all the cells in the functional layer, which results in tissue hypoxia. Cut off from their blood supply, the endometrial glands and stroma in the functional layer start to disintegrate.

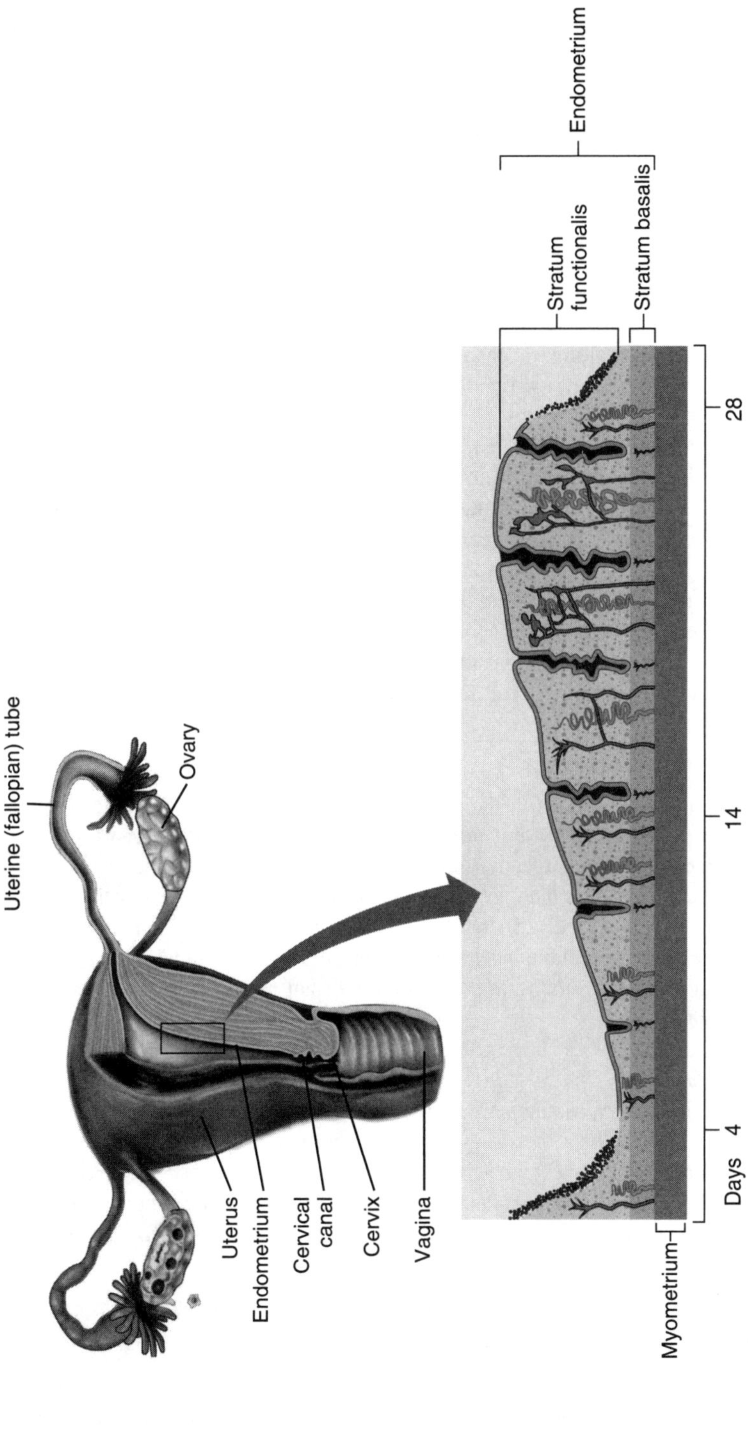

Figure 2-5 Sketch of endometrial layers.

Clinical Applications

- *Progesterone is needed to sustain the endometrium in the luteal phase. Patients taking oral contraceptives who complain of unscheduled spotting and bleeding toward the end of their active combined oral contraceptives may benefit from switching to a formulation with higher levels of progestin in the last days of active pills. Triphasic formulations with increasing progestin content can be helpful in this situation.*

Changes Seen in Menstruation

Menstruation involves extensive inflammatory and vascular changes. The decidualized cells (see p. 25) in the functional layer respond to the drop in progesterone by releasing cytokines, chemokines, chemokine ligands, and adhesive molecules. This triggers an influx of leukocytes that release large quantities of matrix metalloproteinase enzymes along the base of the functional layer. These enzymes cleave the attachments between the two endometrial layers. As patches of the necrotic functional tissue separate from the basal layer, torn edges of veins, arteries, and glands are exposed. Arterial bleeding generally is restricted by vasoconstriction of the spiral arteries in the basal layer, but venous blood loss continues. Without progesterone to quiet myometrial contractions, high local levels of prostaglandins promote uterine contractions to propel the debris and blood toward the cervix and out of the uterine cavity. The process of this separation usually is completed within 24 hours, and regeneration of a new functional layer can start. Bleeding persists until hemostasis is established by typical processes of blood clot formation. Platelet plugs form in the vessels. Fibrin is formed in that platelet matrix and utilizes both the intrinsic and extrinsic clotting pathways to ultimately form a stable clot to halt further blood loss.

Clinical Applications

- *Prostaglandins released in the endometrium (primarily $PGF_2\alpha$) induce the spiral artery vasoconstriction that starts the menstrual phase and triggers uterine contractions. These prostaglandins also are released into the systemic vascular circulation and can cause many of the other complaints that occur with menses, such as headache and nausea. NSAIDs are particularly helpful in reducing many of these diverse symptoms (cramping, heavy bleeding, headache) by adjusting the amount of prostaglandins and the ratio between the different prostaglandin $F_2\alpha$. and prostaglandin E_2.*
- *When ovulation does not occur (as in anovulatory cycling), endometrial sloughing is not synchronous. That is, it does not happen at the same time throughout the endometrium. Instead, individual focal areas of proliferation outgrow their blood supply and slough; bleeding from those sites is only slowly controlled because of higher levels of vasodilating PGE_2 and lower levels of $PGF_2\alpha$. Other areas in the uterine cavity bleed later when their proliferated functional layers outgrow their blood supplies and slough. This can result in prolonged and heavy bleeding (see Chapter 3, Menstrual Disorders).*

Proliferative Phase of the Ovarian-Endometrial Compartment

The proliferative phase follows menses and ends with ovulation. Endometrial regeneration prompted by estrogen is the primary outcome of this phase. After sloughing the

Box 2-3 Why do Humans Menstruate?

Menstruation is very rare in nature. Menstruation in humans has been explained over the centuries in a variety of ways. It was thought to be needed to expel the bacteria acquired from coitus, eliminate unimplanted embryos, relieve "bad humors," or prevent excessively high hemoglobin levels. In fact, the beneficial impacts thought to result from menstruation were used for centuries to justify the practice of bloodletting to treat illness. At other times, it was thought that fertility occurred with menses.[13-15]

Modern experts have recognized that menstruation functionally parallels and is closely linked to the development and delivery of the placenta. But even among mammals that form a placenta, only 84 species (1.6% of all species that form placenta) are known to menstruate. Some of those menstruating species are close to *Homo sapiens*, such as Old World monkeys and most of the New World monkeys. One rodent (spiny mouse), four species of bats, and the elephant shrew round out the total. Dogs have bleeding that precedes ovulation, not bleeding from uterine shedding following an unsuccessful cycle. Menstruation's rarity has raised questions about its biologic role.[15] It may be difficult to understand what evolutionary benefits could possibly accrue from a process that involves so much energy, bleeding, and pain. The answer is that menstruation itself does *not* offer any evolutionary benefit. Menstruation is only the consequence of the process that does provide evolutionary benefits: **spontaneous decidualization**.[16]

Decidualization prepares the uterine lining for implantation and supports the embryo for the first several weeks of gestation. In most species, the conceptus triggers decidualization of the endometrium when it comes into contact with that uterine lining. Furthermore, decidualization only occurs in the area of that contact. In humans, however, decidualization occurs spontaneously before contact with any conceptus, and the process occurs throughout the entire functional layer of the endometrium as it prepares to support the conceptus for months.

Early in the luteal phase in humans, endometrial cells fill with proteins that can be used by the invading embryonic trophoblastic cells as energy sources until the placental exchange can be fully established at the end of the first trimester. Blood vessel formation and growth are prominent during decidualization. Embryos in menstruating species invade much deeper into the endometrium to gain nutrients. However, too deep an invasion must be kept in check because it can threaten the mother's life from massive postpartum hemorrhage. During the luteal phase in humans, there is a large influx of uterine natural killer (uNK) cells to limit the depth of invasion of those embryonic trophoblastic cells into the endometrium. Another potential benefit of spontaneous decidualization is that it may permit some embryo selection by the mother. Decidualized endometrial stromal cells generate a response to impaired embryos and may reject them.[16]

In a failed cycle, the decidualized stroma initiates the process of hypoxic damage (by vasoconstriction of the spiral arteries), and cellular inflammation, which leads to its own destruction and thus prepares for initiation of the next cycle with menstruation as described above.

Data from Jarrell J. The significance and evolution of menstruation. Best Pract Res Clin Obstet Gynaecol. 2018;50:18-26; Coutinho EM, Segal SJ. Is Menstruation Obsolete?. New York. Oxford Universal Press. 1999; Critchley HOD, Babayev E, Bulun SE, Clark S, Garcia-Grau I, Gregersen PK, Kilcoyne A, Kim JJ, Lavender M, Marsh EE, Matteson KA, Maybin JA, Metz CN, Moreno I, Silk K, Sommer M, Simon C, Tariyal R, Taylor HS, Wagner GP, Griffith LG. Menstruation: science and society. Am J Obstet Gynecol. 2020;223:624-664; Okada H, Tsuzuki T, Murata H. Decidualization of the human endometrium. Reprod Med Biol. 2018;17:220-227.

functional layer of the prior cycle, re-epithelialization of the injured endometrial surface occurs rather rapidly. As noted, the process starts even before menstrual bleeding has halted. The repair occurs in a piecemeal fashion, often starting in denuded areas that are next to actively menstruating tissue. The endometrium is rebuilt from the basal layer, which is not affected by swings in progesterone levels since it has abundant progesterone receptors. Because the bases of the endometrial glands lie deep within the basalis layer, they are not destroyed during menstruation. Stem cells and progenitor cells from this basal layer are able to rapidly regenerate all elements of the endometrium, including the glands, stroma, and vascular and immune cells. Epithelial cells in the basal portion of the glands reconstruct the glands and cover the surface of the denuded endometrium. Stromal cells proliferate and start to secrete collagen and ground substance. Spiral arteries lengthen to perfuse the new functional layer. Bone marrow–derived stem and progenitor cells also contribute to rebuilding the endometrial functional layer. However, they differentiate mostly into the endometrial stromal cells.

The large increase in ovarian estrogen secretion in the second half of the proliferative phase causes marked proliferation of cells the endometrial lining, notably of the glands and the connective tissue of the stroma. The endometrial thickness increases from 1–2 mm at the beginning of the cycle to 8–12 mm by the end of the proliferative phase. The spiral arteries lengthen until they reach the full thickness of the endometrium. Synthesis of mRNA and proteins increases, as do the rates of cellular division and cell growth. By the end of the proliferative phase, cellular proliferation and endometrial growth have maximized for a successful cycle. The endometrial glands are straight; their lumens are narrow and contain some glycogen. The stroma has notable edema. Estrogen also increases the contractibility and excitability of the myometrium. During this period, one of the most critical functions of the estrogen is to induce synthesis of progesterone receptors. The proliferative phase ends with ovulation.

Clinical Application

- *Estrogen stimulation allows for continuing endometrial proliferation. Without ovulation, there is no luteal phase and no progesterone dominant phase. In the long run, anovulatory cycling results in continued endometrial proliferation, which is a risk factor for endometrial hyperplasia, for hyperplasia with atypia and, ultimately, for endometrial carcinoma.*

Secretory Phase of the Ovarian–Endometrial Compartment

The secretory phase starts with ovulation and ends with the onset of menses. The primary outcome of this phase is the maturation of the endometrium to allow for successful implantation. With the shift to progesterone production in the ovary following ovulation, distinct changes occur within the endometrium on almost a daily basis. These changes are so prominent that pathologists can determine from a uterine biopsy specimen on which day in an idealized cycle the specimen was obtained. This is called "dating the endometrium." Very importantly, in the secretory phase, virtually all endometrial cellular division (proliferation) stops even though estrogen is still abundant. Proliferation stops because progesterone down-regulates the estrogen receptors on the endometrial cells.

Under the influence of progesterone, the endometrium continues to thicken, but growth in the endometrial thickness comes from hypertrophy of the epithelial cells and increases in vascularity and edema. The endometrium converts into a secretory endometrium. The endometrial stromal cells enlarge and proliferate, becoming loose and edematous. The blood vessels in the functional layer become thickened and highly coiled. The endometrial glands that were tubular and straight become tortuous; their lumens fill with glycoproteins, sugars, and amino acids—all essential nutrients for the survival and growth of the conceptus. Glycogen-rich subnuclear vacuoles divide in the base of the cells lining the glands just after ovulation. As progesterone levels rise, the vacuoles rise toward the glandular lumina. The contents of the vacuoles are released into the endometrial cavity to provide energy to the free-floating blastocyst when it reaches the endometrial cavity several days after fertilization. This energy for the blastocyst is important because implantation does not occur for another 2 to 3 days. With implantation, pregnancy is established.

Prior to implantation, the endometrial stroma cells (ESC) in the functional layer throughout the entire endometrium undergo a dramatic morphologic and functional differentiation called decidualization. The ESCs become rounded, epithelioid-like cells. The uterine glands undergo a secretory transformation. There is an influx of specialized uNK cells. Vascular remodeling takes place to provide maternal blood supply to the growing conceptus. Once decidualized, the ESCs facilitate implantation and provide nutrition to the implanting blastocyst and support the pregnancy. In the decidua, the ESCs also importantly limit the extent of the invasion of the trophoblast cells by forming an extracellular matrix with inhibitory agents that block the enzymes released by the trophoblasts. Decidualized ESCs have direct impacts on local immune response regulation, antioxidant response, and angiogenesis. The uNK cells are important for protecting the conceptus from the maternal immune system. Decidualization plays an important role in promoting placental formation. Failure of this progesterone-induced process of decidualization is associated with infertility, recurrent miscarriage, and uteroplacental disorders.

If implantation into the decidualized endometrium is successful, specialized invading syncytiotrophoblastic cells from the blastocyst produce human chorionic gonadotrophin (hCG). The hCG is absorbed into the maternal circulation. When hCG reaches the ovary, it blocks the involution of the corpus luteum and stimulates the corpus luteum to continue to produce progesterone (as well as estrogen and androgen) to sustain the endometrium and thus, the pregnancy, until the end of the first trimester when the placenta is mature enough to support the pregnancy by itself.

Clinical Applications

- *If the corpus luteum is inadvertently ruptured in the first trimester, supplementary progesterone must be provided to prevent pregnancy loss.*
- *On the other hand, antiprogesterones, such as mifepristone, intentionally block the action of the progesterone. By completely blocking the progesterone receptors, pregnancy loss follows. This is important not only for elective abortion, but also for treatment of early pregnancy loss.*
- *Progesterone causes further enlargement of myometrial cells and significantly suppresses myometrial excitability. As a result, the fundus becomes completely quiescent, which is necessary to permit implantation of the conceptus without triggering uterine contractions that would be expel it.*

- *If pregnancy is not established by cycle day 23, the absence of hCG causes the corpus luteum to involute and circulating levels of progesterone and estrogen to fall. Periodic contractions of the spiral arteries lasting for several hours cause ischemia in the functional layer. After about 2 days of only minimal blood supply, the epithelium of the functional layer is disrupted and the blood vessels rupture. Thus, the superficial functional layer of the endometrium undergoes disintegration. An influx of leukocytes and red blood cell extravasation follows. The menstrual phase of the next cycle starts.*

Summary

The menstrual cycle results from orchestrated signaling between the hypothalamus, the pituitary, the ovaries, and the endometrium for the purpose of establishing pregnancy. By understanding the proper functioning of the system, we can develop techniques to selectively block different steps to control fertility. By understanding the vulnerabilities of the system, we can develop therapies that target the dysfunctions that create fertility challenges and menstrual disorders described in the following chapter.

Author Disclosures—Anita L. Nelson, MD received grant funding for conducting research from Agile Therapeutics, Mylan Pharmaceuticals/Viatris Pharmaceuticals, Organon/Merck, Sagami Rubber Industrie, and Sebela Pharmaceuticals. She has received honoraria for serving as a consultant on advisory boards or speakers bureaus for the following companies: Agile Therapeutics, Bayer HealthCare, Mayne Pharma, Organon/Merck, and TherapeuticsMD.

References

1. Avendaño MS, Vazquez MJ, Tena-Sempere M. Disentangling puberty: novel neuroendocrine pathways and mechanisms for the control of mammalian puberty. Hum Reprod Update. 2017;23:737-63.
2. Nagae M, Uenoyama Y, Okamoto S, et al. Direct evidence that KNDy neurons maintain gonadotropin pulses and folliculogenesis as the GnRH pulse generator. Proc Natl Acad Sci USA. 2021;118:e2009156118.
3. Ruohonen ST, Poutanen M, Tena-Sempere M. Role of kisspeptins in the control of the hypothalamic-pituitary-ovarian axis: old dogmas and new challenges. Fertil Steril. 2020;114:465-74.
4. Anderson RA, Millar RP. The roles of kisspeptin and neurokinin B in GnRH pulse generation in humans, and their potential clinical application. J Neuroendocrinol. 2021 Dec 20:e13081.
5. Harter CJL, Kavanagh GS, Smith JT. The role of kisspeptin neurons in reproduction and metabolism. J Endocrinol. 2018p;238:R173-83.
6. Salem AM. Variation of leptin during menstrual cycle and its relation to the hypothalamic-pituitary-gonadal (HPG) axis: A systematic review. Int J Womens Health. 2021;13:445-58.
7. Liu JH. Hypothalamic amenorrhea: clinical perspectives, pathophysiology, and management. Am J Obstet Gynecol. 1990;163:1732-6.
8. Modi M, Dhillo WS. Neurokinin 3 receptor antagonism: A novel treatment for menopausal hot flushes. Neuroendocrinology. 2019;109:242-248.
9. Maggi R, Cariboni AM, Marelli MM, et al. GnRH and GnRH receptors in the pathophysiology of the human female reproductive system. Hum Reprod Update. 2016;22:358-81.
10. Al-Hendy A, Bradley L, Owens CD, et al. Predictors of response for elagolix with add-back therapy in women with heavy menstrual bleeding associated with uterine fibroids. Am J Obstet Gynecol. 2021;224:72.e1-e50.

11. Baerwald A, Pierson R. Ovarian follicular waves during the menstrual cycle: physiologic insights into novel approaches for ovarian stimulation. Fertil Steril. 2020;114:443-57.
12. Dozortsev DI, Diamond MP. Luteinizing hormone-independent rise of progesterone as the physiological trigger of the ovulatory gonadotropins surge in the human. Fertil Steril. 2020;114:191-9.
13. Jarrell J. The significance and evolution of menstruation. Best Pract Res Clin Obstet Gynaecol. 2018;50:18-26.
14. Coutinho EM, Segal SJ. Is menstruation obsolete? New York, New York: Oxford Universal Press, 1999.
15. Critchley HOD, Babayev E, Bulun SE, et al. Menstruation: science and society. Am J Obstet Gynecol. 2020;223:624-64.
16. Okada H, Tsuzuki T, Murata H. Decidualization of the human endometrium. Reprod Med Biol. 2018;17:220-7.

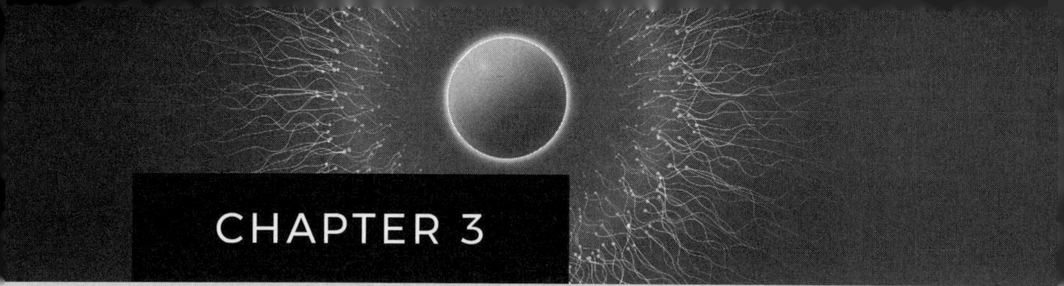

CHAPTER 3

Menstrual Disorders

Anita L. Nelson, MD
Shivika Trivedi, MD, MSc

KEY POINTS

- Menstrual disorders can profoundly affect people's health, fertility, and quality of life.
- The terminology to describe menstrual bleeding and abnormal bleeding patterns has changed in the past decade to allow for clearer communication.
- The PALM-COEIN system is used to classify and describe different etiologies of abnormal uterine bleeding (AUB).
- Understanding the menstrual cycle and the PALM-COEIN classification enables people to understand the mechanisms by which the most appropriate treatments can be utilized to address the various causes of AUB.
- In addition to abnormal bleeding patterns, many suffer from menstrual cramping, mood disorders, and exacerbations of other medical problems at the time of menses.
- Often hormonal contraceptives can help alleviate many menstrual disorders; other treatment options can also be tailored to the patient's individual needs and preferences.

For those born with a uterus, the menstrual cycle is the most fundamental indicator (vital sign) of reproductive health during the reproductive years. As such, it should be assessed and documented at every health care encounter from menarche to menopause. This chapter will review the etiology, evaluation, and treatment of major menstrual disorders, including problems of too much bleeding, too little bleeding, infrequent bleeding, too frequent bleeding, and bleeding that occurs at abnormal times. Then we will discuss menstrually related problems including pain, mood disorders, and systemic problems that develop only during menses or that worsen around the time of menses.

To identify menstrual *disorders*, we must define what is normal and the terminology that should be used to describe menstruation. Fortunately, the Federation of International Gynecologists and Obstetricians (FIGO) has definitively provided all these tools.[1,2] There are four parameters of menstrual cycling that should be recorded at each assessment: the frequency of bleeding, the duration of flow, the volume of flow, and the cycle-to-cycle variability of menses noted over the prior 6 months. All problems associated with or exacerbated during menses should also be noted. **Table 3-1** provides the definitions and the terminology to use to describe different bleeding patterns. These FIGO standards are endorsed by most authorities, with the exception that some still hold that normal menstrual frequency is 28 ± 7 days (21–35 days).

For example, a patient who complains of "irregular bleeding" and reports bleeding episodes every 40 days lasting 8 days with passage of clots would be described in FIGO terms as having infrequent cycling of normal duration with heavy flow. This description is operationally clear and provides a baseline assessment to guide an appropriate evaluation and to measure effectiveness of therapy. While you are developing a differential diagnosis for abnormal bleeding and devising a plan to determine the underlying cause(s), use these terms in the assessment section of the initial visit note.

These FIGO terms have replaced many of the traditional, but far less precise, words that were used in the past (**Table 3-2**). For example, "menorrhagia" was a general term that could have meant heavy bleeding, prolonged bleeding, or even

Table 3-1 Preferred Terminology Used to Assess Menstrual Bleeding

Basic Four Parameters for Menstrual History	Terminology to Use
Frequency of bleeding episodes	Frequent (< 24 days) Normal (24–38 days) Infrequent (> 38 days)
Duration of flow	Normal (≤ 8 days) Prolonged (> 8 days)
Flow volume (this reflects patient's assessment of flow and its impact on quality of life [QOL])	Light Moderate Heavy
Regularity (difference in number of days between the lengths of the longest and the shortest cycles over 6 months)	Normal (≤ 9 days difference) Irregular (≥ 10 days difference)
Terminology for Other Bleeding Patterns	
No bleeding or spotting for > 3 months	Amenorrhea
Bleeding between spontaneous cyclic episodes	Intermenstrual bleeding
Bleeding induced by certain activities	Postcoital/traumatic bleeding
Spontaneous bleeding after menopause	Postmenopausal bleeding
Bleeding that occurs appropriate with use of combined hormonal contraceptives (CHCs)	Scheduled bleeding
Bleeding between scheduled bleeding episodes with CHC use	Unscheduled bleeding

Modified from Munro MG, Critchley HOD, Fraser IS; FIGO Menstrual Disorders Committee. The two FIGO systems for normal and abnormal uterine bleeding symptoms and classification of causes of abnormal uterine bleeding in the reproductive years: 2018 revisions. Int J Gynaecol Obstet. 2018;143:393-408

Table 3-2 Outdated Terminology for Menstrual Bleeding Patterns

Menorrhagia	Polymenorrhagia
Menorrhagia	Oligomenorrhea
Menometrorrhagia	Dysfunctional uterine bleeding

heavy and prolonged bleeding. Since each of those patterns can have different etiologies, different effects, and possibly different treatments, clinicians are strongly encouraged to use the much more complete FIGO terms.

At the initial visit, a comprehensive history (medical, surgical, sexual, medication, and family) and physical examination can suggest specific etiologies for menstrual disorders. Information about age at menarche and obstetrical history complete the snapshot of the patient's menstrual history. However, in practice, a routine menstrual history is often absent from the medical records for nongynecologic visits. Even when women are being admitted to the hospital for profound anemia, clinicians often fail to inquire about menses.[3,4] This omission can easily result in lost opportunities for important interventions or, in other cases, can result in undiagnosed pregnancies.

When obtaining a menstrual history, avoid a checkbox approach. Ask very concrete questions. Self-characterizations of flow and cycling frequency can be very misleading. People who routinely bleed for 10 to 12 days a month may rate those periods as "normal" because that is the only pattern they have experienced. Consider asking the following questions:

- When was the first day of your last period?
- When was the first day of the period before that?
- How many days of bleeding do you usually have?
- Do you ever have spotting or bleeding when you are not on your period?
- On your heaviest flow day, how many sanitary pads/internal protection products do you use?
- Do you ever have to change your protection or empty your menstrual cups more frequently than every 2 hours?
- Do you ever have blood clots, staining, or other accidents because you are not able to contain your flow?

Also consider asking:

- What are your menstrual cramps like?
- Are you able to perform your usual daily activities when you have cramps?
- Do you take any medication or use any other treatments to control the pain?
- How much does that treatment help you?
- What other problems do you have around the time of your period?

It is also important to ask about contraceptive method use, which often can profoundly impact bleeding and the risk of pregnancy. Use of smart phone menstrual cycle tracker apps can enable patients to identify any changes in their cycles early.[5] (For more information, see Chapter 27, Digital Resources for Health and Medical Information.)

Age has a strong influence on bleeding patterns. Recently menarcheal individuals (within 18 to 24 months of the first menses) and those who are perimenopausal have the greatest variability in cycle-to-cycle length. On the other hand, menstrual cycles are most predictable among people in their mid to late 30s. Most of the variability in ovulatory cycle length occurs in the length of the follicular phase; the luteal phase has a relatively fixed duration (13–15 days).

Once the etiology of abnormal bleeding has been identified, the assessment section at the next visit would again list the pattern of abnormal uterine bleeding using the Table 3-1 terms. This entry would then be followed by short-hand documentation of the etiologies identified to explain nongestational abnormal uterine bleeding (AUB) using the FIGO PALM-COEIN classification system.[2,6] In this system, the common causes of abnormal bleeding are categorized into two separate sections: those that are structural or detectable on examination, imaging, or biopsy (PALM) and those that are more functional (COEIN). The individual elements represented by each of those letters are more thoroughly explained later in the section on chronic heavy menstrual bleeding, where the system is most directly applicable.

Abnormal Menstrual Bleeding: Amenorrhea Overview

The most common causes of amenorrhea are pregnancy, lactation, menopause, and contraceptive use. However, about 3% to 4% of cases of amenorrhea are due to other causes, most frequently premature ovarian insufficiency or an extreme version of one of three other conditions: polycystic ovary syndrome (PCOS), hyperprolactinemia, or (functional) hypothalamic amenorrhea ((F)HA). Occasionally, systemic conditions can be associated with primary amenorrhea; these include malignancy, granulomatous diseases, renal failure, thyroid dysfunction, hemochromatosis, and other chronic, debilitating diseases. Accounting for the remaining cases is an exhaustive list of uncommon genetic, anatomic, and enzymatic abnormalities.[7] (See **Figure 3-1** for selective causes of primary and secondary amenorrhea.)

People who never experience menstruation are more likely to have uncommon etiologies than those who stop menstruating after menarche has occurred, but the causes for both primary and secondary amenorrhea are often similar. Reproductive endocrinologists have persuasively argued that the distinction between primary amenorrhea (no menarche) or secondary amenorrhea (cessation of bleeding after menarche) should be eliminated. To evaluate patients for any type of amenorrhea, the Endocrine Society recommends that a comprehensive set of hormonal laboratory tests be obtained initially, including β-human chorionic gonadotropin (β-hCG), free thyroxine (FT4), thyroid-stimulating hormone (TSH), prolactin (PRO), follicle stimulating hormone (FSH), luteinizing hormone (LH), estradiol (E_2), and anti-Müllerian hormone (AMH).[8]

However, most family planning clinics and primary care providers have limited resources and may lack the expertise required to care for the more unusual causes of primary amenorrhea, while the diagnosis and management of secondary amenorrhea is often comfortably within their scope of practice. Therefore, this chapter maintains a distinction between primary amenorrhea and secondary amenorrhea. Readers should be able to recognize and initiate the work up and referrals for the former, but more completely diagnose and treat the latter.

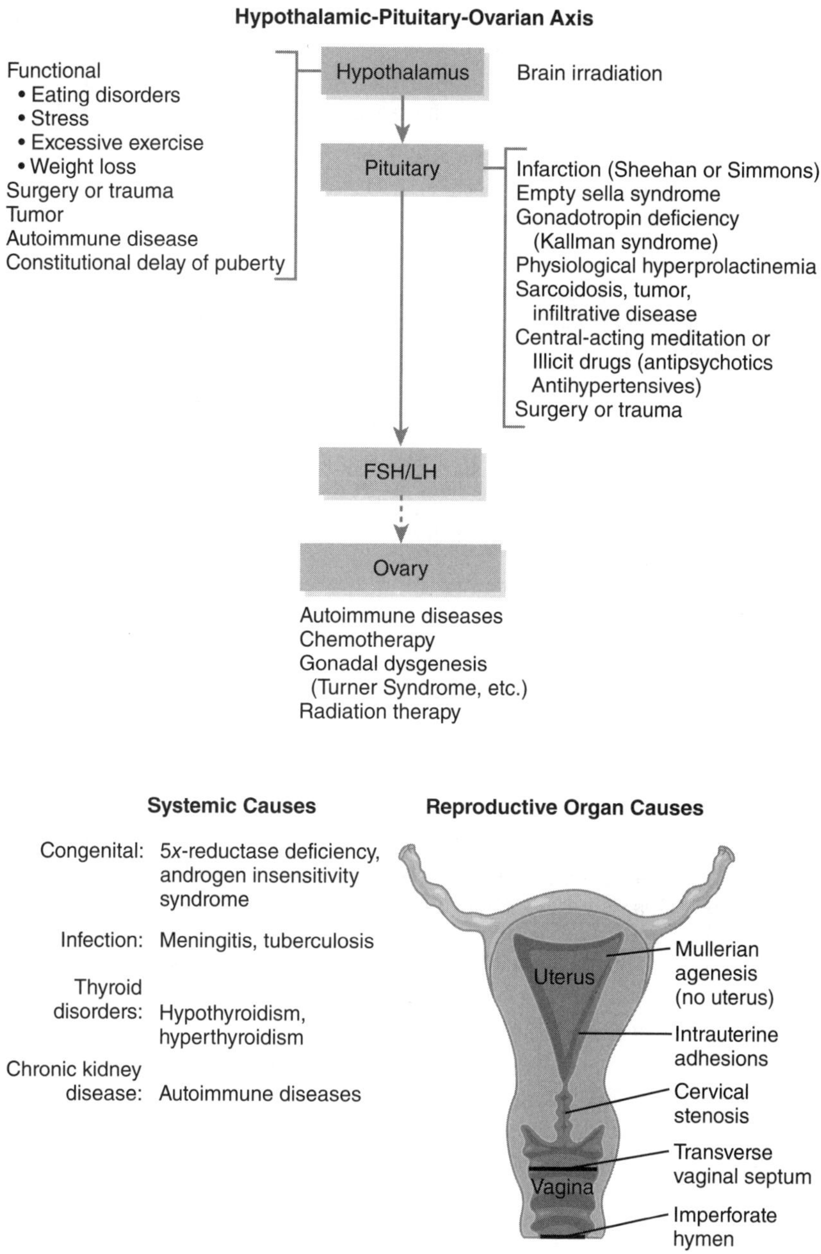

Figure 3-1 Select Causes of Amenorrhea

Primary Amenorrhea (Absence of Menarche)

The first manifestations of puberty are either thelarche (breast budding) or adrenarche (growth of sexual hair). The average age of onset of puberty in girls in the United States is 9.7 years, but normal age of onset ranges from 7 years to 13 years. Despite this great variability in the age of its initiation, once puberty starts, it follows a very predictable progression in time. The first menses (menarche) generally follows thelarche within 2 years. This predictable timeline provides the basis for guidance about *when* the diagnosis of primary amenorrhea should be considered and when a diagnostic work up should be initiated:

- When there has been no adrenarche or thelarche by age 13
- When there has been no menses by age 15
- When adrenarche or thelarche started on time, but menses have not started within 3 years of either event[7]

The differential diagnosis for patients with primary amenorrhea (lack of menarche) includes anatomical, genetic, hormonal, enzymatic, and psychologic causes. Most cases of primary amenorrhea should be referred to reproductive endocrinologists, but nonspecialty providers can often initiate the preliminary evaluation. The work up can be divided into the four following categories based on the presence or absence of breasts and a uterus.

Uterus, no breasts. Patients who have no breasts but have a uterus can be assumed to lack ovarian estrogen production. This ovarian insufficiency can be due to a wide variety of causes, including each of the following:

- Chromosomal abnormalities
  - Turner syndrome, mosaicism, pure gonadal dysgenesis
- Ovarian enzyme deficiency
- Ovarian damage[9,10]
  - Earlier radiation, chemotherapy
- Pituitary or hypothalamic dysfunction
  - Congenital hypogonadotropic hypogonadism (e.g., Kallmann syndrome)

No breasts, no uterus. Patients who have neither breasts nor a uterus are extremely rare. Generally, affected patients have an enzyme deficiency (17,20 desmolase deficiency; 17 alpha-hydroxylase deficiencies in a 46,XY individual) or lack any gonads after birth (but in utero had testicular tissue to prevent the formation of a uterus in the fetus).

Breasts, no uterus. For patients who have no uterus but have normal breast development demonstrating estrogen exposure, there are only a few major possible etiologies, including the following:

- *Androgen insensitivity syndrome.* Patients with this syndrome present with female secondary sexual characteristics, but have a 46,XY chromosomes and bilateral testes (often appearing as inguinal masses). They have male levels of testosterone, to which they are unable to respond. However, they do convert that testosterone peripherally, which explains in their high levels of circulating estrogens. Their testes need to be removed after puberty is complete, but before those organs undergo possible malignant transformation into gonadoblastoma. After diagnosis, patients with androgen insensitivity should be allowed to choose their gender identity as any other person assigned female at birth (AFAB). If they desire children, they will need egg donation and surrogates to carry the pregnancy, or they can adopt.
- *Congenital absence of a uterus* (complete uterine Müllerian agenesis) is found in 10% of cases of primary amenorrhea. Müllerian agenesis is associated with other urogenital malformations, especially kidney and ureteral

abnormalities. Patients with congenital absence of the uterus can use their own eggs if they want to have a child, but must use surrogates to carry the pregnancy.

Breasts, uterus. Most patients with primary amenorrhea have both a uterus and normally developed breasts. Anatomical defects, such as an imperforate hymen, a transverse vaginal septum, or other outflow tract abnormalities, may mask the actual onset of menses. Congenital obstruction of menstrual flow can be ruled out by pelvic examination or imaging studies. In most such obstructive cases, surgical excision can allow normal outflow of menses along the reproductive tract. The remaining evaluations are virtually the same as the evaluations needed for secondary amenorrhea and are described in the following section on secondary amenorrhea.

Secondary Amenorrhea

When patients who have previously menstruated stop menstruating, the first step is to do a pregnancy test. The only exception to this rule would be if the patient were asymptomatic and had consistently used a hormonal contraceptive with a known potential to reduce episodes of bleeding, such as levonorgestrel (LNG) intrauterine contraceptives, depot medroxyprogesterone acetate (DMPA) injections, noncyclic progestin-only pills (POP), or extended-cycle combined hormonal methods. With modern low-dose pills, it is not appropriate to attribute any significant delay in return of menses after pill cessation to "post-pill amenorrhea"; cyclic bleeding should not be delayed by more than 2 to 4 weeks after stopping any hormonal contraceptive method, except DMPA. If the onset of amenorrhea follows a uterine procedure, such as a dilation and curettage (D&C) to treat a septic abortion or postpartum hemorrhage, evaluate the endometrial cavity for adhesions (Asherman syndrome). For amenorrhea following cervical cryotherapy, loop electrosurgical excision procedure (LEEP), or cone biopsy, rule out cervical stenosis.

The question is, how *long* must a someone go without bleeding to be diagnosed as having secondary amenorrhea? Today the diagnosis is most appropriately made for a *regularly cycling* person if there has been no spotting or bleeding for 3 months. "Delayed menses" is used as the diagnosis before then. A patient with a history of *infrequent menses* technically should not be diagnosed as having secondary amenorrhea until bleeding has been absent for twice that patient's expected normal menstrual cycle length. However, that patient would warrant earlier evaluation for infrequent menses (see p. 42).

A lack of uterine bleeding can reflect one of two different endocrine states: a lack of *estrogen* to stimulate growth of the endometrium or a lack of *progesterone* to decidualize the endometrium. Lack of estrogen carries with it the health risks experienced in menopause, such as osteoporosis, early cardiovascular disease, and genitourinary syndrome of menopause (GSM). On the other hand, exposure to estrogen without progesterone significantly increases the risk for endometrial hyperplasia and endometrial cancer. Rarely, in the presence of normal amounts of both estrogen and progesterone, other local factors can suppress the endometrium. For example, relatively high levels of testosterone (as seen in patients with androgen-producing tumors or in transgender men and gender nonconforming individuals on testosterone) can block the ability of estrogen to stimulate endometrial cells. Of course, chronic endometrial suppression by progestins or estrogen-and-progestin combinations in hormonal contraception also results in amenorrhea, but this would not be of clinical concern.

Secondary amenorrhea in reproductive-aged patients not using hormonal contraception can signal problems ranging from problems confined to the reproductive system to systemic medical problems. Even if someone with secondary amenorrhea does not desire fertility, the amenorrhea must be evaluated because the medical problem underlying their lack of bleeding may require treatment.

History and Physical Examination

Take a detailed menstrual history and inquire about vasomotor symptoms. Question the patient about recent changes in weight, acne, hair growth, and cold or heat intolerance. Ask about headaches, galactorrhea, recent pregnancy, recent breastfeeding, recent genital tract procedures or other surgeries (e.g., bariatric surgery), prior chemotherapy or irradiation, eating patterns (diet), psychosocial stressors, and exercise patterns. Chronic illnesses, such as uncontrolled Type 1 diabetes, thyroid dysfunction, end-stage renal disease, AIDS, malabsorption, hepatic failure, Cushing syndrome, sarcoidosis, acromegaly, and craniopharyngiomas, can cause secondary amenorrhea. Also obtain a family history of medical problems—especially endocrine problems—that might influence menstrual cycling.

Take a complete drug history because all classes of medications (prescription, over-the-counter, and street recreational drugs) include some drugs that can induce amenorrhea or infrequent bleeding. Phenothiazine derivatives, phenothiazine-like compounds, haloperidol, selective serotonin reuptake inhibitors (SSRIs), reserpine derivatives, metoclopramide, sulpiride, promazine, cimetidine, verapamil, opioids, diazepam, tricyclic antidepressants, methyldopa, amphetamines, and marijuana can cause amenorrhea. High levels of prolactin can cause amenorrhea; less dramatic elevations in prolactin are associated with infrequent menses (see p. 42). Note that androgenic drugs, sometimes used to improve athletic performance or sexual desire, may be compounded or obtained by patients in unconventional ways. Chemotherapeutic agents and radiation exposure early in life or after menarche can induce early ovarian insufficiency and present as secondary amenorrhea.[9]

On examination, pay close attention to signs of androgen excess (hirsutism, balding, acne, voice changes, hidradenitis suppurativa, and clitoromegaly), insulin resistance (acanthosis nigricans), hypoestrogenism (dry, flattened vaginal mucosa), prolactin excess (galactorrhea), thyroid dysfunction (skin, pulse, and reflex changes), or changes indicating other systemic diseases. Check the patient's index and middle fingers for any signs of calluses on the dorsal surfaces and look for yellow staining on the inner surfaces of teeth, which might suggest induced vomiting associated with eating disorders. Look for behaviors, such as excessive concern with weight or body image, as well as suggestive attitudes, such as perfectionism and stressors.

Laboratory Tests

Some guidelines recommend that a comprehensive panel of serum and imaging tests be ordered all at once, including LH, FSH, estradiol, TSH, prolactin, free testosterone, AMH, and dehydroepiandrosterone sulfate (DHEA-S), as well as pelvic ultrasound.[7] However, it is probably more useful to order laboratory tests that are appropriate for the patient's history, physical exam, immediate fertility desires, and personal and family history, especially in resource-challenged settings. Once pregnancy is ruled out, the most common tests that are needed are TSH and prolactin, although total testosterone or FSH can also be very helpful in certain situations. For example:

- A 35-year-old with secondary amenorrhea, who reports increasing weight and decreased energy, may be best served by first testing TSH.
- A 23-year-old with secondary amenorrhea, who complains of hot flashes and a dry vagina with a history of use of alkylating agents used to treat childhood cancer, should have FSH tested first.[10]
- A 19-year-old with secondary amenorrhea accompanied by progressively worsening, severe hirsutism might need to have levels of 17-α hydroxyprogesterone and total testosterone evaluated to rule out adult-onset congenital adrenal hyperplasia and androgen-producing tumors.
- A 24-year-old nulliparous, hirsute patient with secondary amenorrhea, who desires pregnancy, would most likely benefit from having all these tests done.

Extensive testing may be needed if the results of the first round of testing points toward a specific problem. For example, someone with elevated TSH will need additional testing to determine the cause of the thyroid deficiency. Someone with a significantly elevated prolactin (prolactin $>$ 70 ng/dL) needs to have imaging studies (usually magnetic resonance imaging [MRI]) of the pituitary gland and adjacent areas to rule out pituitary prolactinoma, empty sella syndrome, craniopharyngioma, and other obstructive lesions. The 23-year-old with no bleeding for 8 months, whose FSH is in the postmenopausal range, should have that diagnosis confirmed by repeat testing of FSH and testing of LH and estradiol levels. If both gonadotropins are elevated and estradiol is low, the patient has premature ovarian insufficiency (POI) and is menopausal. POI refers to the loss of ovarian activity before age 40, which leads to hypoestrogenemia that will have life-changing physical and emotional consequences.[11] If there were no history of childhood chemotherapy explaining POI, additional tests would be needed. At age $<$ 30 years, a patient with unexplained POI would need extensive testing to rule out chromosomal abnormalities (most commonly Turner syndrome).[12] For older (30–35 years) patients with new onset POI, testing for thyroid and adrenal antibodies would be needed to rule out other autoimmune endocrinopathies that coexist with POI, which could worsen with time. Patients with POI should also be offered testing for FMR1 gene premutation, which increases the risk of fragile X syndrome in children.[13] Other specialty groups also recommend chromosomal analysis and screening for adrenal antibodies.[13]

Functional Hypothalamic Amenorrhea (FHA)

Two of the most common functional causes of secondary amenorrhea are extreme PCOS and functional hypothalamic amenorrhea (FHA). Each of those conditions presents clinically on a continuum from amenorrhea to subfertility. PCOS is discussed in greater detail in the section on infrequent menses and in the section on heavy menstrual bleeding. FHA deserves more detailed discussion here because it is more likely to present with amenorrhea than is PCOS.[8]

Hypothalamic amenorrhea (HA) can present as primary or secondary amenorrhea. It accounts for 30% of cases of secondary amenorrhea during the reproductive years.[14] Except for rare structural lesions (tumors), most of the cases of hypothalamic amenorrhea result from suppression of the hypothalamic–pituitary–ovarian (HPO) axis by functional causes (FHA). If prolonged, FHA has potential adverse consequences for metabolic, bone, cardiovascular, mental, and reproductive health—all the effects of prolonged hypoestrogenism.[15] Common causes for FHA include disordered eating, weight loss, excessive exercise, and stress. These problems often present in different combinations, but they share the fact that the patient lacks estrogen. An *energy deficit* is the critical factor in both weight loss- and exercise-induced forms of FHA, even if there has been no notable changes in weight with the latter. Low energy directly influences the HPO axis, inducing different clinical presentations in different people. FHA can also occur as a result of abnormalities in gonadotropin-releasing hormone (GnRH) receptors or dynamics induced by chronic disease, malabsorptive illnesses, celiac disease states, severe burns or hyperthyroidism.[14] In the end, FHA is a diagnosis of exclusion.

Closely related to FHA is the *female athlete triad*, which is a medical condition found among physically active women characterized by the following three components:[16]

1. Low energy availability, with or without disordered eating patterns
2. Menstrual dysfunction
3. Low bone density

The female athlete triad can appear at any age, but it can have a more significant impact on the health of adolescents, who have not completed their bone mineral accumulation. Because the consequences of some of these conditions may not be completely reversible, the American College of Obstetrics and Gynecology (ACOG) points out that prevention, early diagnosis, and intervention are all critical. Additionally, ACOG recommends that all patients with FHA should be assessed for components of the triad, and that further investigation be performed if any of them is identified.[16] Hormonal testing can be quite extensive; low levels of FSH, LH, and E_2 are expected. TSH and testosterone should be low-normal, but prolactin should be normal.[15] In addition to those hormonal tests, the work up of FHA also routinely includes complete blood count (CBC), electrolytes, liver and kidney function tests, and sedimentation rate or C-reactive protein tests. MRI is recommended in patients with presumed FHA as well as for other troubling signs or symptoms (e.g., headaches, vomiting, lateralizing neurologic signs, etc.). For teens and adults with more than 6 months of amenorrhea due to FHA, a baseline bone mineral density measurement with dual-energy X-ray absorptiometry (DEXA) is recommended. In young patients with FHA, bone density can range from normal to low. However, osteoporosis should be attributed to FHA only after excluding anatomic and organic pathology.

Treatments for Secondary Amenorrhea

Short-Term Therapies

While blood tests are being analyzed, it is quite reasonable to prescribe someone with secondary amenorrhea a short course of progestin therapy (e.g., medroxyprogesterone acetate [MPA] 10 mg or norethindrone acetate [NETA] 5 mg once daily for 10–12 days) to offset the possible adverse effects that unopposed estrogen may have had on the endometrium. In the past, the result of this so-called *progestin challenge test* was used as part of the work up of amenorrhea. Today, the progestin is considered to be therapeutic, not diagnostic, because the results of the former "progestin challenge test" do not reliably support any diagnosis. The *presence* of withdrawal bleeding after progestin challenge does not necessarily demonstrate prior ovarian estradiol production. Peripheral aromatization of androgens can produce weaker estrogens that can stimulate the endometrium. On the other hand, the *absence* of bleeding after progestin therapy does not reliably verify the absence of ovarian estrogen production. High circulating levels of androgen can block the ability of estrogen to induce endometrial proliferation.

Longer-Term Therapies

If a specific etiology is identified by the work up, therapy should be targeted:

- Prolactinomas without headaches or loss of peripheral vision are generally treated medically with cabergoline or bromocriptine.
- Hypothyroidism is treated with thyroxine replacement.
- Testosterone-producing tumors must be surgically removed.

The care of patients with FHA is best provided by multidisciplinary teams involving, if possible, the patient, an obstetrician-gynecologist, a nutritionist, parents (for minors), a mental health care provider, and, if indicated, sports coaches.[16] It is helpful for the initial clinician to counsel about the diagnosis and outline the care the patient can expect to receive from that team after it has been assembled. The most fundamental step in treating FHA is to correct the energy imbalance; this usually requires behavioral change and weight gain. Generally, these goals can be achieved by any combination of increased caloric consumption, improved nutrition, and/or decreased activity.[16] Cessation of self-induced vomiting or laxative use is also important. Psychological support, such as cognitive behavioral therapy, can contribute greatly to the success of treatment. Use of combined hormonal contraceptives (CHCs) to induce menses or to protect bones is **not** recommended. In fact, a patient with FHA, who does use combined hormonal contraception for birth control, needs to know that those hormones may mask return of spontaneous menses, and that even with CHC use, bone loss may continue until the energy deficit is corrected. These same guidelines say that transdermal estradiol with cyclic oral progestin may be used if menses do not spontaneously resume after a trial of comprehensive therapy. However, current evidence does not support the use of hormonal therapy for the sole purpose of improving bone mass in patients with FHA.[17]

For reproductive-aged patients whose amenorrhea results from other causes of estrogen deficiency, such as premature ovarian insufficiency, ACOG recommends systemic hormone therapy with estrogen and progestin to treat the symptoms and reduce the long-term health risks of hypoestrogenism, as long as there are no contraindications to such therapy.[18] CHCs are usually first-line choices because they are considered to be age-appropriate and might protect patients with premature ovarian insufficiency from the rare (but real) risk of pregnancy. Other patients may prefer postmenopausal hormone therapies.[19] Either therapy should be continued until age 50 or 51 in the absence of developing contraindications.

Patients with persistent secondary amenorrhea due to chronic anovulation require a different approach. They need ongoing *progestin therapy* to mitigate the harmful long-term effects that unopposed estrogen can have on the endometrium. Progestin can be administered *cyclically*, following a variety of protocols. For example, MPA or NETA can be given for the first 10–14 days of each month. CHCs can be given unless there is a contraindication to estrogen, because they are all progestin dominant. Alternatively, eligible patients may prefer to have some degree of *chronic* endometrial suppression using progestin-only methods, such as an LNG intrauterine device, contraceptive injections, the contraceptive implant, or progestin-only pills, or using an extended-cycle CHC.

Abnormal Menstrual Bleeding: Infrequent Menses

Infrequent menstruation is a common problem often caused by milder forms of conditions that cause secondary amenorrhea, such as hypothyroidism, androgen-excess conditions, and obesity. Once pregnancy is ruled out, most of those who have infrequent menses are found to have prolonged anovulation—i.e., estrogen production, but no progesterone. Occasionally, they may experience intermittent estrogen deficiency associated with episodic intermittent strenuous exercise, seasonal sports, periodic extreme stress, severe depression, or perimenopause.

The elements that should be included in the history and physical exam for patients presenting with infrequent menses are almost identical to those outlined for secondary amenorrhea above, except that a more detailed history of recent menstrual bleeding trends is required. Ask about symptoms of ovulation (Mittelschmerz) and moliminal complaints (bloating, cramping, or breast tenderness symptoms that typically herald the onset of menses). Ask about bleeding patterns over time and examine changes in these patterns in the context of events in the patient's life, activities, and changes in weight over time.

Polycystic Ovary Syndrome (PCOS)

PCOS is a complex and multifunctional condition that is the single most frequent endocrine disorder of those born with ovaries and a uterus. It can have reproductive, metabolic, and psychological comorbidities; screening and counseling need to involve all components of the syndrome.[20] Depending upon the PCOS definition used, up to 18% of reproductive-aged patients meet all the criteria for PCOS.[21] With the increasing prevalence of obesity, prevalence estimates of PCOS may be expected to increase substantially in coming years.[22] PCOS is the single most common cause of infertility, and among patients with infertility, it is the single most common antecedent to Type 2 diabetes.[23] Many of those with PCOS have an increased prevalence of traditional cardiovascular risk factors; PCOS may be viewed as a state of lower-grade chronic inflammation.[24] The direct cost of PCOS annually in the United States totals over $8 billion.[23]

The Rotterdam criteria are currently used to diagnose PCOS, although it is recognized that those criteria may overdiagnose PCOS and inflict unnecessary psychological harm.[25,26] The Rotterdam criteria state that, in the absence of other causes (e.g., congenital adrenal hyperplasia, androgen-secreting tumors, Cushing syndrome), adult patients can be diagnosed with PCOS if they meet at least two of the three following criteria:[27]

1. Infrequent menses (< 8 per year)
2. Hyperandrogenism or hyperandrogenemia
3. Polycystic-appearing ovaries

As an aside, adolescents should not be evaluated for PCOS for at least 18 months following menarche, and they should not be diagnosed with PCOS unless they meet *all three* Rotterdam criteria.[21]

PCOS has traditionally been considered to be a condition of androgen excess or, more rarely, of increased androgen sensitivity.[23] Hyperandrogenemia (high normal or slightly elevated levels of free or total testosterone or other androgens) or hyperandrogenism (hirsutism, acne, male-pattern balding) have traditionally been key elements in the clinical presentation.[28] Hirsutism must be distinguished from virilization (e.g., irreversible androgen-induced changes, such as voice deepening, clitoromegaly). According to the Rotterdam criteria, in order to qualify as a polycystic-appearing ovary (PAO), at least one ovary must have at least 12 preantral follicles, each measuring 2 to 9 mm, in any one ultrasound image or have an ovarian volume of ≥ 10 mL.[29] More recently, studies have suggested that age-specific criteria are needed to reflect the expected decrease in ovarian volume and follicle number with increasing age.[30] However, it is important to remember that PAO by itself does not make the diagnosis of PCOS, **because any condition that causes chronic anovulation (such as obesity) will induce polycystic-appearing ovaries**.

One of the most significant new advances made in PCOS has been the recognition that a diagnosis of PCOS by itself may not be very informative. PCOS is a syndrome with a wide range of different clinical presentations, different etiologies, and different long-term health implications. The one clinical problem that all those with PCOS share is decreased fertility, but other potential clinical manifestations of PCOS include menstrual disorders, skin disorders (hirsutism, acne, androgenic alopecia), insulin resistance, metabolic syndrome, nonalcoholic fatty liver disease, sleep apnea, cardiovascular risk factors, endometrial cancer risk factors, and mood disturbances and depression.[29] Pregnancy complications, including miscarriage, gestational diabetes, and premature delivery, occur at higher rates in those with PCOS compared to controls, but the increase in risk is relatively small.[29,31–33]

Individual clinical presentations of PCOS and the clinical implications of PCOS vary greatly by race and ethnicity as well as by the etiology underlying PCOS.[34] To deal with this variety, efforts are underway to describe a series of *phenotypes* within PCOS so that both counseling and therapy may be better individualized to meet the specific needs of those who present with different subtypes of PCOS.[21,34,35] See **Box 3-1** for one proposed classification system.[21,35]

Complicating this situation is the fact that over time, individuals' PCOS phenotypic characteristics can change. Aging affects the impacts of PCOS; decreases are seen in the prevalence of phenotype A over time and even in the prevalence of PCOS itself.[36]

While we await better understanding and definitions for those phenotypes, the most recent ACOG approach to the evaluation and management of PCOS is outlined in this section. However, to provide targeted evaluations and treatments where they may be appropriate, this chapter also suggests individualization of care that may vary from those existing comprehensive clinical guidelines.

Box 3-1 Proposed Phenotypic Categories of PCOS

Phenotype	Manifestations of PCOS
A	Oligo-ovulation, hyperandrogenism, with polycystic appearing ovary(ies)
B	Oligo-ovulation and hyperandrogenism
C	Hyperandrogenism and polycystic appearing ovary(ies)
D	Oligo-ovulation and polycystic appearing ovary(ies)

Data from Hoeger KM, Dokras A, Piltonen T. Update on PCOS: Consequences, challenges, and guiding treatment. J Clin Endocrinol Metab. 2021;106:e1071-e1083; Jamil AS, Alalaf SK, Al-Tawil NG, Al-Shawaf T. Comparison of clinical and hormonal characteristics among four phenotypes of polycystic ovary syndrome based on the Rotterdam criteria. Arch Gynecol Obstet. 2016;2:447-56.

PCOS is a diagnosis of exclusion; other conditions that could explain the signs and symptoms found in PCOS must be excluded by history, physical examination, and appropriate laboratory tests before a patient can be diagnosed with PCOS. For example, rule out pregnancy, thyroid dysfunction, prolactinoma, pituitary or hypothalamic suppression, and medication-induced infrequent menses.

The history should include a description of menstrual patterns over time in conjunction with corresponding estimates of weight, obstetrical history (including prior fertility challenges, gestational diabetes, excessive prenatal weight gain, fetal macrosomia), and history of androgen-related symptoms as well as prior treatments for any of these conditions. Hirsutism is a much more sensitive marker of PCOS than is either acne or alopecia. Family history of endocrine, reproductive, and metabolic disorders is important. On physical examination, take blood pressure, calculate body mass index (BMI), and measure waist circumference. Focus on signs that could either suggest another etiology, such as abnormal deep tendon reflexes (thyroid dysfunction); galactorrhea (prolactinoma); acanthosis nigricans or increased neck circumference (insulin resistance/diabetes); and rapid excessive hair growth, decreased breast tissue, or clitoromegaly (atypical congenital adrenal hyperplasia or androgen-producing tumors); and look for signs that could support the diagnosis of PCOS (acne, hirsutism, androgenic alopecia, acne, skin tags, or hidradenitis suppurativa).[29,37]

ACOG guidelines suggest that a comprehensive panel of tests be performed to evaluate PCOS.[29] (See **Table 3-3** for PCOS screening tests recommended by ACOG.) This list is certainly comprehensive and helpful in a work up for infertility or in a research setting. However, in practice (particularly in less resource-rich areas), those tests may be prohibitively expensive. In the face of clinically apparent nonprogressive hyperandrogenism with acne or hirsutism, the utility of ordering any tests for testosterone or DHEA-S has been questioned.[38] This skepticism may be supported by research implicating androstenedione or 11-oxygenated androgens rather than the classical testosterone as the root cause of PCOS hyperandrogenicity and metabolic risks.[39] Therefore, we may be able to use each individual's history, physical findings, and immediate fertility desires to guide in selecting the more

Table 3-3 PCOS Screening Tests Recommended by ACOG

Evidence of biochemical hyperandrogenemia Total testosterone and sex hormone binding globulin (SHBG) OR Bioavailable/free testosterone
Exclusion of other causes of PCOS symptoms TSH, prolactin 17-hydroxyprogesterone, Consider screening for Cushing or acromegaly
FBS + 2-hour glucose tolerance tests after 75-g glucola load
Fasting lipid panel
Metabolic syndrome evaluation
Ultrasound for ovary appearance and endometrial abnormalities

Modified from American College of Obstetricians and Gynecologists' Committee on Practice Bulletins—Gynecology. ACOG Practice Bulletin No. 194: Polycystic Ovary Syndrome. Obstet Gynecol. 2018;131(6):e157-e171.

essential tests needed in the initial work up. The most common tests that are routinely performed in a family planning clinic would be TSH and, perhaps, prolactin levels if galactorrhea is present. Other diagnostic tests would be ordered only as indicated. For example, a young patient with progressive hirsutism would need a 17-hydroxyprogesterone test for atypical congenital hyperplasia, and perhaps a total testosterone test to rule out an androgen-producing tumor.

Many patients with PCOS have an increased risk of developing prediabetes and diabetes at a younger age.[29] Even after correcting for BMI, those with PCOS, especially with the hyperandrogenic phenotypes, have a four- to fivefold increased risk for developing Type 2 diabetes.[40] Therefore, glucose tolerance testing may be very important for their health, even if it is not part of diagnosing PCOS. The best test is a 2-hour glucose tolerance test with a 75-g glucola load. This test can clearly identify prediabetes (100–125 mg/dL fasting blood glucose, or a 2-hour postprandial glucose level between 140 to 200 mg/dL) as well as overt diabetes (> 126 mg/dL fasting blood glucose or a 2-hour postprandial glucose > 200 mg/dL). Other tests, such as fasting glucose or hemoglobin A1C, can be used instead, but they are less sensitive in diagnosing diabetes and often miss the diagnosis of prediabetes. A substantial percentage of those with PCOS (especially those with BMI > 30 kg/m^2) also have metabolic syndrome, which may also put them at increased risk for future cardiovascular problems.[21] There are considerable racial and ethnic differences in the PCOS metabolic phenotypes that need to be better understood.[41] Patients with PCOS accompanied by obesity or elevated blood pressure benefit from a lipid profile. Also, carefully screen all those with PCOS for depression or anxiety.[21,42]

It is also important to know which tests are *not indicated* to diagnose PCOS. Routine testing for insulin resistance with fasting insulin levels is *not* indicated.[29] This is because there are no commercially available tests that can accurately diagnose insulin resistance and because knowing that a person has insulin resistance does not affect the choice of treatment. Older tests, such as the LH/FSH ratio, are also not relevant. Finally, in the absence of a palpable pelvic mass, it is generally *not* necessary to order a pelvic ultrasound for adult patients who meet the other two criteria for PCOS.

Long-Term PCOS Health Risks by Phenotype

PCOS is a syndrome with variable impacts on long-term health. Monitoring of patients with PCOS should be dynamic because risk factors shift as individuals with PCOS age.[24,36]

While a diagnosis of "PCOS" may not increase long-term risks for cardiovascular disease in all affected patients,[21,43,44] it is clear that the hyperandrogenic anovulatory phenotype A does substantially increase the risk of cardiovascular disease later in life. Similarly, PCOS that is complicated by obesity, tobacco use, dyslipidemia, hypertension, impaired glucose tolerance, overt diabetes, or subclinical vascular disease has been associated with an increase in the risk of heart attack and stroke later in life. Since the prevalence of depression and anxiety are elevated, psychiatric health must also be monitored.[42]

Treatments for PCOS-related problems are discussed with treatments for other causes of infrequent menses.

Other Causes of Unexplained Infrequent Menses

Infrequent menses usually results from anovulation, as noted in the discussion of PCOS. Clinical symptoms such as fatigue, weight gain, constipation, and depressive moods can suggest hypothyroidism; an elevated TSH can confirm the diagnosis and distinguish it from primary depression. Prolactinomas more commonly cause infrequent menses than they do amenorrhea, especially when those pituitary tumors produce prolactin levels in the lower ranges of abnormal. Similarly, marijuana and centrally acting medications, such as lithium and others that interfere with dopamine, modestly raise prolactin levels and can cause infrequent bleeding in their users.[7]

An increasingly common cause of infrequent bleeding during reproductive years is obesity-related anovulation; patients with BMIs > 30 kg/m^2 often have polycystic-appearing ovaries because of chronic anovulation. Technically, criteria 1 and 3 of the Rotterdam definition would qualify them for the diagnosis of PCOS. However, since they have no androgen excess, some experts have objected to labeling these individuals as having PCOS. This issue should be clarified in subsequent refinements of the definition of PCOS, which will recognize different phenotypes within PCOS.

Treatments for Infrequent Menses (Including PCOS)

Treatment of infrequent menses depends upon the underlying etiology, immediate fertility desires, and any other health challenges that are present. Patients with underlying medical problems, such as hyperprolactinemia and hypothyroidism, should receive targeted therapies for those issues, but they should also be provided progestin therapy for endometrial protection until their menses normalize and routine ovulation returns. Contraception during this time is also important, because of episodic ovulation and unannounced return of fertility.

Lifestyle Modifications

The most effective first-line intervention for patients with PCOS who have obesity and who are sedentary is a combination of long-term healthy eating, including a diet rich in fruits, vegetables, fiber, and lean proteins, *and* consistent engagement in physical activity.[29] While short-term studies may suggest superiority of one type of diet over another, there are no long-term studies demonstrating superior outcomes.[45] However, important genetic differences may make some people more resistant to weight loss with diets that may work for other people. Our goal is to support patients in finding a safe diet they can follow over the long term.[29] To lose weight, those with PCOS must maintain low-calorie diets for prolonged periods of time. Reducing their intake to 500 to 600 kcal/day below subsistence level can mean that, without an exercise program, it is calculated that they can consume only 1000–1200 kilocalories a day. To be successful on such stringent diets, patients need significant support in a wide variety of ways. Behavioral therapy support will likely add to success.[46,47]

Exercise is critically important to every weight loss program and to the maintenance of a healthy weight. To lose weight, calories consumed need to be lower than the calories being expended. Exercise helps consume calories, so overly restrictive caloric goals are not necessary. Aerobic exercise by patients with PCOS results in reduction of fasting insulin and insulin resistance.[48] In addition, exercise promotes cardiovascular health, balance, and quality sleep. Sleep disorders associated with obesity or PCOS contribute to insulin resistance, which in turn, increases cardiovascular disease risk. Therefore, *sleep*, *diet*, and *exercise* comprise an interrelated triad of key health-supporting behaviors for patients of all ages. Unfortunately, although most guidelines endorse these approaches, a Cochrane systematic review found most lifestyle interventions may improve free androgen index, weight, and BMI in those with PCOS, but the impact on glucose tolerance was unclear. Most studies in these topics were of low quality and none investigated other outcomes, such as menstrual regulation or live births or miscarriage.[49]

Therapeutic Agents

Choice of therapies in those not seeking immediate pregnancy depends upon the problems PCOS is causing the individual. In general, first-line therapy for those with PCOS not seeking immediate pregnancy is a CHC.[29] The estrogen may help treat acne and hirsutism; the progestin can provide endometrial protection; together those two hormones can provide predictable cyclic bleeding or can safely suppress the frequency of bleeding while providing endometrial protection.[50] Contraceptive patches are indicated only for those with BMI < 30 kg/m^2. Endometrial protection can also be provided by progestin-only methods either locally intrauterine devices (IUDs) or systemically (implants, injections, or oral contraceptives). For those with acne, in general, reduction in acne and hirsutism are considered to be a class effect of all estrogen-containing contraceptives. Maximal therapeutic effect of combined oral contraceptives for treatment of acne is not seen until after 6 months of therapy; up to 2 years of therapy may be needed to maximize the impact of combined oral contraceptives on hirsutism. Generally, CHCs are added to topical therapies (such as drying agents and antibiotics) to treat acne. Use of spironolactone requires the use of other agents to protect against pregnancy (it is a teratogen) and to protect against the abnormal bleeding it can cause. CHCs can meet both needs. Insulin-sensitizing agents in those with impaired glucose tolerance complicating their PCOS are associated with a decrease in circulating androgen levels.[29]

Hirsutism can also be treated topically with eflornithine or may be removed by laser therapy. Combination therapy is superior.[29] Spironolactone is also utilized to reduce androgen stimulation of hair follicle growth. In each case, use of CHCs can complement those therapies. CHCs can also help treat other androgen-excess related conditions, such as hidradenitis suppurativa.

For normoglycemic patients with PCOS who are not seeking pregnancy, routine use of insulin-sensitizing agents is now discouraged by the ACOG.[29] Some experts have recommended dual therapy for subsets of high-risk patients. For example, it might be more effective to combine CHCs and metformin to treat those with findings indicating insulin resistance, such as metabolic syndrome, acanthosis nigricans, or a history of gestational diabetes.[51]

Patients with anovulatory cycling need special attention paid to their reproductive potential. It is optimal if patients are medically prepared for pregnancy because patients with PCOS, especially those with the hyperandrogenic phenotypes, have higher risks for developing gestational diabetes and for requiring cesarean delivery. Their infants are at risk for growth disorders, usually macrosomia.[52,53]

Infertility Treatment

The treatment of infertility in patients with PCOS has changed dramatically over the years. In those with excessive weight, weight loss has always been the first step, because a loss of only 10% to 15% of current weight can restore ovulation to a majority of those with elevated BMIs, but now there are also pharmacologic options to assist them in that effort.[54] If lifestyle interventions are not successful in inducing ovulation, ACOG recommends letrozole for first-line therapy for ovulation induction; insulin-sensitizing agents are not appropriate as sole therapy.[29] Randomized comparative clinical trials have clearly demonstrated that both clomiphene citrate and letrozole as single therapies are superior to extended-release metformin and produce higher rates of ovulation, pregnancy, and live births.[55] Second-line therapies recommended by ACOG for those who do not respond to aromatase inhibitors or clomiphene citrate is ovulation induction with low-dose exogenous gonadotropins or laparoscopic ovarian surgery (drilling).[29] ACOG also recommends combining clomiphene citrate with metformin as a second-line option. Progestin withdrawal prior to ovulation induction does not improve pregnancy rates.[56]

Long-Term Health Promotion

Patients with anovulation-based infrequent menses need *long-term therapies* with a *progestin (with or without estrogen)* to protect their endometrial linings from the long-term effects of unopposed estrogen: endometrial hyperplasia and endometrial carcinoma. Those who are at least 50 pounds overweight have a 10-fold increased risk of endometrial carcinoma. That risk may be due to the fact that they have lower expression of both nuclear and membrane-bound progesterone receptors with their endometrial cells.[57] Progestin can be provided by contraceptive agents or by long-term cyclic progestin therapy.

Patients with hyperandrogenic PCOS and metabolic syndrome or Type 2 diabetes are at higher risk for developing cardiovascular disease (CVD) later in life.[29,43] However, it is not clear that a history of undifferentiated PCOS during the reproductive years will increase the risk of CVD mortality after menopause.[43,44]

Intriguingly, early research has suggested that the fundamental dysfunction with PCOS lies with faulty adipocytes and chronic inflammation; studies have shown that statins may be effective as single agents in normalizing many of the metabolic abnormalities with PCOS (including anovulation) and in providing cardiovascular protection too.[58] Confirmation of these findings may fundamentally alter how some phenotypes of PCOS will be treated in the future.

Attention to psychological health is also important since the prevalence of both depression and anxiety are higher in patients with PCOS.[42,59] Behavioral modification therapy may be a helpful adjunct to weight loss. One good resource for patients with PCOS is the documentary *Scrambled: A Journey Through Polycystic Ovary Syndrome (PCOS)* by Randi Cecchine; another is the PolyCyster website (https://www.polycyster.com/).

Heavy or Prolonged Menstrual Bleeding

Heavy menstrual bleeding (HMB) is a common gynecologic problem affecting 9% to 14% of healthy women, although surveys have found that up to 30% of women consider their bleeding to be excessive.[60] HMB adversely impacts a variety of aspects of a patient's life. Patients with HMB are 45% more likely to use health services and 27% less likely to work. If they do work outside the home, it has been estimated that annual income of those with heavy bleeding is substantially less than those with normal menses.[61]

The prevalence of HMB depends upon how it is defined. The classic definition is the loss of greater than 80 mL of blood per cycle. However, in daily life, the amount of blood loss is very difficult to quantify. Pad counts are not a reliable measure because of differences in product absorbency and in how frequently patients change their pads. Interpretation of hemoglobin levels can be complicated by variations in dietary intake of iron. Blood losses as great as 80 to 120 mL per cycle can occur without causing anemia in patients who consume iron-rich diets and iron supplements. However, by the time a patient does achieve anemia, a considerable amount of menstrual blood will have been lost.

A practical definition of HMB advances the idea that blood loss is excessive not only when it meets the classic objective measure of loss (> 80 mL of blood loss per cycle), but also *when the patient says it is excessive*. This definition illustrates that a *key factor in making a diagnosis of HMB is not only the amount of blood being lost, but how much HMB disrupts one's life*. The National Institute of Health and Care Excellence (NICE) guidelines capture this by defining HMB as "excessive menstrual blood loss, which interferes with the woman's physical, social, emotional, and/or material quality of life, and which can occur alone, or in combination with other symptoms."[62] A patient whose total blood loss is only 60 mL/cycle, but whose flow is so heavy for 2 hours each cycle that it immobilizes that individual, clearly has excessive bleeding. Blood loss so excessive that the patient becomes anemic must be evaluated even if the complaint of heavy bleeding is not volunteered. Another important consideration is that menstrual flow includes much more fluid than just blood. Only about half of the menstrual fluid volume is blood; the rest of the flow is composed of cervical and uterine secretions.[63]

There are two possibly overlapping clinical scenarios that involve nongestational excessive uterine bleeding: acute excessive uterine bleeding and chronic excessive bleeding. It should be noted that "excessive" can reflect either or both heavy or prolonged bleeding episodes.

Acute Excessive Uterine Bleeding

Acute heavy uterine bleeding can present as a life-threatening crisis that often requires immediate therapy even before a precise diagnosis can be confirmed.[3] Rapid pregnancy testing should be performed because pregnancy-related causes of acute heavy bleeding (spontaneous abortion, abruption, placenta previa, etc.) require entirely different interventions. Pelvic examination may identify the source of the bleeding and rule out trauma (lacerations) or other conditions, such as aborting fibroids and expelling IUDs, that require specific procedures.

A CBC is useful to assess the baseline hemoglobin level and platelet count. Low platelet counts can contribute to the active bleeding; elevated platelet counts (thrombocytosis) are relatively common in chronic anemia and increase the risk of venous thromboembolism. If bleeding is very heavy or hemoglobin is low, blood typing and cross matching is prudent. Depending upon the results of the history and physical examination, other common tests include TSH, coagulation studies, iron studies, and pelvic imaging, usually with ultrasound.

Treatments for Acute Excessive Bleeding

Hormonal regimens form the bedrock of virtually all therapies used to arrest acute HMB.[64] Acute nongestational excessive bleeding shares most of the PALM-COIEN etiologies with chronic HMB, but with a few extra conditions to consider. The urgency of the need for therapy will often dictate the speed and the order of the testing that is done.

Actively bleeding patients with severe anemia and those who are hemodynamically unstable often require hospitalization for monitoring, transfusion, and medical or surgical therapy to arrest their hemorrhage. There are few studies that have addressed the efficacy and safety of the classic medical therapies, but intravenous estrogen therapy with conjugated equine estrogen (CEE) 20–25 mg every 3–4 hours for up to 24 hours is often utilized. CEE 2.5 mg orally every 4–6 hours may be offered as an alternative.[65-67] Bleeding should slow in 12–24 hours, at which time a progestin (e.g., MPA 5–10 mg by mouth daily) is added. Doses are reduced and continued for up to a month on an outpatient basis to allow for resolution of anemia. Because of increased risk for venous thromboembolism, high-dose estrogen therapies should be used with caution in patients with reactive thrombocytosis, which is fairly common among those with chronic anemia.[3] Nonsteroidal anti-inflammatory drugs (NSAIDs), tranexamic acid, and iron are added as complementary agents.[68] Antiemetic agents are often helpful with high dose estrogen therapy. Those with coagulation disorders, such as von Willebrand disease, will benefit from targeted therapy such as desmopressin.[69–71] Surgical procedures, such as D&C, uterine packing, tamponade with a uterine balloon, uterine artery embolization, or hysterectomy may be needed in the face of life-threatening hemorrhage, a need for transport of an unstable patient, or if medical therapies fail to correct acute excessive bleeding.[66,67]

Actively bleeding patients who are hemodynamically stable and have hemoglobin above 8 mg/dL are generally treated on an outpatient basis. Clarity has emerged about the safety and efficacy of progestin-only treatments in contrast to the more

Box 3-2 Current First-Line Outpatient Treatment for Acute HMB

Progestin-only regimens are the recommended first-line treatment of acute excessive vaginal bleeding of women who are medically eligible for outpatient therapy:

Medroxyprogesterone acetate (MPA) 10 mg

2 tabs by mouth three times daily for 7 days, followed by 2 tabs by mouth once daily for the next 21 days.

(You may need to add a note to the pharmacist that you really do mean to prescribe these high doses.)[72]

Data from DeVore GR, Owens O, Kase N. Use of intravenous Premarin in the treatment of dysfunctional uterine bleeding--a double-blind randomized control study. Obstet Gynecol. 1982;59:285-91; Borzutzky C, Jaffray J. Diagnosis and Management of Heavy Menstrual Bleeding and Bleeding Disorders in Adolescents. JAMA Pediatr. 2020;174:186-194; Screening and management of bleeding disorders in adolescents with heavy menstrual bleeding: ACOG COMMITTEE OPINION, Number 785. Obstet Gynecol. 2019;134:e71-e83;Connell NT, Flood VH, Brignardello-Petersen R, et al. ASH ISTH NHF WFH 2021 guidelines on the management of von Willebrand disease. Blood Adv. 2021;5:301-325.

traditional "oral contraceptive taper" options.[72] **Box 3-2** outlines the MPA-based therapy that has been shown in the largest prospective randomized trial to be as effective as CHC-based theripies.[72] It suppresses the endometrium for 28 days to allow the hemoglobin to normalize and to provide time for laboratory and imaging studies to be completed so appropriate targeted long-term therapies can be developed.

Because this progestin-only regimen is well tolerated and does not expose patients to any estrogen-related adverse events (e.g., thrombosis, high levels of nausea, vomiting, headache, etc.), it should be considered first-line treatment in the outpatient setting. Experimental work with 48 women found that combination of DMPA 150 IM and oral MPA 20 mg three times daily for 3 days arrested bleeding rapidly and with few side effects, but replication of the study is needed. These progestin-only outpatient therapies are effective for acute heavy bleeding caused by a full range of endometrial pathologies, from endometrial atrophy to hyperplasia.[73]

Other so-called "OC tapers" or short-term, low-dose progestin-only therapies (e.g., MPA 10 mg daily for 10–14 days) are commonly prescribed to treat acute bleeding, especially in emergency department settings. Although these therapies are appropriate to induce bleeding among women who have experienced amenorrhea, no adequate evidence exists to support the effectiveness or safety of any of these regimens to arrest active bleeding. These therapies may arrest current bleeding, but often bleeding returns at the end of the therapy. Appropriate dosing of agents for adequate periods of time are needed to achieve the objectives of stopping bleeding for weeks to enable hemoglobin normalization and to complete any diagnostic testing needed to identify specific causes of bleeding.

Chronic Excessive Bleeding

It is estimated that each year 1.4 million women in the United States are diagnosed with AUB[74] and that nearly 30% of outpatient gynecologic visits are for AUB.[75] As staggering as these numbers are, the true prevalence is likely significantly higher. As noted above, the objective definition of heavy menstrual bleeding is the loss of greater than 80 mL of hemoglobin per cycle. Prolonged bleeding is bleeding that persists for greater than 8 days. Menstrual bleeding can also be classified as excessive if the individuals say that flow adversely affects their quality of life. When a patient experiences an unexplained significant *change* in bleeding patterns, it may also need to be evaluated.

Terminology and Definitions

Chronic AUB refers to abnormalities of menstruation spanning 6 months or more. Abnormal uterine bleeding has a variety of etiologies that must be understood to tailor diagnostic testing and treatment options. The PALM-COEIN classification proposed by the Menstrual Disorders Working Group of FIGO in 2011 and updated in 2018 allows for the standardization of terminology for clinicians. The classification divides etiologies of AUB into structural and nonstructural. The structural abnormalities are further subdivided into categories following the acronym PALM: **P**olyps, **A**denomyosis, **L**eiomyoma, and **M**alignancy and hyperplasia. The etiologies unrelated to structural abnormalities are subdivided into categories following the acronym COEIN: **C**oagulation disorders, **O**vulatory disorders, **E**ndometrial disorders, **I**atrogenic causes, and **N**ot otherwise classified causes.[1]

History and Physical Exam

In the face of heavy bleeding, it is important to inquire about systemic conditions, infections, medications, or coagulation disorders that may be causing heavy or prolonged bleeding. Incorporate principles of trauma-informed care when conducting sensitive physical exams, including breast and pelvic exams. Ask for consent, ensure confidentiality, discuss the presence of a chaperone (giving patients a choice about gender of the chaperone whenever possible), and support the patient's bodily autonomy. Pelvic exams should evaluate for alternative causes of bleeding such as vaginal injury, cervical friability, cervical polyp, or ectropion. Bimanual exam should evaluate the size, shape, and tenderness of the uterus, tubes, and ovaries and assess for any cervical motion tenderness.

Laboratory and Diagnostic Testing

Any reproductively aged patient presenting with AUB should be evaluated for pregnancy with a urine pregnancy test. Depending on the symptoms and signs elucidated during the history and physical exam, a clinician may choose to pursue further testing. If a patient reports symptoms or shows signs of anemia or reports significant blood loss either due to quantity or duration of bleeding, a clinician may choose to evaluate with a CBC. This also allows for comparison after intervention to see if there has been an improvement in blood levels. The actual hemoglobin or hematocrit must be interpreted in the context of a patient. A patient who has had chronic blood loss from heavy menstrual bleeding (HMB) may not exhibit any symptoms despite the hemoglobin being severely low, whereas a patient with acute blood loss may begin to exhibit symptoms at a much higher hemoglobin since their body has not acclimated to the blood loss. A CBC can also diagnose platelet count disorders. Additional laboratory testing may include, when indicated, TSH, cervical cytology, cervicitis testing, and screening for bleeding disorders.

If needed, imaging studies to evaluate for structural uterine pathologies are generally best accomplished by pelvic ultrasound. Sonohysterogram (SHG), also known as saline infusion sonography (SIS), uses a small catheter to slowly instill saline into the uterine cavity while imaging with ultrasound to evaluate for any structural aberrations to the endometrial lining. Occasionally MRI may be of diagnostic value, specifically when evaluating for the presence, size, and distribution of leiomyomas or adenomyosis in the uterus. Diagnostic hysteroscopy is an outpatient procedure that can be performed to directly visualize the uterine cavity for pathology.

Therapies

Long-term, outpatient management of chronic HMB should be tailored to the suspected etiology with an emphasis on improving the patient's quality of life and reproductive goals. Person-centered counseling and shared decision making are paramount in discussing therapeutic options. It is important to discuss the goals of therapy, expected bleeding changes, success rates, and likely side effects to ensure the patient has realistic expectations and the therapy addresses the patient's specific concerns. Patients may have one or more etiologies for their heavy or prolonged bleeding. A full assessment is needed to design the appropriate therapy, but often menstrual suppression is the goal.[50]

Structural Etiologies (PALM) of Chronic Abnormal Uterine Bleeding

Polyps (AUB-P). Uterine polyps are focal endometrial growths, analogous to a skin tag within the uterine cavity. The exact etiology is unknown, but prevalence increases with age, and overall is estimated to be about 8%.[76] Polyps typically present as intermenstrual bleeding (IMB), HMB, or postmenopausal bleeding. Polyps typically will persist until removed.

The gold standard for diagnosing polyps is based on hysteroscopic visualization and guided resection. However, polyps are most often diagnosed using transvaginal ultrasound (TVUS). They appear as hyperechoic lesions within the uterine lumen. Sonohysterogram (SHG) improves diagnostic accuracy and defines the width of the polyp's attachment to the uterine wall. Polyps may be seen as filling defects not only on SHG, but also on HSG. Polyps may also be diagnosed on histologic examination of tissue retrieved from endometrial biopsy.

Although commonly benign, there is a 1% to 3% chance of a polyp being premalignant endometrial intraepithelial neoplasia (EIN), and a 0.5% to 3% chance of a polyp being malignant. The risk of these findings increases with age particularly in those who present with postmenopausal bleeding.[77–79] One randomized controlled trial (RCT) of expectant management versus surgical removal of endometrial polyps did not show any improvement in cyclic blood loss but did show improvements in IMB with surgical removal.[80] The levonorgestrel intrauterine device (LNG-IUD) has been used to prevent the formation of polyps in patients on tamoxifen, but otherwise there is little room for medical management in the treatment of endometrial polyps.[79,81] Hysteroscopic polypectomy is the definitive treatment for endometrial polyps and the most effective way in addressing AUB-P.

Adenomyosis (AUB-A). Adenomyosis is a structural pathology in which the endometrial implants (glands and stroma) are found in the myometrium of the uterus. Risk factors for the development of adenomyosis include increased parity, uterine instrumentation including curettage, cesarean delivery, myomectomy, or abortion. It usually presents as HMB, dysmenorrhea, or infertility. Adenomyosis is definitively diagnosed via histopathology; thus most studies are retrospective following hysterectomy. As imaging techniques have improved, 2-D and 3-D ultrasound are better able to diagnose adenomyosis with higher sensitivity and specificity. However, when older ultrasound was compared to MRI in a meta-analysis, MRI was shown to have superior sensitivity and specificity in making the diagnosis.[82]

Typically, the goal of treating adenomyosis is to improve bleeding and pain symptoms, generally with menstrual suppression.[50] Inducing amenorrhea using continuous combined oral contraceptives (COCs) is one way to alleviate symptoms. LNG-IUD has been demonstrated in several studies to successfully treat bleeding and pain symptoms. An RCT comparing LNG-IUD to hysterectomy looking at short- and long-term effects showed that in the short term, LNG-IUD achieved equivalent improvement in bleeding symptoms and minor superiority in some quality-of-life indicators. In the long term, 72% reported high satisfaction with the LNG-IUD in achieving symptomatic relief and a decrease in uterine volume, while preserving the option for future fertility.[83] In those who do not desire future fertility, hysterectomy is the definitive treatment for pain and bleeding symptoms of adenomyosis.

Leiomyoma (AUB-L). Leiomyomas or uterine fibroids are benign tumors of smooth muscle and fibroblasts. It is estimated that 70% to 80% of women will develop at least one fibroid by age 50, but most are asymptomatic. Approximately 25% of those with fibroids will be clinically symptomatic and require intervention.[84] Fibroids are steroid dependent, expressing estrogen and progesterone receptors, and are thus most prevalent during the premenopausal years and thought to stop growing and even shrink in size following menopause.

Fibroids are classified according to which layer of the uterus they are located—submucosal, intramural, or subserosal in the FIGO Leiomyoma subclassification system (**Figure 3-2**). Rarely, fibroids can become pedunculated and torse or parasitize to other organs, such as the bowel. They can grow retrograde and fill the internal vena cava to reach the heart and lungs (intravenous leiomyomas).

Symptomatic fibroids typically cause bleeding problems or bulk symptoms. Increased endometrial surface area, increased uterine vasculature, changes in uterine contractility, along with possible abnormalities in endometrial angiogenesis and hemostasis lead to the typical bleeding symptoms of heavy menstrual bleeding or prolonged menstrual bleeding often seen with uterine fibroids.[85,86] Increased uterine size and the resultant compression of surrounding structures—bowel, bladder, ureters, vagina, sacrum—leads to bulk symptoms of constipation, abdominal bloating, urinary incontinence/frequency/incomplete emptying, hydronephrosis, dyspareunia, and/or back pain. Fibroids are most commonly diagnosed on physical exam with confirmation via pelvic ultrasound. SHG or SIS can increase sensitivity in differentiating submucosal and intramural fibroids while pelvic MRI may be used for fibroid mapping as part of surgical planning (especially myomectomy). In the absence of significant pelvic pathology, decisions about treatment of leiomyomas should be through shared decision making. The discussion should take into

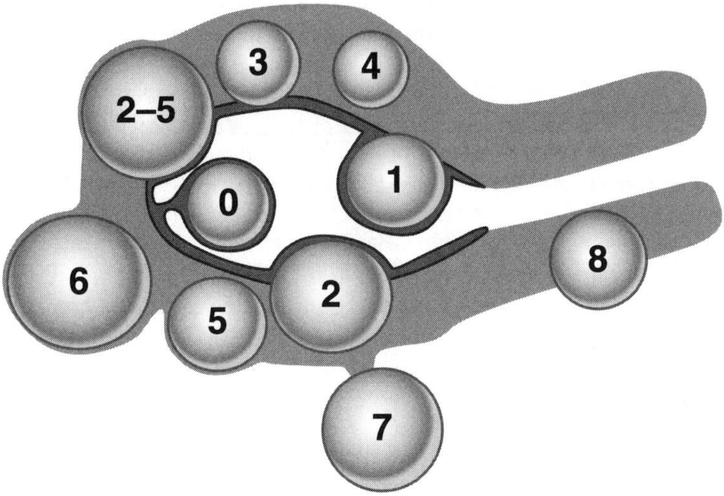

PALM
Polyp
Adenomyosis
Leiomyoma
Malignancy & hyperplasia

Leiomyoma →

Leiomyoma subclassification
Submucous
Other

COEIN
Coagulopathy
Ovulatory dysfunction
Endometrial
Iatrogenic
Not otherwise classified

SM - Submucous	0	Pedunculated intracavitary
	1	<50% intramural
	2	≥50% intramural
	3	Contacts endometrium; 100% intramural
O - Other	4	Intramural
	5	Subserous ≥50% intramural
	6	Subserous <50% intramural
	7	Subserous pedunculated
	8	Other (specify e.g., cervical, parasitic)
Hybrid	Two numbers are listed separated by a hyphen. By convention, the first refers to the relationship with the endometrium while the second refers to the relationship to the serosa. One example is below.	
(contact both the endometrium and the serosal layer)	2–5	Submucous and subserous, each with less than half the diameter in the endometrial and peritoneal cavities, respectively.

Figure 3-2 FIGO Abnormal Uterine Bleeding System

Reproduced from Munro MG, Critchley HOD, Fraser IS; FIGO Menstrual Disorders Committee. The two FIGO systems for normal and abnormal uterine bleeding symptoms and classification of causes of abnormal uterine bleeding in the reproductive years: 2018 revisions. Int J Gynaecol Obstet. 2018;143:393-408.

account a patient's symptoms, threats to their health, reproductive desires, desire to retain their uterus, and quality of life indicators, while ensuring that the clinician adequately addresses the risks and benefits of various treatment modalities.

Table 3-4 Oral NSAID Regimens for Treatment of Chronic Heavy Menstrual Bleeding

Mefenamic Acid
■ 500 mg three times daily for up to first 4–5 days of menses ■ 500 mg three times daily for the first 4–5 days prior to menses to cessation (rarely needed) ■ 500 mg initially; 200 mg four times daily for the first 3–5 days of menses
Naproxen
■ 500 mg at onset and 3–5 hours later; then 500 mg twice daily for up to 5 days ■ 500 mg in AM and 250 mg in PM for 2 days; then 250 mg twice daily for up to 7 days ■ 500 mg; 250 mg four times daily for up to 4 days ■ 550 mg; 275 mg four times daily for up to 5 days
Ibuprofen
■ 600 mg daily or 1200 mg daily (not as effective) ■ 800 mg three times daily for up to 5 days (Norplant trial)

Asymptomatic patients with an incidental finding of uterine fibroids are encouraged to proceed with expectant management, following a description of the typical symptoms in case they develop in the future.

Medications can be used to manage and improve the bleeding symptoms of fibroids without the risks of surgery, while allowing fertility preservation, but are not usually effective in dealing with the bulk symptoms caused by fibroids. Medical management can be divided into nonhormonal and hormonal methods. Nonhormonal methods can always be used as an adjunct to hormonal methods but may also be used in isolation for patients who are not candidates for or desire to avoid hormonal therapies. NSAIDs can be used to improve dysmenorrhea and HMB by blocking prostaglandin synthesis, but careful attention must be paid to dosing.[87] **Table 3-4** displays current recommendations. Tranexemic acid (TXA), an antifibrinolytic agent, is useful for HMB symptoms in that it prevents the breakdown of clot that forms during menstruation to aid in hemostasis, helping to shorten duration of bleeding and quantity of blood loss.[88] In a meta-analysis from 2019, TXA was shown to be more effective in reducing HMB symptoms than NSAIDs alone, but NSAIDs were still found to be better than placebo.[89]

Hormonal medical treatments block or decrease the stimulatory effects of ovarian steroids to decrease fibroid growth and size and to control growth of the endometrium. CHCs help to maintain a thinner endometrial lining. In patients who are not candidates for estrogen-containing therapies, progestin-only methods including pills, injectable depo-medroxyprogesterone, and LNG-IUDs are good options. Until the introduction of GnRH antagonists do with hormonal add-back, the LNG 52 mg IUD was shown to be the most effective medical management for decreasing HMB in patients with fibroids.[90,91] The LNG 52 mg IUD has not been extensively tested in those with large intracavitary components of the fibroids, which may distort its shape and prevent IUD placement. The biggest downside of its use for AUB-L is that there is a greater than threefold increase in the risk of expulsion in patients with fibroid uteri (11% vs 0% to 3%), especially if the fibroids do distort the cavity.[90,91] If contraception is not needed, non-contraceptive progestins can be dosed as "short-cycle" or "long-cycle." "Short-cycle" progestin refers to luteal phase dosing taken for 10 days that induces a scheduled withdrawal bleed. This is particularly useful in those with anovulatory cycling. "Long-cycle" progestin refers to progestin taken for 21 days following one's cycle, with a subsequent scheduled, lighter bleed. Extended cycle progestin therapy is an option to control scheduled bleeding. There are no studies comparing the two regimens nor any that compare progestin pills to placebo to evaluate the efficacy and superior regimen. Additionally, a systematic review of 15 RCTs including over 1000 women showed that "short-cycle" progestin and "long-cycle" progestin were both inferior to TXA and LNG 52 mg IUD.[92,93]

Both the GnRH agonists and the newer GnRH antagonists block pituitary production of the gonadotropins FSH and LH. The suppression of pituitary stimulation leads downstream decreases in sex steroid production from the ovaries. GnRH agonists are limited in the duration of time they can be used due to their hypoestrogenic side effects, including hot flashes, serum lipid abnormalities, and decreased bone mineralization. These symptoms can be mitigated by add-back therapy using norethindrone acetate and/or ethinyl estradiol (or conjugated estrogen) combination therapies. Injectable GnRH agonists can be used in the short term to cause a 30% to 50% reduction in fibroid volume in the first 3–6 months with significant symptomatic improvement in both bulk and bleeding symptoms.[94,95] Because of their limited duration of use (6–12 months maximum), they are typically used as a bridge to an interventional procedure, surgery, or menopause.

GnRH antagonists (elagolix and relugolix) are FDA approved for treatment of HMB due to fibroids for up to 2 years of use. They have faster onset of action and are more convenient in their oral route of administration twice or once daily, respectively, compared to GnRH agonists. Two large RCTs studying the efficacy of elagolix for AUB-L found that over 85% of study participants no longer had HMB (defined as $>$ 80 mL of blood loss per cycle) and nearly half had achieved amenorrhea after 1 year of use.[96,97] Data showed that relugolix had similar improvements in HMB with the same adverse effects when compared to elagolix, but with the added convenience of once daily dosing.[98] In Europe, selective progestin receptor modulators, such as ulipristal acetate, are used in 3-month cycles to treat HMB associated with fibroids.[99]

When medical management has been expended or has failed or when patients experience significant bulk symptoms, interventional procedures or surgery are the next management strategy. Interventional procedures include uterine artery embolization (UAE), radiofrequency ablation, and magnetic-resonance-guided focused ultrasound; surgical management includes myomectomy (hysteroscopic, laparoscopic, robotic-assisted, or abdominal) or hysterectomy. Determination of which intervention or surgery is best for a patient is generally centered around a patient's desire for future fertility or uterine preservation, what symptoms are most bothersome or most dangerous, the likelihood to need reintervention, and the number of years until menopause. Patients desiring future fertility typically pursue myomectomy, especially if the fibroids are distorting or within the uterine cavity. Currently there are insufficient data on pregnancy outcomes following other interventional procedures. In the available literature, reintervention rates for uterine-preserving procedures were lowest for myomectomy (12.2%), then UAE (14.4%), with focused ultrasound having the highest reintervention rates (53.9%).[100] Hysterectomy should be performed with the most minimally invasive approach that is safe and feasible given patient's surgical history, comorbidities, and uterine size as well as the surgeon's experience. Overall, patient satisfaction and quality of life ratings were similar 2–5 years following myomectomy, UAE, and hysterectomy.[101]

Malignancy/Hyperplasia (AUB-M). Between 2012 and 2016, nearly 1 million women were diagnosed with a gynecologic malignancy. Several different gynecologic malignancies may first present with AUB. This may be in the form of postcoital bleeding, IMB, acute bleeding, or postmenopausal bleeding. AUB-M is used for patients with AUB who are diagnosed with a malignancy, premalignancy (CIN, VAIN, EIN), or endometrial hyperplasia.

The underlying cause of endometrial hyperplasia is usually found to be unopposed estrogen, often associated with infrequent cycling during the reproductive years or with obesity or estrogen-alone therapies in the postmenopausal years. Any patient above the age of 45 who presents with AUB or anyone with AUB and prolonged estrogen exposure (obesity, anovulatory cycles from PCOS) should undergo endometrial sampling or ultrasound evaluation to rule out endometrial intraepithelial neoplasia (EIN) and endometrial cancer.[75] Progestin therapies are most effective. The LNG-IUD has been shown to rapidly reverse these cytologic changes and to provide ongoing progestin to protect against recurrence. Oral MPA or megestrol acetate (Megace) have also been used, but the latter should be used with caution in patients with higher BMIs since it increases the risk of deep venous thrombosis. Forty percent of cases of endometrial hyperplasia with atypia have concurrent, but undetected, endometrial carcinoma. For that reason, unless the patient has strong desire for future fertility, hysterectomy is recommended when endometrial hyperplasia with atypia is discovered.

In the most recent epidemiologic surveillance data, endometrial cancer was the most common gynecologic cancer.[102] Endometrial cancer is classified as Type 1 (endometroid adenocarcinoma), which is estrogen-dependent, and Type 2 (clear cell and serous carcinoma), which is not estrogen-dependent. Nearly 50% of Type 1 endometrial cancer is secondary to obesity alone.[102] Endometrial cancers, especially Type 1, most commonly present with AUB.

Cervical cancer was the most common gynecologic cancer in women less than 50 years old.[102] Squamous cell carcinoma caused by persistent human papilloma virus (HPV) infection accounts for about two-thirds of cervical cancer cases, while the remaining one-third are adenocarcinoma.[102] While vaginal cancer is one of the least common type of gynecologic cancer, when it does occur, it is most commonly also squamous cell carcinoma caused by HPV. Cervical and vaginal cancer and their precursor lesions (CIN, VAIN) frequently present with postcoital bleeding. Macroscopic lesions can cause torrential bleeding following penetrative sexual intercourse due to trauma to the highly vascularized tumor.

Nonstructural Etiologies of Chronic Abnormal Uterine Bleeding

Coagulopathy (AUB-C). Coagulopathies refer to any bleeding disorder affecting primary or secondary hemostasis. In the PALM-COEIN system, AUB-C also includes excessive bleeding due to use of anticoagulant medications. Primary hemostasis involves the initial steps of forming a clot (vessel wall, platelets, von Willebrand factor), while secondary hemostasis involves formation of the fibrin-based clot (coagulation factors). It is estimated that up to 20% of women with HMB may have an underlying coagulation disorder and up to 13% have some variant of von Willebrand disease.[103] Approximately half of those with unexplained HMB are thought to have some degree of platelet dysfunction.[104,105]

Von Willebrand disease is the most common bleeding disorder among young people and is due to a decreased quantity or quality of von Willebrand factor (vWF). The disease is generally autosomal dominant. This condition commonly presents at the time of menarche when anovulatory cycles are more common and vWF is at its nadir.[106] Platelet disorders can be inherited or acquired and include abnormalities of aggregation, adhesion, secretion, and signal transduction.[107] Acquired platelet aggregation disorders are the most common cause of coagulopathy in older reproductive-aged women. Finally, acquired medical conditions such as cancer, liver disease, and kidney disease can lead to coagulation abnormalities as well.

AUB-C typically presents as HMB or prolonged bleeding and according to ACOG, all patients presenting with symptoms as described in **Table 3-5** should be screened for underlying disorders of hemostasis. Anyone with a positive screen should be evaluated by a hematologist along with laboratory testing including CBC, prothrombin time (PT), partial thromboplastin time (PTT), vWF, and ristocetin cofactor.[104] AUB-C can also worsen bleeding symptoms caused by structural etiologies of AUB (PALM).

Anticoagulant use is now classified under AUB-C. Increasingly, premenopausal patients are requiring anticoagulation with vitamin K antagonists, antiplatelet therapy, or novel oral anticoagulants (NOAC). Anticoagulation is known to lead to a significant increased risk for HMB and prolonged bleeding.[108,109] Other important drugs to consider are those that interfere with vitamin K synthesis as a side effect, such as the antiseizure medications phenytoin and phenobarbital. Treatment for AUB in this population typically relies on progestin-only methods, especially the LNG-IUD. DMPA can also be used; studies have shown that there is no significantly increased risk for developing a hematoma at the injection site of DMPA in patients using anticoagulants.[110] If surgical intervention is required, endometrial ablation has also been shown to have high satisfaction rates in patients taking anticoagulants. Finally, hysterectomy by the least invasive method may be performed, taking into consideration the precautions to control expected heavy surgical blood losses.

In general, treatment of AUB-C centers around decreasing the number of bleeding episodes and decreasing blood loss volume by addressing the underlying bleeding disorder. Unlike other etiologies of AUB, NSAIDs should be avoided in

Table 3-5 History Suggesting an Underlying Coagulation Disorder

Heavy menstrual bleeding since menarche
One of the following: postpartum hemorrhage, surgery-related bleeding, bleeding associated with dental work
Two or more of the following: Bruising (1 or 2 times/month), epistaxis (1 or 2 times/month), frequent gum bleeding, family history of bleeding symptoms

Modified from ACOG Committee Opinion no. 557: Management of acute abnormal uterine bleeding in nonpregnant reproductive-aged women. Obstet Gynecol. 2013;121:891-896.

treatment of AUB-C as their irreversible effects on platelets can worsen bleeding.[111] As an antifibrinolytic, TXA addresses secondary hemostasis, leading to a significant reduction in menstrual blood loss and improvement in quality-of-life metrics in patients with AUB-C.[104] Hormonal treatments that result in lighter or suppressed menstrual blood loss are also effective in treating AUB-C, especially the LNG-IUD, and continuous COC, and extended use of vaginal rings.[112,113] For patients with von Willebrand disease, desmopressin (DDAVP) is administered nasally to increase plasma factor VIII and the release of endogenous vWF to improve hemostasis. COCS are also known to increase factor VIII and vWF quantities and are used alongside DDAVP to address AUB-C in these patients. TXA has also been shown to improve the efficacy of DDAVP, thereby reducing the dose and frequency required and minimizing dangerous side effects of fluid retention and hyponatremia associated with its use.[114] Surgical interventions in patients with AUB-C are effective; however, they are associated with a greater risk for intraoperative and postoperative (immediate and delayed) hemorrhage. Despite the increased risk of hemorrhage, hysterectomy rates among patients with von Willebrand disease are almost three times greater than age-matched controls.[115]

Ovulatory Disorders (AUB-O). As described in Chapter 2, ovulation is the result of a series of carefully orchestrated events that results in the production of an ovum ready for fertilization and corpus luteum producing progesterone to support a possible pregnancy. During this process, the endometrium is initially exposed to estrogen leading to endometrial proliferation, followed by exposure to estrogen and progesterone that causes secretory changes. Withdrawal of both hormones as the corpus luteum involutes results in shedding of the lining. Anything that derails this series of coordinated events can result in anovulatory cycles along with the associated irregular bleeding and HMB seen in AUB-O. Ovulatory dysfunction can be physiologic, such as during adolescence, perimenopause, or lactation, or it can be pathologic, caused by aberrations at any level in the HPO axis. It can also be caused by other endocrine disorders that affect the HPO axis, such as thyroid disorders and hyperprolactinemia.

In adolescents, the immature HPO axis lacks the formalized hormonal feedback needed for ovulation. This typically resolves within 3 years of menarche.[116] At the other end of the reproductive life span, perimenopausal patients have similar symptoms; however, in periomenopause it is due to the ovaries producing high fluctuations in estrogen and having fewer follicles to release an egg and develop a corpus luteum. As described earlier in this chapter, PCOS is the most common cause of AUB-O in reproductive-aged patients. Unless contraindicated, CHCs can be prescribed to promote regular cycles with predictable scheduled bleeds that are lighter and less painful. While progestin-only methods will not regulate timing of bleeding, they can help to lessen the number of bleeding days and the amount of bleeding, as well as the accompanying cramping, and they protect the endometrium.

Endometrial (AUB-E). AUB that is regular, not due to structural causes, nor due to coagulopathy is attributed to endometrial causes. AUB-E typically presents as HMB or prolonged bleeding and frequently occurs alongside other etiologies of AUB. The cause of AUB-E is not completely understood, and it is considered a diagnosis of exclusion. Bleeding symptoms are thought to be due to abnormalities in prostaglandin synthesis and glucocorticoid metabolism, as well as excessive plasminogen causing premature clot lysis.[117]

Medical treatments for AUB-E were evaluated for reduction in monthly blood loss and quality-of-life improvements in a systematic review and found that all treatments were better than placebo. Treatments for AUB-E evaluated included LNG 52 mg IUDs, COCs, luteal phase progestins (e.g., Provera), mefenamic acid (NSAID), and TXA. LNG 52 mg IUD was more beneficial at blood loss reduction when compared to COCs, luteal phase progestins, and mefenamic acid.[92]

Iatrogenic (AUB-I). Iatrogenic causes of AUB are most associated with medications affecting the HPO axis, the endometrial lining, or coagulation pathways. Contraceptive agents are often associated with bleeding disruptions. Most hormonal treatments for AUB and nearly all contraceptive medications have some associated unscheduled bleeding, especially at initiation.[118] The copper IUD (Cu-IUD) is also associated with unscheduled spotting or bleeding, as well as heavy or prolonged bleeding.[118] More information on the management of these bleeding side effects can be found in the specific chapters discussing each contraceptive method.

Other drugs can also increase menstrual blood loss. Due to its agonist/antagonist nature, tamoxifen affects premenopausal and postmenopausal patients differently; however, AUB is common in both populations.[119] Approximately half of premenopausal patients will become amenorrhoeic or have infrequent menses. Any bleeding in the postmenopausal patient taking tamoxifen should be evaluated promptly. The LNG-IUD has been studied to decrease the risk of uterine pathology for patients taking tamoxifen, generally demonstrating a reduction in hyperplasia and carcinoma.[120] However, LNG-IUD has been shown to increase unscheduled bleeding, especially in the first 2 years of use.[121] Fortunately, most protocols have replaced SERMs with aromatase inhibitors as primary and secondary breast cancer reduction agents, so these days this is not as frequent a problem.

Not Otherwise Classified (AUB-N). AUB-N refers to rare or poorly defined pathologies, or those that do not fit into one of the other AUB categories. Uterine arteriovenous malformations and endometrial pseudoaneurysms may be congenital or iatrogenic following instrumentation of the uterus for D&C. Both are best treated with UAE or hysterectomy in patients who do not desire future fertility.[122] Myometrial hypertrophy is typically identified by uterine weight of more than 200 g, a myometrial thickness above 2 cm, and the absence of an endomyometrial cause of bleeding. Myometrial hypertrophy can impair uterine contraction while also increasing uterine size, leading to increased menstrual bleeding. Myometrial hypertrophy can also be seen overlying cesarean scars, or cesarean scars may result in defects that can collect blood and form an isthmocele.[123] Isthmoceles are diagnosed by transvaginal ultrasound and result in prolonged bleeding. Further study is needed to determine the best medical treatment for these etiologies. Isthmoceles can be surgically repaired via hysteroscopy, laparoscopy, or vaginal surgery. Chronic endometritis that is noninfectious in etiology is sometimes seen in DMPA or IUD users but can also be idiopathic. It typically presents as HMB, irregular bleeding, or prolonged bleeding, typically associated with dysmenorrhea and most often diagnosed clinically based on pain on uterine compression during bimanual exam. The gold standard for diagnosis is endometrial biopsy, but realistically empiric treatment with a 2-week course of doxycycline that shows improvement in bleeding and pain symptoms is typically an easier and more comfortable way of making the diagnosis.[124]

Other Abnormal Uterine Bleeding Patterns

Traumatic Bleeding

Bleeding due to lacerations following injury can appear as external bleeding, but also can be concealed in a variety of hematoma. More common presentations, such as postcoital bleeding or increased or renewed bleeding after removal of tampons, may raise concerns about cervical or vaginal pathology. In younger individuals, the most common cause is cervicitis, usually related to chlamydia, gonorrhea, trichomoniasis, or herpes. In older individuals, benign lesions, such as cervical polyps or vaginal atrophy, and more serious problems, such as cervical carcinoma, classically are associated with this type of bleeding (as noted previously).

Intermenstrual Bleeding

Bleeding between menses is often associated with significant endometrial pathology, such as endometrial hyperplasia or carcinoma. Rarely, reproductive-aged individuals may have midcycle spotting associated with ovulation. Bleeding in those using hormonal contraception technically does not fall into this category (it is called unscheduled bleeding) but relates to the progestational impacts on the endometrium. While it is generally not medically significant, such bleeding and spotting profoundly affects patient quality of life. This is discussed in the AUB-I section and management strategies are individually discussed in the chapters covering each respective contraceptive method.

Menstruation-Related Problems

Painful Menses (Dysmenorrhea)

Greek for painful menstruation, "dysmenorrhea" is classified as *primary dysmenorrhea* (intrinsic without any pelvic pathology and usually of early onset) or *secondary dysmenorrhea* (due to some other physical cause and usually of later onset). Even though the word to describe this problem comes from ancient roots, dysmenorrhea has only recently been recognized as a medical problem. Before the 1970s, there were virtually no scientific articles studying any aspect of the condition. Prevalence now is higher than historical norms because modern contraceptives allow people to limit their numbers of pregnancies or the time spent breastfeeding. Prevalence ranges widely from 17% to 90%. In a study of college students, 84% of those surveyed reported having experienced dysmenorrhea; 9% missed exams due to dysmenorrhea, and 48.7% reported poor satisfaction with their academic performance because of menstrual pain.[125] Many patients with dysmenorrhea also experience nausea, vomiting, diarrhea, headaches, fatigue, or dizziness. Symptoms often vary in severity from cycle to cycle but generally are present each menses throughout the reproductive years. Up to 15% of those with dysmenorrhea suffer symptoms severe enough to cause absenteeism from work, school, and other activities. Estimates are that over 600 million hours or $2 billion annually are lost in the United States due to missed work or reduced productivity at work due to menstrual pain and associated symptoms.[126] It is the most common cause of short-term absenteeism from school in adolescents who menstruate.[127] Despite its high prevalence, dysmenorrhea is frequently underdiagnosed, undertreated, and accepted by patients themselves.

Primary Dysmenorrhea

Primary dysmenorrhea is painful menses without pelvic pathology. Primary dysmenorrhea has physiologic—not psychological—causes. While early investigators believed that dysmenorrhea occurred in "maladjusted women who were intensely rejecting their feminine role and who suffered from deep hostility,"[128] today we understand that the problem is not in the patient's head, but in the uterus. Measurements with intrauterine pressure catheters demonstrate that with primary dysmenorrhea, intrauterine pressures with menstrual contractions are similar to intrauterine pressures seen during the second stage of labor.

With primary dysmenorrhea, the pain is located in the lower abdomen and can radiate to the back, inner thighs, or buttocks. It is described as cramping and of varying intensity, starting just before or at the onset of bleeding and lasting up to 72 hours. Pain peaks 24–36 hours from onset of bleeding. Findings on pelvic exam are normal. Symptoms of primary dysmenorrhea are usually not thought to begin for 6–18 months after menarche when cycles become ovulatory, but some more recent research shows that anovulatory cycles are also associated with primary dysmenorrhea.[129] Progesterone stimulates the production of prostaglandins, via the cyclooxygenase pathway, which are released as the functional layer is sloughed. People with primary dysmenorrhea produce excessive amounts of PGE_2 and $PGF_2\alpha$.[130] Prostaglandin $F_2\alpha$ increases the uterine contractility, which reduces uterine blood flow to the myometrium, causing ischemia and the accumulation of anaerobic metabolites.[131] This directly causes pain and sensitizes afferent nerve fibers in the uterus to other painful stimuli, which augments the patient's perception of pain. In turn, this can increase the risk for the development of chronic pelvic pain.[126] When uterine contractions inject these same prostaglandins into the general circulation, they can cause headache, nausea, vomiting, and diarrhea. Other etiologies of early onset dysmenorrhea, such as structural abnormalities of the uterus (blind horns), cervix (stenotic os), or vagina (transverse septa), can usually be ruled out by a careful pelvic examination and imaging studies.

Physical activity may be an effective treatment for primary dysmenorrhea.[132] Prostaglandin synthetase inhibitors such as NSAIDs are first-line medical therapy for most patients; approximately 80% of those with dysmenorrhea feel relief from cramping pain, backache, headaches, and blood loss with these agents. In some, NSAIDs may cause gastrointestinal symptoms. All currently available NSAIDs are of comparable efficacy and safety, although one meta-analysis suggested that ibuprofen was the most effective over-the-counter medication for dysmenorrhea.[133] In contrast, aspirin is no more effective than placebo for dysmenorrhea and can increase menstrual blood loss. While COX-2 inhibitors also significantly reduce dysmenorrhea, they have been linked to cardiovascular risk and are more expensive, so they are not commonly prescribed for this indication. About 18% of those with dysmenorrhea are unresponsive to NSAIDs.[131]

Menstrual suppression is the most effective medical approach to treating dysmenorrhea, but suppression of ovulation is also associated with decreased menstrual pain.[50,134] NSAIDs and hormonal contraceptives are first-line treatments that can be used independently or in combination.[135,136] Progestin-only methods are helpful. For example, after the third injection, nearly half of DMPA users become amenorrheic and avoid dysmenorrhea entirely. The LNG 52 mg IUDs are also an excellent choice for patients with dysmenorrhea, because menstrual blood loss and duration of bleeding are significantly reduced over time, although expulsion rates are higher among those with dysmenorrhea. Other therapies that have been studied as treatments for dysmenorrhea include vasopressin antagonists,[137] progesterone receptor modulators,[138] dienogest,[139] and sildenafil citrate.[140]

Alternative complementary therapies that have been suggested include dietary supplements, acupuncture, high-frequency transcutaneous electrical nerve stimulation, heat therapy, and self-acupuncture.[136] A recent systematic review studied the effectiveness of a full range of dietary supplements in treating dysmenorrhea, including herbs or other botanicals, vitamins, minerals, enzymes, and amino acids; traditional Chinese medications were excluded. The bottom line was that there is no high-quality evidence to support the effectiveness or safety of any dietary supplement for dysmenorrhea.[141]

Placebo-controlled trials with acupuncture compared to sham procedures have not consistently demonstrated effectiveness.[142] However, many case reports and some placebo-controlled studies have shown that acupuncture reduced pain and related menstrual symptoms. A four-arm dose-finding study without a placebo arm showed that every acupuncture method studied at every intensity reduced menstrual pain intensity and duration.[143] A smart phone app–based self-acupressure therapy was recently found to reduce mean pain intensity more than the usual cure did in a randomized, but not blinded study.[144]

Surgical approaches provide relief for patients who do not respond to medical therapies. Endometrial ablation can reduce dysmenorrhea when it occurs in conjunction with heavy or prolonged menstrual bleeding. Some evidence exists to support the effectiveness of laparoscopic nerve ablation in selected cases. Hysterectomy is the definitive, effective treatment for primary dysmenorrhea when other measures fail.

Secondary Dysmenorrhea

Secondary dysmenorrhea is due to pelvic pathology, most commonly adenomyosis, endometriosis, pelvic adhesions, and neoplasia.[145] Patients with secondary dysmenorrhea also complain of painful uterine cramping with menses but may have other accompanying complaints, such as dyspareunia or nonmenstrual pelvic pain.

As noted above in chronic HMB, *adenomyosis* is the presence of endometrial glands and stroma deep in the myometrium; in *endometriosis*, the endometrial glands and stoma implant outside the uterus on the serosa of the uterus, the fallopian tubes, the ovaries, and the intestines and other peritoneal surfaces. The endometrial cells within these endometriotic implants proliferate early in the cycle and are sloughed at the end of the cycle into the surrounding tissue; this induces intense, usually painful, local inflammation. Long-term, extensive adhesive disease, nodules, or ovarian endometriomas can develop, increasing the likelihood of developing chronic pelvic pain. Endometriosis can also have systemic health impacts due to the chronic inflammatory state it creates.

Guidelines report that both primary and secondary dysmenorrhea are likely to respond to the same medical therapies, so initiation of therapy should not depend on establishing a precise diagnosis.[134] However, the choice of therapy should reflect the desire for fertility. *Menstrual suppression* is usually effective.[50] Progestin-only pills that suppress ovulation (desogestrel) have been found to be better than cyclic combined contraceptive pills.[146] In particular, MPA sold under the trade name

Depo-subQ Provera 104® is an FDA-approved therapy for the treatment of dysmenorrhea associated with endometriosis. The magnitude of pain reduction seen in the clinical trials with Depo-subQ Provera 104 matched the pain score reductions seen with GnRH agonists but had fewer adverse hypoestrogenic impacts.[147] In clinical trials, the LNG 52 mg IUDs were effective in the treatment of dysmenorrhea caused by endometriosis, and also shrunk the size of endometriotic implants, particularly those implants located near the uterus. The contraceptive implant was as effective as DMPA in treating dysmenorrhea associated with endometriosis.[148–150]

Other medications are available to treat dysmenorrhea by inducing amenorrhea, but their use is limited by side effects and cost. GnRH agonists induce amenorrhea and thereby eliminate dysmenorrhea. However, GnRH use is limited to 4–6 months because it causes hypoestrogenic side effects such as vasomotor symptoms (hot flashes), vaginal dryness, and lower bone mineralization. GnRH agonists have been combined with either progestin-only or combined estrogen/progestin add-back therapy for long-term treatment of endometriosis.[151] Danazol, an androgen that was used more frequently in the past to treat endometriosis, effectively induces amenorrhea but can be used for only 4–6 months due to androgenic side effects, such as acne, hirsutism, oily skin, clitoral enlargement, and voice deepening. GnRH antagonist agents with estrogen/progestin add-back (relugolix and elagolix) have been shown to have rapid onset and to provide profound relief for endometriosis-related dysmenorrhea.[152] Other therapies on the horizon, especially for endometriosis-related dysmenorrhea, include selective progesterone (or estrogen) receptor modulators, aromatase inhibitors, immunomodulators, and antiangiogenic agents.[153]

If medical therapies are not effective, or if the patient wants to become pregnant, more definitive surgical approaches may be needed. For example, secondary dysmenorrhea or infertility caused by pelvic scarring may benefit from surgical excision of adhesions, although recurrence of such adhesions is very common. Similarly, excision of endometriotic implants and adenomyosis nodules can help relieve symptoms at least temporarily. Hysterectomy is reserved for treatment of incapacitating dysmenorrhea unresponsive to more conservative measures and is appropriate only for patients who do not desire future childbearing.

Premenstrual Syndrome (PMS) and Premenstrual Dysphoric Disorder (PMDD)

Nearly 90% of cycling people experience some discomfort with their menses. With ovulation, problems with fluid retention, bloating, mood disorders, and breast tenderness are common. In 20% to 30% of menstruating people, these symptoms affect their activities (PMS), and in 1.2% to 6.4%, the problem rises to the level that it qualifies as a psychiatrically defined disorder (PMDD).[154]

Premenstrual Syndrome

Premenstrual syndrome (PMS) is a heterogeneous collection of signs and symptoms that share one common characteristic: a temporal relationship to the menstrual cycle. PMS is the cyclic appearance of at least one symptom during the luteal phase, which abates as menstruation begins and is followed by an entirely symptom-free period.[154] There are many symptoms associated with PMS, including physical symptoms of abdominal bloating, breast tenderness, headaches, and extremity edema, and emotional symptoms of anxiety, depression, confusion, social withdrawal, angry outbursts, and irritability. Other commonly reported manifestations of PMS include fatigue, thirst, appetite changes, and crying spells. According to ACOG, clinically significant PMS can be diagnosed if at least one of the premenstrual symptoms that interferes with work, lifestyle, or interpersonal relationships occurs during the 5 days before the period starts for a minimum of three consecutive cycles. PMS can increase relationship strain, sexual dysfunction, social isolation, work absenteeism, and risk for suicide.[154] Studies have demonstrated that PMS results in poorer self-reported mental and physical health, increased use of health services, and higher health care costs for sufferers.

Premenstrual dysphoric disorder (PMDD) is a more severe form of PMS with a very specific definition. The American Psychiatric Association requires the manifestation of at least five symptoms during the final week before the onset of menses that start to improve after the onset of menses and become minimal or absent in the week following menses (**Table 3-6**).[155] By definition, at least one of the five required symptoms must represent a change in mood that is severe enough to interfere with occupational or social functions for at least two consecutive cycles.

Etiologies of PMS and PMDD

What causes PMS/PMDD? Multiple factors likely are involved. Early investigators suggested that PMS was due to a lack of progesterone,[156] but subsequent research failed to find a difference between PMS sufferers and controls in levels of progesterone or any other major hormones including estradiol, FSH, LH, prolactin, SHBG, or testosterone.[157,158] However, individuals with PMS may be more biologically vulnerable to normal fluctuations in hormone levels than are those without the syndrome.[159] Such sensitive individuals may have a pathologic response to either withdrawal or exposure to allopregnanolone, the agonist to gamma-aminobutyric acid (GABA) and the neurotransmitter that reduces neuronal excitability. Blockage of allopregnanolone reduces premenstrual symptoms in these patients.

Another older hypothesis was that premenstrual disorders are due to a deficit in the function of the serotonin system, because a deficit in the tryptophan or exposure to serotonin receptor antagonist can elicit premenstrual symptoms.[154] Other investigators have hypothesized that PMS may be caused by low beta-endorphin levels, low adrenocorticotropic levels, abnormal prostaglandin production, or endogenous hormone allergies, but again research has not consistently supported any of these hypotheses. Studies of PMS sufferers have also failed to identify deficiencies of magnesium, zinc, vitamin A, vitamin E, thiamine, or vitamin B6.[160] However, association between posttraumatic stress disorder (PTSD) or trauma and PMS/PMDD has been found.[161]

Diagnosis of PMS/PMDD

The differential diagnosis of PMS/PMDD includes other dysthymic and depressive disorders, generalized anxiety disorder, and hypothyroidism. Take a detailed history to begin differentiating among these conditions. Include a careful medical, gynecologic, and psychiatric history. Also ask about diet and exercise. For many individuals, clinical depression and other serious problems worsen premenstrually but never completely abate; patients who do not experience a symptom-free interval do not have PMS or PMDD alone. As many as half of those with self-diagnosed

Table 3-6 Criteria for Premenstrual Dysphoric Disorder

Diagnostic Criteria

A. In the majority of menstrual cycles, at least five symptoms must be present in the final week before the onset of menses, start to *improve* within a few days after the onset of menses, and become *minimal* or absent in the week postmenses.

B. One (or more) of the following symptoms must be present:
   1. Marked affective lability (e.g., mood swings: feeling suddenly sad or tearful, or increased sensitivity to rejection).
   2. Marked irritability or anger or increased interpersonal conflicts.
   3. Marked depressed mood, feelings of hopelessness, or self-deprecating thoughts.
   4. Marked anxiety, tension, and/or feelings of being keyed up or on edge.

C. One (or more) of the following symptoms must additionally be present, to reach a total of *five* symptoms when combined with symptoms from Criterion B above.
   1. Decreased interest in usual activities (e.g., work, school, friends, hobbies).
   2. Subjective difficulty in concentration.
   3. Lethargy, easy fatigability, or marked lack of energy.
   4. Marked change in appetite; overeating; or specific food cravings.
   5. Hypersomnia or insomnia.
   6. A sense of being overwhelmed or out of control.
   7. Physical symptoms such as breast tenderness or swelling, joint or muscle pain, a sensation of "bloating," or weight gain.

   Note: The symptoms in Criteria A-C must have been met for most menstrual cycles that occurred in the preceding year.

D. The symptoms are associated with clinically significant distress or interference with work, school, usual social activities, or relationships with others (e.g., avoidance of social activities; decreased productivity and efficiency at work, school, or home).

E. The disturbance is not merely an exacerbation of the symptoms of another disorder, such as major depressive disorder, panic disorder, persistent depressive disorder (dysthymia), or a personality disorder (although it may co-occur with any of these dis orders).

F. Criterion A should be confirmed by prospective daily ratings during at least two symptomatic cycles.
   Note: The diagnosis may be made provisionally prior to this confirmation.

G. The symptoms are not attributable to the physiological effects of a substance (e.g., a drug of abuse, a medication, other treatment) or another medical condition (e.g., hyperthyroidism).

PMS have other problems that require careful evaluation and may need therapies that may differ from those used to treat PMS. Some patients may have PMDD symptoms as well as an underlying or concomitant psychiatric problem; in one study, 59% of women diagnosed with PMDD also had clinical depression or an anxiety disorder.[162] Those with moderate-to-severe PMDD and PMS are at higher risk of suicide compared to those without premenstrual disturbances and should be routinely screened for suicidal risk.[163]

To diagnose PMS/PMDD, symptoms need to be charted for at least two menstrual cycles to help control for cycle-to-cycle variability. Research studies have validated assessment tools for this purpose, including the Calendar of Premenstrual Experiences (COPE), and the Daily Record of Severity of Problems (DRSP).[154] A patient generally can successfully document menstrually related symptoms by taking notes on a regular calendar or in an app, noting the symptoms experienced each day, along with their severity, and recording the dates of menses. A patient who is overwhelmed by a large number of symptoms can chart the three to five symptoms that are the most profoundly bothersome. Ideally, this chart should also include body weight and, if possible, a record of basal body temperature or home ovulation test results. Ask the patient to document any medications used during this time.

After collecting these data, the patient and clinician should carefully study the pattern of symptoms. Symptoms do not need to recur with equal intensity in each cycle; different symptoms may occur during different cycles. Again, the key to diagnosing PMS/PMDD is the *timing* of symptoms—they must appear in the luteal phase and disappear soon after the onset of menses.

Laboratory tests are generally not needed to diagnose PMS. In some cases, however, the clinician must rule out hypothyroidism, because a patient with low levels of thyroid hormone may present with fatigue, bloating, depression, and irritability. Laboratory testing to measure sex steroid hormone levels is completely unnecessary in the evaluation of PMS or PMDD.

Treatment of Premenstrual Syndromes (PMS)

In a wide range of studies, researchers report that 40% to 94% of patients with PMS will improve in the short term regardless of the treatment used, including a strong placebo effect. This reinforces the need to rely on placebo-controlled studies rather than on case reports or personal testimonials to determine the true efficacy of a particular drug or treatment for PMS.

Treatment requires a comprehensive, individualized approach. Patients choosing to chart their symptoms may experience validation about the diagnosis, and it may provide insight into the problem and provide a way for the patient to have more control. If therapy is initiated, the patient can continue charting to identify which interventions improve symptoms.

According to guidelines, first-line treatments for PMS include exercise, vitamin B6, cognitive behavioral therapy (CBT), hormonal contraceptives with shortened or no hormone-free intervals, and intermittent or continuous selective serotonin reuptake inhibitors (SSRIs).[154,164–166] CBT, typically used for about 12 sessions, is helpful in general and in particular if a patient does not want to use medication.[154] Smoking cessation, limits on alcohol intake, and regular sleep have all been found to be helpful.

Treatment for Premenstrual Dysphoric Disorder (PMDD)

PMDD generally requires medication to deal with its severe symptoms and mood disorders, although some of the measures used for PMS may be added. There are two classes of medications approved by the FDA to treat the physical and emotional symptoms of PMDD. The first is SSRIs. The FDA has specifically approved three SSRIs for treatment of PMDD (fluoxetine, sertraline, and paroxetine). Other SSRIs, like citalopram, have also been shown to be equally effective; that efficacy is likely true for all SSRIs. These agents can be given at low doses continuously (every day) or intermittently (only during the luteal phase) to reduce both the physical and psychological symptoms of PMDD. Research has found that the serotonin and norepinephrine reuptake inhibitor (SNRI) venlafaxine is equally effective.[167] Patients who have severe physical symptoms usually respond better to daily treatment than they do to SSRI use only during the luteal phase. SSRIs should be continued for at least 1 month or (better) 2 months before declaring failure. If one agent is not successful, try another one before abandoning SSRIs as a class, because an individual's response may vary from drug to drug.

Most people tolerate SSRIs without incident, but these medications can cause side effects including nausea, adverse sexual effects, and insomnia. The risk for side effects is related to dose; the use of low-dose SSRIs often provides symptom relief and may minimize side effects. In contrast to experience with SSRIs used for depression, rapid improvement of PMDD symptoms can be noted within a day or two even if SSRIs are taken only during luteal phase. Side effects can develop as rapidly. Clinicians should counsel patients about these potential side effects and inquire about them at follow-up visits.

The other FDA-approved therapy for the symptoms of PMDD is a monophasic oral contraceptive regimen with active pills containing 20 mcg EE and 3 mg drospirenone in a 24/4 formulation. Randomized, prospective, placebo-controlled, double-blinded clinical studies found that this COC reduced both mood disorders and physical complaints of PMDD by about 50%, which was significantly superior to the placebo effect.[168] This is about the same magnitude of response seen with SSRIs.

The clinician must individualize therapy to symptoms and strongly consider referral to a mental health specialist for patients with a PMDD diagnosis meeting DSM-5 criteria. Counseling may be very beneficial for patients with PMDD and their families. Stress management, anger management, self-help support groups, individual and couples therapy, CBT, and light therapy all have been reported to provide relief. Selection depends upon an individual patient's symptoms and ability to access resources.

Menstrual Exacerbation of Other Medical Conditions

Medical conditions commonly worsen during the luteal phase and menses.[169] This may reflect the complex and often poorly understood interplay of hormones with other physiologic processes throughout the body. A classic example is *menstrual migraines*.[170] About 7% to 9% of women with migraine headaches have them only with menses. Another 35% to 40% of migraine sufferers experience worsening of headaches with menses. Menstrual migraines are usually more debilitating, last longer, are more likely to recur, and are less responsive to medical therapies than nonmenstrual migraines.[171,172] One therapeutic approach to menstrual migraines has been to treat prophylactically with standard migraine treatments during at-risk times. Some have recommended menstrual tracking monitors to predict menses more accurately so therapy can be better timed. However, because headaches have been linked to a decline in estrogen levels,[173] another approach has been to suppress menses with extended cycle hormones or to provide estrogen supplementation during bleeding days. The use of estrogen is appropriate only for patients who do not suffer neurologic auras preceding the onset of their migraines and do not suffer worsening of their headaches with estrogen exposure. DMPA or the etonogestrel (ENG) implant, which suppresses ovulation and induces amenorrhea or infrequent menstrual bleeding, would be preferred over an LNG-IUD, which does not control the hormonal cycling. Triptans have also been found to be effective for both acute treatment and for short-term prevention of menstrual migraine.[171]

Patients with *seizure disorders* often experience exacerbations of seizure activity with menstruation. Seizures cluster most frequently right before the onset of menses during a relative drop in estrogen levels. About 40% of menstruating people with epilepsy are affected by catamenial (menses-related) epilepsy.[174] Premenstrual increases in asthma symptoms or deterioration of peak flow measurements have been reported in up to 40% of those with asthma. Catamenial pneumothorax and catamenial hemoptysis have also been reported. Commonly, acne tends to blossom around the time of menses. Less common medical conditions that flare at menses include acute intermittent porphyria, diabetes, inflammatory bowel disease, erythema multiforme, glaucoma, hereditary angioedema, hidradenitis suppurativa, rheumatoid arthritis, hereditary pancreatitis, and multiple sclerosis.

Mental health problems tend to become more symptomatic with menses. Patients with anxiety disorders tend to experience more anxiety and panic attacks as well as higher rates of suicide attempts and psychiatric hospitalizations during menses. Symptoms of obsessive-compulsive disorders have been found to increase before menstruation, and patients with psychotic disorders, including schizophrenia, also tend to suffer more intense symptoms during menses.[175,176] There is some evidence that women with bulimia may experience increased food cravings premenstrually.[177]

Eliminating menses by controlling the endometrium alone (i.e., LNG-IUD use) will be sufficient therapy for some, but may not be adequate for those whose medical conditions fluctuate in response to hormonal cycling. However, it is possible to suppress ovulation with the ENG implant, DMPA, or extended COC use and prevent practically all hormonal fluctuations as well as menstrual-related symptoms. Selection of the appropriate method depends upon patient's preferences, underlying health problems, and specific presentation of symptoms.

Disclosures—Nelson: Grants/Research: Mylan Pharmaceuticals; Myovant Sciences; Organon/Merck & Co.; Sagami Rubber Industries; Sebela Pharmaceuticals; Honoraria/Speakers Bureau: Bayer HealthCare, Mayne Pharma, Organon/Merck, Myovant/Pfizer, TherapeuticsMD; Consultant/Advisory Board: Agile Therapeutics; Bayer Healthcare; Myovant Sciences; Organon; Pfizer; TherapeuticsMD. Trivedi: none.

References

1. Munro MG, Critchley HOD, Fraser IS; FIGO Menstrual Disorders Committee. The two FIGO systems for normal and abnormal uterine bleeding symptoms and classification of causes of abnormal uterine bleeding in the reproductive years: 2018 revisions. Int J Gynaecol Obstet. 2018;144:393-408.
2. Munro MG. Practical aspects of the two FIGO systems for management of abnormal uterine bleeding in the reproductive years. Best Pract Res Clin Obstet Gynaecol. 2017;40:3-22.

3. Nelson AL, Ritchie JJ. Severe anemia from heavy menstrual bleeding requires heightened attention. Am J Obstet Gynecol. 2015;213:97.e1-6.
4. Lam C, Anderson B, Lopes V, Schulkin J, Matteson K. Assessing abnormal uterine bleeding: Are physicians taking a meaningful clinical history? J Womens Health (Larchmt). 2017;26:762-7.
5. Chen KT. Top free menstrual cycle tracking apps for your patients. OBG Management. 2017;29:44-6.
6. Fraser IS, Critchley HO, Broder M, Munro MG. The FIGO recommendations on terminologies and definitions for normal and abnormal uterine bleeding. Semin Reprod Med. 2011;29:383-90.
7. Klein DA, Paradise SL, Reeder RM. Amenorrhea: A systematic approach to diagnosis and management. Am Fam Physician. 2019;100:39-48.
8. Gordon CM, Ackerman KE, Berga SL, et al. Functional hypothalamic amenorrhea: An Endocrine Society clinical practice guideline. J Clin Endocrinol Metab. 2017;102:1413-39.
9. Morgan S, Anderson RA, Gourley C, Wallace WH, Spears N. How do chemotherapeutic agents damage the ovary? Hum Reprod Update. 2012;18:525-35.
10. Chemaitilly W, Li Z, Krasin MJ, et al. Premature ovarian insufficiency in childhood cancer survivors: A report from the St. Jude Lifetime Cohort. J Clin Endocrinol Metab. 2017;102:2242-50.
11. Lambrinoudaki I, Paschou SA, Lumsden MA, Faubion S, Makrakis E, Kalantaridou S, Panay N. Premature ovarian insufficiency: A toolkit for the primary care physician. Maturitas. 2021;147:53-63.
12. Jiao X, Zhang H, Ke H, et al. Premature ovarian insufficiency: phenotypic characterization within different etiologies. J Clin Endocrinol Metab. 2017;102:2281-90.
13. Kirshenbaum M, Orvieto R. Premature ovarian insufficiency (POI) and autoimmunity-an update appraisal. J Assist Reprod Genet. 2019;11:2207-15.
14. Roberts RE, Farahani L, Webber L, Jayasena C. Current understanding of hypothalamic amenorrhoea. Ther Adv Endocrinol Metab. 2020;11:1-12.
15. Sophie Gibson ME, Fleming N, Zuijdwijk C, Dumont T. Where have the periods gone? The evaluation and management of functional hypothalamic amenorrhea. J Clin Res Pediatr Endocrinol. 2020;12(Suppl 1):18-27.
16. ACOG Committee Opinion 702: Female athlete triad. Committee on Adolescent Health Care. Obstet Gynecol. 2017;e160-7.
17. Altayar O, Nofal AA, Leon GC, et al. Treatments to prevent bone loss in functional hypothalamic amenorrhea: A systematic review and meta-analysis. J Endocrine Society. 2017;5:500-11.
18. Committee on Gynecologic Practice. Committee Opinion No. 698: Hormone therapy in primary ovarian insufficiency. Obstet Gynecol. 2017;129:e134-41.
19. Ishizuka B. Current understanding of the etiology, symptomatology, and treatment options in premature ovarian insufficiency (POI). Front Endocrinol (Lausanne). 2021;12:626924.
20. Teede HJ, Misso ML, Costello MF, Dokras A, Laven J, Moran L, Piltonen T, Norman RJ; International PCOS Network. Recommendations from the international evidence-based guideline for the assessment and management of polycystic ovary syndrome. Fertil Steril. 2018;110: 364-79.
21. Hoeger KM, Dokras A, Piltonen T. Update on PCOS: Consequences, challenges, and guiding treatment. J Clin Endocrinol Metab. 2021;106:e1071-83.
22. Yildiz BO, Knochenhauer ES, Azziz R. Impact of obesity on the risk for polycystic ovary syndrome. J Clin Endocrinol Metab. 2008;93162-8.
23. Azziz R. Systemic chronic subclinical inflammation, adipose tissue dysfunction, and polycystic ovary syndrome: three major forces intertwined. Fertil Steril. 2021;116:1147-48.
24. van der Ham K, Louwers YV, Laven JSE. Cardiometabolic biomarkers in women with polycystic ovary syndrome. Fertil Steril. 2022;117:887-96.
25. Fauser BC, Tarlatzis BC, Rebar RW, et al. Consensus on women's health aspects of polycystic ovary syndrome (PCOS): the Amsterdam ESHRE/ASRM-Sponsored 3rd PCOS Consensus Workshop Group. Fertil Steril. 2012;97:28-38.e25.
26. Copp T, Jansen J, Doust J, Mol BW, Dokras A, McCaffery K. Are expanding disease definitions unnecessarily labelling women with polycystic ovary syndrome? BMJ. 2017;358:j3694.
27. The Rotterdam ESHRE/ASRM Sponsored PCOS Consensus Workshop Group. Human Reprod. 2004;19:40-7.
28. Rodriguez Paris V, Bertoldo MJ. The mechanism of androgen actions in PCOS etiology. Med Sci (Basel). 2019;7:89.

29. American College of Obstetricians and Gynecologists' Committee on Practice Bulletins—Gynecology. ACOG practice bulletin no. 194: Polycystic ovary syndrome. Obstet Gynecol. 2018;131:e157-71.
30. Kim HJ, Adams JM, Gudmundsson JA, Arason G, Pau CT, Welt CK. Polycystic ovary morphology: age-based ultrasound criteria. Fertil Steril. 2017;108:548-53.
31. Rees DA, Jenkins-Jones S, Morgan CL. Contemporary reproductive outcomes for patients with polycystic ovary syndrome: A retrospective observational study. J Clin Endocrinol Metab. 2016;101:1664-72.
32. Hart R, Doherty DA. The potential implications of a PCOS diagnosis on a woman's long-term health using data linkage. J Clin Endocrinol Metab. 2015;100:911-9.
33. Guan C, Zahid S, Minhas AS, Ouyang P, Vaught A, Baker VL, Michos ED. Polycystic ovary syndrome: a "risk-enhancing" factor for cardiovascular disease. Fertil Steril. 2022;117:924-35.
34. Chan JL, Kar S, Vanky E, et al. Racial and ethnic differences in the prevalence of metabolic syndrome and its components of metabolic syndrome in women with polycystic ovary syndrome: a regional cross-sectional study. Am J Obstet Gynecol. 2017;217:189.e1-e8.
35. Jamil AS, Alalaf SK, Al-Tawil NG, Al-Shawaf T. Comparison of clinical and hormonal characteristics among four phenotypes of polycystic ovary syndrome based on the Rotterdam criteria. Arch Gynecol Obstet. 2016;2:447-56.
36. van Keizerswaard J, Dietz de Loos ALP, Louwers YV, Laven JSE. Changes in individual polycystic ovary syndrome phenotypical characteristics over time: a long-term follow-up study. Fertil Steril. 2022;117:1059-66.
37. Chen Y, Zheng X, Ma D, et al. Neck circumference is a good predictor for insulin resistance in women with polycystic ovary syndrome. Fertil Steril. 2021;115:753-60.
38. Reid RL, Magee BA. A pragmatic approach to hormonal testing in the assessment of disorders of female reproduction. Intl J Women's Health Wellness. 2016;2:022.
39. O'Reilly MW, Taylor AE, Crabtree NJ, et al. Hyperandrogenemia predicts metabolic phenotype in polycystic ovary syndrome: the utility of serum androstenedione. J Clin Endocrinol Metab. 2014;99:1027-36.
40. Persson S, Elenis E, Turkmen S, Kramer MS, Yong EL, Poromaa IS. Higher risk of type 2 diabetes in women with hyperandrogenic polycystic ovary syndrome. Fertil Steril. 2021;116:862-71.
41. Engmann L, Jin S, Sun F, et al. Racial and ethnic differences in the polycystic ovary syndrome metabolic phenotype. Am J Obstet Gynecol. 2017;216:493.e1-e13.
42. Kerchner A, Lester W, Stuart SP, Dokras A. Risk of depression and other mental health disorders in women with polycystic ovary syndrome: a longitudinal study. Fertil Steril. 2009;91:207-12.
43. Berni TR, Morgan CL, Rees DA. Women with polycystic ovary syndrome have an increased risk of major cardiovascular events: a population study. J Clin Endocrinol Metab. 2021;106:e3369-80.
44. Merz CN, Shaw LJ, Azziz R, et al. Cardiovascular disease and 10-year mortality in postmenopausal women with clinical features of polycystic ovary syndrome. J Womens Health (Larchmt). 2016;25:875-81.
45. Gardner CD, Kiazand A, Alhassan S, et al. Comparison of the Atkins, Zone, Ornish, and LEARN diets for change in weight and related risk factors among overweight premenopausal women: the A TO Z Weight Loss Study: a randomized trial. JAMA. 2007;297:969-77.
46. Lv N, Azar KMJ, Rosas LG, Wulfovich S, Xiao L, Ma J. Behavioral lifestyle interventions for moderate and severe obesity: A systematic review. Prev Med. 2017;100:180-93.
47. Brennan L, Teede H, Skouteris H, Linardon J, Hill B, Moran L. Lifestyle and behavioral management of polycystic ovary syndrome. J Womens Health (Larchmt). 2017;26:836-48.
48. Redman LM, Elkind-Hirsch K, Ravussin E. Aerobic exercise in women with polycystic ovary syndrome improves ovarian morphology independent of changes in body composition. Fertil Steril. 2011;95:2696-9.
49. Lim SS, Hutchison SK, Van Ryswyk E, Norman RJ, Teede HJ, Moran LJ. Lifestyle changes in women with polycystic ovary syndrome. Cochrane Database Syst Rev. 2019;3:CD007506.Pub4.
50. ACOG Clinical Consensus No. 3. General approaches to medical management of menstrual suppression. Am J Obstet Gynecol. 2022;140:528-41.
51. Barbieri RL. Treating polycystic ovary syndrome: start using dual medical therapy. OBG Mgmt. 2017;4:9-13.

52. de Wilde MA, Lamain-de Ruiter M, Veltman-Verhulst SM, et al. Increased rates of complications in singleton pregnancies of women previously diagnosed with polycystic ovary syndrome predominantly in the hyperandrogenic phenotype. Fertil Steril. 2017;108:333-40.
53. Yildiz BO. Approach to the patient: contraception in women with polycystic ovary syndrome. J Clin Endocrinol Metab. 2015;100:794-802.
54. van Oers AM, Mutsaerts MAQ, Burggraaff JM, et al. Cost-effectiveness analysis of lifestyle intervention in obese infertile women. Hum Reprod. 2017;32(7):1418-26.
55. Legro RS, Brzyski RG, Diamond MP, et al. Letrozole versus clomiphene for infertility in the polycystic ovary syndrome. N Engl J Med. 2014;371:119-29.
56. Diamond MP, Kruger M, Santoro N, et al. Endometrial shedding effect on conception and live birth in women with polycystic ovary syndrome. Obstet Gynecol. 2012;119:902-8.
57. Paulson M, Sahlin L, Hirschberg AL. Progesterone receptors and proliferation of the endometrium in obese women with polycystic ovary syndrome-a lifestyle intervention study. J Clin Endocrinol Metab. 2017;102:1244-53.
58. Banaszewska B, Pawelczyk L, Spaczynski RZ, Duleba AJ. Effects of simvastatin and metformin on polycystic ovary syndrome after six months of treatment. J Clin Endocrinol Metab. 2011;96:3493-501.
59. Tay CT, Teede HJ, Hill B, Loxton D, Joham AE. Increased prevalence of eating disorders, low self-esteem, and psychological distress in women with polycystic ovary syndrome: a community-based cohort study. Fertil Steril. 2019;2:353-61.
60. Weisberg E, McGeehan K, Fraser IS. Effect of perceptions of menstrual blood loss and menstrual pain on women's quality of life. Eur J Contracept Reprod Health Care. 2016;21:431-5.
61. Côté I, Jacobs P, Cumming D. Work loss associated with increased menstrual loss in the United States. Obstet Gynecol. 2002;100:683-7.
62. NICE Clinical Guidelines No. 44. Heavy menstrual bleeding: Assessment and management. London: RCOG Press National Institute for Health and Clinical Excellence, 2007. Available at https://www.nice.org.uk/guidance/cg44. Last accessed Sept. 19, 2017.
63. Fraser IS, McCarron G, Markham R, Resta T. Blood and total fluid content of menstrual discharge. Obstet Gynecol. 1985;65:194–8.
64. ACOG Committee on Practice Bulletins-Gynecology. Practice Bulletin No. 128: diagnosis of abnormal uterine bleeding in reproductive-aged women. Obstet Gynecol. 2012;120:197-206.
65. DeVore GR, Owens O, Kase N. Use of intravenous Premarin in the treatment of dysfunctional uterine bleeding--a double-blind randomized control study. Obstet Gynecol. 1982;59:285-91.
66. ACOG Committee Opinion no. 557: Management of acute abnormal uterine bleeding in nonpregnant reproductive-aged women. Obstet Gynecol. 2013;121:891-6.
67. Bofill Rodriguez M, Dias S, Jordan V, et al. Interventions for heavy menstrual bleeding; overview of Cochrane reviews and network meta-analysis. Cochrane Database Syst Rev. 2022;5:CD013180.pub2
68. Bryant-Smith AC, Lethaby A, Farquhar C, Hickey M. Antifibrinolytics for heavy menstrual bleeding. Cochrane Database Syst Rev. 2018;4:CD000249.pub2.
69. Borzutzky C, Jaffray J. Diagnosis and management of heavy menstrual bleeding and bleeding disorders in adolescents. JAMA Pediatr. 2020;174:186-94.
70. Screening and management of bleeding disorders in adolescents with heavy menstrual bleeding: ACOG COMMITTEE OPINION, Number 785. Obstet Gynecol. 2019;134:e71-83.
71. Connell NT, Flood VH, Brignardello-Petersen R, et al. ASH ISTH NHF WFH 2021 guidelines on the management of von Willebrand disease. Blood Adv. 2021;5:301-25.
72. Munro MG, Mainor N, Basu R, Brisinger M, Barreda L. Oral medroxyprogesterone acetate and combination oral contraceptives for acute uterine bleeding: a randomized controlled trial. Obstet Gynecol. 2006;108:924-9.
73. Ammerman SR, Nelson AL. A new progestogen-only medical therapy for outpatient management of acute, abnormal uterine bleeding: a pilot study. Am J Obstet Gynecol. 2013;208:499.e1-5.
74. Matteson KA, Raker CA, Clark MA, Frick KD. Abnormal uterine bleeding, health status, and usual source of medical care: analyses using the medical expenditures panel survey. J Women's Health (Larchmt) 2013; 11:959–65.
75. Spencer CP, Whitehead MI. Endometrial assessment re-visited. Br J Obstet Gynaecol. 1999;7:623-32.

76. Dreisler E, Stampe Sorensen S, Ibsen PH, Lose G. Prevalence of endometrial polyps and abnormal uterine bleeding in a Danish population aged 20-74 years. Ultrasound Obstet Gynecol. 2009;33(1):102-8.
77. Gregoriou O, Konidaris S, Vrachnis N, et al. Clinical parameters linked with malignancy in endometrial polyps. Climacteric. 2009;5:454-8.
78. Wang JH, Zhao J, Lin J. Opportunities and risk factors for premalignant and malignant transformation of endometrial polyps: management strategies. J Minim Invasive Gynecol. 2010;17(1):53-8
79. Ferrazzi E, Zupi E, Leone FP, Savelli L, Omodei U, Moscarini M, et al. How often are endometrial polyps malignant in asymptomatic postmenopausal women? A multicenter study. Am J Obstet Gynecol. 2009;3:235 e1-6
80. Lieng M, Istre O, Sandvik L, Engh V, Qvigstad E. Clinical effectiveness of polyp resection in women with endometrial polyps: randomized controlled trial. J Minim Invasive Gynecol. 2010;3:351-7
81. Clark TH, Stevenson H. Endometrial polyps and abnormal uterine bleeding (AUB-P): What is the relationship, how are they diagnosed and how are the treated? Best Pract Res Clin Obstet Gynaecol. 2017;40:89-104.
82. Abbott JA. Adenomyosis and abnormal uterine bleeding (AUB-A)-pathogenesis, diagnosis, and management. Best Pract Res Clin Obstet Gynaecol. 2017;40:68-81.
83. Sheng J, Zhang WY, Zhang JP, Lu D. The LNG-IUS study on adenomyosis: a 3-year follow-up study on the efficacy and side effects of the use of levonorgestrel intrauterine system for the treatment of dysmenorrhea associated with adenomyosis. Contraception. 2009;3:189-93.
84. Stewart EA, Cookson CL, Gandolfo RA, Schulze-Rath R. Epidemiology of uterine fibroids: a systematic review. BJOG. 2017;10:1501-12
85. Lasmar RB, Lasmar BP. The role of leiomyomas in the genesis of abnormal uterine bleeding (AUB). Best Pract Res Clin Obstet Gynaecol. 2017;40:82-8.
86. Whitaker L, Critchley HO. Abnormal uterine bleeding. Best Pract Res Clin Obstet Gynaecol. 2016;34:54-65.
87. Kashani BN, Centini G, Morelli SS, Weiss G, Petraglia F. Role of Medical management for uterine leiomyomas. Best Pract Res Clin Obstet Gynaecol. 2016;34:85-103.
88. Lukes AS, Moore KA, Muse KN, Gersten JK, Hecht BR, Edlund M, et al. Tranexamic acid treatment for heavy menstrual bleeding: a randomized controlled trial. Obstet Gynecol. 2010; 4:865-75.
89. Bofill Rodriguez M, Lethaby A, Farquhar C. Non-steroidal anti-inflammatory drugs for heavy menstrual bleeding. Cochrane Database Syst Rev. 2019;9:CD000400.pub4.
90. Zapata LB, Whiteman MK, Tepper NK, Jamieson DJ, Marchbanks PA, Curtis KM. Intrauterine device use among women with uterine fibroids: a systematic review. Contraception. 2010;1:41-55.
91. Curtis KM, Tepper NK, Jatlaoui TC, et al. U.S. medical eligibility criteria for contraceptive use, 2016. MMWR Recomm Rep. 2016;3:1-103.
92. Bofill Rodriguez M, Lethaby A, Low C, Cameron IT. Cyclical progestogens for heavy menstrual bleeding. Cochrane Database Syst Rev. 2019 Aug 14;8(8):CD001016.pub3.
93. Zapata LB, Whiteman MK, Tepper NK, Jamieson DJ, Marchbanks PA, Curtis KM. Intrauterine device use among women with uterine fibroids: a systematic review. Contraception. 2010;1:41-55.
94. Olive DL, Lindheim SR, Pritts EA. Non-surgical management of leiomyoma: impact on fertility. Curr Opin Obstet Gynecol. 2004;3:239-43.
95. Lethaby A, Puscasiu L, Vollenhoven B. Preoperative medical therapy before surgery for uterine fibroids. Cochrane Database Syst Rev. 2017;11:CD000547.pub2.
96. Schlaff WD, Ackerman RT, Al-Hendy A, et al. Elagolix for heavy menstrual bleeding in women with uterine fibroids. N Engl J Med. 2020;4:328-340.
97. Simon JA, Al-Hendy A, Archer DF, et al. Elagolix treatment for up to 12 months in women with heavy menstrual bleeding and uterine leiomyomas. Obstet Gynecol. 2020;6:1313-26.
98. Al-Hendy A, Lukes AS, Poindexter AN 3rd, et al. Treatment of uterine fibroid symptoms with relugolix combination therapy. N Engl J Med. 2021;7:630-42.
99. Ghonim M, Magdy R, Sabbour M, Ghonim M, Nabhan A. A systematic review and meta-analysis of ulipristal acetate for symptomatic uterine fibroids. Int J Gynaecol Obstet. 2019;2:141-8.

100. Sandberg EM, Tummers FHMP, Cohen SL, van den Haak L, Dekkers OM, Jansen FW. Reintervention risk and quality of life outcomes after uterine-sparing interventions for fibroids: a systematic review and meta-analysis. Fertil Steril. 2018;4:698-707.e1.
101. Hartmann KE, Fonnesbeck C, Surawicz T, Krishaswami S, Andrews JC, Wilson JE. Management of uterine fibroids. Comparative Effectiveness Review No. 195. Rockville, MD: Agency for Healthcare Research and Quality; 2017. Available at: https://effectivehealthcare.ahrq.gov/products/uterine-fibroids/research-2017. Last accessed Aug. 23, 2022.
102. Centers for Disease Control and Prevention. Gynecologic Cancer Incidence, United States—2012–2016. USCS Data Brief, no 11. Atlanta, GA: Centers for Disease Control and Prevention, US Department of Health and Human Services; 2019.
103. Shankar M, Lee CA, Sabin CA, Economides DL, Kadir RA. von Willebrand disease in women with menorrhagia: a systematic review. BJOG. 2004;111(7):734-40.
104. Kouides PA, Byams VR, Philipp CS, et al. Multisite management study of menorrhagia with abnormal laboratory haemostasis: a prospective crossover study of intranasal desmopressin and oral tranexamic acid. Br J Haematol. 2009;2:212-20
105. Philipp CS, Dilley A, Miller CH, et al. Platelet functional defects in women with unexplained menorrhagia. J Thromb Haemost. 2003;3:477-84.
106. Kadir RA, Economides DL, Sabin CA, Owens D, Lee CA. Variations in coagulation factors in women: effects of age, ethnicity, menstrual cycle and combined oral contraceptive. Thromb Haemost. 1999;5:1456-61.
107. Kadir RA, Sharief LA, Lee CA. Inherited bleeding disorders in older women. Maturitas. 2012;1:35-41.
108. Sjalander A, Friberg B, Svensson P, Stigendal L, Lethagen S. Menorrhagia and minor bleeding symptoms in women on oral anticoagulation. J Thromb Thrombolysis. 2007;1:39-41.
109. Huq FY, Tvarkova K, Arafa A, Kadir RA. Menstrual problems and contraception in women of reproductive age receiving oral anticoagulation. Contraception. 2011;2:128-32.
110. Maas AH, Euler M, Bongers MY, et al. Practice points in gynecardiology: Abnormal uterine bleeding in premenopausal women taking oral anticoagulant or antiplatelet therapy. Maturitas. 2015;4:355-9.
111. Lee CA, Chi C, Pavord SR, Bolton-Maggs PH, et al. The obstetric and gynaecological management of women with inherited bleeding disorders--review with guidelines produced by a taskforce of UK Haemophilia Centre Doctors' Organization. Haemophilia. 2006;4:301-36.
112. hi C, Huq FY, Kadir RA. Levonorgestrel-releasing intrauterine system for the management of heavy menstrual bleeding in women with inherited bleeding disorders: long-term follow-up. Contraception. 2011;3:242-7.
113. Kingman CE, Kadir RA, Lee CA, Economides DL. The use of levonorgestrel-releasing intrauterine system for treatment of menorrhagia in women with inherited bleeding disorders. BJOG. 2004;12:1425-8.
114. Edlund M, Blomback M, Fried G. Desmopressin in the treatment of menorrhagia in women with no common coagulation factor deficiency but with prolonged bleeding time. Blood Coagul Fibrinolysis. 2002;3:225-31.
115. Kirtava A, Drews C, Lally C, Dilley A, Evatt B. Medical, reproductive and psychosocial experiences of women diagnosed with von Willebrand's disease receiving care in haemophilia treatment centres: a case-control study. Haemophilia. 2003;3:292-7.
116. Practice Bulletin no. 136: management of abnormal uterine bleeding associated with ovulatory dysfunction. Obstet Gynecol. 2013;1:176-85.
117. Critchley HO, Maybin JA. Molecular and cellular causes of abnormal uterine bleeding of endometrial origin. Semin Reprod Med. 2011;5:400-9.
118. Hubacher D, Lopez L, Steiner MJ, Dorflinger L. Menstrual pattern changes from levonorgestrel subdermal implants and DMPA: systematic review and evidence-based comparisons. Contraception. 2009;2:113-8.
119. Runowicz CD, Costantino JP, Wickerham DL, et al. Gynecologic conditions in participants in the NSABP breast cancer prevention study of tamoxifen and raloxifene (STAR). Am J Obstet Gynecol. 2011;6:535 e1-5.
120. Dominick S, Hickey M, Chin J, Su HI. Levonorgestrel intrauterine system for endometrial protection in women with breast cancer on adjuvant tamoxifen. Cochrane Database Syst Rev. 2015;12:CD007245.

121. Wong AW, Chan SS, Yeo W, Yu MY, Tam WH. Prophylactic use of levonorgestrel-releasing intrauterine system in women with breast cancer treated with tamoxifen: a randomized controlled trial. Obstet Gynecol. 2013;5:943-50.
122. De Sutter TC, Lohle PN, Boekkooi PF. Severe blood loss days after suction and curettage: consider a pseudoaneurysm. Ned Tijdschr Geneeskd. 2013;26:A6004.
123. Ewies AAA, Zanetto U. Caesarean section scar causes myometrial hypertrophy with subsequent heavy menstrual flow and dysmenorrhea. Med Hypotheses. 2017;108:54-6.]
124. Eckert LO, Thwin SS, Hillier SL, Kiviat NB, Eschenbach DA. The antimicrobial treatment of subacute endometritis: a proof-of-concept study. Am J Obstet Gynecol. 2004;2:305-13.
125. Kamel DM, Tantawy SA, Abdelsamea GA. Experience of dysmenorrhea among a group of physical therapy students from Cairo University: an exploratory study. J Pain Res. 2017;10:1079-85.
126. Ferries-Rowe E, Corey E, Archer JS. Primary dysmenorrhea: Diagnosis and therapy. Obstet Gynecol. 2020;136:1047-58.
127. Kho KA, Shields JK. Diagnosis and management of primary dysmenorrhea. JAMA. 2020 Jan 21;323:268-9.
128. Berry C, McGuire FL. Menstrual distress and acceptance of sexual role. Am J Obstet Gynecol. 1972;114:83–7.
129. Akman AO, Bozdag G, Pehlivantürk-Kizilkan M, Akgul S, Derman O, Kanbur N. Menstrual cycle pain is independent of ovulation in adolescents with primary dysmenorrhea. J Pediatr Adolesc Gynecol. 2021;34:635-42.
130. Sultan C, Gaspari L, Paris F. Adolescent dysmenorrhea. Endocr Dev 2012;22:171-80.
131. Oladosu FA, Tu FF, Hellman KM. Nonsteroidal anti-inflammatory drug resistance in dysmenorrhea: epidemiology, causes, and treatment. Am J Obstet Gynecol. 2018;218:390-400.
132. Matthewman G, Lee A, Kaur JG, Daley AJ. Physical activity for primary dysmenorrhea: a systematic review and meta-analysis of randomized controlled trials. Am J Obstet Gynecol. 2018;219:255.e1-e20.
133. Nie W, Xu P, Hao C, Chen Y, Yin Y, Wang L. Efficacy and safety of over-the-counter analgesics for primary dysmenorrhea: A network meta-analysis. Medicine (Baltimore). 2020;99):e19881.
134. Burnett M, Lemyre M. No. 345-Primary dysmenorrhea consensus guideline. J Obstet Gynaecol Can. 2017;39:585-95.
135. Damm T, Lamvu G, Carrillo J, Ouyang C, Feranec J. Continuous vs. cyclic combined hormonal contraceptives for treatment of dysmenorrhea: a systematic review. Contracept X. 2019;1:100002.
136. McKenna KA, Fogleman CD. Dysmenorrhea. Am Fam Physician. 2021;104(2):164-70.
137. Johnson PS, Ryckmans T, Bryans J, et al. Discovery of PF-184563, a potent and selective V1a antagonist for the treatment of dysmenorrhoea. The influence of compound flexibility on microsomal stability. Bioorg Med Chem Lett. 2011;21:5684-7.
138. Reis FM, Coutinho LM, Vannuccini S, Batteux F, Chapron C, Petraglia F. Progesterone receptor ligands for the treatment of endometriosis: the mechanisms behind therapeutic success and failure. Hum Reprod Update. 2020;26:565-85.
139. Hassanin AI, Youssef AA, Yousef AM, Ali MK. Comparison of dienogest versus combined oral contraceptive pills in the treatment of women with adenomyosis: A randomized clinical trial. Int J Gynaecol Obstet. 2021;154:263-9.
140. Dmitrovic R, Kunselman AR, Legro RS. Sildenafil citrate in the treatment of pain in primary dysmenorrhea: a randomized controlled trial. Hum Reprod. 2013;28:2958-65.
141. Pattanittum P, Kunyanone N, Brown J, et al. Dietary supplements for dysmenorrhoea. Cochrane Database Syst Rev. 2016;3:CD002124.pub2.
142. Smith CA, Armour M, Zhu X, Li X, Lu ZY, Song J. Acupuncture for dysmenorrhoea. Cochrane Database Syst Rev. 2016;4:CD007854.pub3.
143. Armour M, Dahlen HG, Zhu X, Farquhar C, Smith CA. The role of treatment timing and mode of stimulation in the treatment of primary dysmenorrhea with acupuncture: An exploratory randomised controlled trial. PLoS One. 2017;12:e0180177.
144. Blödt S, Pach D, Eisenhart-Rothe SV, et al. Effectiveness of app-based self-acupressure for women with menstrual pain compared to usual care: a randomized pragmatic trial. Am J Obstet Gynecol. 2018;218:227.e1-e9.

145. ACOG Committee Opinion No. 760: Dysmenorrhea and endometriosis in the adolescent. Obstet Gynecol. 2018;132:e249-58.
146. Casper RF. Progestin-only pills may be a better first-line treatment for endometriosis than combined estrogen-progestin contraceptive pills. Fertil Steril. 2017;107:533-6.
147. Crosignani PG, Luciano A, Ray A, Bergqvist A. Subcutaneous depot medroxyprogesterone acetate versus leuprolide acetate in the treatment of endometriosis-associated pain. Hum Reprod. 2006;21:248-56.
148. Margatho D, Carvalho NM, Bahamondes L. Endometriosis-associated pain scores and biomarkers in users of the etonogestrel-releasing subdermal implant or the 52-mg levonorgestrel-releasing intrauterine system for up to 24 months. Eur J Contracept Reprod Health Care. 2020;25:133-40.
149. Ferrero S, Scala C, Ciccarelli S, Vellone VG, Barra F. Treatment of rectovaginal endometriosis with the etonogestrel-releasing contraceptive implant. Gynecol Endocrinol. 2020;36:540-4.
150. Ambacher K, Secter M, Sanders AP. The use of progestin subdermal implants in the management of endometriosis-related pain symptoms and quality of life: a systematic review. Curr Med Res Opin. 2022;38:479-86.
151. Soliman AM, Bonafede M, Farr AM, Castelli-Haley J, Winkel C. Analysis of adherence, persistence, and surgery among endometriosis patients treated with leuprolide acetate plus norethindrone acetate add-back therapy. J Manag Care Spec Pharm. 2016;22:573-87.
152. Donnez J, Dolmans MM. GnRH Antagonists with or without Add-Back Therapy: A new alternative in the management of endometriosis? Int J Mol Sci. 2021;22:11342.
153. Bedaiwy MA, Alfaraj S, Yong P, Casper R. New developments in the medical treatment of endometriosis. Fertil Steril. 2017;107:555-65.
154. Yonkers KA, Simoni MK. Premenstrual disorders. Am J Obstet Gynecol. 2018;218:68-74.
155. Premenstrual Dysphoric Disorder Work Group. Diagnostic and statistical manual of diagnostic and statistical manual of mental disorders. 5th ed. Arlington, VA: American Psychiatric Association, 2013.
156. Dalton K. The premenstrual syndrome and progesterone therapy, 2nd ed. Chicago: Mosby-Year Book Medical Publisher, 1984.
157. Rubinow DR, Hoban MC, Grover GN, et al. Changes in plasma hormones across the menstrual cycle in patients with menstrually related mood disorder and in control subjects. Am J Obstet Gynecol. 1988;158:5-11.
158. Freeman EW, Rickels K, Sondheimer SJ, Polansky M. A double-blind trial of oral progesterone, alprazolam, and placebo in treatment of severe premenstrual syndrome. JAMA. 1995;274:51-7.
159. Schmidt PJ, Nieman LK, Danaceau MA, Adams LF, Rubinow DR. Differential behavioral effects of gonadal steroids in women with and those without premenstrual syndrome. New Engl J Med. 1998;338:209-16.
160. Mira M, Stewart PM, Abraham SF. Vitamin and trace element status in premenstrual syndrome. Am J Clin Nutr. 1988;47:636-41.
161. Perkonigg A, Yonkers KA, Pfister H, Lieb R, Wittchen HU. Risk factors for premenstrual dysphoric disorder in a community sample of young women: the role of traumatic events and posttraumatic stress disorder. J Clin Psychiatry. 2004;65:1314-22.
162. Fava M, Pedrazzi F, Guaraldi GP, Romano G, Genazzani AR, Facchinetti F. Comorbid anxiety and depression among patients with late luteal phase dysphoric disorder. J Anxiety Disorders. 1992;6:325-35.
163. Prasad D, Wollenhaupt-Aguiar B, Kidd KN, de Azevedo Cardoso T, Frey BN. Suicidal risk in women with premenstrual syndrome and premenstrual dysphoric disorder: A systematic review and meta-analysis. J Womens Health (Larchmt). 2021;30:1693-707.
164. Green L, O'Brien P, Panay N, Craig, M. Royal College of Obstetricians and Gynecologists. Management of premenstrual symptoms. BJOG. 2016;124:e73-105.
165. Czajkowska M, Drosdzol-Cop A, Naworska B, et al. The impact of competitive sports on menstrual cycle and menstrual disorders, including premenstrual syndrome, premenstrual dysphoric disorder and hormonal imbalances. Ginekol Pol. 2020;91:503-12.
166. Carlini SV, Deligiannidis KM. Evidence-based treatment of premenstrual dysphoric disorder: A concise review. J Clin Psychiatry. 2020;81:19ac13071.

167. Freeman EW, Rickels K, Yonkers KA, et al. Venlafaxine in the treatment of premenstrual dysphoric disorder. Obstet Gynecol. 2001;98:737-44.
168. Yonkers KA, Brown C, Pearlstein TB, Foegh M, Sampson-Landers C, Rapkin A. Efficacy of a new low-dose oral contraceptive with drospirenone in premenstrual dysphoric disorder. Obstet Gynecol. 2005;106:492-501.
169. Pinkerton JV, Guico-Pabia CJ, Taylor HS. Menstrual cycle-related exacerbation of disease. Am J Obstet Gynecol. 2010;202:221-31.
170. Brandes JL. The influence of estrogen on migraine: a systematic review. JAMA. 2006; 295:1824-30.
171. Nierenburg Hdel C, Ailani J, Malloy M, Siavoshi S, Hu NN, Yusuf N. Systematic review of preventive and acute treatment of menstrual migraine. Headache. 2015;55:1052-71
172. Pavlović JM, Stewart WF, Bruce CA, et al. Burden of migraine related to menses: results from the AMPP study. J Headache Pain. 2015;16:24.
173. Somerville BW. The role of estradiol withdrawal in the etiology of menstrual migraine. Neurology. 1972;22:355-65.
174. Maguire MJ, Nevitt SJ. Treatments for seizures in catamenial (menstrual-related) epilepsy. Cochrane Database Syst Rev. 2019;14(10):CD013225.pub2.
175. Reilly TJ, Sagnay de la Bastida VC, Joyce DW, Cullen AE, McGuire P. Exacerbation of psychosis during the perimenstrual pPhase of the menstrual cycle: Systematic review and meta-analysis. Schizophr Bull. 2020;46:78-90.
176. Sönmez İ, Köşger F. Menstrual cycle in schizophrenic patients: Review with a case. Noro Psikiyatr Ars. 2015;52:417-9.
177. Gladis MM, Walsh BT. Premenstrual exacerbation of binge eating in bulimia. Am J Psychiatry. 1987;144:1592-5.

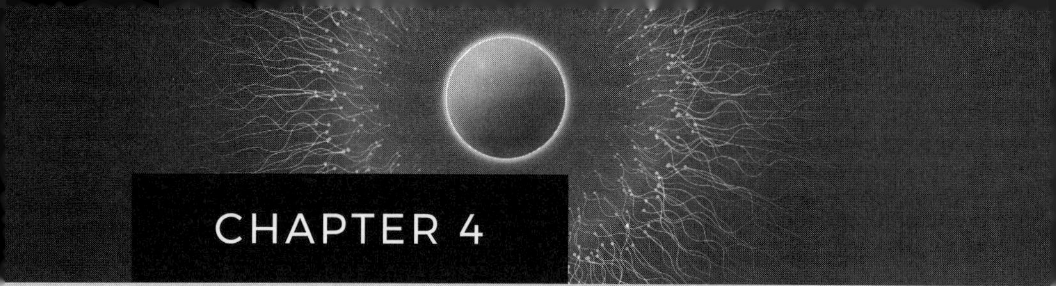

CHAPTER 4

Person-Centered Reproductive Health Conversations and Contraceptive Counseling

Patty Cason, MS, FNP-BC
Joely Pritzker, MS, FNP-C

KEY POINTS

- Sexuality and reproduction are core reflections of the way people express their humanity; decisions regarding sexuality and reproduction are not inherently medical issues.
- Unintended pregnancy has a specific, albeit flawed, public health definition and may not be a clinically relevant concept.
- The various dimensions of reproductive desires and pregnancy preferences—acceptability, plans, intentions, desires, feelings, and the interactions between them—are complex.
- Acceptability rather than intentionality may be a better way to understand an individual's overall attitude about pregnancy.
- Providers can engage in person-centered conversations about patients' reproductive desires and, if appropriate, contraceptive counseling to clarify patients' values and preferences.
- Communication and counseling skills based on a wide variety of strategies from active listening to adult learning principles can be applied to person-centered conversations by using Affirm-Share-Ask (ASA) Cycles. Skills to Operationalize Person-Centered Care begin on p. 92.
- In conversations with patients, talk less, listen, and ask more questions.

Comprehensive sexual and reproductive health rests on the belief that all people can and should have agency over their own sexual and reproductive lives. Indeed, sexuality and reproduction are core reflections of the way people express their humanity. Reproductive Justice[1,2]—a framework and movement developed by Black women activists in the 1990s (see Chapter 1, Reproductive Justice within Reproductive Health Care)—has drawn attention to the need to holistically consider people's sexual and reproductive experiences, including "the human right to maintain personal autonomy, have children, not have children, and parent the children we have in safe and sustainable communities."[3] Part of our role as health care professionals involves helping patients prevent or manage adverse outcomes associated with sex and reproduction, such as sexually transmitted infections, sexual violence, unwanted pregnancy, or negative outcomes of pregnancy. (See Chapter 6, Sexuality and Contraception.) However, people's choices with regard to sexuality and reproduction, while having implications for health and health care needs, are not inherently medical issues.

Many ongoing practices and policies perpetuate inequities and impede efforts to realize Reproductive Justice principles.[4,5] Vulnerable populations experience inadequate access to comprehensive pregnancy care, including prenatal care, abortion, and management of pregnancy of unknown location, miscarriage, and ectopic.[6] The 2022 *Dobbs v. Jackson Women's Health Organization* Supreme Court decision further undermines the core foundation of Reproductive Justice. It is an egregious example of how assaults on human rights inequitably affect long-marginalized communities and individuals.

The legacy of structural and individual racism in sexual and reproductive health care looms large over our current health care landscape.[7-10] Research highlights barriers to on-demand implant and intrauterine device (IUD) removal in the United States and internationally as a salient example of the intersection of structural racism and provider coercion with contraceptive access.[11,12] Progress has been made to rectify some of these harmful practices. While contraceptive initiatives have increasingly moved away from promotion of implants and IUDs to low-income individuals and people of color and toward promotion of full access to all contraceptive options, including on-demand removal,[13-15] countless other opportunities exist to improve practices.[16]

This chapter is designed to give clinicians the tools they need to engage in conversations with patients about their reproductive and sexual health in ways that are trauma-informed and grounded in Reproductive Justice principles. The first section of the chapter reviews person-centered and trauma-informed care. We then address the concept of pregnancy intention as it is understood in the United States and question its relevance to discussions about reproductive desires and contraception. From there, we explore theories grounding the approach to these conversations. The remainder of the chapter recommends tools and counseling skills to achieve person-centered care that is aligned with Reproductive Justice principles.

Person-Centered Care

Health care providers can acknowledge the legacy of racism and prevent future harm by providing nonstigmatizing, antiracist care that regards the individual as a person, not just as a patient. Health care interactions occur within the context, meaning, and values of a person's life. Prioritizing this during your interactions "centers" the patient.[17] Inherent in centering the patient is a clear understanding of our role as providers—to listen as patients identify what they want and then help them get it. We accomplish this by applying principles of patient-centered care, which the National Academy of Medicine (formerly the Institute of Medicine) defines as, "Providing care that is respectful of, and responsive to, individual patient preferences, needs, and values, and ensuring that patient values guide all clinical decisions."[18]

In this chapter, we use the term *person-centered care* to include *patient-centered care*. This aligns with person-first language and language used in the Person-Centered Contraceptive Counseling (PCCC) measure, a new contraceptive quality measure.[19,20] The person-centered communication techniques and Affirm-Share-Ask (ASA) Cycles we recommend can be used by providers with patients during all health care interactions. Many of these skills are also appropriate to use when teaching, training, and communicating with students and colleagues.[21]

A principle of person-centered care is to listen to patients' narratives with respect and trust their lived experiences.[22-28] This involves acknowledging and grappling with the role that the health care system plays in the suffering of individuals and communities.[10,22] Broad structural issues, such as racism, poverty, anti-immigration policies and sentiments, and stigma surrounding sexual minorities, form the context of patients' lives. Issues specific to health care systems—such as policy, reimbursement, metrics, and access to insurance as well as clinic policies, personnel, and intake forms—directly shape patients' access to and experience of how we provide care. These issues are prominent drivers of inequity and the resulting disparities. While outside the scope of this chapter, there is extensive literature representing stories and health care experiences of trans and gender nonconforming individuals, Black Americans, immigrants, refugees, and persons with disabilities, among many others.[29-34] (See Chapter 1, Reproductive Justice within Reproductive Health Care.)

Trauma-informed care acknowledges the pervasiveness of trauma in our society. The goal is to prevent traumatizing or retraumatizing patients by providing sensitive, nonstigmatizing care to all patients regardless of known trauma history.[35] While it is beyond the scope of this chapter to discuss all facets of how to operationalize trauma-informed care, a foundational standard that guides all interactions is to keep the locus of control with the patient as opposed to the provider. Trauma-informed practices include explicit consent during sensitive exams, person-first language, and recommendations in this chapter for provider-patient communication.

Unintended Pregnancy in The United States

Wanted versus unwanted? Planned versus unplanned? Devastating versus a happy surprise? Acceptable versus unacceptable? What exactly is *unintended pregnancy*, and is it a relevant concept? Despite the ubiquitous claim, in the biomedical and social science literature, that unintended pregnancies lead to adverse outcomes, surprisingly little high-quality evidence exists to show a causal link between unintended pregnancy and negative health effects, particularly in high-income countries like the United States.[36] Moreover, what we do know about pregnancy intention is limited by the challenges of accounting for multiple confounding influences.[36,37] Increasingly, scholars and researchers have drawn attention to the problems with focusing on rates of unintended pregnancy as a relevant research and public health measure.[38-41]

From a public health perspective, the term "unintended pregnancy" has a specific meaning. Statistics from the National Survey on Family Growth (NSFG) are a key component of estimates on pregnancy intention. In the NSFG, unintended pregnancy refers to a pregnancy that was reported by the patient as either desired at some future time but not at the time pregnancy occurred, or never desired at any point. Having hovered around 50% for the past decade,[42] the most recent data show a decline in the proportion of pregnancies that were measured as unintended from 49% of all pregnancies in 2006 to 45% in 2011.[43] While national numbers have not been updated since 2011, a 2021 report focused on state level numbers of unintended or "wanted-later" pregnancies.[44] This report examined trends between 2012 and 2017 and highlighted overall declines in unintended or "wanted-later" pregnancies in many states with rates varying greatly between states, spanning 26% of pregnancies in Utah to 44% in New Jersey.

Government agencies and institutional funders use these measurements to direct resources and shape policies based on the notion that unintended pregnancy is a fundamentally undesirable outcome. As a result, public health advocates, researchers, and even clinicians are motivated by the statistic that almost half of all pregnancies in the United States each year are unintended.[43] However, it is challenging to tease apart negative outcomes related to intentionality from those related to poverty, lack of support, and inadequate access to care.[6,45-47]

In addition to these considerations, there are many notable limitations in how unintended pregnancy estimates are calculated.[39] Just a few of them are discussed here. The NSFG is retrospective, which leaves responses vulnerable to recall bias (retrospective bias). This bias can lead to inaccurate recall about intention such that the pregnancy becomes more positively viewed over time, particularly after birth.[48-52] Another limitation is that the NSFG measure is cross-sectional, meaning that it is measured at only a single time point. But descriptions of pregnancy intentions can vary, even over relatively short time periods.[53] And further, combining unwanted and mistimed pregnancies into a single category (unintended) is problematic as they have discrete meanings and implications.[54,55] Finally, by constructing a binary "intended versus unintended" comparison, the NSFG measure leaves little room for pregnancies that were viewed ambivalently, uncertainly, or indifferently.[56]

A more concerning problem from a clinical perspective is conflating the significance of a population level measurement with clinical best practices. **We do not talk about reproductive desires with individuals in order to lower population rates of unintended pregnancy.** We talk about these topics to support people in fulfilling their personal reproductive desires. These desires may or may not include avoiding an unintended pregnancy.

Reproductive Desires

Complexity of Pregnancy Desires

The various dimensions of reproductive desires and pregnancy preferences—acceptability, plans, intentions, desires, feelings, and the interactions between them—are complex. And the nuance inherent in conversations about reproductive desires may seem daunting to clinicians and researchers alike. But acknowledging and valuing the complexity of each individual's values and preferences are vital components of person-centered care.[57,58]

Some people have the inclination and resources to plan a pregnancy and others do not. Planning a pregnancy is not a concept that is resonant or relevant to how many people experience their lives.[59] Some embrace a lack of intention around getting pregnant. There are cultural and religious factors that may strongly shape one's orientation toward pregnancy, including the influence of extended family and the belief that childbearing is determined by fate or a higher power.[60-62]

Understanding prospective pregnancy preferences first requires that we become familiar with concepts beyond timing-based intentions and recognize the pitfalls inherent in considering a "planned pregnancy" the goal. Many people are aware of social norms that encourage waiting until financial, educational, and relationship circumstances are ideal before having a child.[59,63] These circumstances, however, may be unattainable in the near future or, in some cases, ever. Those who do not see their circumstances changing anytime soon may not want to indefinitely delay having a child. Qualitative research reveals how social inequities hinder reproductive autonomy and challenges the widely held belief, which is not evidence-based, that use of contraception, rather than addressing social inequity, is a way out of poverty.[64] Structural factors, like poverty and racism, are significant predictors of future life outcomes, irrespective of when or if people have children.[4,65,66]

Research further demonstrates that the dichotomy of planned versus unplanned pregnancy is often irrelevant to individuals. Acceptability, rather than intentionality, may be a more useful way to characterize an individual's overall attitude about pregnancy, either potential or actual, at a given time.[59,67-70] In assessing the acceptability of a current pregnancy, individuals weigh a combination of personal factors, such as one's health and intimate and family relationships,[71,72] as well as "structural realities (e.g., access to employment, education or capital)."[68]

Acceptability, then—not intentionality—is central.

Other factors that may play into an individual's acceptability of a pregnancy in the near term include:

- Belief that number of children they will have, and the timing of those births, is up to God[59,73,74]
- Self-assessment that there is no good method of contraception for them[26,75]
- Lack of autonomy due to reproductive coercion from an intimate partner[59]
- Simply not wishing to plan and finding the idea of not knowing for sure whether or when a pregnancy will happen exciting or emotionally satisfying[76]

Planning is only one way people discuss their reproductive desires. Some may attach most meaning to their feelings about pregnancy and childbearing— i.e., whether a pregnancy would be greeted with happiness or unhappiness. Others hold ambivalent pregnancy desires (i.e. they simultaneously have some degree of desire for pregnancy and some degree of desire to avoid pregnancy).[60,77] It is not uncommon for people to express feelings toward pregnancy that appear to be at odds with their timing-based intentions.[78,79] Clinicians should not assume such an orientation is ambivalence; it may in fact reflect the nuance inherent in attitudes toward potential parenting or pregnancy.[79] So-called "happy accidents" are an example of this.[70] Further, the qualitative measures used to categorize pregnancy intention frequently misclassify ambivalence.[79]

Those who are indifferent do not express strong desires either to become pregnant or to avoid pregnancy.[77] "If it happens, it happens" is an example of this.[60] When asked about desire for pregnancy over a defined period of time—for example, "in the next year"—people with this orientation are unlikely to express a concrete plan or intention. Providers may incorrectly respond to these individuals with an assumption that they are more motivated to prevent pregnancy than is the case, or that they are experiencing ambivalence that needs to be resolved. Even those who express either a strong desire to avoid pregnancy or to get pregnant in the context of a single clinical encounter may fluctuate in these desires as health, relationships, financial situations, and life opportunities change over time.[53]

While these distinctions are interesting from a theoretical perspective, they are highly relevant to clinical interactions; providers are only able to offer appropriate services when patients express their honest orientation about potential pregnancy. Nondirective conversations about reproductive desires provide an opportunity for the individual to explore and share their attitudes without fear of stigma or judgment.

Conversations about Reproductive Desires

When approached respectfully, any primary care, specialty, or sexual and reproductive health visit is a potential opportunity to explore reproductive desires and offer relevant services.[80] Ask these questions annually for most patients and recognize that some may benefit from more- or less-frequent inquiry based on patient preference and clinical relevance. Visits for emergency contraception, postpartum, third trimester pregnancy, and pregnancy testing when the result is negative present natural opportunities for these conversations.[81-84] Conversations about reproductive desires are also increasingly being incorporated into social service settings, recognizing the importance of meeting people "where they are at" and providing relevant referrals.[85,86] Routine well-child visits are an underutilized opportunity to query parents about reproductive desires and needed services. Positive pregnancy test visits, however, are not the time to discuss theoretical reproductive desires (see Pregnancy Options Counseling, p. 110).

There are various ways to begin these conversations with patients. One approach being researched is to simply ask the patient at the beginning of the visit: "Can I help you with any reproductive services today, such as preventing pregnancy/ birth control or planning for a healthy pregnancy?"[87-89]

Another option is the Self-Identified Need for Contraception (SINC) screening tool (**Figure 4-1**), a standardized needs assessment question[90]: "We ask everyone about their reproductive health needs. Do you want to talk about contraception or pregnancy prevention during your visit today?" SINC is intended to be integrated

Self-Identified Need for Contraception (SINC)
EHR standardized data element

We ask everyone about their reproductive health needs. Do you want to talk about contraception or pregnancy prevention during your visit today?

If **yes**:

- *Mark and refer to provider for contraceptive counseling.*

If **no**:

- Clarification Prompt: "There are a lot of reasons why a person wouldn't want to talk about this, and you don't have to share anything you don't want to. Do any of these apply to you?" *(mark all that apply)*
    - **I'm here for something else**
    - **The question does not apply to me / I prefer not to answer**
    - **I am already using contraception (and what)**
    - **I am unsure or don't want to use contraception**
    - **I am hoping to become pregnant in the near future**

Figure 4-1 SINC Tool

University of California, San Francisco, ASSESSING THE NEED FOR CONTRACEPTIVE SERVICES https://pcrhp.ucsf.edu/sites/g/files/tkssra4126/f/Implementation%20 Guidance_5.7.21.pdf

Box 4-1 Talking about Reproductive Desires

A conversation about reproductive desires:

- Centers a patient's autonomy and agency
- Provides the time and space for the patient to explore attitudes about parenting
- Provides the time and space for the patient to explore the acceptability of a potential pregnancy
- Helps the patient gain clarity about their reproductive preferences
- Helps the patient integrate information relevant to their identified contraceptive preferences
- Directs the provider to offer relevant information, referrals, and services (prepregnancy care, fertility support, contraception)
- Builds rapport and trust by actively listening

into existing workflows and Electronic Health Records and can be asked by a clinician or other members of health center staff.

Providers can also ask directly whether and when someone may want to have a child. This question can be asked either independently or in conjunction with an offer of services. It is efficient to ask about reproductive desires (**Box 4-1**) because if the patient is currently seeking pregnancy, providers should offer a discussion about prepregnancy care (preconception care). By the same token, if a person would like to prevent pregnancy, it is relevant to offer a discussion about contraception. For a patient open to pregnancy, but not actively trying, an offer of both a prepregnancy discussion as well as contraceptive counseling may be appropriate.

The purpose of discussing reproductive desires is NOT:

- For providers to decide for the patient what contraception they "should" use
- To create a concrete plan the patient feels they must commit to
- To resolve the patient's apparent ambivalence

Strategies used to elicit a person's reproductive desires that have been described in the literature are often referred to as a reproductive life plan, a "set of personal goals regarding whether, when, and how to have children based on individual priorities, resources, and values."[91] Discussing a reproductive life plan has been recommended by Centers for Disease Control and Prevention (CDC)[92] for clients receiving contraceptive counseling, pregnancy testing and counseling, basic infertility services, sexually transmitted disease services, and prepregnancy health services. The research discussed earlier in the section entitled Complexity of Pregnancy Desires points to myriad ways the language and perspective of a static "reproductive life plan" is problematic and at odds with key tenets of person-centered care.[36,93,94] Our thinking and approach to this topic continues to evolve as the reproductive and sexual health field further integrates conversations around equity, social determinants of health, and reproductive autonomy into our clinical practices.[8]

The PATH[95] Framework and One Key Question®[96] are two specific examples of person-centered ways to directly ask about reproductive desires. Both strategies are aligned with Office of Population Affairs' (OPA) and CDC's Quality in Family Planning service delivery recommendations.

One Key Question™

One Key Question (OKQ)[96] is a simple way for primary care providers to start conversations about pregnancy desires but can be utilized by all providers, including nonclinical and social service providers. Patients are asked, "Would you like to become pregnant in the next year?" and offered four responses: yes, no, okay either way, unsure. Based on the response, providers ask relevant follow-up questions to understand the need for counseling, clinical services, and/or referrals based on patients' pregnancy desires. Prepregnancy care, contraceptive services, or some combination of the two may be offered. OKQ supports all individuals capable of becoming pregnant, regardless of their sexual orientation or gender identity. OKQ asks a timing-based question with the goal of helping support people to think more concretely about their pregnancy desires in the near future.

OKQ has been identified as a Best Practice by the Association of Maternal and Child Health Programs.[97] Several recent studies have explored the use of OKQ in the provision of contraception and preconception counseling in the clinic setting.[98-103] Additional information about OKQ and how to receive training on it can be found by contacting the nonprofit Power to Decide (www.powertodecide.org).

The PATH Questions

The PATH questions[95,104] give providers inclusive language to facilitate conversations about reproductive desires in a way that is person-centered and builds trust and rapport between people and their health care professionals. They were iteratively developed by this chapter's lead author over many years with input from countless patients and providers. The questions used in the PATH framework are incorporated into the CDC's "A Guide for Taking a Sexual History," a consolidated document offering best practices for engaging in sexual health conversations with patients.[105] They are also included in the CDC's Sexually Transmitted Infections Treatment Guidelines 2021,[106] recommended in the Society for Family Planning clinical recommendations for transgender and gender diverse people,[107] as well as recommended for pediatricians as a way to engage in reproductive health conversations with adolescent clients.[108]

The PATH acronym can help you remember the questions (**Box 4-2**).

While there are three potential PATH Questions, only the question about parenting attitudes, "Do you think you might like to have (more) children at some point?", will be relevant for all patients. The questions about timing and the

Box 4-2 PATH Questions

(PA) Parenting/Pregnancy Attitudes:
Do you think you might like to have (more) children at some point?
(T) Timing:
When do you think that might be?
(H) How important:
How important is it to you to prevent pregnancy (until then)?

importance of pregnancy prevention are only asked when relevant (specific examples discussed later).

Parenting/Pregnancy Attitudes. "Do you think you might like to have (more) children at some point?"

The initial question intentionally addresses attitudes about parenting, not pregnancy. It invites patients to share their thoughts and feelings about having (or not having) children. This allows the question to be asked to anyone, regardless of gender, sexual orientation, or ability to carry a pregnancy.

Including the word "might" in this question encourages patients to clarify their feelings and attitudes in addition to their thoughts about parenting. This first question does not assume that all people want to be parents. For this reason, it is important not to skip over this question and go straight to a timing question. However, if the patient has already mentioned a desire or lack of desire to have (more) children, there is no need to ask this first question.

If the person already has a child or children, ask "Do you think you might like to have more children at some point?"

If the answer to the "Parenting/Pregnancy Attitudes" question is NO, skip the "Timing" question and ask the "How important" question. Examples include:

- "No, I really don't think so; I've really got my hands full with the three I've got!"
- "No, I know it sounds strange, but I've never wanted to have kids."
- "I seriously doubt it. I mean I love my niece, but I think it would be too much to deal with for me."

If the patient answers "Yes" to the "Parenting/Pregnancy Attitudes" question, proceed with the "Timing" question. However, listen carefully to the response to the first question because patients often give an expanded answer.

In the following examples, the person does not want to have a child "any time soon." Therefore, you can skip the "timing" question and proceed to the "How important" question. It is irrelevant to ask about timing if the patient has said they do not desire any (more) children in the future.

- "Yes, I think so. But not until I'm in my thirties."
- "Yes! I definitely want to be a mom someday. I am pretty traditional, and family is one of the most important things in my life, so I want to be married first, which I don't see happening any time soon."

In the following examples, the person actively desires pregnancy and so the provider can offer a conversation about being prepared for a healthy pregnancy. The question "how important is it to you to prevent pregnancy" is irrelevant.

- "Yes, we just started trying!"
- "Absolutely, my wife just had her IUD taken out."

Relevance to Contraception Counseling. If the patient does not desire (more) children ever, it may be appropriate to offer information about permanent contraception (see Chapter 8, Permanent Contraception).

> "Since you've said you are clear that you don't want any more children, would you like to discuss permanent contraceptive options for you or your partner?"

Timing. "When do you think that might be?"

If someone indicates that they are open to parenting at some point, this next question explores their thoughts on timing in an open-ended manner. The question invites individuals to interpret timing in the way that is meaningful to them: in one study, one third of respondents answered with a quantifiable timeline, one third answered with a life event, and another third used some combination of the two.[109] Using this information, the provider then personalizes the conversation.[104]

Use of the words "think" and "might" is also deliberate. These words allow for the possibility that the person has not given the matter a lot of thought. They also do not assume that any response is more correct than any other.

There is no need to press the patient for an exact answer about length of time. The essential information is whether the person is open to parenting now, sometime soon, or no time soon. The length of time until someone would like to parent is relevant when discussing preparation for pregnancy but less relevant when discussing prevention of pregnancy.

Relevance to Contraception Counseling. The "Timing" question is not intended to determine contraceptive choice, because:

- Other than depot medroxyprogesterone acetate (DMPA, sold as DepoProvera), all methods have rapid return to fecundity (see Chapter 11, Injectable Contraceptives).
- Regardless of when they would like to get pregnant in the future, a patient may or may not value potential length of use in a method.
- There is no need to match the potential length of use of a particular method with a patient's reproductive desires. For example, if someone wants to have a child in 3 years, it is not necessary to find a method that will last exactly that long (e.g., a 3-year implant or IUD). Methods with a longer potential length of use than the patient will need can be used for as little time as the patient chooses.

How Important Is It?. "How important is it to you to prevent pregnancy (until then)?"

Before asking about the importance of pregnancy prevention, you must know if pregnancy prevention is relevant. If you do not know the anatomy of the patient's partner(s) or the patient's sexual practices, include a statement such as "I don't want to make any assumptions, but if you ever have sex with someone with whom pregnancy could happen, how important is it to you to prevent pregnancy (until then)?" This provides an opportunity for the patient to share if pregnancy prevention is not a current concern.

By asking "how important," a patient is provided the space to consider the acceptability of potential pregnancy.

The (until then) is a placeholder. Personalize the question using the patient's responses to the "parenting/pregnancy attitudes" and "timing" questions. For example:

- "How important is it to you to prevent pregnancy for the next 5 years?"
- "How important is it to you to prevent pregnancy until you start your treatment program?"
- "How important is it to you to prevent pregnancy until you have your own place?"

- "How important is it to you to prevent pregnancy until your partner gets back?"
- "How important is it to you to prevent pregnancy for the next year until you finish school?"

If no specific timeframe has been provided, or with adolescent patients, "until then" can be used: "How important is it to you to prevent pregnancy *until then*?"

If the patient has said they do not want children, or more children, it is still highly relevant to ask about the importance of pregnancy prevention. Leave off "until then": "How important is it to you to prevent pregnancy?"

Focusing on "to you":

- Invites the patient to consider their feelings and desires, in addition to thoughts about their life circumstance.
- Provides context for preferences regarding the importance of contraceptive efficacy as well as the appropriateness of an offer of prepregnancy counseling or referral.
- For those who consider the acceptability of pregnancy within the context of their family or community, "to you" can be interpreted as plural.

The goal is for both the provider and patient to gain a deeper understanding of whether a pregnancy is or is not acceptable to the patient at this time.

Relevance to Contraception Counseling. This question can inform whether contraceptive effectiveness is a priority for the patient. Providers often assume that effectiveness is the most important attribute of a contraceptive method, but we cannot assume that our patients share this sentiment. Research shows that most people seek effectiveness in their method[110,111] but some do not prioritize effectiveness, or it may be one of several desired qualities.

Examples:

- "I've heard you say it's very important to you to avoid pregnancy until you finish school. Am I correct, then, that one of things you're looking for in your birth control is that it does a good job at preventing pregnancy until you're ready?"
- "I'm hearing you say that it's really important to not have any surprises and that you are sure that you don't want any more kids. Would you like to discuss permanent contraception as well as other highly effective options?"

PATH Questions and Offer of Services. Based on responses to the PATH questions, a provider can easily segue to an offer of a discussion about contraceptive methods and/or an offer to discuss prepregnancy care.

- "Since you've said you'd like to have a child soon, would you like to discuss ways to be prepared for a healthy pregnancy?"
- "It sounds like you are clear that you don't want to have another child anytime soon, so would you like to discuss ways to prevent pregnancy?"
- "I'm hearing you say that ideally, you don't want any more children right now, but if you were to get pregnant, you'd be okay with that. In that case, would you like to talk about ways to prevent pregnancy? We can also discuss ways to be prepared for a healthy pregnancy if it does happen, if you'd like."

The PATH Questions Are Not Gender-Specific. PATH questions can be used verbatim with patients of any gender or sexual orientation.[112] Traditionally, reproductive health conversations have focused on cis-women; PATH is a tool to extend these discussions to cis-men and other individuals who are frequently excluded from such conversations. Research illuminates the benefit of engaging in these conversations with transgender and nonbinary individuals[30] and the need for inclusive questions about reproductive desires.[107] PATH is intentionally gender neutral. Using gender-neutral language allows providers to ask these questions to all clients without having to remember specific wording for different populations. For example, both a trans-man and cis-man can be asked "Do you think you might like to have children at some point?" without any change to the question.

All individuals capable of parenting should be asked about their reproductive desires and deserve the opportunity to explore their thoughts, feelings, and desires with providers willing and able to offer needed information, services, and referrals.

Patient-Facing Tools

Innovative patient-facing tools are another potential way for patients to seek and get the information they need to make fully informed choices and to expand the capacity for more people to receive relevant services. (Refer to Chapter 26 for more on digital resources.)

Patient-facing tools provide platforms for patients to gain the knowledge they need to make informed choices as well as input their medical history and preferences that can be accessed by a provider during a clinical encounter. They do not require interaction with health care providers or staff, though they can be incorporated into clinical visits. We hope that tools like these will facilitate reproductive autonomy by allowing patients to drive more of their health care experiences and access relevant information.

Examples of patient-facing tools include:

- MyPATH[113]
- iCAN[114]
- My Birth Control[115-117]
- PPFA Decision Making[118]
- Bedsider[119]

Contraceptive Counseling: Past, Present, and Future

Contraceptive counseling has undergone a transformation. There is consensus in the current medical literature that providers should support their patients in making decisions about contraception. Providers offer relevant information, help patients identify their preferences in the context of their values, and assist them with choices aligned with these preferences. This shared decision-making approach[120] is an effective way to apply the principles of person-centered care during contraception counseling.[121-124] Following, we briefly describe two ways providers historically have provided contraception counseling and then present a shared decision-making model, which is the preferred approach.

Directive Counseling

Directive counseling is a traditional model[15,125] in which a provider prescribes the same treatment for most patients with similar diagnoses or conditions with little consideration of a patient's unique concerns, preferences, and values. When applying a directive counseling approach to contraception, providers form opinions about what method they believe is best for the patient and counsel accordingly. This may mean that a provider, often unintentionally, offers information in a way that can be coercive and designed to encourage patients to choose more effective methods.[126]

Consumerist Counseling or The "Menu" Approach

In an "informed choice" or consumerist counseling model, providers function as information-givers who are neutral in the decision-making process.[127,128] This can be thought of as a "menu" approach whereby the consumer (patient) is told about every available method without consideration of personal preferences. In this model, the provider does not actively assist the patient in the decision-making process.

This approach places the decision in the hands of the patient, where most providers rightfully believe the decision should rest. However, with the ever-expanding bevy of methods on the menu, the important information about every method is beyond the capacity of the human mind to digest in a single clinical visit. Additionally, providing information on methods that are not in line with a patient's preferences wastes precious visit time. The goal of person-centered counseling is for patients to get the information they need to make an informed choice *given their individual needs and preferences*, and not necessarily to be provided with information on all methods.

Shared Decision Making

Shared decision making as conceptualized in this chapter describes a facilitated (shared) process; however, the decision itself is made by the patient (not shared). A shared decision-making approach is associated with high levels of patient satisfaction in a wide variety of clinical settings,[120,129,130] including contraceptive counseling.[121,123,131,132] It is also grounding principle for informed consent in the clinical setting.[133] Shared decision making has been shown to increase patient engagement in self-care and improve patient outcomes and health status.[134] When applied to contraception counseling, it is associated with increased satisfaction with method choice and continuation.[17]

In this process, the provider:

- Keeps the patient's preferences and values centered in the conversation
- Is aware of their own biases and avoids communicating about and/or being motivated by their own values or preferences
- Asks clarifying questions and actively listens to the responses
- Explains the relevant science in a way that the patient understands and can integrate the information

SKILLS TO OPERATIONALIZE PERSON-CENTERED REPRODUCTIVE AND CONTRACEPTIVE CARE

Careful listening is the most essential skill providers use to center the patient.[21] If we were to winnow down all the skills and recommendations in this chapter, it would be to say, "Talk less, listen, and ask more questions."

Providers use a variety of time-honored communication and counseling skills that stem from an array of theories that we integrate into practical recommendations in this chapter. While specific research on operationalizing person-centered sexual and reproductive health care is limited,[135,136] data on each of the component parts support their utility. We present the ASA Cycle, bringing together most of these person-centered counseling and communication skills into a single digestible concept designed to encourage providers to listen purposefully to their patients and check their own biases continuously.

Grounding many counseling modalities and communication techniques is active listening, first developed by Rogers and Farson in 1957. Active listening foreshadowed shared decision making by highlighting the role of the highly skilled, yet nondirective listener (clinician) and the self-efficacy ascribed to the speaker (patient);

> It is called "active" because the listener has a very definite responsibility. He does not passively absorb the words which are spoken to him. He actively tries to grasp the facts and feelings in what he hears, and he tries, by his listening, to help the speaker work out his own problems.[137]

Other counseling and communication modalities and theories include, "Ask tell ask,"[138,139] motivational interviewing,[140-142] the GATHER technique (**G**reet, **A**sk, **T**ell, **H**elp, **E**xplain, and **R**eturn),[142,143] the SOLER method (**S**it squarely, **O**pen posture, **L**ean forward, **E**ye contact, **R**elax), SURETY (**S**it at an angle, **U**ncross legs and arms, **R**elax, **E**ye contact, **T**ouch, **Y**our intuition),[144] SEGUE (**S**et the stage, **E**licit information, **G**ive information, **U**nderstand the patient's perspective, **E**nd the encounter)[145], health literacy,[146,147] and adult learning principles.[137,148] We highlight communication skills derived from these modalities. There is, however, a critical difference in how these some of the skills are applied and what the goal of the interaction is. For example, motivational interviewing was developed to drive behavior change such as smoking cessation. It is effectively applied during patient interactions with that goal in mind. When applied to preference-sensitive decisions (decisions for which there is clinical equipoise, i.e., no one option that is clinically superior to another), the goal is vastly different. The ASA Cycle skills are applied as tools to facilitate listening, to center the individual, to clarify preferences, and to support decision-making without judgment.

Key Person-Centered Questions

Person-centered questions have broad application and are useful when offering services and having health-related conversations. (See PATH and OKQ sections for examples of key questions about reproductive desires.)

Questions for Small Talk

Intentionally incorporate "small talk" into clinical visits.[149] Patients express the value of small talk for building rapport, instilling trust, and setting them at ease. However, observational research on clinical encounters indicates that small talk does not happen often.[17] Begin a visit with some "small talk" by asking about the patient's life, family, or, if appropriate, work or school. This builds rapport and gathers potentially relevant information for a subsequent conversation about reproductive desires and contraception. Incorporate "small talk" during "down time" during the visit, for example, when bringing the patient back to the room or when preparing the room for an exam or procedure.

Examples of questions to open small talk conversations include:

- "What keeps you busy?" or "How do you spend your time?"[150]
- For patients in an occupational health setting or for those the clinician knows have a job,
  - "What kind of work do you do?"
- For patients seen in a school-based setting or when the clinician knows the patient is a student,
  - "What are you studying?" "How much longer until you are finished with your program? (or high school?)."
- For patients in the office with a child, ask a question relevant to the child's age or about the family.[150]

Questions That Are Open-Ended

"Yes" or "no" questions are appropriate for taking a factual history, such as ensuring no medical contraindications exist for a particular contraceptive method. When the conversation is geared toward helping patients clarify their preferences, open-ended questions, focused on the topic at hand, yield more nuanced information.[23,92,151,152]

Health care providers often think that open-ended questions require significant time to engage in meaningful discussions, particularly when people are not clear about their reproductive desires. These conversations, however, do not need to resolve ambiguity or address all issues that arise in one visit. Patients can identify concrete steps to help them move toward their desires or create an agenda for future visits. A person-centered counseling framework that prioritizes the use of open-ended questions may also uncover other clinically relevant concerns such as interpersonal violence, mental health issues, and economic considerations.

Questions for Obtaining a Nonstigmatizing, Comprehensive Sexual History

The CDC's "A Guide to Taking a Sexual History" provides useful language for providers to obtain an inclusive, comprehensive sexual history (https://www.cdc.gov/std/treatment/sexualhistory.pdf).[105]

Questions for Follow Up

Follow-up questions are an essential, often neglected, part of a clinical conversation and are discussed in detail in the ASA Cycle section.[146]

Questions for Offering Services

Before launching into a conversation, ask a question to allow the patient to accept or decline such a discussion. For example:

- "Given that, would you like to talk about ways to be prepared for a healthy pregnancy?"[153]
- "In that case, would you like to discuss ways to prevent pregnancy?"

Questions for Eliciting Contraceptive Preferences

Ask your patients about their preferences. Patients can make informed choices consistent with their preferences when they know what methods align with what they are seeking. Ask them about characteristics that they do or do not want in their method.[132]

Here are two options for how to ask:

- "Do you have a sense of what is important to you about your method?"[154]
- "Can you tell me something that is important to you about your birth control?"

Including the phrase "Do you have a sense..." or "Can you tell me something..." allows for the likely possibility that no one has asked them that question before and they may need a moment to consider it.

Note that these questions are not:

- "What method are you interested in?" or "What method would you like to start today?" Framed this way, the question could make someone feel as though they are expected to have a formulated answer.
- "What is most important to you about your method?" In this example the person answering is expected to know what is "most" important to them before they have had an opportunity to consider the wide range of things they may be seeking in a contraceptive method. Once a patient has clarified two or more characteristics that are important to them, it may become necessary to ask which is more important if there is not a method that fulfills all the criteria.

When a patient is new to contraception, they may need additional prompting to understand the question. If you sense they are unsure of how to answer, give them 3 or 4 seconds to consider the question. This silence can feel uncomfortable at first, but it gives the patient the time, space, and permission to seriously consider the question. If the patient still doesn't reply or if they ask, "What do you mean?", offer a follow-up statement with examples. "For example, in addition to preventing pregnancy, some methods can help with acne, or some methods help with heavy periods. Are either of those things important to you?" This provides some ideas about potential noncontraceptive benefits. Other prompts could include information about how methods can affect someone's menstrual period or how the methods are used (every time they have sex, daily, monthly, "set it and forget it," etc.). When giving examples, individualize based on what you know about the patient.

For patients with access to all methods of contraception without cost, it is not necessary to address cost or cost effectiveness. But full access to all contraceptive methods is by no means guaranteed. As a result, it may be necessary to address the potential financial strain of contraceptive use when discussing characteristics that are important to the patient.[47]

Table 4-1 Characteristics of Contraceptives With Plain Language Suggestions

Characteristics	Plain Language	Note
Effectiveness	"how well it works to prevent pregnancy"	You will already have a sense of this from their reply to, "How important is it to you to prevent pregnancy?" (Refer to Chapter 5)
Sexual acceptability	"effect on your sexual life/sexuality"	(Refer to Chapter 6)
Effect on the menstrual cycle	"how this method might change your periods"	(Refer to Chapters 2 and 3)
Need for a confidential method ■ This could mean: • Needing to have a bleeding pattern that is unchanged • Avoiding methods that require "supplies"	"Some methods are easier to hide than others." "no change in when your period comes"	It is important to determine in what way they need the method concealed; is a parent or partner monitoring their menses? Is it challenging to store supplies (condoms, pills, etc.)?
Financial considerations for patient/Insurance Coverage		This is only a concern if the patient is un- or underinsured
Return to fecundity	"Once you stop using ___, your ability to get pregnancy goes back to whatever is normal for you, right away."	For all methods except DMPA
Control over discontinuation/ removal	"You can stop using it without a provider visit."	
A foreign object in the body	"This method is placed in your uterus/ arm/vagina."	Use visual and tactile aids. Address concerns by asking for more information. "I hear that a lot. Can you tell me more about what is concerning to you?"
Partner preference	"Is your partner part of this decision?"	

(*continues*)

Table 4-1 Characteristics of Contraceptives With Plain Language Suggestions *(continued)*

Characteristics	Plain Language	Note
Length of (potential) use	"This method is good for **up to** x amount of time."	When addressing potential length of use, add the words, "up to." Length of use does not generally need to be a factor in contraceptive decision making; any method can be used for any length of time; short-acting methods can be used for decades; implants and IUDs are good for "up to" 3–12 years but can be used for any length of time "up to" their expiration. If a patient wants to use a device beyond the effective length of use, they can have it replaced. See Chapters on specific methods
Bleeding profile	"Changes to how your period comes"	See Chapters on specific methods
Side effect	"Something you might notice (or have noticed) when you use this method"	
Noncontraceptive benefit	"Things your birth control can do for you in addition to preventing pregnancy"	
Hormones, whether or not and which ones	"These methods work by using hormones like the ones your body makes."	

Data from Gavin L, Moskosky S, Carter M, et al. Providing quality family planning services: Recommendations of CDC and the U.S. Office of Population Affairs. MMWR Recomm Rep 2014;63(Rr-04):1-54. (In eng).

Affirm-Share-Ask Cycle

ASA Cycles incorporate communication skills that help providers build rapport and trust, center patients in the conversation, provide relevant information in a way that is digestible, and assist patients to integrate information (see **Figure 4-2**).[155,156] This approach can be used repeatedly throughout visits—when sharing new information, responding to misconceptions, and making a recommendation, among many other examples.

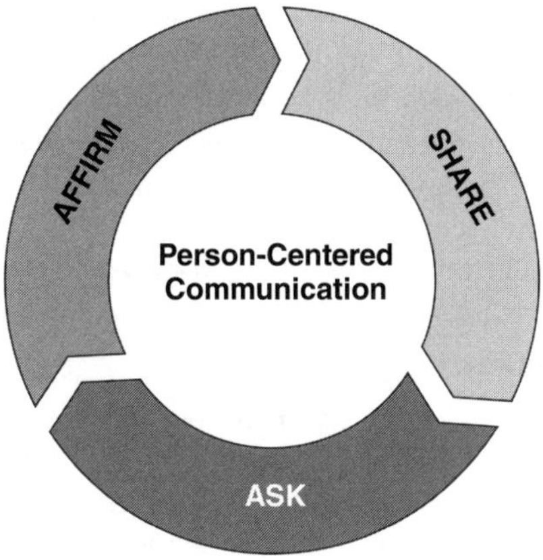

Figure 4-2 Affirm-Share-Ask Cycle

These cycles contain three components:

1. Affirm/acknowledge
2. Share content or information
3. Ask a follow up question

Affirm/Acknowledge

The first component of the ASA Cycle is *Affirm*. When a patient responds to a question, shares information, expresses a feeling, or asks a question, briefly affirm or acknowledge what the person has just said before launching into an explanation. This helps build rapport and trust by showing the patient we are listening and paying attention to them.[92,157] There are different ways to accomplish this—displaying empathy, pointing out a strengths-based positive, finding agreement, or validating. It is essential that your sentiment is authentic and based on your true response to what you have heard.

Empathy

Central to person-centered communication is expressing empathy[23,57,149,158-161]—verbally and nonverbally—by acknowledging and reflecting a patient's feelings. When someone expresses an emotion, acknowledge it.[57] This is respectful, kind, and only takes a few seconds. Communicate that their reaction is understandable and perhaps common to others in similar situations.

Avoid some of the common communications that can create barriers to effectively expressing empathy:

- Underplaying (or overstating) the intensity of the emotion
- Saying "I know how you feel"
- Incorrectly "labeling" someone's feelings

Each of us has our own definitions of what constitutes anger, frustration, anxiety, or sadness and each of us identifies the unique meaning of our own emotions.

To demonstrate empathy, it isn't necessary to label the emotion. This is particularly true with negative emotions like anger or anxiety. For example, it can potentially damage rapport to tell a patient, "I can see that you are angry" at a time when they would have described their feeling as "annoyed." It is only necessary to let them know you care about them and that you are sensitive to what they are expressing. Rather than saying, "you seem angry," or "I can see that this makes you anxious," you can be empathetic in a more general way (**Box 4-3**).

Positive Feedback

Another way to affirm is to notice and point out your patient's health-supporting behaviors or health-related knowledge (**Box 4-4**).[92] This demonstrates that you are paying attention to them as a unique individual and that you are on their side. Avoid giving generic "praise" that is not specific to the individual. People can tell when someone is giving an insincere compliment.

Note that this is not complimenting patients for complying with what a health care provider has told them to do; you are noticing when their behavior supports their health and well-being in a way that is aligned with their own values. By weaving positive feedback into the conversation, patients hear that you respect their perspective.

Examples of Positive Health Supporting Behaviors or Health-Related Knowledge

Notice and point out:

- Insightful questions
- Condom use

Box 4-3 Phrases to Demonstrate Empathy Without Labeling

"I can see that was really concerning to you."
"It seems like that was hard to deal with!"
"That situation must be very difficult to manage"
"I can't even imagine how that must have been for you."
"Wow..."

Box 4-4 Language to Point Out Positives

- "It takes a lot of strength to stand up for yourself like that."
- "It's great you picked up on that."
- "You've clearly thought about this a lot. What do you make of this situation?"
- "That is a great question."
- "It's clear you're interested in protecting yourself."
- "Wow, I wouldn't have thought about that. You're right."
- "I'm impressed that even with all of those challenges, you've been using a condom most of the time."
- "Nursing school? Wow, that's great! We certainly need more people joining our field; welcome!"

- Adherence to a birth control method
- Exercise
- Nutrition improvement
- Smoking cessation
- Ways in which someone is knowledgeable about health-related topics
- If the person is in the field (an RN, MA, dental assistant…)
- If someone is studying biology or science

Validation

Validation is a tool to use when you want to acknowledge a patient's thoughts or opinions.[162,163] This technique is particularly helpful when other forms of acknowledgement would be disingenuous. Example language includes:

- "I hear that all the time."
- "I can understand why you would think that."

Finding Agreement

Finding agreement[164] is a useful tool to address misconceptions. Support self-efficacy by finding agreement or validating when appropriate and then provide clarifying information. Patients often have negative associations with contraception, such as unpleasant side effects and alarming complications. Less frequently, they are aware of noncontraceptive benefits associated with use of contraception. Asking directed questions about a patient's knowledge and beliefs allows an opportunity to share accurate information and to frame the messaging positively when appropriate.

It is not necessary or helpful to disagree with your patient or tell them they are wrong. Finding agreement is one way to affirm, but it requires that you can identify some, perhaps small, kernel of truth in what the patient has said. It is not appropriate to use in situations when you cannot find any point of agreement.

When you find yourself wanting to correct a patient's misinformation, or saying "that's wrong/incorrect," "no," or "but," consider instead the following strategy:

1. Find some kernel of truth in their statement (In other words, a point of agreement!)
2. Say AND. . .
3. Then build on it by adding the information you would like them to know.

Patients frequently go online or to social media to address concerns and answer questions. Your patient may have encountered misinformation about contraception in this way. Rather than immediately correcting the misinformation, you can acknowledge that they were seeking information proactively (i.e., point out the positive) and then share a trusted website like bedsider.org. See **Table 4-2** for examples of ASA cycles.

One particularly perplexing situation is when a patient says that something bad happened to a friend or relative (or even to themselves) that is not scientifically likely or plausible. A strategy that has been shown to resonate with patients is to emphasize that "everyone is different."[165] This readjusts their frame of thinking to allow for the possibility that the "bad outcome" could be a chance occurrence.

Table 4-2 Examples of Affirm within the ASA Cycle

	Affirm	Share	Ask
Addressing side effects "I've been having super heavy periods since I had the copper IUD put in and it's hard to deal with."	"Wow, what a drag. (Empathy) Anyone would find that hard to deal with." (Validation)	"The medications a lot of people use for headaches can lessen the amount of bleeding by half." (See Chapter 10 for information on managing bleeding with IUDs)	"Would you like to hear more about that?" Or "Have you used naproxen sodium or ibuprofen before?"
Responding to misinformation: "I don't want to go on birth control because I really want to have kids someday and I read online that birth control can mess with that."	"I hear that from my patients a lot! (Validation) Going online to find information can be really helpful in a lot of cases. (Positive Feedback) You're right that with one of the methods, the shot, it can take a while for someone's ability to get pregnant to go back to whatever is normal for them." (Agreement)	"With all of the other methods your ability to get pregnant will go back to whatever is normal for you immediately after you stop using it."	"What thoughts do you have about any of those other methods?"

Other potential language to use is "I'm sorry your friend went through that! I haven't heard of that before, and I can tell you it definitely doesn't happen often."[154]

Share Content or Information

The second component of the ASA Cycle is *Share*. Providers share information, reflections, summaries, and recommendations as an integral part of clinical care. (See **Table 4-3**.) How we share directly influences how patients absorb and retain new knowledge.[146,147,170,171]

Person-Centered Patient Education

To make informed choices, patients need to integrate new information into their knowledge base. Learning theory[148,172] tells us that integration requires several steps (**Figure 4-3**). Patients need to:

1. *Hear* the information; listening is hindered if the person is anxious.
2. *Understand* the information, which requires it to have been provided in a language they speak, using terms they know.

3. *Remember* the information, which is more likely if the information is relevant to them.
4. *Process* the information so they can recall it when needed.
5. *Integrate* the new information to make it part the ongoing knowledge base they use when making decisions.

Table 4-3 Examples of Share within the ASA Cycle

	Affirm	Share	Ask
Addressing menstrual concerns: "My mom said it's not healthy not to get my period." (*Note*: at this point you may feel like correcting the patient)	"Your mother is completely right. When you are not using contraception that has hormones in it, it is important to get your period" (Agreement) Or: "Your mother is right. (Agreement) I'm glad you know that it's important to come in if you're not getting your period." (Positive Feedback)	"Interestingly, when someone is using a method that has hormones in it, the hormone keeps the lining of the uterus very thin, and so you don't need to get a regular period to keep the uterus healthy." (Show a diagram of a uterus). The provider could add the following message: Contraceptive hormones actually prevent cancer of the uterus.	"Knowing that, how would it be for you to not get periods?" Or: "Knowing that, how would it be for you not to get your period while using this method?"
Providing information on contraceptive pill use: "What do I do if I miss a pill?"	"I'm so glad you asked that question." (Positive Feedback) Or: "Lots of people ask that that question because many people find it difficult to remember to take a pill every single day." (Validation)	"If you miss one pill, you can take it as soon as you remember. If you don't notice until the next day, you can take two pills together."	"Do you have any medicines or vitamins that you take every day? How is it for you to remember to take them?"

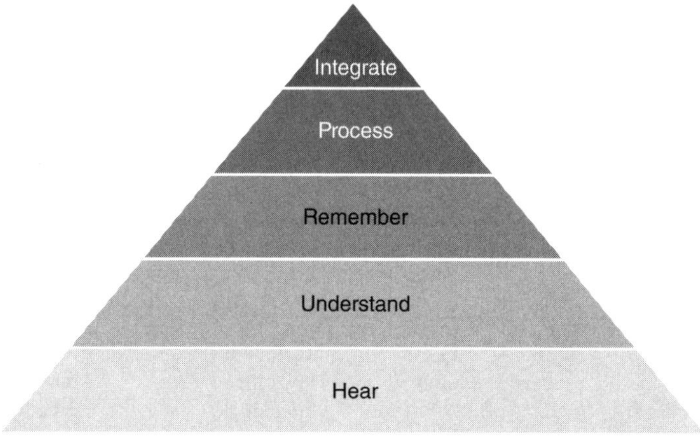

Figure 4-3 Building Blocks of Learning

Box 4-5 Nonverbal Communication[166-169]

People respond to one another's nonverbal communications. Nonverbal communications and suggestions include:

- Sit down to position yourself at or below the patient's level.
- Eye contact:
  - Avoid looking away (toward the electronic medical record, for example) and look in the patient's direction.
  - Return the patient's gaze and look at them when they are speaking. *Note:* Depending on cultural norms, eye contact may be uncomfortable, so it is best to take your cue from the patient's eye contact.
- Lean forward to indicate interest in what the patient is saying.
- Smile in response to positives.
- Use gestures and nods of agreement.
- Use vocal utterances of interest to encourage the patient to continue; mm hmm, huh, ahh, yeah.
- Maintain respectful interpersonal distance; do not invade the patient's personal space during conversations.
- Maintain an open body posture; do not cross your arms.
- Use an expressive tone of voice.
- Convey empathy via facial expressions.
- Moderate your level of speech so that it is audible but not too loud.

Data from Griffith CH, 3rd, Wilson JF, Langer S, Haist SA. House staff nonverbal communication skills and standardized patient satisfaction. J Gen Intern Med 2003;18(3):170-4. DOI: 10.1046/j.1525-1497.2003.10506.x; Versluijs Y, Moore MG, Ring D, Jayakumar P. Clinician facial expression of emotion corresponds with patient mindset. Clin Orthop Relat Res 2021;479(9):1914-1923. DOI: 10.1097/CORR.0000000000001727;Montague E, Xu J, Chen PY, Asan O, Barrett BP, Chewning B. Modeling eye gaze patterns in clinician-patient interaction with lag sequential analysis. Hum Factors 2011;53(5):502-16. DOI: 10.1177/0018720811405986;Riess H, Kraft-Todd G. E.M.P.A.T.H.Y.: a tool to enhance nonverbal communication between clinicians and their patients. Acad Med 2014;89(8):1108-12. DOI: 10.1097/ACM.0000000000000287

Facilitate integration of new knowledge by having the "learner" (patient) interact with the information. When patients are presented with too much information at once, they may forget content or remember it incorrectly. People can integrate large amounts of information in one visit if you break it into digestible pieces. Ask pertinent follow-up questions before sharing more information. This follow-up question or "teach back" is the third component of the ASA Cycle.

The following can help providers share relevant content in a person-centered way:

- **Prioritize essential points.** Avoid giving a pathophysiology lecture. Ask yourself: what is the one thing they really need to know?
- **Highlight important facts** by presenting them first.
- **Individualize the information.** Focus on the needs and knowledge gaps identified during the conversation.[132]
- **Break up the content.** Rather than presenting everything all at once, thread relevant bits throughout the conversation.[132]
- **Follow each bit of information with a question.** The process of thinking about and answering a question requires someone to integrate information.

Visual Aids and Tactile Aids

Many patients are visual learners or tactile learners.[92,142,146,147,173] To facilitate learning, provide visual and tactile aids so that the patient can see, as well as hear, the information and interact with devices or models by touching them. Some examples of these aids include:

- Anatomical drawings, pictures, or three-dimensional models
- Samples of contraceptive methods to hand to patients. This is particularly important for methods that are placed inside someone's body.
- Videos to demonstrate method use, testimonials, basic physiology, etc.
- Handouts to take home

Language Considerations for Patient Education

Health literacy considerations are paramount.[82,170] Table 4-1 gives suggestions for plain language. As health care providers, we are comfortable with use of percentages, relative risk, and absolute risk. Some patients have less understanding of these concepts and may not be able to use the "data" to help inform their decisions if they do not have appropriate context or background. Many patients will better understand relative and absolute risk when framed using natural frequencies (3 people out of 1,000) rather than using percentages (0.3%).[147] When describing relative risk; comparing characteristics such as effectiveness or risk of a particular outcome, use common denominators:

- "If 100 people have unprotected sex for a year, 85 of them will get pregnant, as compared with maybe 1, or none, using an implant."
- "If a person switches from the pill to an IUD, the chance of pregnancy decreases from 7 in 100 to less than 1 in 100."

"Quick Start" Is Person-Centered

Chapters on particular methods in this book recommend "Quick Start."[174-176] This person-centered approach encourages providers to offer timely access to patients' chosen method of contraception, advising them that they can start on the contraceptive method on the day they request it. If it is reasonably certain that a patient is not pregnant (See Box 25-2 "How to be reasonably certain that a person is not pregnant" for further information), offer a Quick Start of the chosen method that day and provide appropriate education on how to initiate that method.

Reflective Listening (Rephrasing)

Reflective listening[21,149,160,177,178] is a person-centered way to respond to patients. It keeps control of the time and focus of the visit by summarizing what has been said and moving the conversation forward. This helpful counseling skill requires some practice, so try it with friends or family before using it with patients. Reflective listening:

- Builds rapport
- Demonstrates that you are listening and that you have heard what is important to them
- Gives patients the opportunity to hear their own priorities, preferences, and desires spoken out loud
- Helps patients clarify what matters to them
- Gives patients the opportunity to correct, clarify, or confirm your reflective listening
- Allows you to be efficient and control the length and focus of the conversation
- Allows you to summarize as the patient moves toward decision making

How to Reflectively Listen (Rephrase). Pay close attention to what a patient says. In addition to listening to the words, pay attention to tone of voice (happy, fearful, negative, concerned), body language (leaning forward, open stance, or arms crossed indicating they are closed off), and facial expression. For example, does the person seem to be excited about the idea of being a parent someday (or having another child), or do they seem put off by the idea?

Reflective listening is ***not*** repeating verbatim what was said. Rephrase what the person has said using different words to capture the essence of what was meant. If you are not clear on a point, use reflective listening to clarify. You can gather pieces of information your patient has mentioned throughout the conversation when you use reflective listening to summarize.

Reflective listening steps:

1. **Begin with:**
   Begin with an introduction like the following: "So I'm hearing you say…", or "It sounds like…", or "Am I right that you…"
2. **Then rephrase:**
   Share your reflection.
3. **Check for accuracy:**
   "Did I get that right?", or "Is that what you mean?", or "Is that correct?", or sometimes just a pause will serve the same effect.

If the patient responds by indicating that you didn't get it right, this is an opportunity to demonstrate humility and show that your priority is understanding the patient more than being right.[177,179] By correcting you, they are actively continuing to clarify their thoughts, feelings, and desires.

The "on the one hand" approach, a specific type of reflective listening, is helpful when the patient's behavior is incongruent or inconsistent with their stated goals. The clinician can help the patient explore what the barrier or obstacle is by mentioning the goal "on one hand" and either the obstacle or the inconsistent behavior "on the other hand." It helps the person gain clarity about what the obstacles are, so that they can make choices consistent with what is most important to them.

Examples:

- "On one hand you've shared a bunch of reasons why you really want to wait until you finish school, and on the other hand, part of you would like to have a baby right now. . . Do I have that right?"
- "It sounds like on the one hand, you would really like to avoid another pregnancy, and on the other hand it's really hard to get into the office for your depo shot every 3 months."
- "So, I hear you saying on one hand that it's important to you to wait until you are ready . . . and it's great hearing about all of your plans; and on the other hand, you had unprotected sex last night?"
- "I'm hearing that on the one hand, you are understandably upset about getting chlamydia again, and on the other hand asking your husband to use condoms feels really uncomfortable for you. Do I have that right?"

Throughout the visit, it helps to intermittently clarify, repeat, or summarize statements and decisions that a patient has made.

Ask A Follow Up Question

The third component of the ASA Cycle is *Ask*.[138,139] Ask a follow up question regarding the content just provided to the patient during the Share portion of the cycle. This assists the patient with integrating new information (See **Table 4-4**.).

Examples of follow-up questions to integrate information:

- "How would it be for you?"
- "Knowing that, what do you think?"
- "Has that ever happened to you before?"
- "How did you manage it?"
- "How would you manage that?"
- "What questions do you have for me about (fill in with the content you just shared)?"
- "Have you experienced anything like that before?"
- "Given that, how would it be for you if …?"

When you want to encourage the patient to ask for information, it is far preferable to ask, "What questions do you have about ____?" rather than, "Do you have any questions?"[142,146]

Teach Back

When you want to check to be sure patients have successfully integrated new information, an excellent strategy is to ask them to repeat back what they heard you say.[21,142,146,147,152] This type of "Ask" is called "teach back." Some providers are concerned

Table 4-4 Examples of Ask within the ASA Cycle

	Affirm	Share	Ask
Reviewing medication use	"I'm sorry you've had to deal with ongoing headaches. (Empathy) And yes, that same medicine (naproxen sodium) that helps with headaches can also help with the heavy periods you've been having with the copper IUD." (Agreement)	"If you want to use that same medicine to help with your heavy periods, you'll take 2 pills in the morning and 2 pills in the evening with food. Start right when you know your period is about to begin."	"I want to be sure I haven't left anything out that I needed to tell you. Can you tell me how you're going to use naproxen sodium?"
Responding to removal requests (Start with this) "I want to take out my IUD/ implant today."	"I understand that you would like your IUD/implant removed." (Agreement)	"I will absolutely do that today" Or "I will absolutely get you scheduled with a provider to remove your IUD."	"Can I ask, what makes you want to remove your IUD/ implant?"
Responding to removal requests due to side effects "I'm really frustrated that I've been on my period nonstop for the last 6 weeks." Part 2 is not relevant, however, if someone wants an IUD/implant removed because they are seeking pregnancy.	"Six weeks, wow. No wonder you feel frustrated." (Empathy)	"I don't know if anyone has talked to you about this before, but there are medications that can help with that." (See Chapter 9, Contraceptive Implant)	"Would you like to hear more about those options before we start getting ready to take this out today?" *Note*: If a patient declines these conversations, accept that they are clear about removal and move on to the removal procedure.

that this can seem awkward or condescending. When implementing "teach back," take full responsibility for the communication. Rather than starting with, "Can you please repeat back to me what we just discussed" try one of the following statements:

- "I would like to be sure that I was as clear as I could be, so can you tell me what someone should do if they forgot to remove the vaginal ring?"
- "We have gone over quite a lot of information and I want to be sure I didn't forget to tell you something important…"
- "I don't always explain things as clearly as I think I have…"

Specific Clinical Circumstances

Barriers to Removal of Implants and IUDs

For the most part, people using implants and IUDs cannot remove the devices themselves, though there is growing literature on the feasibility of IUD self-removal.[180-183] When a patient considers using an implant or IUD, one of the elements they think about is whether they are comfortable deferring control over their reproduction until the device is removed.[11,184] They are also deciding whether or not they can trust the provider's procedural competence, whether there will be a provider willing and able to remove the device on demand, and whether they will have coverage for the cost of the removal.

In many practice settings and communities, patients experience difficulties getting their contraceptive device removed without unnecessary barriers. Providers often express reluctance to remove a device in a timeframe they consider "early."[185] If you are aware of such barriers, discuss those challenges with the patient at the time when they are considering the method or before it is placed and provide potential solutions to address these issues should they arise. Since providers often do not know where someone will be accessing future care, it is reasonable to discuss this issue preemptively with many patients. Sample language to suggest to a patient for use if needed:

- "It is very important to me to have this IUD/implant removed today." (If they are encountering resistance to removal request)
- "Please note in my file that I, the patient, asked for IUD/implant removal and you, the clinician, have refused to remove my IUD/implant." (If a patient has been refused IUD/implant removal)
    - This language is provided by Cherise Scott, CEO & Founder of SisterReach, who notes: "That way the doctor [clinician] is on record refusing to honor the self-determination of the patient, and especially because there is no medical reason an IUD must stay inserted for any reason."[186]

Patients presenting for an IUD or implant removal often have concerns or side effects motivating their desire for removal. Sometimes these can be addressed through education or medical treatment. See **Table 4-5** for examples of language to offer information in a way that does not create barriers to removal.

Obesity and Weight Concerns

Though not always pertinent to conversations about contraception, there are interactions between some contraceptives and weight.[32] People in larger bodies need relevant information about the interaction between weight and contraceptive methods

Table 4-5 Person-Centered Language for Discussing an IUD or Implant

Suggestions for Language	Rationale
Use the words "to place," "placing," or "placement" when referring to an IUD or implant procedure	Using the words "to insert," "inserting," or "insertion" may feel invasive.
Avoid grouping IUDs and implants using the term LARC (long-acting reversible contraception)	Patients generally do not know what the term LARC means. Grouping implants, hormonal IUDs, and copper IUDs together does not help patients learn about the individual methods. While each of these methods is highly effective, each has other characteristics that differentiate them more than group them. These characteristics include hormonal vs. nonhormonal, a range of menstrual effects, and placement in the uterus or subdermally.
Avoid referring to implants and IUDs as the "long-acting" methods	It prioritizes potential length of use as the dominant feature. This may convey an expectation that patients are expected to use the method for the full length of time. It discourages individuals who want to use them for a shorter duration (such as pregnancy spacing). The fact that a device is good for "up to" 3 to 20 years may be an added advantage for some patients but is not necessarily relevant. If the patient identifies length of use as a high priority, then it is appropriate to refer to these methods as "long-acting."
"This [IUD or implant] is good for up to X years (fill in information for the particular method), but if you want to get pregnant before then or you would like it removed for any reason, come in, we will take it out, and your ability to get pregnant will go back to whatever is normal for you."	This phrase: ■ Emphasizes "up to" so that patients know they don't have to use the method for any particular length of time ■ Tells the patient that the method will remain effective for up to a certain amount of time ■ Stresses that the patient has control over removal ■ Points out rapid return to fecundity but does not promise pregnancy; "Goes back to whatever is normal for you" rather than "you can get pregnant right away" ■ Avoids overly medicalized language; "Ability to get pregnant" rather than "return to fecundity (or fertility)"

they are considering. It is not necessary or helpful, however, to proactively tell patients with larger bodies about potential weight interactions with every method until you know their contraceptive preferences. Their preferred methods may not have an interaction with weight. For example, if the patient expresses that effectiveness is a priority to them and they prefer to use contraception that doesn't change the timing of their menstrual period, a nonhormonal IUD may be a good fit. In this case, telling them about the potential for weight gain with DMPA or for decreased effectiveness with a patch is not relevant.

In addition, patients' concerns about potential weight change with contraceptives is common among patients of any weight. Methods associated with weight change or whose efficacy may be affected by physiologic interactions with weight are discussed in the relevant chapter: DMPA in Chapter 11; contraceptive patch in Chapter 12; and emergency contraception in Chapter 18.

Patients with Serious Medical Conditions, Including Substance Abuse Disorders and Mental Illness

People with medical conditions are as likely as the general population to have mistimed or undesired pregnancies.[140,141,187-190] Patients with some medical conditions have an increased risk of an adverse health outcome from pregnancy or associated with use of particular contraceptives. For others, the medical condition itself or the treatment for the condition (such as teratogenic medications) may potentially harm a pregnancy. Outcomes are often better when pregnancy occurs during a period of stability, when a disease is in remission or well controlled.

Patients with complex medical conditions, however, are less likely to be asked about their reproductive desires, especially in the context of specialty care.[191,192] Given that these patients have unique risks for adverse outcomes were they to become pregnant, providers should engage in these conversations more often, not less.[193,194] Conversations about reproductive desires, preparing for a healthy pregnancy, and contraception are complex. (See Chapter 20, Contraception for People with Medical Conditions and Chapter 21, Contraception in the Later Reproductive Years.)

Providers may implicitly or explicitly tell patients "Don't get pregnant," emphasizing the medical risks without exploring reproductive desires, even though many of these patients can have healthy pregnancies. Disease-specific prepregnancy care optimizes outcomes of a potential pregnancy by managing the disease and switching to nonteratogenic medications prior to pregnancy when possible. Without a provider's proactive offer to discuss reproductive desires, however, patients may be reluctant to share their authentic thoughts and feelings about getting pregnant. This has significant consequences. First, if a patient does not share with the provider that they are open to or seeking pregnancy, they would not have the benefit of provider input prior to pregnancy. This sets them up to assume unnecessary risk to achieve their reproductive desires. Conversely, patients may indefinitely defer desired pregnancy because they have not been offered available, nonteratogenic treatment alternatives.

Even providers who are comfortable with shared decision making during interactions about preference-sensitive decisions (decisions for which there is clinical equipoise, i.e., there is not one option that is clinically superior to another) may feel like they should change to a directive counseling approach with a patient who has a medical condition for which there is a clearly superior management choice. A patient's autonomy, however, does not become less important when they become ill or when they have medical conditions that require attention or treatment. In fact, a core goal of the recommendations in this chapter is for patients to have the relevant information they need to make informed choices.

For these reasons, patients with significant medical issues stand to benefit even more from these conversations than would their peers for whom the medical consequences of decisions are less profound. It can be tempting to make assumptions about a patient's feelings and beliefs about the interaction between their medical condition and their reproductive health. Even if you know the important facts about the disease, each patient's reaction to the medical condition is unique. To make informed choices about pregnancy, parenting, their health, and contraceptive use, patients must have specific, accurate, information relevant to their medical condition in the context of their lives, preferences, and values. The ASA Cycle is designed to maximize the likelihood that they will receive, understand, and utilize the needed information.

People with substance use disorder (SUD) and those with mental illness frequently experience discrimination and stigma when interacting with the health care system and health care providers. The consequence of this is a lack of trust that can make honest discussions about reproductive desires, contraception, and prepregnancy care challenging.[195] Providers can work to alleviate this distrust by examining their implicit bias and employing the approaches recommended in this chapter.

We, as providers, often have thoughts about what may be the "better choice" for patients with conditions that confer increased risk with pregnancy. Our professional identity calls us to do what we can to prevent bad outcomes and maximize health. After all, most health care providers went into this work in order help their patients to do just that. The question, then, becomes how to respect the patient's autonomy while not betraying one's professional responsibility. A unique thing a trusted provider can contribute is their individualized medical recommendation. For example, a clear provider recommendation regarding immunization has been shown to be a highly effective way to increase uptake. Make your recommendation during the "Share" portion of the ASA cycle. Some examples:

- "I can see you're excited about having another baby! Someone with diabetes can have a healthy pregnancy, and the best way for you to have a healthy baby is to keep your sugars at **70 to 100 before meals, and less than 120 two hours after eating** [or **A1C less than 6.5** if that is how the patient understands their diabetes] **before you get pregnant**. Knowing that, when are you aiming to get pregnant?"
- "It's wonderful how much this medication has helped your symptoms of _____. I want you to know that if you would like to become pregnant, there is another medicine that I recommend we change you to that would be safe for the baby. **It would be harmful (unsafe) for the baby if you become pregnant on** _____. Do you think you might like to have children at some point?"
- "I'm glad you felt comfortable enough to share with me today that you've been using opiates again recently. I know we talked before about your desire to have another child soon. **I want you to know that stopping opiates or transitioning to medication-assisted treatment like buprenorphine or methadone can help you have the healthiest pregnancy possible.** What are your thoughts on either of those options?"

Pregnancy Options Counseling

In the sections above, we make recommendations for person-centered discussions with individuals about their future reproductive desires—providing the time and

Box 4-6 Recommendations for Counseling Patients With Medical Conditions

- State your medical recommendation in a clear straightforward manner using plain language. Re-state your recommendation as needed with alternative language to help the patient integrate the information.
- Use the skills outlined in this chapter, including "on the one hand" (a form of reflective listening).
- Ask about their feelings, knowledge, and beliefs regarding the interaction between their medical condition and their reproductive health. Demonstrate empathy once they respond.
- Focus on disease-specific patient education about contraception.
- Use follow-up questions frequently.
- Use visual aids and "teach back" about the disease state as well as contraception (as described on pages 103 and 105-106).
- Use nonjudgmental language about the disease state, in particular SUD and mental illness.

space for the patient to consider how, theoretically, parenting may fit into their life. For individuals with a negative pregnancy test, a pregnancy test visit can naturally transition to a conversation about reproductive desires. When someone has a positive pregnancy test, however, this discussion is no longer theoretical. In these situations, questions about future reproductive desires and contraceptive preferences are not relevant.[196-198] Providers will still apply ASA Cycles (that include all the counseling and communication skills described in this chapter) to center the patient during pregnancy options counseling. Chapter 25 describes pregnancy testing and options, and here we address counseling considerations unique to conversations with those who have a positive pregnancy test.

To be effective in providing pregnancy options counseling, it is essential to clarify your own potential bias around abortion, adoption, and whether a person should or should not parent at this time.

When disclosing positive pregnancy test results, use language that avoids confusion:

> "I have the results of your pregnancy test. The test came back positive; that means you are pregnant."[198]

The statement is factual and does not make any assumptions about a person's emotional orientation to the pregnant test results. It also clarifies that "positive" means pregnant, something that not all patients may know.

If a patient does not indicate their next steps on their own, a helpful question for providers to use is:

> "What thoughts do you have about what you might do?"[198]

Like the PATH questions, this question is open-ended and unbiased toward any one option. It allows for the patient to explore their own thoughts. Many providers ask the question, "What do you think you want to do?" While this question can be delivered in a compassionate way, using the word "want" does not always resonate as a person may not want to do any of the options or someone may feel they need to do something they do not want to do.

Additional counseling recommendations when giving positive pregnancy test results and counseling about pregnancy options include:

- Use ASA Cycles
- Respond without judgment
- Demonstrate empathy
- Query about their thoughts/preference without requiring a concrete plan
- Normalize indecision and fluctuating emotions
- Respect when the patient tells you they have made a choice
- Give information consistent with their choice
- Give information without bias
- Sensitively offer to discuss all options when appropriate
- Watch for reproductive coercion/intimate partner violence
- Assess for support systems
- Have tissues within patient's reach

When giving positive pregnancy test results and counseling about pregnancy options, **avoid**:

- Making assumptions about how someone will respond emotionally to the positive pregnancy test result
- Proactively asking about:
    - "What happened"
    - Past adherence to contraception
    - What a patient may have "done wrong" with use of contraception
- Asking about future reproductive desires
- Proactively discussing future contraception (see exceptions below)
- Discussing options or providing referrals that are counter to what the patient has clearly stated as their preference, i.e.:
    - Stressing that continuing the pregnancy is an option when someone has clearly stated they will seek an abortion
    - Reminding someone that abortion is an option when they have expressed a clear desire to continue the pregnancy

Some topics may or may not be relevant to discuss during these visits. For example, when a patient gets pregnant while using a contraceptive method, it may be tempting to the provider to try to figure out what went wrong. That inquiry is usually not germane. If the patient has questions about the method failure, focus on overall typical-use pregnancy rates, not on individual behaviors (refer to Chapter 5 on efficacy to learn more about pregnancy rates on various contraceptive methods). Methods fail, not people. It is also generally unnecessary to proactively bring up future contraception use unless there is a need to plan ahead—for example, if the patient wants to start an oral contraceptive pill (OCP) after a medication abortion or have an IUD or implant placed immediately post-abortion. (See Chapter 9, Contraceptive Implant and Chapter 10, Intrauterine Devices [IUDs].)

A patient may have had sex with more than one person in the timeframe during which they think they got pregnant. In these cases, it may be important to the patient to figure out precisely when they got pregnant, as it may affect their decision making about the current pregnancy. Providers can use their clinical knowledge to help determine likely dates of conception. This is a useful time to implement ASA Cycles to operationalize respectful, nonjudgmental care.

For patients who are unsure of their decision or plan to seek abortion, review local access to abortion services as well as relevant gestational age limits. Unless a patient has stated a clear choice to continue the pregnancy, it is critical to assess gestational age so patients know whether or not abortion is a viable option. Sometimes 24 hours is the difference between a patient being able to terminate or having to continue an unacceptable pregnancy (see Chapter 26, Abortion).

Summary

A person-centered framework aligned with Reproductive Justice principles values patients' lived experiences and trusts them to make the best reproductive choices for themselves. Applying such an approach works to actively counter (re-)traumatization of patients seeking reproductive and sexual health services. Thoughts, feelings, desires, and actions around parenting and pregnancy are complex, variable, and nuanced. To operationalize person-centered care, this chapter recommends key questions about reproductive desires and contraceptive preferences. It also asks providers to actively listen to the patient's responses to those questions. Affirm-Share-Ask Cycles help providers center the patient, optimize communication, and maximize the potential for the patient to retain and apply new knowledge to make informed choices.

Author Disclosures—Cason: Creator of and trainer for the PATH Questions, PATH Framework, and ASA Cycle; Consultant and trainer for Sebela; Nexplanon trainer for Organon; Pritzker: Trainer for the PATH Framework; Co-creator of ASA Cycle; Nexplanon trainer for Organon; Speaker bureau for Merck unbranded talk on counseling

Additional resources: https://www.envisionsrh.com/; https://www.path-framework.com/

References

1. Ross L, Solinger R. Reproductive justice: An introduction. Oakland, CA: University of California Press, 2017.
2. Ross L. Radical reproductive justice: foundations, theory, practice, critique. New York City: The Feminist Press at The City University of New York, 2017.
3. SisterSong. Reproductive justice. (https://www.sistersong.net/reproductive-justice).
4. Downey MM, Gómez AM. Structural competency and reproductive health. AMA J Ethics. 2018;20(3):211-23. DOI: 10.1001/journalofethics.2018.20.3.peer1-1803.
5. Foster KE, Johnson CN, Carvajal DN, et al. Dear white people. Ann Fam Med. 2021;19(1):66-9. DOI: 10.1370/afm.2634.
6. Foster DG. The turnaway study: ten years, a thousand women, and the consequences of having—or being denied—an abortion. New York: Scribner, 2020.
7. Thompson TM, Young YY, Bass TM, et al. Racism runs through it: Examining the sexual and reproductive health experience of Black women in the south. Health Aff. 2022;41(2):195-202. DOI: 10.1377/hlthaff.2021.01422.
8. Dehlendorf C, Akers AY, Borrero S, et al. Evolving the preconception health framework: A call for reproductive and sexual health equity. Obstet Gynecol. 2021;137(2):234-9. DOI: 10.1097/aog.0000000000004255.
9. Gomez AM, Wapman M. Under (implicit) pressure: young Black and Latina women's perceptions of contraceptive care. Contraception. 2017;96(4):221-6. DOI: 10.1016/j.contraception.2017.07.007.
10. Owens DC. Medical bondage: Race, gender, and the origins of American gynecology. Athens, GA: University of Georgia Press, 2017.
11. Amico JR, Bennett AH, Karasz A, Gold M. "She just told me to leave it": Women's experiences discussing early elective IUD removal. Contraception. 2016;94(4):357-61. DOI: 10.1016/j.contraception.2016.04.012.

12. Pearlson G, Gomez AM, Dehlendorf C, Prata N, Kerns J. A randomized trial of the effects of patient race, socioeconomic status, and parity on provider response to request for iud removal after six months of use. Contraception. 2020;102(4):292. DOI: https://doi.org/10.1016/j.contraception.2020.07.067.
13. Bryson A, Koyama A, Hassan A. Addressing long-acting reversible contraception access, bias, and coercion: supporting adolescent and young adult reproductive autonomy. Curr Opin Pediatr. 2021;33(4):345-353. DOI: 10.1097/mop.0000000000001008.
14. Holt K, Reed R, Crear-Perry J, Scott C, Wulf S, Dehlendorf C. Beyond same-day long-acting reversible contraceptive access: a person-centered framework for advancing high-quality, equitable contraceptive care. Am J Obstet Gynecol. 2020;222(4, Supplement):S878.e1-6. DOI: https://doi.org/10.1016/j.ajog.2019.11.1279.
15. Brandi K, Fuentes L. The history of tiered-effectiveness contraceptive counseling and the importance of patient-centered family planning care. Am J Obstet Gynecol. 2020;222(4s):S873-7. DOI: 10.1016/j.ajog.2019.11.1271.
16. Mann ES, Chen AM, Johnson CL. Doctor knows best? Provider bias in the context of contraceptive counseling in the United States. Contraception. 2021 DOI: 10.1016/j.contraception.2021.11.009.
17. Dehlendorf C, Henderson JT, Vittinghoff E, et al. Association of the quality of interpersonal care during family planning counseling with contraceptive use. Am J Obstet Gynecol. 2016;215(1):78.e1-9. DOI: 10.1016/j.ajog.2016.01.173.
18. Insitute of Medicine. Crossing the quality chasm: A new health system for the 21st century. Washington, DC: The National Academies Press, 2001.
19. Dehlendorf C, Fox E, Silverstein IA, et al. Development of the Person-Centered Contraceptive Counseling scale (PCCC), a short form of the Interpersonal Quality of Family Planning care scale. Contraception. 2021;103(5):310-5. DOI: 10.1016/j.contraception.2021.01.008.
20. University of California San Francisco. Person-Centered Contraceptive Counseling Measure. (https://pcccmeasure.ucsf.edu).
21. Links MJ, Watterson L, Martin P, O'Regan S, Molloy E. Finding common ground: meta-synthesis of communication frameworks found in patient communication, supervision and simulation literature. BMC Med. Educ. 2020;20(1):45. DOI: 10.1186/s12909-019-1922-2.
22. Logan RG, Daley EM, Vamos CA, Louis-Jacques A, Marhefka SL. "When is health care actually going to be care?" The lived experience of family planning care among young Black women. Qual Health Res 2021;31(6):1169-82. DOI: 10.1177/1049732321993094
23. Pinto RZ, Ferreira ML, Oliveira VC, et al. Patient-centred communication is associated with positive therapeutic alliance: a systematic review. J Physiother. 2012;58(2):77-87. DOI: 10.1016/S1836-9553(12)70087-5.
24. Tancman S, HaCohen N, Lazarus G, Solt I, Sagi-Dain L. Silent voices that must be heard - women's perceptions of gynecologic examinations. J Psychosom Obstet Gynaecol. 2021:1-8. DOI: 10.1080/0167482X.2020.1864727.
25. Raja S, Hasnain M, Hoersch M, Gove-Yin S, Rajagopalan C. Trauma informed care in medicine: current knowledge and future research directions. Fam Community Health. 2015;38(3):216-26. DOI: 10.1097/FCH.0000000000000071.
26. Gomez AM, Arteaga S, Aronson N, Goodkind M, Houston L, West E. No perfect method: Exploring how past contraceptive methods influence current attitudes toward intrauterine devices. Arch Sex Behav. 2020;49(4):1367-78. DOI: 10.1007/s10508-019-1424-7.
27. Gagliardi AR, Kim C, Jameel B. Physician behaviours that optimize patient-centred care: Focus groups with migrant women. Health Expect. 2020;23(5):1280-8. DOI: 10.1111/hex.13110.
28. Carvajal DN, Zambrana RE. Challenging stereotypes: A counter-narrative of the contraceptive experiences of low-income Latinas. Health Equity. 2020;4(1):10-6. DOI: 10.1089/heq.2019.0107.
29. Gomez AM, Hooker N, Olip-Booth R, Woerner P, Ratliff GA. "It's being compassionate, not making assumptions": Transmasculine and nonbinary young adults' experiences of "women's" health care settings. Womens Health Issues. 2021;31(4):324-31. DOI: 10.1016/j.whi.2021.02.008.
30. Gomez AM, Đỗ L, Ratliff GA, Crego PI, Hastings J. Contraceptive beliefs, needs, and care experiences among transgender and nonbinary young adults. J Adolescent Health. 2020;67(4):597-602. DOI: https://doi.org/10.1016/j.jadohealth.2020.03.003.

31. Chalmiers MA, Karaki F, Muriki M, Mody SK, Chen A, Thiel de Bocanegra H. Refugee women's experiences with contraceptive care after resettlement in high-income countries: A critical interpretive synthesis. Contraception. 2021;108:7-18. DOI: 10.1016/j.contraception.2021.11.004.
32. Boyce TM, Neiterman E. Women in larger bodies' experiences with contraception: a scoping review. Reprod Health. 2021;18(1):89. DOI: 10.1186/s12978-021-01139-2.
33. Horner-Johnson W, Klein KA, Campbell J, Guise JM. "It would have been nice to have a choice": Barriers to contraceptive decision-making among women with disabilities. Womens Health Issues. 2022;32(3):261-7. DOI: 10.1016/j.whi.2022.01.001.
34. Wu J, Braunschweig Y, Harris LH, Horner-Johnson W, Ernst SD, Stevens B. Looking back while moving forward: a justice-based, intersectional approach to research on contraception and disability. Contraception. 2019;99(5):267-71. DOI: 10.1016/j.contraception.2019.01.006.
35. Substance Abuse and Mental Health Services Administration. SAMHSA's Concept of Trauma and Guidance for a Trauma-Informed Approach. HHS Publication No. (SMA) 14-4884. Rockville, MD: Substance Abuse and Mental Health Services Administration; 2014.
36. Gipson JD, Koenig MA, Hindin MJ. The effects of unintended pregnancy on infant, child, and parental health: a review of the literature. Stud Fam Plann. 2008;39(1):18-38. DOI: 10.1111/j.1728-4465.2008.00148.x.
37. Kost K, Lindberg L. Pregnancy intentions, maternal behaviors, and infant health: investigating relationships with new measures and propensity score analysis. Demography. 2015;52(1):83-111. DOI: 10.1007/s13524-014-0359-9.
38. Kost K, Zolna M. Challenging unintended pregnancy as an indicator of reproductive autonomy: a response. Contraception. 2019;100(1):5-9. DOI: 10.1016/j.contraception.2019.04.010.
39. Potter JE, Stevenson AJ, Coleman-Minahan K, et al. Challenging unintended pregnancy as an indicator of reproductive autonomy. Contraception. 2019;100(1):1-4. DOI: 10.1016/j.contraception.2019.02.005.
40. Aiken AR, Borrero S, Callegari LS, Dehlendorf C. Rethinking the pregnancy planning paradigm: Unintended conceptions or unrepresentative concepts? Perspect Sex Reprod Health. 2016;48(3):147-51. DOI: 10.1363/48e10316.
41. Dehlendorf C, Reed R, Fox E, Seidman D, Hall C, Steinauer J. Ensuring our research reflects our values: The role of family planning research in advancing reproductive autonomy. Contraception. 2018;98(1):4-7. DOI: 10.1016/j.contraception.2018.03.015.
42. Finer LB, Zolna MR. Shifts in intended and unintended pregnancies in the United States, 2001-2008. Am J Public Health. 2014;104 Suppl 1(Suppl 1):S43-8. DOI: 10.2105/ajph.2013.301416.
43. Finer LB, Zolna MR. Declines in unintended pregnancy in the United States, 2008-2011. N Engl J Med. 2016;374(9):843-52. DOI: 10.1056/NEJMsa1506575.
44. Kost K, Maddow-Zimet I, Little A. Pregnancies and pregnancy desires at the state level: Estimates for 2017 and trends since 2012. New York: Guttmacher Institute, 2021.
45. Moseson H, Mahanaimy M, Dehlendorf C, Gerdts C. "…Society is, at the end of the day, still going to stigmatize you no matter which way": A qualitative study of the impact of stigma on social support during unintended pregnancy in early adulthood. PLoS One. 2019;14(5):e0217308. DOI: 10.1371/journal.pone.0217308.
46. Moseson H, Dehlendorf C, Gerdts C, Vittinghoff E, Hiatt RA, Barber J. No one to turn to: Low social support and the incidence of undesired pregnancy in the United States. Contraception. 2018;98(4):275-80. DOI: 10.1016/j.contraception.2018.06.009.
47. Lyons S, Arcara J, Deardorff J, Gomez AM. Financial strain and contraceptive use among women in the United States: Differential effects by age. Womens Health Issues. 2019;29(2):153-60. DOI: 10.1016/j.whi.2018.12.006.
48. Koenig MA, Acharya R, Singh S, Roy TK. Do current measurement approaches underestimate levels of unwanted childbearing? Evidence from rural India. Popul Stud (Camb). 2006;60(3):243-56. DOI: 10.1080/00324720600895819.
49. Rosenzweig MR, Wolpin KI. Maternal expectations and ex post rationalizations: The usefulness of survey information on the wantedness of children. J Human Resourc. 1993;28(2):20529. DOI: 10.2307/146201.
50. Joyce T, Kaestner R, Korenman S. On the validity of retrospective assessments of pregnancy intention. Demography. 2002;39(1):199-213. DOI: 10.1353/dem.2002.0006.

51. Miller WB. Relationships between the intendedness of conception and the wantedness of pregnancy. J Nerv Ment Dis. 1974;159(6):396-406. DOI: 10.1097/00005053-197412000-00002.
52. Bankole A, Westoff CF. The consistency and validity of reproductive attitudes: evidence from Morocco. J Biosoc Sci. 1998;30(4):439-55. DOI: 10.1017/s0021932098004398.
53. Jones RK, Tapales A, Lindberg LD, Frost J. Using longitudinal data to understand changes in consistent contraceptive use. Perspect Sex Reprod Health. 2015;47(3):131-9. DOI: 10.1363/47e4615.
54. Center for Disease Control and Prevention (CDC) National Center for Health Statistics (NHCS). National Survey of Family Growth (NSFG). (https://www.cdc.gov/nchs/nsfg/about_nsfg.htm).
55. Bachrach CA, Newcomer S. Intended pregnancies and unintended pregnancies: distinct categories or opposite ends of a continuum? Fam Plann Perspect. 1999;31(5):251-2. (In eng).
56. Santelli J, Rochat R, Hatfield-Timajchy K, et al. The measurement and meaning of unintended pregnancy. Perspect Sex Reprod Health. 2003;35(2):94-101. DOI: 10.1363/3509403.
57. Nyhof BB, Jameel B, Dunn S, et al. Identifying strategies to implement patient-centred care for women: Qualitative interviews with women. Patient Educ Couns. 2020;103(7):1422-7. DOI: 10.1016/j.pec.2020.02.008.
58. Callegari LS, Borrero S, Reiber GE, et al. Reproductive life planning in primary care: A qualitative study of women veterans' perceptions. Womens Health Issues. 2015;25(5):548-54. DOI: 10.1016/j.whi.2015.05.002.
59. Borrero S, Nikolajski C, Steinberg JR, et al. "It just happens": a qualitative study exploring low-income women's perspectives on pregnancy intention and planning. Contraception. 2015;91(2):150-6. DOI: 10.1016/j.contraception.2014.09.014.
60. Manze MG, Watnick D, Romero D. A qualitative assessment of perspectives on getting pregnant: the Social Position and Family Formation study. Reprod Health. 2019;16(1):135. DOI: 10.1186/s12978-019-0793-7.
61. Manze MG, Romero DR, De P, Hartnett J, Roberts L. The association of pregnancy control, emotions, and beliefs with pregnancy desires: A new perspective on pregnancy intentions. PLoS One. 2021;16(3):e0249032. DOI: 10.1371/journal.pone.0249032.
62. Hernandez ND, Chandler R, Nava N, et al. Young adult US-born Latina women's thoughts, feelings and beliefs about unintended pregnancy. Cult Health Sex. 2020;22(8):920-36. DOI: 10.1080/13691058.2019.1642517.
63. Manze MG, Watnick D, Besthoff C, Romero D. Examining women's and men's ideal criteria before forming families. J Fam Stud. 2022;28(1):239-54. DOI: 10.1080/13229400.2019.1702079.
64. Gomez AM, Arteaga S, Freihart B. Structural inequity and pregnancy desires in emerging adulthood. Arch Sex Behav. 2021;50(6):2447-58. DOI: 10.1007/s10508-020-01854-0.
65. Reeves R, Rodrigue E, Gold E. Following the success sequence? Success is more likely if you're white. Washington, DC: Brookings Institution; 2015. (https://www.brookings.edu/research/following-the-success-sequence-success-is-more-likely-if-youre-white/).
66. Geronimus AT. Damned if you do: culture, identity, privilege, and teenage childbearing in the United States. Soc Sci Med. 2003;57(5):881-93. DOI: 10.1016/s0277-9536(02)00456-2.
67. Arteaga S, Caton L, Gomez AM. Planned, unplanned and in-between: the meaning and context of pregnancy planning for young people. Contraception. 2019;99(1):16-21. DOI: 10.1016/j.contraception.2018.08.012.
68. Gomez AM, Arteaga S, Ingraham N, Arcara J, Villaseñor E. It's not planned, but is it okay? The acceptability of unplanned pregnancy among young people. Womens Health Issues. 2018;28(5):408-414. DOI: 10.1016/j.whi.2018.07.001.
69. Yeatman S, Smith-Greenaway E. Women's health decline following (some) unintended births: A prospective study. Demographic Research 2021;45(17):547-576. (https://www.demographic-research.org/volumes/vol45/17/45-17.pdf).
70. Aiken AR, Dillaway C, Mevs-Korff N. A blessing I can't afford: factors underlying the paradox of happiness about unintended pregnancy. Soc Sci Med. 2015;132:149-55. DOI: 10.1016/j.socscimed.2015.03.038.
71. Arcara J, Arteaga S, Burny I, Gómez AM. Changes in expectation of relationship permanence, pregnancy acceptability and desire, and contraceptive use over time among young Latino/a

women and men: An exploratory analysis. Contraception. 2021;103(1):19-25. DOI: 10.1016/j.contraception.2020.09.006.

72. Arteaga S, Downey MM, Freihart B, Gómez AM. "We kind of met in-between": A qualitative analysis of young couples' relationship dynamics and negotiations about pregnancy intentions. Perspect Sex Reprod Health. 2020;52(2):87-95. DOI: 10.1363/psrh.12136.
73. Casterline JB, El-Zeini LO. The estimation of unwanted fertility. Demography. 2007;44(4):729-45. DOI: 10.1353/dem.2007.0043.
74. Rodriguez AL, Arcara J, Deardorff J, Gomez AM. The association between religiosity and pregnancy acceptability among Latino/a young adults: does generational status matter? Cult Health Sex. 2020;22(2):184-200. DOI: 10.1080/13691058.2019.1581260.
75. Downey MM, Arteaga S, Villaseñor E, Gomez AM. More Than a destination: Contraceptive decision making as a journey. Womens Health Issues. 2017;27(5):539-45. DOI: 10.1016/j.whi.2017.03.004.
76. Higgins JA, Hirsch JS, Trussell J. Pleasure, prophylaxis and procreation: a qualitative analysis of intermittent contraceptive use and unintended pregnancy. Perspect Sex Reprod Health. 2008;40(3):130-7. DOI: 10.1363/4013008.
77. Miller WB, Barber JS, Gatny HH. The effects of ambivalent fertility desires on pregnancy risk in young women in the USA. Popul Stud (Camb). 2013;67(1):25-38. DOI: 10.1080/00324728.2012.738823.
78. Aiken AR, Potter JE. Are Latina women ambivalent about pregnancies they are trying to prevent? Evidence from the Border Contraceptive Access Study. Perspect Sex Reprod Health. 2013;45(4):196-203. DOI: 10.1363/4519613.
79. Gómez AM, Arteaga S, Villaseñor E, Arcara J, Freihart B. The Misclassification of ambivalence in pregnancy intentions: A mixed-methods analysis. Perspect Sex Reprod Health. 2019;51(1):7-15. DOI: 10.1363/psrh.12088.
80. Srinivasulu S, Falletta KA, Bermudez D, et al. Primary care providers' responses to pregnancy intention screening challenges: community-based participatory research at an urban community health centre. Fam Pract. 2019;36(6):797-803. DOI: 10.1093/fampra/cmz027.
81. Dam A, Yeh PT, Burke AE, Kennedy CE. Contraceptive values and preferences of pregnant women, postpartum women, women seeking emergency contraceptives, and women seeking abortion services: A systematic review. Contraception. 2021 DOI: 10.1016/j.contraception.2021.10.007.
82. Gavin L, Pazol K, Ahrens K. Update: Providing quality family planning services - Recommendations from CDC and the U.S. Office of Population Affairs, 2017. MMWR Morb Mortal Wkly Rep. 2017;66(50):1383-1385. DOI: 10.15585/mmwr.mm6650a4.
83. Biggs MA, Kimport K, Mays A, Kaller S, Berglas NF. Young women's perspectives about the contraceptive counseling received during their emergency contraception visit. Womens Health Issues. 2019;29(2):170-5. DOI: 10.1016/j.whi.2018.09.004.
84. Sznajder K, Carvajal DN, Sufrin C. Patient perceptions of immediate postpartum long-acting reversible contraception: A qualitative study. Contraception. 2020;101(1):21-5. DOI: 10.1016/j.contraception.2019.09.007.
85. Every Body Texas. No wrong door. (https://www.everybodytexas.org/what-we-do/current-projects/no-wrong-door).
86. Public Health Solutions. Partnership to advance integrated referrals (PAIR). (https://www.healthsolutions.org/community-work/sexual-reproductive-health/capacity-building-program/).
87. Jones HE, Calixte C, Manze M, et al. Primary care patients' preferences for reproductive health service needs assessment and service availability in New York federally qualified health centers. Contraception. 2020;101(4):226-30. DOI: 10.1016/j.contraception.2019.12.003.
88. Manze MG, Calixte C, Romero DR, et al. Physician perspectives on routine pregnancy intention screening and counseling in primary care. Contraception. 2020;101(2):91-6. DOI: 10.1016/j.contraception.2019.11.004.
89. Manze MG, Romero DR, Sumberg A, Gagnon M, Roberts L, Jones H. Women's perspectives on reproductive health services in primary care. Fam Med. 2020;52(2):112-9. DOI: 10.22454/FamMed.2020.492002.
90. University of California Person-Centered Reproductive Health Program. SINC-based eCQM. (https://pcrhp.ucsf.edu/sincbasedeCQMs).

91. Morse JE, Moos MK. Reproductive life planning: Raising the questions. Matern Child Health J. 2018;22(4):439-44. DOI: 10.1007/s10995-018-2516-z.
92. Gavin L, Moskosky S, Carter M, et al. Providing quality family planning services: Recommendations of CDC and the U.S. Office of Population Affairs. MMWR Recomm Rep. 2014;63(Rr-04):1-54.
93. Callegari LS, Aiken ARA, Dehlendorf C, Borrero S. Reproductive life planning and patient-centered care: Can the inconsistencies be reconciled? Matern Child Health J. 2019;23(7):869-70. DOI: 10.1007/s10995-019-02734-3.
94. Morse JE, Moos M-K. Authors' response, "Reproductive Life planning and patient-centered care: Can the inconsistencies be reconciled?". Matern Child Health J. 2019;23(7):871. DOI: 10.1007/s10995-019-02742-3.
95. The PATH Framework. (https://www.path-framework.com).
96. Murray CC. One Key Question: Putting women first. Power to Decide; 2019. (https://powertodecide.org/news/one-key-question-putting-women-first).
97. Association of Maternal and Child Health Programs. Best Practice-One Key Question. (https://www.amchpinnovation.org/database-entry/one-key-question/).
98. Stulberg DB, Dahlquist IH, Disterhoft J, Bello JK, Hunter MS. Increase in contraceptive counseling by primary care clinicians after implementation of One Key Question® at an urban community health center. Matern Child Health J. 2019;23(8):996-1002. DOI: 10.1007/s10995-019-02754-z.
99. Stulberg DB, Datta A, White VanGompel E, Schueler K, Rocca CH. One Key Question® and the Desire to Avoid Pregnancy Scale: A comparison of two approaches to asking about pregnancy preferences. Contraception. 2020;101(4):231-6. DOI: 10.1016/j.contraception.2019.12.010.
100. Song B, White VanGompel E, Wang C, et al. Effects of clinic-level implementation of One Key Question® on reproductive health counseling and patient satisfaction. Contraception. 2021;103(1):6-12. DOI: 10.1016/j.contraception.2020.10.018.
101. Gawron LM, Simonsen S, Millar MM, Lewis-Caporal J, Patel S, Simmons RG. Pregnancy risk screening and counseling for women veterans: Piloting the One Key Question in the Veterans Healthcare Administration. South Med J. 2021;114(3):150-5. DOI: 10.14423/smj.0000000000001218.
102. Thorman A, Engle A, Brintz B, et al. Quantitative and qualitative impact of One Key Question on primary care providers' contraceptive counseling at routine preventive health visits. Contraception. 2022;109:73-9. DOI: 10.1016/j.contraception.2022.01.004.
103. Ferketa M, Schueler K, Song B, Carlock F, Stulberg DB, White VanGompel E. Facilitators of and barriers to successful implementation of the One Key Question® pregnancy intention screening tool. Women's Health Rep. 2022;3(1):326-34. DOI: 10.1089/whr.2021.0100.
104. Geist C, Aiken AR, Sanders JN, et al. Beyond intent: exploring the association of contraceptive choice with questions about Pregnancy Attitudes, Timing and How important is pregnancy prevention (PATH) questions. Contraception. 2019;99(1):22-6. DOI: 10.1016/j.contraception.2018.08.014.
105. U.S. Centers for Disease Control and Prevention. A guide to taking a sexual history. (https://www.cdc.gov/std/treatment/sexualhistory.pdf).
106. Workowski KA, Bachmann LH, Chan PA, et al. Sexually transmitted infections treatment guidelines, 2021. MMWR Recomm Rep. 2021;70(4):1.
107. Bonnington A, Dianat S, Kerns J, et al. Society of Family Planning clinical recommendations: Contraceptive counseling for transgender and gender diverse people who were female sex assigned at birth. Contraception. 2020;102(2):70-82. DOI: 10.1016/j.contraception.2020.04.001.
108. Wilkinson TA, Maslowsky J, Berlan ED. The pediatrician in the post-Roe landscape. JAMA Pediatr. 2022;176(10):967-8. DOI: 10.1001/jamapediatrics.2022.2868.
109. Valdez-Barkwill M. Reproductive goals and academic goals: Knowledge, attitudes, and perceptions of women in community college. Northridge, California: California State University; 2019.
110. Lessard LN, Karasek D, Ma S, et al. Contraceptive features preferred by women at high risk of unintended pregnancy. Perspect Sex Reprod Health. 2012;44(3):194-200. DOI: 10.1363/4419412.
111. Madden T, Secura GM, Nease RF, Politi MC, Peipert JF. The role of contraceptive attributes in women's contraceptive decision making. Am J Obstet Gynecol. 2015;213(1):46.e1-6. DOI: 10.1016/j.ajog.2015.01.051.

112. Carpenter E, Everett BG, Greene MZ, Haider S, Hendrick CE, Higgins JA. Pregnancy (im) possibilities: identifying factors that influence sexual minority women's pregnancy desires. Soc Work Health Care. 2020;59(3):180-98. DOI: 10.1080/00981389.2020.1737304.
113. Callegari LS, Nelson KM, Arterburn DE, et al. Development and pilot testing of a patient-centered web-based reproductive decision support tool for primary care. J Gen Intern Med. 2021;36(10):2989-99. DOI: 10.1007/s11606-020-06506-6.
114. Now IICA. Start Quiz. (https://ican4all.org/start-quiz/).
115. Dehlendorf C, Fitzpatrick J, Fox E, et al. Cluster randomized trial of a patient-centered contraceptive decision support tool, My Birth Control. Am J Obstet Gynecol. 2019;220(6):565.e1-12. DOI: 10.1016/j.ajog.2019.02.015.
116. Dehlendorf C, Reed R, Fitzpatrick J, Kuppermann M, Steinauer J, Kimport K. A mixed-methods study of provider perspectives on My Birth Control: a contraceptive decision support tool designed to facilitate shared decision making. Contraception. 2019;100(5):420-3. DOI: 10.1016/j.contraception.2019.08.001.
117. Holt K, Kimport K, Kuppermann M, Fitzpatrick J, Steinauer J, Dehlendorf C. Patient-provider communication before and after implementation of the contraceptive decision support tool My Birth Control. Patient Educ Couns. 2020;103(2):315-20. DOI: https://doi.org/10.1016/j.pec.2019.09.003.
118. Planned Parenthood. Which birth control is right for me? (https://tools.plannedparenthood.org/bc/birth_control_quiz).
119. Bedsider. (https://www.bedsider.org/birth-control).
120. Fried TR. Shared decision making--finding the sweet spot. N Engl J Med. 2016;374(2):104-6. DOI: 10.1056/NEJMp1510020.
121. Chen M, Lindley A, Kimport K, Dehlendorf C. An in-depth analysis of the use of shared decision making in contraceptive counseling. Contraception. 2019;99(3):187-91. DOI: 10.1016/j.contraception.2018.11.009.
122. American College of Obstetricians Gynecologists' Committee on Health Care for Underserved Women CEEWGCoE. Patient-centered contraceptive counseling: ACOG Committee Statement Number 1. Obstet Gynecol. 2022;139(2):350-3. DOI: 10.1097/AOG.0000000000004659.
123. Dehlendorf C, Grumbach K, Schmittdiel JA, Steinauer J. Shared decision making in contraceptive counseling. Contraception. 2017;95(5):452-5. DOI: 10.1016/j.contraception.2016.12.010.
124. Zapata LB, Pazol K, Dehlendorf C, et al. Contraceptive counseling in clinical settings: An updated systematic review. Am J Prev Med. 2018;55(5):677-90. DOI: 10.1016/j.amepre.2018.07.006.
125. Madden T, Mullersman JL, Omvig KJ, Secura GM, Peipert JF. Structured contraceptive counseling provided by the Contraceptive CHOICE Project. Contraception. 2013;88(2):243-9. DOI: 10.1016/j.contraception.2012.07.015.
126. Moskowitz E, Jennings B. Directive counseling on long-acting contraception. Am J Public Health. 1996;86(6):787-90. DOI: 10.2105/ajph.86.6.787.
127. Dehlendorf C, Kimport K, Levy K, Steinauer J. A qualitative analysis of approaches to contraceptive counseling. Perspect Sex Reprod Health. 2014;46(4):233-40. DOI: 10.1363/46e2114.
128. Upadhyay UD. Informed choice in family planning. Helping people decide. Popul Rep J. 2001(50):1-39.
129. Barry MJ, Edgman-Levitan S. Shared decision making--pinnacle of patient-centered care. N Engl J Med. 2012;366(9):780-1. DOI: 10.1056/NEJMp1109283.
130. Carvajal DN, Gioia D, Mudafort ER, Brown PB, Barnet B. How can primary care physicians best support contraceptive decision making? A qualitative study exploring the perspectives of Baltimore Latinas. Womens Health Issues. 2017;27(2):158-66. DOI: 10.1016/j.whi.2016.09.015.
131. American College of Obstetrics and Gynecologists. Informed consent and shared decision making in obstetrics and gynecology: ACOG Committee Opinion, Number 819. Obstet Gynecol. 2021;137(2):e34-41. DOI: 10.1097/aog.0000000000004247.
132. Fox E, Reyna A, Malcolm NM, et al. Client preferences for contraceptive counseling: A systematic review. Am J Prev Med. 2018;55(5):691-702. DOI: 10.1016/j.amepre.2018.06.006.
133. American College of Obstetricians and Gynecologists' Committee on Health Care for Underserved Women, Contraceptive Equity Expert Work Group, and Committee on Ethics.

Patient-centered contraceptive counseling: ACOG Committee Statement Number 1. Obstet Gynecol. 2022;139(2):350-3. DOI: 10.1097/aog.0000000000004659.
134. Shay LA, Lafata JE. Where is the evidence? A systematic review of shared decision making and patient outcomes. Med Decis Making. 2015;35(1):114-31. DOI: 10.1177/0272989x14551638.
135. Gagliardi AR, Dunn S, Foster A, et al. How is patient-centred care addressed in women's health? A theoretical rapid review. BMJ Open. 2019;9(2):e026121. DOI: 10.1136/bmjopen-2018-026121.
136. Carvajal DN, Klyushnenkova E, Barnet B. Latina contraceptive decision-making and use: The importance of provider communication and shared decision-making for patient-centered care. Patient Educ Couns. 2021;104(9):2159-64. DOI: 10.1016/j.pec.2021.03.006.
137. Rogers C, Farson R. Active listening. Eastford, Connecticut: Martino Publishing; 2015.
138. Gaster B, Edwards K, Trinidad SB, Gallagher TH, Braddock CH, 3rd. Patient-centered discussions about prostate cancer screening: a real-world approach. Ann Intern Med. 2010;153(10):661-5. DOI: 10.7326/0003-4819-153-10-201011160-00010.
139. Hahn SR, Bradt P, Hewett KA, Ng DB. Physician-patient communication about overactive bladder: Results of an observational sociolinguistic study. PLoS One. 2017;12(11):e0186122. DOI: 10.1371/journal.pone.0186122.
140. Miller WR, Rollnick S. Motivational interviewing: Helping people change. 3rd ed. New York, NY: Guilford Press; 2013.
141. Miller WR, Rose GS. Toward a theory of motivational interviewing. Am Psychol. 2009;64(6):527-37. DOI: 10.1037/a0016830.
142. Rinehart W, Rudy S, Drennan M. GATHER guide to counseling. Popul Rep J. 1998(48):1-31. (https://www.ncbi.nlm.nih.gov/pubmed/10096107).
143. Moghadam FS, Mahmoodi Z, Kabir K, Mirabi P, Yazdkhasti M. Effectiveness of a multidimensional group counseling program based on the GATHER approach on the quality of life in surgically menopausal women. J Menopausal Med. 2019;25(3):130-41. DOI: 10.6118/jmm.19200.
144. Stickley T. From SOLER to SURETY for effective non-verbal communication. Nurse Educ Pract. 2011;11(6):395-8. DOI: 10.1016/j.nepr.2011.03.021.
145. Makoul G. The SEGUE Framework for teaching and assessing communication skills. Patient Educ Couns. 2001;45(1):23-34. DOI: 10.1016/s0738-3991(01)00136-7.
146. Sudore RL, Schillinger D. Interventions to improve care for patients with limited health literacy. J Clin Outcomes Manag. 2009;16(1):20-9. (https://www.ncbi.nlm.nih.gov/pubmed/20046798).
147. Health Literacy Universal Precautions Toolkit, 2nd Edition. Agency for Healthcare Research and Quality. September 2020 (https://www.ahrq.gov/health-literacy/improve/precautions/toolkit.html).
148. Knowles MS, Holton EF III, Swanson RA. The adult learner: The definitive classic in adult education and human resource development (8th ed.). Philadelphia, Pennsylvania: Routledge; 2015.
149. Hashim MJ. Patient-centered communication: Basic skills. Am Fam Physician. 2017;95(1):29-34. (https://www.ncbi.nlm.nih.gov/pubmed/28075109).
150. Hanyok LA, Hellmann DB, Rand C, Ziegelstein RC. Practicing patient-centered care: the questions clinically excellent physicians use to get to know their patients as individuals. Patient. 2012;5(3):141-5. DOI: 10.2165/11599530-000000000-00000.
151. Committee Opinion No. 710: Counseling Adolescents About Contraception. Obstet Gynecol. 2017;130(2):e74-80. DOI: 10.1097/aog.0000000000002234.
152. Makoul G. Essential elements of communication in medical encounters: the Kalamazoo consensus statement. Acad Med. 2001;76(4):390-3. DOI: 10.1097/00001888-200104000-00021.
153. Reproductive Health National Training Center. Client-centered reproductive goals and counseling flow chart. (https://rhntc.org/resources/client-centered-reproductive-goals-and-counseling-flow-chart).
154. Christine Dehlendorf MD, MAS. Personal Communication. July 29, 2017.
155. Danna K, Angel A, Kuznicki J, Lemoine L, Lerma K, Kalamar A. Leveraging the client-provider interaction to address contraceptive discontinuation: A scoping review of the evidence that links them. Glob Health Sci Pract. 2021;9(4):948-63. DOI: 10.9745/ghsp-d-21-00235.

156. Gilligan C, Powell M, Lynagh MC, et al. Interventions for improving medical students' interpersonal communication in medical consultations. Cochrane Database Syst Rev 2021;2:CD012418. DOI: 10.1002/14651858.CD012418.pub2.
157. Dang BN, Westbrook RA, Njue SM, Giordano TP. Building trust and rapport early in the new doctor-patient relationship: a longitudinal qualitative study. BMC Med. Educ 2017;17(1):32. DOI: 10.1186/s12909-017-0868-5.
158. Mercer SW, Reynolds WJ. Empathy and quality of care. Br J Gen Pract. 2002;52 Suppl:S9-12. (https://www.ncbi.nlm.nih.gov/pubmed/12389763).
159. Schrooten I, de Jong MD. If You Could Read My Mind: The role of health care providers' empathic and communicative competencies in clients' satisfaction with consultations. Health Commun. 2017;32(1):111-8. DOI: 10.1080/10410236.2015.1110002.
160. Buffington A, Wenner P, Brandenburg D, Berge J, Sherman M, Danner C. The art of listening. Minn Med. 2016;99(6):46-8. (https://www.ncbi.nlm.nih.gov/pubmed/28858459).
161. Zeh S, Christalle E, Zill JM, Harter M, Block A, Scholl I. What do patients expect? Assessing patient-centredness from the patients' perspective: an interview study. BMJ Open. 2021;11(7):e047810. DOI: 10.1136/bmjopen-2020-047810.
162. Filler T, Dunn S, Grace SL, Straus SE, Stewart DE, Gagliardi AR. Multi-level strategies to tailor patient-centred care for women: qualitative interviews with clinicians. BMC Health Serv Res. 2020;20(1):212. DOI: 10.1186/s12913-020-05082-z.
163. Filler T, Foster AM, Grace SL, Stewart DE, Straus SE, Gagliardi AR. Patient-centered care for women: Delphi consensus on evidence-derived recommendations. Value Health. 2020;23(8):1012-9. DOI: 10.1016/j.jval.2020.03.017.
164. Higgins K, Nesbitt C. Improvisation theater exercises: A novel approach to teach communication skills. J Nurs Educ. 2021;60(2):116-9. DOI: 10.3928/01484834-20210120-12.
165. Anderson N, Steinauer J, Valente T, Koblentz J, Dehlendorf C. Women's social communication about IUDs: a qualitative analysis. Perspect Sex Reprod Health. 2014;46(3):141-8. DOI: 10.1363/46e1814.
166. Griffith CH, 3rd, Wilson JF, Langer S, Haist SA. House staff nonverbal communication skills and standardized patient satisfaction. J Gen Intern Med. 2003;18(3):170-4. DOI: 10.1046/j.1525-1497.2003.10506.x.
167. Versluijs Y, Moore MG, Ring D, Jayakumar P. Clinician facial expression of emotion corresponds with patient mindset. Clin Orthop Relat Res. 2021;479(9):1914-23. DOI: 10.1097/CORR.0000000000001727.
168. Montague E, Xu J, Chen PY, Asan O, Barrett BP, Chewning B. Modeling eye gaze patterns in clinician-patient interaction with lag sequential analysis. Hum Factors. 2011;53(5):502-16. DOI: 10.1177/0018720811405986.
169. Riess H, Kraft-Todd G. E.M.P.A.T.H.Y.: A tool to enhance nonverbal communication between clinicians and their patients. Acad Med. 2014;89(8):1108-12. DOI: 10.1097/ACM.0000000000000287.
170. Schillinger D, Duran ND, McNamara DS, Crossley SA, Balyan R, Karter AJ. Precision communication: Physicians' linguistic adaptation to patients' health literacy. Sci Adv. 2021;7(51):eabj2836. DOI: 10.1126/sciadv.abj2836.
171. Williams N, Ogden J. The impact of matching the patient's vocabulary: a randomized control trial. Fam Pract. 2004;21(6):630-5. DOI: 10.1093/fampra/cmh610.
172. Ormrod JE. Human learning. Sixth edition. Boston, Massachusetts: Pearson; 2012.
173. Pazol K, Zapata LB, Dehlendorf C, Malcolm NM, Rosmarin RB, Frederiksen BN. Impact of Contraceptive education on knowledge and decision making: An updated systematic review. Am J Prev Med. 2018;55(5):703-15. DOI: 10.1016/j.amepre.2018.07.012.
174. Westhoff C, Kerns J, Morroni C, Cushman LF, Tiezzi L, Murphy PA. Quick start: novel oral contraceptive initiation method. Contraception. 2002;66(3):141-5. DOI: 10.1016/s0010-7824(02)00351-7.
175. Westhoff C, Heartwell S, Edwards S, et al. Initiation of oral contraceptives using a quick start compared with a conventional start: a randomized controlled trial. Obstet Gynecol. 2007;109(6):1270-6. DOI: 10.1097/01.AOG.0000264550.41242.f2.
176. Morgan IA, Zapata LB, Curtis KM, Whiteman MK. Health care provider attitudes about the safety of "Quick Start" initiation of long-acting reversible contraception for adolescents. J Pediatr Adolesc Gynecol. 2019;32(4):402-8. DOI: 10.1016/j.jpag.2019.01.007.

177. Ruberton PM, Huynh HP, Miller TA, Kruse E, Chancellor J, Lyubomirsky S. The relationship between physician humility, physician-patient communication, and patient health. Patient Educ Couns. 2016;99(7):1138-45. DOI: 10.1016/j.pec.2016.01.012.
178. Wadhwa A, Mahant S. Humility in medical practice: a qualitative study of peer-nominated excellent clinicians. BMC Med Educ. 2022;22(1):88. DOI: 10.1186/s12909-022-03146-8.
179. Huynh HP, Dicke-Bohmann A. Humble doctors, healthy patients? Exploring the relationships between clinician humility and patient satisfaction, trust, and health status. Patient Educ Couns. 2020;103(1):173-9. DOI: 10.1016/j.pec.2019.07.022.
180. Amico JR, Stimmel S, Hudson S, Gold M. "$231 . . . to pull a string!!!" American IUD users' reasons for IUD self-removal: An analysis of internet forums. Contraception. 2020;101(6):393-8. DOI: 10.1016/j.contraception.2020.02.005.
181. Amico JR, Bennett AH, Karasz A, Gold M. Taking the provider "out of the loop:" patients' and physicians' perspectives about IUD self-removal. Contraception. 2018;98(4):288-91. DOI: 10.1016/j.contraception.2018.05.021.
182. Stimmel S, Hudson SV, Gold M, Amico JR. Exploring the experience of IUD self-removal in the United States through posts on internet forums. Contraception. 2022;106:34-8. DOI: 10.1016/j.contraception.2021.10.013.
183. Broussard K, Becker A. Self-removal of long-acting reversible contraception: A content analysis of YouTube videos. Contraception. 2021;104(6):654-8. DOI: 10.1016/j.contraception.2021.08.002.
184. Gomez AM, Mann ES, Torres V. 'It would have control over me instead of me having control': intrauterine devices and the meaning of reproductive freedom. Critical Public Health. 2018;28(2):190-200. DOI: 10.1080/09581596.2017.1343935.
185. Amico JR, Bennett AH, Karasz A, Gold M. "I wish they could hold on a little longer": physicians' experiences with requests for early IUD removal. Contraception. 2017;96(2):106-10. DOI: 10.1016/j.contraception.2017.05.007.
186. Scott C. Personal Communication. February 15, 2022.
187. Kang MM, Guetterman TC, Prussack JK, Ursu A, Wu JP. Contraceptive care for women with medical conditions: A qualitative study to identify potential best practices for primary care physicians. Fam Med. 2019;51(7):559-66. DOI: 10.22454/FamMed.2019.499467.
188. Charron E, Tahsin F, Balto R, et al. Provider perspectives of barriers to contraceptive access and use among women with substance use disorders. Women's Health Issues. 2021;32(2):P165-72. DOI: https://doi.org/10.1016/j.whi.2021.11.010.
189. Bhakta J, Bainbridge J, Borgelt L. Teratogenic medications and concurrent contraceptive use in women of childbearing ability with epilepsy. Epilepsy Behav. 2015;52(Pt A):212-7. DOI: 10.1016/j.yebeh.2015.08.004.
190. Schonewille NN, Rijkers N, Berenschot A, Lijmer JG, van den Heuvel OA, Broekman BFP. Psychiatric vulnerability and the risk for unintended pregnancies, a systematic review and meta-analysis. BMC Pregnancy Childbirth. 2022;22(1):153. DOI: 10.1186/s12884-022-04452-1.
191. Tanner AE, Chambers BD, Philbin MM, et al. The intersection between women's reproductive desires and HIV care providers' reproductive health practices: A mixed methods analysis. Matern Child Health J. 2018;22(9):1233-9. DOI: 10.1007/s10995-018-2603-1.
192. Birru Talabi M, Clowse MEB, Schwarz EB, Callegari LS, Moreland L, Borrero S. Family planning counseling for women with rheumatic diseases. Arthritis Care Res. (Hoboken) 2018;70(2):169-174. DOI: 10.1002/acr.23267.
193. Gipson JD, Bornstein M, Berger A, Rocca CH. Desire to avoid pregnancy and contraceptive use among female methadone patients in Los Angeles. Contraception. 2021;103(5):322-7. DOI: 10.1016/j.contraception.2021.01.019.
194. Wolgemuth T, Stransky OM, Chodoff A, Kazmerski TM, Clowse MEB, Birru Talabi M. Exploring the Preferences of women regarding sexual and reproductive health care in the context of rheumatology: A qualitative study. Arthritis Care Res (Hoboken). 2021;73(8):1194-200. DOI: 10.1002/acr.24249.
195. Charron E, Mayo RM, Heavner-Sullivan SF, et al. "It's a very nuanced discussion with every woman": Health care providers' communication practices during contraceptive counseling for

patients with substance use disorders. Contraception. 2020;102(5):349-55. DOI: https://doi.org/10.1016/j.contraception.2020.09.002.

196. French VA, Steinauer JE, Kimport K. What women want from their health care providers about pregnancy options counseling: A qualitative study. Womens Health Issues. 2017;27(6): 715-20. DOI: 10.1016/j.whi.2017.08.003.
197. Nobel K, Ahrens K, Handler A, Holt K. Patient-reported experience with discussion of all options during pregnancy options counseling in the US South. Contraception. 2022;106:68-74. DOI: 10.1016/j.contraception.2021.08.010.
198. Perrucci A. Decision assessment and counseling in abortion care: Philosophy and practice. Lanham, Maryland: Rowman & Littlefield; 2012.

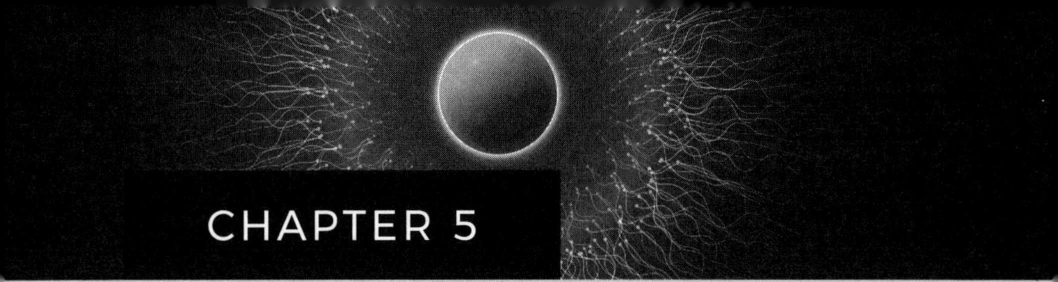

CHAPTER 5

Effectiveness, Safety, and Comparative Side Effects

Sarah E.K. Bradley, PhD, MHS
Chelsea B. Polis, PhD
Elizabeth A. Micks, MD, MPH
Markus J. Steiner, PhD, MSPH

KEY POINTS

Effectiveness:

- More than 1 million pregnancies occur every year in the United States among people using contraception.
- Contraceptive effectiveness is one of several key factors that most people consider when choosing their method of contraception.
- When discussing contraceptive effectiveness in the context of comprehensive person-centered counseling, grouping methods into three effectiveness categories can be useful to facilitate understanding:
  - The category with the most highly effective methods includes intrauterine devices (IUDs), contraceptive implants, and permanent contraception, which entail the lowest risk of pregnancy with either perfect or typical use (< 1%); this very low risk applies to all users.
  - Methods in the second effectiveness category include injectables, pills, patches, and rings. These also have a very low risk of pregnancy when used correctly and consistently (< 1% with perfect use), but with typical use, these methods have pregnancy rates between 4% and 7%, with variability influenced by age, coital frequency, and many other factors.
  - Methods in the third effectiveness category include condoms (internal and external), diaphragm, withdrawal, sponge, fertility awareness–based methods, spermicides/vaginal pH regulators, and the cervical cap. These methods have the highest pregnancy rates during both perfect use (≥ 2%) and typical use (≥ 8%) with even greater variability for individual user.
    - However, limited, moderate-quality evidence suggests that some specific fertility awareness–based methods may be as effective as the second category of methods.

- The simultaneous use of two different methods can lower pregnancy risk and, if a condom is one of the methods, can also reduce the risk of transmission of sexually transmitted infections.

Safety:

- While all medications and devices have risks and benefits, in the vast majority of cases, pregnancy confers a greater risk than use of a contraceptive method. Screening for personal health risk factors, as well as discussing reproductive desires, is important when selecting a contraceptive method.

Side Effects:

- Contraceptive side effects, including changes in bleeding patterns, are a major cause of method nonuse, dissatisfaction, and discontinuation. Beneficial side effects, or noncontraceptive benefits, may motivate individuals to use a method consistently.

Individuals must weigh many factors when deciding which contraceptive method or methods they will use. The best method of contraception for an individual or couple is one that is safe and that is consistent with their preferences for particular contraceptive characteristics, their reproductive desires, and their values. Contraceptive decision making can be challenging. A method that is not effective for an individual or couple can lead to an unintended pregnancy. A method that is not safe for the user can lead to unacceptable health risks. A method with intolerable side effects, or that does not fit well into the individual's life, is not likely to be used correctly or consistently, increasing the risk of failure, and will detract from the user's general well-being.

Most people will use a variety of contraceptive methods throughout their lives. When choosing a method or methods, individuals' choices are based on many factors, with side effects/safety and effectiveness being mentioned most frequently, followed by ease/frequency/duration of use, and other factors, according to a recent systematic review by the World Health Organization (WHO).[1] Other factors include access, reversibility, timing of the return of fecundity after discontinuation, positive contribution to sex or at least noninterference in sex, menstrual bleeding changes, costs, ability for discreet use, and other characteristics. Through counseling, you can help your client choose the method best suited to their priorities. (See Chapter 4, Person-Centered Reproductive Health Conversations and Contraceptive Counseling.)

Information on levels and trends in contraceptive use in the United States is based on the National Surveys of Family Growth (NSFG), periodic surveys conducted by the National Center for Health Statistics in which people who self-identify as female ages 15 to 49 are interviewed about topics related to childbearing, family planning, and maternal and child health. Among the 72.7 million women of reproductive age (ages 15 to 49), about 65% (47 million) were using some method of contraception, according to the most recently available NSFG, collected in 2017–2019.[2] Among the 35% (25.2 million) who were not currently using a method, about one-fifth were sexually active and not seeking pregnancy. The remaining four-fifths had had a hysterectomy, were trying to become pregnant, were pregnant, were interviewed within 6 weeks after the completion of a pregnancy, or had not had intercourse during the 3 months prior to the survey.[3] Most sexually active women not seeking pregnancy use a contraceptive method, but between 6% and 17% of all women not seeking pregnancy (~5.1 million) are not using any contraceptive method.[4-6]

Today, the most popular contraceptive methods in the United States are fallopian tube surgery (previously referred to as female sterilization;13.2 million), oral contraceptive pills (10.1 million), external (formerly referred to as male) condoms (6.1 million), intrauterine devices (IUDs; 6 million), vas surgery (formerly referred to as male sterilization; 4.1 million), withdrawal (also called coitus interruptus; 2.7 million), and implants (1.7 million) (**Table 5-1**). Fewer than 1 million women use rings, patches, or methods in the combined category of diaphragms, cervical caps,

Table 5-1 Number of US Women 15–49 Using Each Method and Percent Using Among Women at Risk of Unintended Pregnancy

Method	Number of women 15–49, in millions*	% Using among sexually active women not seeking pregnancy†
Fallopian tube surgery (Female sterilization)	13.2	23.9
Oral contraceptive pill	10.1	16.4
Male (external) condom	6.1	13.2
IUD	6.1	12.0
Vas surgery (Male sterilization)	4.1	8.5
Withdrawal	2.7	5.8
Implant	1.5	2.6
Injectable (Depo-Provera)	1.4	2.1
Fertility awareness–based method‡	1.2	2.6
Emergency contraception	1.0	0.2
Contraceptive vaginal ring	0.6	1.2
Transdermal patch	0.2	0.4
Other method§	0.1	0.2
No method	25.2	11.0

*"Contraceptive users" does not restrict to those who have been sexually active in the previous 3 months. Table shows only most effective method used at last sex.

†"Sexually active women not seeking pregnancy" includes all women who report sexual activity in the previous 3 months; are not currently pregnant, seeking to become pregnant, or postpartum; and are not noncontraceptively sterile.

‡Fertility awareness–based methods include periodic abstinence, cervical mucus tests, temperature tests, or calendar rhythm.

§Includes diaphragm, female condom, cervical cap, spermicides, and other methods.

Modified from https://www.guttmacher.org/fact-sheet/contraceptive-method-use-united-states; data derived from the 2017–2018 National Survey of Family Growth.

spermicides, and internal (formerly referred to as female) condoms, though data do not reflect the several new methods that have become available since these data were collected.

The most recent information on contraceptive use by age is from the 2015–2017 NSFG. We believe these patterns likely hold in the most recent data, as the overall method mix has not substantially changed.[3] The contraceptive methods women use differ substantially by age, as shown in **Figure 5-1**. Almost three-quarters of adolescents 15–19 use pills (45%), implants (16%), or injectables (12%), while fewer than 10% of women over age 40 use these methods. The vast majority (79%) of women 45–49 who are using contraception rely on permanent methods: fallopian tube surgery (61%) or vas surgery (18%). Condom use is highest among women in their 20s and early 30s (18% to 20%), and slightly lower among 15- to 19-year-olds (14%). Use of withdrawal (7% to 11%) and fertility awareness–based methods (FABMs) (2% to 4%) are also highest among women 20–34. Fewer than 1% of women in any age group report other coitally dependent methods, including the diaphragm, sponge, or spermicides, as their most effective method.[5]

Use of the external (male) condom, withdrawal, FABMs, and "other" methods is greater than indicated in Table 5-1, because some people use these methods in

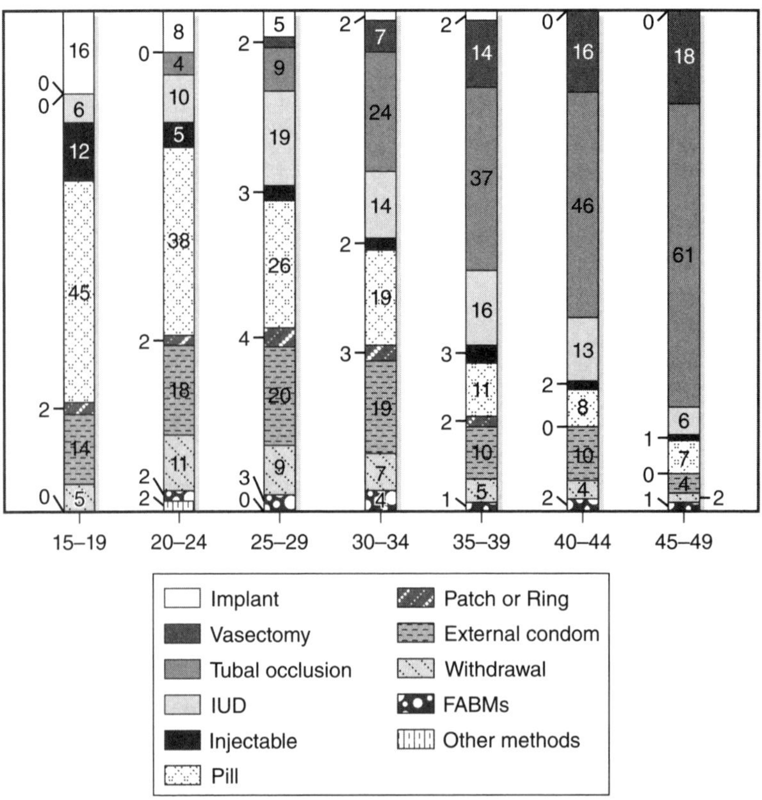

Figure 5-1 Method mix among all women using contraception by age.

Data from Kavanaugh ML, Pliskin E. Use of contraception among reproductive-aged women in the United States, 2014 and 2016. F S Rep 2020;1(2):83-93. (In eng). DOI: 10.1016/j.xfre.2020.06.006.

addition to another method. In the NSFG, women were asked to report all contraceptive methods used in the current month for any reason (for protection against either pregnancy or STIs). When more than one method was reported, only the most effective method is coded as the current method. The most recent data available on multiple method use come from the 2013–2015 NSFG.[7] When data on the most effective method used was recoded to capture all use of the external condom in the month of interview, the fraction using external condoms among all users 15–44 at risk rises by 48%, from 14.5% to 21.4%. When the data are recoded to capture all use of withdrawal, the fraction using withdrawal rises by 96%, from 8.1% to 15.8%. The percentage using FABMs increases 48%, from 2.2% to 3.2%.

Couples' use of the mix of methods shown in Table 5-1 resulted in an estimated 1.2 million pregnancies in 2017, 21% of the total (5.7 million) pregnancies occurring that year. The 11% of people sexually active, not seeking pregnancy but not using contraception resulted in an additional 1.4 million pregnancies (25% of total pregnancies). People actively seeking pregnancies accounted for only slightly over half (54%) of the total pregnancies. Nearly half (46%) of pregnancies were reported to be mistimed (wanted later) or unwanted (not wanted at any time), resulting in 2.6 million unintended pregnancies per year.[8] Thirty-seven percent of these pregnancies occurred among individuals who reported using contraception.[8-10]

Effectiveness: "How Well Will It Work?"

"How well will it work?" is a question frequently asked about any method of contraception. Although this question cannot be answered with certainty for any specific couple, clinicians and counselors can help clients understand something of the difficulty of quantifying effectiveness. In this chapter, we use the term ***efficacy*** to refer to data on how well a method works with perfect (consistent) use of that method. Efficacy reflects how well a method prevents pregnancy in clinical trials when study participants use the method correctly and consistently as defined by the manufacturer's instructions. We use the term ***effectiveness*** to indicate how well a method works with actual, real-life, typical use. Effectiveness varies according to many factors including the intrinsic efficacy of the method, whether the method is easy to use correctly, and user characteristics such as age and frequency of intercourse. These factors can vary significantly in different populations. Our current understanding of the literature on contraceptive efficacy during perfect use and effectiveness during typical use is summarized in **Table 5-2**.

It is useful to distinguish between measures of contraceptive effectiveness and measures of the risk of pregnancy during contraceptive use. Many people, including clinicians and clients, prefer positive rather than negative statements; instead of the negative statement that 20% of individuals using a method become pregnant during their first year of use, they prefer the alternative positive statement that the method is 80% effective. Strictly speaking that is not correct; it does not follow that the method is 80% effective, because it is not true that 100% of these individuals would have become pregnant if they had not been using contraception. However, no study can ascertain the proportion who would have become pregnant had they not used the contraceptive method under investigation. Our best estimate of the probability of pregnancy during 1 year of intercourse with no contraception is 85% (see No Method Section on p. 144). Therefore, we focus attention on pregnancy rates or probabilities of pregnancy during contraceptive use, which are directly measurable. When the risk

Table 5-2 Percentage of Users Becoming Pregnant During the First Year of Contraceptive Use in the United States (Perfect Use and Typical Use) and Internationally (Typical Use)*

Method	% of Users Experiencing an Unintended Pregnancy within the First Year of Contraceptive Use			Effectiveness Category
	Perfect Use[a]	Typical Use, United States[b]	Typical Use, International Population-based Survey Estimates[c]	
Implant	0.1	0.1	**0.3**	Category 1 < 1 pregnancy per 100 women in 1 year with either perfect or typical use
Vas surgery	0.1	0.15		
Fallopian tube surgery	0.5	0.5		
Intrauterine contraceptives				
LNG-releasing IUDs[d]	0.3	0.4		
Copper-bearing IUD	0.6	0.8	**1**	
Depot-medroxyprogesterone Acetate (DMPA, DepoProvera) Injectable	0.2	**4**	**2**	Category 2 1–7 pregnancies per 100 women in 1 year with typical use
Oral contraceptive pills (combined or progestin-only)	0.3	**7**	**6**	
Transdermal patches	0.3	**7**		
Contraceptive vaginal rings	0.3	**7**		
Fertility awareness–based methods[e]				This group of methods spans effectiveness Categories 2 and 3.
Sensiplan	0.4	2		
Natural Cycles		7		
Clue	3	8		
Standard Days	5	13		
Billings	3	23		
Calendar rhythm	NA	**15**	**19**	

Method	% of Users Experiencing an Unintended Pregnancy within the First Year of Contraceptive Use			Effectiveness Category
	Perfect Use[a]	Typical Use, United States[b]	Typical Use, International Population-based Survey Estimates[c]	
External (male) condom	2	**13**	**9**	Category 3 More than 8 pregnancies per 100 women in 1 year with typical use
Sponge (both parous and nulliparous)[f]	12	17		
Diaphragm[g]	16	17		
Withdrawal	4	**20**	**17**	
Internal (female) condom	5	21		
Vaginal pH regulator (Phexxi)	12	21		
Spermicides	16	21		
Cervical cap (FemCap)	22	22		
No method[h]	85	85		

Emergency contraceptives: Use of emergency contraceptive pills or placement of an IUD after unprotected intercourse substantially reduces the risk of pregnancy. (See Chapter 10 Intrauterine Devices [IUDs]).

Lactational Amenorrhea Method: LAM is a highly effective, temporary method of contraception.[i] (See Chapter 17, Coitus Interruptus [Withdrawal, the Pull-Out Method].)

[a] Among couples who initiate use of a method (not necessarily for the first time) and who use it perfectly (both consistently and correctly) for the first year, the percentage who experience an accidental pregnancy if they do not stop use for any other reason. Most estimates in this column come from clinical data; see text for the derivation of the estimate for each method.
[b] Among couples who initiate use of a method (not necessarily for the first time), the percentage who experience an accidental pregnancy during the first year of typical use if they do not stop use for any reason other than pregnancy. Estimates of the probability of pregnancy during the first year of typical use for withdrawal, the male condom, the pill, and Depo-Provera are taken from the 2006–2010 National Survey of Family Growth (NSFG) corrected for under-reporting of abortion. See text for the derivation of estimates for the other methods.
[c] Among couples who initiate use of a method (not necessarily for the first time), the percentage who experience an accidental pregnancy during the first year if they do not stop use for any reason other than pregnancy. Estimates in this column are based on population-based Demographic and Health Survey data from 15 countries, not adjusted for under-reporting of abortion. All estimates in this column are calculated using life tables. See text for details.
[d] For details rates for specific LNG-releasing IUDs, see text.
[e] Multiple FABMs exist with varying features; a subset are shown here. See Chapter 15, Fertility Awareness-Based Methods, for additional detail.
[f] Estimates are for all sponge users. For nulliparous women, the typical-use pregnancy rate is 14% and the perfect use pregnancy rate is 9%. For parous women, the typical use pregnancy rate is 27% and the perfect use pregnancy rate is 20%.
[g] With spermicidal cream or jelly.
[h] This estimate represents the percentage who would become pregnant within 1 year without using contraception. See text.
[i] However, to maintain effective protection against pregnancy, another method of contraception must be used as soon as menstruation resumes, the frequency or duration of breastfeeds is reduced, bottle feeds are introduced, or the baby reaches 6 months of age.
***Bold** estimates are from population-based surveys.

is framed as the probability of *not* becoming pregnant, i.e., 100 minus the pregnancy rate, this may be good marketing, but it overestimates the true effectiveness because no population is certain to conceive during 1 year of not using contraception.

Data Sources and Methods for Estimating Contraceptive Effectiveness

Pregnancy rates during contraceptive use come from two different types of studies: (1) analyses of population-based survey data like the NSFG, which samples the total US population to reflect the actual experience of a representative sample of contraceptive users with differing demographic characteristics, and (2) clinical trials, which enroll a select group of individuals whose experiences may not be generalizable to the wider population. Both typical- and perfect-use pregnancy rates can theoretically be measured in clinical trials. However, for methods with a sufficiently large number of users, experts generally rely on—and we have used whenever available—typical-use rates calculated with survey data for several reasons, beyond the generalizability issues mentioned above. First, population-based survey data capture the lived experiences of contraceptive users outside a clinical setting. These real-world estimates are the most relevant for patients interested in understanding how effective contraceptive methods would be for them. Second, the behavior of people in clinical trials is most likely affected by frequent contact with investigators and study staff, particularly for methods that are highly user-dependent. Such frequent "reminders" about their contraceptive use may make trial participants more likely to use the method correctly and consistently than they would outside of a trial setting, potentially biasing pregnancy rates downward.

Population-based survey estimates are not without their flaws. The two largest sources of population-based contraceptive effectiveness data—the NSFG in the US, and the Demographic and Health Surveys (DHS) internationally—are surveys that collect data retrospectively. These surveys ask respondents about their current contraceptive use, recent pregnancies and births, and then ask respondents to think back about which contraceptive method they were using each month for the past 2 to 3 years (NSFG) or 5 to 6 years (DHS). Retrospective data collection, especially about events that occurred far in the past, is potentially subject to recall bias, both intentional and unintentional.[11-13] If interviewees do not accurately recall the dates of their contraceptive use and reasons for discontinuation, including discontinuation because they became pregnant, typical-use pregnancy rates could be inaccurate. Additionally, researchers expect respondents to omit at least some pregnancies that occurred during contraceptive use, and especially those pregnancies that resulted in induced abortion. For this reason, pregnancy rates estimated from NSFG data are often adjusted for under-reporting of abortion.[*14]

Pregnancy rates from population-based surveys and those from clinical trial data are sometimes calculated differently. The "gold standard" is to use single-decrement

---

[*] US-based estimates, drawn from NSFG data, are adjusted for under-reporting of abortion using additional data from a survey of US abortion patients. Such adjustment for abortion is not currently feasible for DHS data, due to limitations in estimation of abortion in many international settings.

Evidence suggests that more than half of abortions are not reported in NSFG data.[15] If interviewees are less likely to report episodes of contraceptive use that ended in a preg-

life-table methods that calculate the cumulative incidence of pregnancy among a group of contraceptive method users, beginning from method initiation and continuing through the 12th full month of use for a 1-year pregnancy rate.[19] Life tables allow for inclusion of varying durations of contraceptive use without introducing the problems associated with the Pearl Index (see below). These life-table rates are statistically unbiased and standardized to represent the experience of an average user within the study sample during 1 year of use. This approach is used with all estimates presented in this chapter.

Many clinical trials use an approximation of the life table method called a Pearl Index which, despite its well-known shortcomings, remains the standard method used by the US Food and Drug Administration (FDA) to analyze clinical trial data. The Pearl Index is calculated by simply dividing the number of pregnancies during contraceptive use by the number of years of exposure to the risk of pregnancy contributed by all participants in the study.[†] This measure can be misleading when one

---

nancy that was then aborted, pregnancy rates during contraceptive use will be too low. Researchers who use NSFG data to produce typical-use pregnancy rates therefore make adjustments to attempt to counteract such under-reporting. To adjust the most recent estimates of pregnancy rates presented in Table 5-2, researchers used information from the 2008 Abortion Patient Survey (APS), a nationally representative survey of abortion patients that includes information on contraceptive use at the time of pregnancy.[16] Briefly, researchers apply weights to the few episodes of contraceptive use that are reported to end in pregnancy followed by abortion, "weighting up" those contraceptive episodes to reflect the likely number of abortions after failures that occurred in each subpopulation (for details see Sundaram et al.[17]).

The correction for under-reporting of abortion may produce estimates that are too high because patients in abortion clinics (surveys of whom provided the information for the correction) tend to over-report use of a contraceptive method at the time they became pregnant (social desirability bias). Moreover, those interviewed for the NSFG also might over-report use of a contraceptive method at the time of an unintended pregnancy that led to a live birth. Evidence for this suspicion is provided by uncorrected first-year probabilities of pregnancy of 3.7% for the IUD and 2.3% for the implant (methods with little or no scope for user error) in the 1995 NSFG; these probabilities are much higher than rates observed in clinical trials of these methods.[18] Such overreporting of contraceptive use is unsurprising; individuals may feel less stigmatized in acknowledging an unintended pregnancy if reported as stemming from contraceptive failure versus from contraceptive nonuse. Thus, biases in opposite directions affect these estimates. Pregnancy rates based on the NSFG alone would tend to be too low because induced abortions (and contraceptive failures leading to induced abortions) are under-reported, but they would tend to be too high because contraceptive failures leading to live births are over-reported. We reason that the former bias is the more important one.

In many countries where the DHS works, induced abortions are illegal. There is likely underreporting of failures terminated in abortion in international survey data too, but because no comparable data source to the APS exists internationally, there is no similar adjustment made to DHS-based pregnancy rate estimates.

† Specifically, the calculations for the Pearl Index are:

- If a study used monthly intervals, the formula is: (# of pregnancies / # of months of exposure) × 1200.
- If a study used cycle intervals, the formula is: (# of pregnancies / # of cycles of exposure) × 1300.

wishes to compare pregnancy rates obtained from studies with different durations of exposure to the risk of pregnancy during contraceptive use. The likelihood of pregnancy declines over time because those most likely to become pregnant do so at earlier durations of contraceptive use and exit from observation. Those still using contraception after long durations are increasingly less likely to become pregnant, so an investigator could (wittingly or unwittingly) drive the reported pregnancy rate toward zero by running the trial "forever."[‡]

Because estimates for different contraceptive methods in this chapter come from studies with different durations of exposure (e.g., 6 months, seven cycles, 1 year), and the purpose is to enable readers to compare estimates across contraceptive methods, we do not use any Pearl Index estimates in this chapter. We instead focus on life-table measures of pregnancy during contraceptive use, and use standard methods to extrapolate from shorter durations to a standard 12-month time period, so pregnancy rates for each contraceptive method can appropriately be compared to each other (see details under each specific method heading, below). These life-table measures are easy to interpret and control for the distorting effects of varying durations of use. Ideally, we would present perfect-use rates from clinical data and typical-use rates calculated with life tables from population-based survey data for all contraceptive methods. However, only five methods (injectables/DMPA, oral contraceptive pills, external condoms, calendar rhythm method, and withdrawal) had enough users in the most recent NSFG analyzed for contraceptive effectiveness to allow population-based estimates of typical-use pregnancy rates.[17,21] We therefore base the estimates for many of the remaining methods on clinical studies because there is no US-based alternative. In a few instances where robust data are not available from either NSFG or US-based clinical trials, we simply use the best available information (see below). We also include a column of typical-use pregnancy rates using international data from the DHS, which provides both a range of estimates across different populations, and the ability to produce population-based rates for seven contraceptive methods due to larger sample sizes.

Perfect Use

In the first column of Table 5-2, we provide estimates of the probabilities of pregnancy during the first year of perfect use. A method is used perfectly when it is used consistently and correctly as defined by a specified set of rules. For many methods in the third category, perfect use requires correct use at every act of intercourse. Some perfect-use pregnancy rates reported in the literature have been calculated incorrectly and are too low[22] (see Interpretation of Effectiveness Data, p. 135). We expect that our understanding of efficacy during perfect use will be enhanced by additional studies.

---

‡ For example, two investigators using the NSFG could obtain Pearl Index pregnancy rates of 7.5 and 4.4 per 100 woman-years of exposure for the condom.[20] One (who got 4.4) allowed each study subject to contribute a maximum of 5 years of exposure while the other (who got 7.5) allowed each study subject to contribute only 1 year. Which investigator is incorrect? Neither. The two rates are simply not comparable.

Typical Use

In the second column of Table 5-2, we provide estimates of the probabilities of pregnancy (adjusted for under-reporting of abortion in the NSFG) during the first year of typical use of each method in the United States. Pregnancy rates during typical use reflect how effective methods are for the average person who does not always use methods correctly or consistently. Typical use does not imply that a contraceptive method was always used. In the NSFG and in most clinical trials, people are "using" a contraceptive method if they consider themselves to be using that method. Typical use of the condom could include actually using a condom only occasionally, and a person could report that they are "using" oral contraception even though they sometimes forget to take pills. In short, *use*—which is identical to *typical use*—is a very elastic concept that depends on an individual's perception.

The third column shows first-year typical-use pregnancy rates from international survey data. These data provide additional population-based survey estimates of typical use across a wide variety of populations from 15 countries in Asia, Eastern Europe, Latin America and the Caribbean, the Middle East, and sub-Saharan Africa selected for their relatively high calendar data quality.[23] Estimates generally align with, though are slightly lower than, estimates from NSFG data for contraceptive methods that can be measured with both data sources, as expected given that DHS-based estimates cannot be adjusted for under-reporting of abortion. The exception is for calendar rhythm, in which the DHS-based estimate is higher. This column also provides the only population-based survey estimates of pregnancy rates during implant and copper-bearing IUD use.

Interpretation of Effectiveness Data

In Table 5-2, we have relied on life table estimates derived from population-based studies wherever possible. Perfect-use estimates are almost exclusively from clinical trials. Typical-use estimates from population-based surveys are highlighted in bold in column two. We encourage readers to consider the unbolded, clinical-trial typical-use estimates to generally be lower than pregnancy rates that truly occur in a population. The differences between clinical-trial and population-based estimates can be assumed to be larger for methods in the second, and especially the third category, which are easier than methods in the first category to use incorrectly or inconsistently.

Given the challenges and utility of communicating point estimates of the various methods (see Pitfalls and Challenges of Communicating Pregnancy Risk, p. 153), many experts prefer to group methods into meaningful categories.[14] **Figure 5-2** uses the typical-use pregnancy rates to group contraceptive methods into categories, has been empirically tested both domestically[24] and internationally[25] for comprehensibility and adopted by the WHO,[26] and may be a useful counseling tool as part of comprehensive person-centered counseling (Chapter 4).[27]

Given the shameful history of some in the medical establishment coercively using permanent contraception, IUDs, and implants, there is near-universal agreement that providers should prioritize patient preference and avoid promoting particular methods or exclusively prioritizing contraceptive effectiveness during counseling. Promoting methods and directing patients toward any particular method damages trust and causes harm. Tiered effectiveness charts are a valuable visual aid to use during counseling to clarify comparative effectiveness. However, contraceptive

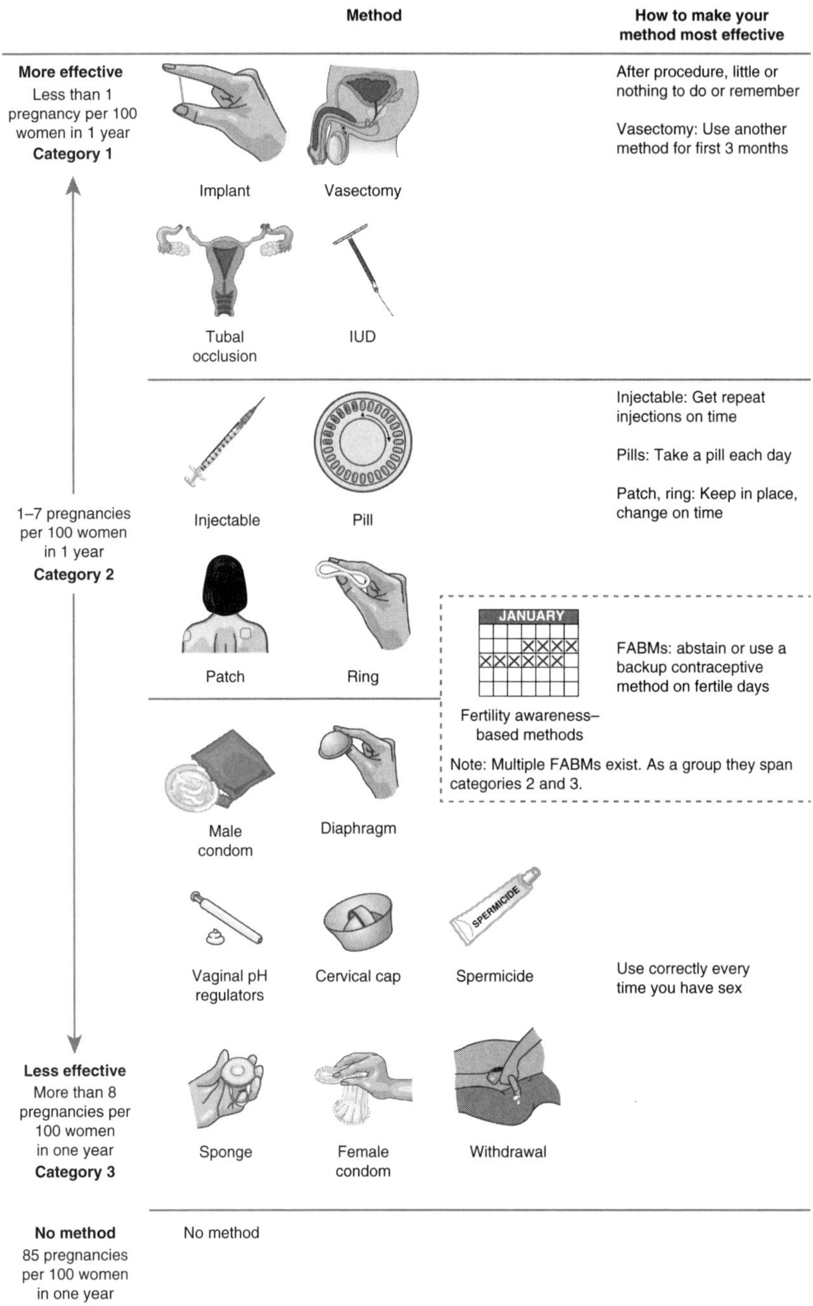

Figure 5-2 Effectiveness Categories

counseling based on tiered effectiveness can prioritize effectiveness to an extreme that is coercive and undermines patient autonomy. Counseling on effectiveness should always accompany thorough discussions of other key characteristics important to an individual patient. Figure 5-2 is not meant to be the sole visual aid used during contraceptive counseling but rather a useful tool for clients interested in the effectiveness offered by various methods.

Methods in the top category have typical-use pregnancy rates below 1% and the perfect-use rates are nearly identical (< 1%) because they do not require the individual to "actively" use the method regularly (monthly, daily, or with every act of intercourse). Importantly, the methods have similarly low pregnancy rates regardless of the population studied, statistical approach employed, or data source and thus apply to all users of these methods.

Methods in the second category have typical-use pregnancy rates between 1% and 7% but substantially lower pregnancy rates during perfect use (< 1%) illustrating these methods are highly effective if used correctly and consistently. Different sociodemographic subgroups can have widely varying typical-use pregnancy rates. For example, in the NSFG analysis by Fu et al., the rate for oral contraceptive pills ranged from 3.3% to 48.4% among different demographic groups.[28] The overall typical-use pregnancy rates for second category methods are not applicable to any one user and may not be useful to focus on during counseling; rather, their utility lies in grouping methods into categories.[14]

Finally, methods in the third category all have typical-use pregnancy rates above 8% and are generally not highly effective (≥ 2%) even if used correctly and consistently. Again, none of the rates are applicable to any one user for counseling purposes but are sufficiently robust and useful for categorization, which is helpful to illustrate differences in comparative effectiveness.[14]

As a group, FABMs span categories 2 and 3, so are indicated as such in Table 5-2 and Figure 5-2.

Data Sources and Derivation for Effectiveness Estimates of Individual Contraceptive Methods

To update pregnancy rates for this chapter, we relied heavily on the approach and literature review of previous editions of this text. For pregnancy rates reported in population-based surveys we contacted investigators working with the current round of NSFG to make sure no additional pregnancy rate analyses have been published since the analysis referenced in the last edition.[8] We added population-based rates from a 15-country peer-reviewed paper published in 2019. For clinical trial data, we searched for systematic reviews as well as individual studies published since the last edition, and contacted authors of individual chapters to ensure we were basing our analysis on the most recent literature. We reviewed clinical trial data for several new methods of contraception, including the segesterone acetate and ethinyl estradiol vaginal ring (Annovera), the drospirenone-only pill (Slynd), a vaginal pH regulator (Phexxi), and the levonorgestrel and ethinyl estradiol transdermal patch (Twirla). We aimed to provide the best estimates of pregnancy rates for each major contraceptive category (e.g., oral contraceptive pills, levonorgestrel-releasing IUDs, contraceptive vaginal rings) rather than separate effectiveness estimates for every hormonal formulation and dosing regimen. The source and derivation for each estimate are described by contraceptive method category below, with additional details provided in Appendix B: Method Efficacy Tables, which is included in the eBook (indicated by **B-** before the table number).

Perfect Use of Contraceptive Implant, DMPA Injectable, and Oral Contraceptive Pills, and Typical use of Contraceptive Implant. Information about the contraceptive implant Nexplanon is taken from studies of Implanon because the dose of etonogestrel is the same and no new efficacy studies were required for approval. Implanon failures are rare (**Table B-15**).[29] We took the pregnancy rate during typical use of Implanon (0.1%) from a multicenter study,[30] and set the probability during perfect use equal to that during typical use. In that same study, Jadelle, a two-rod contraceptive implant containing levonorgestrel and available in many countries outside the United States, had a 0% typical-use pregnancy rate in the first year and both implants had the identical cumulative typical-use 3-year pregnancy rate of 0.4%. In another recent trial comparing Jadelle to Levoplant, another two-rod implant containing levonorgestrel available outside the United States, both products had zero pregnancies during the first year of use.[31] The typical-use estimate of 0.3 in the third column reflects the real-life experience of several thousand women and is the best estimate we have of the (very low) implant pregnancy rate in the general population.[23]

The perfect-use pregnancy rate estimate of 0.2% for depot-medroxyprogesterone acetate (DMPA) is the weighted average of the results from the seven trials of the 150-mg intramuscular dose (90-day or 3-month) and the two trials of the 104-mg subcutaneous dose shown in **Table B-13**.[32-39] These trials yield a pregnancy rate estimate for perfect rather than typical use either because participants late for an injection were discontinued or because all pregnancies reported occurred during actual use (after one injection but before the next was scheduled). In the two trials of DMPA-SC, there were no reported pregnancies during perfect use in either study.[53,54]

Although the lowest reported pregnancy rate for the combined pill during typical use is 0% (**Table B-12**), more recent studies indicate that pregnancies do occur, albeit rarely, during perfect use.[40,41] Hence, we set the perfect-use estimate for the pill at the very low level of 0.3%. Perfect-use pregnancy rates for progestin-only pill formulations are generally slightly higher than those for combined pills (see **Table B-11**), though differences may not be statistically significant.[42] Whether the progestin-only pill is less effective than the combined pill during perfect use is unknown.

Typical and Perfect Use of Permanent Contraception. The weighted average of the results from the nine vasectomy studies in **Table B-17** analyzed with life-table procedures is a 0.02% partner pregnancy rate (perfect use) in the year following the procedure.[43-51] In eight of these studies, pregnancies occurred after the ejaculate had been declared to be sperm-free. This perfect-use estimate of 0.02% is undoubtedly too low, because clinicians are understandably hesitant to publish articles describing their surgical failures and journals would be reluctant to publish an article documenting poor surgical technique. The difference between typical-use and perfect-use pregnancy rates for vasectomy would depend on the frequency of unprotected intercourse after the procedure had been performed but before the ejaculate had been certified to be sperm-free. We kept the estimates the authors of previous editions of this text "arbitrarily set" at 0.15% for typical use and 0.10% for perfect use.

For current methods of fallopian tube surgery, there is almost no possibility of user error. Hysteroscopic methods are more subject to user error but are not currently available in the United States. The typical- and perfect-use pregnancy rate estimates (both 0.5%) are the pooled results from the US Collaborative Review of Sterilization, a prospective study of 10,685 individuals undergoing fallopian tube surgery (see **Table B-18**).[52] We are less concerned about publication bias with tubal than with vas surgery for permanent contraception because the largest studies of tubal surgery are based on prospective, multicenter clinical trials, not retrospective reports from one investigator. An increasing proportion of surgeons are favoring bilateral salpingectomy compared to other methods of tubal surgery in recent years, primarily due to evidence that a significant proportion of ovarian cancers originate in the distal fallopian tube.[53] Large prospective efficacy studies have not been performed; however, presumably this method is more effective than other methods of female permanent contraception.[54]

Typical and Perfect Use of Intrauterine Devices. All typical-use and perfect-use pregnancy rates for the hormonal formulations are low, below 1%, and to reinforce our caution not to put any emphasis on the differences among these very small probabilities, we have generalized the estimates to the average across the four formulations: 0.3 for perfect use and 0.4 for typical use. The formulation-specific rates are described below and in **Table B-14**.

The estimate for typical use of the copper-bearing IUD (0.8%) is taken directly from the largest study for Paragard.[55] Typical-use estimates for Mirena (52 mg LNG) (0.7%) and Skyla (13.5 mg LNG) (0.4%), come from the largest studies of these methods.[56,57] The typical-use estimates for Kyleena (19.5 mg LNG) (0.2%) and Liletta (52 mg LNG) (0.1%) are taken from the only studies of these methods.[57,58]

Perfect-use rates for IUDs are calculated for devices that remain in position, excluding pregnancies that occurred after expulsion. The estimate for perfect use of the Paragard (0.6%) was obtained by removing the pregnancies that resulted when the device was not known to be in situ from the numerator of the pregnancy rate.[59] The perfect-use estimates for Mirena (0.5%), Skyla (0.3%), and Kyleena (0.2%) were derived under the assumption that the same proportions of pregnancies during contraceptive use occurred when the device had been expelled (25%). No differences in the typical-use and perfect-use estimates for Kyleena are apparent due to the fact that only one significant digit is shown. The perfect-use rate for Liletta (0.1%) was obtained by removing the one pregnancy that occurred after an expulsion. None of these studies focused on postpartum or postabortion IUD placements, which have higher expulsion rates.[60,61]

Typical Use of DMPA Injectable, Oral Contraceptive Pills, External (Male) Condom, and Withdrawal. Our estimates of the probability of pregnancy during the first year of typical use for DMPA (4%), the oral contraceptive pill (7%), the external (male) condom (12.6%), and withdrawal (20%) are derived from the 2006–2010 NSFG corrected for under-reporting of abortion.[17] These current estimates are generally lower than the previous estimates derived from the 2002 NSFG (also corrected for abortion under-reporting), except withdrawal (19.9% vs. 18.4%). The most notable change in the estimated probability of pregnancy is for the male condom (12.6% vs. 17.4%).[62]

The NSFG does not ask for brand of pill; thus, combined and progestin-only pills cannot be distinguished. However, since use of the combined oral contraceptive (COC) pill is far more common than use of the progestin-only pill (POP), the results from the NSFG overwhelmingly reflect typical use of COCs.[63] The pregnancy rates of progestin-only pills may be higher than that for combined pills since northindrone-containing progestin-only pills are probably less forgiving of nonadherence to the dosing schedule. (See Chapter 9, Contraceptive Implant.) However, DRSP-containing POPs suppress ovulation and are more forgiving of inconsistent pill use.[64]

Typical and Perfect Use of the Contraceptive Patch and Vaginal Ring. The typical-use (7%) and perfect-use (0.3%) estimates for transdermal patches (Xulane and Twirla) and contraceptive vaginal rings (NuvaRing and Annovera) were set equal to those for combination hormonal pills. It is possible that the patch and ring will prove to have lower pregnancy rates than the pill during typical use because of better adherence with the dosing schedule. However, such superior efficacy has not been demonstrated in randomized trials. Two large-scale systematic reviews and meta-analyses of randomized trials found no significant differences in efficacy between the patch, ring, and COCs,[65] nor between the ring and COCs.[66] Formulations of the patch (2.6 mg levonorgestrel and 2.3 mg ethinyl estradiol; Twirla) and the 13-cycle ring (delivering 0.15 mg segesterone acetate and 0.013 mg ethinyl estradiol per day; Annovera) that have become available since these systematic reviews were conducted so far do not show efficacy profiles that are substantially different than the formulations included in the reviews. Note that patches are restricted to use among people with body mass index (BMI) < 30. (See the section on differences in effectiveness by body weight, p. 151.)

Typical and Perfect Use of Fertility Awareness-Based Methods (FABMs). Numerous kinds of FABMs exist; each relies upon tracking different indicators (for example, day of menstrual cycle, or cervical secretions, or basal body temperature, or urinary hormones, or some combination of these) and using different rules for interpreting that information. Typical-use pregnancy rates for most individual FABMs are challenging to estimate in national surveys in the United States given relatively few users of each. Furthermore, several clinical trials have used inappropriate methodological approaches for calculating perfect-use pregnancy rate estimates. A systematic review published in 2018 identified at least 14 different FABMs for which published evidence exists[67]; additional FABMs have also come onto the market since then. As it would be impractical to list all FABMs in summary Table 5-2, we list a subset of FABMs (Sensiplan, Natural Cycles, Clue, Standard Days Method, Billings Ovulation method, and calendar rhythm); detail on effectiveness for other FABMs is available in Chapter 15.

Probabilities of pregnancy during typical and perfect use for Sensiplan (2% typical use; 0.4% perfect use), the Standard Days method (13% typical use; 5% perfect use), and the Billings Ovulation Method (23% typical use; 3% perfect use) are taken from the only clinical studies of these methods that also contain correctly computed perfect-use pregnancy rate estimates, and which were rated moderate quality in the 2018 systematic review.[68-70] The only study on Clue Birth Control,[71] and three of four studies on Natural Cycles,[72-75] have not yet been formally assessed for quality in a systematic review. For Clue, we use pregnancy rates used by the FDA (8% typical use and 3% perfect use). For Natural Cycles, we use the typical-use lifetable-derived pregnancy rate of 7% used by the FDA, which also aligns with two recently published studies.[74,75] There is no published lifetable perfect-use estimate for Natural Cycles; the Pearl Index estimate cited by the FDA is 1.8.[76]

Estimates for calendar rhythm are derived from population-based surveys. In the 2006–2010 NSFG, among women who report using either "rhythm or safe period by calendar" or "safe period by temperature or cervical mucus test, natural family planning," over 80% of observations were for "rhythm or safe period by calendar," and 15% are expected to experience pregnancy while using one of these FABMs during the first year of use (after adjustment for under-reporting of abortion).[17] This specific 15% estimate was unpublished, because the 257 observations did not meet the prespecified minimum of 50 observations at each month for the first 12 months. It is substantially lower than the estimate derived from the previous (2002) NSFG (24%)[68]; it is unclear if this change relates to instability in the estimates given the small number of women reporting use of these methods, to improved use of these methods between the two survey periods, or to other factors. The international estimate of 19% is based on a sample of 7,859 women, and is not adjusted for under-reporting of abortion.

Perfect Use of the External (Male) Condom. Our estimate of the probability of pregnancy during a year of perfect use of the external condom is based on results from the only three studies of the external condom meeting modern standards of design, execution, and analysis.[77-79] In each study, couples were randomly assigned to use either a latex condom or a polyurethane condom. All three studies reported pregnancy rates during consistent use but only one reported pregnancy rates during perfect use[78]; in that study the six-cycle probability of pregnancy during perfect use (0.7%) was 70% of that (1%) during typical use. We assumed that in the other two studies the six-cycle probability of pregnancy during perfect use would also be 70% during typical use, assumed that the pregnancy rate per cycle during perfect use would be constant, extrapolated a 1-year probability from the six-cycle probability reported for the latex condom in each trial, and took as our estimate the median (2%, also the mean) of those three estimates. This estimate is consistent with an estimate based on studies of condom breakage and slippage.[80] Under the assumption that 1.5% of condoms break or slip off the penis and that individuals have intercourse twice a week, then about 1.5% of users relying on this method would experience condom breaks during the half-week that they are at risk of pregnancy during each cycle. The per-cycle probability of conception would be reduced by 98.5%, from 0.1358 to only 0.0020, if a condom failure results in no protection whatsoever against pregnancy, so that about 2.6% of users at risk for pregnancy would become pregnant each year.[81] Unfortunately, breakage and slippage rates did not accurately predict pregnancy rates during consistent use in one clinical trial of the latex and polyurethane external (male) condom,[77] and estimates of condom breakage and slippage during intercourse or withdrawal vary substantially across studies in developed countries, from a low of 0.6% among commercial sex workers in Nevada's legal brothels[80] to a high of 7.2% among monogamous couples in North Carolina.[82]

Typical and Perfect Use of the Sponge. Our estimates of the probabilities of pregnancy during the first year of typical and perfect use of the sponge correspond with results of a reanalysis of data from a clinical trial in which participants were randomly assigned to use the diaphragm or sponge.[83] The probability of pregnancy during typical use was 17%. The probability of pregnancy during typical use among parous users (27.4%) was twice as high as that among nulliparous users (14.0%). The results indicate that within the first year of perfect use, the range of pregnancy rates with sponge use will be 11.4% to 12.0% among all users, 19.4% to 20.5% among parous users, and 9.0% to 9.5% among nulliparous users. We take as our estimate the midpoints of these ranges: 12%, 20%, and 9%, respectively.[84]

Typical and Perfect Use of the Diaphragm. Results are based on the only clinical trial of the Caya diaphragm (formerly called SILCS), used with contraceptive gel.[85] That study estimated a 6-month probability of pregnancy during typical use of 10.4%; from this we extrapolated a 12-month probability of 17.4% under the assumption that the probability of pregnancy during the second 6 months is 75% of that in the first 6 months (the median of the four estimates for the sponge, cap, and diaphragm).[86] During perfect use, we extrapolated the six-cycle probability of 7.9% to a 13-cycle probability of 16.3%, under the assumption that the per-cycle probability remains constant under perfect use. Unlike the sponge and cervical cap, effectiveness of the diaphragm does not appear to vary between parous and nulliparous users.[84]

The only other diaphragms currently available in the United States are Milex: Arcing and Omniflex. These are made of silicone and have been available in the United States since the late 1970s; before that time, diaphragms were made of latex. There are no published efficacy studies. The latest estimate of the probability of pregnancy during typical use of the Ortho (now discontinued) and Milex diaphragms is based on the 1995 NSFG; use of the Ortho diaphragm has virtually disappeared, and would not reflect the experience of current users of Milex.[28] A recent systematic review found no differences in effectiveness between newer and older types of diaphragms [87]

Perfect Use of Withdrawal. Our estimate of the proportion becoming pregnant during a year of perfect use of withdrawal (4%) is simply a guess based on the reasoning that the risk of pregnancy resulting from pre-ejaculatory fluid is modest. Although three studies found no motile sperm in the pre-ejaculate,[88-90] the most recent study did not replicate this result, perhaps because the samples were examined within 2 minutes of production.[91] In that study, 37% of participants produced pre-ejaculatory samples that contained motile sperm, and the sperm concentration and the percentage of motile sperm were similar in an individual's pre-ejaculatory and ejaculatory specimens. However, the volume of the pre-ejaculate and therefore, the actual number of sperm, in the pre-ejaculate was low.

Typical and Perfect Use of the Internal (Female) Condom. The typical-use pregnancy rate estimate for the internal (female) condom is based on the results of a 6-month clinical trial of the FC condom, formerly called Reality condom; 12.4% of study participants in the United States experienced a pregnancy during the first 6 months of use.[86] We extrapolated the 12-month probability of pregnancy for users of FC condoms in the United States (21%) under the assumption that the probability of pregnancy during the second 6 months is 75% of that in the first 6 months.[86] The probability of pregnancy during 6 months of perfect use of FC by US participants who met the adherence criteria stipulated in the study protocol was 2.6%. Those who reported fewer than four acts of intercourse during the month prior to any follow-up visit, who did not use at every act of intercourse, who at any time reported not following the instructions, or who used another method of contraception were censored (results not included in calculations) at the beginning of the first interval where nonadherence was noted.[92] Under the assumption that the probability of pregnancy in the second 6 months of perfect use would be the same, the probability of pregnancy during a year of perfect use would be 5.1%. There have been no efficacy trials of the currently used second version of the internal condom (the FC2 female condom).

Typical and Perfect Use of Vaginal pH Regulators (Phexxi). Phexxi, a vaginal pH regulator consisting of lactic acid, citric acid, and potassium bitartrate (called Amphora in clinical trials), was approved by the FDA in 2020 for contraception. The sole published clinical study included 1,834 participants assigned to use 5-mg pre-filled vaginal applicators of the drug and found a seven-cycle typical-use pregnancy rate of 13.7%.[93] We extrapolate this to a 13-cycle pregnancy rate of 21% using the assumption that the per-cycle rate for cycles 8–13 is 75% of that for cycles 1–7.[86] There are no peer-reviewed estimates of perfect-use pregnancy rates with Phexxi, at the time of this writing. The Phexxi health care provider website refers to seven-cycle perfect use pregnancy rate of 6.7%.[94] Using the standard assumption that the per-cycle pregnancy rate during perfect use would be constant, we calculate a 13-cycle perfect-use pregnancy rate of 11.9%.

Typical and Perfect Use of Spermicides. Our estimate of the proportion of users becoming pregnant during a year of typical use of spermicides (21%) is based on a randomized National Institutes of Health (NIH) trial of five spermicides.[95] We extrapolated a 1-year pregnancy probability from the 6-month pregnancy probability reported for each method by assuming the probability of pregnancy in the second 6 months would be 75% of that in the first 6 months,[86] and took as our estimate the mean of the four estimates of products still marketed (excluding the 52.5 mg gel).

Our estimate of the proportion becoming pregnant during 1 year of perfect use of spermicides (16%) is based on the same NIH trial of five spermicides.[95] We assumed that the pregnancy rate per cycle during perfect use would be constant, extrapolated a 1-year pregnancy probability from the six-cycle pregnancy probability reported for each method, and took as our estimate the mean of the four estimates of products still marketed (excluding the 52.5 mg gel). Our estimate is considerably higher than would be expected from the extensive literature on the contraceptive efficacy of spermicides.

Six studies outside the United States,[96-101] in addition to several US studies,[22] have yielded very low probabilities of pregnancy during the first year of typical use of spermicides, much lower than any estimates for barriers with spermicides. The efficacy literature on spermicides in general is dominated by studies of suppositories, foams, and film; high spermicide efficacy is documented only in these studies. There are few studies of creams and gels used alone, and those with the lowest pregnancy rates are more than 30 years old (**Table A-3**). We consider it likely that the spermicide studies suffer from flaws in analysis or design that are not apparent in the brief published descriptions. For example, an FDA advisory committee was openly skeptical of one German study:[96] "the way in which the survey was designed and the manner in which the various incentives were offered" (physicians reportedly received a fee for completing *q* data forms) "would clearly make the data resulting from the survey unacceptable to any scientific group or regulatory agency."[102,103]

The first clinical trial of Emko vaginal foam is also one of the few studies to compute separate pregnancy rates for cycles in which the product was used at every act of intercourse and for cycles in which unprotected intercourse occurred.[104] The design of that trial was also quite sophisticated. Study participants were randomly assigned to six groups. Each group used three different spermicidal products for three cycles each. The six groups represented all possible permutations of orders of use of the three products. If the pregnancy rate for three cycles of consistent use (not perfect use, which requires both consistent *and* correct use) of Emko vaginal foam is extrapolated, then the implied proportion becoming pregnant in the first year of consistent use is 8.9%.

A randomized clinical trial comparing the efficacy of a film and a foaming tablet—the first trial of spermicides conducted according to modern standards of design, execution, and analysis—supports the conclusion that the pregnancy rate with spermicides is considerably higher than was previously thought.[105] In that trial, 6-month probabilities of pregnancy during consistent use were 28% for the tablet and 24% for the film, probabilities that were nearly identical to those during typical use and about the same as the 12-month probability of pregnancy during typical use of spermicides in the 2002 NSFG (the most recent estimate).[106]

Typical and Perfect Use of the Cervical Cap. The typical- and perfect-use pregnancy rates of the FemCap, the only cervical cap currently on the market in the United States, come from the Phase II/III randomized trial of 841 participants.[107] The study found a Kaplan-Meier 6-month typical use pregnancy rate of 13.5. We extrapolated to a 12-month typical use pregnancy rate of 22.3, under the assumption that the rate for months 7–12 is 75% of the rate for months 1–6.[86] The same study calculated a six-cycle perfect-use life-table pregnancy rate of 11.1. We extrapolated this to a 13-cycle perfect use pregnancy rate, under the standard assumption that the pregnancy rate during perfect use is constant, of 22%.

The cervical cap comes in different sizes for different parity/delivery status. Pregnancy rates (only available for typical use) appear to vary with parity, based on an unpublished study referenced in the FDA product insert. Nulligravid study participants using the 22-mm cap experienced a 14% pregnancy rate. The same rate of 14% was found among parous individuals who delivered nonvaginally, using a 26-mm cap. Parous individuals with vaginal birth(s) were assigned a 30-mm cap; their pregnancy rate during typical use was 29%.[108] A recent systematic review found no differences in effectiveness between newer and older types of cervical caps.[87]

No Method. Our estimate of the percentage of individuals becoming pregnant among those not using contraception is based on populations not using contraception (Hutterites), and on individuals in clinical studies who stopped using contraceptives because they wanted to conceive. **Table A-2** summarizes the studies of the 12-month probability of pregnancy among these individuals. None of these is ideal for our needs, since all but one were studies of those planning a pregnancy after stopping contraceptive use. What we want is an estimate of the fraction of individuals now using contraception who would become pregnant if contraception simply vanished and people did not alter their sexual behavior. Perhaps the most relevant is the study among Hutterites, an Anabaptist sect that does not use contraception, in which the estimate is 88.8%.[109] However, this is an estimate of pregnancies leading to the first live birth among married cisgender women who reported no fetal losses. The proportion would be higher if those with fetal losses were included. However, this group of women was young, with a median age at marriage of 21, so presumably having a higher-than-average rate of fertility. Therefore, we arbitrarily lowered our pregnancy rate estimate to 85%. This estimate is certainly on the high end of the range of plausible estimates: 80%, 75%, and 70% are also plausible.

Available evidence in the United States suggests that only 40% to 60% of individuals at risk for pregnancy who do not use contraception (but who still wish to avoid pregnancy) become pregnant within 1 year.[62,110] However, such individuals are almost certainly self-selected for low fecundity, low frequency of intercourse, or perhaps they report no contraceptive use with a method but they are in fact preventing pregnancy with nonpenetrative sex or intermittently avoiding intravaginal contact with sperm during fertile times. They may not use contraception because, in part, they are aware that they are unlikely to conceive based on prior experiences of not getting pregnant despite not using contraception. The probability of pregnancy of 85%, therefore, is our best guess of the fraction of individuals currently using reversible methods of contraception who would become pregnant within 1 year if they were to discontinue contraception but not otherwise change their behavior. Individuals who have regular unprotected intercourse for a year without achieving pregnancy are clinically defined as infertile (but by no means are they necessarily incapable of pregnancy or childbearing).

Effectiveness Over Time

We focus attention on the first-year probabilities of pregnancy solely because probabilities for longer durations are generally not available. There are three main points to remember about the effectiveness of contraceptive methods over time.

First, the risk of pregnancy during either perfect or typical use of a method should remain constant over time *for an individual with a specific partner*, providing that underlying fecundity and frequency of intercourse do not change (both fecundity and coital frequency do generally decline as individuals age, but we assume they are held constant when calculating risk over the first year of use). It is possible, however, that the risk of pregnancy could decline during typical use of certain methods because the individual learns to use the method correctly and consistently.

Second, in contrast, the risk of pregnancy during typical use of a method will decline over time *for a group of users*, primarily because those users who are most prone to fail do so early, due to higher fecundity, incorrect or inconsistent method use, and/or higher coital frequency, leaving a pool of contraceptive users who may be at lower risk. This decline will be far less pronounced among users of those methods with little or no margin for imperfect use. The risk of pregnancy during perfect use for a group of users should decline as well, but this decline will not be as pronounced as that during typical use, because only the relatively more fecund and those with higher coital frequency are selected out early. For these reasons, the probability of becoming pregnant during the second year of use of a contraceptive method will be lower than the probability of becoming pregnant during the first year of use.[111]

Third, probabilities of pregnancy accumulate over time. Suppose that 10%, 6%, and 4% of people using a method become pregnant during years 1, 2, and 3, respectively. The probability of not becoming pregnant within 3 years is calculated by multiplying the probabilities of *not becoming pregnant* for each of the 3 years: 0.90 times 0.94 times 0.96, which equals 0.81. Thus, the percentage becoming pregnant within 3 years is 19% (= 100% – 81%).

The *differences* among probabilities of pregnancy for various methods will increase over time. For example, consider the typical-use pregnancy estimates for the diaphragm (17%) with Phexxi (21%), a difference of 4 percentage points. Assuming that the typical-use pregnancy rates for a group of individuals decline by 2 percentage points each year, after 3 years, an estimated 39% of diaphragm users will have become pregnant, compared to an estimated 47% of Phexxi users. After 3 years, the difference in pregnancy rates between methods has doubled to 8 percentage points.

The number of pregnancies (contraceptive failures) in a lifetime have been calculated using previous NSFG surveys. Based on data reported in 1995, the typical woman who used reversible methods of contraception continuously from age 15 to age 45 would experience 1.8 pregnancies. Increased use of more effective methods of contraception will reduce this number; however, given that probabilities of pregnancy during contraceptive use accumulate over time, this figure will never be zero.

Simultaneous Use of Methods

Using two different methods at once dramatically lowers the risk of pregnancy, provided they are used consistently. If one of the methods is a condom, protection from sexually transmitted infection (STI) is an added benefit. It is worth noting that none of the methods in category 1 or 2 provides protection against STIs; patients who wish to effectively prevent both pregnancy and STI transmission may want to use a barrier and another method simultaneously. For example, perfect use of both condoms and spermicides together is highly effective for pregnancy prevention and protects against STIs. The probabilities of pregnancy during the first year of perfect use of external (male) condoms and spermicides are estimated to be 2% and 16%, respectively, in Table 5-2. It is reasonable to assume that during perfect use, the contraceptive mechanisms of condoms and spermicides operate independently, since lack of independence during typical use would most likely be due to imperfect use (either use both methods or use neither). The annual probability of pregnancy during simultaneous perfect use of condoms and spermicides would be 0.3%,[§] about the same as that achieved by the oral contraceptive pill (0.3%) during perfect use.[81]

Nearly one in five (18%) contraceptive users reported simultaneous use of at least two contraceptive methods at last sex.[112] Dual method use is an important strategy that can improve effectiveness, especially for patients who prefer not to use methods in category 1 or 2. During the postpartum period, counseling should also highlight the potential for dual method use with Lactational Amenorrhea Method (LAM).

Factors that Influence Reported Effectiveness

Our understanding of contraceptive effectiveness is influenced by four primary factors: (1) the inherent efficacy of the method when used correctly and consistently (perfect use), (2) the attributes of the method that facilitate or interfere with correct and consistent use (leading to imperfect use), (3) characteristics of the user, and (4) the quality of published evidence.

---

§ The probabilities multiply, thus the calculation is 1– (1 – 2% × 16%) = 0.3%.

Inherent Method Efficacy

Inherent method efficacy refers to how effective the method is when used perfectly. Methods in the top category are inherently highly effective and user-independent: there is little for the user to do (or not do) that would affect method effectiveness. The inherent efficacy of combined hormonal contraceptives and injectables is also quite high, but these methods are user-dependent, requiring the user to repeatedly use the method on a daily, weekly, monthly, or every 3-month schedule. Methods in the third category have both lower inherent efficacy and are completely user-dependent, requiring correct use at each coital act.

Imperfect Use

Imperfect use refers to any use that is not consistent with the manufacturer's instructions. After inherent efficacy, imperfect use has the greatest effect on the probability of pregnancy while using a method. Examples of imperfect use include missed pills, delayed start of a new pack of pills, missed injections, or incorrect placement of a diaphragm. Reproductive desires are complex, nuanced, and change over time; some individuals may prefer not to get pregnant but do not have strong motivation to prevent pregnancy or use their methods correctly and consistently; some have ambivalence about pregnancy at a given moment, leading them to not use their method for a specific act of intercourse. Many factors that can result in imperfect use are often outside of an individual's control. Individuals may not receive adequate instructions or may receive incorrect information from a health care provider. Others may act on misinformation provided on social media platforms or by friends. There are many systemic issues that can lead to imperfect use, including barriers in obtaining contraceptive refills and lack of access to a health care provider.[113]

User Characteristics

Characteristics of the user can affect both inherent method efficacy and imperfect use. The pregnancy rate for any method will vary by user characteristics, but the impact will be greatest for methods with the highest pregnancy rates during typical use, either because the method has less inherent efficacy or because it is hard to use consistently or correctly. This section reviews several important user characteristics that impact contraceptive effectiveness, but this is not an exhaustive list. Less common factors, such as drug interactions and medical conditions, can also be important to consider for an individual.[114]

Age. Many studies have found that pregnancy rates decline with age, meaning contraceptive effectiveness essentially increases.[19,23,106,115,116] This association is certainly driven by biological fecundity and coital frequency, both of which usually decline with age (see Frequency of Intercourse). The decrease in pregnancy rates with increasing age may also reflect older users' increased familiarity with and ability to correctly use contraceptive methods. Because of these fertility rates decline with increasing age, those over age 35 are often excluded from calculations of method efficacy in clinical trials.

Figure 5-3, which comes from a multicountry study using DHS data collected from women ages 15–49 in 15 low- and middle-income countries, demonstrates the substantially higher pregnancy rates among the youngest compared to older

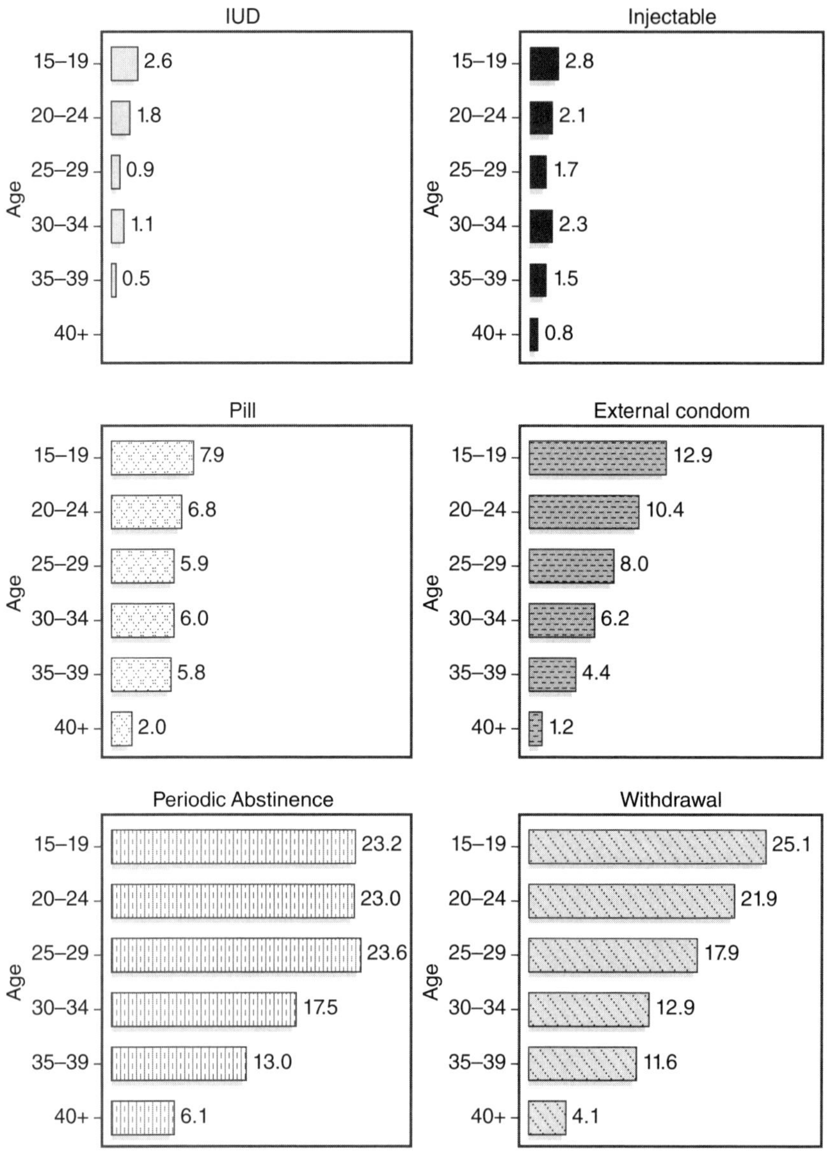

Figure 5-3 Typical-use 12-month pregnancy rates by age and contraceptive method from demographic and health surveys.

Reproduced from Bradley SEK, Polis CB, Bankole A, Croft T. Global Contraceptive Failure Rates: Who Is Most at Risk? Stud Fam Plann 2019;50(1):3-24. (In eng). DOI: 10.1111/sifp.12085.

users, a pattern that holds across contraceptive methods.[23,117] Individuals aged 15–19 consistently experience the highest rates of pregnancy, and women older than 40 the lowest. Differences in pregnancy rates by age for users of the same method are substantial: 12.9% of condom users aged 15–19 experienced pregnancy in 1 year of use, more than 10 times the rate of women aged 40 and older (1.2%). The pregnancy rate for pill users is 8% for 15- to 19-year-olds, compared to 2% for users older than 40. Periodic abstinence users (which comprise calendar and other fertility awareness–based methods) ages 15–19 experienced a 23.2% pregnancy rate, almost four times higher than the 6.1% of women in their 40s. Withdrawal users aged 15–19 have rates that are six times higher, compared to women in their 40s: 25% versus 4%. Though these are not US-based data, these patterns by age are largely consistent with multiple other US-based studies including those based on the NSFG, which has a smaller sample size that precludes analysts from calculating detailed age-specific rates.[17,19,28,106,110]

Frequency of Intercourse. Among those who use a method consistently and correctly (perfect users), the most important user characteristic that determines the risk of pregnancy is frequency of exposure to that risk through penile-vaginal intercourse. As definitions for intercourse vary widely, here we use this term generally to indicate actions with the potential for sperm to enter the uterus and fallopian tube(s). In a study in which users were randomly assigned to either the diaphragm or the sponge, diaphragm users who had intercourse four or more times a week became pregnant in the first year twice as frequently as those who had intercourse fewer than four times a week.[83] In that clinical trial, among women who used the diaphragm at every act of intercourse, only 3.4% of those who had intercourse fewer than three times a week became pregnant in the first year, compared with 9.7% of those who had intercourse three or more times per week. Coital frequency for many people is strongly associated with age, declining as individuals and their partners grow older and with relationship duration.[118]

Biologic Fecundity. The probability of conception per coital act decreases substantially with age.[119-121] The decline in ovarian reserve is moderate until a woman reaches her late thirties.[119] Risk of tubal factor infertility also increases with age among women who are exposed to STIs such as gonorrhea and chlamydia. The biologic fecundity and sperm quality of partners also decline with age.[122,123] Regular menstrual cycles are one proxy measure for fecundity. Women with regular cycles were 7.2 times as likely as women with irregular cycles (one or more cycles < 17 days or > 43 days) to become pregnant while using the internal (female) condom.[124]

Social Determinants of Health Such as Race and Income. Several studies have found higher pregnancy rates during contraceptive use among Black and Hispanic users compared to non-Hispanic White individuals.[17,28,106] For example, in the most recent analysis of NSFG data, Black condom users experienced pregnancy at more than twice the rate of White users (20.7 versus 8.7 pregnancies per 100 women, respectively).[17] Pregnancy rates during contraceptive use are also frequently found to be associated with poverty, with women in families with low incomes experiencing higher rates.[17,23,28,106] These findings likely reflect differences in health care access, lower quality care, negative experiences with and lack of trust in health care providers, and many other barriers experienced by contraceptive users in these groups. In addition, individuals have varying levels of motivation to prevent pregnancy yet often do not feel supported in expressing their nuanced reproductive desires that may seem incongruent or ill advised to their provider. Hence, an individual may be categorized as, for example, a "condom user" but in fact may not feel a strong need to consistently protect against pregnancy. This person could be erroneously categorized as experiencing a pregnancy while using contraception or as having an unintended pregnancy even though becoming pregnant is acceptable to (but perhaps not actively sought by) them. (See Chapter 4, Person-Centered Reproductive Health Conversations and Contraceptive Counseling.)

Access to Reproductive Health Services. Multiple studies have shown strong associations between access to reproductive health services, including insurance, and contraceptive use and continuation.[5,125] Patients cannot use methods consistently and correctly if they face transportation or cost barriers returning to clinics for repeat injections, to pharmacies for pills, and/or stores for condoms. Cost may also be a barrier to selecting certain methods, especially implants and IUDs, if patients cannot access sufficient insurance. Social norms, provider biases, dispensing patterns, and prohibitive policies and guidelines are also factors that can hinder access to reproductive health services.

User Motivation. Contraceptive users who are highly motivated to avoid pregnancy may be more likely to use a method consistently and correctly.[126,127] However, even if a current pregnancy would be unacceptable to someone, they would not have a reason to take steps to avoid pregnancy if they did not perceive that they are at risk of becoming pregnant.[128,129] Motivation to avoid pregnancy often changes over time and is related to the complex attitudes people have regarding pregnancy and their perceived risk of becoming pregnant in their specific circumstances. Pregnancy desires are not binary and cannot be accurately categorized within the limited designations of "intended" or "unintended"; a person can be relatively indifferent and report that they are not seeking pregnancy, yet if they were to become pregnant it would be acceptable to them (or they would be happy). Ambivalence can also arise depending on an individual's relationship, financial, or social situation including cost of childcare and missed career opportunities.

One study documenting the impact of user motivation comes from a comparison of perfect-and typical-use pregnancy rates with pregnancy rates observed among women using isotretinoin, which is effective in treating severe acne but is also teratogenic. To minimize pregnancies among women undergoing treatment, the manufacturer and the FDA implemented a pregnancy prevention program. Among 76,149 participants who reported using contraception, 268 became pregnant, yielding a rate of 3.6 per 1,000 20-week courses of therapy;[130] this rate, if constant for a year, would be equivalent to an annual probability of pregnancy of 0.9%. The estimated annual probabilities of pregnancy were 0.8%, 2.1%, and 2.6% among those who reported using oral contraceptives, diaphragms, and condoms, respectively. Thus, individuals using diaphragms achieved lower rates of pregnancy than we estimate would occur during perfect use, and those using condoms and oral contraceptives experienced about the same pregnancy rates that would be expected during perfect use. Pregnancy rates for individuals using any of these three methods, however, were substantially below rates generally observed during typical use; this finding would appear to indicate that users' understanding of the teratogenic risks of isotretinoin substantially enhanced correct and consistent use. It is also possible that participants in this study had lower than average fecundity (because acne is a marker for excess androgen production associated with anovulation[131]), that they lowered their coital frequency during treatment, or that they under-reported their number of pregnancies (and abortions).

Body Weight. Clinicians and patients often raise concerns that weight may decrease the efficacy of hormonal contraceptive methods. Pharmacokinetic data indicate differences associated with obesity, such as increased metabolic rate and volume of distribution, affecting time to achieve therapeutic contraceptive hormone levels and steady state hormone levels.[132] Unfortunately, early clinical trials for hormonal methods excluded participants with overweight and obesity due to the potential for greater venous thromboembolism (VTE) risk, limiting data on efficacy. For most hormonal contraceptive methods, effectiveness does not appear to be significantly associated with weight, despite small differences in hormone levels.[133] However, the levonorgestrel and ethinyl estradiol transdermal patches are contraindicated and should not be used in individuals with a BMI over 30 kg/m^2, given increased pregnancy risk in clinical trials.[134] Data on the effectiveness of the oral contraceptive pill among participants with a BMI > 30 kg/m^2 versus individuals of normal weight are inconsistent, with some studies showing an increase in pregnancy risk[135,136] and others showing no difference.[137] Body weight also affects medical comorbidities that are important to consider when determining which methods of contraception are safe for an individual.[114] Concerns about weight gain may also influence choice of methods.[138]

Quality of Published Evidence

When the published evidence is of poor quality, we cannot rely on it to help inform contraceptive decision making. The reasons for poor quality data range from simple arithmetical mistakes to improper design or execution or analysis of studies to outright fraud.[22]

Fraud. One well-documented instance of fraud involved the Dalkon shield. In a two-page article published in the *American Journal of Obstetrics and Gynecology*, a first-year probability of pregnancy of 1.1% was presented and the claim made that "only the combined type of oral contraceptive offers slightly greater protection."[139] It was not revealed by the researcher that some participants had been instructed to use spermicides as an adjunctive method to reduce the risk of pregnancy, nor that he was part-owner of the Dalkon Corporation. Furthermore, he never subsequently revealed (except to the A.H. Robins Company, which bought the shield from the Dalkon Corporation but did not reveal this information either) that as the original trial matured, the first-year probability of pregnancy more than doubled.[140]

Discrepancies in Presentation of Information. When comparing contraceptive method effectiveness, researchers compare typical-use to typical-use rates (or perfect-use to perfect-use rates). Similarly, effectiveness data presented in counseling tools and advertisements should use a standard 12-month rate used for all other methods to avoid confusing providers and clients alike. At the time of this writing, Phexxi's advertising presents a seven-cycle rate, rather than the 12-month or 13-cycle rate used by all other contraceptive methods, which has in some cases led to an erroneous understanding of Phexxi's effectiveness. The "health care professionals" portion of the Phexxi website, in very small font, states: "The effectiveness rates described above should not be compared to other contraceptive methods with different trial designs and study duration beyond 7 cycles".[141] However, the consumer-facing portion of the Phexxi website does not provide any information explaining the rates are from a seven-cycle study and should not be compared to pregnancy rates of other methods that present annual pregnancy rates. As a result, several articles and websites have drawn incorrect conclusions based on the comparison. For example, a STEPS New Drug Review article compares the seven-cycle Phexxi pregnancy rates with a table of 1-year rates for other methods and assumes Phexxi is comparable in effectiveness to condoms (which are more effective, at 13% typical use).[142] If the 1-year 21% typical-use rate estimate was included in the table, Phexxi would be equal to other spermicides.

Other manufacturers, including those of basal body temperature mini-computer Daysy® have also made claims about effectiveness that were not based on a standard 1-year prospective methodology used in other studies.[143,144]

What Gets Published. The incentives to conduct research on contraceptive failure vary widely from method to method. Many studies of the pill and IUD exist because companies wishing to market them must conduct clinical trials to demonstrate their efficacy. In contrast, few studies of withdrawal exist because there is no financial reward for investigating this method. Moreover, researchers face differing incentives to report unfavorable results. The vasectomy literature is filled with short articles by clinicians who have performed 500 or 1,000 or 1,500 vasectomies. When they report pregnancies (pregnancy is seldom mentioned in discussions of vasectomy "failures," which focus on the continued presence of sperm in the ejaculate), their pregnancy rates are invariably low. Likewise, drug companies do not commonly publicize their failures. Even if investigators prepared reports describing failures, journal editors may not be likely to publish them. Current requirements to register trials (e.g., clinicaltrials.gov) aim to decrease publication bias.

Analytical Pitfalls

Several analytical pitfalls can snare investigators. Three of the most common are (1) comparing trials with different frequency of pregnancy testing, (2) the incorrect calculation of method failure rates, and (3) failure to follow up participants in a trial. Other, more technical, errors that have biased reported results are discussed in other publications.[145,146]

Inconsistent Frequency of Pregnancy Testing Across Studies. In population-based surveys and in older clinical trials, individuals reported whether they became pregnant in a specific month. By contrast, in some recent clinical trials, sensitive pregnancy tests were administered every month and whenever the participant had symptoms. The number of pregnancies (and hence the pregnancy rate) therefore increased because early pregnancy losses not clinically noted by the study participant are added to the number of observed pregnancies. More frequent pregnancy testing in the more recent contraceptive trials has resulted in higher pregnancy rates than would otherwise have been obtained and makes the results not comparable to those from older trials and population-based surveys.

Incorrect Calculation of Pregnancy Rates. Some studies separate pregnancies occurring during perfect and imperfect use to calculate "method" and "user" failure rates. Some investigators have calculated these rates incorrectly.

By convention, pregnancies that occur during a month in which a method was used improperly are classified as user failures (even though, logically, a pregnancy might be due to failure of the method, if it was used correctly on some occasions and incorrectly on others), and pregnancies that occurred with correct and consistent use are classified as method failures. But investigators do not always separate the exposure (the denominator in the calculation of failure rates) into these two groups.

For example, suppose that two method failures and eight user failures occur during 100 woman-years of exposure to the risk of pregnancy. Then the common calculation is that the user failure rate is 8% and the method failure rate is 2%; the sum of the two is the overall failure rate of 10%. By definition, however, method failures can occur only during perfect use and user failures cannot occur during perfect use. If there are 50 years of perfect use and 50 years of imperfect use in the total of 100 years of exposure, then the method failure rate would be 4% and the user failure rate would be 16%. The difference between the two rates (here 12%) provides a measure of how forgiving of imperfect use the method is. However, if investigators do not inquire about perfect use except when a pregnancy occurs, the proper calculations cannot be performed.

Loss to Follow-up. The standard assumption made at the time of analysis is that individuals who are lost to follow-up (LFU) experience pregnancy at the same rate as those who are observed. This assumption is probably innocuous when the proportion LFU is small. But in many studies the proportion LFU may be 20% or higher, so that what really happens to these individuals could drastically affect the estimate of the proportion becoming pregnant. Our strong suspicion is that those who are LFU are more likely to experience pregnancy than are those who remain in the trial. For example, one study found that the pregnancy rate for calendar rhythm rose from 9.4 to 14.4 per 100 woman-years of exposure as a result of resolution of cases LFU.[147]

Pitfalls and Challenges of Communicating Pregnancy Risk

Most people seeking contraception believe effectiveness is one of the most important factors—often the most important factor—when choosing a contraceptive method or methods.[148-152] Yet general knowledge about absolute and relative effectiveness is often low, and patients may underestimate the effectiveness of IUDs and implants, and overestimate the effectiveness of other methods.[153] People need correct information on effectiveness and relative effectiveness to make an individual informed choice. Yet, not all patients prioritize effectiveness and it is coercive for providers to overemphasize effectiveness based on their own priorities rather than on the priorities, preferences, and values of the individual patient.

Striking the right balance as well as the exact messaging around contraceptive effectiveness is challenging. The overall estimated perfect use and typical use pregnancy rates derived from US studies do not pertain to any individual in the US (or elsewhere), but rather represent the average effect of the mix of characteristics found in the population studied.[14] Moreover, the statistical approach used to estimate these rates as well as quality of the data make these estimates rather crude.

Keep these key points in mind when counseling about contraceptive effectiveness:

1. **Methods in category 1 are highly effective for all users**. Use of the top-category methods—IUDs, implant, vas surgery, and fallopian tube surgery—entails the lowest risk of pregnancy, and this very low risk applies to all users.
2. **Correct and consistent use of most other contraceptive methods results in a low risk of pregnancy**. However, effectiveness for individual users of these methods (Categories 2 and 3) varies substantially by age, coital frequency, and other characteristics that are often associated with each other.
3. **Counseling tools may help communicate pregnancy risks associated with different methods**. Tables of numeric risks, such as Table 5-2, are likely to be more useful for health care providers than patients. Informational graphics that group effectiveness rates into categories (Figure 5-2) may lead to more informed contraceptive choices for clients interested in method effectiveness by demonstrating relative effectiveness to potential users.
4. **Using two methods at once dramatically lowers the risk of pregnancy**, provided they are used consistently and in appropriate combination (e.g., two condoms should not be used at the same time). If one of the methods is a condom, protection from STI acquisition and transmission is an added benefit.
5. **No method of contraception is 100% effective**. Clients are sometimes told that pregnancies occurring during contraceptive use are their own fault because they did not use the method correctly or consistently. Contraceptive methods are imperfect and can fail even the most diligent user.

Safety

In general, contraceptives pose few serious health risks to the majority of users. Moreover, the use of contraceptive methods, including hormonal methods, is generally far safer than pregnancy. This fact may not be well understood: one study found that 75% of women believed COCs were at least as hazardous to a woman's health as pregnancy.[154] Contraceptive failure (pregnancy) is associated with risk: an individual must assess the likelihood of contraceptive failure and the dangers that a pregnancy would pose. Depending on where a person lives, they may face risks associated with delayed or unsafe abortion, or risks associated with pregnancy continuation and childbirth. These risks are all affected by an individual's health and sociocultural circumstances. Thus, people in many lower-income countries with higher pregnancy-related mortality rates will experience an even greater relative health advantage in using contraceptive methods. As people age, they are more likely to have health problems that can complicate pregnancy. Nonetheless, use of hormonal or device-based contraceptive methods (IUDs and implants), and permanent contraception, may entail potential risks.

Major Health Risks

Some contraceptive options, such as fertility awareness–based methods, are not associated with any serious health risks (beyond those associated with pregnancy via method failure). When it comes to the most serious outcome of all—death—the absolute level of risk is extraordinarily low for most people, and lower than the risks associated with pregnancy and birth. Other major health risks, such as blood clots, cancer, anaphylactic reactions, or serious infections, are uncommon. People with underlying medical conditions may have greater health risks from contraception, yet also may have greater health risks from pregnancy. The US Medical Eligibility for Contraceptive Use provides information about the safe use of contraception for individuals with selected medical conditions. (See Appendix A: Summary Chart of US Medical Eligibility Criteria for Contraceptive Use available at the end of the book.)

Risk of Death with Combined Oral Contraceptive Use

Studies using data from the 1990s and earlier compared mortality among users and users of COCs. Some early studies found increased mortality risks among older users and smokers, and especially users who were in both groups.[155,156] Many early studies were based on older formulations using far higher doses of hormones (specifically ethinyl estradol) than found in pills used today. More recent large-scale analyses have found no increase in all-cause mortality associated with oral contraceptive use either in the short term or in the long term.[157-160]

Comparing Risks of Contraceptive Use to Risks of Pregnancy

It may be useful to weigh the low risks associated with COCs and permanent contraception against the risks associated with carrying a pregnancy to term and delivery. The risk of death associated with COC use is 0.06 in 100,000 among nonsmoking users aged 15–34, and 3 in 100,000 for those aged 35 to 44; for smokers aged 15–34, the risk is 1.7 in 100,000.[156] The risk of death among those undergoing fallopian tube surgery for permanent contraception is 1.5 in 100,000.[161]

The most recent data available, from 2019, show an increasing maternal mortality rate in the United States.[162] Among all women, there were 20.1 deaths due to maternal causes for every 100,000 live births. Risks are substantially higher for Black women and older women. The maternal mortality rate for non-Hispanic Black women was 44 deaths per 100,000 live births, 2.5 times the rate for non-Hispanic White women (17.9) and 3.5 times the rate for Hispanic women (12.6). Maternal mortality rates also increased with maternal age, from 12.6 for women younger than age 25, to 19.9 for those aged 25–39, and 75.5 for those aged 40 and older. The mortality risk for women aged 40 and older was 6 times higher than the rate for women younger than age 25.

The risk of death associated with legal abortion is low, approximately 0.6 in 100,000; this varies by gestational age and method (medication or surgical).[163,164] However, the risks of unsafe abortion are substantially greater. The risk of death is 55 per 100,000 unsafe abortions worldwide, accounting for 70,000 deaths per year.[165] As access to abortion is restricted, the proportion of individuals seeking unsafe abortion increases.

Cardiovascular Disease

Use of combined hormonal contraceptives (CHCs), including COCs, the patch, and vaginal ring, as well as injectable contraceptives, are associated with an increased risk of arterial and venous thromboembolism (ATE and VTE). The most serious thrombotic events, myocardial infarction (MI) and stroke, are extremely rare and much less common than deep venous thrombosis (DVT). Smoking significantly increases the risk of MI, especially in users older than age 35. However, evidence is mixed regarding an increased risk of MI among CHC users of any age who do not smoke and do not have hypertension or diabetes.[166,167] The risk of stroke in normotensive nonsmokers younger than age 35 may not be increased by use of CHCs,[155,168] except potentially in those with certain medical conditions such as migraines with aura.[169] The risk of VTE is increased by certain contraceptive methods (two-to fourfold for DMPA, two-to sixfold for COCs, and higher for patches and vaginal rings),[170,171] but the absolute risk is low, ranging from 2 events per 10,000 woman-years among those aged 15 to 19, to 7 events per 10,000 woman-years among those aged 45 to 49.[172,173]

Cancer

Many clients have concerns about the effect of hormonal contraception on cancer risk. COCs are the best studied, as they were the first hormonal method available in the United States. Given that cancer incidence increases with age, and clients potentially use hormonal contraception for several decades, methods must be available on the market for long periods of time before researchers can identify increases in risk, especially when those increases are small.

At the population level, the net effect of COC use across all cancers is neutral,[174-177] and ever-users of COCs have a significantly lower death rate from all cancers than do never-users.[158] Use of COCs (and presumably the patch and ring as well) protects users against cancers of the endometrium and ovary. Longer duration of use increases that protection. A comprehensive review concluded that use of COCs is associated with an increased risk of cancer of the cervix and liver, an increased risk of breast cancer in young women (equivalent to the risk with pregnancy), and a decreased risk of colorectal cancer.[174] The risk of death is lower among ever-users of COCs than never-users for colorectal,[158,176] uterine,[157,158] ovarian,[157,158] and lymphatic and hematopoietic[176] cancer. Moreover, COC use has neither a harmful nor a beneficial effect on breast cancer mortality.[157,158,178]

Fewer studies have evaluated cancer risk among users of progestin-only methods of contraception (including POPs, injectables, implants, and levonorgestrel-releasing IUDs). Use of injectable contraception, and likely other progestin-only methods, substantially reduces the risk of endometrial cancer.[179] Though some studies have identified an increased risk of breast cancer for some progestin-only methods,[180-184] a 2016 systematic review concluded that progestin-only methods of contraception do not appear to increase the risk of breast cancer.[185]

See individual method chapters for more information on method-specific health risks, and a summary of risks associated with each contraceptive method in **Table 5-3**.

Goals For Communicating About Safety

Providers should prioritize the following in communicating about the safety of contraceptive options:

1. **Users must be offered information on both the risks and benefits of contraceptive option(s) that align with their preferences**. It is essential to provide detailed information regarding any potential risks and contraceptive benefits as part of person-centered contraceptive counseling.
2. **Be clear about cancer risks and benefits.** While the risks of certain cancers may be increased with the use of hormonal contraception, recent large-scale

Table 5-3 Summary of Major Risks, Bleeding Pattern Changes, Side Effects/Noncontraceptive Benefits, and Return to Fecundity[a]

Method	Major Risks	Bleeding Pattern Changes	Selected Side Effects and Noncontraceptive Benefits	Return to Ability to Conceive
Permanent contraception (vas surgery, Fallopian tube surgery)	Anesthetic or surgical complications; if pregnancy occurs after tubal surgery, high risk of ectopic. Risk of regret.	None	Pain at surgical site. Tubal surgery reduces risk of ovarian cancer (particularly salpingectomy) and may protect against pelvic inflammatory disease (PID).	None
Progestin implant	Problems with removal if inserted too deeply. Extremely rare: migration, infection at implant site.	Irregular bleeding or spotting, may range from amenorrhea to frequent bleeding	Mood changes, increased acne. Decreases dysmenorrhea, can be used to treat endometriosis.	May be delayed by up to 2 cycles
Intrauterine devices	Expulsion (and subsequent risk of pregnancy), perforation, embedment, infection, anemia (with copper-bearing IUD). If pregnancy occurs, higher risk of ectopic.	Irregular bleeding or spotting, increased bleeding with copper-bearing IUD; less bleeding or amenorrhea with levonorgestrel-releasing IUD	Levonorgestrel-releasing IUD: Hormonal side effects. Decreased dysmenorrhea, decreased anemia, can be used to treat endometriosis, and can provide progestin for hormone therapy. Copper-bearing IUD: Increased dysmenorrhea, heavier menses.	May be delayed by up to 2 cycles
Injectable	Injection site reactions, decreased bone mineral density, cardiovascular complications.	Irregular bleeding or spotting, amenorrhea (increases over time)	Weight gain, adverse effects on lipids. Decreased anemia. May protect against ovarian and endometrial cancers.	Delayed up to 12 months (DMPA-SC); 5–8 cycles for DMPA-IM)

(continues)

Table 5-3 **Summary of Major Risks, Bleeding Pattern Changes, Side Effects/Noncontraceptive Benefits, and Return to Fecundity**[a]

(continued)

Method	Major Risks	Bleeding Pattern Changes	Selected Side Effects and Noncontraceptive Benefits	Return to Ability to Conceive
Combined hormonal contraception (pill, patch, and vaginal ring)	Cardiovascular complications (stroke, heart attack, blood clots); hepatic adenomas; increased risk of breast, cervical, and liver cancer diagnosis	Reduces menstrual bleeding; irregular bleeding and spotting especially with extended or continuous use	Nausea, headaches, breast tenderness, melasma; decreases dysmenorrhea, decreases anemia and cyclic mood problems (PMS or PMDD); reduces acne, and protects against ovarian, endometrial, and colorectal cancer. Can be used to treat endometriosis. Ability to schedule bleeding.	May be delayed 3–4 cycles
Progestin-only pill	None known	Irregular bleeding or spotting	Increased acne.	
External condom	Anaphylactic reaction to latex	None	Protects against STIs, including HIV. May reduce sexual pleasure, delays premature ejaculation.	Immediate
Internal condom	None known	None	Protects against STIs, including HIV. May affect sexual pleasure.	Immediate
Abstinence	None known	None	Prevents STIs, including HIV, if anal and oral intercourse are avoided as well	Immediate

Diaphragm, sponge	Vaginal and urinary tract infections, toxic shock syndrome	None	Vaginal discomfort, vaginal irritation, vaginal discharge if left in too long, allergy to spermicides.	Immediate
Spermicides	Vaginal and urinary tract infections; possible increase in susceptibility to HIV/AIDS acquisition if exposed to positive partner. N-9 can denude vaginal epithelium	None	N-9 can denude vaginal epithelium and cause vaginal irritation, allergy.	Immediate
Phexxi	Urinary tract, bladder, or kidney infections; yeast infection, bacterial vaginosis	None	Vaginal itching, burning, pain. Painful urination. May positively affect sexual pleasure.	Immediate
Fertility awareness–based methods	None known	None	Users have knowledge about the functioning of their body; adaptability of the method to trying to conceive if reproductive desires change.	Immediate
Lactational Amenorrhea Method (LAM)	None known	None	Breast/chestfeeding provides excellent nutrition for infants.	May be delayed for duration of breast/chestfeeding
Withdrawal	None known	None	None known	Immediate

[a]Among healthy women with no concurrent medical condition.

analyses have found no increase in the short-term or long-term in all-cause mortality associated with contraceptive use. Hormonal contraception can reduce risk of endometrial and other cancers.

3. **Compare risks of using contraception with pregnancy risks**. In general, the potential health risks inherent in pregnancy, abortion, and delivery are far greater than those for using a contraceptive method, including hormonal methods. Poor access to maternity and abortion care may increase the health risks associated with pregnancy occurring during contraceptive use.

Comparative Side Effects

Side effects are the most frequent reason for method discontinuation or switching.[186-190] Often, the possibility of side effects influences whether an individual selects a certain method. Do not dismiss the important role that concerns about side effects play for an individual assessing whether to initiate or continue using a method. See Table 5-3 for a summary of side effects for each contraceptive method.

The vast majority of contraceptive studies are not placebo-controlled, and many do not have an appropriate comparison group to determine rates of various side effects attributable to a method. Placebo-controlled studies of COCs have shown no significant difference in the frequency of most nonspecific side effects,[191] but it should be noted that these studies are not large enough to encompass the full range of variations in patients' lived experiences. Patients reporting side effects that are not typically associated with their contraceptive method may want to explore whether the symptom(s) may be caused by factors other than the contraceptive method—for instance, other medications, health conditions, or social factors. However, it is not effective to attempt to talk someone out of symptoms that they have experienced first-hand, and it is coercive to try to convince them to continue a method with which they are not satisfied.

There are some side effects, such as bleeding and skin changes, that should be proactively brought up with the potential user. Offering anticipatory guidance about side effects and potential management options gives users the information they need, were they to experience side effects. Some researchers have argued (based on three randomized controlled trials that found similar levels of reported side effects between oral contraceptives and placebo pills) that anticipatory counseling about side effects may increase the probability that they will experience that side effect.[191] However, people who wish to discontinue using a method due to side effects must be supported in doing so, even if the clinician does not believe that the side effect is harmful or related to the method. Clinicians have an important role to play in respecting patient autonomy, helping clients feel heard, and helping them choose another method, if desired.

Bleeding Pattern Changes With Hormonal Methods and the Copper IUD

All hormonal methods, and the copper-bearing IUD, are associated with menstrual changes. Substantial variability exists in terms of how users respond to such changes, and they play a substantial role in patient satisfaction, contraceptive discontinuation, and unmet need.[192] Some of these changes, such as lighter or no periods associated with levonorgestrel-releasing IUDs, injectables, and continuous use of CHCs and POPs, may be considered "side benefits" and are desired by some patients.

Those who want regular periods may not appreciate these changes and may prefer methods like CHCs with hormone-free intervals that enable one to schedule bleeding to resemble regular periods. Some will prefer to maintain their natural menstrual pattern with a copper IUD, a method associated with heavier periods.

Delayed Ability to Conceive

Desiring pregnancy is an often-cited reason for discontinuing contraception and delayed ability to conceive may be considered a serious side effect by some people. A recent prospective cohort study of 17,954 women trying to conceive suggested that people discontinuing injectables had the longest delay in return of normal fecundity (five to eight menstrual cycles), followed by patch users (four cycles), oral contraceptive pills (OCPs) and ring users (four cycles), and IUD and implant users (two cycles), with little to no long-term effects on fecundity.[193] Delayed conception is most likely to occur with DMPA (IM and SC). DMPA-SC prescribing information advises that the delay may be 1 year or longer based on internal data from 15 study participants.[194] More recent data support this substantial delay when discontinuing DMPA-SC.[195] DMPA-IM prescribing information provides a median time-to-pregnancy of 10 months after discontinuation.[196] A secondary metabolite of DMPA is stored in the adipose tissue and is biologically active; users with more adipose tissue have longer time to return of fertility. Delayed return to conception after contraceptive discontinuation may be greater among some individuals, including those living with HIV.[197] On the other hand, some individuals will experience immediate return to their normal fecundity patterns. People discontinuing a method who want to maintain protection against pregnancy should be reminded to begin another method immediately.

Changes in Sexual Desire and Function

Clients commonly express concern about sexual side effects. Potential effects on sexuality can include changes in desire, vaginal lubrication, pleasure, and orgasm. Physical sensations such as decreased penile sensitivity, pressure on vaginal walls, or uterine cramping may be caused by mechanical methods such as condoms, the diaphragm, or IUDs.[198-200] (See Chapter 6, Sexuality and Contraception.) DMPA can create a hypoestrogenic milieu that can cause the user to experience dryness in their vagina, especially when used by those who are chestfeeding.

Noncontraceptive Benefits

When a contraceptive side effect is considered positive, it is referred to as a "noncontraceptive benefit" or "something your birth control can do for you in addition to preventing pregnancy." Reduction in endometrial cancer risk is a noncontraceptive benefit of hormonal contraceptives, for instance. In some cases, whether a particular side effect is positive or negative depends on the user.

Noncontraceptive benefits can be major considerations when an individual selects a contraceptive method (see Table 5-3). Adolescents may opt for a CHC to help improve their acne or reduce dysmenorrhea, and an increasing proportion of people opt for a levonorgestrel-releasing IUD to reduce or eliminate menstrual blood loss. In many cases, noncontraceptive benefits can help patients decide between two or more suitable methods. Awareness that a method of contraception has noncontraceptive benefits may also increase the likelihood of satisfaction with continued use of that method. In addition to counseling on risks, make it a practice to tell your clients about the potential noncontraceptive benefits of the various methods:

- **Reducing the risk of STIs** may be an important factor as an individual selects a contraceptive method. Any person who may be at risk of acquiring STIs has the contraceptive benefit of STI prevention with external or internal condoms, either alone or with another method. Because condoms reduce the risk of STIs that cause pelvic inflammatory disease, which can lead to infertility, they protect future fertility.
- Fertility awareness methods help users **learn about their menstrual physiology**. This knowledge can also help someone achieve a pregnancy.
- Several contraceptive methods treat **heavy menstrual bleeding**. They also decrease dysmenorrhea and are first-line treatments for endometriosis. Hormonal methods all contain a progestin and so can be used to protect the endometrium for individuals who are anovulatory, have polycystic ovarian syndrome, or are on hormone therapy.
- COCs, and presumably the patch and vaginal ring, can **improve acne and premenstrual dysphoric disorder (PMDD) and premenstrual syndrome (PMS)**. These CHC methods may improve bone health in women with low estrogen levels related to premature ovarian insufficiency. Higher-dose pills (those with 30–35 mcg ethinyl estradiol), DMPA injection, and implants may protect against functional ovarian cysts.

Table 5-3 summarizes major risks, bleeding pattern changes, selected side effects/contraceptive benefits, and return to fecundity for each contraceptive method.

Goals For Communicating About Side Effects

Side effects, particularly changes in bleeding pattern, are a major cause of method discontinuation. Some clients wish to hear about treatment options or the likelihood of the side effect improving over time. When management options are available, providing a treatment someone can try on their own in advance can reduce dissatisfaction with their method. Providers should prioritize the following in communicating about side effects:

1. Support individuals who report that they are experiencing side effects in learning about management options and in choosing whether to continue their method or select a new method.
2. Discuss noncontraceptive benefits when counseling about side effects. Noncontraceptive benefits may help individuals decide to use a particular method and increase patient satisfaction with their method choice.
3. Support a client's decision to discontinue a method for any reason (particularly a method that a user is unable to remove without assistance from a health care provider, such as an implant or IUD).

Author disclosures: Bradley: none; Polis: none; Steiner: none; Micks: none.

Acknowledgments: James Trussell, PhD, Abigail RA Aiken, MD, MPH, PhD, and Katherine A. Guthrie, FRCOG, FFSRH for previous editions of this chapter. We note the essential contributions of James Trussell to multiple previous editions of *Contraceptive Technology* and to much of the seminal research on contraceptive effectiveness.

References

1. Yeh PT, Kautsar H, Kennedy CE, Gaffield ME. Values and preferences for contraception: A global systematic review. Contraception. 2022;111:3-21. DOI: 10.1016/j.contraception.2022.04.011.
2. Guttmacher Institute. Contraceptive use in the United States by method. May 2021. (https://www.guttmacher.org/fact-sheet/contraceptive-method-use-united-states).
3. Personal communication with Megan Kavanaugh. 2022 April 5.
4. Frederiksen BN, Ahrens K. Understanding the extent of contraceptive non-use among women at risk of unintended pregnancy, National Survey of Family Growth 2011-2017. Contracept X. 2020;2:100033. DOI: 10.1016/j.conx.2020.100033.
5. Kavanaugh ML, Pliskin E. Use of contraception among reproductive-aged women in the United States, 2014 and 2016. F S Rep 2020;1(2):83-93. DOI: 10.1016/j.xfre.2020.06.006.
6. Mosher W, Jones J, Abma J. Nonuse of contraception among women at risk of unintended pregnancy in the United States. Contraception. 2015;92(2):170-6. DOI: 10.1016/j.contraception.2015.05.004.
7. Polis CB, Jones RK. Multiple contraceptive method use and prevalence of fertility awareness based method use in the United States, 2013-2015. Contraception. 2018;98(3):188-92. DOI: 10.1016/j.contraception.2018.04.013.
8. Personal communication with Jonathan Bearak. 2022 April 12.
9. Bearak JM, Popinchalk A, Beavin C, et al. Country-specific estimates of unintended pregnancy and abortion incidence: a global comparative analysis of levels in 2015-2019. BMJ Glob Health. 2022;7(3):e007151. DOI: 10.1136/bmjgh-2021-007151.
10. Guttmacher Institute. United States country profile. (https://www.guttmacher.org/geography/northern-america/united-states).
11. Callahan RL, Becker S. The reliability of calendar data for reporting contraceptive use: evidence from rural Bangladesh. Stud Fam Plann. 2012;43(3):213-22. DOI: 10.1111/j.1728-4465.2012.00319.x.
12. Bradley SEK, Winfrey W, Croft TN. Contraceptive use and perinatal mortality in the DHS: An assessment of the quality and consistency of calendars and histories. Rockville, Maryland, USA: ICF International; 2015.
13. Althubaiti A. Information bias in health research: definition, pitfalls, and adjustment methods. J Multidiscip Healthc. 2016;9:211-7. DOI: 10.2147/JMDH.S104807.
14. Steiner MJ. Contraceptive effectiveness: what should the counseling message be? JAMA. 1999;282(15):1405-7. DOI: 10.1001/jama.282.15.1405.
15. Jones RK, Kost K. Underreporting of induced and spontaneous abortion in the United States: an analysis of the 2002 National Survey of Family Growth. Stud Fam Plann. 2007;38(3):187-97. DOI: 10.1111/j.1728-4465.2007.00130.x.
16. Jones RK, Finer LB, Singh S. Characteristics of U.S. abortion patients, 2008. New York: Guttmacher Institute, 2010.
17. Sundaram A, Vaughan B, Kost K, et al. Contraceptive failure in the United States: Estimates from the 2006-2010 National Survey of Family Growth. Perspect Sex Reprod Health. 2017;49(1):7-16. DOI: 10.1363/psrh.12017.
18. Trussell J, Vaughan B. Contraceptive failure, method-related discontinuation and resumption of use: results from the 1995 National Survey of Family Growth. Fam Plann Perspect. 1999;31(2):64-72, 93.
19. Schirm AL, Trussell J, Menken J, Grady WR. Contraceptive failure in the United States: the impact of social, economic and demographic factors. Fam Plann Perspect. 1982;14(2):68-75.
20. Trussell J, Menken J. Life table analysis of contraceptive failure. In: Hermalin AI EB, ed. The role of surveys in the analysis of family planning programs. Liege (Belgium): Ordina Editions; 1982:537-71.
21. Personal communication with Aparna Sundaram and Barbara Vaughan. 2016 Oct 6.
22. Trussell J, Kost K. Contraceptive failure in the United States: a critical review of the literature. Stud Fam Plann. 1987;18(5):237-83.
23. Bradley SEK, Polis CB, Bankole A, Croft T. Global Contraceptive failure rates: Who is most at risk? Stud Fam Plann. 2019;50(1):3-24. DOI: 10.1111/sifp.12085.

24. Steiner MJ, Dalebout S, Condon S, Dominik R, Trussell J. Understanding risk: a randomized controlled trial of communicating contraceptive effectiveness. Obstet Gynecol. 2003;102(4): 709-17. DOI: 10.1016/s0029-7844(03)00662-8.
25. Steiner MJ, Trussell J, Mehta N, Condon S, Subramaniam S, Bourne D. Communicating contraceptive effectiveness: A randomized controlled trial to inform a World Health Organization family planning handbook. Am J Obstet Gynecol. 2006;195(1):85-91. DOI: 10.1016/j.ajog.2005.12.053.
26. World Health Organization and Johns Hopkins Bloomberg School of Public Health. Family planning - A global handbook for providers. Center for Communication Programs; 2018.
27. Lopez LM, Steiner M, Grimes DA, Hilgenberg D, Schulz KF. Strategies for communicating contraceptive effectiveness. Cochrane Database Syst Rev. 2013(4):CD006964. DOI: 10.1002/14651858.CD006964.pub3.
28. Fu H, Darroch JE, Haas T, Ranjit N. Contraceptive failure rates: new estimates from the 1995 National Survey of Family Growth. Fam Plann Perspect. 1999;31(2):56-63.
29. Graesslin O, Korver T. The contraceptive efficacy of Implanon: a review of clinical trials and marketing experience. Eur J Contracept Reprod Health Care. 2008;13 Suppl 1:4-12. DOI: 10.1080/13625180801942754.
30. Bahamondes L, Brache V, Meirik O, et al. A 3-year multicentre randomized controlled trial of etonogestrel- and levonorgestrel-releasing contraceptive implants, with non-randomized matched copper-intrauterine device controls. Hum Reprod. 2015;30(11):2527-38. DOI: 10.1093/humrep/dev221.
31. Steiner MJ, Brache V, Taylor D, et al. Randomized trial to evaluate contraceptive efficacy, safety and acceptability of a two-rod contraceptive implant over 4 years in the Dominican Republic. Contracept X. 2019;1:100006. DOI: 10.1016/j.conx.2019.100006.
32. Mishell DR, el-Habashy MA, Good RG, Moyer DL. Contraception with an injectable progestin. A study of its use in postpartum women. Am J Obstet Gynecol. 1968;101(8):1046-53. DOI: 10.1016/0002-9378(68)90346-3.
33. Multinational comparative clinical trial of long-acting injectable contraceptives: norethisterone enanthate given in two dosage regimens and depot-medroxyprogesterone acetate. Final report. Contraception. 1983;28(1):1-20. DOI: 10.1016/s0010-7824(83)80002-x.
34. Schwallie PC, Assenzo JR. Contraceptive use--efficacy study utilizing medroxyprogesterone acetate administered as an intramuscular injection once every 90 days. Fertil Steril. 1973;24(5): 331 9. DOI: 10.1016/s0015-0282(16)39669-8.
35. Scutchfield FD, Long WN, Corey B, Tyler CW. Medroxyprogesterone acetate as an injectable female contraceptive. Contraception. 1971;3:21-35.
36. Sangi-Haghpeykar H, Poindexter AN, Bateman L, Ditmore JR. Experiences of injectable contraceptive users in an urban setting. Obstet Gynecol. 1996;88(2):227-33. DOI: 10.1016/0029-7844(96)00194-9.
37. Said S, Omar K, Koetsawang S, et al. A multicentred phase III comparative clinical trial of depot-medroxyprogesterone acetate given three-monthly at doses of 100 mg or 150 mg: 1. Contraceptive efficacy and side effects. World Health Organization Task Force on Long-Acting Systemic Agents for Fertility Regulation. Special Programme of Research, Development and Research Training in Human Reproduction. Contraception. 1986;34(3):223-35. DOI: 10.1016/0010-7824(86)90004-1.
38. Jain J, Jakimiuk AJ, Bode FR, Ross D, Kaunitz AM. Contraceptive efficacy and safety of DMPA-SC. Contraception. 2004;70(4):269-75. DOI: 10.1016/j.contraception.2004.06.011.
39. Kaunitz AM, Darney PD, Ross D, Wolter KD, Speroff L. Subcutaneous DMPA vs. intramuscular DMPA: a 2-year randomized study of contraceptive efficacy and bone mineral density. Contraception. 2009;80(1):7-17. DOI: 10.1016/j.contraception.2009.02.005.
40. Hernádi L, Marr J, Trummer D, De Leo V, Petraglia F. Efficacy and safety of a low-dose combined oral contraceptive containing drospirenone 3 mg and ethinylestradiol 20 mcg in a 24/4-day regimen. Contraception. 2009;80(1):18-24. DOI: 10.1016/j.contraception.2009.01.016.
41. Kroll R, Reape KZ, Margolis M. The efficacy and safety of a low-dose, 91-day, extended-regimen oral contraceptive with continuous ethinyl estradiol. Contraception. 2010;81(1):41-8. DOI: 10.1016/j.contraception.2009.07.003.

42. Palacios S, Colli E, Regidor PA. Multicenter, phase III trials on the contraceptive efficacy, tolerability and safety of a new drospirenone-only pill. Acta Obstet Gynecol Scand. 2019;98(12):1549-57. DOI: 10.1111/aogs.13688.
43. Alderman PM. The lurking sperm. A review of failures in 8879 vasectomies performed by one physician. JAMA. 1988;259(21):3142-4. DOI: 10.1001/jama.259.21.3142.
44. Moss WM. A comparison of open-end versus closed-end vasectomies: a report on 6220 cases. Contraception. 1992;46(6):521-5. DOI: 10.1016/0010-7824(92)90116-b.
45. Philp T, Guillebaud J, Budd D. Complications of vasectomy: review of 16,000 patients. Br J Urol. 1984;56(6):745-8. DOI: 10.1111/j.1464-410x.1984.tb06161.x.
46. One thousand vasectomies. Br Med J. 1973;4(5886):216-21. DOI: 10.1136/bmj.4.5886.216.
47. Kase S, Goldfarb M. Office vasectomy. Review of 500 cases. Urology. 1973;1(1):60-2. DOI: 10.1016/0090-4295(73)90115-5.
48. Klapproth HJ, Young IS. Vasectomy, vas ligation and vas occlusion. Urology. 1973;1(4):292-300. DOI: 10.1016/0090-4295(73)90273-2.
49. Schmidt SS. Vasectomy. JAMA. 1988;259(21):3176.
50. Marshall S, Lyon RP. Variability of sperm disappearance from the ejaculate after vasectomy. J Urol. 1972;107(5):815-7. DOI: 10.1016/s0022-5347(17)61147-9.
51. Jamieson DJ, Costello C, Trussell J, et al. The risk of pregnancy after vasectomy. Obstet Gynecol. 2004;103(5 Pt 1):848-50. DOI: 10.1097/01.AOG.0000123246.11511.e4.
52. Peterson HB, Xia Z, Hughes JM, Wilcox LS, Tylor LR, Trussell J. The risk of pregnancy after tubal sterilization: findings from the U.S. Collaborative Review of Sterilization. Am J Obstet Gynecol. 1996;174(4):1161-8; discussion 1168-70. DOI: 10.1016/s0002-9378(96)70658-0.
53. Powell CB, Alabaster A, Simmons S, et al. Salpingectomy for sterilization: Change in practice in a large integrated health care system, 2011-2016. Obstet Gynecol. 2017;130(5):961-7. DOI: 10.1097/AOG.0000000000002312.
54. Mills K, Marchand G, Sainz K, et al. Salpingectomy vs tubal ligation for sterilization: a systematic review and meta-analysis. Am J Obstet Gynecol. 2021;224(3):258-65.e4. DOI: 10.1016/j.ajog.2020.09.011.
55. Sivin I, Stern J. Long-acting, more effective copper T IUDs: a summary of U.S. experience, 1970-75. Stud Fam Plann. 1979;10(10):263-81.
56. Heinemann K, Reed S, Moehner S, Minh TD. Comparative contraceptive effectiveness of levonorgestrel-releasing and copper intrauterine devices: the European Active Surveillance Study for Intrauterine Devices. Contraception. 2015;91(4):280-3. DOI: 10.1016/j.contraception.2015.01.011.
57. Nelson A, Apter D, Hauck B, et al. Two low-dose levonorgestrel intrauterine contraceptive systems: a randomized controlled trial. Obstet Gynecol. 2013;122(6):1205-13. DOI: 10.1097/AOG.0000000000000019.
58. Eisenberg DL, Schreiber CA, Turok DK, et al. Three-year efficacy and safety of a new 52-mg levonorgestrel-releasing intrauterine system. Contraception. 2015;92(1):10-6. DOI: 10.1016/j.contraception.2015.04.006.
59. Personal communication with Sivin, I. (Center for Biomedical Research, Population Council). Email to: James Trussell (Office of Population Research, Princeton University). 1992.
60. Bednarek PH, Creinin MD, Reeves MF, et al. Immediate versus delayed IUD insertion after uterine aspiration. N Engl J Med. 2011;364(23):2208-17. DOI: 10.1056/NEJMoa1011600.
61. Averbach SH, Ermias Y, Jeng G, et al. Expulsion of intrauterine devices after postpartum placement by timing of placement, delivery type, and intrauterine device type: a systematic review and meta-analysis. Am J Obstet Gynecol. 2020;223(2):177-88. DOI: 10.1016/j.ajog.2020.02.045.
62. Vaughan B, Trussell J, Kost K, Singh S, Jones R. Discontinuation and resumption of contraceptive use: results from the 2002 National Survey of Family Growth. Contraception. 2008;78(4):271-83. DOI: 10.1016/j.contraception.2008.05.007.
63. Hall KS, Trussell J. Types of combined oral contraceptives used by US women. Contraception. 2012;86(6):659-65. DOI: 10.1016/j.contraception.2012.05.017.
64. Regidor PA, Colli E. Drospirenone 4 mg in a 24/4 regimen maintains inhibition of ovulation even after a 24-h delay pill intake - Pharmacological aspects and comparison to other progestin-only pills. Eur Rev Med Pharmacol Sci. 2022;26(6):1994-9. DOI: 10.26355/eurrev_202203_28348.

65. Lopez LM, Grimes DA, Gallo MF, Stockton LL, Schulz KF. Skin patch and vaginal ring versus combined oral contraceptives for contraception. Cochrane Database Syst Rev. 2013(4):CD003552. DOI: 10.1002/14651858.CD003552.pub4.
66. López-Picado A, Lapuente O, Lete I. Efficacy and side-effects profile of the ethinylestradiol and etonogestrel contraceptive vaginal ring: a systematic review and meta-analysis. Eur J Contracept Reprod Health Care. 2017;22(2):131-46. DOI: 10.1080/13625187.2017.1287351.
67. Peragallo Urrutia R, Polis CB, Jensen ET, Greene ME, Kennedy E, Stanford JB. Effectiveness of fertility awareness-based methods for pregnancy prevention: A systematic review. Obstet Gynecol. 2018;132(3):591-604. DOI: 10.1097/AOG.0000000000002784.
68. Arévalo M, Jennings V, Sinai I. Efficacy of a new method of family planning: the Standard Days Method. Contraception. 2002;65(5):333-8. DOI: 10.1016/s0010-7824(02)00288-3.
69. Trussell J, Grummer-Strawn L. Further analysis of contraceptive failure of the ovulation method. Am J Obstet Gynecol. 1991;165(6 Pt 2):2054-9. DOI: 10.1016/s0002-9378(11)90581-x.
70. Frank-Herrmann P, Heil J, Gnoth C, et al. The effectiveness of a fertility awareness based method to avoid pregnancy in relation to a couple's sexual behaviour during the fertile time: a prospective longitudinal study. Hum Reprod 2007;22(5):1310-9. DOI: 10.1093/humrep/dem003.
71. Jennings V, Haile LT, Simmons RG, Spieler J, Shattuck D. Perfect- and typical-use effectiveness of the Dot fertility app over 13 cycles: results from a prospective contraceptive effectiveness trial. Eur J Contracept Reprod Health Care 2019;24(2):148-53. DOI: 10.1080/13625187.2019.1581164.
72. Berglund Scherwitzl E, Gemzell Danielsson K, Sellberg JA, Scherwitzl R. Fertility awareness-based mobile application for contraception. Eur J Contracept Reprod Health Care 2016;21(3):234-41. DOI: 10.3109/13625187.2016.1154143.
73. Berglund Scherwitzl E, Lundberg O, Kopp Kallner H, Gemzell Danielsson K, Trussell J, Scherwitzl R. Perfect-use and typical-use Pearl Index of a contraceptive mobile app. Contraception. 2017;96(6):420-5. DOI: 10.1016/j.contraception.2017.08.014.
74. Pearson JT, Chelstowska M, Rowland SP, et al. Natural Cycles app: contraceptive outcomes and demographic analysis of UK users. Eur J Contracept Reprod Health Care 2021;26(2):105-10. DOI: 10.1080/13625187.2020.1867844.
75. Pearson JT, Chelstowska M, Rowland SP, et al. Contraceptive effectiveness of an FDA-cleared birth control App: Results from the Natural Cycles U.S. Cohort. J Womens Health (Larchmt). 2021;30(6):782-8. DOI: 10.1089/jwh.2020.8547.
76. Natural Cycles. US FDA-approved product information.
77. Frezieres RG, Walsh TL, Nelson AL, Clark VA, Coulson AH. Evaluation of the efficacy of a polyurethane condom: results from a randomized, controlled clinical trial. Fam Plann Perspect. 1999;31(2):81-7.
78. Walsh TL, Frezieres RG, Peacock K, Nelson AL, Clark VA, Bernstein L. Evaluation of the efficacy of a nonlatex condom: results from a randomized, controlled clinical trial. Perspect Sex Reprod Health. 2003;35(2):79-86.
79. Steiner MJ, Dominik R, Rountree RW, Nanda K, Dorflinger LJ. Contraceptive effectiveness of a polyurethane condom and a latex condom: a randomized controlled trial. Obstet Gynecol. 2003;101(3):539-47. DOI: 10.1016/s0029-7844(02)02732-1.
80. Albert AE, Warner DL, Hatcher RA, Trussell J, Bennett C. Condom use among female commercial sex workers in Nevada's legal brothels. Am J Public Health 1995;85(11):1514-20. DOI: 10.2105/ajph.85.11.1514.
81. Kestelman P, Trussell J. Efficacy of the simultaneous use of condoms and spermicides. Fam Plann Perspect. 1991;23(5):226-7, 232.
82. Steiner M, Piedrahita C, Glover L, Joanis C. Can condom users likely to experience condom failure be identified? Fam Plann Perspect. 1993;25(5):220-3, 226.
83. Edelman DA, McIntyre SL, Harper J. A comparative trial of the Today contraceptive sponge and diaphragm. Am J Obstet Gynecol. 1984;150(7):869-76. DOI: 10.1016/0002-9378(84)90465-4.
84. Trussell J, Strickler J, Vaughan B. Contraceptive efficacy of the diaphragm, the sponge and the cervical cap. Fam Plann Perspect. 1993;25(3):100-5, 135.
85. Schwartz JL, Weiner DH, Lai JJ, et al. Contraceptive efficacy, safety, fit, and acceptability of a single-size diaphragm developed with end-user input. Obstet Gynecol. 2015;125(4):895-903. DOI: 10.1097/AOG.0000000000000721.

86. Trussell J, Sturgen K, Strickler J, Dominik R. Comparative contraceptive efficacy of the female condom and other barrier methods. Fam Plann Perspect. 1994;26(2):66-72.
87. Lindh I, Othman J, Hansson M, Ekelund AC, Svanberg T, Strandell A. New types of diaphragms and cervical caps versus older types of diaphragms and different gels for contraception: a systematic review. BMJ Sex Reprod Health. 2021;47(3):e12. DOI: 10.1136/bmjsrh-2020-200632.
88. Ilaria G, Jacobs JL, Polsky B, et al. Detection of HIV-1 DNA sequences in pre-ejaculatory fluid. Lancet. 1992;340(8833):1469. DOI: 10.1016/0140-6736(92)92658-3.
89. Pudney J, Oneta M, Mayer K, Seage G, Anderson D. Pre-ejaculatory fluid as potential vector for sexual transmission of HIV-1. Lancet. 1992;340(8833):1470. DOI: 10.1016/0140-6736(92)92659-4.
90. Zukerman Z, Weiss DB, Orvieto R. Does preejaculatory penile secretion originating from Cowper's gland contain sperm? J Assist Reprod Genet. 2003;20(4):157-9. DOI: 10.1023/a:1022933320700.
91. Killick SR, Leary C, Trussell J, Guthrie KA. Sperm content of pre-ejaculatory fluid. Hum Fertil (Camb). 2011;14(1):48-52. DOI: 10.3109/14647273.2010.520798.
92. Farr G, Gabelnick H, Sturgen K, Dorflinger L. Contraceptive efficacy and acceptability of the female condom. Am J Public Health. 1994;84(12):1960-4. DOI: 10.2105/ajph.84.12.1960.
93. Thomas MA, Chappell BT, Maximos B, Culwell KR, Dart C, Howard B. A novel vaginal pH regulator: results from the phase 3 AMPOWER contraception clinical trial. Contracept X. 2020;2:100031. DOI: 10.1016/j.conx.2020.100031.
94. Phexxi Product Website: Efficacy and Safety. (https://hcp-phexxi.com/efficacy_and_safety).
95. Raymond EG, Chen PL, Luoto J, Group ST. Contraceptive effectiveness and safety of five nonoxynol-9 spermicides: a randomized trial. Obstet Gynecol. 2004;103(3):430-9. DOI: 10.1097/01.AOG.0000113620.18395.0b.
96. Brehm H, Haase W. Die alternative zur hormonalen kontrazeption? Med Welt. 1975;26:1610-7. (In German.).
97. Dimpfl J, Salomon W, Schicketanz KH. Die spermizide barriere. Sexualmedizin. 1984;13:95-8. (In German.).
98. Florence N. Das kontrazeptive vaginal-suppositorium: ergebnisse einer klinischen fünfjahresstudie. Sexualmedizin. 1977;6:385-6. (In German.).
99. Godts P. Klinische prüfung eines vaginalem antikonzipiens. Ars Medici. 1973;2:589-93. (In German.).
100. Iizuka R, Kobayashi T, Kawakami S, et al. [Clinical experience of vaginal contraceptive film containing the spermicide, polyoxyethylene nonylphenyl ether (C-film Study Group) (authors' transl)]. Nihon Funin Gakkai Zasshi. 1980;25(2):64-8. (In Japanese).
101. Salomon W, Haase W. Intravaginale kontrazeption. Sexualmedizin. 1977;6:198-202. (In German.).
102. Over-the-Counter Contraceptives and Other Vaginal Drug Products Review Panel (Elizabeth B. Connell, Chairman). Encare Oval. Memorandum to Food and Drug Administration Commissioner Donald Kennedy, February 9, 1978.
103. Stewart FH, Stewart G, Guest FJ, Hatcher RA. My body, my health: the concerned woman's guide to gynecology. New York: John Wiley & Sons, 1979.
104. MEARS E. Chemical contraceptive trial. II. J Reprod Fertil 1962;4:337-43. DOI: 10.1530/jrf.0.0040337.
105. Raymond E, Dominik R. Contraceptive effectiveness of two spermicides: a randomized trial. Obstet Gynecol. 1999;93(6):896-903. DOI: 10.1016/s0029-7844(99)00002-2.
106. Kost K, Singh S, Vaughan B, Trussell J, Bankole A. Estimates of contraceptive failure from the 2002 National Survey of Family Growth. Contraception. 2008;77(1):10-21. DOI: 10.1016/j.contraception.2007.09.013.
107. Mauck C, Callahan M, Weiner DH, Dominik R. A comparative study of the safety and efficacy of FemCap, a new vaginal barrier contraceptive, and the Ortho All-Flex diaphragm. The FemCap Investigators' Group. Contraception 1999;60(2):71-80. DOI: 10.1016/s0010-7824(99)00068-2.
108. FemCap. US FDA-approved product information.
109. Sheps MC. An analysis of reproductive patterns in an American isolate. Population Studies. 1965;19(1):65-80.

110. Grady WR, Hayward MD, Yagi J. Contraceptive failure in the United States: estimates from the 1982 National Survey of Family Growth. Fam Plann Perspect. 1986;18(5):200-9.
111. Polis CB, Bradley SEK, Bankole A, Onda T, Croft T, Singh S. Contraceptive failure rates in the developing world: An analysis of demographic and health survey data in 43 Countries. Guttmacher Institute, 2016. (https://www.guttmacher.org/sites/default/files/report_pdf/contraceptive-failure-rates-in-developing-world_1.pdf).
112. Kavanaugh ML, Pliskin E, Jerman J. Use of concurrent multiple methods of contraception in the United States, 2008 to 2015. Contracept X. 2021;3:100060. DOI: 10.1016/j.conx.2021.100060.
113. Steenland MW, Rodriguez MI, Marchbanks PA, Curtis KM. How does the number of oral contraceptive pill packs dispensed or prescribed affect continuation and other measures of consistent and correct use? A systematic review. Contraception. 2013;87(5):605-10. DOI: 10.1016/j.contraception.2012.08.004.
114. Curtis KM, Tepper NK, Jatlaoui TC, et al. U.S. Medical Eligibility Criteria for Contraceptive Use, 2016. MMWR Recomm Rep 2016;65(3):1-103. DOI: 10.15585/mmwr.rr6503a1.
115. Sivin I, Schmidt F. Effectiveness of IUDs: a review. Contraception 1987;36(1):55-84. DOI: 10.1016/0010-7824(87)90061-8.
116. Vessey M, Lawless M, Yeates D. Efficacy of different contraceptive methods. Lancet. 1982; 1(8276):841-2. DOI: 10.1016/s0140-6736(82)91885-2.
117. The Demographic and Health Surveys (DHS) Program. USAID. (https://dhsprogram.com/).
118. Trussell J, Westoff CF. Contraceptive practice and trends in coital frequency. Fam Plann Perspect. 1980;12(5):246-9.
119. Menken J, Trussell J, Larsen U. Age and infertility. Science 1986;233(4771):1389-94. DOI: 10.1126/science.3755843.
120. Wesselink AK, Rothman KJ, Hatch EE, Mikkelsen EM, Sørensen HT, Wise LA. Age and fecundability in a North American preconception cohort study. Am J Obstet Gynecol. 2017; 217(6):667.e1-667.e8. DOI: 10.1016/j.ajog.2017.09.002.
121. Rothman KJ, Wise LA, Sørensen HT, Riis AH, Mikkelsen EM, Hatch EE. Volitional determinants and age-related decline in fecundability: a general population prospective cohort study in Denmark. Fertil Steril 2013;99(7):1958-64. DOI: 10.1016/j.fertnstert.2013.02.040.
122. Kühnert B, Nieschlag E. Reproductive functions of the ageing male. Hum Reprod Update 2004;10(4):327-39. DOI: 10.1093/humupd/dmh030.
123. Matorras R, Matorras F, Expósito A, Martinez L, Crisol L. Decline in human fertility rates with male age: a consequence of a decrease in male fecundity with aging? Gynecol. Obstet Invest 2011;71(4):229-35. DOI: 10.1159/000319236.
124. Steiner MJ, Hertz-Picciotto I, Raymond E, Trussell J, Wheeless A, Schoenbach V. Influence of cycle variability and coital frequency on the risk of pregnancy. Contraception 1999;60(3): 137-43. DOI: 10.1016/s0010-7824(99)00073-6.
125. Skiles MP, Cunningham M, Inglis A, et al. The effect of access to contraceptive services on injectable use and demand for family planning in Malawi. Int Perspect Sex Reprod Health. 2015;41(1):20-30. DOI: 10.1363/4102015.
126. LaCross A, Smaldone A, Angelson J. Ambivalence Toward Pregnancy as an Indicator for Contraceptive Nonuse: A Systematic Review and Meta-Analysis. J Midwifery Womens Health. 2019;64(4):385-394. DOI: 10.1111/jmwh.12969.
127. Higgins JA, Popkin RA, Santelli JS. Pregnancy ambivalence and contraceptive use among young adults in the United States. Perspect Sex Reprod Health. 2012;44(4):236-43. DOI: 10.1363/4423612.
128. Polis CB, Zabin LS. Missed conceptions or misconceptions: perceived infertility among unmarried young adults in the United States. Perspect Sex Reprod Health. 2012;44(1):30-8. DOI: 10.1363/4403012.
129. Gemmill A. Perceived Subfecundity and Contraceptive Use Among Young Adult U.S. Women. Perspect Sex Reprod Health. 2018;50(3):119-127. DOI: 10.1363/psrh.12072.
130. Mitchell AA, Van Bennekom CM, Louik C. A pregnancy-prevention program in women of childbearing age receiving isotretinoin. N Engl J Med 1995;333(2):101-6. DOI: 10.1056/NEJM199507133330206.

131. Wierman ME. Hyperandrogenic Anovulation: Differential Diagnosis and Evaluation. Endocrinol Metab Clin North Am 2021;50(1):1-10. DOI: 10.1016/j.ecl.2020.12.003.
132. Edelman AB, Cherala G, Munar MY, et al. Prolonged monitoring of ethinyl estradiol and levonorgestrel levels confirms an altered pharmacokinetic profile in obese oral contraceptives users. Contraception. 2013;87(2):220-6. DOI: 10.1016/j.contraception.2012.10.008.
133. Lopez LM, Bernholc A, Chen M, et al. Hormonal contraceptives for contraception in overweight or obese women. Cochrane Database Syst Rev.. 2016(8):CD008452. DOI: 10.1002/14651858.CD008452.pub4.
134. TWIRLA (levonorgestrel and ethinyl estradiol) transdermal system. US FDA approved product information. (https://www.accessdata.fda.gov/drugsatfda_docs/label/2020/204017s000lbl.pdf).
135. Yamazaki M, Dwyer K, Sobhan M, et al. Effect of obesity on the effectiveness of hormonal contraceptives: an individual participant data meta-analysis. Contraception. 2015;92(5):445-52. DOI: 10.1016/j.contraception.2015.07.016.
136. Edelman A, Trussell J, Aiken ARA, Portman DJ, Chiodo JA, Garner EIO. The emerging role of obesity in short-acting hormonal contraceptive effectiveness. Contraception. 2018;97(5):371-7. DOI: 10.1016/j.contraception.2017.12.012.
137. Trussell J, Schwarz EB, Guthrie K. Obesity and oral contraceptive pill failure. Contraception. 2009;79(5):334-8. DOI: 10.1016/j.contraception.2008.11.017.
138. Gallo MF, Lopez LM, Grimes DA, Carayon F, Schulz KF, Helmerhorst FM. Combination contraceptives: effects on weight. Cochrane Database Syst Rev. 2014(1):CD003987. DOI: 10.1002/14651858.CD003987.pub5.
139. Davis HJ. The shield intrauterine device. A superior modern contraceptive. Am J Obstet Gynecol. 1970;106(3):455-6. DOI: 10.1016/0002-9378(70)90375-3.
140. Mintz M. At any cost: corporate greed, women, and the Dalkon shield. New York: Pantheon Books, 1985.
141. Phexxi Product Website. (https://phexxi.com/).
142. Steinberg J, Lynch SE. Lactic acid, citric acid, and potassium bitartrate (Phexxi) vaginal gel for contraception. Am Fam Physician. 2021;103(10):628-9.
143. Polis CB. Published analysis of contraceptive effectiveness of Daysy and DaysyView app is fatally flawed. Reprod Health. 2018;15(1):113. DOI: 10.1186/s12978-018-0560-1.
144. Haslett E. "It's a Wild West": the scientist who took on the multi-billion femtech industry. (https://www.newstatesman.com/the-business-interview/2022/04/its-a-wild-west-the-scientist-who-took-on-the-multi-billion-femtech-industry).
145. Trussell J, Hatcher RA, Cates W, Stewart FH, Kost K. A guide to interpreting contraceptive efficacy studies. Obstet Gynecol. 1990;76(3 Pt 2):558-67.
146. Trussell J. Methodological pitfalls in the analysis of contraceptive failure. Stat Med. 1991; 10(2):201-20. DOI: 10.1002/sim.4780100206.
147. Tietze C, Poliakoff SR, Rock J. The clinical effectiveness of the rhythm method of contraception. Fertil Steril. 1951;2(5):444-50. DOI: 10.1016/s0015-0282(16)30664-1.
148. Stanback J, Steiner M, Dorflinger L, Solo J, Cates W. WHO tiered-effectiveness counseling is rights-based family planning. Glob Health Sci Pract. 2015;3(3):352-7. DOI: 10.9745/GHSP-D-15-00096.
149. Snow R, Garcia S, Kureshy N, et al. Attributes of contraceptive technology: women's preferences in seven countries. In: Berer M, Cottingham J, eds. Beyond Acceptability: Users' Perspectives on Contraception: Reproductive Health Matters for the World Health Organization; 1997:36-48.
150. Lessard LN, Karasek D, Ma S, et al. Contraceptive features preferred by women at high risk of unintended pregnancy. Perspect Sex Reprod Health. 2012;44(3):194-200. DOI: 10.1363/4419412.
151. Madden T, Secura GM, Nease RF, Politi MC, Peipert JF. The role of contraceptive attributes in women's contraceptive decision making. Am J Obstet Gynecol. 2015;213(1):46.e1-6. DOI: 10.1016/j.ajog.2015.01.051.
152. Donnelly KZ, Foster TC, Thompson R. What matters most? The content and concordance of patients' and providers' information priorities for contraceptive decision making. Contraception. 2014;90(3):280-7. DOI: 10.1016/j.contraception.2014.04.012.

153. Eisenberg DL, Secura GM, Madden TE, Allsworth JE, Zhao Q, Peipert JF. Knowledge of contraceptive effectiveness. Am J Obstet Gynecol. 2012;206(6):479.e1-9. DOI: 10.1016/j.ajog.2012.04.012.
154. Nelson AL, Shabaik S, Xandre P, et al. Perceptions of health risks associated with pregnancy compared to oral contraceptive use. Contraception. 2019;100(3):193-5. DOI: 10.1016/j.contraception.2019.04.008.
155. Haemorrhagic stroke, overall stroke risk, and combined oral contraceptives: results of an international, multicentre, case-control study. WHO Collaborative Study of Cardiovascular Disease and Steroid Hormone Contraception. Lancet. 1996;348(9026):505-10.
156. Schwingl PJ, Ory HW, Visness CM. Estimates of the risk of cardiovascular death attributable to low-dose oral contraceptives in the United States. Am J Obstet Gynecol. 1999;180(1 Pt 1):241-9. DOI: 10.1016/s0002-9378(99)70182-1.
157. Vessey M, Painter R, Yeates D. Mortality in relation to oral contraceptive use and cigarette smoking. Lancet. 2003;362(9379):185-91. DOI: 10.1016/S0140-6736(03)13907-4.
158. Hannaford PC, Iversen L, Macfarlane TV, Elliott AM, Angus V, Lee AJ. Mortality among contraceptive pill users: cohort evidence from Royal College of General Practitioners' Oral Contraception Study. BMJ 2010;340:c927. DOI: 10.1136/bmj.c927.
159. Charlton BM, Rich-Edwards JW, Colditz GA, et al. Oral contraceptive use and mortality after 36 years of follow-up in the Nurses' Health Study: prospective cohort study. BMJ 2014;349:g6356. DOI: 10.1136/bmj.g6356.
160. Nur U, El Reda D, Hashim D, Weiderpass E. A prospective investigation of oral contraceptive use and breast cancer mortality: findings from the Swedish women's lifestyle and health cohort. BMC Cancer 2019;19(1):807. DOI: 10.1186/s12885-019-5985-6.
161. Escobedo LG, Peterson HB, Grubb GS, Franks AL. Case-fatality rates for tubal sterilization in U.S. hospitals, 1979 to 1980. Am J Obstet Gynecol. 1989;160(1):147-50. DOI: 10.1016/0002-9378(89)90108-7.
162. Hoyert D. Maternal mortality rates in the United States, 2019. NCHS Health E-Stats. 2021. DOI: https://doi.org/10.15620/cdc:103855.
163. Raymond EG, Grimes DA. The comparative safety of legal induced abortion and childbirth in the United States. Obstet Gynecol. 2012;119(2 Pt 1):215-9. DOI: 10.1097/AOG.0b013e31823fe923.
164. Zane S, Creanga AA, Berg CJ, et al. Abortion-related mortality in the United States: 1998-2010. Obstet Gynecol. 2015;126(2):258-65. DOI. 10.1097/AOG.0000000000000945.
165. Shah I, Ahman E. Unsafe abortion: global and regional incidence, trends, consequences, and challenges. J Obstet Gynaecol Can 2009;31(12):1149-58.
166. Lewis MA. Myocardial infarction and stroke in young women: what is the impact of oral contraceptives? Am J Obstet Gynecol. 1998;179(3 Pt 2):S68-77. DOI: 10.1053/ob.1998.v179.a93122.
167. Lidegaard Ø, Løkkegaard E, Jensen A, Skovlund CW, Keiding N. Thrombotic stroke and myocardial infarction with hormonal contraception. N Engl J Med. 2012;366(24):2257-66. DOI: 10.1056/NEJMoa1111840.
168. Ischaemic stroke and combined oral contraceptives: results of an international, multicentre, case-control study. WHO Collaborative Study of Cardiovascular Disease and Steroid Hormone Contraception. Lancet. 1996;348(9026):498-505.
169. Horton LG, Simmons KB, Curtis KM. Combined hormonal contraceptive use among obese women and risk for cardiovascular events: A systematic review. Contraception. 2016;94(6):590-604. DOI: 10.1016/j.contraception.2016.05.014.
170. James AH. Pregnancy, contraception and venous thromboembolism (deep vein thrombosis and pulmonary embolism). Vasc Med. 2017;22(2):166-9. DOI: 10.1177/1358863X17690601.
171. Tepper NK, Whiteman MK, Marchbanks PA, James AH, Curtis KM. Progestin-only contraception and thromboembolism: A systematic review. Contraception. 2016;94(6):678-700. DOI: 10.1016/j.contraception.2016.04.014.
172. Lidegaard Ø, Løkkegaard E, Svendsen AL, Agger C. Hormonal contraception and risk of venous thromboembolism: national follow-up study. BMJ 2009;339:b2890. DOI: 10.1136/bmj.b2890.

173. Heinemann LA, Dinger JC. Range of published estimates of venous thromboembolism incidence in young women. Contraception. 2007;75(5):328-36. DOI: 10.1016/j.contraception.2006.12.018.
174. Burkman R, Schlesselman JJ, Zieman M. Safety concerns and health benefits associated with oral contraception. Am J Obstet Gynecol. 2004;190(4 Suppl):S5-22. DOI: 10.1016/j.ajog.2004.01.061.
175. Hannaford PC, Selvaraj S, Elliott AM, Angus V, Iversen L, Lee AJ. Cancer risk among users of oral contraceptives: cohort data from the Royal College of General Practitioners' oral contraception study. BMJ 2007;335(7621):651. DOI: 10.1136/bmj.39289.649410.55.
176. Iversen L, Sivasubramaniam S, Lee AJ, Fielding S, Hannaford PC. Lifetime cancer risk and combined oral contraceptives: the Royal College of General Practitioners' Oral Contraception Study. Am J Obstet Gynecol. 2017;216(6):580.e1-9. DOI: 10.1016/j.ajog.2017.02.002.
177. Vessey M, Yeates D, Flynn S. Factors affecting mortality in a large cohort study with special reference to oral contraceptive use. Contraception. 2010;82(3):221-9. DOI: 10.1016/j.contraception.2010.04.006.
178. Wingo PA, Austin H, Marchbanks PA, et al. Oral contraceptives and the risk of death from breast cancer. Obstet Gynecol. 2007;110(4):793-800. DOI: 10.1097/01.AOG.0000284446.22251.6e.
179. Mueck AO, Seeger H, Rabe T. Hormonal contraception and risk of endometrial cancer: a systematic review. Endocr Relat Cancer 2010;17(4):R263-71. DOI: 10.1677/ERC-10-0076.
180. Li CI, Beaber EF, Tang MT, Porter PL, Daling JR, Malone KE. Effect of depo-medroxyprogesterone acetate on breast cancer risk among women 20 to 44 years of age. Cancer Res 2012;72(8):2028-35. DOI: 10.1158/0008-5472.CAN-11-4064.
181. Urban M, Banks E, Egger S, et al. Injectable and oral contraceptive use and cancers of the breast, cervix, ovary, and endometrium in black South African women: case-control study. PLoS Med. 2012;9(3):e1001182. DOI: 10.1371/journal.pmed.1001182.
182. Soini T, Hurskainen R, Grénman S, Mäenpää J, Paavonen J, Pukkala E. Cancer risk in women using the levonorgestrel-releasing intrauterine system in Finland. Obstet Gynecol. 2014;124(2 Pt 1):292-9. DOI: 10.1097/AOG.0000000000000356.
183. Soini T, Hurskainen R, Grénman S, Mäenpää J, Paavonen J, Pukkala E. Impact of levonorgestrel-releasing intrauterine system use on the cancer risk of the ovary and fallopian tube. Acta Oncol 2016;55(11):1281-4. DOI: 10.1080/0284186X.2016.1175660.
184. Kaunitz AM. Depot medroxyprogesterone acetate contraception and the risk of breast and gynecologic cancer. J Reprod Med 1996;41(5 Suppl):419-27.
185. Samson M, Porter N, Orekoya O, et al. Progestin and breast cancer risk: a systematic review. Breast Cancer Res Treat 2016;155(1):3-12. DOI: 10.1007/s10549-015-3663-1.
186. Huber LR, Hogue CJ, Stein AD, et al. Contraceptive use and discontinuation: findings from the contraceptive history, initiation, and choice study. Am J Obstet Gynecol. 2006;194(5):1290-5. DOI: 10.1016/j.ajog.2005.11.039.
187. Rothschild CW, Richardson BA, Guthrie BL, et al. Contributions of side effects to contraceptive discontinuation and method switch among Kenyan women: a prospective cohort study. BJOG 2021;129(6):926-37. DOI: 10.1111/1471-0528.17032.
188. Beesham I, Bosman S, Beksinska M, Scoville CW, Smit J, Nanda K. Contraceptive method preference and reasons for contraceptive discontinuation among women randomized to intramuscular depot medroxyprogesterone acetate, a copper intrauterine device or a levonorgestrel implant: Findings from Durban, South Africa. Contraception. 2022;108:37-43. DOI: 10.1016/j.contraception.2021.11.002.
189. Tolley E, Loza S, Kafafi L, Cummings S. The impact of menstrual side effects on contraceptive discontinuation: findings from a longitudinal study in Cairo, Egypt. Int Fam Plan Perspect 2005;31(1):15-23. DOI: 10.1363/3101505.
190. Sato R, Elewonibi B, Msuya S, Manongi R, Canning D, Shah I. Why do women discontinue contraception and what are the post-discontinuation outcomes? Evidence from the Arusha Region, Tanzania. Sex Reprod Health Matters 2020;28(1):1723321. DOI: 10.1080/26410397.2020.1723321.
191. Grimes DA, Schulz KF. Nonspecific side effects of oral contraceptives: nocebo or noise? Contraception. 2011;83(1):5-9. DOI: 10.1016/j.contraception.2010.06.010.

192. Polis CB, Hussain R, Berry A. There might be blood: a scoping review on women's responses to contraceptive-induced menstrual bleeding changes. Reprod Health. 2018;15(1):114. DOI: 10.1186/s12978-018-0561-0.
193. Yland JJ, Bresnick KA, Hatch EE, et al. Pregravid contraceptive use and fecundability: prospective cohort study. BMJ 2020;371:m3966. DOI: 10.1136/bmj.m3966.
194. DEPO-SUBQ PROVERA 104. US FDA-approved product information.
195. Taylor DJ, Halpern V, Brache V, Bahamondes L, Jensen JT, Dorflinger LJ. Ovulation suppression following subcutaneous administration of depot medroxyprogesterone acetate. Contracept X. 2022;4:100073. DOI: 10.1016/j.conx.2022.100073.
196. Depo Provera CI. US FDA approved product information. (https://www.accessdata.fda.gov/drugsatfda_docs/label/2010/020246s036lbl.pdf).
197. Gemmill A, Bradley SEK, van der Poel S. Reduced fecundity in HIV-positive women. Hum Reprod 2018;33(6):1158-66. DOI: 10.1093/humrep/dey065.
198. Malmborg A, Persson E, Brynhildsen J, Hammar M. Hormonal contraception and sexual desire: A questionnaire-based study of young Swedish women. Eur J Contracept Reprod Health Care 2016;21(2):158-67. DOI: 10.3109/13625187.2015.1079609.
199. Boozalis A, Tutlam NT, Chrisman Robbins C, Peipert JF. Sexual desire and hormonal contraception. Obstet Gynecol. 2016;127(3):563-72. DOI: 10.1097/AOG.0000000000001286.
200. Both S, Lew-Starowicz M, Luria M, et al. Hormonal contraception and female sexuality: Position statements from the European Society of Sexual Medicine (ESSM). J Sex Med. 2019;16(11):1681-95. DOI: 10.1016/j.jsxm.2019.08.005.

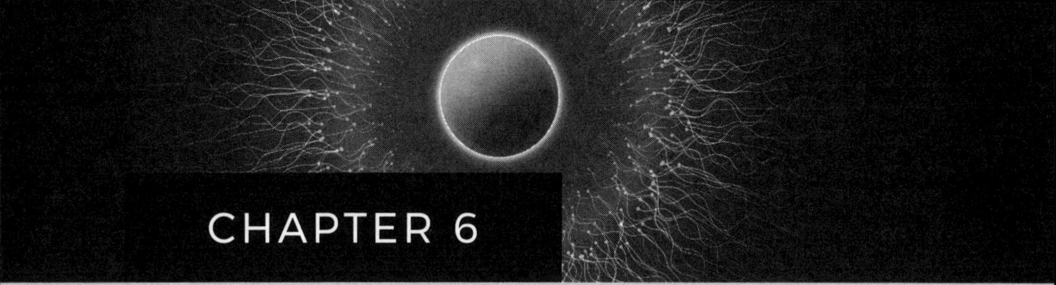

CHAPTER 6

Sexuality and Contraception

Jenny A. Higgins, PhD, MPH
Patty Cason, MS, FNP-PC
Jessica N. Sanders, PhD, MSPH

KEY POINTS

- Sexual and reproductive health involves the positive aspects of sexuality and not merely the prevention of unwanted pregnancy, STIs, and sexual violence.
- People use contraception in sexual contexts, so to provide the best contraceptive care, health care providers should invite patients to frame their contraceptive needs in the context of their sexuality and sexual expressions.
- Sexual activity can have physical, emotional, and social benefits.
- Sex can also involve coercion, violence, and trauma that undermine reproductive autonomy, contraceptive use, and sexual well-being.
- The sexual acceptability of contraception, which involves physiologic, psychological, and dyadic elements, can influence contraceptive preferences, satisfaction, and use over time.
- While many similarities exist across methods, individual methods can be associated with different aspects of sexual acceptability due to mechanism of action, side effects, and other factors.
- Evidence suggests that contraceptive methods can improve many individuals' sex lives, while a smaller percentage of users report sexual detractions.
- Providers can take advantage of a number of tools when addressing sexual acceptability of various contraceptives.

People don't have sex to use contraception. Rather, people overwhelmingly use contraception so they can engage in the pleasures and other benefits of sexual expression without experiencing unwanted pregnancy. Almost all contraceptive use takes place within sexual contexts and sexual relationships. However, contraceptive clinical care rarely addresses these sexual contexts of patients' lives, and many providers remain underinformed about contraception's impact on sex and, in turn, sex's impact on contraception. These phenomena not only undermine person-centered contraceptive care but also fail to help contraceptive clients maximize their full sexual and reproductive health potential.[1] This chapter tries to address this gap by focusing on the sexual acceptability of contraception, which refers to how contraceptive methods affect sexual experiences and well-being.

Sexual and reproductive health entails not merely the ability to avoid unwanted pregnancy, sexually transmitted infections (STIs), or sexual violence; it also requires the opportunity for sexual flourishing, including a pleasurable, unstigmatized, and satisfying sex life. The World Health Organization,[2] the American Sexual Health Association,[3] and major research outlets[4] have all underscored the salience of sexual flourishing in relation to optimal sexual and reproductive health. The World Association for Sexual Health commissioned a recent Declaration on Sexual Pleasure, underscoring that sexual pleasure is integral to broader health, well-being, and rights.[5] Moreover, social advocates worldwide have argued that sexual pleasure is critical not only to overall health but also to gender equity.[6,7] Integrating this full spectrum of sexual pleasure, well-being, and equity into contraceptive care can help providers align person-centered care with reproductive health outcomes.[8]

Two additional reasons underscore why a positive approach to sexuality, including consideration of sexual acceptability, should matter to contraceptive care providers. First, addressing the notion that the way sex feels matters to patients could have positive if not revolutionary effects on contraceptive satisfaction, use over time, and thus, individuals' ability to avoid unwanted pregnancy. It would acknowledge patients as sexual agents versus targets of contraceptive programs. Second, patients, including adolescents,[9,10] *want* us to care about their sexuality, even though many are uncomfortable initiating such topics themselves.[11] One study found that 93% of surveyed patients would welcome the question of "how is your sexuality these days?" during a primary care visit.[12] Providers also believe that addressing sexual well-being is an important part of holistic care, but most feel insufficiently trained or ill-prepared to do so;[13] thus, few providers inquire or follow up on sexual issues.[14,15]

In this chapter, after reminding readers of some of the benefits of a satisfying sex life, we describe the various components of sexual acceptability and document sexual acceptability's associations with contraceptive preferences, satisfaction, and use over time. Then, method by method, we review the literature examining connections between people's sexual experiences and contraceptive acceptability and practices. We conclude with resources and recommendations to assist practitioners in addressing sexuality and sexual acceptability during clinical encounters.

Gender and Sexual Identities

Our field now widely recognizes that contraceptive clients are hardly limited to cisgender women; people with myriad gender identities use contraception. Sexual identity is also a critical consideration in sex-positive contraceptive care. Research reveals that upward of one-in-three contraceptive clients identifies as something other than exclusively[16] heterosexual. Of course, people with diverse gender and sexual identities are not defined solely by those identities, but these identities may influence their experiences with contraception.[17] Pleasurable sexual expression and the sexual acceptability of contraception matters to contraceptive users of all gender and sexual identities.

Substantively, understandings of gender diversity in relationship to contraceptive care demand awareness of the following: reproductive health care isn't about "women" but people; many families don't have a mom and/or a dad; and reproductive organs and hormones don't have a gender.[18] Commitment to gender diversity also brings logistical implications for contraceptive care, including: waiting areas and patient-facing elements of clinical spaces should feel welcoming to diverse genders; and providers at all levels of the health care system should solicit and use the correct names and pronouns for each patient, not just for those thought or known to be gender diverse.

Sex Brings Both Benefits and Harms

As providers, we have the opportunity to promote sexual well-being not only as a desirable outcome in itself but also for its connection to better physical, emotional, and relationship health.[19-21] Sexual activity that is noncoercive, wanted, and pleasurable, either partnered or solo, confers a variety of health and relationship benefits.[22,23] Overall well-being, quality of life, and even happiness are greater among those fortunate individuals who enjoy a satisfying sexual life.[24-30] While these associations are often more correlational than causal, it's helpful to become familiar with some of the health and social advantages of pleasurable sexual activity.

For example, a recent study demonstrated the positive, even protective, effect that consistent partnered sexual activity can have on anxiety, depression, and relationship stress by examining sexual experiences during the COVID-19 pandemic.[31] Sexual activity is a method of low-impact, regular exercise[32] and is excellent for cardiovascular health, reducing risk of fatal coronary events with no increased risk of stroke.[33,34] Perhaps most striking is the longevity advantage.[35-39] People who have consistent, satisfying sex and who experience orgasm throughout their life don't just feel younger—they live longer. Sex has relational benefits, too. Satisfying coupled sex is causally associated with healthier and satisfying relationships and with relationships that are more likely to remain intact.[40-44]

Sex also benefits a variety of reproductive health outcomes. For example, exposure to a partner's semen for 6 months prior to conception is associated with a decreased risk of preeclampsia; coitus during in vitro fertilization cycles improves the chance of pregnancy; and contrary to previous assumptions, both coitus and orgasm in late pregnancy are associated with a reduced risk of preterm delivery.[45-47] Sexual frequency is associated with a later age of natural menopause and less genitourinary syndrome of menopause.[48,49] Data show remarkable benefits from all types of sex and intimate touch for mental health,[21,50] cognition,[51,52] and even the ability to treat migraine and cluster headache[53] in many people. Ejaculation has been shown to reduce symptoms of Parkinson disease[54] and risk of prostate cancer.[55,56] And if you have atopy, kissing your romantic partner can reduce allergic skin wheal responses.[57]

In other words, there are good clinical reasons to invest in patients' pleasure and to encourage conversations and openness about sex during clinical encounters.

However, people have unequal access to sexual pleasure and well-being—a phenomenon called "erotic inequity."[58] Gender is one example of how sociocultural systems enable, or fail to enable, positive aspects of sexuality. Research on the orgasm gap indicates that in heterosexual relationships, people with penises are much more likely to have orgasms than people with clitorises,[59] despite nearly identical abilities to achieve orgasm while masturbating. Poverty can constrain sexual expression, with financial scarcity associated with significantly lower reports of sexual satisfaction and functioning.[58] Discrimination such as homophobia and transphobia also undermine sexual flourishing.[60,61] Fighting for social equity and justice is a critical way to support and promote positive sexual health. The recently integrated tenets of the Reproductive Justice framework (see Chapter 1, Reproductive Justice within Reproductive Health Care) include the right to sexual pleasure, the freedom to express one's own gender, and access to health care and body positivity.[62]

Sexism, homophobia, and transphobia within our society also greatly affect people's *negative* sexual experiences, including sexual violence and coercion. The United Nations estimates that 35% of women worldwide have experienced either physical and/or sexual intimate partner violence or sexual violence by a nonpartner at some point in their lives,[63] and reported rates from the United States are virtually identical.[64] Patriarchy, misogyny, and gender-based power differences all drive greater rates of sexual violence and reproductive coercion among women, both cis and trans, compared to cisgender men.[65,66] However, people of all gender identities experience sexual violence and its attendant, harmful sequelae. People with queer and gender-diverse identities are also at significantly elevated risk of sexual violence.[67,68] These negative sexual experiences affect patient reproductive health, including inconsistent contraceptive use, risk of STIs, sexual dysfunction, and other unwanted sexual outcomes.

Thus, providers must consider the possibility that sexual trauma shapes many of their patients' sexual experiences. Moreover, patients' interactions with the medical establishment can also serve as a source of (re)trauma, especially for trans and gender-nonconforming individuals. Sexual and reproductive health care providers can reduce the likelihood of such harmful interactions with patients by learning about and providing care that is trauma-informed. Such trauma must be carefully considered and addressed in patient care related to the sexual acceptability of contraception.[69] Traumatic events are common in patients' lives and have deep and long-lasting effects on physical and mental health, including sexual health. Trauma-informed care focuses on principles of safety, transparency, and collaboration, and it prioritizes efforts to keep the locus of control with the patient, in effort to avoid retraumatizing patients. Chapters 4 and 22 feature more information on person-centered, trauma-informed care.

The Importance of The Sexual Acceptability of Contraception

Just as sex can bring both benefits and harms, contraception can both positively and negatively influence people's sex lives. For example, protection against pregnancy can lead to a type of sexual disinhibition that may improve people's sexual experiences.[70] Reduced vaginal bleeding can also facilitate more frequent or enjoyable sex. However, side effects such as increased bleeding, unpredictable spotting or bleeding, breast tenderness, or headaches can detract from sexual experiences or keep people from having the type of sex they would like at the time they would like to. Some hormonal mechanisms, especially those that suppress ovulation, can reduce libido. Other methods such as external condoms can reduce one or both partners' pleasure, a dyadic phenomenon that can have an impact on sexual expression.

Gendered expectations about sexuality and birth control—for example, that women are charged with being responsible for sex, contraception, and relationships, and can face serious social consequences if they transgress—can also influence people's sexual experiences.[71] Given that contraceptives can affect sexual influences through physiologic, dyadic, and cultural experiences, "a holistic approach is needed to understand the complexity of aspects related to women's *[sic]* sexuality and their link with contraception."[72]

However, a central but often overlooked aspect of the acceptability of contraceptive products is *sexual acceptability,* or how contraceptive methods influence sexual experiences,[70] which has subsequent, direct implications for contraceptive practices.[70] Research already suggests that patients may reject or discontinue methods that detract from their own or their partner's sexual experiences.[73] Contraceptive methods are only effective if used, and they must be designed to fit patients' sexual lives rather than vice versa. Sexual acceptability plays a role in patient satisfaction with contraception used for noncontraceptive benefits, as well as for people who do not engage in penetrative sexual activity.

As the method-by-method section below indicates, a now-sizable body of contraception literature documents various aspects of sexual acceptability.[70] However, much of this research still has shortcomings. In addition to study design limitations,[74] including cross-sectional versus longitudinal designs, most studies assign research participants particular methods, whereas in real-life clinical practice, patients select their own desired methods.

Further, the bulk of existing studies have taken a narrow, predominantly physiologic approach to assessing sexual acceptability.[75] Researchers have primarily used the Female Sexual Function Index, or FSFI, which captures domains such as

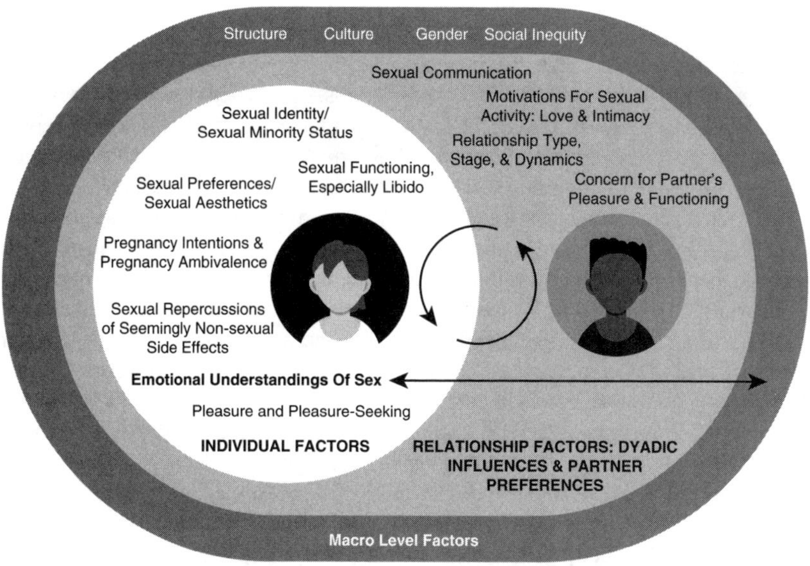

Figure 6-1 Dalessandro, Thorpe, and Sanders' Revised Model of the Sexual Acceptability of Contraception

Reproduced from Dalessandro C, Thorpe R, Sanders J. "For Me, It's Having Something Meaningful": Women's Emotional Understandings of Sex and the Sexual Acceptability of Contraception. J Sex Res 2021;0(0):1–12.

lubrication, libido, and orgasm.[76,77] These physiologic phenomena are important but fail to account for other domains of sexual acceptability such as psychological disinhibition, sexual aspects of side effects such as bleeding and cramping, and people's perceptions of whether their methods affect sexuality. Signs also indicate that measures of sexual function have few significant associations with people's sexual experiences of contraception. A 2020 meta-analysis of contraception and sexual dysfunction observed no significant, negative associations between contraceptive use and sexual arousal, lubrication, orgasm, satisfaction, or pain.[78] The researchers did find significant associations between contraceptive use and desire.

Notably, investigators in the studies above found that patients' perceptions of their method's sexual impact were strikingly similar across methods. This similarity suggests two things. First, on average, no particular methods appear significantly more likely than others to improve, or detract from, users' sexual experiences. Thus, providers should not recommend one method as more sexually acceptable than another, and they should recognize that patients as a group can have significantly different sexual experiences with a given method. Second, we cannot predict which users will experience which sexual effects with which methods. The key is to impart to patients the importance of their sexual experiences with their methods, encouraging and supporting method change when their method makes their sex life worse.

Researchers are finding ways to improve the study of sexual acceptability, including the use of more multifaceted measures. In a recent longitudinal study[73] of over 2,000 new-start contraceptive users selecting one of six reversible methods, investigators collected information on sexual functioning,[77] sexual satisfaction,[79] menstrual-related changes,[80] and whether, and how, participants' contraceptive method had affected their sex life in the past month (from "a lot worse" to "a lot better").

Participants in the study reported no significant changes in sexual functioning or sexual satisfaction scores.[81] However, at 1 month, over half (53%) of participants said their new method improved their sex life (26% "improved a lot"; 27% "improved a little"); 17% said it made their sex life worse (14% "a little worse"; 3% "a lot worse"); and 30% reported no sexual effect. In other words, even when their sexual functioning and satisfaction measures remain stable, a significant proportion of contraceptive users perceive sexual effects—mostly positive sexual effects—of their methods. These findings were similar in a study of 159 new-start IUD and implant users.[82]

To establish a more multifaceted measure of contraceptive sexual acceptability, investigators evaluated the study's multiple scales and items for validity and reliability and reduced them a 10-item contraceptive sexual acceptability scale.[83] While not yet tested in clinical settings, this scale is intended for future use in research and clinical care.

Of course, method selection precedes any actual contraceptive use. Research also indicates that contraceptive clients value sexual-related characteristics when selecting a new method.[81,84] In one US study of 382 participants, the most frequently desired contraceptive feature was "does not interfere with the pleasure of sex," which was selected by more respondents than "is 99% effective without having to do anything" (87% versus 74%, respectively).[85] In another study of family planning and abortion clinic patients, 68% of 1,783 participants said it was "extremely important" that a "method doesn't detract from my sexual enjoyment."[86] In their development of a contraceptive decision-making aid, Jamin et al. found that "effect on sexual pleasure," "effect on intimacy/spontaneity/libido," and "level of sexual activity" emerged as key factors influencing contraceptive choice.[87]

Research indicates that sexual acceptability influences contraceptive use over time—perhaps more so than all other factors. A prospective study in the United

States followed 100 new combined oral contraceptive users for 1 year. Among those 47% of patients who stopped using their pills over the course of the study, decreased sexual thoughts and decreased psychosexual arousal were the strongest predictors of discontinuation. In the heretofore-mentioned study of over 2,000 new-start contraceptive users,[73] sexual acceptability had the largest measured effect on continuation[73] over time. Contraceptive users' perceptions that their new method negatively affected their sex lives were strongly associated with discontinuation by 6 months—more robustly than other adverse effects such as increases in bleeding and physical or mood-related changes. For example, participants whose method made their sex lives "a lot worse" had 3.3 increased odds of discontinuation by 6 months relative to those whose method improved their sex life "a lot."

However, contraceptive continuation is rarely the best way, and certainly not the only way, to measure success in contraceptive care. Researchers and providers often focus on contraceptive continuation or "adherence," but "satisfaction" is a more person-centered outcome that better captures users' actual experiences of their contraceptive method.[88] Many people report contraceptive nonuse or inconsistent use because of method dissatisfaction. While relatively little research examines the method characteristics and other factors most strongly associated with satisfaction, preliminary research suggests that sexual acceptability can play a key role.

In a study of over 1,800 new-start contraceptive clients, researchers found that users' perceived impact of their method on their sex life in the first month strongly predicted satisfaction at 3 months, whereas factors such as mood-related side effects (e.g., depression) or changes in sexual functioning did not significantly predict contraceptive satisfaction.[89,90] Compared with patients in this study who said their contraceptive method made their sex life "a lot" worse in the first month of use, patients whose method improved their sex life "a lot" had a 7.7 times increased odds of greater satisfaction at 3 months. To a much lesser degree, experiencing less or no bleeding was significantly associated with increased satisfaction, whereas worsening of physical side effects (e.g., breast tenderness) was linked to decreased satisfaction.

Before describing method-specific research on sexual acceptability, we wish to underscore once again the strong similarity across methods in terms of users' sexual experiences. For example, levonorgestrel IUD users appear no more likely than users of combined oral contraceptives or injectables to report that their method has improved or detracted from their sex life.[81] Patients should be supported in finding methods that are most acceptable to them at various points in their lives,[85,91,92] sexually and otherwise. People differ in what they desire in a contraceptive method and what helps them feel sexually well. Providers and researchers alike should prioritize support both for people's contraceptive satisfaction and for their sexual well-being.

Method-Specific Research on Sexual Acceptability

Hormonal Methods

Combined Hormonal Methods

Significant debate surrounds which hormones (estrogen, progesterone, testosterone, or oxytocin)[98] exert the greatest influence on sexual functioning, and how or even if hormonal changes are really that important relative to contraceptive users' subjective experiences of their sexuality. The standard, albeit controversial, explanation for how combined hormonal contraceptives (CHCs)—that is, patches, pills, and rings—influence sexual functioning, including desire, primarily involves the role of androgens. Given that CHCs inhibit luteinizing hormone and that one of the mechanisms of action is suppression of ovulation, they will also decrease ovarian production of testosterone. Adding exogenous estrogen often raises the amount of sex hormone–binding globulin (SHBG), which contributes to declines in levels of free testosterone.[93] While most studies do show an increase in SHBG as well as a decrease in total and free testosterone in CHC users, the majority of those studies do *not* demonstrate a negative impact on libido.[94] Some researchers, however, have concluded that lower levels of free testosterone contribute to lowered libido in CHC users, particularly given that non-contraception-focused trials suggest that the addition of exogenous testosterone may improve libido significantly more than placebo.[95] As a result, some researchers have been studying the effects of "androgen-restored contraception," which supplements combined oral contraceptives with testosterone.[96] Phase II trials suggest that, in some users, adding testosterone may decrease combined oral contraceptives' negative effects on sexual functioning.[97]

Though testosterone decreases are perhaps the most popular explanation for how CHCs affect users' sexual functioning, testosterone research itself can be marred by possible confounders that bias the interpretation of findings.[99] In those not using hormonal contraception, different levels of endogenous androgens among individuals do not correlate with differences in sexual functioning or libido. No particular androgen level is predictive of "low" sexual function,[100] and patients vary in the degree to which they are sensitive to these hormonal changes[101] or the degree to which lowered testosterone has any clear effect on sexual interest.[102]

We urge caution regarding assumptions that androgens always contribute directly to increased sexual desire—or that CHC use results in universal changes to sexual libido. Encouragingly, evidence suggests that CHC users who experience issues with libido or arousal may find relief when switching to a different hormonal formulation, particularly one with a progestin that has more androgenic characteristics.[103,104]

We wish to note that almost no long-term data specifically document the sexual effects of transmasculine people using testosterone. This scenario creates a different landscape of sexual issues, including effects on libido and lubrication. Future research in this area must attend to such individuals.

Combined Hormonal Oral Contraceptives. Most research on combined oral contraceptives (COCs) and sexuality examines libido. Several reviews have found reports of both increased and decreased libido with COC use.[105-107] A systematic review of 36 studies and 13,000 people documented no significant associations between COCs and sexual desire.[94] These reviews also noted the lack of high-quality studies on this topic. Few studies are randomized and placebo-controlled, and fewer meet every single standard for high-quality reporting of randomized clinical trials (CONSORT[108] guidelines). One well-designed trial demonstrated a decrease in libido in COC users compared to placebo in a sample of women in Scotland (higher baseline libido) but not in a sample of women in the Philippines (lower baseline libido).[109] A prospective study in the United States followed new-start COC users for 1 year.[110] Researchers found that decreased sexual thoughts and decreased psychosexual arousal were the strongest predictors of COC discontinuation over time.

Many people using COCs experience no negative sexual functioning outcomes.[111,112] Birth control pills can also relieve dysmenorrhea and lighten menstrual bleeding, two potential sexual benefits for many individuals and couples. COCs can mitigate negative effects of health conditions such as endometriosis and polycystic ovary syndrome (PCOS) that adversely affect sexuality. Other positive sexual outcomes associated with COCs for some individuals include improvements in hirsutism and acne.[113] However, other aspects of COC use, such as breakthrough bleeding, breast tenderness,[114] and vaginal dryness,[115] are likely to detract from sexual acceptability for those patients who experience such side effects.[116]

Vaginal Rings. Vaginal rings offer an effective, user-controlled contraceptive option. Current FDA-approved combined hormonal vaginal rings include the monthly option and a newer ring designed for 1 year of use.

A recent 2020 systematic review found high user satisfaction across ring users ranging between 80% and 90%.[117] Continuation rates averaged 54% across studies, similar to COCs (55%), depot-medrozyprogesterone acetate, (57%) and combined hormonal patches (49%), but lower than IUDs and implants (86%).[106] Additionally, studies that assessed contraceptive satisfaction and continuation strongly suggest that people who associated the method with positive sexual attributes were more likely to continue using it over time.[66,101] Interestingly, a randomized, controlled trial on extended regimens and continuous cycling found that continuation was higher for individuals using shorter and standard cycling protocols than for those who were assigned to longer intervals and continuous cycling. This finding may be related to the sexual impact of unpredictable bleeding.[105]

The *mechanics* of the ring may also affect its sexual acceptability, for both users and their partners. Use of the ring requires touching one's genitals, which necessitates an element of sexual self-comfort, although some patients are more comfortable having their partner place the ring. Ring-related sexual events, such as feeling the ring inside the vagina, or interference with or expulsion during sex, have been associated with higher rates of discontinuation. On the other hand, the overwhelming majority of partners reported that they never felt the ring during sex, expressed no change in sexual sensations, or reported that being able to feel the ring did not bother them or disrupt sex.[118] Across studies, less than one-third of contraceptive ring users or their sexual partners expressed concerns regarding sexual discomfort with the ring during intercourse.[117]

As with any hormonal method, ring users experience adverse hormone-related experiences such as unfavorable bleeding, nausea, headache, breast tenderness, and vaginal discomfort.[119] However, compared to COC users, ring users in one study reported comparatively fewer issues with vaginal dryness.[120] Extended-cycle use (63 days followed by hormone-free interval) has been associated with improvements in Italian women's dyspareunia, sexual function, sexual distress, and quality of life.[119] Highly satisfied ring users in one US study reported fewer side effects than with pills, no detection of the ring during normal use, and either no change or an increase in sexual pleasure and/or sexual frequency; these satisfied users were more likely to continue using the ring.[121]

Conversations with patients who are interested in using a vaginal ring may include discussions designed to increase their knowledge of lower genital tract anatomy and to explore their level of comfort with putting their finger in their vagina. Providers can anticipate and respond to patient concerns about the ring expelling or getting lost during sex, and offer alternative strategies to help make ring placement more acceptable—for example, placing the ring while showering or using a clean empty tampon applicator to help with placement. Clarifying expectations around bleeding profiles, including the potential for spotting with continuous cycling, can start a conversation about how that aligns with their sexual preferences and can support sexually informed, person-centered contraceptive counseling.

Transdermal Contraceptive Patch. While the transdermal patch is a less frequently used method, with 1% of contraceptive users reporting current use and 10% ever use, this method has a number of desirable characteristics for certain patients.[122]

There are limited data on the sexual acceptability of transdermal contraceptive patches, and the number of users were exceedingly small in some of the larger prospective studies, such as the HER Salt Lake Contraceptive Initiative.[123] But in a comparison of ring and patch users, one study found that patch users reported slight increases in FSFI scores 3 months after initiation; however, these changes are not likely to be clinically significant.[124] The fact that the transdermal patch is visible to others, particularly sexual partners, may render some users uncomfortable. On the other hand, additional communication about the patch between partners may enhance intimacy. Providers may also encounter patient concerns that the patch will come off during sexual activity, and they can underscore this event's strong unlikeliness.

Progestin-Only Methods

Progestin-Only Pills. Studies that specifically examine the progestin-only pill (POP) and sexual acceptability are limited. Existing data suggest that, on average, the POP has little or no negative impact on sexual interest or activity.[109] However, individuals who recently delivered and are breastfeeding may have noncontraceptive-related factors affecting their sexual experiences. In a prospective study of new-start contraceptive users who were not recently postpartum, 2% selected a POP at enrollment. At follow-up, 12% reported some sexual detraction due to their method, 31% reported sexual improvement, and 57% reported no impact on their sex life.[125]

Hormonal IUDs. More people than ever before are using IUDs for highly effective pregnancy prophylaxis as well as for noncontraceptive benefits such as reduction in menstrual bleeding. Currently 7.8% of all people using contraception in the United States have an IUD, equating to about 4.4 million individuals.[126] Just over three-quarters of IUD users select a hormonal IUD versus a copper nonhormonal IUD.[127]

Over the last few years, a rapidly growing body of literature has documented the sexual acceptability of hormonal IUDs as users start and continue the method for extended durations (up to 7 years). Studies have more commonly associated use of a hormonal IUD with positive or neutral sexual effects versus negative ones. However, one review identified mixed results, a lack of US studies, and potential methodological limitations.[128] A prospective US study addressed some of these gaps by documenting sexual acceptability using a variety of sexuality measures among people initiating an IUD or implant method. Investigators controlled for baseline sexual functioning, relationship length, general health and well-being, and other factors that can influence sexuality.[82] Measured after both 1 and 3 months of use, the total FSFI scores and New Sexual Satisfaction Scale scores among new IUD and implant users did not differ from baseline. However, participants *were* significantly more likely to report perceived improvements (versus detractions) to their sexual lives. For example, at one month, 41% of women indicated their new hormonal IUD had improved their sex life in the last 4 weeks, compared to 15% reporting their method had made their sex life worse. By 3 months, 40% of women still reported improvements. Among those reporting sexual detractions due to their contraceptive method, 88% said they had experienced an increase in vaginal bleeding. Perceived sexual improvements were strongly associated with the ability to "let go" in sex and with one's sense of control over pregnancy prevention, suggesting that many people may be able to enjoy sexual activity more when the threat of pregnancy is reduced. And a more recent assessment of changes in sexual functioning after 2 years of use found no negative declines in sexual functioning scores over that time.[129]

A US-based qualitative study of the sexual acceptability of IUDs revealed mostly positive themes such as increased sexual disinhibition due to the method's high contraceptive efficacy, greater allowance for sexual spontaneity compared to condoms, and psychosocial benefits of no or fewer synthetic hormones compared to other hormonal methods.[71] These sexual themes connected to users' method satisfaction and nonusers' openness to the method. Nonusers' most frequently cited sexual concern about IUDs was the potential for their partner to feel or be "poked" by the string. Another qualitative study revealed similar string troubles; IUD users reported that one's partner's ability to feel IUD strings during sex put a "damper" on sexual experiences.[71] (See the Tools and Resources section on p. 191 for suggestions on how to speak to patients about this concern.)

Individuals' preferences for, and responses to, menstrual bleeding changes with IUD use also affect sexual acceptability. For patients preferring little to no menstrual bleeding, a levonorgestrel IUD may be particularly enticing, as blood flow decreases significantly (up to 90% at 1 year for 52-mg devices) in the vast majority of users.[130] Chapter 10 on IUDs describes bleeding profiles for each of the IUD types. The bleeding profile associated with the hormonal IUD is likely to increase sexual acceptability of this method, though some people prefer monthly periods.

In sum, while studies demonstrate mostly positive effects of IUDs on patients' sexuality, sexual acceptability will vary according to the characteristics of each IUD, including which dose of levonorgestrel is in the device or if it contains no hormones. Most importantly, sexual acceptability of IUDs will be shaped by individual user preferences for particular characteristics, including bleeding preferences, comfort with an object inside the body, and tolerance for hormone-related side effects for people using hormone-containing devices.

Progestin-Only Injectable Contraceptive. Sexual acceptability of the injectable contraceptive, depot-medroxyprogesterone acetate (DMPA), depends largely on an individual's response to high-dose progestin. Evidence suggests the high dose of progestin in DMPA inhibits not only ovulation but also ovarian production of estradiol, which decreases endogenous estrogen levels. A recent study of sexual acceptability of various contraceptive methods, including DPMA, found varied impacts on sexual experiences. Users on average reported reduced satisfaction with their level of arousal and overall sexual functioning; however, overall reports of perceived impact of DMPA on sexual experiences were largely neutral or positive, with 13% reporting a negative impact, 51% reporting no perceived impact, and 36% reporting a positive impact on their sex lives.[125]

Other studies have documented decreased libido with DMPA use, with one reporting that up to 21% of users reporting reductions in sexual desire (compared to only 8% reporting increases).[131] The latter study also found that 20% of women using DMPA reported breast tenderness and 9% experienced sexual pain, perhaps due to the hypoestrogenic effect on vaginal tissue. DMPA has also been associated with negative changes in mood and is highly correlated with weight gain, with a subset of users experiencing large increases in weight. However, 49% of DMPA users report not having experienced weight gain in the first 6 months of use. In this same cohort, two-thirds (66%) experienced no bleeding or less bleeding than before.[132] All of these factors combined could shape DMPA users' sexual well-being.

To better understand the experiences with DMPA use, Gubrium[76] conducted qualitative interviews with 34 US women, highlighting that side effects are not experienced in isolation, but rather as a constellation of factors including weight gain, changes in body image, unpredictable bleeding, and emotionality, all of which affect users' intimate relationships and interactions with sexual partners. This study underscores the social and not merely physical impacts of contraceptives on users and their sexual selves. Taken together, these factors can enact changes in sexual desire or libido, thus contributing in important and understudied ways to the sexual acceptability of this contraceptive method. Again, given varied user preferences and experiences, it becomes critical to assess the preferences and experience of the patient in front of you.

The Progestin-Only Subdermal Implant (Nexplanon). Use of subdermal contraceptive implants is growing across the United States, especially in adolescent and young adult populations.[133,134] The implant must be placed by a trained provider but does not require a vaginal exam or intrauterine placement. These attributes are preferred by many individuals who are uncomfortable with or prefer to avoid pelvic exams or who have past sexual or gynecologic trauma. Given its high efficacy and "set-it-and-forget-it" mode of administration, the implant has many of the sexual benefits of IUDs, particularly enhanced sexual disinhibition. However, the unpredictable and sometimes unfavorable bleeding associated with the implant may detract from sexual experiences. Studies suggest that 20% to 25% of implant users report frequent or prolonged bleeding sometime within the first year of use. However, at least one-third (32% to 42%) of users experience amenorrhea, and an additional 20% experience minimal bleeding, which translates into over half of users experiencing minimal to no bleeding.[135,136] The perceived impact of bleeding patterns on sexual acceptability is variable as reduced bleeding is highly desired by many users, while a smaller group of users may find amenorrhea concerning.

A variety of other possible implant side effects, including headaches, acne, or mood changes, may indirectly decrease sexual acceptability. The implant reliably suppresses ovulation, so some users will experience reductions in sexual interest that often occur during the ovulatory period. Implant use has also been associated with positive sexual outcomes. One study reported significantly higher FSFI scores measuring arousal, orgasm, satisfaction, and pain after 3 months of Nexplanon use compared to baseline assessments, and these higher scores persisted at 6 months.[112] Though 2% to 9% of new implant users across several studies reported libido loss, these figures are smaller than those seen in studies of oral contraceptives and other hormonal methods.[135-137]

Another prospective assessment of new-start implant users demonstrated little change in sexual functioning or sexual satisfaction scores across methods, but found varied reports of changes in perceived sexual impacts reported by implant users across 1, 3, and 6 months of use. One-in-seven users (15%) reported that their method had a negative impact on their sex lives, 46% reported no noticeable change, and 40% reported some positive sexual impact.[125] Despite variation in how individuals perceived the method affected their sexual experiences, the perception of sexual impact closely mirrored the overall satisfaction with the method over time.[90] Once again, these findings highlight the importance of person-centered approaches to contraceptive care, especially as it pertains to sexual experiences and sexual acceptability.

Postcoital Contraception

Postcoital contraception, also known as emergency contraception (EC), includes oral levonorgestrel and an oral antiprogestin. Both the copper IUD and the levonorgestrel IUD are also highly effective forms of contraception that can be initiated following unprotected intercourse for people who do not want to become pregnant and wish to initiate an IUD.[138] (We include this umbrella category of methods in the "hormonal methods" section even though copper IUDs do not contain synthetic hormones.) As of 2015, about one-quarter (23%) of sexually active US women between the ages of 15 and 44 reported ever having used oral EC.[139]

Data on the sexual acceptability of these methods used after sex is limited; however, general acceptability around EC seems favorable. A clinical consideration is the potential for irregular bleeding during the EC cycle to negatively affect an individual's sex life. Qualitative research has shown that some people, depending on life stage, partner, and other factors, can enjoy sex more when the risk of pregnancy is present in the heat of the moment, even if a child isn't truly wanted.[140] The distinction of emergency or postcoital contraception versus anticipatory or ongoing contraception may also influence sexual acceptability. However, literature is lacking on this psychological and emotional component of the sexual acceptability of contraception specific to time-sensitive settings. Additionally, advance provision may also influence the convenience of oral EC and therefore users' confidence in the method, which could in turn affect the perceived impact on their sex lives.[141]

Nonhormonal Methods

Permanent Contraception

Tubal Ligation. Fallopian tube surgery is the most common method of contraception in the United States.[142] Despite the widespread prevalence of this method, few recent studies assess its sexual acceptability. However, the literature suggests that, for most people, there is little negative impact and potentially positive impacts on patients' sexual function after the procedure.[143]

Before undergoing tubal surgery, some individuals report concerns about losing their femininity, sexual desirability, or their desire for sex, though few may actually experience these outcomes after the procedure.[144] Subsequent sexual disinhibition due to high contraceptive efficacy may counteract potential negative sexual effects. Tubal ligation has no effect on ovulation and thereby no effect on potential increases in libido during the ovulatory period. Especially after a reproductive lifetime of trying to prevent unwanted pregnancy, many patients may enjoy the psychological and sexual freedoms of no longer having to actively engage in contraceptive practices and/or experience regular contraceptive side effects. Celebrating the high sexual acceptability of fallopian tube surgery, particularly if done in tandem with in-depth counseling for sexual concerns, may prove beneficial for clients seeking permanent contraception.

Vas Surgery. Vas surgery, widely known as vasectomy, is highly effective and safe, and many argue that it is underutilized. Compared to tubal surgery, vas surgery is is effective, safe, and arguably underutilized. However, the ratio of vas surgeries to tubal surgeries in the United States is one to three,[142] and in many countries, vas surgery is rarely, if ever, performed. This comparatively lower use of vas surgery pertains at least in part to widespread concerns, documented in the United States and abroad, related to "loss of manhood" and potential interference with erection and ejaculation.[145,146]

Highlighting the rapid return to full sexual function after the procedure and addressing individuals' concerns and misconceptions make it more likely that someone interested in permanent contraception has the correct information they need to make an informed choice. Providers engaging in these conversations should strive to hear fully the individual's specific concerns and questions before offering clarifying science and facts meant to address those concerns. Techniques for addressing patient's misinformation and concerns about contraception are described in detail in Chapter 4. Vas surgery is associated with few sexual side effects and may promote better sexual outcomes both at the individual level and couple level.[147] In a study of Austrian couples, while people who had received vas surgery reported no changes in sexual function after 6 months, their *partners* reported improved sexual functioning.[148] Shared responsibility for pregnancy prevention is psychologically appealing to many. It is easy to imagine sexual benefits for a couple when the partner with sperm assumes responsibility for contraception after the partner who is capable of pregnancy has shouldered the burden of pregnancy prevention up to that point. Dominant cultural narratives suggest that pregnancy prevention is the sole or foremost responsibility of the person with the biological capacity for pregnancy, but these gendered assumptions can come with both psychological and physical costs.[149]

Copper IUD

Copper IUDs have many of the same sexual benefits of hormonal IUDs. Qualitative research on the sexual acceptability of both types of IUDs revealed mostly positive themes such as increased sexual disinhibition due to the method's high contraceptive efficacy and greater allowance for sexual spontaneity compared to condoms.

Compared to hormonal IUDs, copper IUDs have the added psychosexual and physiologic benefits of no synthetic hormones, which some clients desire, and which means no effects on ovulation. Many patients prefer to feel themselves cycle and ovulate naturally. During ovulation, people are more likely to masturbate and more likely to initiate sexual activity with a partner,[150] so use of a method that does not suppress ovulation can have a sexual benefit. On the other hand, the sexual acceptability of copper IUDs may be thwarted for patients who experience increases in amount of blood, unscheduled bleeding, or cramping with the device.[82]

In a 2014 systematic review of people's sexual experiences with IUDs, use of both hormonal and nonhormonal IUDs was more commonly associated with positive or neutral sexual effects than with negative ones.[128] However, the review identified mixed results, a lack of US studies, and potential methodological limitations. Two prospective US studies addressed some of these gaps by documenting sexual acceptability using a variety of sexuality measures and controlling for baseline factors. In both studies, investigators found that among copper IUD users (as well as hormonal IUD users), sexual functioning and satisfaction scores did not change over the first 3 months of use, but people were significantly more likely to report that their IUDs led to improvements versus detractions to their sexual lives.[81,82] For example, among 572 new-start copper IUD users, 58% said their method had improved their sex life in the first 3 months of use (31% improved a lot, 28% improved a little), compared to 29% reporting no sexual change and only 13% reporting a negative sexual change (2% "made my sex life much worse, 11% "made my sex life a little worse"[81]). Reports of positive sexual effects with copper IUDs were greater than all other methods in the study, although this difference was not statistically significant.

In sum, while studies demonstrate mostly positive effects of copper IUDs on patients' sexuality, this method's sexual acceptability will vary according to individual user characteristics, including bleeding preferences, comfort with an object inside the body, and desire for a nonhormonal method.

Pre-Sex and During-Sex Methods

External Condoms. Though external condoms help prevent STIs, they also play an enormous role in pregnancy prevention. At least one in three penile–vaginal sex acts among individuals aged 15–44 in the United States involves the use of external condoms,[151] and approximately 10% of all US contraceptive users report external condoms as their primary method.[142] Studies have documented that condoms can reduce pleasure and sensation for people with penises.[152] Research has also documented condom-associated erection loss.[153] As expected, the people who report these condom-related sexual detractions are significantly less likely to use them.[154,155]

Research has been slower to document the sexual experiences with external condoms among people with vaginas, but recent years have witnessed new research into this area. These studies demonstrate that people with vaginas, like people with penises, can also experience reductions of pleasure and sensation with condom use, especially when used in the absence of exogenous lubricants.[154,156] Findings on condoms and sexual acceptability exhibit far more similarities than differences across bodies and genders. (Exceptions include the following: people with penises can be more likely to report "fit and feel" issues with external condoms, and people with vaginas can be more likely to report condom-related discomfort or pain, particularly in association with reduced lubrication.[157]) Most notably, although people with penises may be somewhat more likely to say that condoms diminish their physical pleasure,[158,159] the associations between such pleasure attitudes and actual condom practices may be just as strong if not stronger for people with vaginas.[160]

That said, given cultural emphasis on the pleasure of the person with the penis, cisgender women's perceptions of their *partners'* experiences with condoms play a strong role in their use.[69,71]

Researchers have been developing external condoms with erectogenic gel, a substance designed to increase penile firmness, erection duration, and overall pleasure. A randomized controlled trial in Vietnam found that the group using erectogenic condoms, including their partners, had significantly higher quality of sexual experience scores[161] compared to the control group. Those using the novel condoms also reported greater sensations of "naturalness" during intercourse. Chemically enhanced external condoms may be an appealing new option for more pleasurable sexual experiences.

Contraceptive care providers should start with the assumption that at least some of their patients experience reductions in pleasure and sensation when using external condoms. Clients should be encouraged to try a variety of condom types, sizes, and personal (sexual) lubricants. Sexual lubricants, either with or without condoms, may help overcome sexual discomfort and lackluster sexual satisfaction.

On the psychosexual side, some people perceive external condoms as a barrier to intimacy and trust, which can lead to a waning of condom use as a relationship develops,[162] and that sexual motivations pertaining to love (versus, say, pleasure or fun) can undercut the likelihood of condom use.

That said, as with any contraceptive method, external condoms offer many positives in terms of sexual acceptability, and many patients strongly prefer and trust this method. Protection against STIs can greatly improve people's sexual experiences by way of enhanced sexual disinhibition. Many couples benefit relationally and sexually when the person with the penis takes part in pregnancy prevention. Sexual activity profiles such as lower-frequency intercourse and/or multiple concurrent sexual partnerships may make condoms especially suitable. Other positive sexual aspects of external condoms include (if desired) prolonged intercourse, as well as less mess and easier cleanup after sexual activity. Refer to Chapter 14 for more information on external condoms.

Some public health campaigns and programs have shown promise integrating pleasure into condom promotion, especially for communities and populations disproportionately burdened by STIs. A recent systematic review and meta-analysis of such programs found that sexual and reproductive health interventions that incorporated focus on pleasure had significant, positive effects on information about, attitudes toward, and use of condoms.[163] Contraceptive providers can similarly integrate sexual pleasure considerations into their work with patients.

Internal Condoms. Other than external condoms, internal condoms are the only currently available contraceptive method that helps prevent both pregnancy and STIs. Although less popular than their external counterparts, they provide vital dual-prevention prophylaxis[164,165]—especially for resource-limited communities and countries with relatively high rates of HIV, where their use has been the most promoted by public health officials and policy makers.[166]

Studies suggest that internal condoms can be sexually acceptable to many people with vaginas by way of enhanced level of lubrication, greater pleasure and sensation than external condoms, clitoral stimulation from the outer ring, capacity to comfortably accommodate all penis sizes, and ability to place it prior to penetrative sexual activity. Indeed, users' experiences of greater pleasure and sexual sensations helped predict longer-term use of internal condoms among 255 users in Brazil.[167] Since the internal condom does not rely on a penile erection, it can be placed at any time—a significant benefit in couples where erectile difficulties are present.[164,168] Internal condoms also have the potential for increased sexual agency since they are controlled by the person with the vagina, and this psychological phenomenon could also enhance sexual acceptability. However, not all people's sexual experiences with this device are positive, and—just as with external condoms—an obstacle to more internal condom use is the perception that it interferes with sexual satisfaction and pleasure for both partners.[169,170]

The internal condom requires comfort putting something inside the vagina. Some people may not like or feel comfortable with genital touching or penetrating the introitus with their fingers, so this method may not be well-suited for everyone. Prolonging sexual activity prior to intercourse or enlisting a partner's help with placement could increase intimacy and encourage both partners' active engagement in external condom use.

Withdrawal. The family planning community sometimes overlooks withdrawal as a method of contraception. However, withdrawal is commonly practiced the world over, both as a sole or additional method. As Chapter 17 on coitus interruptus describes, the majority of sexually experienced people in the United States have used withdrawal at some point. In a study of 4,634 adult US women, Jones et al. found that 33% reported any use of withdrawal in the last 30 days.[171]

Withdrawal is associated with a variety of sexual implications. It can interrupt sexual flow, requires climax awareness and control on the part of the person with semen for effective use, and can interfere with pleasure for both partners. In a study of family planning patients in Turkey, researchers found that women who reported use of coitus interruptus had the highest levels of sexual dysfunction in the sample,[172] although of course a variety of other underlying factors may help explain this phenomenon. On the other hand, withdrawal may be sexually preferable to condoms, especially since it does not share condoms' profile of reducing sensation or making erections more difficult to maintain.[173-176] In one nationally representative study of US young adults, those who reported that condoms can reduce their pleasure had significantly greater odds of having used withdrawal at their last penile–vaginal sexual encounter.[174] Particularly if couples want to engage in additional pregnancy prevention (that is, dual or even triple method use), withdrawal may provide a more sexually acceptable "double-up option" than condoms if STI risk is mininal. For psychosexual reasons, other couples may prefer extra-vaginal ejaculation versus ejaculation inside the vagina. Other sexual benefits of this method include partners' involvement in pregnancy prevention and its free and immediate availability to those engaging in infrequent sexual activity.

Vaginal Spermicides

Nonoxynol 9 (N-9) is the active ingredient in all products labeled as spermicides in the United States. This holds true for all delivery systems: gels, creams, film, foam, and sponges. N-9 is a surfactant spermicide that can cause local toxic effects on vaginal epithelium, including inflammatory responses and potential ulceration of the vaginal mucosa,[177] particularly when used frequently. N-9 can disrupt the normal vaginal flora and increase risk of STI and HIV transmission.[178] These attributes could cause adverse sexual effects both by causing vaginal discomfort in some users and by decreasing trust in the method for users who are aware of these the potential risks. On the plus side, this method can offer additional vaginal lubrication.

Phexxi

As Chapter 16 documents, Phexxi is a hormone-free vaginal pH modulator that works as a contraceptive when the gel is placed into the vagina prior to penile–vaginal intercourse. It is not a spermicide and contains no nonoxynol 9; it works by maintaining a normal, low (acidic) pH in the vagina when semen (which has a high pH) is deposited into the vagina. Keeping the pH low reduces sperm motility.

Due to its recent introduction to the market, few larger studies document its sexual acceptability. However, phase III clinical trials suggest several positive sexual aspects of the method, with a greater proportion of users reporting positive (45%) versus negative (17%) sexual changes due to the method in the 4 weeks of use.[179] Factors that may contribute to strong sexual acceptability include additional lubrication from the gel, which was initially approved as a sexual lubricant and can reduce vaginal dryness, tightness, and discomfort. The ability to use it on demand may enhance some people's sexual lives. Potential sexual drawbacks may include the taste of the gel, which has a vinegar-like flavor and could thus affect oral sex—for example, the partner of the person with the clitoris may be less likely to perform oral sex if the taste is a turn-off.

This method can be combined with other contraceptive methods as an add-on or as a lubricant to increase effectiveness, thereby enhancing sexual disinhibition brought about by trust in the effectiveness of one's method. When used as a sexual lubricant to mitigate the vaginal dryness with the use of internal or external condoms, it can increase both effectiveness of the method and sexual acceptability. Sexual activity patterns may play a role here as well. Those who only occasionally have penile–vaginal intercourse may sexually prefer this method; longer-acting methods, particularly those with exogenous hormones, may seem like overkill if one is only engaging in sporadic sexual activity.

Fertility Awareness–Based Methods

The contraceptive field has paid some increased attention to fertility awareness–based methods (FABM) in recent years as the FDA approved the first contraceptive mobile medical application using FABM algorithms in mid-2018.[180] Natural Cycles and other FABM methods require individuals to use physiologic data to determine fertility and then make decisions about sexual activity on fertile days to align with their reproductive goals of avoiding (or achieving or risking) pregnancy.[181] Research on FABM continues to be limited in the contraceptive literature, despite the United Nations' estimate that 41 million couples worldwide use some form of these methods. Data from 2013–2017 indicate that the estimated prevalence of FABM use in the United States has increased from 2.2% to 3.4% among people using contraception.[182,183] Additionally, about one-quarter of FABM users combine FABM techniques with condoms or postcoital contraception.[125,182]

A systematic review on FABM highlighted increased bodily awareness and self-control as common positive experiences among users of FABM. Particularly given the necessity of couple participation with these methods, couple factors are likely to influence uptake and sexual acceptability. Many couples may choose FABM based on their preference for a method that feels "natural," facilitation of skin-to-skin contact, or lack of hormonal influences. However, unless people use a secondary method (condoms, withdraw, or postcoital contraception) during the fertile window, these methods may limit spontaneous sexual activity. A small group of FABM users were included in the HER Salt Lake study.[123] FABM users reported increased satisfaction with their arousal, sexual functioning, and ability to emotionally open up during sex, as well as overall satisfaction with their sex life. Over a 3-year period, 13% of 73 FABM users reported sexual detraction as a result their method, 49% reported no impact, and 38% reported that their method improved their sex life. Overall, the average contraceptive sexual acceptability score was similar to other methods in the study.[125] Clinical considerations around FABM include ensuring adequate knowledge about how to use the method and options for back-up methods. (See Chapter 15, Fertility Awareness–Based Methods.)

TOOLS AND RESOURCES FOR PROVIDING PERSON-CENTERED CARE IN CONVERSATIONS ABOUT PATIENTS' SEXUALITY AND SEXUAL ACCEPTABILITY OF CONTRACEPTION

Conversing With Patients About Sexuality and Contraception

Some providers may be reluctant to bring up sexuality and pleasure if they feel unprepared to adequately handle patient concerns and questions. Providers are not expected to have an exhaustive knowledge of treatments for sexual disorders nor all the details or the precise current nomenclature surrounding the universal array of sexual practices their patients prefer. However, providers *should* be able to present their patients with accurate information regarding the sexual aspects of each contraceptive method.

It is essential not to make assumptions about any aspect of an individual's sexuality and to take a sexual history nonjudgmentally with a genuine desire to understand. Taking an inclusive sexual history that is respectful and nonjudgmental can build rapport and trust. Even if the provider "gets it wrong" (e.g., by misunderstanding what it means when a cis woman identifies as asexual), the patient will still feel safe and respected as the clinician prioritizes understanding. To "get it right," the provider listens closely as the patient responds to focused, open-ended questions designed to clarify the patient's goals, risks, and priorities. Providers who become comfortable having open conversations about sex and asking direct, open-ended questions that are focused on potential concerns and knowledge gaps can provide valuable education and relevant suggestions.

We offer contraceptive care providers an array of tools and resources to facilitate their interactions with patients. Here are the fundamentals:

- Include sexuality in discussions about contraception.
- Ask at least one question about the impact of their contraceptive method(s) on their sex life.
- Consider and address possible sexual effects, both positive and negative, when providing information about contraceptive methods.
- Ask questions that clarify what, if any, specific contraceptive sexual effects are of concern or are important to an individual.
- Explore whether sexual side effects led to discontinuation of methods in the past.
- With gender-diverse and sexual-identity-diverse patients, inquire respectfully how their identities may influence their sexual experiences (and other experiences) of their methods so you can provide the best care possible.
- Offer education about sexual anatomy when appropriate.
- Familiarize yourself with clinical pearls for erotizing safer sex and mitigating potential adverse sexual effects of contraceptive methods.

Sexuality changes across the lifespan. Life changes and events such as menarche, sexual experiences, childbearing, and menopause affect one's sexuality. Various life situations, relational factors, and medical conditions also bring benefits and challenges to one's sexuality. Providers can help patients navigate the impact these transitions and life experiences have on their sexuality by proactively asking about sexual effects. Addressing the sexual effects of contraceptives within the context of the person's life focuses the conversation on the unique concerns of the individual.

Boxes 6-1 through **6-4** present selected suggestions for engaging in person-centered conversations with patients about their sexuality and the sexual impact and acceptability of their contraception, as well as language and questions for initiating the conversation, questions for taking a sexual history recommended by the CDC, and sample questions for proactively asking about sexuality at various life stages or with medical conditions or in specific life circumstances.[184,185] These questions are designed to be inclusive of all genders, sexual orientations, and practices without being judgmental or stigmatizing. (See Chapter 19, Contraception After Pregnancy; Chapter 20, Contraception for People with Medical Conditions; and Chapter 21, Contraception in the Later Reproductive Years.)

Box 6-1 A script with questions to introduce the topic of sexuality, including sexual acceptability of contraception, with your patients.

At this point in the visit, I generally ask some questions regarding your sexual life. Will that be okay? (Some people don't want to talk about their sexual life with me, and that's okay, too.) I ask these questions to all my patients. These questions are as important as the questions about other areas of your physical and mental health. Like the rest of our visits, this information is kept in strict confidence unless you or someone else is being hurt or is in danger.

1. Do you have a sense of what might be important to you about how your contraceptive method affects your sex life?

2. Some people notice that their contraceptive method affects their sexual life, sometimes in good ways and sometimes in ways they don't like. Have you ever noticed any effects on your sexual life from using a contraceptive at any point?
3. Are there particular things that are important to you, or things I should keep in mind, as you decide what type of contraception might fit best with your sexuality and your current sex life?
4. Is the sex that you're having good for you? Is there anything that would make it better?
5. What questions do you have about ____? (Fill in based on what the patient has already shared.)

Box 6-2 Selected questions from the CDC's A Guide to Taking a Sexual History.

The 5 Ps: Partners, Practices, Protection from STIs, Past history of STIs, and Pregnancy intention

1. **Partners.**
   The "old" question was: "Do you have sex with men, women, or both?" This approach is problematic because the gender of the partner does not necessarily correlate with the genitalia that will be in contact with other genitalia during sex. When assessing what STI- and pregnancy-related services should be offered, the relevant information is about body parts, not gender.
   The new questions address what body parts are involved when they have partnered sex and what body parts of their partner(s) are involved.
   Are you currently having sex of any kind—oral, vaginal, or anal—with anyone? (Are you having sex?)
   - (If no) Have you ever had sex with another person?
   - (If yes) In recent months, how many sex partners have you had?
   - What is/are the gender(s) of your sex partner(s)? (Notice that this question is asked only as a follow-up question.)
   - Do you or your partner(s) currently have other sex partners?
2. **Practices.**
   - What kind of sexual contact do you have (or have you had)?
     - Vaginal sex (penis in the vagina)?
     - Anal sex (penis in rectum/anus)?
     - Oral sex (mouth on penis, vagina, or anus)?
3. **Protection from STIs.** (See Chapter 23.)
4. **Past history of STIs.** (See Chapter 23.)
5. **Pregnancy intention.** Chapter 4 describes in detail the questions about pregnancy intentions in the context of person-centered conversations about reproduction and contraceptive choice.

For people using condoms for pregnancy prevention, STI protection, or both, two excellent, gender-neutral questions that can lead to discussions about the sexual impact of condom use are: "What parts of your body are covered by a condom during sex? What parts of your partner's body?"

Data from Reno H, Park I, Workowski K, Machefsky A, Bachmann L. A Guide to Taking a Sexual History [Internet]. 2022 [cited 2022 Feb 11]; Available from: https://www.cdc.gov/std/treatment/sexualhistory.htm.

Box 6-3 Examples of prompts when exploring the effects life stages or situations or medical conditions may have on sexuality.

Normalize and validate. For example:

- "For many people at this time in their life, ____ (difficulty with orgasm, pain, decreased interest in sex, etc.) can be a problem. I would be happy to discuss these or other issues with you. If I can't answer your question, I'll find someone who can."
- "Many of my patients (individualize; for example: who have diabetes, as they get older, or who have a new baby, etc.) notice a change in (or have difficulty with) ____."
- "It's not uncommon for people ____ (around menopause, who have young children, etc.) to have that problem."
- "Would you like to discuss anything else going on in your life that has affected your relationship to sex?"

Offer Education about Sexual Anatomy

Many people have not had comprehensive, sex-positive sexual education and are unfamiliar with sexual anatomy, particularly anatomy of the pleasure center (clitoris) for female-bodied people. Many people think of the clitoris as the small nub beneath the clitoral hood. In fact, anatomic dissection; imaging with ultrasound, MRI, and F-MRI; and histologic studies demonstrate that in addition to this small tip (called the glans), the clitoris is made up of a neck and body (shaft), legs (crura), a large bulbs of erectile tissue (clitoral bulbs or vestibular bulbs), and a neural plexus across much of the introitus and lower vagina.[192-195] During embryonic development, the clitoris develops from the same tissue that would become a penis in a body with XY chromosomes, including both the shaft and glans. The size of clitoral erections can range from 10 to 20 cm (4–7.9 inches), with the clitoral body itself extending from 2 to 4 cm (0.8–1.6 inches) and attaining a width of from 1 to 2 cm (0.39–0.79 inch). When stimulated, the crura can swell to 5 to 9 cm (2–3.5 inches), and the bulbs' length can vary from 3 to 7 cm (1.2–2.8 inches). **Figure 6-2** depicts the entire clitoris and labels the various parts. All parts of the clitoris are capable of being highly responsive to arousal and touch.

When Is It a Sexual Dysfunction?

The standard for diagnosing sexual dysfunction is that *distress* is a diagnostic criterion.[189,190] Sexual dysfunction involves a complex interaction of psychological, interpersonal, social, cultural, physiologic, and gender-influenced processes. Definitions, classification systems, and nomenclature for each sexual disorder/dysfunction vary somewhat between the *Diagnostic and Statistical Manual of Mental Disorders*, Fifth Edition (DSM-5; American Psychiatric Association, 2013), the International Classification of Diseases, 11th Revision (ICD-11), and professional societies such as the Fourth International Consultation in Sexual Medicine, the International Society for the Study of Women's Sexual Health, and the World Association of Sexual Health in conjunction with the World Health Organization. Common to all classification systems for sexual dysfunction are diagnostic criteria requiring that the signs

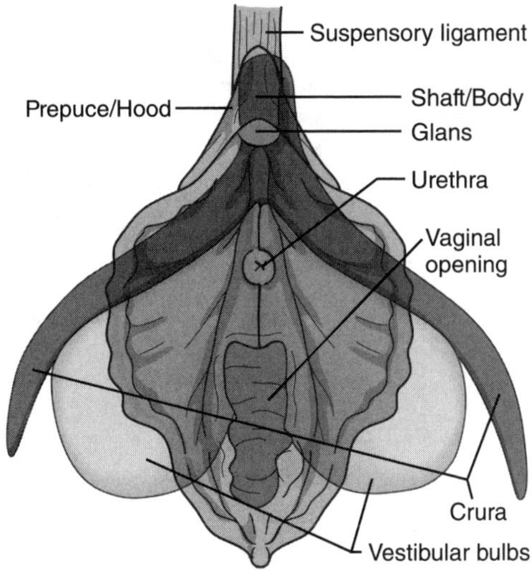

Figure 6-2 The Clitoris

Box 6-4 Clinical pearls for erotizing safer sex and mitigating potential adverse sexual effects of contraceptive methods.

IUD strings:

- Leave the strings long enough to cover the posterior lip of the cervix to allow it to be tucked back under the cervix. This is usually 3–4 cm or longer. Short strings are more likely to stick straight out and poke the partner's penis.
- Cut strings straight across rather than at an angle. Strings cut at an angle will have sharper, pointed tips that are more likely to poke the partner's penis.

Vaginal rings:

- Anticipate and respond to patient concerns about the ring expelling or getting lost during sex, and offer alternative strategies to help make ring placement more acceptable—for example, placing the ring while showering or using a clean, empty tampon applicator to help with placement.

Transdermal patches:

- For patients concerned that the patch will come off during sexual activity, underscore the exceedingly low chance of this event occurring.

Condoms:

- Encourage patients to use personal lubricant that is compatible with the condom material. Adding lubricant vaginally and to the outside of the condom once it is correctly positioned on the erect penis can increase pleasure and decrease sensations of dryness.
- Some people may wish to add a few drops of personal lubricant inside the external condom to create movement within the area around the upper portion of the penis to increase pleasure.

and symptoms cause clinically significant distress in the individual. This diagnostic criterion is clinically relevant when deciding when it is appropriate to offer intervention based on a diagnosis of sexual dysfunction.

If clinically significant distress were not a criterion, a large percentage of the population would be diagnosed with sexual dysfunction or disorder. For example, in a sample of cis women, 31% of 741 women self-identified a lack of sexual interest, but only 10% identified that a lack of sexual interest was a problem usually or always.[191] The ICD-11 emphasizes that there is no normative standard for sexual activity. If the individual is not distressed by their sexual experience, even if it is different from what may be satisfying to other people or from what is considered normative, a sexual dysfunction should not be diagnosed.

Unusual Sexual Practices (Paraphilia)

It is important to briefly consider paraphilic "disorders," which refer to mental health distress associated with sexual arousal or sexual expression derived from atypical sources.

Providers engaging in open conversations about sex and pleasure with their patients will encounter terms and descriptions of sexual behaviors, practices, and preferences that are unfamiliar, and in some cases, even alarming. Sexual practices labeled by the DSM-5 as "paraphilias" (mental disorders) in some generations and cultures are considered normative in others.[186,187] For example, until fairly recently, standard medical approaches diagnosed homosexuality as a paraphilia, and some societies and communities still considered homosexuality deviant. Health care providers are human beings who live in a society with cultural customs and norms that dictate what is considered acceptable or "normal" behavior.[188] Since providers interact with patients through that cultural lens, it is a given that they bring their cultural bias to clinical encounters.

Providers need to interact nonjudgmentally with patients, but it is not a simple task to distinguish between sexual practices that are harmful and those that are merely unconventional, so they need both to be vigilant about bias and to apply clear parameters for what constitutes a mental disorder or dangerous sexual practice. Is the sexual practice consensual? Does a particular behavior put the person or their partner(s) at risk? If so, is that a risk they understand and are willing to take? Is the behavior potentially coercive or causing harm to someone else? Is the person distressed by their behavior or interest? As a general rule, unless the answer to one of these questions is yes, the practice can be thought of as sexual arousal or sexual expression derived from atypical sources rather than pejoratively labeled as sexual perversion or sexual deviance, or diagnosed as a paraphilia.

The DSM-5 helps health care providers distinguish between atypical sexual interests and mental disorders that involve those interests. Most people with atypical sexual interests do *not* have a mental disorder. To be diagnosed with a paraphilic disorder, DSM-5 requires that people have one or more of the following diagnostic criteria:

- Feel personal distress about their interest, including distress resulting from society's disapproval
- Have a sexual desire or behavior that involves another person's psychological distress, injury, or death
- Have a desire for sexual behaviors involving unwilling persons or persons unable to give legal consent

People who engage in consensual but perhaps atypical sexual behavior not meeting these diagnostic criteria should not be inappropriately labeled with a mental disorder.

Resources

For Providers Offering Referrals for People with Sexual Concerns

Patients who need more in-depth counseling for treatment can be referred to a qualified sex therapist; such therapists can be located via the American Association of Sexuality Educators (www.aasect.org). The American Physical Therapy Association (APTA)'s section specializing in pelvic health is an excellent source of referrals for those with dyspareunia and a variety of vulvar and vaginal pain issues (https://aptapelvichealth.org/).

Providers who would like more information on diagnosis and treatment of sexual problems and concerns can refer to the following:

- The leading clinical reference and text in the field, originally developed by the late Sandra Leiblum: *Principles and Practice of Sex Therapy*.[196]
- Volume 10, issue 1 of the *Journal of Sexual Medicine* (2013) contains standard operating procedures for diagnosis and treatment of each sexual dysfunction/disorder.

For Both Nonproviders and Providers Interested in Learning More about Sexuality, Pleasure, Sexual Health, and Contraception

The Pleasure Project (https://thepleasureproject.org/) is an international education and advocacy organization working to eroticize safer sex. The project offers an array of resources to support sex positivity and pleasure, such as demonstrating the art of erotic condom use. The Project provides training and consultancy for providers who want to take a more sex-positive and pleasure-based approach to their work including an extensive, free, on-line trainer toolkit with exercises to "Mix Pleasure *with* Prevention."

Bedsider (https://www.bedsider.org/) has a wide variety of resources about contraception and includes extensive sections on sex and relationships and on sexual health.

Author Disclosures—Higgins: none; Cason: Nexplanon trainer for Organon and clinical trainer and consultant for Sebela and Speaker's Bureau Merck; Sanders: consultant for Bayer Pharmaceuticals (Dr. Sanders' Division of Family Planning receives research funding from Bayer Women's Health Care, Merck & Co. Inc., Cooper Surgical, Sebela Pharmaceuticals, Femasys, and Medicines 360)

References

1. Higgins JA, Hirsch JS. The Pleasure deficit: Revisiting the "sexuality connection" in reproductive health. Perspect Sex Reprod Health. 2007;39(4):240-7.
2. Sexual health [Internet]. [cited 2021 May 12]; Available from: https://www.who.int/westernpacific/health-topics/sexual-health

3. ASHA Homepage [Internet]. [cited 2021 May 12]; Available from: https://www.ashasexualhealth.org/
4. Landers S, Kapadia F. The public health of pleasure: Going beyond disease prevention. Am J Public Health. 2020;110(2):140-1.
5. Ford JV, Corona E, Cruz M, et al. The World Association for Sexual Health's declaration on sexual pleasure: A technical guide. Int J Sex Health. 2022;0(0):1-31.
6. CNN EA. These women are making sexual pleasure a gender equality priority [Internet]. CNN. [cited 2022 Feb 3]; Available from: https://www.cnn.com/2021/09/03/africa/women-sexual-pleasure-gender-equality-as-equals-intl-cmd/index.html
7. Why pleasure should be part of the solution [Internet]. The Pleasure Project (website). 2021 [cited 2022 Feb 3]; Available from: https://thepleasureproject.org/blog/pleasure-news-views/2021/why-pleasure-should-be-part-of-the-solution/
8. Philpott A, Larsson G, Singh A, Zaneva M, Gonsalves L. How to navigate a blindspot: Pleasure in sexual and reproductive health and rights programming and research. Int J Sex Health. 2021;33(4):587-601. https://doi.org/10.1080/19317611.2021.1965690
9. Hoopes AJ, Benson SK, Howard HB, Morrison DM, Ko LK, Shafii T. Adolescent perspectives on patient-provider sexual health communication: A qualitative study. J Prim Care Community Health. 2017;8(4):332-7.
10. Fuzzell L, Fedesco HN, Alexander SC, Fortenberry JD, Shields CG. "I just think that doctors need to ask more questions": Sexual minority and majority adolescents' experiences talking about sexuality with health care providers. Patient Educ Couns. 2016;99(9):1467-72.
11. Berman L, Berman J, Felder S, et al. Seeking help for sexual function complaints: what gynecologists need to know about the female patient's experience. Fertil Steril. 2003;79(3):572-6.
12. Zéler A, Troadec C. Doctors talking about sexuality: What are the patients' feelings? Sex Med. 2020;8(4):599-607.
13. Haboubi NHJ, Lincoln N. Views of health professionals on discussing sexual issues with patients. Disabil Rehabil. 2003;25(6):291-6.
14. Logan RG, Daley EM, Vamos CA, Louis-Jacques A, Marhefka SL. "When is health care actually going to be care?" The lived experience of family planning care among young Black women. Qual Health Res. 2021;31(6):1169-82.
15. Maurice W, Bowman M. Sexual medicine in primary care. St. Louis: Mosby Year Book; 1999.
16. Everett BG, Sanders JN, Myers K, Geist C, Turok DK. One in three: challenging heteronormative assumptions in family planning health centers. Contraception. 2018;98(4):270-4.
17. Higgins JA, Carpenter E, Everett BG, Greene MZ, Haider S, Hendrick CE. Sexual minority women and contraceptive use: complex pathways between sexual orientation and health outcomes. Am J Public Health. [Internet] 2019 [cited 2022 Feb 8];109(12). Available from: https://ajph.aphapublications.org/doi/full/10.2105/AJPH.2019.305211
18. Pulice-Farrow L, Lindley L, Gonzalez KA. "Wait, what is that? A man or woman or what?": Trans microaggressions from gynecological healthcare providers. Sex Res Soc Policy. [Internet] 2022 [cited 2022 Feb 23]; Available from: https://doi.org/10.1007/s13178-021-00675-7
19. Jannini EA, Fisher WA, Bitzer J, McMahon CG. Controversies in sexual medicine: Is sex just fun? how sexual activity improves health. J Sex Med. 2009;6(10):2640-8.
20. Gianotten WL, Alley JC, Diamond LM. The health benefits of sexual expression. Int J Sex Health. 2021;0(0):1-16.
21. Diamond LM, Huebner DM. Is good sex good for you? Rethinking sexuality and health. Soc Personal Psychol Compass 2012;6(1):54-69.
22. Levin RJ. Sexual activity, health and well-being – the beneficial roles of coitus and masturbation. Sex Relatsh Ther. 2007;22(1):135-48.
23. Hogarth H, Ingham R. Masturbation among young women and associations with sexual health: An exploratory study. J Sex Res. 2009;46(6):558-67.
24. Anderson RM. Positive sexuality and its impact on overall well-being. Bundesgesundheitsblatt Gesundheitsforschung Gesundheitsschutz 2013;56(2):208-14.
25. Buczak-Stec E, König H-H, Hajek A. The link between sexual satisfaction and subjective well-being: a longitudinal perspective based on the German Ageing Survey. Qual Life Res. 2019;28(11):3025-35.

26. Flynn KE, Lin L, Bruner DW, et al. Sexual satisfaction and the importance of sexual health to quality of life throughout the life course of U.S. adults. J Sex Med. 2016;13(11):1642-50.
27. Lee DM, Vanhoutte B, Nazroo J, Pendleton N. Sexual health and positive subjective well-being in partnered older men and women. J Gerontol Ser B. 2016;71(4):698-710.
28. Davison SL, Bell RJ, LaChina M, Holden SL, Davis SR. The relationship between self-reported sexual satisfaction and general well-being in women. J Sex Med. 2009;6(10):2690-7.
29. Loewenstein G, Krishnamurti T, Kopsic J, McDonald D. Does increased sexual frequency enhance happiness? J Econ Behav Organ. 2015;116:206-18.
30. Muise A, Schimmack U, Impett EA. Sexual frequency predicts greater well-being, but more is not always better. Soc Psychol Personal Sci. 2016;7(4):295-302.
31. Mollaioli D, Sansone A, Ciocca G, et al. Benefits of sexual activity on psychological, relational, and sexual health during the COVID-19 breakout. J Sex Med. 2021;18(1):35-49.
32. Frappier J, Toupin I, Levy JJ, Aubertin-Leheudre M, Karelis AD. Energy expenditure during sexual activity in young healthy couples. PLoS One. 2013;8(10):e79342.
33. Drory Y. Sexual activity and cardiovascular risk. Eur Heart J. Suppl 2002;4:H13-8.
34. Ebrahim S, May M, Shlomo YB, et al. Sexual intercourse and risk of ischaemic stroke and coronary heart disease: the Caerphilly study. J Epidemiol Community Health. 2002;56(2):99-102.
35. Seldin DR, Friedman HS, Martin LR. Sexual activity as a predictor of life-span mortality risk. Personal Individ Differ. 2002;33(3):409-25.
36. Buettner D. The blue zones: 9 Lessons for living longer from the people who've lived the longest. National Geographic Books; 2012.
37. Weeks D, James J. Secrets of the superyoung. New York: Berkley Books; 1998.
38. Cao C, Yang L, Xu T, et al. Trends in sexual activity and associations with all-cause and cause-specific mortality among US adults. J Sex Med. 2020;17(10):1903-13.
39. Palmore EB. Predictors of the longevity difference: A 25-year follow-up. Gerontologist. 1982;22(6):513-8.
40. Heiman JR, Long JS, Smith SN, Fisher WA, Sand MS, Rosen RC. Sexual satisfaction and relationship happiness in midlife and older couples in five countries. Arch Sex Behav. 2011;40(4): 741-53.
41. Muise A, Giang E, Impett EA. Post sex affectionate exchanges promote sexual and relationship satisfaction. Arch Sex Behav. 2014;43(7):1391-402.
42. Triscoli C, Croy I, Olausson H, Sailer U. Touch between romantic partners: Being stroked is more pleasant than stroking and decelerates heart rate. Physiol Behav. 2017;177:169-75.
43. Fallis EE, Rehman US, Woody EZ, Purdon C. The longitudinal association of relationship satisfaction and sexual satisfaction in long-term relationships. J Fam Psychol. 2016;30(7):822-31.
44. Yeh H-C, Lorenz FO, Wickrama KAS, Conger RD, Elder Jr. GH. Relationships among sexual satisfaction, marital quality, and marital instability at midlife. J Fam Psychol. 2006;20(2):339-43.
45. Robertson SA, Sharkey DJ. Seminal fluid and fertility in women. Fertil Steril. 2016;106(3):511-9.
46. Sayle AE, Savitz DA, Thorp JM, Hertz-Picciotto I, Wilcox AJ. Sexual activity during late pregnancy and risk of preterm delivery. Obstet Gynecol. 2001;97(2):283-9.
47. Tan PC, Andi A, Azmi N, Noraihan MN. Effect of coitus at term on length of gestation, induction of labor, and mode of delivery. Obstet Gynecol. 2006;108(1):134-40.
48. Leiblum S, Bachmann G, Kemmann E, Colburn D, Swartzman L. Vaginal atrophy in the postmenopausal woman: The importance of sexual activity and hormones. JAMA 1983;249(16): 2195-8.
49. Arnot M, Mace R. Sexual frequency is associated with age of natural menopause: results from the Study of Women's Health Across the Nation. R Soc Open Sci 2020;7(1):191020.
50. Gianotten WL. The (mental) health benefits of sexual expression [Internet]. In: Lew-Starowicz M, Giraldi A, Krüger THC, editors. Psychiatry and sexual medicine: A comprehensive guide for clinical practitioners. Cham: Springer International Publishing; 2021 [cited 2022 Feb 2]. p. 57-70. https://doi.org/10.1007/978-3-030-52298-8_6
51. Saunders B, Riesel A, Klawohn J, Inzlicht M. Interpersonal touch enhances cognitive control: A neurophysiological investigation. J Exp Psychol Gen. 2018;147(7):1066-77.
52. Wright H, Jenks RA, Demeyere N. Frequent sexual activity predicts specific cognitive abilities in older adults. J Gerontol Ser B. 2019;74(1):47-51.

53. Hambach A, Evers S, Summ O, Husstedt IW, Frese A. The impact of sexual activity on idiopathic headaches: An observational study. Cephalalgia. 2013;33(6):384-9.
54. Picillo M, Palladino R, Erro R, et al. The PRIAMO study: active sexual life is associated with better motor and non-motor outcomes in men with early Parkinson's disease. Eur J Neurol. 2019;26(10):1327-33.
55. Jian Z, Ye D, Chen Y, Li H, Wang K. Sexual activity and risk of prostate cancer: A dose-response meta-analysis. J Sex Med. 2018;15(9):1300-9.
56. Rider JR, Wilson KM, Sinnott JA, Kelly RS, Mucci LA, Giovannucci EL. Ejaculation frequency and risk of prostate cancer: updated results with an additional decade of follow-up. Eur Urol 2016;70(6):974-82.
57. Kimata H. Kissing selectively decreases allergen-specific IgE production in atopic patients. J Psychosom Res. 2006;60(5):545-7.
58. Higgins J, Lands M, Ufot M, McClelland S. Socioeconomics and erotic inequity: A theoretical overview and narrative review of associations between poverty, socioeconomic conditions, and sexual wellbeing. J Sex Res. 2022;59(8):940-56. doi: 10.1080/00224499.2022.2044990.
59. Mahar EA, Mintz LB, Akers BM. Orgasm equality: Scientific findings and societal implications. Curr Sex Health Rep. 2020;12(1):24-32.
60. Kumar P. Introduction to the special theme: Erotic marginality and erotic justice. 2018;2:16.
61. Collins D, Talcott M. 'A new language that speaks of change just as it steps toward it': Transnationalism, erotic justice and queer human rights praxis. Sociol Compass. 2011;5(7):576-90.
62. Kalra A. Activist and Prof. Loretta Ross speaks about reproductive justice [Internet]. Dly Northwest. 2021 [cited 2022 Feb 8]; Available from: https://dailynorthwestern.com/2021/10/28/campus/activist-and-prof-loretta-ross-speaks-about-reproductive-justice/
63. Facts and figures: Ending violence against women [Internet]. UN Women. [cited 2022 Feb 3]; Available from: https://www.unwomen.org/en/what-we-do/ending-violence-against-women/facts-and-figures
64. Preventing sexual violence [Internet]. 2021 [cited 2022 Feb 3]; Available from: https://www.cdc.gov/violenceprevention/sexualviolence/fastfact.html
65. Smith SG, Zhang X, Basile KC, et al. The National Intimate Partner and Sexual Violence Survey: 2015 Data Brief — Updated Release. Atlanta, GA: National Center for Injury Prevention and Control, Centers for Disease Control and Prevention. https://www.cdc.gov/violenceprevention/pdf/2015data-brief508.pdf
66. Grace KT, Anderson JC. Reproductive coercion: A systematic review. Trauma Violence Abuse 2018;19(4):371-90.
67. Peitzmeier SM, Malik M, Kattari SK, et al. Intimate partner violence in transgender populations: Systematic review and meta-analysis of prevalence and correlates. Am J Public Health. 2020;110(9):e1-14.
68. McCauley HL, Silverman JG, Decker MR, et al. Sexual and reproductive health indicators and intimate partner violence victimization among female family planning clinic patients who have sex with women and men. J Womens Health. 2015;24(8):621-8.
69. Higgins JA, Hirsch JS. Pleasure, power, and inequality: Incorporating sexuality into research on contraceptive use. Am J Public Health. 2008;98(10):1803-13.
70. Higgins JA, Smith NK. The sexual acceptability of contraception: reviewing the literature and building a new concept. J Sex Res. 2016;53(4-5):417-56.
71. Dalessandro C, Thorpe R, Sanders J. "For me, it's having something meaningful": Women's emotional understandings of sex and the sexual acceptability of contraception. J Sex Res. 2021; 59(4):445-56. doi: 10.1080/00224499.2021.1958194.
72. Caruso S, Fava V, Rapisarda AMC. Contraception and sexuality [Internet]. In: Meriggiola MC, Gemzell-Danielsson K, editors. Female and male contraception. Cham: Springer International Publishing; 2021 [cited 2022 Feb 14]. p. 31-43. https://doi.org/10.1007/978-3-030-70932-7_4
73. Higgins JA, Kramer RD, Everett B, Wright KQ, Turok DK, Sanders JN. Association between patients' perceptions of the sexual acceptability of contraceptive methods and continued use over time. JAMA Intern Med. 2021;181(6):874-6.
74. Bancroft J, Graham CA. The varied nature of women's sexuality: Unresolved issues and a theoretical approach. Horm Behav. 2011;59(5):717-29.

75. Both S, Lew-Starowicz M, Luria M, et al. Hormonal contraception and female sexuality: position statements from the European Society of Sexual Medicine (ESSM). J Sex Med. 2019;16(11): 1681-95.
76. Gubrium A. "I've lost my mojo, baby." Sex Res Soc Policy. 2011;8(4):321-34.
77. Isidori AM, Pozza C, Esposito K, et al. Development and validation of a 6-item version of the Female Sexual Function Index (FSFI) as a diagnostic tool for female sexual dysfunction. J Sex Med. 2010;7(3):1139-46.
78. Huang M, Li G, Liu J, Li Y, Du P. Is there an association between contraception and sexual dysfunction in women? A systematic review and meta-analysis based on Female Sexual Function Index. J Sex Med. 2020;17(10):1942-55.
79. Štulhofer A, Buško V, Brouillard P. Development and bicultural validation of the new sexual satisfaction scale. J Sex Res. 2010;47(4):257-68.
80. Negriff S, Dorn LD, Hillman JB, Huang B. The measurement of menstrual symptoms: Factor structure of the menstrual symptom questionnaire in adolescent girls. J Health Psychol. 2009; 14(7):899-908.
81. Higgins JA, Kramer RD, Wright KQ, Everett B, Turok DK, Sanders JN. Sexual functioning, satisfaction, and well-being among contraceptive users: A three-month assessment from the HER Salt Lake Contraceptive Initiative. J Sex Res. 2021; 59(4):435-44. DOI: 10.1080/00224499.2021.1873225.
82. Higgins JA, Sanders JN, Palta M, Turok DK. Women's sexual function, satisfaction, and perceptions after starting long-acting reversible contraceptives. Obstet Gynecol. 2016;128(5):1143-51.
83. Sanders JN, Kean J, Zhang C, et al. Measuring the Sexual acceptability of contraception: psychometric examination and development of a valid and reliable prospective instrument. J Sex Med. 2022;S1743-6095(21)00824-9.
84. Higgins JA, Wright KQ, Turok DK, Sanders JN. Beyond safety and efficacy: sexuality-related priorities and their associations with contraceptive method selection. Contracept X. 2020;2: 100038.
85. Gomez AM, Clark JB. The relationship between contraceptive features preferred by young women and interest in IUDs: An exploratory analysis. Perspect Sex Reprod Health. 2014;46(3): 157-63.
86. Jackson AV, Karasek D, Dehlendorf C, Foster DG. Racial and ethnic differences in women's preferences for features of contraceptive methods. Contraception. 2016;93(5):406-11.
87. Jamin CG, Häusler G, Lobo Abascal P, et al. Development and conceptual validation of a questionnaire to help contraceptive choice: CHLOE (Contraception: HeLping for wOmen's choicE). Eur J Contracept Reprod Health Care. 2017;22(4):286-90.
88. Dehlendorf C, Reed R, Fox E, Seidman D, Hall C, Steinauer J. Ensuring our research reflects our values: The role of family planning research in advancing reproductive autonomy. Contraception. 2018;98(1):4-7.
89. Moreau C, Cleland K, Trussell J. Contraceptive discontinuation attributed to method dissatisfaction in the United States. Contraception. 2007;76(4):267-72.
90. Kramer RD, Higgins JA, Everett B, Turok DK, Sanders JN. A prospective analysis of the relationship between sexual acceptability and contraceptive satisfaction over time. Am J Obstet Gynecol. [Internet] 2021 [cited 2022 Jan 31]; Available from: https://www.sciencedirect.com/science/article/pii/S0002937821011091
91. Dehlendorf C, Levy K, Kelley A, Grumbach K, Steinauer J. Women's preferences for contraceptive counseling and decision making. Contraception. 2013;88(2):250-6.
92. Lessard LN, Karasek D, Ma S, et al. Contraceptive features preferred by women at high risk of unintended pregnancy. Perspect Sex Reprod Health. 2012;44(3):194-200.
93. Devineni D, Skee D, Vaccaro N, et al. Pharmacokinetics and pharmacodynamics of a transdermal contraceptive patch and an oral contraceptive. J Clin Pharmacol. 2007;47(4):497-509.
94. Pastor Z, Holla K, Chmel R. The influence of combined oral contraceptives on female sexual desire: A systematic review. Eur J Contracept Reprod Health Care. 2013;18(1):27-43.
95. Braunstein GD. Androgen insufficiency in women. Growth Horm IGF Res. 2006;16:109-17.
96. Zimmerman Y, Foidart J-M, Pintiaux A, et al. Restoring testosterone levels by adding dehydroepiandrosterone to a drospirenone containing combined oral contraceptive: II. Clinical effects. Contraception. 2015;91(2):134-42.

97. van Lunsen RHW, Zimmerman Y, Coelingh Bennink HJT, et al. Maintaining physiologic testosterone levels during combined oral contraceptives by adding dehydroepiandrosterone: II. Effects on sexual function. A phase II randomized, double-blind, placebo-controlled study. Contraception. 2018;98(1):56-62.
98. Salonia A, Nappi RE, Pontillo M, et al. Menstrual cycle-related changes in plasma oxytocin are relevant to normal sexual function in healthy women. Horm Behav. 2005;47(2):164-9.
99. van Anders SM, Goldey KL, Bell SN. Measurement of testosterone in human sexuality research: methodological considerations. Arch Sex Behav. 2014;43(2):231-50.
100. Davis SR, Davison SL, Donath S, Bell RJ. Circulating androgen levels and self-reported sexual function in women. JAMA 2005;294(1):91-6.
101. Warnock JK, Clayton A, Croft H, Segraves R, Biggs FC. ORIGINAL RESEARCH—WOMEN'S SEXUAL HEALTH: Comparison of androgens in women with hypoactive sexual desire disorder: Those on combined oral contraceptives (COCs) vs. those not on COCs. J Sex Med. 2006;3(5):878-82.
102. Graham CA, Bancroft J, Doll HA, Greco T, Tanner A. Does oral contraceptive-induced reduction in free testosterone adversely affect the sexuality or mood of women? Psychoneuroendocrinology 2007;32(3):246-55.
103. Strufaldi R, Pompei LM, Steiner ML, et al. Effects of two combined hormonal contraceptives with the same composition and different doses on female sexual function and plasma androgen levels. Contraception. 2010;82(2):147-54.
104. Shahnazi M, Bayatipayan S, Khalili AF, et al. Comparing the effects of the second-and third-generation oral contraceptives on sexual functioning. Iran J Nurs Midwifery Res. 2015;20(1):47.
105. Schaffir J. Hormonal contraception and sexual desire: A critical review. J Sex Marital Ther 2006;32(4):305-14.
106. Davis AR, Castaño PM. Oral contraceptives and libido in women. Annu Rev Sex Res. 2004; 15(1):297-320.
107. Burrows LJ, Basha M, Goldstein AT. The effects of hormonal contraceptives on female sexuality: A review. J Sex Med. 2012;9(9):2213-23.
108. Moher D, Schulz KF, Altman DG. The CONSORT statement: revised recommendations for improving the quality of reports of parallel-group randomised trials. Lancet. 2001;357(9263): 1191-4.
109. Graham CA, Ramos R, Bancroft J, Maglaya C, Farley TMM. The effects of steroidal contraceptives on the well-being and sexuality of women: A double-blind, placebo-controlled, two-centre study of combined and progestogen-only methods. Contraception. 1995;52(6):363-9.
110. Sanders SA, Graham CA, Bass JL, Bancroft J. A prospective study of the effects of oral contraceptives on sexuality and well-being and their relationship to discontinuation. Contraception. 2001;64(1):51-8.
111. Witting K, Santtila P, Jern P, et al. Evaluation of the Female Sexual Function Index in a population based sample from Finland. Arch Sex Behav. 2008;37(6):912-24.
112. Di Carlo C, Gargano V, De Rosa N, Tommaselli GA, Sparice S, Nappi C. Effects of estradiol valerate and dienogest on quality of life and sexual function according to age. Gynecol Endocrinol. 2014;30(12):925-8.
113. Göretzlehner G, Waldmann-Rex S, Schramm GAK. Extended cycles with the combined oral contraceptive chlormadinone acetate 2 mg/ethinylestradiol 0.03 mg. Clin Drug Investig. 2011;31(4):269-77.
114. Roumen FJME. The contraceptive vaginal ring compared with the combined oral contraceptive pill: a comprehensive review of randomized controlled trials. Contraception. 2007; 75(6):420-9.
115. Sabatini R, Cagiano R. Comparison profiles of cycle control, side effects and sexual satisfaction of three hormonal contraceptives. Contraception. 2006;74(3):220-3.
116. Littlejohn KE. "It's those pills that are ruining me": Gender and the social meanings of hormonal contraceptive side effects. Gend Soc. 2013;27(6):843-63.
117. Delvaux T, Jespers V, Benova L, van de Wijgert J. Acceptability and satisfaction of contraceptive vaginal rings in clinical studies: A systematic review and narrative synthesis. Front Glob Womens Health. 2021;2:799963.

118. Guida M, Di Spiezio Sardo A, Bramante S, et al. Effects of two types of hormonal contraception—oral versus intravaginal—on the sexual life of women and their partners. Hum Reprod. 2005;20(4):1100-6.
119. Caruso S, Cianci S, Malandrino C, Cicero C, Lo Presti L, Cianci A. Quality of sexual life of women using the contraceptive vaginal ring in extended cycles: Preliminary report. Eur J Contracept Reprod Health Care. 2014;19(4):307-14.
120. Roumen FJ. Review of the combined contraceptive vaginal ring, NuvaRing®. Ther Clin Risk Manag. 2008;4(2):441-51.
121. Huang Y, Merkatz R, Zhu H, Roberts K, Sitruk-Ware R, Cheng L. The free perinatal/postpartum contraceptive services project for migrant women in Shanghai: effects on the incidence of unintended pregnancy. Contraception. 2014;89(6):521-7.
122. NSFG - Listing C - Key Statistics from the National Survey of Family Growth [Internet]. 2019 [cited 2022 Feb 14]; Available from: https://www.cdc.gov/nchs/nsfg/key_statistics/c.htm
123. Sanders JN, Myers K, Gawron LM, Simmons RG, Turok DK. Contraceptive method use during the community-wide HER Salt Lake Contraceptive Initiative. Am J Public Health. 2018; 108(4):550-6.
124. Gracia CR, Sammel MD, Charlesworth S, Lin H, Barnhart KT, Creinin MD. Sexual function in first-time contraceptive ring and contraceptive patch users. Fertil Steril. 2010;93(1): 21-8.
125. Sanders J, Carter G, Everett B, Turok D, Higgins J. 2022. Sexual acceptability of common FDA-approved contraceptive methods in the US. Unpublished Manuscript. ASCENT Center for Reproductive Health, The University of Utah School of Medicine. Salt Lake City, UT.
126. Hubacher D, Kavanaugh M. Historical record-setting trends in IUD use in the United States. Contraception. 2018;98(6):467-70.
127. King LA, Michels KA, Graubard BI, Trabert B. Trends in oral contraceptive and intrauterine device use among reproductive-aged women in the US from 1999 to 2017. Cancer Causes Control CCC 2021;32(6):587-95.
128. Sanders JN, Smith NK, Higgins JA. The intimate link: A systematic review of highly effective reversible contraception and women's sexual experience. Clin Obstet Gynecol. 2014;57(4): 777-89.
129. He YR, Li Y, Ma L, Wei SS, Wu HY, Huang J. [Effects of LNG-IUS on sexual function and sexual quality in women of childbearing age]. Zhonghua Yi Xue Za Zhi 2020;100(16):1255-9. [in Chinese].
130. Bastianelli C, Farris M, Benagiano G. Use of the levonorgestrel-releasing intrauterine system, quality of life and sexuality. Experience in an Italian family planning center. Contraception. 2011;84(4):402-8.
131. Gholamitabar TM, Moslemi L, Esmaelzadeh S, Bijani A. Comparison of side effects and marital satisfaction between the women taking cyclofem and depo-medroxyprogesterone contraceptive ampoules. Afr J Pharm Pharmacol. 2012;6(26):1933-7.
132. Sanders J, Carter G, Everett B, Turok D, Higgins J. 2022. Frequency of menstrual symptoms and contraceptive side effects in new-start contraceptive users in the HER Salt Lake Study. Unpublished Manuscript. ASCENT Center for Reproductive Health, The University of Utah School of Medicine.
133. Tyson N, Lopez M, Merchant M, Postlethwaite D. Subdermal Contraceptive implant insertion trends and retention in adolescents. J Pediatr Adolesc Gynecol. 2021;34(3):348-54.
134. Kavanaugh ML, Jerman J. Contraceptive method use in the United States: trends and characteristics between 2008, 2012 and 2014. Contraception. 2018;97(1):14-21.
135. Duvan Cİ, Gözdemir E, Kaygusuz İ, Kamalak Z, Turhan NÖ. Etonogestrel contraceptive implant (Implanon): analysis of patient compliance and adverse effects in the breastfeeding period. J Turk Ger Gynecol Assoc. 2010;11(3):141-4.
136. Gezginc K, Balci O, Karatayli R, Colakoglu MC. Contraceptive efficacy and side effects of Implanon®. Eur J Contracept Reprod Health Care. 2007;12(4):362-5.
137. Aisien AO, Enosolease ME. Safety, efficacy and acceptability of Implanon a single rod implantable contraceptive (etonogestrel) in University of Benin Teaching Hospital. Niger J Clin Pract. [Internet] 2010 [cited 2022 Feb 14];13(3). Available from: https://www.ajol.info/index.php/njcp/article/view/59796

138. Turok DK, Gero A, Simmons RG, et al. Levonorgestrel vs. copper intrauterine devices for emergency contraception. N Engl J Med. 2021;384(4):335-44.
139. Use of emergency contraception in the United States [Internet]. Guttmacher Institute; 2020 [cited 2022 Feb 14]. Available from: https://www.guttmacher.org/fact-sheet/use-emergency-contraception-united-states
140. Higgins JA, Hirsch JS, Trussell J. Pleasure, prophylaxis and procreation: A qualitative analysis of intermittent contraceptive use and unintended pregnancy. Perspect Sex Reprod Health. 2008;40(3):130-7.
141. Rocca CH, Schwarz EB, Stewart FH, Darney PD, Raine TR, Harper CC. Beyond access: Acceptability, use and nonuse of emergency contraception among young women. Am J Obstet Gynecol. 2007;196(1):29.e1-6.
142. Daniels K, Abma JC. Current contraceptive status among women aged 15-49: United States, 2017-2019. NCHS Data Brief. 2020;(388):1-8.
143. ACOG. Treatment of menorrhagia and sexual function. ACOG Clin Rev 2008;13:7.
144. Schaffir J, Fleming M, Waddell V. Patient perceptions regarding effect of gynecological surgery on sexuality. J Sex Med. 2010;7(2 pt 1):826-31.
145. Shih G, Dubé K, Sheinbein M, Borrero S, Dehlendorf C. He's a real man: A qualitative study of the social context of couples' vasectomy decisions among a racially diverse population. Am J Mens Health. 2013;7(3):206-13.
146. Bunce A, Guest G, Searing H, et al. Factors affecting vasectomy acceptability in Tanzania. Int Fam Plan Perspect. 2007;33(1):13-21.
147. Yang F, Dong L, Zhang X, et al. Vasectomy and male sexual dysfunction risk. Medicine (Baltimore). 2020;99(37):e22149.
148. Mohamad Al-Ali B, Shamloul R, Ramsauer J, et al. The effect of vasectomy on the sexual life of couples. J Sex Med. 2014;11(9):2239-42.
149. Littlejohn KE. Just get on the pill: The uneven burden of reproductive politics. Oakland, California: University of California Press; 2021.
150. Caruso S, Agnello C, Malandrino C, Lo Presti L, Cicero C, Cianci S. Do hormones influence women's sex? Sexual activity over the menstrual cycle. J Sex Med. 2014;11(1):211-21.
151. Higgins JA, Smith NK, Sanders SA, et al. Dual method use at last sexual encounter: a nationally representative, episode-level analysis of US men and women. Contraception. 2014;90(4):399-406.
152. Randolph ME, Pinkerton SD, Bogart LM, Cecil H, Abramson PR. Sexual pleasure and condom use. Arch Sex Behav. 2007;36(6):844-8.
153. Sanders SA, Hill BJ, Crosby RA, Janssen E. Correlates of condom-associated erection problems in young, heterosexual men: Condom fit, self-efficacy, perceptions, and motivations. AIDS Behav. 2014;18(1):128-34.
154. Crosby R, Milhausen R, Yarber WL, Sanders SA, Graham CA. Condom 'turn offs' among adults: an exploratory study. Int J STD AIDS. 2008;19(9):590-4.
155. Hensel DJ, Stupiansky NW, Herbenick D, Dodge B, Reece M. Sexual pleasure during condom-protected vaginal sex among heterosexual men. J Sex Med. 2012;9(5):1272-6.
156. Fennell J. "And isn't that the point?": pleasure and contraceptive decisions. Contraception. 2014;89(4):264-70.
157. Crosby RA, Milhausen RR, Mark KP, Yarber WL, Sanders SA, Graham CA. Understanding problems with condom fit and feel: An important opportunity for improving clinic-based safer sex programs. J Prim Prev. 2013;34(1):109-15.
158. Kaneko N. Association between condom use and perceived barriers to and self-efficacy of safe sex among young women in Japan. Nurs Health Sci. 2007;9(4):284-9.
159. Trμen B, Gravningen K. The use of protection for sexually transmitted infections (STIs) and unwanted pregnancy among Norwegian heterosexual young adults 2009. Sex Cult. 2011;15(2): 195-212.
160. Higgins JA, Wang Y. The role of young adults' pleasure attitudes in shaping condom use. Am J Public Health. 2015;105(7):1329-32.
161. Gallo MF, Nguyen NC, Luff A, et al. Effects of a novel erectogenic condom on men and women's sexual pleasure: Randomized controlled trial. J Sex Res. 2022;59(9):1133-9.

162. Sanders SA, Reece M, Herbenick D, Schick V, Dodge B, Fortenberry JD. Condom use during most recent vaginal intercourse event among a probability sample of adults in the United States. J Sex Med. 2010;7(s5):362-73.
163. Zaneva M, Philpott A, Singh A, Larsson G, Gonsalves L. What is the added value of incorporating pleasure in sexual health interventions? A systematic review and meta-analysis. PLoS One. 2022;17(2):e0261034.
164. Mathenjwa T, Maharaj P. 'Female condoms give women greater control': A qualitative assessment of the experiences of commercial sex workers in Swaziland. Eur J Contracept Reprod Health Care. 2012;17(5):383-92.
165. Naidu UM. Perceptions around second generation female condoms: Reporting on women's experiences. 2013 [cited 2022 Feb 9]; Available from: https://researchspace.ukzn.ac.za/handle/10413/9935
166. Peters AJ, van Driel FT, Jansen WH. Silencing women's sexuality: global AIDS policies and the case of the female condom. J Int AIDS Soc. 2013;16(1):18452.
167. Telles Dias PR, Souto K, Page-Shafer K. Long-term female condom use among vulnerable populations in Brazil. AIDS Behav. 2006;10(1):67-75.
168. Mack N, Grey TG, Amsterdam A, Williamson N, Matta CI. Introducing female condoms to female sex workers in Central America. Int Perspect Sex Reprod Health. 2010;36(3):149-56.
169. Okunlola MA, Morhason-Bello IO, Owonikoko KM, Adekunle AO. Female condom awareness, use and concerns among Nigerian female undergraduates. J Obstet Gynaecol. 2006; 26(4):353-6.
170. Sobze Sanou M, Fokam J, Guetiya Wadoum R, et al. Condom perception and prevention of HIV/AIDS infection in Cameroon: appraisal of knowledge, attitudes and practices among level one students of the University of Dschang. Ig E Sanita Pubblica. 2013;69(2):183-94.
171. Jones RK, Lindberg LD, Higgins JA. Pull and pray or extra protection? Contraceptive strategies involving withdrawal among US adult women. Contraception. 2014;90(4):416-21.
172. Sahin B, Sel G, Sahin B, Hatirnaz S. Comparison of sexual function scale scores in women according to the contraception method used as part of family planning strategy in Turkey. Clin Exp Obstet Gynecol. 2021;48(2):347.
173. Freundl G, Sivin I, Batár I. State-of-the-art of non-hormonal methods of contraception: IV. Natural family planning. Eur J Contracept Reprod Health Care. 2010;15(2):113-23.
174. Higgins JA, Wang Y. Which young adults are most likely to use withdrawal? The importance of pregnancy attitudes and sexual pleasure. Contraception. 2015;91(4):320-7.
175. Ortayli N, Bulut A, Ozugurlu M, Çokar M. Why withdrawal? Why not withdrawal? Men's perspectives. Reprod Health Matters. 2005;13(25):164-73.
176. Whittaker PG, Merkh RD, Henry-Moss D, Hock-Long L. Withdrawal attitudes and experiences: A qualitative perspective among young urban adults. Perspect Sex Reprod Health. 2010;42(2):102-9.
177. Stafford MK, Ward H, Flanagan A, et al. Safety study of nonoxynol-9 as a vaginal microbicide: Evidence of adverse effects. J Acquir Immune Defic Syndr Hum Retrovirol 1998;17(4): 327-31.
178. Xia M, Yang M, Wang Y, et al. dl-Mandelic acid exhibits high sperm-immobilizing activity and low vaginal irritation: A potential non-surfactant spermicide for contraception. Biomed Pharmacother. 2020;126:110104.
179. Thomas MA, Culwell KR, Mollan SG, Howard B. Sexual satisfaction with a vaginal pH regulator (EVO100): Results from the Amprevence clinical trial. Fertil Steril. 2020;114(3):e12-3.
180. Health C for D and R. FDA allows marketing of first direct-to-consumer app for contraceptive use to prevent pregnancy [Internet]. FDA. 2020 [cited 2022 Feb 10]; Available from: https://www.fda.gov/news-events/press-announcements/fda-allows-marketing-first-direct-consumer-app-contraceptive-use-prevent-pregnancy
181. Simmons RG, Jennings V. Fertility awareness-based methods of family planning. Best Pract Res Clin Obstet Gynaecol. 2020;66:68-82.
182. Polis CB, Jones RK. Multiple contraceptive method use and prevalence of fertility awareness based method use in the United States, 2013-2015. Contraception. 2018;98(3):188-92.
183. Brewer M, Stevens L. Use of fertility awareness-based methods of contraception: Evidence from the National Survey of Family Growth, 2013-2017. Contraception. 2021;104(2):183-7.

184. Reno H, Park I, Workowski K, Machefsky A, Bachmann L. A guide to taking a sexual history [Internet]. 2022 [cited 2022 Feb 11]; Available from: https://www.cdc.gov/std/treatment/sexualhistory.htm
185. Workowski K, Bachmann L, Chan P, et al. Sexually transmitted infections treatment guidelines, 2021 [Internet]. 2021 [cited 2022 Feb 11]; Available from: https://www.cdc.gov/std/treatment-guidelines/default.htm
186. Moser C. DSM-5, Paraphilias, and the paraphilic disorders: Confusion reigns. Arch Sex Behav. 2019;48(3):681-9.
187. Waldura JF, Arora I, Randall AM, Farala JP, Sprott RA. Fifty shades of stigma: Exploring the health care experiences of kink-oriented patients. J Sex Med. 2016;13(12):1918-29.
188. Joyal CC, Cossette A, Lapierre V. What exactly is an unusual sexual fantasy? J Sex Med. 2015;12(2):328-40.
189. McCabe MP, Sharlip ID, Atalla E, et al. Definitions of sexual dysfunctions in women and men: A consensus statement From the Fourth International Consultation on Sexual Medicine 2015. J Sex Med. 2016;13(2):135-43.
190. Parish SJ, Cottler-Casanova S, Clayton AH, McCabe MP, Coleman E, Reed GM. The evolution of the female sexual disorder/dysfunction definitions, nomenclature, and classifications: A Review of DSM, ICSM, ISSWSH, and ICD. Sex Med Rev 2021;9(1):36-56.
191. McCabe MP, Goldhammer DL. Demographic and psychological factors related to sexual desire among heterosexual women in a relationship. J Sex Res. 2012;49(1):78-87.
192. Pauls RN. Anatomy of the clitoris and the female sexual response. Clin Anat 2015;28(3):376-84.
193. Buisson O, Foldes P, Paniel B-J. Sonography of the clitoris. J Sex Med. 2008;5(2):413-7.
194. O'connell HE, DeLANCEY JOL. Clitoral anatomy in nulliparous, healthy, premenopausal volunteers using unenhanced magnetic resonance imaging. J Urol 2005;173(6):2060-3.
195. Abdulcadir J, Dewaele R, Firmenich N, et al. In vivo imaging-based 3-dimensional pelvic prototype models to improve education regarding sexual anatomy and physiology. J Sex Med. 2020;17(9):1590-602.
196. Hall KSK, Binik YM. Principles and practice of sex therapy, sixth edition. Guilford Publications; 2020.

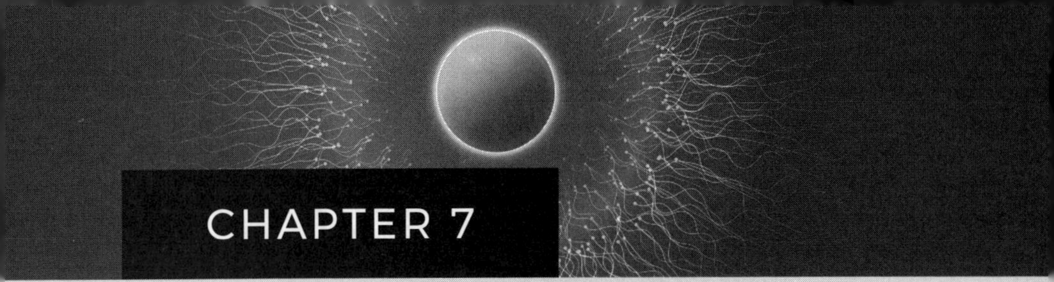

CHAPTER 7

Abstinence and Sexual Health: What Every Clinician Needs to Know

John Santelli, MD, MPH
Samuel Master, DO
Melissa Kottke, MD, MPH, MBA

KEY POINTS

- Abstinence from sexual intercourse (oral, anal, and/or vaginal) can be a healthy choice at any life stage. Abstinence is a personal decision that may evolve over time. It can include limits set by an individual regardless of their gender or sexuality.
- Sexual activity should always be mutually agreed upon. Verbal, affirmative, and ongoing consent is essential for any sexual activity. Sexual coercion is unhealthy at any age.
- With perfect use, abstinence from penile–vaginal sex prevents pregnancy. In real-life practice, abstinence from penile–vaginal sexual intercourse appears to be relatively ineffective against pregnancy and sexually transmitted infections (STIs), as abstinence intentions can fail. A back-up method should be planned.
- Avoiding penile–vaginal sex may not fully prevent STIs given transmission is variable (for example, may involve skin-to-skin contact) according to organism and activity.
- The health care provider should offer anticipatory guidance: assessing relationship history and sexual practices, screening for sexual coercion, providing counseling about pregnancy and STI risk, and providing support for patient choices and the development of healthy and satisfying sexuality.

Individuals at every life stage may pass through periods of abstinence from sexual intercourse. This chapter addresses several aspects related to abstinence: definitions of abstinence, sexual rights and sexual expression, the demography of abstinence and sexual behaviors including same-sex behaviors, the relationship of sex and marriage, the effectiveness of abstinence in preventing pregnancy and STIs, sexual assault, clinical assessment and counseling, clinicians and comprehensive sexuality education, user instructions for abstinence, and web-based resources for adolescent and adult patients. This chapter draws from studies that were restricted to binary classifications of "male" and "female" in their methodology. We acknowledge that this does not represent the fullness of gender expression and sexuality. We will use the terms self-identified (SI) females and self-identified (SI) males throughout and will utilize more inclusive terminology when possible.

Definitions of Abstinence

There is a lack of common and clinical consensus about what abstinence entails. Some people define abstinence as refraining from all sexual behavior, including masturbation. Some define abstinence as refraining from sexual behavior involving genital contact or refraining from penetrative sexual practices. Still others offer different definitions. Understanding how people define abstinence for themselves has important clinical implications, so these terms need careful exploration.

For some people, and in many older studies, only penile penetration of the vagina is considered sexual intercourse, and abstinence is conventionally defined as not engaging in penile–vaginal intercourse. However, persons who are abstaining from penile–vaginal sex may engage in a variety of other sexual behaviors. Many adolescents do not consider oral sex or mutual masturbation to be sex. In a study of high-school students who consider themselves never to have had sex, 30% had practiced heterosexual masturbation of or by a partner, 9% had engaged in fellatio (oral–penile contact) with ejaculation, and 10% had engaged in cunnilingus (oral–vulvar contact).[1] This definition also falls short, given its ableist and cis-heteronormative underpinnings. A study of lesbian, gay, or bisexual individuals identified similar variation in what was considered sex, with some specifying penetration, others describing oral–genital/anal contact, and some seeing a disconnect with the idea of sexual debut altogether, referring to the "inapplicability of virginity to queer populations."[2]

Most people have a more expansive view of sexual expression, and other activities give them pleasure and meaning. While allowing that individuals have personal definitions of abstinence, it is important to also understand a person's risk for pregnancy and STIs given their sexual behaviors. For purposes of contraception, abstinence may be defined as refraining from penile–vaginal sex. For purposes of protection from STIs, abstinence should be defined as refraining from those acts that could result in transmission of an STI and development of disease or continued transmission. These other sexual acts (particularly oral and anal sex) vary greatly in their STI risk.

In this chapter, we define *primary abstinence* as occurring when a person has never had sexual intercourse (oral, anal, or vaginal) with another person regardless of that person's gender identity.

Sexual Rights and Sexual Expression

A large group of experts convened by the World Health Organization and the World Association for Sexology to address the state of sexual health globally suggested that "Sexual health is a state of physical, emotional, mental and social well-being in relation to sexuality; it is not merely the absence of disease, dysfunction or infirmity. Sexual health requires a positive and respectful approach to sexuality and sexual relationships, as well as the possibility of having pleasurable and safe sexual experiences, free of coercion, discrimination, and violence. For sexual health to be attained and maintained, the sexual rights of all persons must be respected, protected and fulfilled."[3]

Sexual rights must also include the right to abstain from specific sexual practices and to feel satisfaction in that choice. All individuals should be supported to explore the range of sexual expression they find acceptable and pleasurable, if they so desire. (See Chapter 4, Person-Centered Reproductive Health and Contraceptive Counseling, and Chapter 6, Sexuality and Contraception.)

Being able to choose to engage, or not engage, in a wide array of sexual activities is central to sexual health and sexual rights. Individuals should be supported in exploring their individual preferences and priorities for sexual activities. Verbal and affirmative consent should be established between partners prior to engaging in sexual activity. Consent should be obtained every time, for every type of activity. This open communication between partners, where agreement about sexual activities is verbally confirmed, can ensure that an individual's boundaries and desires are respected. Further, ongoing communication with partners is very important because comfort levels and consent can change or be withdrawn at any time.

Demographics of Abstinence, Sexual Behaviors, and Marriage

Data in this section include new analyses from the 2015–2019 National Survey of Family Growth (NSFG, **Tables 7-1** and **7-2**)[4] and data from published studies that used a variety of datasets. Sexual behaviors in these surveys are generally dichotomized into sex with same and opposite sex partners, although this dichotomization is problematic. We define abstinence as not engaging in oral, anal, and vaginal sex. The NSFG provides population-representative data for the United States but provides limited data on lesbian, gay, or bisexual persons and no data on transgender people.

Primary abstinence is very common among the youngest teens. Primary abstinence among SI females in the United States for 2015–2019 declines from 75% at age 15 to 21% at age 19 to 10% at age 20–24, and less than 1% after age 35 (Table 7-1).[4] Among SI males, primary abstinence declines from 77% at age 15, 25% at 19, 14% at age 20–24, and about 1% after age 35 (Table 7-2).[4]

When oral, anal, and penile–vaginal sex are examined separately, we find that all three increase with age during the teen years and into the 20s for SI females and males; the same is true for same-sex sexual intercourse. Among adults over 25, > 85% of SI females and > 90% of SI males have had oral sex (Table 7-1 and Table 7-2).[4] Anal sex is less common than oral sex and penile–vaginal sex and generally initiated later. Among 25- to 44-year-olds, anal sex is reported by about one-third of SI females and almost one-half of SI males (Tables 7-1 and 7-2).[4]

While abstinence-until-marriage (AUM) has been a policy goal in the United States, sex and marriage have become increasingly disconnected over time. Marriage rates have decreased steadily in United States over the past 50 years and the median age at first marriage have risen considerably. Among SI females, the median age at first marriage rose from 20.3 in 1960 to 28.6 in 2021; among SI males, the

Table 7-1 Percentage of US self-identified females age 15–44 who report primary abstinence, secondary abstinence, ever having oral, anal or vaginal sex, ever married, and abstinence until marriage.

	Age									
	15	**16**	**17**	**18**	**19**	**20–24**	**25–29**	**30–34**	**35–39**	**40–44**
N	332	393	397	402	370	1556	1950	1923	1607	1358
Primary Abstinence	74.3	56.1	49.7	35.6	21.4	10.2	4.9	1.3	0.3	0.5
Ever had sexual intercourse, same or opposite sex	25.2	43.9	50.3	64.4	78.6	89.8	95.1	98.7	99.7	99.5
Ever had sexual intercourse, same sex	10.4	8.8	14.7	15.5	22.7	22.5	22.4	21.5	17.2	17.0
Ever had oral sex	19.2	35.5	43.0	55.3	71.7	84.3	87.3	89.3	90.8	85.2
Ever had penile–vaginal sex^	10.1	28.0	33.8	56.1	70.0	83.7	92.5	97.5	99.0	98.7
Ever had anal sex^	2.5	4.7	5.5	13.5	19.8	31.3	37.8	43.0	38.6	36.0
Ever married^	0.0	0.0	0.0	1.1	0.9	13.3	40.9	65.3	75.3	80.4
Ever had premarital sex, if never married	25.2	43.9	50.5	64.0	78.4	88.3	91.9	96.4	98.6	97.5
Secondary Abstinence	24.1	8.3	12.8	7.3	5.4	6.4	4.6	4.4	7.5	10.6
Notes:										

The NSFG asks about same-sex and opposite-sex partners, but certain behaviors are asked only of opposite-sex partners.
^ Indicates that the measure is limited to heterosexual partners.

Definitions:

Primary abstinence is defined as never having had oral, vaginal, or anal sexual contact, including same- and opposite-sex sexual contact.
Ever had sexual intercourse includes ever having had oral, vaginal, or anal sexual contact, including same- and opposite-sex sexual contact.
Oral sex includes same- or opposite-sex partners.
Penile–vaginal anal sex includes sexual intercourse with the opposite sex.
Ever married includes only opposite-sex partners (i.e., only heterosexual marriage).
Premarital sex is defined as ever had oral, penile–vaginal, or anal sex if not heterosexually married.
Secondary abstinence is defined as not having had oral, vaginal, or anal sexual contact in the 12 months prior to interview among females who have ever had sexual intercourse.

Data from Thompson J, Lindberg L, Maddow-Zimet I. Special analyses of the 2015-2019 National Survey of Family Growth. February 2022.

Table 7-2 **Percentage of US self-identified males age 15–44 who report primary abstinence, secondary abstinence, ever having oral, anal, or vaginal sex, ever married, and abstinence until marriage.**

	Age									
	15	**16**	**17**	**18**	**19**	**20-24**	**25-29**	**30-34**	**35-39**	**40-44**
N	352	363	397	428	378	1306	1465	1518	1301	1104
Primary Abstinence	76.9	61.8	46.5	33.8	24.9	14.4	4.4	2.2	1.4	0.6
Ever had sexual intercourse, same or opposite sex	23.1	38.2	53.5	66.2	75.1	85.6	95.6	97.8	98.6	99.4
Ever had sexual intercourse, same sex	4.7	1.7	2.1	4.2	4.0	6.7	8.5	7.1	7.4	6.5
Ever had oral sex	15.9	32.0	44.4	58.3	68.2	79.6	91.0	91.3	92.1	92.8
Ever had penile–vaginal sex^	10.2	20.6	37.6	56.9	64.9	81.7	92.7	96.5	96.9	98.6
Ever had anal sex	5.0	4.4	5.9	13.5	13.1	30.8	44.1	50.2	51.3	47.7
Ever married^	0.0	0.0	0.0	0.2	1.0	9.2	33.1	53.2	72.7	82.0
Ever had premarital sex, if never married	23.1	38.2	53.5	66.1	74.9	84.2	93.4	95.2	94.9	96.8
Secondary Abstinence	19.5	14.6	9.2	10.4	16.3	9.6	7.8	6.6	5.9	5.6

Notes:

The NSFG asks about same-sex and opposite-sex partners, but certain behaviors are asked only of opposite-sex partners.
^ Indicates that the measure is limited to heterosexual partners.

Definitions:

Primary abstinence is defined as never having had oral, vaginal, or anal sexual contact, including same- and opposite-sex sexual contact.

Ever had sexual intercourse includes ever having had oral, vaginal, or anal sexual contact, including same- and opposite-sex sexual contact.

Oral and anal sex includes same- or opposite-sex partners.

Penile–vaginal includes sexual intercourse with the opposite sex.

Ever married includes only opposite-sex partners (i.e., only heterosexual marriage).

Premarital sex is defined as ever had oral, penile–vaginal, or anal sex if not heterosexually married.

Secondary abstinence is defined as not having had oral, vaginal, or anal sexual contact in the 12 months prior to interview among males who have ever had sexual intercourse.

Data from Thompson J, Lindberg L, Maddow-Zimet I. Special analyses of the 2015-2019 National Survey of Family Growth. February 2022.

median age rose from 22.8 to 30.4, over the same period.[5] Abstinence outside of marriage has declined over time in the United States, from about half of women born in the 1930s and early 1940s to about 1 in 9 among SI women born between the mid-1960s and the early 1980s.[6] Today, more than 90% of unmarried people report premarital sex by age 30 and 95% to 99% report premarital sex by age 44 (Tables 7-1 and 7-2).[4] Marriage itself is rare among adolescents (< 1% before age 20) and rises steadily through the 20s and 30s (Tables 7-1 and 7-2).[4]

Rates of sexual activity among US teens have changed considerably over the past 60 years. From the mid-1960s through about 1990, the median age for first penile–vaginal sex declined from age 19 to age 17. (By comparison, the median age for first penile–vaginal sex in much of the developed world is between 17.5 and 18.5 years for SI females and between 16.5 and 18.5 years for SI males).[7] In the United States, the percentage of SI adolescent females (15 to 19 years of age) who reported penile–vaginal sex declined from 51% in 1988 to 43% in 2006-2010 to 42% in 2015-17; among SI adolescent males, the percentages reporting sex with an opposite sex partner declined from 60% in 1988 to 46% in 2002 to 38% in 2015-17.[8,9]

Most lesbian, gay, bisexual, transgender, and questioning/queer (LGBTQ) youth also initiate sexual activity in their teens and early 20s. Among SI women, ever having had same-sex sexual intercourse rises from 10% at age 15 to 23% at age 20–24 (Table 7-1[4]). Among SI men, ever having had same-sex sexual intercourse increases from 5% at age 15 to 7% at ages 20–24. LGBTQ youth may also engage in penile–vaginal sex, which puts them at risk for unintended pregnancy and STIs.[10–12] Further, development of sexual identity may be gradual or fluid over time. Stigmatization may also influence partner choice. It is important for the clinician to elicit a comprehensive and inclusive sexual health history to assess risk. (See Chapters 4, 6, and 22 for more information on obtaining a sexual history.)

Secondary abstinence occurs when individuals who have ever had sexual intercourse (oral, anal, or vaginal) abstain from sex for a period of time. Secondary abstinence over the prior 12 months is common among younger teens but less common among adults (4% to 10% between age 20 and 44 years, Tables 7-1 and 7-2[4]). Many of these secondary abstainers are not currently in a relationship or are not having sex for a variety of reasons. While some may choose long-term abstinence, others may not. Thus, clinical counseling with patients practicing secondary abstinence should address renewed sexual activity, contraception, and protection from STIs.

Effectiveness

As an action, abstinence prevents pregnancy or STI at the moment of abstaining. As an ongoing contraceptive method, abstinence should *in theory* be highly effective. However, "typical use" efficacy of abstinence in preventing pregnancy has not been reported (See Chapter 5, Effectiveness, Safety, and Comparative Side Effects). *In practice*, abstinence intentions can change or fail, particularly for adolescents.[13] Some primary abstainers do not anticipate first penile–vaginal sex; many report, "It just happened."[14] Programs to promote abstinence until marriage among youth are generally not effective (see below). Abstinence intentions among youth (*primary abstainers*) as exemplified by "virginity" pledges generally provide, at best, short-term benefits in delaying initiation of penile–vaginal sex and may increase initiation of other sexual activity.[15] Likewise, *secondary abstainers* may see intentions to abstain changed by situational factors such as a non-supportive partner or the development of a new romantic relationship. Clinician counseling can respectfully address these issues, and clinicians can suggest that abstainers have access to a back-up method to prevent pregnancy. Abstinence may be used in conjunction with fertility awareness–based methods (FABM) where penile–vaginal sex is avoided during known fertile periods to prevent pregnancy. Perfect and typical use estimates of FABM efficacy are detailed in Chapter 15, Fertility Awareness–Based Methods.

Abstinence from penile–vaginal sex may reduce the risk of some STIs but may not fully eliminate risk. In considering STI risk, it is important to understand that most people engage in a variety of sexual behaviors with the same partner. These practices include mutual masturbation, oral–genital/anal sex, digital–genital/anal play, and penile–anal sex. The risk of STI transmission varies considerably with the specific STI organism and specific behaviors. Among these behaviors, penile–anal sex carries considerably greater risk for transmission of HIV. For HIV, oral sex is generally safer than vaginal sex, which in turn is safer than anal sex. However, STIs that infect epithelial tissue, including herpes simplex virus (HSV) and human papillomavirus (HPV) can be transmitted via oral–genital contact and digital–genital contact, and HPV may cause oral or vulvovaginal cancer. HSV type-1 is also readily transmitted via kissing and is especially common with oral–genital contact. HPV may be transmitted via digital–genital contact, and with insertive sex toys. (See Chapter 23, Reproductive Tract Infections.)

Sexual Assault

Not all sexual activity is voluntary, and abstinence may be undercut by sexual assault. Screening and counseling regarding sexual coercion and assault are important aspects of reproductive health care. Sexual coercion and sexual assault happen at every age, and they have implications on an individual's ability to rely on abstinence to prevent pregnancy and STIs. Among young SI females age 18 to 24 years who first had sex as a teenager, about 1 in 10 report that their first sex was not voluntary; 13% report that they did not want it to happen the first time, and 52% report having mixed feelings.[8] In the United States, 44% of SI females have experienced violent sexual contact in their lifetimes and 21% report experiencing attempted or completed rape (forced or alcohol/drug-facilitated oral, anal, or vaginal penetration); among these, 82% experienced their first rape before the age of 25 and 43% before the age of 18 years. Among SI males, 18% have experienced unwanted sexual contact in their lifetimes.[16] Individuals who are younger age, SI female gender, nonheterosexual, and transgender experience rape and sexual assault at higher rates. Partner factors, such as unequal power dynamics and prior experience of violence within the relationship, are also associated with higher risk.[17,18] Adolescents who have initiated sex before the age of 13 are at increased risk for their first sexual experience to have been sexual assault and are also at an increased risk for sexual assault later in life.[19] Those who have already experienced sexual assault may have different counseling and clinical needs in reference to their sexual health, contraception, and other protective and preventive care. Those who have experienced sexual violence should be offered counseling and referrals, as indicated.

Clinical Assessment and Counseling Regarding Abstinence

Conversations about healthy sexuality, reproductive desires, and risk should be patient (person)-centered, individually tailored, and have foundations in explicit consent and satisfaction. (See Chapter 4, Person-Centered Reproductive Health Conversations and Contraceptive Counseling) Clinicians can help patients understand the possible benefits of abstinence across the life course and pragmatically discuss how to integrate it into a given circumstance.

Abstaining from sexual activity has a number of benefits. It has no medical or hormonal side effects. There are no eligibility requirements or contraindications. Further, it is always available, without a prescription, co-pay, or other external barrier. Abstinence does not have a time bound. It can be used for years, months, days, or just for right now.

The definition of abstinence may be unique for an individual. Understanding an individual's personal definition of abstinence, along with their goals for use of abstinence, is an opportunity to enhance counseling and education.

For those who choose abstinence, your role as care provider is to understand the individual's long- and short-term goals, to support healthy choices and counsel about risks associated with different choices, to teach negotiation and planning skills to achieve goals for establishing or maintaining abstinence, and to provide counseling and referrals as needed. Reaffirm that participating in sexual activities is not a requirement for being a fulfilled human. (See Chapter 6, Sexuality and Contraception.)

Contraception. When the goal of abstinence is to avoid pregnancy, then all forms of sexual expression are available except for penile–vaginal sex. Because opportunities may arise for having sex and because intentions may change, educate all persons who may engage in penile–vaginal sex about the other methods of contraception and safer sex available to them, including the following:

- Effective over-the-counter products, including emergency contraception
- Prescription methods
- Safer-sex practices
- Options for managing an unintended pregnancy

STI protection. In clinical assessment and counseling for STI risk, understand the scope of sexual activity and body parts the individual is using for any sexual activity. Also, consider infection risk from partner factors (e.g., multiple partners, exchange sex, substance use) and the community prevalence of specific STIs.[20] The most important risk factor for becoming infected with an STI is having sexual contact with an infected partner. A person's history of recent STI, multiple sexual partners, or one's partner(s) having multiple partners are predictors of becoming infected. Because most people engage in other sexual activities with the same partner with whom they engage in penile–vaginal sex, evaluate whether these behaviors add additional risk beyond that posed by penile–vaginal sex. Clinical counseling should focus on reducing STI risks, which may include reduced number of partners, mutual STI screening, STI screening of all exposed body parts, and use of internal/external condoms, dental dams, or other barriers to inhibit STI transmission during oral and anal sex. The care provider's role is to offer factual, explicit guidance on safer-sex options. (See Chapter 23, Reproductive Tract Infections.)

Lack of partner. Patients may be abstinent if they lack a partner or their partner decides to become abstinent. Clinicians can proactively address the possibility of masturbation or other ways to fulfill their sexual needs, if they so desire. They may also benefit from counseling (couples or individual) if abstinence is a dissatisfying situation. (For more information, see Chapter 6, Sexuality & Contraception.)

Medical reasons. There are few medical situations that warrant encouraging abstinence from penile–vaginal sex, but some include the following:

- Known or suspected STI, which also calls for avoiding other sexual practices that transmit body fluids such as semen, cervical-vaginal secretions, and blood
- Postoperative pain or tenderness, such as from episiotomy, hemorrhoidectomy, vasectomy, and other procedures
- Dyspareunia or other pelvic pain (While providers may not encourage abstinence in these circumstances, it is important to explore if pain with sex is a reason for the choice of abstinence. It is the provider's role to identify the source of pain and to try to resolve the symptoms. For example, pain may be secondary to pelvic, vaginal, or urinary tract infection, which require urgent diagnosis and treatment.)
- Certain pregnancy conditions such as placenta previa and pre-term labor
- Immediately postpartum (Though this is a common recommendation, the data to support it are lacking and people should be supported in following their own timeline in most instances.)
- Immediately post-myocardial infarction, recommendations should be individualized
- Other physical conditions when one is not healthy enough for sex

Sex problems. Therapy may be beneficial for a variety of physical, emotional, and relational sexual problems for an individual or a dyad. Therapy may include exploration of avenues of sexual gratification other than genital contact. (See Chapter 6, Sexuality and Contraception.)

Clinician Roles in Supporting Comprehensive Sexuality Education Programs

Sexuality education is important for promoting sexual health and an informed use of abstinence. Thus, as a clinician, you have an important role to play in supporting young people's access to medically accurate, developmentally appropriate, and evidence-based sexuality education. Health professional and professional associations have been crucial supporters of comprehensive sexuality education—in schools, in churches and communities, and online.[13] Clinicians have been strong and steady supporters of sex education as they often see the consequences of sexual ignorance and misinformation. Informed young people are better able to understand medical advice and to practice effective pregnancy and STI prevention.

Comprehensive sexuality education has been shown to have multiple positive behavioral outcomes, including helping youth delay initiation of intercourse, reduce STI risk, and improve contraceptive use.[21,22] *In contrast, abstinence-only-until-marriage (AOUM) programs have generally been a colossal failure, providing virtually no behavioral benefit.*[13] Federal sexuality education policy since 1981 has funded a variety of AOUM, aka sexual risk avoidance, programs, which have emphasized abstaining from all sexual contact (through a cis/heteronormative lens); from 1981 to 2019, the US government provided $2.2 billion for AOUM programs, including $110 million in FY2019.[23] Two meta-analyses of abstinence interventions and comprehensive intervention by the Centers for Disease Control and Prevention- (CDC-) sponsored Task Force on Community Preventive Services found "insufficient evidence" for the effectiveness of abstinence interventions in terms of behavioral impact on sexual initiation and other sexual behaviors.[21] In contrast, the Task Force found evidence of effectiveness and recommended comprehensive risk-reduction interventions for adolescents to promote behaviors that prevent or reduce the risk of pregnancy, HIV, and other STIs. Moreover, AOUM programs often promote misinformation about sexual health and contraception.[13] A state-level evaluation of AOUM from 1998–2016 found that federal funding has had no effect on adolescent birthrates.[24] By restricting access to health promotion and life-saving information, AOUM programs violate the principles of medical ethics and human rights. Clinicians should support science-based policies and oppose policies promoting ideas that are medically inaccurate and ineffective.

Comprehensive sexuality education should contain clear and trauma-informed messages about the health benefits and health risks of both abstinence and sexual activity. Young people who are not ready for sex need the social skills to refuse unwanted sexual advances—information they can use to protect themselves throughout their adult lives, including during periods of abstinence and sexual activity.

The internet has become an important source for information on sexual health. Help guide patients and parents/guardians to websites that provide accurate and useful information by providing information in the office about these and providing social endorsement for their use. See below for a listing of helpful websites and apps.

USER INSTRUCTIONS FOR ABSTINENCE—FOR CONTRACEPTION OR STI PROTECTION*

1. **Abstinence from sexual intercourse can have many benefits**. It is free, always available, has no medical side effects, and can be used throughout the life course.
2. **Abstinence can reduce the risk of pregnancy and STIs**. The reduced risk depends upon how abstinence is defined and practiced, and the mode of STI transmission.
3. **Decide in advance** which sexual activities interest you and that you consent to and discuss these with your partner or partners. Seek clarity about which sexual activities interest them and what they consent to. Seek agreement. Communicate with clarity and confidence.
4. **Avoid high-pressure sexual situations**. Avoid drinking to excess and using drugs that may cloud judgment and decision making.
5. **You can choose to engage in different sexual activities, including abstaining from penile–vaginal sex**, even if you have had sex in the past, as well as

* These instructions are intended to guide providers in educating patients in how to use their method.

if you have had sex in the past with a partner who may expect that your past actions dictate your current actions.

6. **Learn more** about your body, sexual health, contraception, and how to keep yourself healthy.
   Medically accurate and reliable online resources include:
   - American Sexual Health Association—www.ashasexualhealth.org/sexual-health
   - CDC—www.cdc.gov/sexualhealth
   - National Coalition for Sexual Health—https://nationalcoalitionforsexualhealth.org
   - Planned Parenthood—https://www.plannedparenthood.org/learn
   - The Pleasure Project—https://thepleasureproject.org/

   Good resources specifically for young people can be found at:
   - Ask Alice www.goaskalice.columbia.edu
   - Sex, Etc. www.sexetc.org
   - Scarleteen www.scarleteen.com
   - Bedsider www.bedsider.org
   - Young Women's Health https://youngwomenshealth.org/
   - Young Men's Health https://youngmenshealthsite.org/
7. **Learn about contraception and safer sex**, so you will be ready if you change your mind. Always keep condoms on hand.
8. **Refrain from penile–vaginal sex if** you do not have a contraceptive method available and you do not want to become pregnant.
9. **Learn about emergency contraception** in case you have unprotected or underprotected penile–vaginal sex. Emergency contraceptive pills or placement of an intrauterine device after unprotected intercourse substanially reduces the risk of pregnancy. If you need information about emergency contraception, see Chapter 18, Emergency Contraception.

Author Disclosures—Santelli: none; Master: none; Kottke: Receives research support from Merck/Organo.

Acknowledgements—A special thanks to Julia Thompson and Laura D. Lindberg for running the special analyses of the 2015-2019 National Survey of Family Growth in Tables 7-1 and 7-2. And a big thanks to Nao Haba for her help with the references.

References

1. Schuster MA, Bell RM, Kanouse DE. The sexual practices of adolescent virgins: genital sexual activities of high school students who have never had vaginal intercourse. Am J Public Health. 1996;86(11):1570–6.
2. Gillespie I, Armstrong H, Ingham R. Exploring reflections, motivations, and experiential outcomes of first same-sex/gender sexual experiences among lesbian, gay, bisexual, and other sexual minority individuals. J Sex Res. 2021;59(1):26-38.
3. World Health Organization, Department of Reproductive Health and Research. Defining sexual health: Report of a technical consultation on sexual health, 28–31 January 2002. Geneva: WHO, 2006.
4. Thompson J, Lindberg L, Maddow-Zimet I. Special analyses of the 2015-2019 National Survey of Family Growth. February 2022.
5. The U.S. Census Bureau. Historical marital status tables [Internet]. United States Census Bureau. November 2021. Available from: https://www.census.gov/data/tables/time-series/demo/families/marital.html. Accessed April 15, 2022.

6. Wu LL, Martin SP, England P, Mark NDE. Sexual abstinence in the United States: Cohort Trends in abstaining from sex while never married for U.S. women born 1938 to 1983. Socius. 2020;6:1-3.
7. Wellings K, Collumbien M, Slaymaker E, et al. Sexual behaviour in context: a global perspective. Lancet. 2006;368(9548):1706-28.
8. Abma JC, Martinez GM, Mosher WD, Dawson BS. Teenagers in the United States: sexual activity, contraceptive use, and childbearing, 2002. National Center for Health Statistics. Vital Health Stat 23. 2004;(24):1-48.
9. Martinez GM, Abma JC. Sexual activity and contraceptive use among teenagers aged 15-19 in the United States, 2015-2017. NCHS Data Brief. No 366. Hyattsville, MD: National Center for Health Statistics, 2020.
10. Coker TR, Austin SB, Schuster MA. The health and health care of lesbian, gay, and bisexual adolescents. Annu Rev Public Health. 2010;31:457-77.
11. Elia JP, Eliason MJ. Dangerous omissions: Abstinence-only-until-marriage school-based sexuality education and the betrayal of LGBTQ youth. Am J Sex Educ. 2010;5(1):17-35.
12. Everett BG, Turner B, Hughes TL, Veldhuis CB, Paschen-Wolff M, Phillips G. Sexual orientation disparities in pregnancy risk behaviors and pregnancy among sexually active teenage girls: Updates from the Youth Risk Behavior Survey. LGBT Health. 2019;6(7):342-9.
13. Santelli JS, Kantor LM, Grilo SA, et al. Abstinence-only-until-marriage: An updated review of U.S. policies and programs and their impact. J Adolesc Health. 2017;61(3):273-80.
14. Rosenthal SL, Von Ranson KM, Cotton S, Biro FM, Mills L, Succop PA. Sexual initiation: predictors and developmental trends. Sex Transm Dis. 2001;28(9):527-32.
15. Bearman PS, Brückner H. Promising the future: Virginity pledges and first intercourse. Am J Sociol. 2001;106(4):859-912.
16. Smith SG, Zhang X, Basile KC, et al. The National Intimate Partner and Sexual Violence Survey: 2015 Data Brief — Updated Release. Atlanta, GA: National Center for Injury Prevention and Control, Centers for Disease Control and Prevention; 2018, 32.
17. Tharp AT, Simon TR, Saul J. Preventing violence against children and youth. J Safety Res. 2012;43(4):291-8.
18. Carey KB, Durney S, Shepardson RL, Carey MP. Incapacitated and forcible rape of college women: Prevalence across the first year. J Adolesc Health. 2015;56(6):678-80.
19. Centers for Disease Control and Prevention. Violence prevention, risk and protective factors [Internet]. 2022. Available from: https://www.cdc.gov/violenceprevention/sexualviolence/riskprotectivefactors.html. Accessed April 12, 2022.
20. American College of Obstetricians and Gynecologists. Addressing health risks of noncoital sexual activity. Committee Opinion No. 582. Obstet Gynecol. 2013;122(6):1378-82. DOI: 10.1097/01.AOG.0000438963.23732.80. Available from: https://www.acog.org/en/clinical/clinical-guidance/committee-opinion/articles/2013/12/addressing-health-risks-of-noncoital-sexual-activity. Accessed 4/15/2022.
21. Chin HB, Sipe TA, Elder R, et al. The effectiveness of group-based comprehensive risk-reduction and abstinence education interventions to prevent or reduce the risk of adolescent pregnancy, human immunodeficiency virus, and sexually transmitted infections: two systematic reviews for the Guide to Community Preventive Services. Am J Prev Med. 2012;42(3):272-94.
22. Kirby D. Emerging answers 2007: New research findings on programs to reduce teen pregnancy. Washington, DC: Power to Decide (formerly The National Campaign to Prevent Teen and Unplanned Pregnancy); 2007. Available from: https://powertodecide.org/what-we-do/information/resource-library/emerging-answers-2007-new-research-findings-programs-reduce. Accessed April 15, 2022.
23. Sexuality Information and Education Council of the United States (SIECUS). A history of abstinence-only-until-marriage (AOUM) funding [Internet]. 2019. Available from: https://siecus.org/wp-content/uploads/2019/05/AOUM-Funding-History-Report-5.2019.pdf. Accessed April 15, 2022.
24. Fox AM, Himmelstein G, Khalid H, Howell EA. Funding for abstinence-only education and adolescent pregnancy prevention: Does state ideology affect outcomes? Am J Public Health. 2019;109(3):497-504.

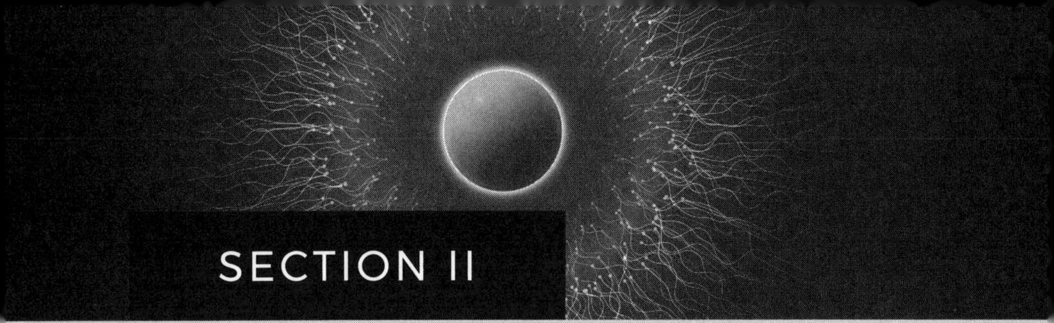

SECTION II

Methods

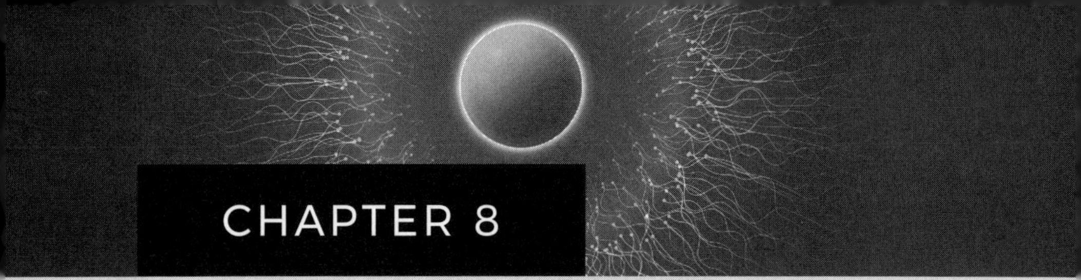

CHAPTER 8

Permanent Contraception

Jewel A. Brown, MD
Melody Y. Hou, MD, MPH

KEY POINTS

- Permanent contraception is one of the safest, most effective, and most cost-effective contraceptive methods.
- Permanent contraception is the most widely used method of family planning in the world in both developed and developing countries.
- Current approved permanent contraception includes fallopian tube and vas deferens surgery.
- Patients should be advised that these procedures should be considered permanent.
- Achieving pregnancy after permanent contraception is expensive, requiring either assisted reproductive technology (such as in vitro fertilization, or IVF) or highly technical surgery, and results cannot be guaranteed.
- Permanent contraception does not provide any protection against sexually transmitted infections (STIs), including human immunodeficiency virus (HIV).

Fallopian tube and vas deferens (vas) surgery are safe and effective permanent methods of contraception. (See Chapter 5, Effectiveness, Safety, and Comparative Side Effects.)

Permanent contraception continues to be the most commonly used method in the United States at 23.7% among individuals using a contraceptive method who were interviewed for the National Survey of Family Growth (NSFG) in 2017–2019.[1]

No medical condition should prohibit permanent contraception, although some conditions and circumstances may require certain surgical precautions. A couple considering permanent contraception should be advised on both fallopian tube and vas deferens surgery as well as nonsurgical, yet highly effective, options. In the United States, the most common approaches for fallopian tube surgery are laparotomy, at time of cesarean delivery or immediately postpartum, and laparoscopy, performed in the interval period (occurring at least 6 weeks postpartum). The Essure and Adiana systems were hysteroscopic transcervical methods of interval tubal surgery that were manufactured from 2002–2019 and 2009–2012, respectively, and are no longer available.

Culdoscopy, which involves introducing a camera into the rectovaginal pouch through an incision in the posterior vaginal cul-de-sac, is no longer recommended due to its higher complication rate. Hysterectomy also confers permanent contraception, but performing this major surgery solely for contraception is discouraged due to its risk of morbidity compared to other permanent contraception methods.

Vas surgery is one of the safest and most effective family planning methods. The no-scalpel approach under local anesthesia is the most common method of vas surgery throughout the world and is the most common nondiagnostic procedure performed by urologists in the United States. Vas surgery is the fifth most commonly used contraceptive method at 5.6% among patients aged 15–44 years in the NSFG 2017–19, following tubal surgery (18.1%), oral contraceptive pills (14%), long-acting reversible contraception such as intrauterine devices and implants (10.4%), and male condom (8.4%).[1]

Vas surgery is more effective than tubal occlusive methods in preventing pregnancy. It is a safer and faster procedure, the recovery time is shorter than any tubal surgery, and it costs one-fourth as much.[2,3] Despite its cost-effectiveness, vas surgery lags far behind tubal surgery as the permanent contraceptive method of choice in the United States; tubal surgery is chosen nearly four times more than vas surgery for permanent contraception.[1,4] The most common reasons that couples choose vas surgery are favorable reports from peers and recommendations by a clinician.[5] The most common sources of anxiety for patients who choose vas surgery are anticipated pain and fear of the unknown.[6]

Mechanism of Action

Tubal and vas surgery blocks fertilization by cutting or occluding the fallopian tubes or vas deferens, or removing the fallopian tubes entirely, to prevent the sperm and egg from uniting (**Figure 8-1**).

Advantages

Permanent contraception is ideal for patients who do not desire future fertility. (See Chapter 4, Person-Centered Reproductive Health Conversations and Contraceptive Counseling.) Advantages include the following:

- Permanence
- High effectiveness
- High acceptability
- Safety
- Quick recovery
- Lack of significant long-term side effects
- Protective effect against ovarian cancer with tubal surgery
- Long-term cost-effectiveness (vas surgery is the most cost-effective of all contraceptive methods)
- No need to buy anything
- No need for partner compliance
- Removal of contraceptive burden from the partner
- No need to interrupt coitus
- Privacy of choice

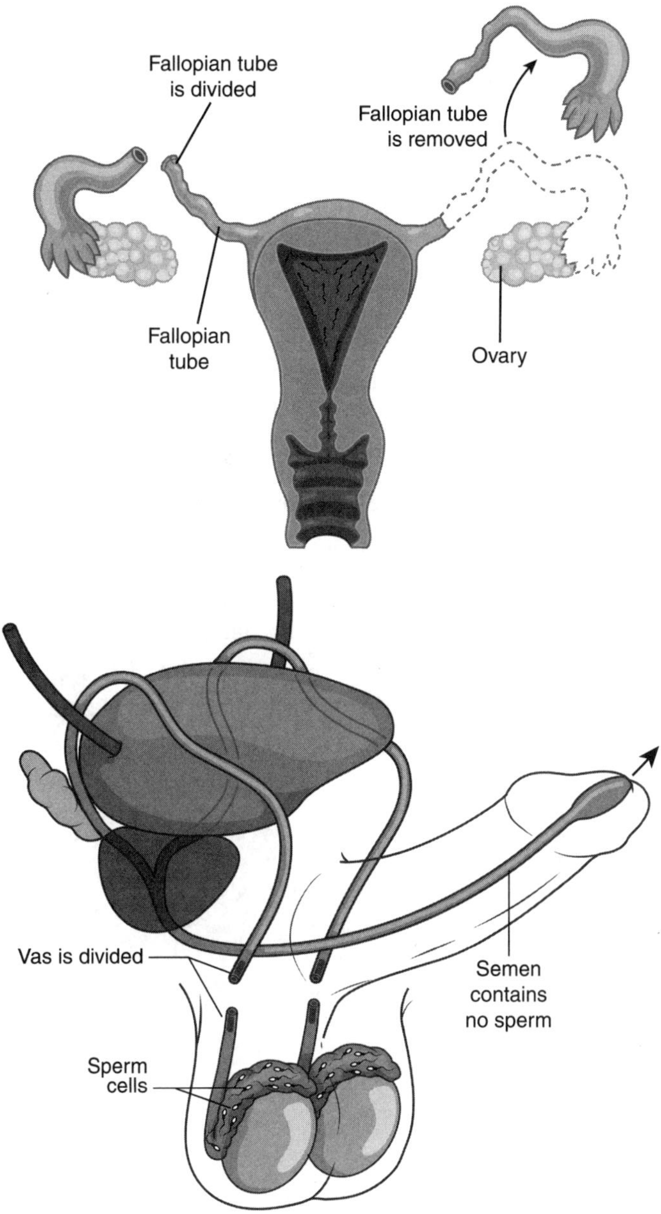

Figure 8-1 Mechanism of action for vas surgery and tubal surgery.

Reproduced from EngenderHealth. No-Scalpel Vasectomy Curriculum. 2nd ed. New York: EngenderHealth; 2007.

Disadvantages

Permanent contraception is not recommended for patients who are unsure of their desire for future fertility. Other disadvantages include the following:

- Restoring fertility after permanent contraception is possible but difficult. It is expensive, requiring either costly assisted reproductive technology (such as in vitro fertilization [IVF] or intracytoplasmic sperm injection [ICSI]) or highly technical surgical reversal, and results cannot be guaranteed

- All surgical procedures carry some risk specific to the nature of the surgery and anesthetic used
- Effect of vas surgery and transcervical tubal surgery is not immediate, and these cannot provide dependable contraception until procedure success is confirmed
- Risk of regret may be high among some groups of patients
- Need for trained provider, procedure room (aseptic conditions), assistants, medications, and surgical equipment
- Expense at the time of the procedure
- Higher probability of pregnancy being ectopic if tubal occlusion method fails
- Lack of protection against sexually transmitted infections (STIs), including HIV

FALLOPIAN TUBE SURGERY

Table 8-1 lists fallopian tube surgery approaches and available methods.

Table 8-1 Fallopian Tube Surgery Approaches and Available Methods

Approach	Occlusion Method	Advantages	Disadvantages
Interval Tubal Surgery			
Laparoscopy	■ Complete salpingectomy ■ Silicone bands ■ Titanium or spring clips ■ Bipolar electrocoagulation	■ 2–3 small incisions ■ Less pain than from mini-laparotomy ■ Low complication rate ■ Short recovery time	■ Need for specialist with method-specific training necessary ■ Necessary equipment is often difficult to obtain and maintain ■ Need a fully equipped operating and recovery room with trained staff
Suprapubic mini-laparotomy	■ Complete salpingectomy ■ Ligation techniques ■ Silicone bands ■ Titanium or spring clips	■ Local or general anesthesia ■ Incision site usually not visible (below pubic hairline)	■ Difficult technique if the patient is obese, the uterus immobile, or the tubes have adhesions ■ Recovery can be more painful than with laparoscopy

Approach	Occlusion Method	Advantages	Disadvantages
Postpartum Tubal Surgery			
Infraumbilical mini-laparotomy	■ Complete salpingectomy ■ Ligation techniques ■ Titanium or spring clip	■ Convenience ■ Lower costs ■ Ease of surgery ■ Does not necessarily extend hospital stay beyond that for a normal delivery	■ Counseling must occur prior to labor*
Cesarean delivery	■ Complete salpingectomy ■ Ligation techniques ■ Titanium or spring clips	■ Convenience ■ Lower costs ■ Anatomy fully visible	■ Cesarean delivery should not be performed solely to occlude the tubes ■ Other disadvantages from infraumbilical mini-laparotomy apply
Postabortion Tubal Surgery			
Laparoscopy	■ Complete salpingectomy ■ Silicone bands ■ Titanium or spring clips ■ Bipolar electrocoagulation	■ Convenience ■ Patient motivation	■ Need for careful counseling with consideration of risk of regret* ■ If using general anesthesia, may increase the amount of blood loss with the abortion procedure
Suprapubic mini-laparotomy	■ Complete salpingectomy ■ Ligation techniques ■ Titanium or spring clips	Same as above	Same as above

* See Chapter 4, Person-Centered Reproductive Health Conversations and Contraceptive Counseling.

Effectiveness

Tubal surgery is far more effective than short-term user-dependent reversible contraceptive methods, such as oral contraceptives, condoms, and injectable methods (See Chapter 5, Effectiveness, Safety, and Comparative Side Effects.) Failure rates of tubal surgery are roughly comparable to those of long-acting reversible methods, such as the contraceptive implants and intrauterine devices (IUDs), which are described in Chapters 9 and 10. The World Health Organization (WHO) and Centers for Disease Control and Prevention (CDC) place permanent contraception in the top tier of contraceptive effectiveness. The overall first-year typical-use failure rates are 0.5% for fallopian tube surgery and 0.15% for vas surgery (Table 5-2).

In 1996, the CDC conducted the Collaborative Review of Sterilization (CREST), a large, prospective, multicenter observational study of over 10,000 patients undergoing transabdominal tubal occlusion surgery in the United States who were followed for up to 14 years. The study demonstrated that transabdominal tubal occlusion surgery is highly effective.[7] Analysis of CREST data found that the 5-year cumulative probability of failure of aggregated surgical methods was 13 per 1,000 procedures.[7] The risk of failure persists for years after the procedure, and varies by several factors, including patient age at the time of surgery and surgical technique (see Approaches and Techniques, p. 235). Patients were more likely to have a contraceptive failure the younger they were at the time of surgery. Postpartum partial salpingectomy had the lowest 5-year and 10-year cumulative pregnancy rates (6.3 per 1,000 and 7.5 per 1,000 procedures, respectively). The highest 10-year cumulative pregnancy rates were found in patients younger than 28 years who had tubal occlusion with bipolar coagulation, at 54 pregnancies per 1,000 patients.[7] The results of the CREST study should be interpreted in context; the study included certain transabdominal occlusion methods for which surgical techniques were still evolving, and it did not evaluate the titanium clip, which was introduced in the United States in 1996 after the study was completed. According to the Royal College Working Party on Sterilization in 1999, efficacy of the titanium clip is comparable to other occlusion methods with a crude failure rate of 2 to 3 per 1,000 patients.[8] However, postpartum use of the titanium clip may have a higher failure rate compared to postpartum partial salpingectomy.[9-11]

To date, no randomized controlled studies directly compare pregnancy rates for bilateral total salpingectomy with that of bilateral tubal occlusion. No cases of spontaneous pregnancy have been reported after total bilateral salpingectomy when surgery was performed for the purpose of permanent contraception, although four cases of spontaneous pregnancies have occurred after a total bilateral salpingectomy was completed for other indications (hydrosalpinx, pelvic inflammatory disease, and ectopic pregnancy).[12] We believe that the risk of pregnancy following total salpingectomy would likely be the same and possibly the lowest of all the methods of tubal surgery. With its comparable safety and likely greater efficacy and cancer prevention (see Cancer Prevention, p. 231), total bilateral salpingectomy should be considered the preferred tubal method for permanent contraception when appropriate.

Two transcervical permanent contraceptive systems approved by the Food and Drug Administration (FDA), Essure and Adiana, relied on the hysteroscopic placement of devices in the proximal portion of the fallopian tubes that initiated physiologic fibrosis within the tubal lumen to cause occlusion. Both systems retain FDA approval, although their manufacturers discontinued making Adiana in April 2012 and Essure in January 2019. In both systems, successful bilateral device placement in the tubes is essential for effectiveness. Long-term effectiveness has not been directly assessed for either transcervical system, but Markov modeling suggests that these methods for transcervical sterilization are less effective than laparoscopic occlusion.[13,14]

Intrauterine Pregnancy

Intrauterine pregnancy following transabdominal tubal surgery carries no known added risk to the patient or the fetus. Pregnancy outcomes are unclear with Essure left in-situ. A portion of the Essure coils trails into the uterine cavity, but trailing coils appear to shorten and become completely encapsulated in tissue on follow-up hysteroscopy. Clinical trials show that pregnancy rates are inferior when Essure is used to block hydrosalpinges prior to IVF than when laparoscopic salpingectomy is performed.[20-22] The extended follow-up of patients in the Phase III trial for Essure found no pregnancies among the 449 patients who completed all 5 years of follow-up, so outcome data of spontaneous intrauterine pregnancies are limited to case publications or postmarketing reports to FDA. Miscarriage, ectopic pregnancy, abortion, and successful delivery have all been reported with transcervical procedures,[17,18,23-25] but these are insufficient to estimate rates of pregnancy outcomes following these procedures.

Ectopic Pregnancy

The overall risk of ectopic pregnancy in patients using permanent contraception is significantly lower than that of the general population, since the risk of becoming pregnant with permanent contraception is very low. However, if a patient becomes pregnant following tubal surgery for permanent contraception, the risk of that pregnancy being ectopic is high. An analysis of CREST data found that roughly 30% of pregnancies following tubal occlusion were ectopic pregnancies.[26] The risk of ectopic pregnancy varies with the method of tubal surgery. The 10-year cumulative probability of ectopic pregnancy after transabdominal tubal occlusion by all methods was 7.3 per 1,000 procedures. For the titanium clip and silicone band, the 10-year cumulative probabilities were, respectively, 8.5 and 7.3 per 1,000 procedures. Postpartum partial salpingectomy had the lowest risk of ectopic pregnancy at 1.5 per 1,000 procedures. The risk of ectopic pregnancy did not diminish with the length of time since the tubal surgery but did vary inversely with the age of the patient. The probability of ectopic pregnancy was greater for patients who initiated permanent contraception using these occlusion methods before age 30 than for patients 30 years or older. Young patients who had bipolar tubal coagulation had a 10-year cumulative probability of ectopic pregnancy of 31.9 per 1,000 procedures.[26] The rate of ectopic pregnancy following complete salpingectomy is unknown. However, since most ectopic pregnancies occur in the distal end of the fallopian tube, the rate of ectopic pregnancies following removal of the entire tube should be virtually zero. All four of the spontaneous pregnancies following bilateral salpingectomy documented in case reports were intrauterine.[12]

There are no equivalent data on ectopic pregnancy risk for transcervical procedures, although there have been reports of ectopic pregnancies in Adiana trials and in postmarketing surveillance after Essure placement.[19,27]

Safety

Tubal surgery is a safe method of contraception. Death from transabdominal tubal surgery is extremely rare. Mortality rates in the United States have been estimated at 1 to 4 deaths per 100,000 procedures; most deaths in the United States have been associated with anesthetic complications.[28-31] In the CREST study, no deaths were reported among 9,475 patients who underwent interval laparoscopic tubal surgery.[32]

Major complications from transabdominal tubal occlusion are also uncommon, estimated to be 0.9 to 1.6 per 100 procedures, with no difference in major morbidity between mini-laparotomy and laparoscopy.[33,34] The types of complications vary by surgical procedure, anesthesia, and whether energy is used for tubal occlusion.[33] Intraoperative complications include damage to bowel, bladder, or major vessels. Rarely, laparotomy and/or blood transfusion may be required to manage these events. Postoperative complications include wound infection and prolonged pelvic or abdominal pain. Risk factors for complications during transabdominal tubal occlusion include previous abdominal or pelvic surgery and obesity.[32]

Complete salpingectomy is a relatively new option for routine permanent contraception and not just for individuals with a history of ovarian cancer. Long-term safety data for routine use are unavailable. A 2021 review that included five randomized controlled studies compared bilateral tubal ligation versus bilateral salpingectomy and found no differences between pre- or postoperative complications, wound infection, surgical blood loss, or length of hospital stay.[34]

No randomized trials compare safety outcomes of transcervical permanent contraception to transabdominal procedures.[33] Complications of transcervical methods include pregnancy as described prior and tubal perforation, which was reported in 1% to 3% of Essure cases, with Essure devices found in the intraperitoneal cavity in 0.5% to 3% of patients. No perforations were reported during the Adiana trial.[35,36] Potential hysteroscopic-related complications include infection, bleeding, uterine perforation, injury to surrounding organs, hypervolemia, and hyponatremia.[35,36] Compared with laparoscopic procedures, claims data indicate that transcervical permanent contraception is associated with more claims for repeat procedures and abnormal uterine bleeding, but fewer claims for procedural complications and pelvic and abdominal pain.[37] However, patients are increasingly requesting Essure device removal for a variety of reasons, including unintended pregnancy, chronic pain, menstrual disorders, nickel hypersensitivity, or improper placement diagnosed after imaging.[38]

Special Issues

Ovarian Function

Several studies evaluated the vascular effects of tubal occlusion and subsequent ovarian function, as well as possible long-term outcomes such as menopausal symptoms. A prospective study of patients undergoing laparoscopic tubal occlusion using bipolar coagulation showed no change in ovarian function or reserve compared to a matched control group who did not undergo tubal occlusion.[39] Another prospective study of mini-laparotomy and laparoscopic tubal surgery found no difference in uterine or ovarian blood flow or ovarian hormone secretion after 6 months.[40] Likewise, complete salpingectomy had a similar effect on ovarian reserve as tubal ligation at cesarean delivery, with no differences in anti-Müllerian hormone levels before or after surgery.[41]

Despite relatively strong evidence that ovarian function is not affected by tubal occlusion, tubal occlusion may be associated with menopausal symptoms such as hot flushes, although age at menopause does not appear affected.[42-45]

Cancer Prevention

Transabdominal tubal surgery has a protective effect against ovarian cancer that persists over many years.[46-48] The specific tubal surgery technique used is often not mentioned in the literature. A large case-control study showed tubal surgery was associated with a 39% reduction in the risk of ovarian cancer irrespective of technique. The risk remained low up to 25 years after surgery.[46] Results of a cohort study of more than 65,000 Danish patients not only showed an overall decrease in the risk of ovarian cancer, but also a reduced rate of endometrial cancer, although the association was not as strong.[47]

The protective effect of transabdominal tubal surgery on ovarian cancer risk extends to carriers of the *BRCA1* mutation.[49,50] The risk reduction does not appear to include carriers of *BRCA2*, although this may be due to the small sample size.[50] Combined oral contraceptive (COC) use, especially long-term use, confers more protection in *BRCA1* carriers, but the combination of COCs and tubal surgery offered greater protection than either method alone, conferring a risk reduction of 72%.[50]

The biological mechanism for ovarian cancer reduction in patients who have undergone transabdominal tubal ligation surgery is unknown. However, increasing evidence indicate the distal end of the fallopian tube is the main site of origin of high-grade serous ovarian carcinoma.[51] While occlusive techniques are estimated to lower a patient's lifetime risk of ovarian cancer by 24% to 36%, primarily by reducing the incidence of endometrioid and clear cell carcinoma, bilateral salpingectomy may create an overall 49% reduction in ovarian cancer that includes a decrease in serous carcinoma.[52-54] The transition to complete salpingectomy instead of only segmental occlusion has occurred because of this potential reduction of ovarian cancer risk for all individuals and not just those at high risk. The American College of Obstetricians and Gynecologists now recommends opportunistic complete salpingectomy during hysterectomy and salpingectomy over tubal occlusion procedures for permanent contraception.[55] An educational initiative promoting opportunistic salpingectomy for ovarian cancer reduction that took place in British Columbia, Canada was followed by an increase in salpingectomy for permanent contraception and at the time of hysterectomy in that region.[56] The majority of surveyed obstetricians and gynecologists in the United States now perform salpingectomy at the time of hysterectomy and for permanent contraception for cancer reduction risk.[57]

Studies generally show no to mild protective association between tubal occlusion and breast cancer. One prospective cohort study of 619,199 patients suggested an inverse association between tubal surgery and breast cancer mortality (RR, 0.82), with a stronger benefit related to younger age at time of surgery (RR among women before age 35, 0.69).[58] However, data from the Nurses' Health Study, the Cancer and Steroid Hormone Study, and the Cancer Prevention Study II Nutrition Cohort yielded no overall association with breast cancer risk.[59,60]

Menstrual Abnormalities

The long-term health effects of tubal surgery on menstrual pattern appear to be negligible. Reported menstrual disturbances following tubal surgery, known as post-tubal ligation syndrome, are likely due to inaccurate recall of previous menstrual patterns, weight changes, and pre-surgery use of hormonal contraceptives that can mask underlying menstrual dysfunction.[61-67] Although 2% to 4% of patients in the Essure and Adiana trials reported a disturbance in their menstrual patterns, the relationship of menstrual abnormalities to transcervical permanent contraception is unclear, with the same confounders as for other tubal occlusion procedures.[35,36]

Sexuality

Studies of sexuality found no detrimental long-term effects from permanent contraception. The CREST study found that interval tubal surgery was not likely to change sexual interest or pleasure.[68] The majority of patients who had changes in libido or sexual pleasure reported positive effects. Another study found an increase in coital frequency after 1 year among women who had permanent contraception as compared with women not using permanent contraception.[68,69]

Postablation Tubal Sterilization Syndrome (PATSS)

Postablation tubal sterilization syndrome (PATSS), in which menstrual blood trapped in the cornua or proximal tube causes painful distention, has an incidence of 8% to 33%.[70] Endometrial ablation is an option for treatment of abnormal uterine bleeding. Although patients have reduced fertility after an ablation, they should still be advised not to undergo ablation unless they have completed childbearing due to the increased risk of abnormal placentation, spontaneous abortion, and preterm delivery in a subsequent pregnancy.[71] Permanent birth control is thus an appealing contraceptive option for these patients. However, after ablation, endometrial tissue can persist or regenerate in the cornual regions of the uterine cavity, even when the remaining cavity may be reduced in size or completely obliterated by the procedure.[72] Patients who have both endometrial ablation and tubal surgery may later develop retrograde bleeding from persistent endometrial tissue in the cornua and in isolated areas of the myometrium that can lead to PATSS.[70,73] Treatment may require hysterectomy.[74]

Although no longer on the market, many patients still have Essure devices in place. It is important to note that performing ablation after transcervical procedures carries risk. The stainless steel core of in-situ Essure devices may conduct energy during global radiofrequency ablation, causing damage to surrounding organs.[17] The theoretical risk for global thermal methods and endometrial resection under direct visualization should be less than that of global radiofrequency ablation, but safety data are limited.[75,76] Although transcervical permanent birth control occludes the tubes more proximally than transabdominal procedures, PATSS can still occur following transcervical procedures and ablation.[77]

Chronic Pelvic Pain

Transabdominal tubal surgery does not seem to be associated with an increased risk of chronic pelvic pain if prior contraceptive use and previous menstrual patterns are considered.[61-63,65,67] Younger patients with preexisting reports of menstrual dysfunction may be at increased risk following transabdominal surgery.[61]

Pelvic pain is the most common complaint after Essure placement.[78] In a retrospective study of 458 patients who underwent Essure placement, the incidence of acute pelvic pain after the procedure was 8.1%. By 3 months after the procedure,

4.2% of patients reported continued pain.[79] Most patients who experience pelvic pain after Essure will report pain within the first month after Essure placement, but an additional 19.2% reported the onset of pain between 1 and 12 months and 30.8% reported pain beginning 12 months or later.[80] The varying latency period documented in case reports and series about pain after Essure placement supports this finding, indicating that patients may still develop pain related to Essure placement months or years after the procedure.[81,82] Patients with a history of chronic pain, who had been excluded from the device approval trials, are more likely to report pain after hysteroscopic occlusion (OR 6.81; 95% CI 2.95–15.73).[79] A prospective observational study of 80 patients with reported pelvic pain demonstrated short- and medium-term improvement in quality of life as well as reduction in pelvic pain following laparoscopic removal of Essure.[83]

Following Adiana, 6% of the 635 patients who participated in the clinical trial reported cramping unrelated to menses; 5% reported dysmenorrhea, 3% reported pelvic pain, and 1% reported dyspareunia.[36] There are no published data documenting incidence of chronic pelvic pain following Adiana, but some patients have reported chronic pelvic pain in the FDA device experience database.[84]

Risk of Future Hysterectomy

Although there is no known biological mechanism for tubal permanent contraception to increase the risk for hysterectomy, a strong association exists between transabdominal procedures and hysterectomy (RR, 1.6–4.4).[65,85,86] Patients who undergo tubal surgery appear to be 4.4 times more likely to undergo hysterectomy than those whose partners underwent vasectomy.[85] However, the majority of patients do not undergo subsequent hysterectomy; the cumulative probability of undergoing hysterectomy 14 years after tubal occlusion in the CREST study was 17%.[87] Increased risk was associated with a presurgery history of menstrual or other benign gynecologic disorders, such as endometriosis.[87] There are no data yet on the rate of hysterectomy following transcervical procedures, although case reports of hysterectomy due to pain or other complaints have been published.[88,89]

Regret

Most patients who choose tubal surgery as a contraceptive method never regret their decision. However, because of relationship changes and other life events, regret is always possible. Patients who undergo tubal surgery at age 30 or younger are at greater risk for regret.[90-92] The cumulative probability of regret over 14 years of follow-up in the CREST study was 12.7%.[90] However, the probability of regret was 20.3% for patients aged 30 years or younger at the time of surgery, compared with 5.9% for patients older than 30 years at the time of surgery. For all patients in the CREST study, the rate of regret following interval procedures within 1 year of delivery was 17.6%, compared to 17.8% following postpartum tubal ligation after vaginal delivery and 16.1% following cesarean delivery. The cumulative probability of regret diminished steadily with the interval between delivery and surgery.[90] Immediate postabortion procedures were not associated with increased regret when compared with interval procedures after abortion.[90,93,94]

Analysis of the data from the CREST study showed the 14-year cumulative probability of requesting reversal information was 14.3%, but in patients younger than 24 years who underwent tubal surgery, the request for reversal information was as high as 40.4%.[92,94] The number of patients who requested information about IVF was not documented, nor the number of patients who initiated reversal or IVF.

Risk factors for increased regret include having received less preoperative information about the procedure, having had less access to information about or support for other contraceptive methods, and having made the decision under pressure from a spouse or because of a medical indication.[92,95,96] Younger patients are at greater risk for regret given the longevity of their future fertility and the opportunity for life events such as relationship changes or the death of a child.

The presence of strong risk factors for regret should not be used to restrict or delay tubal surgery but should indicate the need for careful counseling. (See Chapter 4, Person-Centered Reproductive Health Conversations and Contraceptive Counseling.) Nulliparity and age are not contraindications, and a nulliparous or young patient seeking permanent contraception should not be required to undergo a mental health evaluation due to a clinician's concern for this risk of patient regret.

Desire for Pregnancy Following Tubal Occlusion

Permanent contraception should be considered irreversible, but some patients will have a change in personal circumstance and later desire to bear children. Assisted reproductive technologies such as IVF and microsurgical tubal reversal are options for a patient who desires pregnancy following tubal surgery, but success is not guaranteed. There are no randomized controlled trials comparing the success rates and costs of IVF with surgical reversal.

The choice between IVF and tubal surgery reversal for pregnancy is dependent on multiple factors, including the method of tubal surgery, the age of the patient at the time of treatment, severity of the tubal damage, remaining tubal length, and other fertility factors. With careful case selection and meticulous surgical technique, reasonable pregnancy rates of 12% to 69% can be achieved following microsurgical reversal of tubal occlusion.[97,98]

Patients should be aware that surgical reversal carries operative and anesthesia risks. Ectopic pregnancy is more common among pregnancies occurring after surgical reversal of tubal surgery than IVF. Published ectopic pregnancy rates following surgical reversal range from 4% to 8%.[98] Nonetheless, tubal occlusion reversal may be appealing for younger patients, those who desire more than a single additional pregnancy, or those who are not comfortable with IVF. Both IVF and reversal surgery are costly and often are not covered by health insurance. Finally, patients undergoing tubal reversal surgery may have the need for future contraception. In a large Canadian study, 23% of patients obtaining tubal reversal following tubal ligation went on to obtain a subsequent method of permanent contraception.[99]

There are limited data on outcomes after reversal of transcervical tubal occlusion. Issues with reversal of transcervical procedures include the location of the implants within the tubal cornual junction rather than the tube itself, and the tissue ingrowth into the implants. One reversal technique that has resulted in successful pregnancies is removing the devices and reimplanting the tube into the uterus (tubouterine implantation).[100,101] IVF implantation and pregnancy outcomes are unknown with Essure left in situ, since a portion of the coils trail into the uterine cavity. Although there are case reports of successful IVF pregnancies following transcervical tubal occlusion, studies show that using Essure to block hydrosalpinges prior to IVF is inferior to laparoscopic salpingectomy in ongoing pregnancy rates.[20-22,102,103] A successful pregnancy with IVF following device removal has been reported, but outcome data are still lacking.[104]

Tubal Occlusion Device Removal

Patients may request tubal occlusion device removal for reasons other than regret or desired fertility. Clinicians should conduct careful history-taking, examination, imaging, and testing to eliminate other causes of the patient's complaints before attributing the symptoms to the devices. Removal of transabdominal devices such as clips and rings can be done via laparoscopic salpingectomy. However, removal of transcervical devices that lie at the tubal cornual junction is more challenging.[38] Treatment options for patients who request Essure device removal include leaving the devices in place with medical management of the presenting complaints, surgical removal of devices, or hysterectomy. Case reports and case series describe successful surgical removal of Essure devices using hysteroscopic removal, laparoscopic salpingectomy or salpingostomy, and wedge resection.[38,80,105-107] Outcomes after Essure device removal are generally favorable, with most patients reporting improvement in pelvic pain and nickel hypersensitivity reactions after Essure removal.[80] However, clinicians should caution patients that their specific complaints may not resolve after removal.[108] There are no published case reports documenting removal for Adiana.

Providing Tubal Surgery: Approaches and Techniques

Timing

Tubal surgery can be performed postpartum (at the time of cesarean delivery or shortly after vaginal delivery), after spontaneous or therapeutic abortion, or as an interval procedure (unrelated in time to a pregnancy). The timing of the procedure influences both the surgical approach and the method of tubal surgery.

Postpartum Tubal Surgery

Approximately half of all permanent tubal procedures are performed in the postpartum period. Postpartum tubal surgery is performed after 10% of all hospital deliveries in the United States.[109] Tubal surgery may be done at the time of cesarean delivery or via mini-laparotomy following vaginal delivery and should not extend the patient's hospital stay. Institutional barriers may create delays that prevent fulfillment of postpartum tubal surgery requests. Since subsequent unintended pregnancy occurs in nearly 50% of patients not receiving their requested postpartum tubal surgery, hospital procedures should prioritize these procedures in the immediate postpartum period.[109]

Postpartum mini-laparotomy should be done in a medically stable patient prior to the onset of significant uterine involution (within 1 to 2 days following delivery).[110] In the presence of unexpected medical or obstetric complications, consider postponing tubal surgery to the interval time period.

Interval Tubal Surgery

In the United States, approximately half of all tubal surgeries are performed as interval procedures.[110] Although transabdominal tubal surgery can be done at any time during the menstrual cycle, performing the procedure during the patient's follicular phase reduces the likelihood of concurrent (luteal phase) pregnancy, as does the patient's use of an effective method of contraception before the procedure. Highly sensitive urine pregnancy tests can detect pregnancies as early as 1 week after fertilization.[111]

Postabortion Tubal Surgery

Tubal surgery, either laparoscopically or via mini-laparotomy, following uncomplicated first and second trimester abortions can be provided without added risk over interval procedures.[112]

Options for Approach

Laparoscopy

Laparoscopy is the most common approach to interval tubal surgery and is usually performed as an outpatient procedure (**Figure 8-2**). Laparoscopy provides the opportunity to better visualize the abdominal and pelvic organs, results in small incision

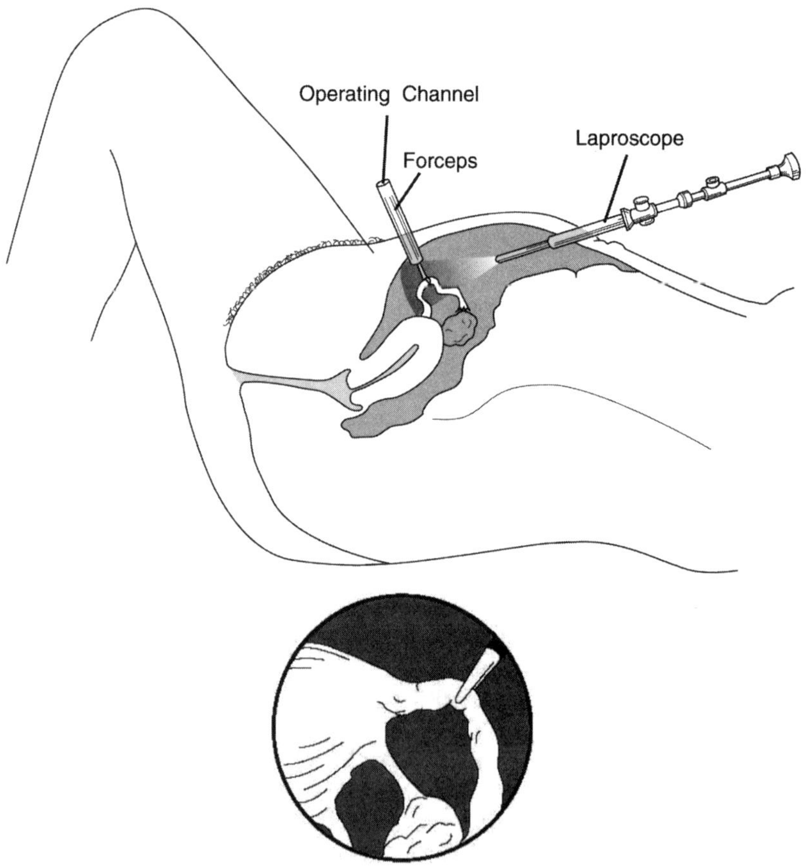

Figure 8-2 Laparoscopic tubal surgery approach.

scars, and allows a rapid return to full activity for the patient (**Figure 8-3**). The disadvantages of laparoscopy include the special training and equipment required.

Choice of Laparoscopic Method. The choice of tubal surgery method depends on the provider's training and experience, the patient's medical history including prior abdominal or uterine surgery, and availability of supplies (**Figure 8-4**).

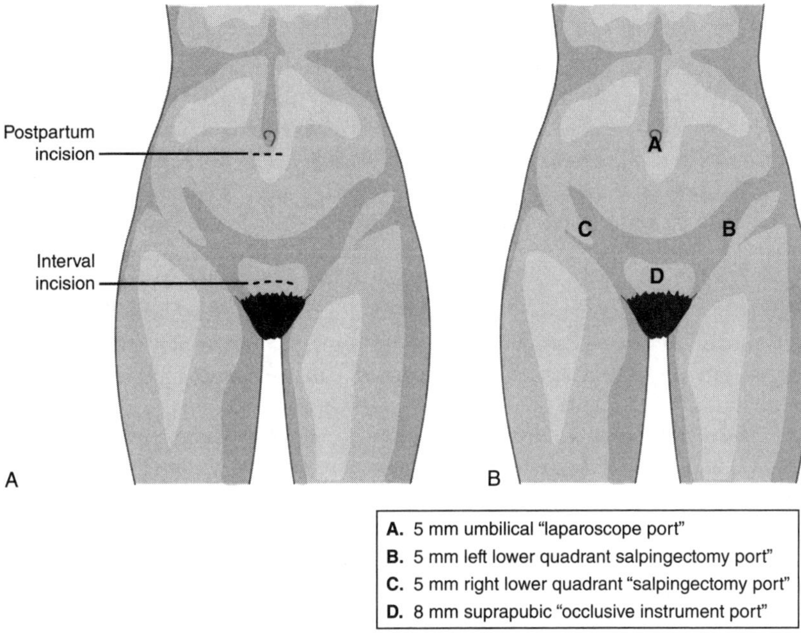

Figure 8-3 Laparoscopic and postpartum and interval mini-laparotomy incision site and size.

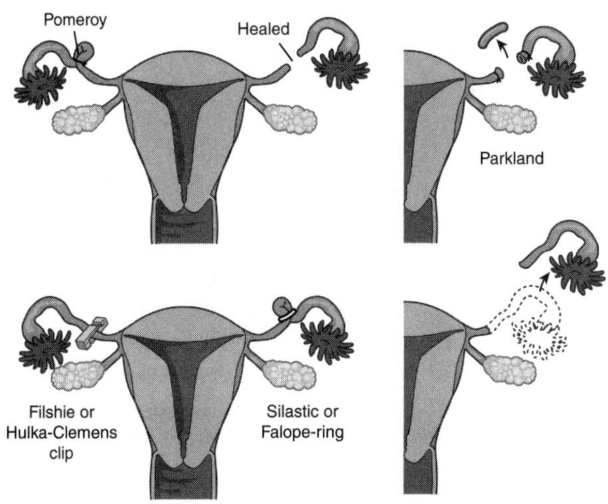

Figure 8-4 Possible tubal surgery techniques.

Electrocoagulation. Electrocoagulation for tubal occlusion is used exclusively with laparoscopic procedures.[113] Unipolar electrocoagulation is not recommended because of the increased risk of thermal bowel injury.[114] At least 3 cm of the isthmic portion of the tube must be coagulated using sufficient energy to achieve maximum efficacy.[115] Use of a resistance meter to measure the decreasing electric current across the desiccating tissue to zero to indicate complete coagulation during bipolar coagulation is more accurate than simple visualization, and is associated with improved effectiveness.[115] Ectopic pregnancy rates are substantially higher with electrocoagulation methods than with other occlusion methods. In the CREST study, the risk of ectopic pregnancy for patients who underwent permanent birth control by bipolar coagulation before the age of 30 years was 27 times higher than for those patients who had a postpartum partial salpingectomy (31.9 vs. 1.2 ectopic pregnancies per 1,000 procedures).[26]

Mechanical devices. Mechanical occlusion devices commonly used with laparoscopic procedures in the United States include the silicone band (Falope Ring), the spring clip (Hulka-Clemens clip), and the titanium clip (Filshie clip). All require special applicators and are most effective when used to occlude normal-appearing tubes. None of these methods involves risk of electrical injury.[116,117] While tubal occlusion by ring or clip should always be considered a permanent method, these devices typically destroy less of the fallopian tube than electrocoagulation methods, making future reversal efforts more likely to succeed.[113]

The silicone band was first developed in the 1970s in pursuit of a safer, nonthermal method. Two centimeters of tube is contained in a constricted loop following application. This method can lacerate the tube or surrounding vessels, and application may be more difficult when tubal abnormalities are present, such as adhesions, edema, or hydrosalpinx. The silicone band is one of the most commonly used tubal occlusion devices worldwide, with a cumulative 10-year failure rate in the CREST study at 33.2 per 1,000 procedures.[26] Postoperative pain was reported twice as often by patients receiving silicone bands than those receiving electrocoagulation.[33]

The spring clip was developed at the same time as the silicone band and was introduced in the United States in 1972. The hinged spring-loaded plastic clip with interlocking teeth is loaded in a special applicator and applied perpendicular to the tube across the isthmus, destroying less than 1 cm of tissue. The cumulative 10-year failure rate in the CREST study for the spring clip was 52.1 per 1,000 procedures.[26]

The titanium clip was approved in 1996. It is a hinged, locking clip made of titanium with a silicone rubber lining, which expands to keep the tube compressed as it flattens. It destroys 5 mm of tube and has a higher efficacy than the spring clip.[116,118] The titanium clip requires a special applicator for interval laparoscopic tubal surgery and for postpartum tubal occlusion.[118,119] The titanium clip has a similar safety and efficacy profile as other occlusion devices; data from the United Kingdom demonstrate a crude failure rate of 2 to 3 in 1,000 patients.[120] Studies do not support routine application of multiple clips per tube.[121,122] If a clip is misfired so that the tube is not occluded, a second one may be placed as close to the first as possible to reduce the risk of hydrosalpinx formation between the two clips.[122]

Although use of loop ligation for laparoscopic tubal occlusion, similar to the Pomeroy technique (see Mini-laparotomy: Ligation, below), has been described as a teaching model for gynecology residents, its effectiveness is not known.[123-126]

Salpingectomy. Although no clinical trials evaluate its effectiveness, laparoscopic salpingectomy is conceptually 100% effective at preventing pregnancy.[127] Salpingectomy gained in popularity because of increasing evidence showing a reduction in ovarian cancer with this approach.[52-54] Limited available evidence suggests that laparoscopic salpingectomy takes approximately 6 minutes longer to complete than mechanical occlusion methods, with no increased risk of immediate or short-term complication rates.[124]

Mini-laparotomy

In the United States, mini-laparotomy is the most common approach for postpartum procedures prior to involution of the uterus. A small 2- to 3-cm incision is made just inferior to the umbilicus, allowing easy access to the fallopian tubes (Figure 8-3). Mini-laparotomy requires only basic surgical instruments and training. In developing countries where laparoscopy is not available, suprapubic mini-laparotomy is frequently used for nonpostpartum tubal surgery.[110]

Choice of Mini-laparotomy Method

Ligation and partial salpingectomy. Tubal surgery at the time of cesarean delivery or postpartum or interval mini-laparotomy is usually performed by ligation and resection of a portion of both fallopian tubes. A variety of partial salpingectomy techniques have been described, including the Pomeroy and Parkland methods (Figure 8-4).[110] The most common method used is a variation of the Pomeroy method using plain catgut, which degrades more rapidly than the original chromic suture type and thus decreases the risk of recanalization (**Figure 8-5**). The Parkland method involves creating a window through the mesosalpinx using electrocautery or scissors. Suture is then placed through the window and tied on either side to ligate a 1- to 2-cm segment of fallopian tube above the mesosalpinx. The segment is then excised using scissors.[110]

Irving and Uchida methods involve ligating and excising a segment of the tube and burying the proximal end either in the myometrium (Irving) or in the mesosalpinx (Uchida). Occasionally the distal end is also buried in the mesosalpinx, although it is more frequently left exposed. The Irving and Uchida methods are seldom used in the United States, although failures with these methods are extremely rare.[110]

Total salpingectomy. Salpingectomy can be safely performed at the time of cesarean delivery or via postpartum or interval mini-laparotomy. Several studies have found that postpartum salpingectomy has a slightly longer operating time than postpartum partial salpingectomy (one study showed an increase of 11 minutes).The studies also demonstrated similar blood loss and short-term complication rates.[34,128-130]

Mechanical devices. Mechanical occlusion with titanium clips or silicon bands is most often performed laparoscopically; however, these devices may be used at the time of cesarean delivery or postpartum interval mini-laparotomy. Some

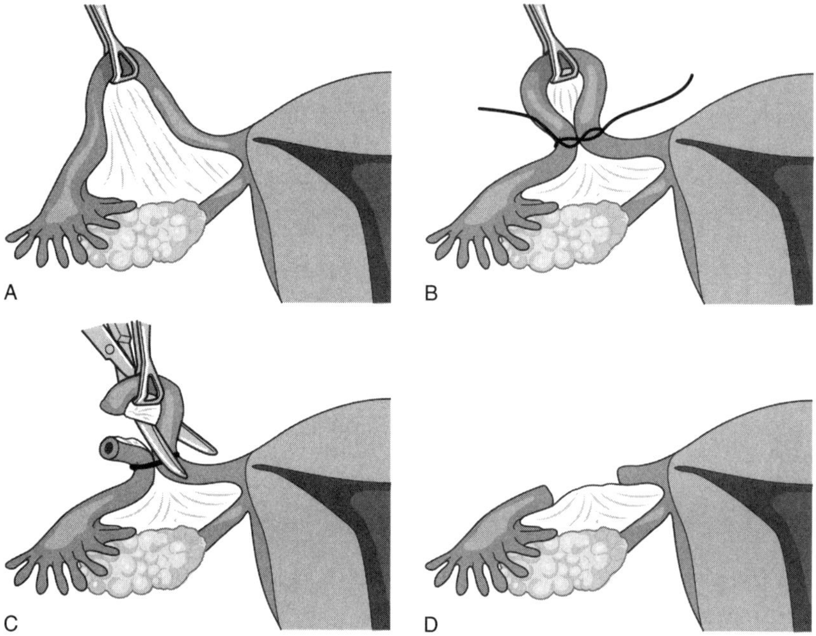

Figure 8-5 Modified Pomeroy technique.

studies have found decreased operative time with titanium clip placement compared to partial salpingectomy, although failure rates may be higher.[9-11] One study that investigated the use of the silicone band compared to the Pomeroy technique at the time of cesarean delivery demonstrated no difference in complications or pregnancy rates between the two methods.[131] Surgeons should be aware that more edematous peripartum fallopian tubes may pose more of a challenge to proper placement of titanium clips or silicone bands.

Hysteroscopy

As previously mentioned, no transcervical method is currently available for use, but some patients still have these devices in place. The transcervical approach to tubal occlusion involved accessing the fallopian tubes via the cervix using a hysteroscope. The Essure device was a flexible device consisting of two concentric metal coils (**Figure 8-6**).[35] The nitinol (nickel-titanium) outer coil, which ends in platinum markers, anchored the device in the tubal lumen; the inner stainless steel coil anchored synthetic polyethylene terephthalate (PET) fibers, which caused a benign inflammatory response. The inflammation stimulated growth of fibrous tissue, which occluded the tubes over the subsequent few weeks. The Adiana procedure applied low radiofrequency energy to the proximal portion of the fallopian tube to create a superficial lesion and placed a small silicone matrix in the damaged area. The resulting fibrotic reaction would occlude the tube by infiltrating the matrix.[132] Clinicians required special training to perform these hysteroscopic procedures, which could only be done as an interval procedure. The procedure could be provided under local anesthesia, with or without sedation, in a properly equipped physician's office.

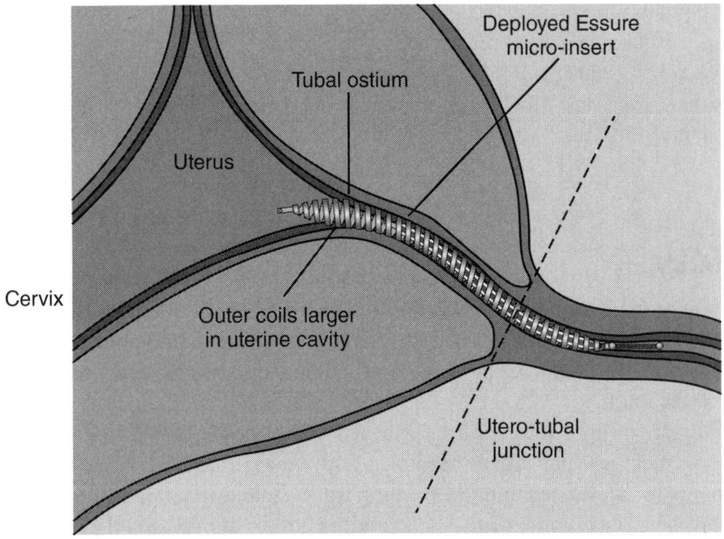

Figure 8-6 Hysteroscopic placement of Essure device within the tubal lumen.

Successful placement was not guaranteed, and the procedure may be abandoned due to abnormal findings at the time of hysteroscopy or from failed attempts to place one or both devices.[35] Patients relied on an alternate method of contraception while tubal ingrowth was occurring until success was confirmed. Procedure success could be confirmed at least 3 months following the transcervical procedure using modified hysterosalpingogram (HSG) to evaluate the lack of free peritoneal dye spillage from the fallopian tubes.[35] Essure success could also be confirmed by transvaginal ultrasound to evaluate device retention and location.[35]

VAS SURGERY

Effectiveness

Permanent contraception, along with intrauterine devices and implants, are in the WHO and CDC's top tier of contraceptive effectiveness. The overall first-year typical use failure rate for permanent contraception is 0.15% for vas surgery and 0.5% for tubal surgery. (See Chapter 5, Effectiveness, Safety, and Comparative Side Effects.)

Vas surgery is not immediately effective. Once the vas is divided, time and ejaculations are needed to clear the sperm from the reproductive tract, and azoospermia or rare nonmotile sperm (RNMS) must be confirmed before vas surgery can be deemed successful.[133-135] Approximately 25% to 50% of pregnancies after vas surgery occur during the period following surgery but before sperm are cleared.[131-133] True vas surgery failure results from errors in surgical technique, such as incorrect identification and division of structures at the time of surgery (such as occluding one vas twice without occluding the other); a rare, unrecognized congenital duplication of the vas; or spontaneous recanalization of the divided vas.

The rate of pregnancy in partners of patients who have documented azoospermia after vas surgery is approximately 1 in 2,000.[128,134,135] The rate of failure to achieve azoospermia or RNMS after vas surgery, which then requires repeat surgery, is less than 1%. The CREST study included 573 patients whose partners underwent vas surgery, and found that the cumulative probability of failure per 1,000 procedures was 7.4 at 1 year after surgery and 11.3 at 2, 3, and 5 years later.[136]

Safety

Vas surgery is a very safe method of contraception. Mortality due to the procedure itself is extremely rare, at 0.5 death per 100,000 patients undergoing the surgery worldwide. No deaths have been reported in the United States using contemporary surgical techniques.[137-140]

The rate of immediate postoperative complications is low. About 1% to 2% of patients experience hematoma formation and wound infection.[141-151] The relationship between surgical technique and complication rate is unclear, but higher-volume surgeons have fewer immediate postoperative complications than other clinicians.[152] Significant morbidity such as Fournier's gangrene is limited to very rare case reports.[153]

Extensive research has identified no significant long-term physical or mental health effects with vas surgery. Studies have consistently shown no adverse effects of vas surgery on cardiovascular disease, stroke, dementia, prostate or testicular cancer, and a variety of other conditions.[153] The American Urological Association states that clinicians do not need to routinely discuss these conditions during presurgical counseling because vas surgery is not a risk factor for these conditions.[140]

Special Issues

Chronic Scrotal Pain

Approximately 1% to 2% of patients undergoing vas surgery will develop severe chronic unilateral or bilateral scrotal pain or discomfort that interferes with quality of life and prompts patients to seek treatment.[154] Also known as postvasectomy pain syndrome, this diagnosis is defined as at least 3 months of chronic, intermittent scrotal pain following vas surgery, in contrast to acute postprocedure pain which typically resolves 2 to 4 weeks postprocedure.[155] Chronic scrotal pain can have a delayed onset of months or years, unrelated to patient demographics or operative techniques.[156,157] Nearly 15% of patients have some scrotal discomfort following vas surgery, but only 1% to 2% report chronic pain causing regret or having a negative impact on their lives.[156,158] The pathophysiology of chronic scrotal pain after vas surgery is poorly understood, but may be related to epididymal or vas congestion, back-pressure–induced epididymal blowout, sperm granuloma formation, or scrotal and spermatic cord nerve injury.[159-161] Conservative therapy such as scrotal support and rest, nonsteroidal anti-inflammatory drugs, tricyclic antidepressants, or gabapentin is sufficient treatment in most cases. If medical treatment fails, clinicians may consider spermatic cord nerve block, excision of site granulomas, epididymectomy or vasovasotomy, micro-denervation of the spermatic cord, or ultimately orchiectomy.[162] Very few men ever require surgical treatment for chronic scrotal pain following their vasectomy. According the American Urological Association (AUA), information about the low risk of severe, chronic scrotal pain is essential in presurgical counseling.[140]

Sexual Function

Many patients are concerned about erectile dysfunction, reduced orgasmic sensation, decreased semen volume, reduced libido, decreased genital sensation, or diminished sexual pleasure following vas surgery. Large numbers of studies consistently show that sexual function remains unaffected by vas surgery, and surgery does not lead to impotence, other sexual difficulties, or reduction in the amount of semen ejaculated. Multiple studies have shown an increase in frequency or improvement in sexual satisfaction in half or more of patients and decrease in frequency of intercourse and sexual habits in only 5% of men.[6,163,164]

Anti-sperm Antibodies

Anti-sperm antibodies appear in 50% to 80% of men following vas surgery, compared to only 8% to 21% of men in the general population.[165,166] Multiple studies have shown no evidence of adverse health consequences, including immunologic diseases, from anti-sperm antibodies.[167-169] The only possible clinical significance of anti-sperm antibodies is that very high levels may impair fertility after vas surgery reversal, which occurs infrequently.[167] The interpretation and clinical relevance of different types of anti-sperm antibody tests are controversial, and the presence of a specific antibody class may have more significance than titer level.[168,169] Presence of serum anti-sperm antibodies should not be considered a contraindication for vasectomy reversal.

Regret

Most patients who have vas surgery do not regret their decision; however, because of relationship changes and other life events, regret is always possible. The 1% to 2% risk of regret among patients after vas surgery is lower than the reported regret among patients after tubal surgery.[169,170] Partners of patients who have had vas surgery may have slightly higher rates of regret at 6% to 8% compared to those patients themselves, but this rate is similar to patients who had tubal surgery.[91,171] Regret following vas surgery is more common among patients who, at the time of the surgery, were younger than 30 years old, were in an unstable marriage, had no or very young children, or made the decision for permanent contraception during a time of financial crisis or for reasons related to a pregnancy.[172,173] The most commonly reported reason for regret was the desire for more children, due to changing their mind, having a new partner, or losing a child.[174-176] Another reason for patient dissatisfaction or regret includes feeling that a problem or complication following vas surgery was caused by the surgery itself. However, 80% to 100% of patients having vas surgery would recommend it to others.[140]

The presence of strong risk factors for regret should not restrict or delay vas surgery but should indicate the need for careful counseling (see Chapter 4, Person-Centered Reproductive Health Conversations and Contraceptive Counseling.) Age and lack of biological children are not contraindications, and patients seeking permanent contraception should not be required to undergo a mental health evaluation due to a clinician's concern for patient regret.

Desire for Pregnancy Following Vas Surgery

Permanent contraception should be considered permanent, but some patients will have a change in personal circumstance and later desire children. Assisted reproductive technologies and microsurgical vas surgery reversal are options for a patient who desires a pregnancy following vas surgery, but success is not guaranteed.[177]

The longer the interval between vas surgery and reversal, the less likely the patient will be fertile after the reversal. Pregnancy rates are less than 50% when reversal is performed more than 10 to 15 years after vas surgery.[176,178,179] Other factors that affect the success of vas surgery reversal include the skill of the surgeon, type of vas surgery originally performed, levels of anti-sperm antibodies, age of the partner, and partial obstruction of the vas after the reversal surgery that prevents movement of sperm through the vas.[180] After microsurgical reversal, the percentage of patients with sperm in the ejaculate is 75% to 100%.[176,181] However, presence of sperm in the ejaculate does not guarantee pregnancy. Reported pregnancy rates following microsurgical reversal range from 38% to 89%.[176,177,179,181] Finally, individuals undergoing vas reversal surgery may need future contraception.

Assisted reproductive technologies are a good option for patients who want children but do not want a vas surgery reversal or who already underwent unsuccessful reversal surgeries. Sperm can be retrieved from the epididymis or the testis and then used for ICSI with IVF. Pregnancy rates per attempt following ICSI with IVF using epididymal or testicular sperm are reported to be 17% to 36%.[182] Data are conflicting on whether longer time elapsed between vas surgery and ICSI reduces the chance of pregnancy.[183-186]

Vas surgery reversal should be the first choice for patients who had vas surgery but now wish to have children, even for patients who have failed a previous reversal attempt.[178,184,187] Vas surgery reversal has the same if not better pregnancy rates and is less costly than ICSI using epididymal sperm.[186,187,190] However, both assisted reproductive technologies and reversal surgery are expensive and are often not covered by health insurance. Factors in deciding whether to have a reversal or ICSI with IVF should not only include cost but also the age and fertility of the partner and the number of children desired.

Vas Surgery: Approaches and Techniques

Options for Approach

The two key steps in vas surgery are to isolate the vas, then occlude the vas. Immediate postoperative complications such as pain, bleeding, and infection are related to the method of isolation, whereas success of vas surgery is related to occlusion method.

Vas Isolation

There are two methods for vas isolation: conventional vasectomy and minimally invasive vasectomy (MIV), which includes no-scalpel vasectomy (NSV). Standard of care is MIV for vas isolation. Conventional vasectomy involves skin incisions 1.5 to 3 cm long that are made with a scalpel and then closed with suture. No special instruments are used to dissect and grasp the vas (**Figure 8-7**). MIV creates skin openings of < 1 cm using special instruments, with minimal dissection around the vas. NSV was the first MIV technique, developed in 1974 in China to make vasectomy a more acceptable method of contraception. In this method, the clinician places a vas ring clamp around the vas, perivasal tissue, and overlying skin before making the skin opening with the vas dissector.[188] The clinician will then use the vas ring clamp and dissector to isolate the vas before elevating, dividing, and occluding the ends of

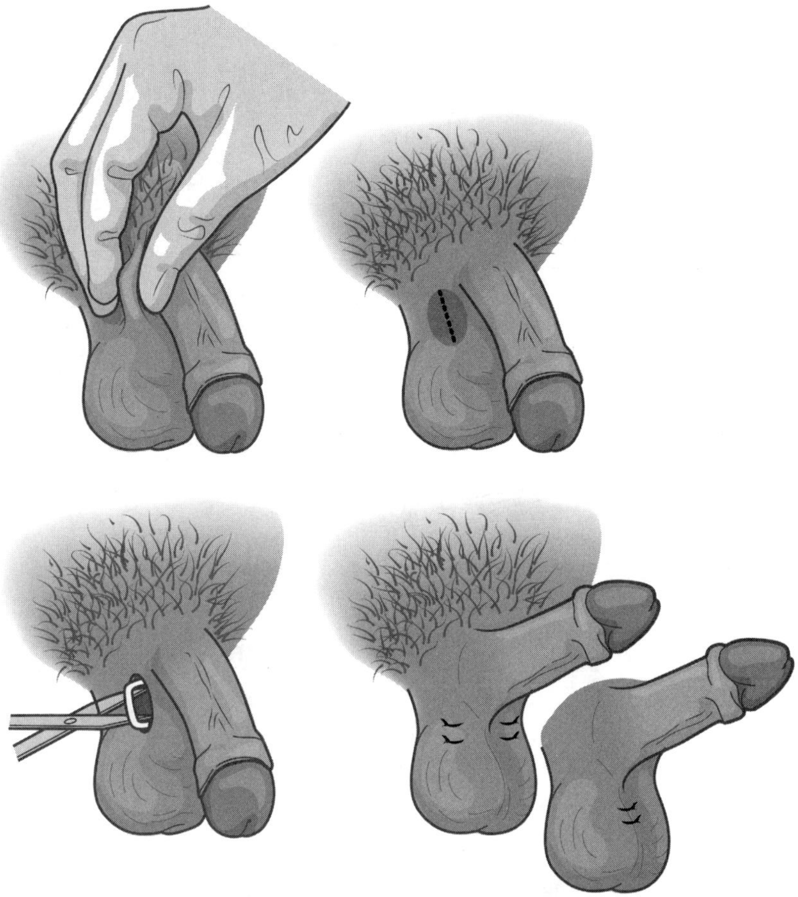

Figure 8-7 Conventional vasectomy.

vas. The skin opening is left to heal by secondary intent unless suturing is necessary (**Figure 8-8**).[188] A detailed description can be found at www.engenderhealth.org (*No-Scalpel Vasectomy: An Illustrated Guide For Surgeons*).[189]

NSV has less bleeding, hematoma formation, infection, postoperative pain, and a shorter operation time compared to conventional vasectomy. If a single midline opening is used, the clinician must insure that both vas are occluded, rather than one vas occluded twice.[190] Several modifications to the NSV approach regarding finger placement, timing and placement of skin openings, and instrument design are published in the literature, although these variants should be referred to as MIV methods.[191-194]

Vas Occlusion

Once the vas is isolated, it is completely divided in nearly all occlusion techniques, with or without excision of a vas segment (division/excision) and with or without blockage of at least one end of the divided vas. Methods of blockage include ligation, application of clips, chemical occlusion, thermal or electrocautery, fascial interposition, or a combination of these.

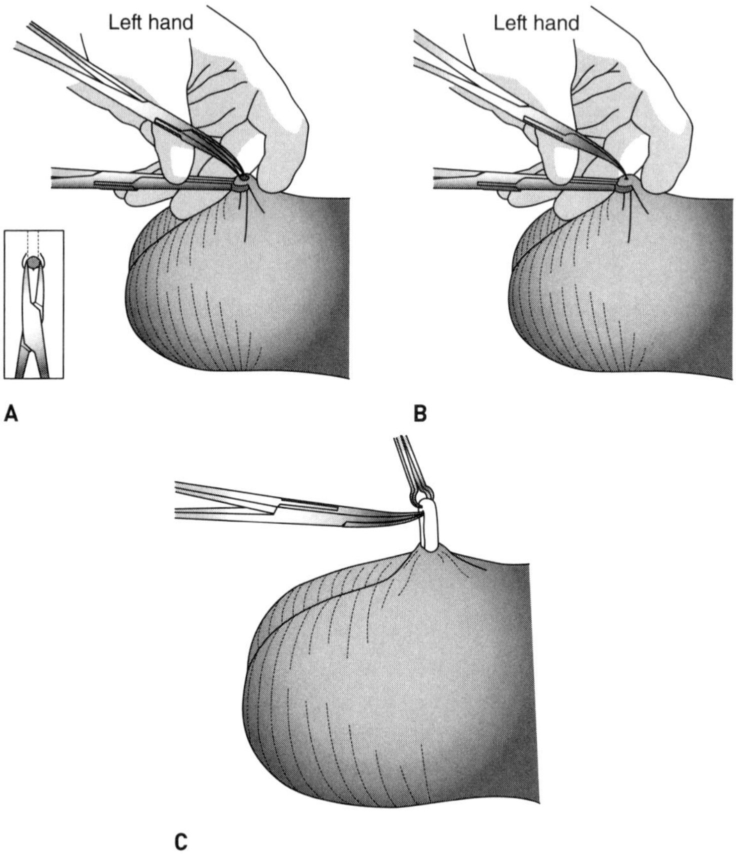

Figure 8-8 No-scalpel vasectomy. **A.** Inserting both tips of the vas dissector into the puncture site. **B.** Spreading the tissues to make a skin opening twice the diameter of the vas. **C.** Grasping a partial thickness of the elevated vas.

Reproduced from EngenderHealth. No-scalpel vasectomy: an illustrated guide for surgeons. 3rd ed. New York: EngenderHealth; 2003.

Ligation occludes the vas with ligatures or clips placed 1 cm apart, with division/excision of the vas length between.[2] Mucosal cautery involves electrocautery to the mucosa of the cut ends of the vas to destroy the luminal mucosa with minimal damage to the muscle layers. Cautery induces fibrosis to occlude the lumen; sparing the muscular layer decreases the risk of the cauterized portion sloughing off and the vas recanalizing.[141,195,196] Fascial interposition places a layer of internal spermatic fascia between the two divided ends, over the testicular or the abdominal end, and usually used with other techniques such as ligation and division/excision or mucosal cautery.[196,197] Folding and suturing each divided vas end on itself to prevent the cut ends from facing each other is not recommended.

Open-ended vasectomy involves division/excision followed by fascial interposition to cover the abdominal end of the divided vas. Theoretically, the open ends may minimize pressure and damage to the epididymis and increase success rates for vas surgery reversal.[198] Fascial interposition is necessary with this technique to prevent recanalization.

There are no well-designed randomized trials comparing these practices, except for one trial showing that simple ligation and division of the vas is more likely to fail compared to using fascial interposition.[2,197] One study investigating an intra-vas device of urethane filled with nylon thread showed lower success compared with no-scalpel vasectomy.[199]

The AUA identified the following three division methods having data demonstrating excellent contraceptive and occlusive effectiveness, with failure rates consistently $\leq 1\%$ in large numbers across different studies (**Figure 8-9**):[140]

1. Mucosal cautery with fascial interposition, without ligatures or clips
2. Mucosal cautery without fascial interposition and without ligatures or clips
3. Open-ended vasectomy, using mucosal cautery and fascial interposition on the abdominal end of the vas

Only one method, the Marie Stopes International technique, does not divide the vas but instead occludes it by using extended monopolar electrocautery to destroy 2.5 to 3 cm of the vas.[200] This method is not used in the United States but is considered a reasonable vas surgery technique by AUA.[140]

Data show no benefit of excising a short vas segment over no excision. If excision is performed, routine histological examination of the excised vas segments is not required, since a postvasectomy semen analysis (PVSA) will confirm success.[140] However, if the surgeon suspects that the excised structure is not a section of vas, histology may be helpful for identification.

Providing Permanent Contraception

Counseling

A significant consideration for counseling a patient on permanent contraception is the permanence of the procedure. Respect for a patient's autonomy, including a dialogue about the patient's reproductive desires and wishes, should be the primary concern during this discussion.[201]

The factors contributing to an individual's decision about permanent contraception vary. Each patient needs to weigh the risks, benefits, effectiveness, and side effects of the various contraceptive options available to them. (See Chapter 4, Person-Centered Reproductive Health Conversations and Contraceptive Counseling and Chapter 5, Effectiveness, Safety, and Comparative Side Effects.) Racial disparities have been identified in tubal surgery rates, which is mediated through an association with unintended pregnancy history (see Chapter 1, Reproductive Justice within Reproductive Health Care).[202]

Counseling should address the following:

1. **Provide choices.** Present alternative options of highly effective contraception available such as long-acting, reversible methods such as the contraceptive implant or IUDs.
2. **Assess the patient's understanding of the procedure, including risk of failure.** Although awareness of permanent contraception is widespread in the United States, review the procedures, their effectiveness, and their risks with your patients to minimize misconceptions. Inform patients that permanent contraception is not 100% successful and that failure can occur, even years after the procedure was performed. Inform patients that if pregnancy does occur after tubal surgery, there is a significant risk of ectopic pregnancy. Discuss the need for postprocedural contraception following transcervical tubal surgery or

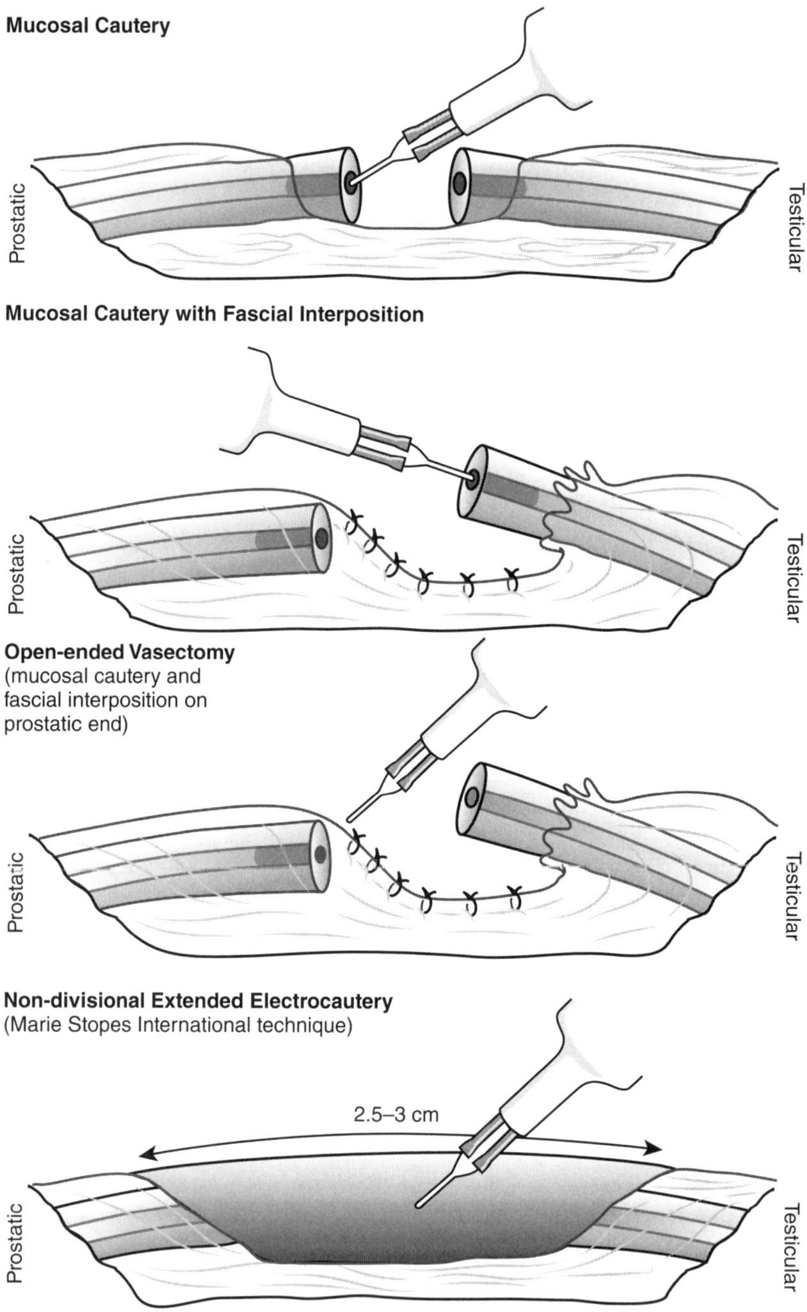

Figure 8-9 Recommended vas occlusion techniques.

Modified from Sharlip ID, Belker AM, Honig S, et al. Vasectomy: AUA guideline. J Urol 2012;188(6):2482–91. DOI:10.1016/j.juro.2012.09.080. https://www.auajournals.org/doi/10.1016/j.juro.2012.09.080

vas surgery until occlusion is confirmed (see Affirm/Share/Ask [ASA] Cycle in Chapter 4 to optimize patient education).

3. **Facilitate the decision-making process.** Give the patient sufficient time to make a thoughtful, informed decision about a permanent method of contraception, especially patients having immediate postpartum or postabortion (spontaneous or induced) procedures or when there are financial, marital, or sexual problems. Address risk factors for regret with both the patient and partner if appropriate. The patient should decide they want a permanent method well before delivery or a pregnancy-related event or procedure.
4. **Discuss STI prevention.** Permanent contraception will not provide protection against STIs, including HIV. Condom use will be necessary if the patient is at risk of such infections. (See Chapter 23, Reproductive Tract Infections, Including HIV and Other Sexually Transmitted Infections.)

Informed Consent and Policy/Legal Issues

Informed consent is a process to ensure that a person can give consent, is fully informed about a surgical procedure and its consequences, and can make a voluntary decision. Provide information on permanent contraception in a language that the patient can easily understand. Patients must always sign or mark an informed consent form indicating that they understand the type of operation and intended permanence, possibility of failure, and risks and benefits, including the option to decline permanent contraception without loss of medical or financial benefits. The surgeon or authorized representative must also sign the form. Written informed consent should document, but not substitute for, the provider's active involvement in the patient's informed decision to proceed with permanent contraception. Ensure that the patient has knowingly and freely requested the procedure. Understand that the federally mandated consent for permanent birth control does not replace surgical consent.

Knowledge of federal, state, and local, or institutional guidelines is important in the counseling and consent process. Some states have requirements about the consent process and its documentation, even if private funding is used.

- Strict adherence to informed consent procedures is mandatory prior to permanent contraception.[203]
- Partner or spousal consent is not legally required in the United States.[204]
- Patients using Medicaid funds for permanent birth control must be age 21 or older and mentally competent; they must wait 30 days after signing a valid consent document before receiving a permanent contraception procedure. In cases of premature delivery, patients must have signed their consent document (https://opa.hhs.gov/sites/default/files/2020-07/consent-for-sterilization-english-updated-large.pdf) 72 hours prior to delivery. Consent cannot be given when a patient is seeking or obtaining an abortion; is in active labor or childbirth; under the influence of alcohol or other drugs; or is institutionalized in a correctional facility, mental hospital, or other rehabilitative facility. Consent documents are invalid 180 days after signing.[204]
- Patients whose procedures are funded by private insurance may not have the same restrictions as those using Medicaid funds, including age restrictions and waiting periods.

Federal guidelines that impose a waiting period for patients using Medicaid funds for permanent birth control, while initially developed to protect patients of vulnerable populations from involuntary procedures, have been called into question because they often unfairly restrict access for the very populations that they intend to protect. Particularly in the immediate postpartum period, timing of informed consent and availability of signed forms at the time of desired permanent tubal surgery can be a barrier to care. Approximately 24% to 44% of postpartum tubal surgery requests are not fulfilled because of Medicaid policy barriers.[205,206] Patients using private insurance do not face the same logistical hurdles to obtaining a permanent procedure.

Health care providers, policy makers, and the public should be aware of the ethical and legal issues involved in providing voluntary permanent contraception to those who may not be able to give informed consent.[207] When patients have limited mental capacity, the provider should consult with the patient's family, caregivers, and often institutional ethics committees to balance patient autonomy with what is understood to be in the best interests of the patient.[201] If an individual clinician or institution will not provide permanent contraception due to personal beliefs or institutional policy, the patient should be informed and referred elsewhere for care in a timely manner.[201]

Preoperative Screening

Take a preoperative history and perform a physical exam with attention to potential issues that may complicate surgery. Patients undergoing tubal surgery may have anesthetic or surgical issues, such as severe respiratory disease or a complicated history of abdominal surgeries. Since vas surgery is a nonabdominal surgery performed under local anesthesia, absolute surgical contraindications are rare. However, localized problems may make vas surgery more difficult to perform, such as inguinal hernia, large hydrocele or varicocele, and cryptorchidism.[141] Order any standard preoperative laboratory tests per the surgeon's practice or institution's policies or pertinent to the patient's medical condition relevant to surgery, such as a blood type, complete blood count, pregnancy test, or serum glucose level.

Anesthesia, Pain Management, and Antibiotics

The most frequently used anesthesia approaches for tubal surgery in the United States are short-acting general anesthesia for interval tubal procedures and regional anesthesia for postpartum procedures.[208] Tubal surgery can also be performed safely under local anesthesia.[110]

For patients undergoing transabdominal procedures under local anesthesia, application of lidocaine 1% solution to the tubal surface may provide additional pain control.[119] If postabortion tubal surgery is planned, use a single-anesthetic approach to minimize additional risk.

Vas surgery is performed under local anesthesia alone in nearly all patients seeking vas surgery. Some patients whose anatomy may lead to a particularly difficult surgery or who are unable to tolerate the procedure under local anesthesia may benefit from oral or intravenous sedation or general anesthesia, although risks of anesthesia increase with deeper sedation. Topical anesthesia applied by the clinician to the surgical site is optional, but infiltration of local anesthesia into the skin and perivasal tissue should always be used.[140] Clinicians should administer local anesthetic using their smallest available needle, between 24- and 32-gauge, to minimize pain from the spermatic cord block.

All anesthetic methods need the attention of a trained professional who carefully monitors the patient and the drugs used. For more complete information on anesthetic techniques and regimens, visit www.engenderhealth.org.[209]

Routine prophylactic antibiotics are not indicated for vas surgery or laparoscopic tubal surgery.[140,210] Tubal surgery at time of cesarean delivery does not require any additional prophylactic antibiotic coverage beyond the recommended antibiotic regiment for cesarean deliveries. Providers may consider use of cefazolin for laparotomy procedures that do not involve entry into bowel or vagina.[210]

Managing Problems and Follow-Up

Major complications from permanent contraception are uncommon. Fewer than 3% of vas surgery cases require medical attention,[2] and the risk of 1% to 3.5% of tubal surgery complications vary by type of procedure and anesthesia used.[32,116,117]

Tubal surgery risks include general surgical risks, such as hemorrhage, infection, and the risk of death from anesthesia. These risks can be reduced by careful screening, use of local anesthesia or light sedation, close monitoring of vital signs, careful aseptic surgical technique, and early recognition with aggressive management. Vas surgery risks such as vasovagal reaction, lidocaine toxicity, and excessive bleeding are unusual and can generally be prevented if appropriate guidelines and procedures are followed. Most postoperative complications, including swelling of the scrotum, bruising, pain, and minor bleeding under the skin, are minor and subside within 1 or 2 weeks. Scrotal support, mild pain medication, and local application of cold therapy are usually sufficient for treatment. More significant complications such as heavy bleeding, hematoma, or infection are quite rare, and a routine postoperative visit specifically to examine the scrotum is not necessary. No patient should leave the recovery room after a permanent contraception procedure without both verbal and clear written instructions for follow-up, including 24-hour contact information for concerns or emergencies, immediate self-care, and a follow-up visit to confirm success if applicable.

Successful vas surgery must be confirmed with a PVSA that shows azoospermia or RNMS (≤ 100,000 nonmotile sperm/mL).[205] All patients have motile and functional sperm in the ejaculate after surgery for some period of time, which can range from weeks to months based on factors such as frequency of ejaculation, patient age and anatomy, and surgical technique.[140,211-213] Timing of the PVSA may be based on postoperative time or number of postsurgery ejaculations. The optimal time will minimize the number of PVSAs needed to establish success but still allow a patient to stop using other forms of contraception as soon as possible after surgery, which ranges from 1 week to 3 months. If motile sperm are still seen on PVSA at 6 months after vas surgery, the vas surgery should be considered a failure and repeat surgery considered.[140] In resource-poor settings, where semen analysis may not be available or practical to confirm success, patients should be advised to use another form of contraception for at least 12 weeks after surgery to minimize the chance of pregnancy.[197,214,215]

USER INSTRUCTIONS

Preoperative Instructions for Surgery

1. Be completely sure of your decision for permanent contraception. Know what it means to you and your family that this is a permanent procedure. You can change your mind at any time before the operation.

2. Before surgery while you are home, clip (not shave) all the hair from around the planned surgical area. Wash the area thoroughly to remove all loose hairs.
3. If you intend on having sedation or general anesthesia, do not eat or drink anything as instructed prior to your procedure.
4. If you intend on having sedation or general anesthesia, bring someone who can accompany you home after the procedure.
5. For vas surgery, bring a pair of tight-fitting underwear or an athletic supporter to support the scrotum and minimize swelling.

Postoperative Instructions

1. Avoid strenuous physical exercise for 1 week. Strenuous exercise means physical exertion such as lifting or straining that could bring pressure to the pelvis. When you resume strenuous activity, stop if it is uncomfortable.
2. If you have vas surgery, use scrotal support for at least 2 days (e.g., wearing brief-style underwear) to reduce pain. If possible, keep a cold pack on the scrotum for at least 4 hours to reduce the chances of swelling, bleeding, and discomfort. You may discontinue the scrotal support once you're comfortable without it.
3. If you have vas surgery, avoid ejaculation and activities that may rub or put pressure on the scrotum (such as bicycle riding) for 1 week after vas surgery to allow the surgical sites to heal and to allow occlusion for methods that occlude the vas using mucosal cautery.[140]
4. Take one or two analgesic tablets at 4- to 6-hour intervals if you need them for pain. (Note to provider: name and dose should be specified.) Do not use aspirin, since it may promote bleeding. If you have vas surgery, you will probably have some mild pain and swelling in the scrotal region, the scrotum may be somewhat discolored, and you may notice blood in your ejaculate during the first month or two after surgery. These conditions will resolve on their own and do not mean anything is wrong.
5. You may bathe 24 hours after surgery but avoid putting tension on the incision and do not rub or irritate the incision for 1 week. Pat dry the incision site after bathing.
6. Stitches will dissolve and do not require removal. (Note to provider: this instruction must be modified if nonabsorbable sutures are used.)
7. If you don't have any bothersome discomfort, you may return to nonphysical work. You may return to more strenuous activities after 1 week.
8. Watch for the symptoms listed in **Table 8-2**.
9. If you are scheduled for a postoperative visit, please attend the visit.
10. If you have vas surgery, please return to your clinician for the confirmatory test in 3 months so the success of the procedure can be assessed. Use condoms or other contraceptive method until you know that you are not releasing sperm in your ejaculate.
11. If you have tubal surgery and think you are pregnant at any time in the future, return to the clinic immediately. Although pregnancy after tubal surgery is rare, chances are increased that it will be an ectopic pregnancy (outside the uterus) if it does occur. This can be a dangerous life-threatening condition and must be treated immediately.

Table 8-2 Symptoms to Watch For After Vas Surgery

Condition	Action
Temperature: > 100.4 degrees Fahrenheit	Contact your provider immediately
Fainting: Fainting spells	Contact your provider immediately
Pain: Pain that is persistent, severe, and/or increasing after 12 hours	If unrelieved by analgesic, contact your provider immediately
Incision site issues	
Bleeding or spotting from incision sites	Put pressure on the area for 10 minutes If condition continues or worsens, contact provider
Pus or discharge from incision sites	Contact your provider immediately
Stitch in wound	Contact your provider—most stitches will dissolve or fall out, but any permanent suture must be removed by your provider
Vas surgery: Scrotal swelling greater than twice normal size	Contact your provider
Vas surgery: Groin nodules larger than a nickel, painful and tender	Contact your provider

Methods in Development

Although tubal surgery via traditional culdoscopy is no longer recommended due to higher complications rates compared to laparoscopic methods,[3] investigators are adapting a new technique called transvaginal natural orifice transluminal endoscopic surgery (V-NOTES) for tubal surgery. In V-NOTES, entry into the peritoneal cavity is achieved with a colpotomy followed by placement of a retractor bag and a specialized platform to allow for insufflation. Specialized trocars are placed onto the platform, through which a camera and instruments can complete the planned procedure. This device and technique have been used for salpingectomy and salpingo-oophorectomy at time of vaginal hysterectomy[216] and surgical management of ectopic pregnancy.[217,218] A current clinical trial is comparing V-NOTES with traditional laparoscopy for elective bilateral salpingectomy.[219]

Currently no transcervical permanent contraception options are commercially available, but a new transcervical permanent contraceptive system called FemBloc® is in development.[220,221] Similar to previous transcervical procedures, FemBloc® induces scarring and occlusion of the fallopian tubes by delivering a small volume of a liquid biopolymer (polyglycolic acid, which is used in absorbable sutures) to the proximal portions of the fallopian tubes. Successful occlusion of the fallopian tubes must be confirmed at least 3 months following the procedure.[221] Another transcervical method under early investigation is intrauterine 5% polidocanol foam (PF), which had 100% fallopian tube occlusion in baboon studies.[222]

Developments in vasectomy have focused on easier reversibility. Vasalgel™ is a nonhormonal male contraceptive comprised mainly of styrene-alt-maleic acid (SMA acid), which is injected into the vas deferens to fill the lumen as a hydrogel polymer, preventing sperm passage. If reversibility is desired, sodium bicarbonate can be injected in the vas deferens to dissolve the hydrogel. Animal studies have shown efficacy in vas deferens occlusion and reversibility, with sperm concentrations and mobility returning to baseline at a 6-month follow-up.[223,224]

Disclosures—Brown: none; Hou: none

Acknowledgements—The authors would like to thank Drs. Danielli Roncari, Amy E. Pollock, and several other colleagues for their contributions to prior versions of this chapter over the many editions.

References

1. Daniels K, Abma JC. Current contraceptive status among women aged 15–49: United States, 2017–2019. NCHS Data Brief. 2020;(388):1-8.
2. Cook LA, Van Vliet HA, Lopez LM, Pun A, Gallo MF. Vasectomy occlusion techniques for male sterilization. Cochrane Database Syst Rev. 2014;(3):CD003991.
3. Trussell J, Lalla AM, Doan QV, Reyes E, Pinto L, Gricar J. Cost effectiveness of contraceptives in the United States. Contraception. 2009;79(1):5-14.
4. Daniels K, Daugherty J, Jones J, Mosher W. Current contraceptive use and variation by selected characteristics among women aged 15-44: United States, 2011-2013. Natl Health Stat Rep. 2015;(86):1-14.
5. Thompson B, MacGillivray I, Fraser C. Some factors in the choice of male or female sterilisation in Aberdeen. J Biosoc Sci. 1991;23(3):359-63.
6. Sandlow JI, Westefeld JS, Maples MR, Scheel KR. Psychological correlates of vasectomy. Fertil Steril. 2001;75(3):544-8.
7. Peterson HB, Xia Z, Hughes JM, Wilcox LS, Tylor LR, Trussell J. The risk of pregnancy after tubal sterilization: findings from the U.S. Collaborative Review of Sterilization. Am J Obstet Gynecol. 1996;174(4):1161-8; discussion 1168-70.
8. Shaw R, Russell I, Settatree R, Templeton A, Filschie GM, Argent VP. Male and female sterilization: evidence based guidelines No. 4. London: Royal College of Obstetricians and Gynaecologists; 1999.
9. Kohaut BA, Musselman BL, Sanchez-Ramos L, Kaunitz AM. Randomized trial to compare perioperative outcomes of Filshie clip vs. Pomeroy technique for postpartum and intraoperative cesarean tubal sterilization: a pilot study. Contraception. 2004;69(4):267-70.
10. Madari S, Varma R, Gupta J. A comparison of the modified Pomeroy tubal ligation and Filshie clips for immediate postpartum sterilisation: A systematic review. Eur J Contracept Reprod Health Care. 2011;16(5):341-9.
11. Rodriguez MI, Edelman AB, Kapp N. Postpartum sterilization with the titanium clip: a systematic review. Obstet Gynecol. 2011;118(1):143-7.
12. Baltus T, Brown J, Molakatalla S, Kapurubandara S. Spontaneous pregnancy after totalling bilateral salpingectomy: A systematic review of literature. J Minim Invasive Gynecol. 2021;S1553-4650(21)01177-8.
13. Gariepy AM, Creinin MD, Schwarz EB, Smith KJ. Reliability of laparoscopic compared with hysteroscopic sterilization at 1 year: a decision analysis. Obstet Gynecol. 2011;118(2 Pt 1):273-9.
14. Gariepy AM, Creinin MD, Smith KJ, Xu X. Probability of pregnancy after sterilization: a comparison of hysteroscopic versus laparoscopic sterilization. Contraception. 2014;90(2):174-81.
15. la Chapelle CF, Veersema S, Brolmann HA, Jansen FW. Effectiveness and feasibility of hysteroscopic sterilization techniques: a systematic review and meta-analysis. Fertil Steril. 2015;103(6):1516-25 e1-3.

16. Hurskainen R, Hovi SL, Gissler M, et al. Hysteroscopic tubal sterilization: a systematic review of the Essure system. Fertil Steril. 2010;94(1):16-9.
17. Smith RD. Contemporary hysteroscopic methods for female sterilization. Int J Gynaecol Obstet. 2010;108(1):79-84.
18. Dhruva SS, Ross JS, Gariepy AM. Revisiting Essure: toward safe and effective sterilization. N Engl J Med. 2015;373(15):e17.
19. Walter JR, Ghobadi CW, Hayman E, Xu S. Hysteroscopic sterilization with Essure: summary of the U.S. Food and Drug Administration actions and policy implications for postmarketing surveillance. Obstet Gynecol. 2017;129(1):10-9.
20. Kerin JF, Munday D, Ritossa M, Rosen D. Tissue encapsulation of the proximal Essure micro-insert from the uterine cavity following hysteroscopic sterilization. J Minim Invasive Gynecol. 2007;14(2):202-4.
21. Dreyer K, Lier MC, Emanuel MH, et al. Hysteroscopic proximal tubal occlusion versus laparoscopic salpingectomy as a treatment for hydrosalpinges prior to IVF or ICSI: an RCT. Hum Reprod. 2016;31(9):2005-16.
22. Barbosa MW, Sotiriadis A, Papatheodorou SI, Mijatovic V, Nastri CO, Martins WP. High miscarriage rate in women treated with Essure(R) for hydrosalpinx before embryo transfer: a systematic review and meta-analysis. Ultrasound Obstet Gynecol. 2016;48(5):556-65.
23. Munro MG, Nichols JE, Levy B, Vleugels MP, Veersema S. Hysteroscopic sterilization: 10-year retrospective analysis of worldwide pregnancy reports. J Minim Invasive Gynecol. 2014;21(2):245-51.
24. Hitzerd E, Schreuder HW, Vleugels MP, Veersema S. Twelve-year retrospective review of unintended pregnancies after Essure sterilization in the Netherlands. Fertil Steril. 2016;105(4):932-7.
25. Chudnoff SG, Nichols JE, Levie M. Hysteroscopic Essure inserts for permanent contraception: extended follow-up results of a phase III multicenter international study. J Minim Invasive Gynecol. 2015;22(6):951-60.
26. Peterson HB, Xia Z, Hughes JM, Wilcox LS, Tylor LR, Trussell J. The risk of ectopic pregnancy after tubal sterilization. U.S. Collaborative Review of Sterilization Working Group. N Engl J Med. 1997;336(11):762-7.
27. FDA approves new female sterlization device. FDA Talk Pap. 2002;T02-41:1-2.
28. Escobedo LG, Peterson HB, Grubb GS, Franks AL. Case-fatality rates for tubal sterilization in U.S. hospitals, 1979 to 1980. Am J Obstet Gynecol. 1989;160(1):147-50.
29. Peterson HB, DeStefano F, Rubin GL, Greenspan JR, Lee NC, Ory HW. Deaths attributable to tubal sterilization in the United States, 1977 to 1981. Am J Obstet Gynecol. 1983;146(2):131-6.
30. Hulka JF, Phillips JM, Peterson HB, Surrey MW. Laparoscopic sterilization: American Association of Gynecologic Laparoscopists' 1993 membership survey. J Am Assoc Gynecol Laparosc. 1995;2(2):137-8.
31. Peterson HB, Hulka JF, Phillips JM, Surrey MW. Laparoscopic sterilization. American Association of Gynecologic Laparoscopists 1991 membership survey. J Reprod Med. 1993;38(8):574-6.
32. Jamieson DJ, Hillis SD, Duerr A, Marchbanks PA, Costello C, Peterson HB. Complications of interval laparoscopic tubal sterilization: findings from the United States Collaborative Review of Sterilization. Obstet Gynecol. 2000;96(6):997-1002.
33. Lawrie TA, Kulier R, Nardin JM. Techniques for the interruption of tubal patency for female sterilisation. Cochrane Database Syst Rev. 2016;(8):CD003034.
34. Yang M, Du Y, Hu Y. Complete salpingectomy versus tubal ligation during cesarean section: a systematic review and meta-analysis. J Matern Fetal Neonatal Med. 2021;34(22):3794-802.
35. Bayer HealthCare Pharmaceuticals I. Essure permanent birth control: instructions for use. 2002;
36. Hologic. Adiana permanent contraception: instructions for use. 2009.
37. Gariepy AM, Lewis C, Zuckerman D, et al. Patient-Centered Safety Outcomes After Hysteroscopic Compared With Laparoscopic Sterilization. Obstet Gynecol. 2022;139(3):423-32.
38. Albright CM, Frishman GN, Bhagavath B. Surgical aspects of removal of Essure microinsert. Contraception. 2013;88(3):334-6.
39. Carmona F, Cristobal P, Casamitjana R, Balasch J. Effect of tubal sterilization on ovarian follicular reserve and function. Am J Obstet Gynecol. 2003;189(2):447-52.
40. Cevrioglu AS, Degirmenci B, Acar M, et al. Examination of changes caused by tubal sterilization in ovarian hormone secretion and uterine and ovarian artery blood flow rates. Contraception. 2004;70(6):467-73.

41. Ganer Herman H, Gluck O, Keidar R, et al. Ovarian reserve following cesarean-delivery with salpingectomy versus tubal ligation - a randomized trial. Am J Obstet Gynecol. 2017;
42. Whiteman MK, Miller KP, Tomic D, Langenberg P, Flaws JA. Tubal sterilization and hot flashes. Fertil Steril. 2004;82(2):502-4.
43. Wyshak G. Menopausal symptoms and psychological distress in women with and without tubal sterilization. Psychosomatics. 2004;45(5):403-13.
44. Ozkaya E, Gokmen O, Tosun A, et al. Unfavorable lipid profile and higher frequency of hot flashes during perimenopausal years after fallopian tube ligation. Gynecol Endocrinol. 2013;29(6):559-62.
45. Nichols HB, Baird DD, DeRoo LA, Kissling GE, Sandler DP. Tubal ligation in relation to menopausal symptoms and breast cancer risk. Br J Cancer. 2013;109(5):1291-5.
46. Green A, Purdie D, Bain C, et al. Tubal sterilisation, hysterectomy and decreased risk of ovarian cancer. Survey of Women's Health Study Group. Int J Cancer. 1997;71(6):948-51.
47. Kjaer SK, Mellemkjaer L, Brinton LA, Johansen C, Gridley G, Olsen JH. Tubal sterilization and risk of ovarian, endometrial and cervical cancer. A Danish population-based follow-up study of more than 65 000 sterilized women. Int J Epidemiol. 2004;33(3):596-602.
48. Irwin KL, Weiss NS, Lee NC, Peterson HB. Tubal sterilization, hysterectomy, and the subsequent occurrence of epithelial ovarian cancer. Am J Epidemiol. 1991;134(4):362-9.
49. McGuire V, Felberg A, Mills M, et al. Relation of contraceptive and reproductive history to ovarian cancer risk in carriers and noncarriers of BRCA1 gene mutations. Am J Epidemiol. 2004;160(7):613-8.
50. Narod SA, Sun P, Ghadirian P, et al. Tubal ligation and risk of ovarian cancer in carriers of BRCA1 or BRCA2 mutations: a case-control study. Lancet. 2001;357(9267):1467-70.
51. George SH, Garcia R, Slomovitz BM. Ovarian cancer: the fallopian tube as the site of origin and opportunities for prevention. Front Oncol. 2016;6:108.
52. Cibula D, Widschwendter M, Zikan M, Dusek L. Underlying mechanisms of ovarian cancer risk reduction after tubal ligation. Acta Obstet Gynecol Scand. 2011;90(6):559-63.
53. Yoon SH, Kim SN, Shim SH, Kang SB, Lee SJ. Bilateral salpingectomy can reduce the risk of ovarian cancer in the general population: a meta-analysis. Eur J Cancer. 2016;55:38-46.
54. Castellano T, Zerden M, Marsh L, Boggess K. Risks and benefits of salpingectomy at the time of sterilization. Obstet Gynecol Surv. 2017;72(11):663-8.
55. American College of Obstetricians and Gynecologists. Committee Opinion No. 620: Salpingectomy for ovarian cancer prevention. Obstet Gynecol. 2015;125(1):279-81.
56. McAlpine JN, Hanley GE, Woo MM, et al. Opportunistic salpingectomy: uptake, risks, and complications of a regional initiative for ovarian cancer prevention. Am J Obstet Gynecol. 2014;210(5):471 e1-11.
57. Jones NL, Schulkin J, Urban RR, et al. Physicians' perspectives and practice patterns toward opportunistic salpingectomy in high- and low-risk women. Cancer Invest. 2017;35(1):51-61.
58. Calle EE, Rodriguez C, Walker KA, Wingo PA, Petrelli JM, Thun MJ. Tubal sterilization and risk of breast cancer mortality in US women. Cancer Causes Control. 2001;12(2):127-35.
59. Eliassen AH, Colditz GA, Rosner B, Hankinson SE. Tubal sterilization in relation to breast cancer risk. Int J Cancer. 2006;118(8):2026-30.
60. Gaudet MM, Patel AV, Sun J, Teras LR, Gapstur SM. Tubal sterilization and breast cancer incidence: results from the cancer prevention study II nutrition cohort and meta-analysis. Am J Epidemiol. 2013;177(6):492-9.
61. Gentile GP, Kaufman SC, Helbig DW. Is there any evidence for a post-tubal sterilization syndrome? Fertil Steril. 1998;69(2):179-86.
62. Bhiwandiwala PP, Mumford SD, Feldblum PJ. Menstrual pattern changes following laparoscopic sterilization with different occlusion techniques: a review of 10,004 cases. Am J Obstet Gynecol. 1983;145(6):684-94.
63. DeStefano F, Perlman JA, Peterson HB, Diamond EL. Long-term risk of menstrual disturbances after tubal sterilization. Am J Obstet Gynecol. 1985;152(7 Pt 1):835-41.
64. Rivera R, Gaitan JR, Ruiz R, et al. Menstrual patterns and progesterone circulating levels following different procedures of tubal occlusion. Contraception. 1989;40(2):157-69.
65. Rulin MC, Davidson AR, Philliber SG, Graves WL, Cushman LF. Long-term effect of tubal sterilization on menstrual indices and pelvic pain. Obstet Gynecol. 1993;82(1):118-21.

66. Sahwi S, Toppozada M, Kamel M, Anwar MY, Ismail AA. Changes in menstrual blood loss after four methods of female tubal sterilization. Contraception. 1989;40(4):387-98.
67. Thranov I, Hertz JB, Kjer JJ, et al. Hormonal and menstrual changes after laparoscopic sterilization by Falope-rings or Filshie-clips. Fertil Steril. 1992;57(4):751-5.
68. Costello C, Hillis SD, Marchbanks PA, Jamieson DJ, Peterson HB. The effect of interval tubal sterilization on sexual interest and pleasure. Obstet Gynecol. 2002;100(3):511-7.
69. Shain RN, Miller WB, Holden AE, Rosenthal M. Impact of tubal sterilization and vasectomy on female marital sexuality: results of a controlled longitudinal study. Am J Obstet Gynecol. 1991;164(3):763-71.
70. Tam T, Elgar C, Jirschele K, Lombard E. Post-ablation tubal sterilization syndrome (PATSS) following Novasure endometrial ablation: two case reports and a review of literature. J Minim Invas Gynecol. 2012;19(6 Suppl):S112-3.
71. Lo JS, Pickersgill A. Pregnancy after endometrial ablation: English literature review and case report. J Minim Invas Gynecol. 2006;13(2):88-91.
72. McCausland AM, McCausland VM. Frequency of symptomatic cornual hematometra and postablation tubal sterilization syndrome after total rollerball endometrial ablation: a 10-year follow-up. Am J Obstet Gynecol. 2002;186(6):1274-80; discussion 1280-3.
73. Webb JC, Bush MR, Wood MD, Park GS. Hematosalpinx with pelvic pain after endometrial ablation confirms the postablation-tubal sterilization syndrome. J Am Assoc Gynecol Laparosc. 1996;3(3):419-21.
74. Kreider SE, Starcher R, Hoppe J, Nelson K, Salas N. Endometrial ablation: is tubal ligation a risk factor for hysterectomy. J Minim Invasive Gynecol. 2013;20(5):616-9.
75. Donnadieu AC, Fernandez H. The role of Essure sterilization performed simultaneously with endometrial ablation. Curr Opin Obstet Gynecol. 2008;20(4):359-63.
76. Valle RF, Valdez J, Wright TC, Kenney M. Concomitant Essure tubal sterilization and Thermachoice endometrial ablation: feasibility and safety. Fertil Steril. 2006;86(1):152-8.
77. Chaves KF, Merriman AL, Hassoun J, Cedó Cintrón LE, Zhao Z, Yunker AC. Post-ablation tubal sterilization syndrome: Does route of sterilization matter? Contraception. 2021;S0010-7824(21)00414-5.
78. Al-Safi ZA, Shavell VI, Hobson DT, Berman JM, Diamond MP. Analysis of adverse events with Essure hysteroscopic sterilization reported to the Manufacturer and User Facility Device Experience database. J Minim Invas Gynecol. 2013;20(6):825-9.
79. Yunker AC, Ritch JM, Robinson EF, Golish CT. Incidence and risk factors for chronic pelvic pain after hysteroscopic sterilization. J Minim Invas Gynecol. 2015;22(3):390-4.
80. Casey J, Aguirre F, Yunker A. Outcomes of laparoscopic removal of the Essure sterilization device for pelvic pain: a case series. Contraception. 2016;94(2):190-2.
81. Jain P, Clark TJ. Removal of Essure(R) device 4 years post-procedure: a rare case. J Obstet Gynaecol. 2011;31(3):271-2.
82. Mahmoud MS, Fridman D, Merhi ZO. Subserosal misplacement of Essure device manifested by late-onset acute pelvic pain. Fertil Steril. 2009;92(6):2038 e1-3.
83. Chene G, Cerruto E, Moret S, et al. Quality of life after laparoscopic removal of Essure® sterilization devices. Eur J Obstet Gynecol Reprod Biol X. 2019;3:100054.
84. U. S. Food and Drug Administration. MAUDE - Manufacturer and User Facility Device Experience.
85. Hillis SD, Marchbanks PA, Tylor LR, Peterson HB. Higher hysterectomy risk for sterilized than nonsterilized women: findings from the U.S. Collaborative Review of Sterilization. Obstet Gynecol. 1998;91(2):241-6.
86. Goldhaber MK, Armstrong MA, Golditch IM, Sheehe PR, Petitti DB, Friedman GD. Long-term risk of hysterectomy among 80,007 sterilized and comparison women at Kaiser Permanente, 1971-1987. Am J Epidemiol. 1993;138(7):508-21.
87. Hillis SD, Marchbanks PA, Tylor LR, Peterson HB. Tubal sterilization and long-term risk of hysterectomy: findings from the United States Collaborative Review of Sterilization. Obstet Gynecol. 1997;89(4):609-14.
88. Sills ES, Dalton MM. Referrals for complications following hysteroscopic sterilisation: characteristics associated with symptomatic patients after the Essure procedure. Eur J Contracept Reprod Health Care. 2016;21(3):227-33.

89. Hou MY. Discordant relationship between Essure microinsert position and tubal occlusion. BMJ Case Rep. 2016;2016.
90. Hillis SD, Marchbanks PA, Tylor LR, Peterson HB. Poststerilization regret: findings from the United States Collaborative Review of Sterilization. Obstet Gynecol. 1999;93(6):889-95.
91. Jamieson DJ, Kaufman SC, Costello C, Hillis SD, Marchbanks PA, Peterson HB. A comparison of women's regret after vasectomy versus tubal sterilization. Obstet Gynecol. 2002;99(6):1073-9.
92. Schmidt JE, Hillis SD, Marchbanks PA, Jeng G, Peterson HB. Requesting information about and obtaining reversal after tubal sterilization: findings from the U.S. Collaborative Review of Sterilization. Fertil Steril. 2000;74(5):892-8.
93. Wilcox LS, Chu SY, Eaker ED, Zeger SL, Peterson HB. Risk factors for regret after tubal sterilization: 5 years of follow-up in a prospective study. Fertil Steril. 1991;55(5):927-33.
94. Wilcox LS, Chu SY, Peterson HB. Characteristics of women who considered or obtained tubal reanastomosis: results from a prospective study of tubal sterilization. Obstet Gynecol. 1990;75(4):661-5.
95. Neuhaus W, Bolte A. Prognostic factors for preoperative consultation of women desiring sterilization: findings of a retrospective analysis. J Psychosom Obstet Gynaecol. 1995;16(1):45-50.
96. Boring CC, Rochat RW, Becerra J. Sterilization regret among Puerto Rican women. Fertil Steril. 1988;49(6):973-81.
97. Lee DM, Patton PE. Tubal surgery and treatment of infertility. In: Sciarra JJ, editor. Gynecology & Obstetrics. Philadelphia: Lippincott Williams & Wilkins; 2004.
98. van Seeters JA, Chua SJ, Mol BW, Koks CA. Tubal anastomosis after previous sterilization: a systematic review. Hum Reprod Update. 2017;1-13.
99. Trussell J, Guilbert E, Hedley A. Sterilization failure, sterilization reversal, and pregnancy after sterilization reversal in Quebec. Obstet Gynecol. 2003;101(4):677-84.
100. Monteith CW, Berger GS. Normal pregnancy after outpatient tubouterine implantation in patient with Adiana sterilization. Fertil Steril. 2011;96(1):e45-6.
101. Monteith CW, Berger GS, Zerden ML. Pregnancy success after hysteroscopic sterilization reversal. Obstet Gynecol. 2014;124(6):1183-9.
102. Ng KYB, Cheong Y. Hydrosalpinx - Salpingostomy, salpingectomy or tubal occlusion. Best Pract Res Clin Obstet Gynaecol. 2019;59:41-7.
103. Xu B, Zhang Q, Zhao J, Wang Y, Xu D, Li Y. Pregnancy outcome of in vitro fertilization after Essure and laparoscopic management of hydrosalpinx: a systematic review and meta-analysis. Fertil Steril. 2017;108(1):84-95.e5.
104. Salem SA, Peck AC, Salem RD, Sills ES. Can laparoscopic removal of Essure device before embryo transfer correct poor reproductive outcome pattern in IVF? A case report. Clin Exp Obstet Gynecol. 2014;41(2):219-22.
105. Lannon BM, Lee SY. Techniques for removal of the Essure hysteroscopic tubal occlusion device. Fertil Steril. 2007;88(2):497 e13-4.
106. Hur HC, Mansuria SM, Chen BA, Lee TT. Laparoscopic management of hysteroscopic Essure sterilization complications: report of 3 cases. J Minim Invas Gynecol. 2008;15(3):362-5.
107. Thiel J, Suchet I, Tyson N, Price P. Outcomes in the ultrasound follow-up of the Essure micro-insert: complications and proper placement. J Obstet Gynaecol Can. 2011;33(2):134-8.
108. Brito LG, Cohen SL, Goggins ER, Wang KC, Einarsson JI. Essure surgical removal and subsequent symptom resolution: case series and follow-up survey. J Minim Invas Gynecol. 2015;22(5):910-3.
109. American College of Obstetricians and Gynecologists. Committee Opinion No. 530: Access to postpartum sterilization. Obstet Gynecol. 2012;120(1):212-5.
110. Peterson HB, Warshaw JS, Pollack AE, Levy BS. Tubal sterilization. In: Jones HW, Rock JA, editors. Te Linde's operative gynecology. Philadelphia: Lippincott Williams & Wilkins; 2015.
111. Kasliwal A, Farquharson RG. Pregnancy testing prior to sterilisation. BJOG. 2000;107(11):1407-9.
112. Akhter HH, Flock ML, Rubin GL. Safety of abortion and tubal sterilization performed separately versus concurrently. Am J Obstet Gynecol. 1985;152(6 Pt 1):619-23.
113. American College of Obstetricians and Gynecologists. Practice Bulletin No. 133: Benefits and risks of sterilization. Obstet Gynecol. 2013;121(2 Pt 1):392-404.

114. Peterson HB, Ory HW, Greenspan JR, Tyler CW. Deaths associated with laparoscopic sterilization by unipolar electrocoagulating devices, 1978 and 1979. Am J Obstet Gynecol. 1981;139(2):141-3.
115. Peterson HB, Xia Z, Wilcox LS, Tylor LR, Trussell J. Pregnancy after tubal sterilization with bipolar electrocoagulation. U.S. Collaborative Review of Sterilization Working Group. Obstet Gynecol. 1999;94(2):163-7.
116. Dominik R, Gates D, Sokal D, et al. Two randomized controlled trials comparing the Hulka and Filshie clips for tubal sterilization. Contraception. 2000;62(4):169-75.
117. Sokal D, Gates D, Amatya R, Dominik R. Two randomized controlled trials comparing the tubal ring and Filshie clip for tubal sterilization. Fertil Steril. 2000;74(3):525-33.
118. Sterilization device to offer ease of use. Contracept Technol Update. 1996;17:53-64.
119. Update on female sterilization. Contracept Rep. 1996;7(3):13-4.
120. Kulier R, Boulvain M, Walker D, Candolle G, Campana A. Minilaparotomy and endoscopic techniques for tubal sterilisation. Cochrane Database Syst Rev. 2004;(3):CD001328.
121. Chi IC. Use of multiple clips for tubal occlusion in interval laparoscopic sterilization: circumstances and consequences. Contraception. 1994;50(5):409-16.
122. Subair O, Uku A, Amu O. Hydrosalpinx complicating routine double clip sterilisation. J Obstet Gynaecol. 2004;24(8):942-3.
123. Fox MD, Long CA, Meeks GR, Jutras ML, Cowan BD. Laparoscopic Pomeroy tubal ligation as a teaching model for residents. J Reprod Med. 1994;39(11):862-4.
124. Westberg J, Scott F, Creinin MD. Safety outcomes of female sterilization by salpingectomy and tubal occlusion. Contraception. 2017;95(5):505-8.
125. Murray JE, Hibbert ML, Heth SR, Letterie GS. A technique for laparoscopic pomeroy tubal ligation with endoloop sutures. Obstet Gynecol. 1992;80(6):1053-5.
126. Thomas AG, Dottino P, Brodman M, Friedman F. Laparoscopic Pomeroy tubal ligation in a residency training program. J Am Assoc Gynecol Laparosc. 1994;1(4 Pt 1):321-4.
127. Creinin MD, Zite N. Female tubal sterilization: the time has come to routinely consider removal. Obstet Gynecol. 2014;124(3):596-9.
128. Roeckner JT, Sawangkum P, Sanchez-Ramos L, Duncan JR. Salpingectomy at the time of cesarean delivery: A systematic review and meta-analysis. Obstet Gynecol. 2020;135(3):550-7.
129. Shinar S, Blecher Y, Alpern S, et al. Total bilateral salpingectomy versus partial bilateral salpingectomy for permanent sterilization during cesarean delivery. Arch Gynecol Obstet. 2017;295(5):1185-9.
130. Danis RB, Della Badia CR, Richard SD. Postpartum permanent sterilization: Could bilateral salpingectomy replace bilateral tubal ligation? J Minim Invasive Gynecol. 2016;23(6):928-32.
131. Basava L, Roy P, Anusha Priya V, Srirama S. Falope rings or modified Pomeroy's technique for concurrent tubal sterilization. J Obstet Gynaecol India. 2016;66(Suppl 1):198-201.
132. Herbst SJ, Evantash EG. Clinical performance characteristics of the Adiana® System for permanent contraception: The first year of commercial use. Rev Obstet Gynecol. 2010;3(4): 156-62.
133. Philp T, Guillebaud J, Budd D. Complications of vasectomy: review of 16,000 patients. Br J Urol. 1984;56(6):745-8.
134. Davies AH, Sharp RJ, Cranston D, Mitchell RG. The long-term outcome following "special clearance" after vasectomy. Br J Urol. 1990;66(2):211-2.
135. Alderman PM. The lurking sperm. A review of failures in 8,879 vasectomies performed by one physician. JAMA. 1988;259(21):3142-4.
136. Jamieson DJ, Costello C, Trussell J, Hillis SD, Marchbanks PA, Peterson HB. The risk of pregnancy after vasectomy. Obstet Gynecol. 2004;103(5 Pt 1):848-50.
137. Grimes DA, Satterthwaite AP, Rochat RW, Akhter N. Deaths from contraceptive sterilization in Bangladesh: rates, causes, and prevention. Obstet Gynecol. 1982;60(5):635-40.
138. Grimes DA, Peterson HB, Rosenberg MJ, et al. Sterilization-attributable deaths in Bangladesh. Int J Gynaecol Obstet .1982;20(2):149-54.
139. Khairullah Z, Huber DH, Gonzales B. Declining mortality in international sterilization services. Int J Gynaecol Obstet. 1992;39(1):41-50.
140. Sharlip ID, Belker AM, Honig S, et al. Vasectomy: AUA guideline. Linthicum, MD: 2012.

141. Labrecque M, Dufresne C, Barone MA, St-Hilaire K. Vasectomy surgical techniques: a systematic review. BMC Med. 2004;2:21.
142. Klapproth HJ, Young IS. Vasectomy, vas ligation and vas occlusion. Urology. 1973;1(4):292-300.
143. Hieu DT, Luong TT, Anh PT, Ngoc DH, Duong LQ. The acceptability, efficacy and safety of quinacrine non-surgical sterilization (QS), tubectomy and vasectomy in 5 provinces in the Red River Delta, Vietnam: a follow-up of 15,190 cases. Int J Gynaecol Obstet. 2003;83 Suppl 2: S77-85.
144. Kendrick JS, Gonzales B, Huber DH, Grubb GS, Rubin GL. Complications of vasectomies in the United States. J Fam Practice. 1987;25(3):245-8.
145. Kjersgaard AG, Thranov I, Rasmussen OV, Hertz J. Male or female sterilization: a comparative study. Fertil Steril. 1989;51(3):439-43.
146. Rees RW. Vasectomy: problems of follow up. Proc R Soc Med. 1973;66(1 Pt 1):52-4.
147. Sobrero AJ, Kohli KL. Two years' experience of an outpatient vasectomy service. Am J Public Health. 1975;65(10):1091-4.
148. Arellano Lara S, Gonzalez Barrera JL, Hernandez Ono A, Moreno Alcazar O, Espinosa Perez J. No-scalpel vasectomy: review of the first 1,000 cases in a family medicine unit. Arch Med Res. 1997;28(4):517-22.
149. de los Rios Osorio J, Castro Alvarez EA. [Analysis of 5000 vasectomies at a family planning clinic in Medellin-Colombia]. Arch Esp Urol. 2003;56(1):53-60.
150. Kumar V, Kaza RM, Singh I, Singhal S, Kumaran V. An evaluation of the no-scalpel vasectomy technique. BJU Int. 1999;83(3):283-4.
151. Sokal D, McMullen S, Gates D, Dominik R. A comparative study of the no scalpel and standard incision approaches to vasectomy in 5 countries. J Urol. 1999;162(5):1621-5.
152. EngenderHealth. Male sterilization. In: Contraceptive sterilization: global issues and trends. New York: EngenderHealth; 2002. p. 161-77.
153. Lema VM. Fournier's gangrene complicating vasectomy. East Afr Med J. 2003;80(9):492-6.
154. Valencic M. Re: Granitsiotis P, Kirk D. Chronic testicular pain: an overview. Eur Urol. 2004;45:430-6 [Letter]. Eur Urol. 2005;47(5):720.
155. Tan WP, Levine LA. An overview of the management of post-vasectomy pain syndrome. Asian J Androl. 2016;18(3):332-7.
156. Leslie TA, Illing RO, Cranston DW, Guillebaud J. The incidence of chronic scrotal pain after vasectomy: a prospective audit. BJU Int. 2007;100(6):1330-3.
157. Nangia AK, Myles JL, Thomas AJ. Vasectomy reversal for the post-vasectomy pain syndrome: a clinical and histological evaluation. J Urol. 2000;164(6):1939-42.
158. Manikandan R, Srirangam SJ, Pearson E, Collins GN. Early and late morbidity after vasectomy: a comparison of chronic scrotal pain at 1 and 10 years. BJU Int. 2004;93(4):571-4.
159. Christiansen CG, Sandlow JI. Testicular pain following vasectomy: a review of postvasectomy pain syndrome. J Androl. 2003;24(3):293-8.
160. Granitsiotis P, Kirk D. Chronic testicular pain: an overview. Eur Urol. 2004;45(4):430-6.
161. Chen TF, Ball RY. Epididymectomy for post-vasectomy pain: histological review. Br J Urol. 1991;68(4):407-13.
162. Levine LA, Hoeh MP. Evaluation and management of chronic scrotal content pain. Curr Urol Rep. 2015;16(6):36.
163. Smith A, Lyons A, Ferris J, Richters J, Pitts M, Shelley J. Are sexual problems more common in men who have had a vasectomy? A population-based study of Australian men. J Sex Med. 2010;7(2 Pt 1):736-42.
164. Hofmeyr DG, Greeff AP. The influence of a vasectomy on the marital relationship and sexual satisfaction of the married man. J Sex Marital Ther. 2002;28(4):339-51.
165. Ghazeeri GS, Kutteh WH. Autoimmune factors in reproductive failure. Curr Opin Obstet Gynecol. 2001;13(3):287-91.
166. Gubin DA, Dmochowski R, Kutteh WH. Multivariant analysis of men from infertile couples with and without antisperm antibodies. Am J Reprod Immunol. 1998;39(2):157-60.
167. Lea IA, Adoyo P, O'Rand MG. Autoimmunogenicity of the human sperm protein Sp17 in vasectomized men and identification of linear B cell epitopes. Fertil Steril. 1997;67(2):355-61.
168. Helmerhorst FM, Finken MJ, Erwich JJ. Antisperm antibodies: detection assays for antisperm antibodies: what do they test? Hum Reprod. 1999;14(7):1669-71.

169. Hjort T. Antisperm antibodies. Antisperm antibodies and infertility: an unsolvable question? Hum Reprod. 1999;14(10):2423-6.
170. Shain RN. Psychosocial consequences of vasectomy in developed and developing countries. In: Goldsmith A, Spieler JM, Sciearra J, Zatuchni GI, editors. Male contraception: advances and future prospects. Philadelphia: Harper and Row; 1986. p. 34-53.
171. Pitaktepsombati P, Janowitz B. Sterilization acceptance and regret in Thailand. Contraception. 1991;44(6):623-37.
172. Holman CD, Wisniewski ZS, Semmens JB, Rouse IL, Bass AJ. Population-based outcomes after 28,246 in-hospital vasectomies and 1,902 vasovasostomies in Western Australia. BJU Int. 2000;86(9):1043-9.
173. Potts JM, Pasqualotto FF, Nelson D, Thomas AJ, Agarwal A. Patient characteristics associated with vasectomy reversal. J Urol. 1999;161(6):1835-9.
174. Ehn BE, Liljestrand J. A long-term follow-up of 108 vasectomized men. Good counselling routines are important. Scand J Urol Nephrol. 1995;29(4):477-81.
175. Miller WB, Shain RN, Pasta DJ. The pre- and poststerilization predictors of poststerilization regret in husbands and wives. J Nerv Ment Dis. 1991;179(10):602-8.
176. Belker AM, Thomas AJ, Fuchs EF, Konnak JW, Sharlip ID. Results of 1,469 microsurgical vasectomy reversals by the Vasovasostomy Study Group. J Urol. 1991;145(3):505-11.
177. Tanrikut C, Goldstein M. Obstructive azoospermia: a microsurgical success story. Semin Reprod Med. 2009;27(2):159-64.
178. Donovan JF, DiBaise M, Sparks AE, Kessler J, Sandlow JI. Comparison of microscopic epididymal sperm aspiration and intracytoplasmic sperm injection/in-vitro fertilization with repeat microscopic reconstruction following vasectomy: is second attempt vas reversal worth the effort? Hum Reprod. 1998;13(2):387-93.
179. Practice Committee of the American Society for Reproductive Medicine. Vasectomy reversal. Fertil Steril. 2004;82 Suppl 1:S194-8.
180. Nagler HM, Jung H. Factors predicting successful microsurgical vasectomy reversal. Urol Clin North Am. 2009;36(3):383-90.
181. Lee HY. A 20-year experience with vasovasostomy. J Urol. 1986;136(2):413-5.
182. Pollack AP, Barone MA. Reversing vasectomy. In: Sciarra JJ, editor. Gynecology & obstetrics. Philadelphia: Lippincott Williams & Wilkins; 2000.
183. Borges EJ, Rossi-Ferragut LM, Pasqualoto FF, Rocha CC, Iaconelli AJ. Different intervals between vasectomy and sperm retrieval interfere in the reproductive capacity from vasectomized men. J Assist Reprod Genet. 2003;20:33-7.
184. Kolettis PN, Thomas AJ. Vasoepididymostomy for vasectomy reversal: a critical assessment in the era of intracytoplasmic sperm injection. J Urol. 1997;158(2):467-70.
185. Fuchs EF, Burt RA. Vasectomy reversal performed 15 years or more after vasectomy: correlation of pregnancy outcome with partner age and with pregnancy results of in vitro fertilization with intracytoplasmic sperm injection. Fertil Steril. 2002;77(3):516-9.
186. Sukcharoen N, Sithipravej T, Promviengchai S, Chinpilas V, Boonkasemsanti W. No differences in outcome of surgical sperm retrieval with intracytoplasmic sperm injection at different intervals after vasectomy. Fertil Steril. 2000;74(1):174-5.
187. Pasqualotto FF, Lucon AM, Sobreiro BP, Pasqualotto EB, Arap S. The best infertility treatment for vasectomized men: assisted reproduction or vasectomy reversal? Rev Hosp Clin Fac Med Sao Paulo. 2004;59(5):312-5.
188. Li SQ, Goldstein M, Zhu J, Huber D. The no-scalpel vasectomy. J Urol. 1991;145(2):341-4.
189. EngenderHealth. No-scalpel vasectomy: an illustrated guide for surgeons. 3rd ed. New York: EngenderHealth; 2003.
190. Cook LA, Pun A, Gallo MF, Lopez LM, Van Vliet HA. Scalpel versus no-scalpel incision for vasectomy. Cochrane Database Syst Rev. 2014;(3):CD004112.
191. Chen KC. A novel instrument-independent no-scalpel vasectomy - a comparative study against the standard instrument-dependent no-scalpel vasectomy. Int J Androl. 2004;27(4):222-7.
192. Jones JS. Percutaneous vasectomy: a simple modification eliminates the steep learning curve of no-scalpel vasectomy. J Urol. 2003;169(4):1434-6.
193. Marmar JL, Kessler S, Hartanto VH. A minimally invasive vasectomy with the no suture, inline method for vas occlusion. Int J Fertil Womens Med. 2001;46(5):257-64.

194. Moon HJ. Minimally invasive vas surgery using a newly designed double-ringed clamp. World J Urol. 2010;28(2):205-8.
195. Barone MA, Irsula B, Chen-Mok M, Sokal DC. Effectiveness of vasectomy using cautery. BMC Urol. 2004;4:10.
196. Sokal D, Irsula B, Chen-Mok M, Labrecque M, Barone MA. A comparison of vas occlusion techniques: cautery more effective than ligation and excision with fascial interposition. BMC Urol. 2004;4(1):12.
197. Sokal D, Irsula B, Hays M, Chen-Mok M, Barone MA. Vasectomy by ligation and excision, with or without fascial interposition: a randomized controlled trial [ISRCTN77781689]. BMC Med. 2004;2:6.
198. Shapiro EI, Silber SJ. Open-ended vasectomy, sperm granuloma, and postvasectomy orchialgia. Fertil Steril. 1979;32(5):546-50.
199. Song L, Gu Y, Lu W, Liang X, Chen Z. A phase II randomized controlled trial of a novel male contraception, an intra-vas device. Int J Androl. 2006;29(4):489-95.
200. Black T, Francome C. Comparison of Marie Stopes scalpel and electrocautery no-scalpel vasectomy techniques. J Fam Plann Reprod Health Care. 2003;29(2):32-4.
201. American College of Obstetricians and Gynecologists. Committee Opinion No. 695: Sterilization of women: ethical issues and considerations. Obstet Gynecol. 2017;129(4):e109-16.
202. Borrero S, Moore CG, Qin L, et al. Unintended pregnancy influences racial disparity in tubal sterilization rates. J Gen Intern Med. 2010;25(2):122-8.
203. Soderstrom R. Clinical challenges: share warning information, court case teaches. Contracept Technol Update. 1981;2:8-9.
204. Department of Health and Human Services. Title 42 Chapter 1 Subchapter D Part 50 Subpart B: Sterilization of persons in federally assisted family planning projects. Code of Federal Regulations; 2004.
205. Borrero S, Zite N, Potter JE, Trussell J, Smith K. Potential unintended pregnancies averted and cost savings associated with a revised Medicaid sterilization policy. Contraception. 2013;88(6):691-6.
206. Wolfe KK, Wilson MD, Hou MY, Creinin MD. An updated assessment of postpartum sterilization fulfillment after vaginal delivery. Contraception. 2017;96(1):41-6.
207. American College of Obstetricians and Gynecologists. Committee Opinion No. 371: Sterilization of women, including those with mental disabilities. Obstet Gynecol. 2007;110(1):217-220.
208. American Society of Anesthesiologists. Practice guidelines for obstetric anesthesia. An updated report by the American Society of Anesthesiologists rask force on obstetric anesthesia and the society for obstetric anesthesia and perinatology. Anesthesiology. 2007;106(4):843-63.
209. EngenderHealth. Minilaparotomy for female sterilization: An illustrated guide for providers. New York: EngenderHealth; 2003.
210. Prevention of Infection After Gynecologic Procedures: ACOG Practice Bulletin, Number 195. Obstet Gynecol. 2018;131(6):e172.
211. Poddar AK, Roy S. Disappearance of spermatozoa from semen after vasectomy. J Popul Res. 1976;3(2):61-70.
212. Richardson DW, Aitken RJ, Loudon NB. The functional competence of human spermatozoa recovered after vasectomy. J Reprod Fertil. 1984;70(2):575-9.
213. Labrecque M, St-Hilaire K, Turcot L. Delayed vasectomy success in men with a first postvasectomy semen analysis showing motile sperm. Fertil Steril. 2005;83(5):1435-41.
214. Barone MA, Nazerali H, Cortes M, Chen-Mok M, Pollack AE, Sokal D. A prospective study of time and number of ejaculations to azoospermia after vasectomy by ligation and excision. J Urol. 2003;170(3):892-6.
215. World Health Organization. Selected practice recommendations for contraceptive use. 3rd ed. Geneva: World Health Organization; 2016.
216. Mat E, Kale A, Gundogdu EC, Basol G, Yildiz G, Usta T. Transvaginal natural orifice endoscopic surgery for extremely obese patients with early-stage endometrial cancer. J Obstet Gynaecol Res. 2021;47(1):262-9.
217. Lamblin G, Chene G, Mansoor A, Katuta C, Bouvet L, Nohuz E. Ectopic pregnancy management by V-NOTES technique. J Gynecol Obstet Hum Reprod. 2021;50(5):102073.

218. Kaya C, Alay I, Cengiz H, et al. Conventional laparoscopy or vaginally assisted natural orifice transluminal endoscopic surgery for adnexal pathologies: A paired sample cross-sectional study. J Investig Surg Off J Acad Surg Res. 2020;1-6.
219. Yassa M. The use of vNOTES approach in elective bilateral salpingectomy for sterilization as a cancer prevention strategy [Internet]. clinicaltrials.gov; 2021 [cited 2021 Nov 1]. Available from: https://clinicaltrials.gov/ct2/show/NCT04809428
220. Femasys Inc. Pilot bi-lateral tubal occlusion trial for female permanent contraception [Internet]. clinicaltrials.gov; 2020 [cited 2021 Nov 4]. Available from: https://clinicaltrials.gov/ct2/show/NCT03067272
221. Products & Candidates - Femasys Inc. [Internet]. [cited 2021 Nov 5];Available from: https://www.femasys.com/Pipeline
222. Slayden OD, Hanna CA, Mishler E, Jensen JT. Advances in permanent contraception: intrauterine administration of combined polidocanol plus doxycycline foam stimulates permanent fallopian tube occlusion in baboons. Fertil Steril. 2018;110(4):e3-4.
223. Waller D, Bolick D, Lissner E, Premanandan C, Gamerman G. Azoospermia in rabbits following an intravas injection of Vasalgel™. Basic Clin Androl. 2016;26:6.
224. Waller D, Bolick D, Lissner E, Premanandan C, Gamerman G. Reversibility of Vasalgel™ male contraceptive in a rabbit model. Basic Clin Androl. 2017;27:8.

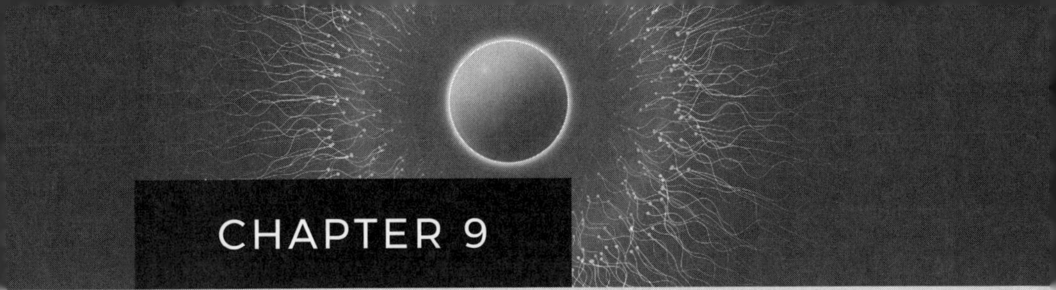

CHAPTER 9

Contraceptive Implant

Melissa J. Chen, MD, MPH
Melissa C. Matulich, MD, MAS

KEY POINTS

- The US implant (Nexplanon) is the most effective reversible option for pregnancy prevention.
- The implant is a convenient and safe contraceptive option with few medical contraindications to use.
- Bleeding concerns are the most common side effect of implant use that leads to discontinuation of the method.
- Both placement and removal of the implant can be accomplished quickly.
- Same day placement is very feasible, even in busy practices.

Contraceptive implants are reversible and potentially long-acting contraception characterized by low failure rates due to decreased reliance on user actions to maintain effectiveness. Historically, Norplant®, which consisted of six Silastic capsules containing crystalline levonorgestrel (LNG), was the first widely used contraceptive implant system. However, due to placement and removal difficulties with this product, Norplant® production ceased in the United States (US) in 2002 and worldwide in 2008. Since then, several other implants have been developed. Another LNG-releasing implant is the two-rod system containing 150 mg LNG total (75 mg in each rod), which include Jadelle®, approved for 5 years, and Sino-implant II (Levoplant®), approved for 3 years. While Jadelle is approved by Food and Drug Administration (FDA) in the US, it is not marketed in the US; both brands of LNG-releasing implants are only available internationally.

Nexplanon®, a single-rod system releasing etonogestrel (ENG), is indicated by the FDA to provide contraception for up to 3 years and is the only implant currently available in the US. This product is a soft, flexible white rod made of ethylene vinyl acetate that measures 4 cm in length and 2 mm in diameter. ENG is an active metabolite of desogestrel, which is a progestin with low androgenic impacts. Desogestrel is found in commonly used combined oral contraceptives (COC), such as Mircette® and Ortho-Cept®.

Nexplanon features several design improvements to its predecessor, Implanon®. Specifically, the inclusion of barium sulfate renders the implant radiopaque to help with its localization using X-ray, and the one-hand applicator was developed to decrease the risk of deep placement that had been reported with Implanon's trocar applicator. As with Implanon, clinicians who wish to provide Nexplanon to their patients must complete formal training in placement and removal of the implant, as required by the FDA.[1]

Mechanisms of Action

The ENG implant prevents pregnancy through inhibition of ovulation and blocking fertilization through cervical mucus thickening.

Prior research determined that ENG concentrations of at least 90 pg/mL were sufficient for ovulation suppression.[2] In pharmacokinetic evaluations of the ENG implant, serum ENG concentrations increased to concentrations associated with ovulation inhibition within 8 hours after implant placement and reached maximum serum concentration (C_{max}) in about 4 days.[3] To determine how long ovulation was reliably suppressed, investigators evaluated follicular development, endometrial thickness, and serum concentrations of 17 b-estradiol and progesterone twice weekly for 3 years. They found that the ENG implant universally suppressed ovulation for 30 months. Between 30 and 36 months, 3% of users showed some evidence of ovulation, but no pregnancies occurred because the thickened cervical mucus prevented sperm entry into the upper genital tract.[3] Of note, subsequent studies have revealed significant interindividual differences in serum levels, with some participants having up to 14-fold difference between the extremes.[4] The difference was attributed to differences in drug metabolism and might have impacts on bleeding patterns (see Disadvantages and Cautions, p. 269).

Effectiveness

Implants are in the top tier of contraceptive efficacy, demonstrating similar failure rates with both typical use and correct use. Of 100 participants, 0.1 become pregnant with typical use and 0.1 with correct and consistent use.[5] The package label reports a failure rate of 0.38 per 100 participants based on an analysis of 11 international clinical trials.[6] This estimate is based on six pregnancies that were likely conceived in the 14 days after implant removal, as no pregnancies were reported while the implant was in place.[6] (See Chapter 5, Effectiveness, Safety, and Comparative Side Effects.)

Duration of Use

The current product label for the ENG implant indicates that the implant must be removed by the end of the third year. For those who desire a longer period of use, labeling recommends that this implant be removed and replaced by a new unit.[6]

However, several studies have investigated extended use of the ENG implant and found continued effectiveness beyond 3 years. In a follow-up of the CHOICE study (based in St. Louis, Missouri, US), researchers followed 291 participants who wanted to use their implants past 3 years; 223 (77%) participants and 102 (35%) used the implant for an additional 12 months and 24 months, respectively. There were no pregnancies that occurred during 2 years of extended use.[7] In an international seven-country study, 390 participants consented to continue the ENG implant beyond 3 years with 311 and 204 participants who completed 4 years and 5 years of implant use, respectively.[8] No pregnancies occurred during the 2 years of additional follow-up. Extended use of the contraceptive implant has multiple benefits, such as fewer placements and removals for those who desire a longer period of use, potentially less burden on the health care system, and decreased costs.[8] Based on the evidence for extended use, the American College of Obstetricians and Gynecologists (ACOG) published Practice Bulletin 186 in November 2017 to indicate that, "the etonogestrel implant is effective for at least 4 years."[9] Limited data for effectiveness in the fifth year among individuals with a body mass index (BMI) greater than 30 mg/kg^2 preclude recommendations for extended use to 5 years for all users. A clinical trial is currently ongoing to evaluate the contraceptive efficacy, bleeding patterns, and safety of extending use of the ENG implant to obtain FDA approval for an additional 24 months (NCT#04626596).

Advantages

Safety

The contraceptive implant is one of the safest options available. Because the implant contains no estrogen, users do not have an increased risk of venous thromboembolism, stroke, or acute myocardial infarction.[10] (See Chapter 12, Combined Hormonal Contraceptives [CHCs].) Metabolic safety studies also suggest that the implant induces changes consistent with a *lower risk* of insulin resistance and dyslipidemia compared with baseline risk prior to implant use.[11,12]

Virtually every person seeking contraception (even those with serious medical conditions) is eligible for ENG implant use based on the 2016 Centers for Disease Control and Prevention (CDC) US Medical Eligibility Criteria (MEC).[13] The US MEC lists only one Category 4 condition contraindicating initiation of the ENG implant (i.e., current or recent breast cancer within 5 years) and few category 3 conditions that require further discussion with the patient about the severity of the condition and ability to use alternative methods (e.g., systemic lupus erythematosus with positive or unknown antiphospholipid antibodies, unexplained abnormal vaginal bleeding, past breast cancer, hepatocellular adenoma, and hepatoma). Most common medical conditions, such as hypertension, diabetes, and migraine headaches are *not* contraindications to implant use.

Highly Effective

Implants are the most effective reversible option for pregnancy protection, even more effective than the protection provided by an intrauterine device (IUD).[5,8] With typical use, the implant is essentially as effective as it is with correct and consistent use because there are few things that can reduce its efficacy (see Disadvantages and Cautions).

Convenience

Once the implant has become active (≤ 7 days) after placement, users do not need any additional visits to the clinic or pharmacy for resupply or to follow specific instructions to maintain contraceptive protection. This convenience makes the implant a particularly attractive option for patients who desire a method that requires little effort on their part. Furthermore, the implant can be placed postpartum before discharge home and directly after an abortion (See Special Issues or Populations).

Discreet

The implant is palpable, but it should not be visibly detected except for the small skin puncture scar near the base of the implant. This method does not require obtaining or concealing supplies, and it also cannot be detected during intercourse.

High Rates of Continuation

Implant continuation rates are overall high, regardless of the clinical setting. In an international clinical trial, the continuation rate was 89.5% at the end of 1 year.[5] Overall, 1-year continuation rates in US populations ranged from 76.0% using retrospective claims data to 89.7% in an outpatient pediatric setting.[14-16] Continuation rates are also higher at 3 years at 56.4% with implant use compared with 28.1–33.2% with pill, patch, ring, or injectable options.[17]

Menstrual-Related Benefits

While bleeding irregularities are the most common reason for implant removal (see Disadvantages and Cautions), up to 20% of patients with normal menstrual cycles at baseline reported amenorrhea with continued use at 1 year.[18] Most patients had infrequent bleeding, or less than three episodes of bleeding in a 90-day reference period.[18] Dysmenorrhea also improved with implant use, with 80.7% of those with baseline dysmenorrhea experiencing a decrease in their symptoms during the study period.[18]

In addition to pregnancy prevention, patients have used the ENG implant for addressing various menstrual-related issues, such as treatment of endometriosis pain, menstrual suppression, endometrial protection, and reduction in ovarian cyst formation, particularly corpus luteal cysts.[19-23]

Rapid Return of Fecundity

After removal of the implant, there is a rapid return to fecundity, with the exception of age-related declines in fecundity. Serum ENG concentrations are undetectable within 1 week of implant removal and most clinical trial participants resumed normal menses after implant removal.[3,24] Among those not using contraception, 13.8% became pregnant within 3 months of implant removal.[25]

Does Not Require Examinations or Tests Prior to Initiation

According to the 2016 CDC Selected Practice Recommendations (SPR) for Contraceptive Use, no examinations or tests are needed before implant initiation, decreasing barriers for patients who prefer to avoid or clinicians who do not routinely perform pelvic examination.[26] According to these guidelines, a routine pregnancy test is also not necessary, as long as the clinician is reasonably certain that the patient is not pregnant based on the criteria listed in the CDC SPR.[26]

Ease of Integrating Implant Services into Various Health Care Settings

After completing the mandatory clinical training, health care providers from all types of clinical backgrounds can offer the implant to their patients. This method does not require specialized equipment for routine initiation and removal, such as an examination table with stirrups or instrument sterilization process. The ability to integrate implant services into various clinical settings potentially decreases barriers for patients who do not have ready access to specialists. In an observational study of ENG implant placement and removal-related events among US health care providers, nurse practitioners, general practitioners, physician assistants, and nurses performed over half of the placements.[27]

Disadvantages and Cautions

Procedure-Related Risks

Implant placement and removal are relatively simple procedures that are performed in clinic. Minor risks associated with both the placement and removal procedures include erythema (0.3%), hematoma (3.0%), bruising (2.0%), pain (1.0%), and swelling (0.7%).[6,28] Infection occurs in less than 1% of procedures; in a trial with the updated applicator, no infections were reported in 301 placements.[28] Rare complications include pain or paresthesia from neural compression or damage, superficial venous thrombosis from vascular compression, and distant implant migration.[29] The risk of deep implant placement occurs in less than 1% (0.1–0.9%) of procedures and may lead to the inability to palpate the implant at the time of desired removal.[1,27,30] Nonpalpable implants result in a more challenging removal procedure, which is discussed in more detail below. Other removal-specific complications include breaking the implant, fibrosis, and adherence of the implant to underlying tissues.[31] In a large US prospective cohort study known as the Nexplanon Observational Risk Assessment (NORA) study, 14 per 1,000 removals were reported by providers as difficult due to fibrotic tissue, requirement of multiple attempts for removal, migration, or deep position.[27]

Nonpalpable Implants

Nonpalpable implants are defined as implants that cannot be identified by palpation at the time of requested removal or during contraceptive surveillance. Nonpalpable implants are estimated to occur in 1 per 1,000 removals and can be related to deep placement at time of insertion or influenced by patient weight changes.[1,27] Nonpalpable implants can be further characterized as suprafascial (above the fascia) or subfascial (below the fascia).[32] Nonpalpable suprafascial implants are more difficult to locate and remove than those appropriately placed beneath the skin, but they typically do not pose significant threat to nearby neurovascular structures located below the fascia. If the implant is localized below the fascia, or is suspected to be, removal becomes even more complicated as these implants can be located near neurovascular structures or even within the body of the muscle. Clinicians should counsel patients that in these circumstances, referral to an experienced provider is essential for implant localization and removal. (See Difficult Removals on p. 280

for discussion of removal techniques.) One very rare complication of nonpalpable subfascial implants is distant migration. This complication is estimated to occur in just over 1 patient per million implants sold.[33] When migration occurs, it is usually limited to less than several centimeters from the original placement site towards the ipsilateral axilla; however, there are a few case reports that describe intravascular placement resulting in migration to the thoracic cavity via the pulmonary artery.[34-36] These reports prompted the change in instructions for implant placement: *clinicians are now advised to avoid placement in the biceps groove, no matter how superficial that placement might be, and placement over the triceps area is specifically recommended.*

Unpredictable Bleeding

With the suppression of ovulation and the progestin effects on the endometrium, implant users often have unpredictable bleeding patterns that range from no bleeding to frequent or prolonged spotting or bleeding. In the US trials, approximately 11.1% to 14.4% of users asked for early implant removal because of bleeding complaints.[6,18,31] While it is not possible to anticipate the bleeding pattern for any particular user, reanalysis of clinical studies has revealed some general patterns. In the first 3 months of use, about one-third of implant users experienced favorable bleeding patterns (0 to 28 spotting or bleeding days), which usually continued over the next 2 years of use. In the second 3 months, another one-third developed favorable patterns. However, after 6 months of use, one-third still experienced bleeding patterns that were identified as unfavorable (e.g., frequent or prolonged bleeding).[37] Some studies suggest that unfavorable bleeding patterns may be more common among users with lower BMIs and that patients switching from combined hormonal contraception are less likely to have heavy or prolonged bleeding during the early transitional months.[37] In general, prolonged bleeding (uninterrupted episode lasting more than 14 days in one 90-day reference period) or frequent bleeding (more than five episodes in one 90-day reference period) occurs more frequently in the early months of implant use, perhaps related to higher ENG levels.[4]

Several other analyses about bleeding patterns can be helpful when counseling interested candidates. In 75% of 90-day reference periods, the number of spotting or bleeding days was less than or the same as what participants had experienced with their normal cycles, but those spotting or bleeding days occurred at unpredictable intervals.[37] Amenorrhea occurred in 19% of participants between 3 and 6 months, 24% of participants between 9 and 12 months, and 17% of participants near the 2 year mark.[6] (See Chapter 4, Person-Centered Reproductive Health Conversations and Contraceptive Counseling.)

Other Potential Hormone-Related Side Effects

A systematic review of several clinical studies reported that the most commonly reported complaints over a 3-year period of implant use were headache (15.5%), perceived weight increase (11.8%), acne (12%), breast pain (10.2%), emotional lability (5.8%), and abdominal pain (5.2%).[18,31] Interestingly, comparative trials have demonstrated that implant users did not have any differences in weight gain or body composition changes compared with copper IUD users.[38,39] The ability of postpartum users with BMI > 25 kg/m^2 to lose weight by 6 months was also not statistically different from postpartum patients who used nonhormonal contraceptive methods.[40]

Acne deserves special mention. In a US clinical trial, 16% of users reported development of acne while using the implant. However, of patients who reported baseline acne at the time of implant placement, 60% noted improvement of acne while using the implant.[18] Of note, many new implant users switch from combined hormonal contraceptives, which inherently improve acne. Therefore, it is difficult to know if reported increases in acne are related to initiation of the implant or cessation of combined hormonal contraceptives.

Pregnancy Issues

Failure of the implant to prevent pregnancy is rare but has occurred. An Australian postmarketing surveillance program received 218 reports of pregnancies over the first 3 years after Implanon introduction, of which five were ectopic.[41] Only 13 pregnancies were attributed to failure of the method. Other pregnancies had occurred before insertion (luteal phase pregnancy) or resulted from failure to insert the implant properly.[41] Drug–drug interactions should always be investigated.

The absolute risk of ectopic pregnancy is low due to the implant's high contraceptive efficacy. However, should the method fail, the ectopic pregnancy risk may theoretically be increased because progestins slow ciliary motion within the fallopian tube. According to a large retrospective cohort study, the incidence of ectopic pregnancy during implant use was 2.0 per 10,000 woman-years, which is significantly lower than the incidence in patients who recently discontinued a prescription contraceptive (20.6 per 10,000 woman-years) or those who either had never used a contraceptive or did so more than 12 months prior to this study (10.3 per 10,000 woman-years).[42] Regardless, if the implant fails, localization of the pregnancy is important given the theoretical increased risk of ectopic pregnancy.

Lack of Protection Against Sexually Transmitted Infections

Implants do not provide protection against sexually transmitted infections (STIs). Condom use may be lower in implant users as patients no longer see the need for additional forms of contraception due to the implant's high efficacy.[43-47] Patients at risk for STI transmission should be counseled to use condoms, pre-exposure prophylaxis (PrEP), and available vaccines. (See Chapter 23, Reproductive Tract Infections Including HIV and other Sexually Transmitted Infections.)

Special Issues or Populations

Efficacy in Users with Body Mass Index (BMI) ≥ 30 kg/m^2

In US clinical trials, only participants whose weights were less than 30% above their ideal body weights were enrolled in the initial studies for FDA approval. As a result, the product labeling states that the effectiveness of the ENG implant is not known in those with higher BMIs.[6] Since those original clinical trials, many studies have investigated the pharmacokinetics and efficacy of the implant in users with BMI ≥ 30 kg/m^2.[48-51]

Early pharmacokinetic studies showed that ENG concentrations were lower in obese compared to normal weight participants at various time points up to 6 months after implant placement.[48] However, follow-up studies found that ENG concentrations were comparable across BMI categories in normal weight, overweight, and obese participants with implants in place for more than 1 year, and none of the participants had a serum ENG concentration less than 90 pg/mL.[49] In a subanalysis of serum ENG concentrations among participants using the implant past 3 years, the median ENG concentration was 188.3 pg/mL (range 75.9–520.9 pg/mL) and 167.8 pg/mL (range 72.5–470.5 pg/mL) at the end of 3 and 4 years, respectively, which were not significantly different from the median serum ENG concentrations in the other weight categories.[50]

The CHOICE study has provided robust data about the efficacy, safety, and continuation rates of users of all ages and of all BMIs. In that study, investigators found no significant difference in failure rates among implant users with different BMI categories. Among 1,377 women-years of implant use, there was one pregnancy that occurred in an obese participant with BMI 30.7 kg/m^2 at enrollment. Overall, the cumulative implant failure rates were 0.00 per 100 woman-years in normal and overweight participants and 0.23 per 100 woman-years in obese participants.[51] The investigators commented that the one pregnancy that occurred could have been related to a luteal phase pregnancy as the participant was transitioning from COC to implant use.[51] In follow-up studies examining extended implant use, zero pregnancies occurred among the 291 participants, of whom 23.0% were overweight and 51.9% were obese.[7]

Based on the available evidence, the implant may be offered as a first-line contraceptive method to candidates of all BMIs.[13]

Drugs that Impact Efficacy

Implant efficacy relies on adequate systemic levels of ENG, which makes this method susceptible to drug–drug interactions. The most significant threat comes from drugs that increase activity of the hepatic cytochrome P-450 enzyme system that promotes metabolic clearance of ENG. (See Medication Interactions and the Impact on COC Effectiveness in Chapter 12.) Anticonvulsants are important because they are used as treatment for a broad array of clinical indications in addition to epilepsy, such as several nonepileptic neurologic and psychiatric conditions.[52] One small study found that the median ENG concentrations before and after carbamazepine coadministration were 158.1 pg/mL and 50.9 pg/mL, respectively ($p=.005$), and in 8 of 10 participants the ENG concentration was below the threshold for ovulatory suppression.[52] These findings call into question the effectiveness of this method when using carbamazepine or other drugs with similar pharmacologic effects. Herbal remedies such as St. John's Wort may have similar effects as well. For up to 30 days after the user has taken the last dose of St. John's Wort, hepatic enzyme activity can remain increased. Studies of St. John's Wort with implants are not directly available, but St. John's Wort showed a pattern of small to moderate induction of metabolism of contraceptive steroids, including progestin.[53] Ritonavir-boosted protease inhibitors can suppress circulating ENG after 2 years of implant use, so implant replacement at that time might be prudent to avoid an ENG drop below therapeutic levels. Case reports of pregnancies in people with human immunodeficiency virus (HIV) using efavirenz have raised issues about this antiretroviral agent as well.[54] However, in combination with lopinavir, neither ritonavir nor efavirenz impaired the efficacy of the implant.[55] Discuss medications—both prescription and nonprescription supplements—with patients considering the implant and remind them of the potential for deleterious drug–drug interactions when they rely on the implant for pregnancy prevention.

Table 9-1 **Potential Adverse Drug—Drug Interactions: Nexplanon Product Labeling versus US MEC**

Drugs and Herbal Products Listed on Product Labeling[6]	Drugs and Herbal Products Listed in US MEC[13]*
Aprepitant	
Barbiturates	Barbiturates
Bosentan	
Carbamazepine	Carbamazepine
Efavirenz	
Felbamate	
Griseofulvin	
Oxcarbazepine	Oxcarbazepine
Phenytoin	Phenytoin
Rifampin	Rifampin
Rifabutin	Rifabutin
Rufinamide	
St. John's Wort	St. John's Wort
Topiramate	Topiramate
	Fosamprenavir
	Primidone

All of the listed drugs are Category 2 or 2 for either initiation or continuation on the US MEC 2016.
Data from Product labeling etonogestrel implant. https://www.accessdata.fda.gov/drugsatfda_docs/label/2019/021529s018lbl.pdf; Curtis KM, Tepper NK, Jatlaoui TC, et al. U.S. Medical Eligibility Criteria for Contraceptive Use, 2016. MMWR Recomm Rep 2016;65(3):1-104. DOI: 10.15585/mmwr.rr6503a1.

Table 9-1 contrasts two listings of the drugs and herbal products that reduce ENG levels: one listing is from the implant product labeling[6] and the other is from the US MEC.[13] The current US MEC categorizes the listed medications as category 2. Given the study findings suggesting reduced circulating ENG concentrations with these medications, clinicians should engage in shared decision making with patients about the risks and benefits of implant initiation if the patient is taking any of the listed medications.

Postabortion Placement

Surgical Abortion. Implants can be placed at any time after an abortion, including immediately after the abortion.[26] With surgical abortion (i.e., dilation and curettage [D&C] and dilation and evacuation [D&E]), there are no medical contraindications to same-day postabortion implant initiation. Same-day placement may be more convenient for some people as this option eliminates another visit to a health care facility and increases the likelihood of using the method. In a randomized trial comparing immediate versus delaying placement by 2–4 weeks following a D&E procedure, 100% of participants in the immediate group had the implant placed versus 42.7% in the delayed treatment group. Furthermore, more patients who had same-day implant placement were still using the implant at 6 months postprocedure (54.8% versus 25.3%).[56] Prospective cohort studies comparing immediate and interval implant after abortion found that 1-year continuation rates were similar.[57,58]

Medication Abortion. While placing an implant at the initial visit for medication abortion increases convenience for users, concurrent initiation of a progestin contraception and mifepristone, an antiprogestin, raises concerns about increasing medication abortion failures. Initial small pilot and cohort studies did not find an increase in medication abortion failure with immediate implant placement at time of mifepristone.[59-62] Two subsequent larger randomized trials confirmed these findings. In one study, 3.9% of those in the immediate implant group and 3.8% in the interval placement group required surgery to complete the abortion. Despite more participants starting the implant in the immediate group compared with interval placement (100% vs. 83.3%), pregnancies at 6 months were no different between groups.[63] In the other study, 5.8% in the immediate implant group and 4.0% in the interval placement group had a surgical intervention after medication abortion, with the risk difference within the margin of equivalence.[64] Implant placement rates were higher in the immediate group compared with interval group (98.9% versus 71.6%), and there were fewer pregnancies at 6 months in the immediate group (0.8% versus 3.8%).[64] Given these findings, clinicians can discuss immediate implant placement as an option during the initial medication abortion visit instead of routinely delaying contraception initiation until the follow-up visit.[65]

Postpartum Placement and Lactation. Delaying contraception initiation until the postpartum visit can be a barrier for patients who are unable to return to a health care facility after delivery. Several studies have shown an increase in implant initiation and decrease in rapid repeat pregnancies in those who had an implant placed before hospital discharge compared with those who were scheduled to return to the office for implant placement.[66-68] (See Chapter 19, Contraception After Pregnancy.)

For those who desire to breastfeed, this earlier implant placement might raise concerns of potentially negative effects on lactation or infant health. After delivery of the placenta, decreasing progesterone levels trigger lactogenesis II, or onset of copious milk production, which occurs 2 to 3 days after delivery.[69] Starting a progestin contraceptive method during this time could potentially interfere with lactogenesis II, and ultimately with overall breastfeeding ability.[70] To address this concern, multiple randomized trials have compared breastfeeding and infant outcomes with immediate and interval implant placement demonstrating no difference in time to lactogenesis II, breast milk volume, infant growth, and exclusive breastfeeding rates.[71-75] Based on the available evidence, the CDC MEC assigns implant initiation at less than 21 days postpartum as category 2, or a condition for which the advantages of using the method generally outweigh the theoretical or proven risks.[13]

While the evidence to date is reassuring regarding lactation outcomes, clinicians should be aware that studies primarily included participants who had healthy, term infants and previous breastfeeding experience. Furthermore, while there were no differences in exclusive breastfeeding rates between the immediate and interval implant groups, the reported rates at 3 and 6 months are lower than expected, which brings into question the population enrolled (e.g., how much did participants desire to breastfeed?). Accordingly, these results cannot be extrapolated directly to people who have risk factors for lactation difficulty (e.g., preterm birth, delivery of multiples) or prioritize breastfeeding success above contraception.

Vulnerable Populations. The long-acting potential and excellent contraceptive efficacy of contraceptive implants have clear patient and public health benefits. However, these same characteristics have facilitated use of these implants for coercive and discriminatory practices in the US. Between 1991 and 1994, 13 states introduced legislation that offered financial incentives for implant placement to patients receiving public assistance, although to our knowledge these measures were not passed and therefore were not implemented.[76,77] Seven states introduced bills attempting to mandate Norplant® use in targeted communities, including patients seeking abortion services, people with more than two children on welfare, people who used substances during pregnancy, and at the time of legal sentencing. According to some judges, legal sentencing was reduced if the person agreed to have the implant placed. Additionally, some Medicaid programs previously funded implant insertion but not removal.[76] Although these coercive practices may seem like something of the past, coercive provider behaviors, philosophies, and biases unfortunately still exist. Clinicians are enthusiastic about the multiple benefits of the implant; however, users will request removal of the implant for various reasons and it is imperative that clinicians respect this request.[78] Outside of clinical trials, no removal is "early" if it is what the user desires. (See Chapter 4, Person-Centered Reproductive Health Conversations and Contraceptive Counseling.) Implant discontinuation has typically required clinician interactions, and frustration with barriers to implant removal has been well-documented.[79,80] As a result, some users have resorted to self-removal of the implant.[81]

Patients must be in control of their contraception at all times. Therefore, if a person has concerns about the implant, they may seek counseling or reassurance, but if implant removal is desired, then clinicians should promptly remove the implant. As providers, we should continue to celebrate all the benefits that contraceptive implants provide, and we should support programs that increase access to both placement and desired removals and maintain caution when counseling patients by acknowledging prior reproductive injustices and reflecting on our own implicit biases.

Providing the Method

Requirements for Implant Providers

All clinicians who wish to provide the ENG contraceptive implant must attend an FDA-approved, company-sponsored training program to ensure proficiency in placement and removal of implants in artificial models. Completing this training enables clinicians to order implants from the distributors. Of course, providers should be familiar with the anatomy of the arm for both placement and removal.

Counseling and Informed Consent

When counseling a potential user about the implant, provide information about the benefits of the implant, the expected bleeding pattern changes, the hormone-related potential side effects, and the risks associated with placement and removal procedures. (See Chapter 4, Person-Centered Reproductive Health Conversations and Contraceptive Counseling.) The FDA specifies that in order to give informed consent, those considering the implant should read the product information provided within the product labeling.

Timing of Initiation

The implant can be initiated when the clinician can be reasonably certain that the patient is not pregnant based on the criteria listed in the US CDC SPR.[26] A routine urine pregnancy test is not necessary; a negative pregnancy test does not exclude the possibility of a luteal phase pregnancy if an individual does not meet the criteria to reasonably exclude pregnancy (see Chapter 25, Pregnancy Testing). In these circumstances, the clinician and patient can engage in shared decision making about the risks and benefits of starting the implant that day.

The importance of a single visit protocol for implant placement has been highlighted in several studies. In the CHOICE study, those who had delayed initiation of the implant or IUD had a 60% increase in risk of unintended pregnancy compared with those who got same-day placement. Delays for implant placement in that study were as long as 16 weeks.[82] In another study with a two-visit protocol for implant or IUD initiation in an adolescent and young adult population, about two-thirds had their contraceptive device order completed.[83] The most common reason for not completing an order was the patient not returning for a follow-up appointment or completing the necessary consent or device-specific ordering forms. For those who did not complete their order, 28% had a pregnancy during the study period, of which 15% occurred between the first and second appointments.[83]

The incidence of luteal phase pregnancy was < 1% in a study that offered same-day placement in any patient with a negative pregnancy test, regardless of timing within menstrual cycle or recent contraceptive use.[84] After counseling, if a patient chooses same-day implant initiation, it is reasonable for the patient to check a urine pregnancy test about 2 weeks after the implant is placed. No other examinations or tests are needed prior to implant initiation.[26]

There is no need for back-up contraception after the implant is placed if a patient is within the first 5 day of menses, 7 days after a miscarriage or abortion, or 21 days postpartum if not breastfeeding, or meets criteria for lactational amenorrhea method (see Chapter 19, Contraception After Pregnancy).[26] If placed at any other time point, the clinician should recommend using a backup method for 7 days.

Implant Placement Principles

Proper placement technique is essential for safe and satisfactory use of the implant. Not only does superficial placement under the skin avoid complications related to deep placement, but also facilitates easier future removal. Please note, **the new instructions for placement state that the implant should not be placed in the biceps groove**, as had been previously advised, but over the triceps muscle starting 8 to 10 cm distal to the medial epicondyle.[6]

Practical Tips on Implant Placement and Removal

Implant Placement. The steps for implant placement are reviewed in **Video 9-1**. Formal training, which is required prior to being able to order and use the implant, stresses the following points:

1. Assess for the possibility of pregnancy prior to placement.
2. Select a site for the implant in the inner aspect of the preferred upper arm (usually the nondominant arm), just below the skin in the subcutaneous tissue about 8–10 cm from the medial epicondyle overlying the triceps muscle mass and avoiding the biceps groove.
3. Placement using all the steps should be under direct visualization.
4. Skin should be cleansed and numbed prior to placement.
5. Check the applicator to make sure an implant is visible inside the insertion needle.
6. Initial insertion of the needle through the skin should be performed with no greater than a 30° angle, just enough of an angle to slide the bevel of the needle under the skin, at which point the angle of the inserter should be adjusted to be parallel to the skin (this should help avoid deep placement).
7. Applying countertraction to the skin distal to where the implant is being placed facilitates advancement of the needle.
8. Lifting or tenting the skin while advancing the needle will also avoid deep placement.
9. Ensure the needle has been advanced completely before pulling back on the purple lever to release the implant.
10. Always confirm appropriate superficial placement by palpation; preferably both patient and provider will palpate the implant, but occasionally the patient will decline.
11. If the implant cannot be identified by palpation immediately after placement:
    a. Check the applicator to make sure the implant was deployed.
    b. If the implant was deployed, remove the implant and start over.
    c. Consider imaging if unable to remove or truly palpate the implant.

Implant Removal

Palpable Rods. Steps for removal of palpable implants are reviewed in **Video 9-2**.

- To visualize the implant, the package labeling says to mark skin over each end of the implant.
- **BUT** this can create tattoos if the marked skin is punctured.
- **SO** it is much easier to clean the entire area with betadine, and while the betadine is still wet, drag the wooden part of a sterile Q-tip along the skin from the upper to the lower edge of the area along the axis of the arm. This will scrape the betadine off the skin overlying the implant and reveal its presence on the skin like the negative of a photo (**Figure 9-1**).

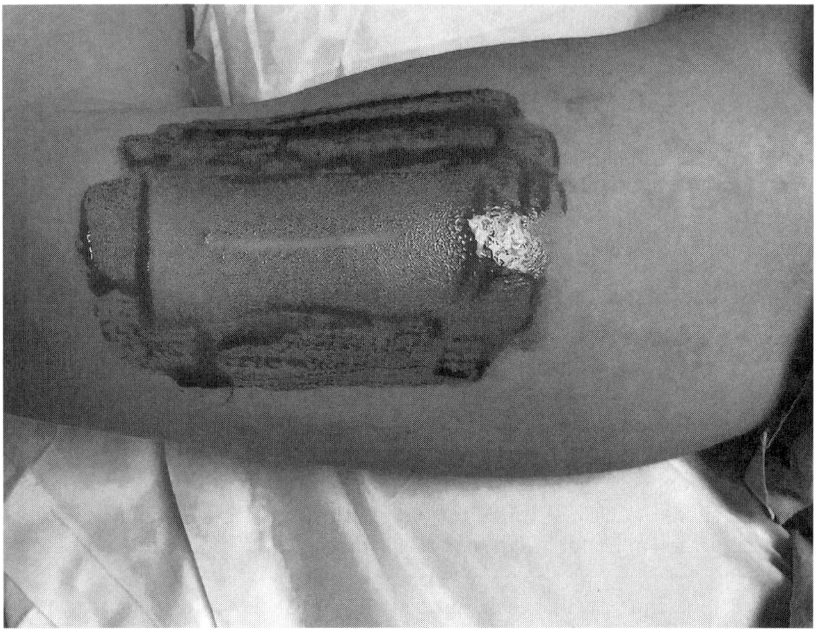

Figure 9-1 Betadine stripping technique to visualize implant for removal.

- Place the anesthesia at the distal tip of the implant and just underneath it (**Figure 9-2**).
- *Always* keep the implant stabilized under pressure with the distal tip of the implant pressing up against the skin when you are removing the implant. To get the implant positioned for removal, follow these steps.
  - Press with the ring finger of your nondominant hand down on the proximal tip of the implant. Press down to the floor and towards the elbow.
  - Drag the thumb of your nondominant hand from the top of the implant along its length to tighten the skin overlying the implant. Then pull your thumb laterally (toward yourself) to expose the distal tip of the implant under tension.
  - Do not move your fingers holding the implant in place until the implant is completely out of the arm.
  - Make your incision with your dominant hand: incise the skin **longitudinally (not perpendicular to the axis of the implant)** about 2–3 mm starting just over tip of the implant, cutting through the fibrous sheath to expose the distal end of the implant. (See **Figure 9-3**.)
  - Put the scalpel down.
  - Remove the implant by popping the implant out through the incision and grasping it with your thumb and index finger[85] or with forceps (See **Figure 9-4**.)
- The procedure should take less than 30 seconds.

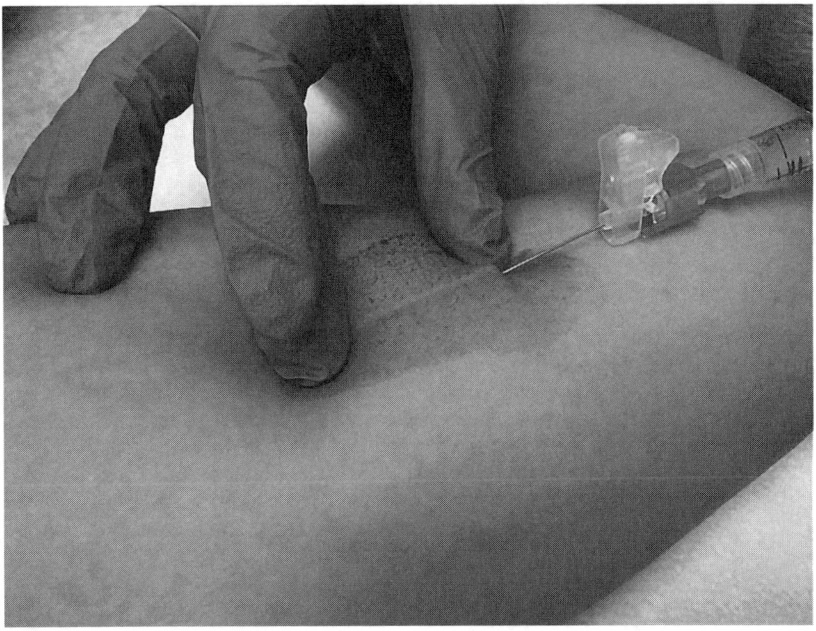

Figure 9-2 Maintain pressure on implant during anesthetic infusion below implant.

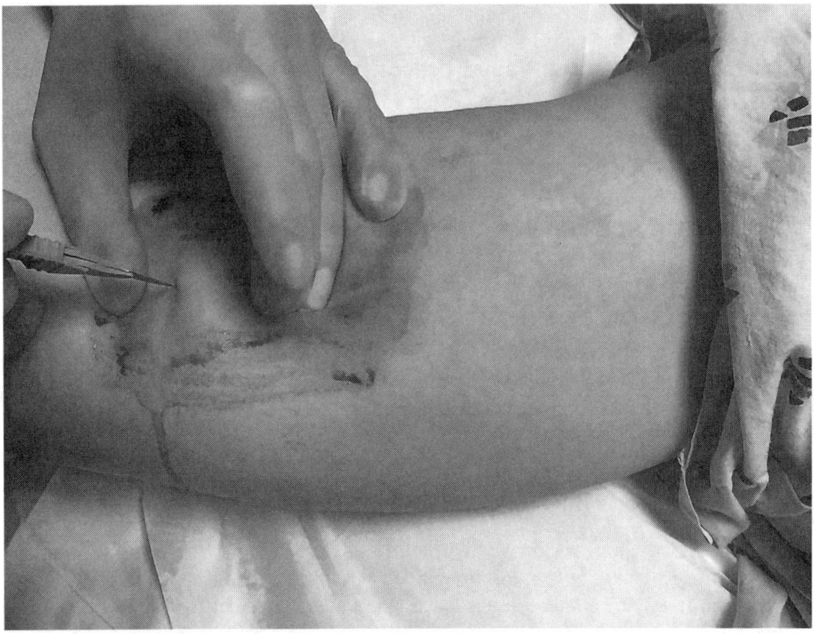

Figure 9-3 Maintain pressure to stabilize implant during vertical incision for removal.

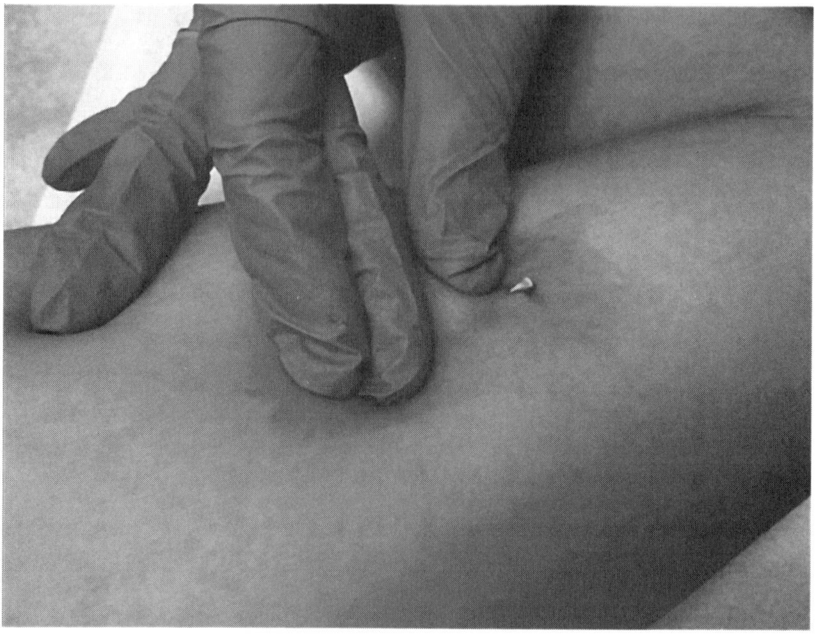

Figure 9-4 Maintain pressure on implant to enable it to pop out once fibrous tissue is incised.

Difficult Removals

Localization of Deeply Placed or Nonpalpable Implants. *Always* know exactly where the implant is before you try to remove it.[86]

If you have *any* trouble palpating the full length of the implant, STOP. Apply lubricant (KY jelly) and repeat the exam. Rock the proximal and distal ends like a teeter-totter to identify the tips of the implant. If you cannot palpate the implant, perform imaging to localize it. A sample algorithm for localization of radiopaque contraceptive implants is shown in **Figure 9-5**.[87] Ultrasound is usually the most effective imaging tool (**Figures 9-6** and **9-7**). A CT or an MRI can help define in which tissue the implant is located, though not as effectively as ultrasound. An X-ray may help identify that the Nexplanon implant is present in the arm but is not helpful in localization for removal (**Figure 9-8**). If you cannot localize the implant or do not feel comfortable performing the removal, refer the patient for removal to a more experienced provider.

> Throughout the US, there are many Centers of Excellence with the ability to accept referrals of patients with nonpalpable implants as well as those in whom the removal may be challenging, regardless of insurance coverage. For general advice and support for nonpalpable implants, visit https://www.organonconnect.com/nexplanon/professional-resources/

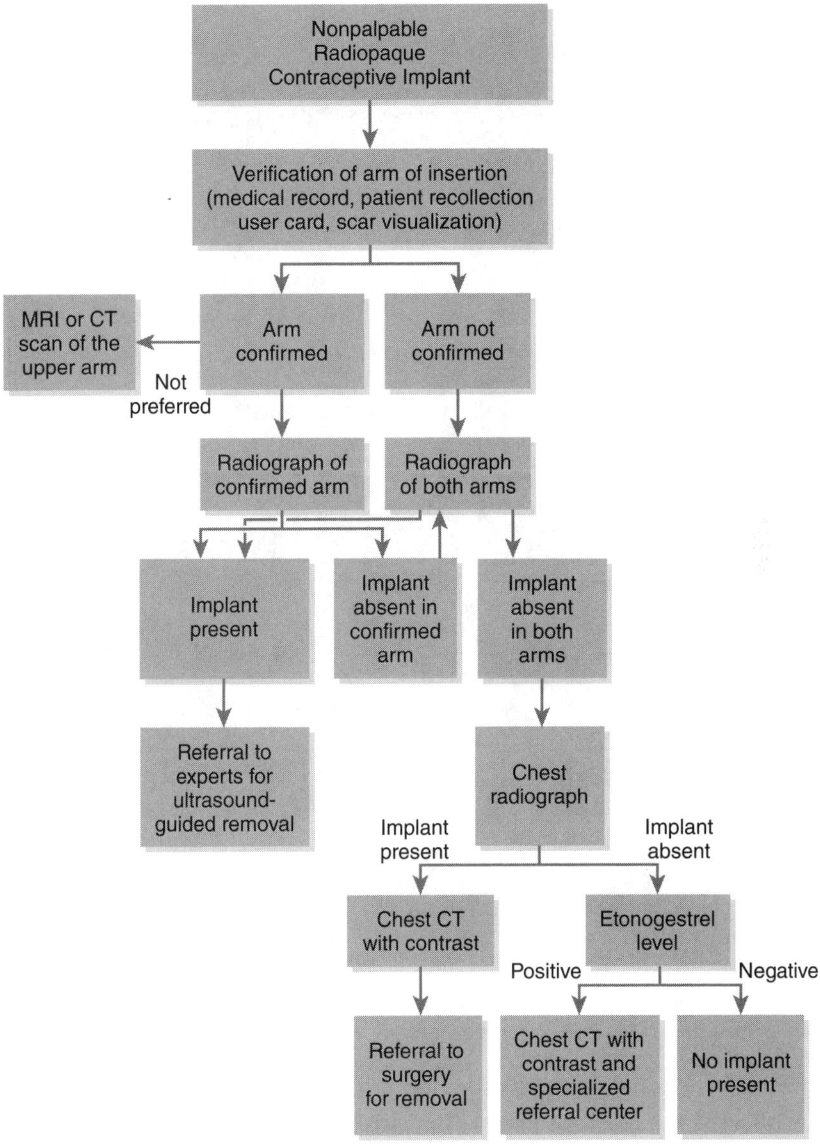

Figure 9-5 Algorithm for localization of radiopaque contraceptive implant.

Reproduced from Kwal J, Maguire K, Carugno J. Localization and management of nonpalpable radiopaque contraceptive implant. Contraception 2022;106: page 4

- Tip: If the implant moves with muscle contraction, it is likely within the muscle.[88] To localize the implant with ultrasound, use a linear array transducer with at least 10 mHz (15 or 18 mHz is preferred).[89]
- Place the transducer at right angles to the implant.
- Find the echogenic shadow cast by the implant (the "eclipse sign").

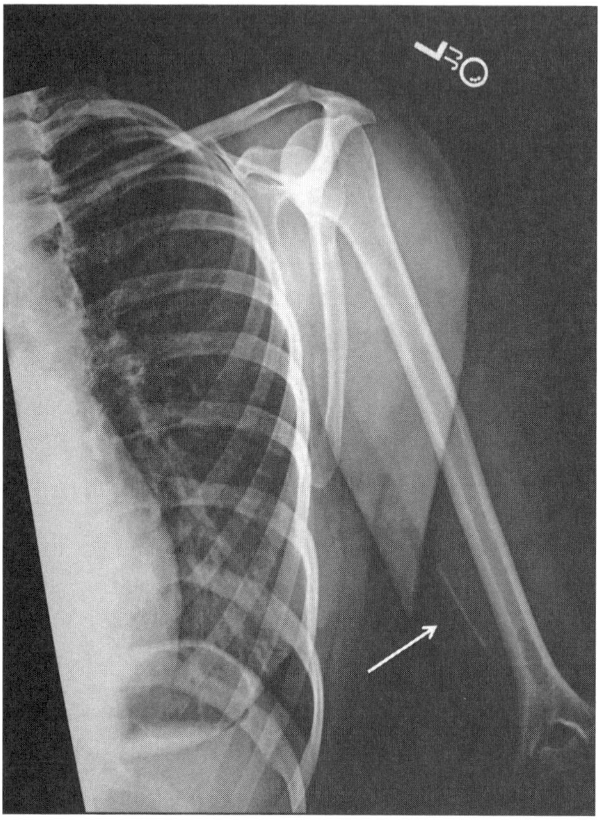

Figure 9-6 Radiograph examination showing presence of implant.

Reproduced from Chen MJ, Creinin MD. Removal of a nonpalpable etonogestrel implant with preprocedure ultrasonography and modified vasectomy clamp. Obstet Gynecol 2015;126(5):935-938. DOI: 10.1097/AOG.0000000000001082

- The implant will be at the top of that shadow.
- Rotate the transducer along the length of the implant to see where it is closest to the skin.
- Identify if the implant is above or below the fascia.
- If below the fascia, turn on the Doppler flow to see if there are any adjacent vessels (and nerves) near the implant. It is important to avoid these to prevent hemorrhage and nerve damage.

Removal Techniques Available for Deeply Placed or Nonpalpable Implants. Deeply placed implants can be removed as outpatient procedures by those with additional training and imaging tools. Here are some of the options:

- Removal under real-time ultrasound guidance has been shown to be quite effective.[90-92] The best approach to the implant is identified by ultrasound imaging. The implant can be localized with ultrasound and the skin can be marked just prior to clinic or surgical removal.[32,89,93] Under guidance (if needed), anesthesia can be placed through the overlying skin and along the track from

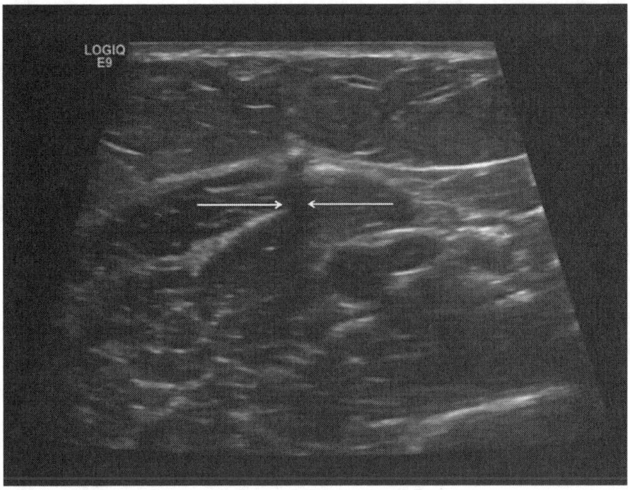

Figure 9-7 Ultrasound showing posterior acoustic shadow of implant.

Reproduced from Chen MJ, Creinin MD. Removal of a nonpalpable etonogestrel implant with preprocedure ultrasonography and modified vasectomy clamp. Obstet Gynecol 2015;126(5):935-938. DOI: 10.1097/AOG.0000000000001082

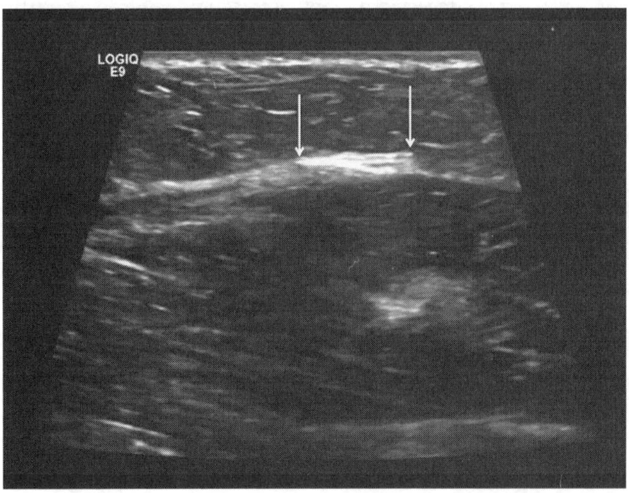

Figure 9-8 Ultrasound showing longitudinal view of the implant.

Reproduced from Chen MJ, Creinin MD. Removal of a nonpalpable etonogestrel implant with preprocedure ultrasonography and modified vasectomy clamp. Obstet Gynecol 2015;126(5):935-938. DOI: 10.1097/AOG.0000000000001082

the skin to the implant and beneath the implant. Make a longitudinal incision in the overlying skin and a track through the subcutaneous tissue and (if needed) through the fascia down to the implant. The implant and its fibrous sheath are grasped with a Norgrasp or modified vasectomy clamp and elevated out of the incision. The fibrous sheath is incised, and the implant is maneuvered out. Steps for removal of nonpalpable implant removal are shown in **Video 9-3**.

- A hook wire can be placed beneath implant under ultrasound guidance to guide the dissection to the implant.[92]
- Fluoroscopy can be used to localize the implant and guide removal in combination with ultrasound if necessary.[94]

Occasionally patients and providers will need to work with other surgical specialists for removal in the operating room if the implant is found to be close to neurovascular structures or the clinic procedure fails at removal.[32,95]

Tips On Placing a New Implant After Removal of Prior One

- Infuse anesthesia along the tract in which the new implant will be placed.
- If the prior implant was correctly positioned over the triceps muscle, the new implant can be placed through the removal incision (technique described here):
  - Slide the tip of the introducer into the incision while holding the introducer *parallel* to floor. Do *not* approach the skin at the 20 to 30° angle. Insert the implant flat to avoid deep placement of the new implant.
- Do not use the removal incision if overlying the bicipital groove or if prior implant not in the correct position.
- Consider using a separate incision if the patient has a BMI of less than 30 kg/m^2 based on a study that suggested possible association between reinsertion through a removal incision and subfascial placement in nonobese individuals.[32]

Managing Problems and Follow-Up

Follow-up visits after implant placement are not routinely needed, but always reassure users that if they have any problems or questions, you will see them promptly.

Managing Unfavorable Bleeding

It is important to recognize that counseling patients about the range of possible bleeding pattern changes can be influential prior to implant initiation. Providing patients with tools and ideas to deal with the prolonged or heavy bleeding episodes may decrease frustration they may have with potential bothersome bleeding and improve satisfaction. Counseling can also include the information that higher levels of ENG are associated with unfavorable bleeding patterns and that over time these unfavorable patterns often resolve.[4] Also a prophylactic prescription for NSAIDs to use as needed for prolonged or heavy bleeding episodes can be considered. (See below for details related to this regimen, and refer to Chapter 4 on Person-Centered Reproductive Health Conversations and Contraceptive Counseling.)

An evaluation is suggested for patients with bothersome or unexpected bleeding, especially if other concerning symptoms develop (e.g., nausea, vomiting, pain, temperature intolerance, etc.) or if the bleeding patterns change part way through implant use. Once pregnancy and other gynecologic or endocrine problems such as infection, thyroid abnormalities, polyps, fibroids, and malignancy are ruled out as causes of unfavorable bleeding, reassurance can be helpful. Review the patient's bleeding patterns to see if there has been improvement over time, as this is often the case. Treatment options that have been tested for unfavorable or bothersome bleeding with progestin-only methods are listed in **Box 9-1**. Since the circulating levels of ENG are low, the addition of combined hormonal contraceptives to control bothersome heavy or prolonged bleeding or spotting is generally well tolerated. Monophasic combined oral contraceptives can be given cyclically or continuously (using only active pills). The vaginal ring may be especially useful in treating unfavorable bleeding because it provides continuous, steady levels of hormonal support.[96] Typically, relief occurs within 2 weeks of combined hormonal contraception use, but bothersome bleeding usually returns after cessation of the treatment; therefore, some patients may choose to continue combination hormonal therapy for 2 to 3 months or even longer to experience more relief.[97,98] No serious adverse events occurred in a 6-month study evaluating simultaneous use of the ENG implant with combined oral contraceptives, and the frequency of reported side effects did not increase.[99] Another multicenter trial is underway evaluating simultaneous use for 12 months (NCT#04423055). However, some may prefer implant removal if short-term interventions do not provide them adequate relief, and patient autonomy in these situations should always be respected. Before starting a combined hormonal method, providers should ensure the patient does not have any contraindications to exogenous estrogen use (see Chapter 12, Combined Hormonal Contraceptives [CHCs].)

Pregnancy

When a patient is diagnosed with pregnancy with an implant in place and chooses to continue the pregnancy, we recommend that the implant be removed because it

Box 9-1 Practice tips: How to control bothersome bleeding with progestin-only implant.

Preplacement counseling and reassurance during use is important. (See Chapter 4, Person-Centered Reproductive Health Conversations and Contraceptive Counseling.)

- All treatments stop current bleeding episodes only. Recurrence is common.[100]
- Assess for contraindications to any of the following medical therapies before initiation.
- Hormonal therapies
  - Any monophasic combination pill (consider ethinyl estradiol dose of 30–35 mcg).
    - Short term—daily for 14 days or cyclic/continuous use for up to 3 months.[97,98]
    - Longer term—cyclic/continuous use for 6 months and potentially beyond.[99]
  - NuvaRing—1 ring for up to 35 days; extended cycle use.
  - Estrogen only (conjugated equine estrogen 1.25 mg or estradiol 2 mg) daily for 1–2 weeks.[100]
  - High-dose cyclic progestin (medroxyprogesterone acetate 10 mg twice daily or norethindrone 5 mg twice daily) for 21 days.[101]
  - Tamoxifen 10 mg twice daily for 7–190 days.[102,103]

(continues)

Box 9-1 Practice tips: How to control bothersome bleeding with progestin-only implant. *(continued)*

- Ulipristal acetate 15 mg daily for 7 days.[104]
  - This dose may not be easily available clinically.
- Mifepristone 50 mg once monthly
  - Benefit with levonorgestrel contraceptive implant but minimal short-term benefit and no long-term benefit over placebo in ENG implant users.[105,106]
  - Access to this medication is challenging and use of this antiprogesterone medication may compromise contraceptive efficacy.[105]
  - Mifepristone in combination with ethinyl estradiol or doxycycline is more effective in terminating an episode of bleeding than doxycycline alone or in combination with ethinyl estradiol, or placebo.[105]

■ Nonhormonal therapies

- Ibuprofen 800 mg 3 times a day for up to 5 days or naproxen 500 mg 2 times a day for up to 5 days to stop heavy or prolonged bleeding.[107-109]
  - Can provide counseling about NSAIDs or prophylactic prescription after implant placement.
  - Treatment can be repeated if problem bleeding returns.
- Tranexamic acid 650 mg three times a day for up to 5 days.[110]
- Doxycycline 100 mg twice daily for 5 days.
  - This treatment was initially found to be more effective than placebo in reducing bleeding and spotting, but this benefit was not replicated in a larger trial.[105]

Data from Hou MY, McNicholas C, Creinin MD. Combined oral contraceptive treatment for bleeding complaints with the etonogestrel contraceptive implant: a randomised controlled trial. Eur J Contracept Reprod Health Care 2016;21(5): 361-6. DOI: 10.1080/13625187.2016.1210122; Guiahi M, McBride M, Sheeder J, Teal S. Short-term treatment of bothersome bleeding for etonogestrel implant users using a 14-day oral contraceptive pill regimen: a randomized controlled trial. Obstet Gynecol 2015;126(3):508-513. DOI: 10.1097/AOG.0000000000000974; Chen MJ, Hsia JK, Creinin MD. Etonogestrel implant use in women primarily choosing a combined oral contraceptive pill: A proof-of-concept trial. Contraception 2018;97(6):533-537. DOI: 10.1016/j.contraception.2018.02.009; Zigler RE, McNicholas C. Unscheduled vaginal bleeding with progestin-only contraceptive use. Am J Obstet Gynecol 2017;216(5):443-450. DOI: 10.1016/j.ajog.2016.12.008; Mansour D, Bahamondes L, Critchley H, Darney P, Fraser IS. The management of unacceptable bleeding patterns in etonogestrel-releasing contraceptive implant users. Contraception 2011;83(3):202-10. DOI: 10.1016/j.contraception .2010.08.001; Simmons KB, Edelman AB, Fu R, Jensen JT. Tamoxifen for the treatment of breakthrough bleeding with the etonogestrel implant: a randomized controlled trial. Contraception 2017;95(2):198-204. DOI: 10.1016/j.contraception.2016 .10.001; Abdel-Aleem H, Shaaban OM, Amin AF, Abdel-Aleem AM. Tamoxifen treatment of bleeding irregularities associated with Norplant® use. Contraception 2005;72(6):432-7. DOI: 10.1016/j.contraception.2005.05.015; Phaliwong P, Taneepanichskul S. The effect of mefenamic acid on controlling irregular uterine bleeding second to Implanon use. J Med Assoc Thai 2004;87 Suppl 3:S64-8. https://www.ncbi.nlm.nih.gov/pubmed/21213495; Diaz S, Croxatto HB, Pavez M, Belhadj H, Stern J, Sivin I. Clinical assessment of treatments for prolonged bleeding in users of Norplant® implants. Contraception 1990;42(1):97-109. DOI: 10.1016/0010-7824(90)90094-c; Abdel-Aleem H, d'Arcangues C, Vogelsong KM, Gaffield ML, Gulmezoglu AM. Treatment of vaginal bleeding irregularities induced by progestin only contraceptives. Cochrane Database Syst Rev 2013(10):CD003449. DOI: 10.1002/14651858.CD003449.pub5; Phupong V, Sophonsritsuk A, Taneepanichskul S. The effect of tranexamic acid for treatment of irregular uterine bleeding secondary to Norplant® use. Contraception 2006;73(3):253-6. DOI: 10.1016/j.contraception.2005.09.012; Zigler RE, Madden T, Ashby C, Wan L, McNicholas C. Ulipristal acetate for unscheduled bleeding in etonogestrel implant users: A randomized controlled trial. Obstet Gynecol 2018;132(4):888-894. DOI: 10.1097/AOG.0000000000002810; Weisberg E, Hickey M, Palmer D, et al. A pilot study to assess the effect of three short-term treatments on frequent and/or prolonged bleeding compared to placebo in women using Implanon. Hum Reprod 2006;21(1):295-302. DOI: 10.1093/humrep/dei273; Cheng L, Zhu H, Wang A, Ren F, Chen J, Glasier A. Once a month administration of mifepristone improves bleeding patterns in women using subdermal contraceptive implants releasing levonorgestrel. Hum Reprod 2000;15(9):1969-72. DOI: 10.1093/humrep/15.9.1969.

provides no benefits during pregnancy. Additionally, patients can be reassured that there is no evidence of increased birth defects with ENG exposure during pregnancy. If the patient terminates the pregnancy and wishes to continue to use the implant, it is prudent to determine why the implant failed in the first place. If a cause can be identified and corrected (such as use of a drug that diminished the implant's effectiveness), then continued reliance on the implant for contraception can be appropriate. If the implant was placed during the luteal phase (after conception and before detection of the pregnancy was possible), clinicians can also discuss with patients about maintaining the same implant if the patient decides not to continue the pregnancy.

Other Problems

Infection at the implant site can be treated with oral antibiotics while the implant remains in place or can be removed pending severity of infection and shared decision making with the patient. If the trial of oral antibiotics does not resolve the infection, or if the infection evolves into a more systemic infectious process, prompt removal should then occur. Pressure dressings can reduce bruising and can prevent enlargement of hematomas. Mild allergic reactions or local irritation usually resolve spontaneously; if bothersome to patient, topical steroids can also be used for treatment. Local superficial venous thrombosis following placement can usually be managed with warm compresses and NSAIDs after neurologic involvement has been ruled out. Rapid removal is recommended whenever neural compression is suspected. Involve neurologists if any neurologic deficits are suspected. If the implant is thought to be in the thoracic cavity, consult with pulmonary specialists.

USER INSTRUCTIONS*

Before you decide to use the Nexplanon implant, be sure to read the FDA-approved product information in case you have any questions that you want to discuss with your clinician during the informed consent process. You can get up-to-date information from your clinician or from websites such as Bedsider.org (see Chapter 27, Digital Resources for Health and Medical Information).

*These instructions are intended to guide providers in educating patients in how to use their method.

1. The contraceptive implant is one of the most effective reversible options for preventing pregnancy. Once the implant is placed, there are no other contraception visits needed until you decide to remove the implant or you have any side effects from using the implant that you want to discuss with the clinician.
2. With the implant, most people notice that their periods change. In general, periods become lighter with time, but people can have all kinds of different bleeding patterns at the beginning. Some people have no bleeding, some have spotting or light bleeding, while others may even experience heavier bleeding or bleeding that goes on for a long time. If you experience spotting or bleeding that bothers you, talk with your clinician about the options that are available to treat the abnormal spotting or bleeding.

3. Some people may experience side effects when using the implant, such as acne, weight changes, and mood changes. If you think these changes may be related to the implant and they do not improve, you can talk with your clinician about what options are available.
4. The implant is placed just under your skin on the inside of your arm. During the implant placement, your clinician will cleanse your skin, apply a numbing medicine, and then place the implant after the skin is numb. The procedure usually takes about 30 seconds.
5. Because you have a nick in your skin, some people may have bruising or even a collection of blood under your skin called a hematoma. Clinicians generally place a wrap on your arm after implant placement to decrease the bruising. There is a very small chance of getting an infection on the skin, a blood clot in the vein, or nerve damage from the implant placement. In very rare cases, the implant may migrate, or move to a different location. You can always touch your arm to make sure that the implant is still in place.
6. If you want to have the implant removed, the clinician will first feel for the implant underneath the skin, cleanse your skin, apply a numbing medicine, and then make a very small cut on the skin after the skin is numb to take out the implant. This usually takes a few minutes. Once the implant is taken out, the hormone from the implant leaves your body very quickly. That means that your ability to get pregnant goes back to whatever is normal for you immediately. For those who do not want to become pregnant, you can have a new implant placed at that time if you want it or you can discuss other options to prevent pregnancy with your clinician if you are interested.
7. The implant is very good at preventing pregnancy for at least 4 years. But that does not mean you have to use it for that whole time! You can keep the implant for the whole 4 years if that is what you want to do, or you can have it taken out at any time before that! You can have it taken out because you want to get pregnant, you don't like it, or for any reason at all—or just because you change your mind—it is your body!

Methods in Development

While subdermal implants are already considered one of the most convenient options due to the efficacy and potential for long-term use, there are several methods in development that may further increase user convenience. Currently, patients are advised to see a clinician for implant placement and for removal. Biodegradable implant systems can provide users with a long-acting, effective contraceptive method that will not require a clinician visit for removal. This method could potentially reduce patient barriers to implant removal, such as access to a trained clinician, appointment availability, and ability to coordinate logistics to attend a health care visit. A Phase 1 study is planned to evaluate the pharmacokinetics, removability, safety, and tolerability of pellets containing ENG, known as Casea S (NCT#05174884). Another avenue of innovation is in the development of multipurpose technologies (MPTs) to address both pregnancy and infection prevention. The only products currently on market that fit this class of products are condoms. While condoms have multiple advantages, including prevention of STIs, this method also has disadvantages that preclude widespread use (see Chapter 16, On-Demand Internal Methods and Chapter 14, External ["Male"] Condoms).

A potential MPT in preclinical development is an implant system releasing ENG or LNG for contraception and tenofovir alafenamide or islatravir for prevention of HIV.[111]

Author Disclosures—Matulich: Research grant from Merck (Organon); Chen: None

Acknowledgment—Thank you to Anita Nelson, MD, Diana Crabtree, MD, Jaclyn Grentzer, MD, MSCI and Elizabeth Raymond, MD MPH, who were all contributing authors to the prior editions of the contraceptive implant chapters.

References

1. Creinin MD, Kaunitz AM, Darney PD, et al. The US etonogestrel implant mandatory clinical training and active monitoring programs: 6-year experience. Contraception. 2017;95(2): 205-210. DOI: 10.1016/j.contraception.2016.07.012.
2. Diaz S, Pavez M, Moo-Young AJ, Bardin CW, Croxatto HB. Clinical trial with 3-keto-desogestrel subdermal implants. Contraception. 1991;44(4):393-408. DOI: 10.1016/0010-7824(91)90030-j.
3. Makarainen L, van Beek A, Tuomivaara L, Asplund B, Coelingh Bennink H. Ovarian function during the use of a single contraceptive implant: Implanon compared with Norplant®. Fertil Steril. 1998;69(4):714-21. DOI: 10.1016/s0015-0282(98)00015-6.
4. Lazorwitz A, Aquilante CL, Dindinger E, Harrison M, Sheeder J, Teal S. Relationship between etonogestrel concentrations and bleeding patterns in contraceptive implant users. Obstet Gynecol. 2019;134(4):807-813. DOI: 10.1097/AOG.0000000000003452.
5. Bahamondes L, Brache V, Meirik O, et al. A 3-year multicentre randomized controlled trial of etonogestrel- and levonorgestrel-releasing contraceptive implants, with non-randomized matched copper-intrauterine device controls. Hum Reprod. 2015;30(11):2527-38. DOI: 10.1093/humrep/dev221.
6. Merck Sharpe & Dohme B.V. Nexplanon® product information sheet. 2018. Available from: https://www.accessdata.fda.gov/drugsatfda_docs/label/2019/021529s018lbl.pdf).
7. McNicholas C, Swor E, Wan L, Peipert JF. Prolonged use of the etonogestrel implant and levonorgestrel intrauterine device: 2 years beyond Food and Drug Administration-approved duration. Am J Obstet Gynecol. 2017;216(6):586 e1-586 e6. DOI: 10.1016/j.ajog.2017.01.036.
8. Ali M, Akin A, Bahamondes L, et al. Extended use up to 5 years of the etonogestrel-releasing subdermal contraceptive implant: comparison to levonorgestrel-releasing subdermal implant. Hum Reprod. 2016;31(11):2491-2498. DOI: 10.1093/humrep/dew222.
9. Committee on Practice Bulletins-Gynecology, Long-Acting Reversible Contracepton Work Group. Practice Bulletin No. 186: Long-Acting Reversible Contraception: Implants and Intrauterine Devices. Obstet Gynecol. 2017;130(5):e251-e269. DOI: 10.1097/AOG.0000000000002400.
10. Tepper NK, Whiteman MK, Marchbanks PA, James AH, Curtis KM. Progestin-only contraception and thromboembolism: A systematic review. Contraception. 2016;94(6):678-700. DOI: 10.1016/j.contraception.2016.04.014.
11. Villas-Boas J, Vilodre LC, Malerba H, Pontremoli Salcedo M, Foresti Jimenez M, El Beitune P. Metabolic safety of the etonogestrel contraceptive implant in healthy women over a 3-year period. Eur J Obstet Gynecol Reprod Biol. 2016;202:51-4. DOI: 10.1016/j.ejogrb.2016.04.025.
12. Oderich CL, Wender MC, Lubianca JN, Santos LM, de Mello GC. Impact of etonogestrel-releasing implant and copper intrauterine device on carbohydrate metabolism: a comparative study. Contraception. 2012;85(2):173-6. DOI: 10.1016/j.contraception.2011.05.018.
13. Curtis KM, Tepper NK, Jatlaoui TC, et al. U.S. Medical Eligibility Criteria for Contraceptive Use, 2016. MMWR Recomm Rep. 2016;65(3):1-103. DOI: 10.15585/mmwr.rr6503a1.
14. Peterson AM, Brown A, Savage A, Dempsey A. Prevalence of early discontinuation and associated factors among a retrospective cohort of etonogestrel contraceptive implant users. Eur J Contracept Reprod Health Care. 2019;24(6):475-479. DOI: 10.1080/13625187.2019.1666361.

15. Law A, Liao L, Lin J, Yaldo A, Lynen R. Twelve-month discontinuation rates of levonorgestrel intrauterine system 13.5 mg and subdermal etonogestrel implant in women aged 18-44: A retrospective claims database analysis. Contraception. 2018. DOI: 10.1016/j.contraception.2018.04.006.
16. Berlan E, Mizraji K, Bonny AE. Twelve-month discontinuation of etonogestrel implant in an outpatient pediatric setting. Contraception. 2016;94(1):81-6. DOI: 10.1016/j.contraception.2016.02.030.
17. Diedrich JT, Zhao Q, Madden T, Secura GM, Peipert JF. Three-year continuation of reversible contraception. Am J Obstet Gynecol. 2015;213(5):662 e1-8. DOI: 10.1016/j.ajog.2015.08.001.
18. Funk S, Miller MM, Mishell DR, Jr., et al. Safety and efficacy of Implanon, a single-rod implantable contraceptive containing etonogestrel. Contraception. 2005;71(5):319-26. DOI: 10.1016/j.contraception.2004.11.007.
19. Ambacher K, Secter M, Sanders AP. The use of progestin subdermal implants in the management of endometriosis-related pain symptoms and quality of life: a systematic review. Curr Med Res Opin. 2022;38(3):479-486. DOI: 10.1080/03007995.2022.2031144.
20. Grandi G, Barra F, Ferrero S, et al. Hormonal contraception in women with endometriosis: a systematic review. Eur J Contracept Reprod Health Care. 2019;24(1):61-70. DOI: 10.1080/13625187.2018.1550576.
21. Frances Fei Y, Ernst SD, Dendrinos ML, Quint EH. Satisfaction with hormonal treatment for menstrual suppression in adolescents and young women with disabilities. J Adolesc. 2021;69(3):482-488. DOI: 10.1016/j.jadohealth.2021.01.031.
22. Hou MY, Davis SL, Ponzini MD, et al. Complex family planning and pediatric hematology oncology integrated clinic for young people with blood disorders and heavy or abnormal menstrual bleeding. Contraception. 2022;108:69-72. DOI: 10.1016/j.contraception.2021.12.014.
23. Buyers E, Sass AE, Severn CD, Pyle L, Cree-Green M. Twelve-month continuation of the etonogestrel implant in adolescents with polycystic ovary syndrome. J Pediatr Adolesc Gynecol. 2021;34(1):33-39. DOI: 10.1016/j.jpag.2020.08.017.
24. Bennink HJ. The pharmacokinetics and pharmacodynamics of Implanon, a single-rod etonogestrel contraceptive implant. Eur J Contracept Reprod Health Care 2000;5 Suppl 2:12-20. Available from: https://www.ncbi.nlm.nih.gov/pubmed/11246602.
25. Croxatto HB, Urbancsek J, Massai R, Coelingh Bennink H, van Beek A. A multicentre efficacy and safety study of the single contraceptive implant Implanon. Implanon Study Group. Hum Reprod 1999;14(4):976-81. DOI: 10.1093/humrep/14.4.976.
26. Curtis KM, Jatlaoui TC, Tepper NK, et al. U.S. Selected Practice Recommendations for Contraceptive Use, 2016. MMWR Recomm Rep. 2016;65(4):1-66. DOI: 10.15585/mmwr.rr6504a1.
27. Reed S, Do Minh T, Lange JA, Koro C, Fox M, Heinemann K. Real world data on Nexplanon(R) procedure-related events: final results from the Nexplanon Observational Risk Assessment study (NORA). Contraception. 2019;100(1):31-36. DOI: 10.1016/j.contraception.2019.03.052.
28. Mommers E, Blum GF, Gent TG, Peters KP, Sordal TS, Marintcheva-Petrova M. Nexplanon, a radiopaque etonogestrel implant in combination with a next-generation applicator: 3-year results of a noncomparative multicenter trial. Am J Obstet Gynecol. 2012;207(5):388 e1-6. DOI: 10.1016/j.ajog.2012.08.002.
29. Brown M, Britton J. Neuropathy associated with etonogestrel implant insertion. Contraception 2012;86(5):591-3. DOI: 10.1016/j.contraception.2012.05.014.
30. Mansour D, Walling M, Glenn D, et al. Removal of non-palpable etonogestrel implants. J Fam Plann Reprod Health Care. 2008;34(2):89-91. Available from: https://www.ncbi.nlm.nih.gov/pubmed/18413020.
31. Darney P, Patel A, Rosen K, Shapiro LS, Kaunitz AM. Safety and efficacy of a single-rod etonogestrel implant (Implanon): results from 11 international clinical trials. Fertil Steril. 2009;91(5):1646-53. DOI: 10.1016/j.fertnstert.2008.02.140.
32. Matulich MC, Chen MJ, Schimmoeller NR, et al. Referral center experience with nonpalpable contraceptive implant removals. Obstet Gynecol. 2019;134(4):801-806. DOI: 10.1097/AOG.0000000000003457.
33. Rowlands S, Mansour D, Walling M. Intravascular migration of contraceptive implants: two more cases. Contraception. 2017;95(2):211-214. DOI: 10.1016/j.contraception.2016.07.015.

34. Diego D, Tappy E, Carugno J. Axillary migration of Nexplanon(R): Case report. Contraception. 2017;95(2):218-220. DOI: 10.1016/j.contraception.2016.11.002.
35. Gallon A, Fontarensky M, Chauffour C, Boyer L, Chabrot P. Looking for a lost subdermal contraceptive implant? Think about the pulmonary artery. Contraception 2017;95(2):215-217. DOI: 10.1016/j.contraception.2016.11.004.
36. Choi JH, Kim HY, Lee SS, Cho S. Migration of a contraceptive subdermal device into the lung. Obstet Gynecol Sci. 2017;60(3):314-317. DOI: 10.5468/ogs.2017.60.3.314.
37. Mansour D, Korver T, Marintcheva-Petrova M, Fraser IS. The effects of Implanon on menstrual bleeding patterns. Eur J Contracept Reprod Health Care. 2008;13 Suppl 1:13-28. DOI: 10.1080/13625180801959931.
38. Vickery Z, Madden T, Zhao Q, Secura GM, Allsworth JE, Peipert JF. Weight change at 12 months in users of three progestin-only contraceptive methods. Contraception. 2013;88(4):503-8. DOI: 10.1016/j.contraception.2013.03.004.
39. Silva Dos Santos PN, Madden T, Omvig K, Peipert JF. Changes in body composition in women using long-acting reversible contraception. Contraception. 2017;95(4):382-389. DOI: 10.1016/j.contraception.2016.12.006.
40. Griffin L, Hammond C, Liu D, Rademaker AW, Kiley J. Postpartum weight loss in overweight and obese women using the etonogestrel subdermal implant: a pilot study. Contraception. 2017;95(6):564-570. DOI: 10.1016/j.contraception.2017.02.020.
41. Harrison-Woolrych M, Hill R. Unintended pregnancies with the etonogestrel implant (Implanon): a case series from postmarketing experience in Australia. Contraception. 2005;71(4):306-8. DOI: 10.1016/j.contraception.2004.10.005.
42. Raine-Bennett T, Fassett MJ, Chandra M, et al. Ectopic pregnancy prevention: Further evidence of benefits of prescription contraceptives. Contraception. 2022;105:19-25. DOI: 10.1016/j.contraception.2021.09.007.
43. Bastow B, Sheeder J, Guiahi M, Teal S. Condom use in adolescents and young women following initiation of long- or short-acting contraceptive methods. Contraception. 2018;97(1):70-75. DOI: 10.1016/j.contraception.2017.10.002.
44. Lemoine J, Teal SB, Peters M, Guiahi M. Motivating factors for dual-method contraceptive use among adolescents and young women: a qualitative investigation. Contraception. 2017;96(5):352-356. DOI: 10.1016/j.contraception.2017.06.011.
45. McNicholas CP, Klugman JB, Zhao Q, Peipert JF. Condom use and incident sexually transmitted infection after initiation of long-acting reversible contraception. Am J Obstet Gynecol. 2017;217(6):672 e1-672 e6. DOI: 10.1016/j.ajog.2017.09.009.
46. Rattray C, Wiener J, Legardy-Williams J, et al. Effects of initiating a contraceptive implant on subsequent condom use: A randomized controlled trial. Contraception. 2015;92(6):560-6. DOI: 10.1016/j.contraception.2015.06.009.
47. Steiner RJ, Pampati S, Kortsmit KM, Liddon N, Swartzendruber A, Pazol K. Long-acting reversible contraception, condom use, and sexually transmitted infections: A systematic review and meta-analysis. Am J Prev Med. 2021;61(5):750-760. DOI: 10.1016/j.amepre.2021.04.032.
48. Mornar S, Chan LN, Mistretta S, Neustadt A, Martins S, Gilliam M. Pharmacokinetics of the etonogestrel contraceptive implant in obese women. Am J Obstet Gynecol. 2012;207(2):110 e1-6. DOI: 10.1016/j.ajog.2012.05.002.
49. Morrell KM, Cremers S, Westhoff CL, Davis AR. Relationship between etonogestrel level and BMI in women using the contraceptive implant for more than 1 year. Contraception. 2016; 93(3):263-5. DOI: 10.1016/j.contraception.2015.11.005.
50. McNicholas C, Maddipati R, Zhao Q, Swor E, Peipert JF. Use of the etonogestrel implant and levonorgestrel intrauterine device beyond the U.S. Food and Drug Administration-approved duration. Obstet Gynecol. 2015;125(3):599-604. DOI: 10.1097/AOG.0000000000000690.
51. Xu H, Wade JA, Peipert JF, Zhao Q, Madden T, Secura GM. Contraceptive failure rates of etonogestrel subdermal implants in overweight and obese women. Obstet Gynecol. 2012;120(1):21-6. DOI: 10.1097/AOG.0b013e318259565a.
52. Lazorwitz A, Davis A, Swartz M, Guiahi M. The effect of carbamazepine on etonogestrel concentrations in contraceptive implant users. Contraception. 2017;95(6):571-577. DOI: 10.1016/j.contraception.2017.03.004.

53. Berry-Bibee EN, Kim MJ, Tepper NK, Riley HE, Curtis KM. Co-administration of St. John's wort and hormonal contraceptives: a systematic review. Contraception. 2016;94(6):668-677. DOI: 10.1016/j.contraception.2016.07.010.
54. Leticee N, Viard JP, Yamgnane A, Karmochkine M, Benachi A. Contraceptive failure of etonogestrel implant in patients treated with antiretrovirals including efavirenz. Contraception. 2012;85(4):425-7. DOI: 10.1016/j.contraception.2011.09.005.
55. Vieira CS, Bahamondes MV, de Souza RM, et al. Effect of antiretroviral therapy including lopinavir/ritonavir or efavirenz on etonogestrel-releasing implant pharmacokinetics in HIV-positive women. J Acquir Immune Defic Syndr. 2014;66(4):378-85. DOI: 10.1097/QAI.0000000000000189.
56. Cowett AA, Ali R, Cooper MA, Evans M, Conzuelo G, Cremer M. Timing of etonogestrel implant insertion after dilation and evacuation: A randomized controlled trial. Obstet Gynecol. 2018;131(5):856-862. DOI: 10.1097/AOG.0000000000002590.
57. Mark A, Sonalkar S, Borgatta L. One-year continuation of the etonogestrel contraceptive implant in women with postabortion or interval placement. Contraception. 2013;88(5):619-23. DOI: 10.1016/j.contraception.2013.05.009.
58. Madden T, Eisenberg DL, Zhao Q, Buckel C, Secura GM, Peipert JF. Continuation of the etonogestrel implant in women undergoing immediate postabortion placement. Obstet Gynecol. 2012;120(5):1053-9. DOI: http://10.1097/AOG.0b013e3182632cd6
59. Sonalkar S, Hou MY, Borgatta L. Administration of the etonogestrel contraceptive implant on the day of mifepristone for medical abortion: a pilot study. Contraception. 2013;88(5):671-3. DOI: 10.1016/j.contraception.2013.07.008.
60. Park J, Robinson N, Wessels U, Turner J, Geller S. Progestin-based contraceptive on the same day as medical abortion. Int J Gynaecol Obstet. 2016;133(2):217-20. DOI: 10.1016/j.ijgo.2015.08.025.
61. Barros Pereira I, Carvalho RM, Graca LM. Intra-abortion contraception with etonogestrel subdermal implant. Eur J Obstet Gynecol Reprod Biol. 2015;185:33-5. DOI: 10.1016/j.ejogrb.2014.11.025.
62. Church E, Sengupta S, Chia KV. The contraceptive implant for long acting reversible contraception in patients undergoing first trimester medical termination of pregnancy. Sex Reprod Health. 2010;1(3):105-9. DOI: 10.1016/j.srhc.2010.02.002.
63. Raymond EG, Weaver MA, Tan YL, et al. Effect of immediate compared With delayed insertion of etonogestrel implants on medical abortion efficacy and repeat pregnancy: A randomized controlled trial. Obstet Gynecol.2016;127(2):306-12. DOI: 10.1097/AOG.0000000000001274.
64. Hognert H, Kopp Kallner H, Cameron S, et al. Immediate versus delayed insertion of an etonogestrel releasing implant at medical abortion-a randomized controlled equivalence trial. Hum Reprod.2016;31(11):2484-2490. DOI: 10.1093/humrep/dew238.
65. Schmidt-Hansen M, Hawkins JE, Lord J, et al. Long-acting reversible contraception immediately after medical abortion: systematic review with meta-analyses. Hum Reprod Update. 2020;26(2):141-160. DOI: 10.1093/humupd/dmz040.
66. Wu M, Eisenberg R, Negassa A, Levi E. Associations between immediate postpartum long-acting reversible contraception and short interpregnancy intervals. Contraception. 2020;102(6):409-413. DOI: 10.1016/j.contraception.2020.08.016.
67. Cohen R, Sheeder J, Arango N, Teal SB, Tocce K. Twelve-month contraceptive continuation and repeat pregnancy among young mothers choosing postdelivery contraceptive implants or postplacental intrauterine devices. Contraception. 2016;93(2):178-83. DOI: 10.1016/j.contraception.2015.10.001.
68. Tocce KM, Sheeder JL, Teal SB. Rapid repeat pregnancy in adolescents: do immediate postpartum contraceptive implants make a difference? Am J Obstet Gynecol. 2012;206(6):481 e1-7. DOI: 10.1016/j.ajog.2012.04.015.
69. Lawrence R, Lawrence R. Breastfeeding: A Guide for the Medical Profession. 9th ed. Philadelphia, PA: Elsevier, 2022.
70. Brownell E, Howard CR, Lawrence RA, Dozier AM. Delayed onset lactogenesis II predicts the cessation of any or exclusive breastfeeding. J Pediatr 2012;161(4):608-14. DOI: 10.1016/j.jpeds.2012.03.035.

71. Gurtcheff SE, Turok DK, Stoddard G, Murphy PA, Gibson M, Jones KP. Lactogenesis after early postpartum use of the contraceptive implant: a randomized controlled trial. Obstet Gynecol. 2011;117(5):1114-1121. DOI: 10.1097/AOG.0b013e3182165ee8.
72. Braga GC, Ferriolli E, Quintana SM, Ferriani RA, Pfrimer K, Vieira CS. Immediate postpartum initiation of etonogestrel-releasing implant: A randomized controlled trial on breastfeeding impact. Contraception. 2015;92(6):536-42. DOI: 10.1016/j.contraception.2015.07.009.
73. Carmo L, Braga GC, Ferriani RA, Quintana SM, Vieira CS. Timing of etonogestrel-releasing implants and growth of breastfed infants: A randomized controlled trial. Obstet Gynecol. 2017;130(1):100-107. DOI: 10.1097/AOG.0000000000002092.
74. Averbach S, Kakaire O, McDiehl R, Dehlendorf C, Lester F, Steinauer J. The effect of immediate postpartum levonorgestrel contraceptive implant use on breastfeeding and infant growth: a randomized controlled trial. Contraception. 2019;99(2):87-93. DOI: 10.1016/j.contraception.2018.10.008.
75. Phillips SJ, Tepper NK, Kapp N, Nanda K, Temmerman M, Curtis KM. Progestogen-only contraceptive use among breastfeeding women: a systematic review. Contraception. 2016;94(3): 226-52. DOI: 10.1016/j.contraception.2015.09.010.
76. Ross L, Solinger R. Reproductive Justice: An Introduction. 1st ed. Oakland, CA: University of California Press, 2017.
77. Gold RB. Some lawmakers continue to promote contraceptive use in return for welfare. State Reprod Health Monit 1995;6(1):3, 6. Available from: https://www.ncbi.nlm.nih.gov/pubmed/12289005.
78. Poleon S, Thompson EL. Reasons for intent to discontinue and remove long-acting reversible contraceptives: National Survey of Family Growth 2017-2019. J Womens Health (Larchmt). 2022;31(5):733-740. DOI: 10.1089/jwh.2021.0272.
79. Amico JR, Bennett AH, Karasz A, Gold M. "She just told me to leave it": Women's experiences discussing early elective IUD removal. Contraception 2016;94(4):357-61. DOI: 10.1016/j.contraception.2016.04.012.
80. Amico JR, Bennett AH, Karasz A, Gold M. "I wish they could hold on a little longer": physicians' experiences with requests for early IUD removal. Contraception. 2017;96(2):106-110. DOI: 10.1016/j.contraception.2017.05.007.
81. Broussard K, Becker A. Self-removal of long-acting reversible contraception: A content analysis of YouTube videos. Contraception. 2021;104(6):654-658. DOI: 10.1016/j.contraception.2021.08.002.
82. Reeves MF, Zhao Q, Secura GM, Peipert JF. Risk of unintended pregnancy based on intended compared to actual contraceptive use. Am J Obstet Gynecol. 2016;215(1):71 e1-6. DOI: 10.1016/j.ajog.2016.01.162.
83. Wilkinson TA, Edmonds BT, Cheng ER. Outcomes of a two-visit protocol for long acting reversible contraception for adolescents and young adults. Contraception. 2022;105:33-36. DOI: 10.1016/j.contraception.2021.07.107.
84. Richards M, Teal SB, Sheeder J. Risk of luteal phase pregnancy with any-cycle-day initiation of subdermal contraceptive implants. Contraception 2017;95(4):364-370. DOI: 10.1016/j.contraception.2017.01.010.
85. Pymar HC, Creinin MD, Schwartz JL. “Pop-out” method of levonorgestrel implant removal. Contraception. 1999;59(6):383-7. DOI: 10.1016/s0010-7824(99)00048-7.
86. Pearson S, Stewart M, Bateson D. Implanon NXT: Expert tips for best-practice insertion and removal. Aust Fam Physician 2017;46(3):104-108. Available from: https://www.ncbi.nlm.nih.gov/pubmed/28260268).
87. Kwal J, Maguire K, Carugno J. Localization and management of nonpalpable radiopaque contraceptive implant. Contraception. 2022;106:3-5. DOI: 10.1016/j.contraception.2021.10.002.
88. Biskamp C, Kauffman RP. Arm flexion during ultrasound assists localization of an intramuscular etonogestrel contraceptive implant. Contraception. 2016;93(3):273-5. DOI: 10.1016/j.contraception.2015.11.004.
89. Chen MJ, Creinin MD. Removal of a nonpalpable etonogestrel implant With preprocedure ultrasonography and modified vasectomy clamp. Obstet Gynecol. 2015;126(5):935-938. DOI: 10.1097/AOG.0000000000001082.

90. Persaud T, Walling M, Geoghegan T, Buckley O, Stunell H, Torreggiani WC. Ultrasound-guided removal of Implanon devices. Eur Radiol. 2008;18(11):2582-5. DOI: 10.1007/s00330-008-1055-1.
91. Nelson AL, Sinow RM. Real-time ultrasonographically guided removal of nonpalpable and intramuscular Norplant® capsules. Am J Obstet Gynecol. 1998;178(6):1185-93. DOI: 10.1016/s0002-9378(98)70321-7.
92. Nouri K, Pinker-Domenig K, Ott J, Fraser I, Egarter C. Removal of non-palpable Implanon(R) with the aid of a hook-wire marker. Contraception. 2013;88(4):577-80. DOI: 10.1016/j.contraception.2013.05.002.
93. Vollans SR, Grainger A, O'Connor P, Limb D. Hormone-releasing contraceptive implants: our experience of complex removals using preoperative ultrasound. Contraception. 2015;92(1):81-3. DOI: 10.1016/j.contraception.2015.03.015.
94. Guiahi M, Tocce K, Teal S, Green T, Rochon P. Removal of a Nexplanon implant located in the biceps muscle using a combination of ultrasound and fluoroscopy guidance. Contraception. 2014;90(6):606-8. DOI: 10.1016/j.contraception.2014.06.030.
95. Mastey N, Matulich MC, Uhm S, et al. US referral center experience removing nonpalpable and difficult contraceptive implants with in-office ultrasonography: A case series. Contraception. 2021;103(6):428-430. DOI: 10.1016/j.contraception.2021.01.018.
96. van den Heuvel MW, van Bragt AJ, Alnabawy AK, Kaptein MC. Comparison of ethinylestradiol pharmacokinetics in three hormonal contraceptive formulations: the vaginal ring, the transdermal patch and an oral contraceptive. Contraception. 2005;72(3):168-74. DOI: 10.1016/j.contraception.2005.03.005.
97. Hou MY, McNicholas C, Creinin MD. Combined oral contraceptive treatment for bleeding complaints with the etonogestrel contraceptive implant: a randomised controlled trial. Eur J Contracept Reprod Health Care. 2016;21(5):361-6. DOI: 10.1080/13625187.2016.1210122.
98. Guiahi M, McBride M, Sheeder J, Teal S. Short-term treatment of bothersome bleeding for etonogestrel implant users using a 14-day oral contraceptive pill regimen: A randomized controlled trial. Obstet Gynecol. 2015;126(3):508-513. DOI: 10.1097/AOG.0000000000000974.
99. Chen MJ, Hsia JK, Creinin MD. Etonogestrel implant use in women primarily choosing a combined oral contraceptive pill: A proof-of-concept trial. Contraception. 2018;97(6):533-537. DOI: 10.1016/j.contraception.2018.02.009.
100. Zigler RE, McNicholas C. Unscheduled vaginal bleeding with progestin-only contraceptive use. Am J Obstet Gynecol. 2017;216(5):443-450. DOI: 10.1016/j.ajog.2016.12.008.
101. Mansour D, Bahamondes L, Critchley H, Darney P, Fraser IS. The management of unacceptable bleeding patterns in etonogestrel-releasing contraceptive implant users. Contraception. 2011;83(3):202-10. DOI: 10.1016/j.contraception.2010.08.001.
102. Simmons KB, Edelman AB, Fu R, Jensen JT. Tamoxifen for the treatment of breakthrough bleeding with the etonogestrel implant: a randomized controlled trial. Contraception. 2017;95(2):198-204. DOI: 10.1016/j.contraception.2016.10.001.
103. Abdel-Aleem H, Shaaban OM, Amin AF, Abdel-Aleem AM. Tamoxifen treatment of bleeding irregularities associated with Norplant® use. Contraception. 2005;72(6):432-7. DOI: 10.1016/j.contraception.2005.05.015.
104. Zigler RE, Madden T, Ashby C, Wan L, McNicholas C. Ulipristal acetate for unscheduled bleeding in etonogestrel implant users: A randomized controlled trial. Obstet Gynecol. 2018;132(4):888-894. DOI: 10.1097/AOG.0000000000002810.
105. Weisberg E, Hickey M, Palmer D, et al. A pilot study to assess the effect of three short-term treatments on frequent and/or prolonged bleeding compared to placebo in women using Implanon. Hum Reprod. 2006;21(1):295-302. DOI: 10.1093/humrep/dei273.
106. Cheng L, Zhu H, Wang A, Ren F, Chen J, Glasier A. Once a month administration of mifepristone improves bleeding patterns in women using subdermal contraceptive implants releasing levonorgestrel. Hum Reprod. 2000;15(9):1969-72. DOI: 10.1093/humrep/15.9.1969.
107. Phaliwong P, Taneepanichskul S. The effect of mefenamic acid on controlling irregular uterine bleeding second to Implanon use. J Med Assoc Thai. 2004;87 Suppl 3:S64-8. (https://www.ncbi.nlm.nih.gov/pubmed/21213495).

108. Diaz S, Croxatto HB, Pavez M, Belhadj H, Stern J, Sivin I. Clinical assessment of treatments for prolonged bleeding in users of Norplant® implants. Contraception. 1990;42(1):97-109. DOI: 10.1016/0010-7824(90)90094-c.
109. Abdel-Aleem H, d'Arcangues C, Vogelsong KM, Gaffield ML, Gulmezoglu AM. Treatment of vaginal bleeding irregularities induced by progestin only contraceptives. Cochrane Database Syst Rev. 2013(10):CD003449. DOI: 10.1002/14651858.CD003449.pub5.
110. Phupong V, Sophonsritsuk A, Taneepanichskul S. The effect of tranexamic acid for treatment of irregular uterine bleeding secondary to Norplant® use. Contraception. 2006;73(3):253-6. DOI: 10.1016/j.contraception.2005.09.012.
111. Li L, Gatto GJ, Brand RM, et al. Long-acting biodegradable implant for sustained delivery of antiretrovirals (ARVs) and hormones. J Control Release. 2021;340:188-199. DOI: 10.1016/j.jconrel.2021.10.021.

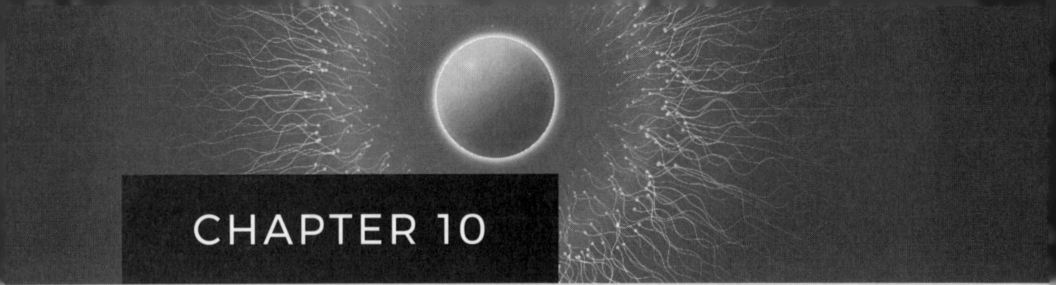

CHAPTER 10

Intrauterine Devices (IUDs)

Nicole Economou, MD, MPH
Biftu Mengesha, MD, MAS
Eleanor Bimla Schwarz, MD, MS*

KEY POINTS

- IUDs are among the safest, most convenient, and well-liked methods of contraception.
- IUDs are the most commonly used reversible contraceptives in the world.
- IUDs are over 20 times more effective than pills and at least as effective as permanent contraception.
- IUDs are among the most cost-effective contraceptives available.
- IUDs are safe for adolescents and nulliparous individuals.
- IUDs are promptly reversible and pose virtually no risk to future fertility.
- Levonorgestrel IUDs reduce dysmenorrhea, anemia, and risk of endometrial cancer.
- IUDs are the most effective form of emergency contraception.

Intrauterine devices (IUDs) are among the most effective, safest, and well-liked methods of contraception available. IUDs are broadly categorized as nonhormonal IUDs and hormonal IUDs. While pharmaceutical companies have introduced various acronyms for IUDs in marketing materials, this has led to confusion in classification of devices and as a result, the World Health Organization and other professional societies have recommended standard nomenclature when referring to IUDs, including discontinuing the use of terms such as "intrauterine systems (IUS)."[1]

Worldwide, the IUD is the most commonly used reversible method of contraception.[2] In China, Korea, and Vietnam, IUDs are used by over 40% of married women of reproductive age; in Europe, 6% to 16% of such women use IUDs.[2] The United States (US) has been slower to adopt intrauterine contraception, and in 2002, only 2% of US contraceptive users chose an IUD.[3] However, by 2016 the

* Authors contributed equally to this manuscript.

prevalence of use grew to 18%.[4] It is estimated that 40% of US family planning clinicians use an IUD for their personal contraceptive needs.[5]

Widespread use of IUDs in the United States was historically limited by negative publicity; misinformation about the risks of ectopic pregnancy, infection, and subsequent infertility; misconceptions about the mechanism of action; lack of clinician training; and fears of litigation.[6] In the 1970s, only 10% of US contraceptive users chose IUDs.[7] Research from this period associated IUDs, particularly the Dalkon Shield, with an increased risk of pelvic inflammatory disease (PID)[8] and septic abortion, and use of IUDs subsequently fell until the first part of the 21st century.[9] In addition, in the 1970s, it was not possible to test for asymptomatic chlamydia. As such, early studies of the associations between IUDs and PID suffered from methodological flaws; data on modern IUDs show no increase in PID in new IUD users.[10,11]

The IUDs available in the 1970s differed from modern IUDs in design and efficacy. Early IUDs were inert (plastic only) and had 1-year failure rates of 2%[12] to 9%,[13,14] while modern IUDs have copper or LNG added to a polyethylene frame; these additions improve contraceptive efficacy by an order of magnitude.[13] Modern IUDs have monofilament threads that have not been associated with infections[15] or other adverse outcomes in comparison to the Dalkon Shield, which had a polyfilamentous thread. In recent years, a number of new IUDs have been introduced to the US and international markets. All available IUDs are safer and more effective than oral contraceptives. When cost is an issue, Liletta is noteworthy as a low-cost option. Otherwise, the primary difference among currently available IUDs is their effect on menstrual bleeding patterns and potential duration of use.

IUD use in the US has also been impacted by a range of sociopolitical structures that have adversely impacted communities of color, individuals with low income or who receive government financial benefits, individuals with disabilities, and those in the carceral system, all of whom have experienced contraceptive coercion. A person-centered, noncoercive approach to contraceptive counseling and provision of IUDs is critical to advancing reproductive justice. (See Chapter 4, Person-centered Reproductive Health Conversations and Contraceptive Counseling.) Unfortunately, injustices in reproductive control date to the founding of the US. More recent enthusiasm for long-acting contraceptive methods have included problematic programs requiring individuals receiving welfare benefits to use high-efficacy contraceptive methods.[16] There also have been reports of clinicians downplaying IUD side effects and discouraging removal within the first year of use.[17] IUDs have been promoted as a "cure" for poverty,[18,19] reminiscent of eugenic policies and laws in the 20th century. Additional concerns have been raised that clinicians disproportionately counsel low-income patients to consider an IUD if they are Black than if they are White[20] and recommend long-acting methods to those from socially marginalized groups.[21] Family planning clinicians striving to serve our communities must be mindful of this painful context. The possibility of self-removal by the user is an important difference between IUDs and the other highly effective reversible contraceptive, the subdermal implant. Awareness of the option of IUD self-removal remains less common than it should be.[22]

IUD Options in the United States

As of 2022, there are five IUDs available in the United US (see **Table 10-1**). All of these are made of polyethylene with barium sulfate added to create X-ray visibility and can be safely imaged using MRI.[23] The copper IUD is highly echogenic on

Table 10-1 Characteristics of IUDs Available in the United States in 2023

	Copper 380 mm^2 IUD (Paragard)	LNG 52 mg IUD (Mirena)	LNG 52 mg IUD (Liletta*)	LNG 19.5 mg IUD (Kyleena)	LNG 13.5 mg IUD (Skyla†)
Contains	380 mm^2 copper	52 mg LNG	52 mg LNG	19.5 mg LNG	13.5 mg LNG
LNG release/day (1st year)	0 mcg	20 mcg	20 mcg	12 mcg	8 mcg
Evidence-based use	**12-20 years[24,25]**	**8 years[26]**	**8 years[26]**	**5 years[27]**	**3 years[27]**
FDA-labeled use	10 years	8 years	8 years	5 years	3 years
FDA approval year	1984	2000	2015	2016	2013
LNG serum concentration over 3 years of use[21]	0 ng/L	218 ng/L	218 ng/L	114 ng/L	74.3 ng/L
Approximate placement tube diameter	4.40 mm	4.40 mm	4.80 mm	3.80 mm	3.80 mm
Size of frame (mm)	32 × 36	32 × 32	32 × 32	28 × 30	28 × 30
Silver ring on T	No	No	No	Yes	Yes
Thread color	White	Brown	Blue	Blue	Brown
Ovulatory cycles (%)	All (No change from baseline)	45% at 1 year 75% at 4 years[28]	45% at 1 year 75% at 4 years[28]	Almost all (Almost no change from baseline)	Almost all (Almost no change from baseline)
Amenorrhea at 1 year	0% (No change from baseline)	15%[29] to 24%[30]	15%[29] to 24%[30]	13%[30]	6%[31]
Amenorrhea at 2 years	0% (No change from baseline)	10%[30] to 26%[32]	10%[30] to 26%[32]	20%[33]	10%[31]

(continues)

Table 10-1 Characteristics of IUDs available in the United States in 2023 *(continued)*

	Copper 380 mm^2 IUD (Paragard)	LNG 52 mg IUD (Mirena)	LNG 52 mg IUD (Liletta*)	LNG 19.5 mg IUD (Kyleena)	LNG 13.5 mg IUD (Skyla†)
1st year Pearl Index (95% CI)	0.7[34]	0.19[35]	0.15 (0.02–0.55)[36]	0.16 (0.02–0.58)[27]	0.48 (0.13–1.23)[31]
Lifetime Pearl Index (95% CI)	0.52 (0.42–0.64)[37]	0.06 (0.04–0.09)[37]	0.06 (0.04–0.09)[37]	0.29 (0.16–0.50)[27]	0.9 (0.4–1.9)[31]
Need for backup contraception[32] after placement‡	None	0–7 days^[38]	0–7 days^[38]	7 days	7 days

*Marketed as Levosert in the UK

†Marketed as Jaydess in Asia

‡Unless placed postabortion, postpartum, or within 7 days of beginning last menstrual period

^Can be used for emergency contraception with shared decision making with patients

"Data from Gomez AM, Fuentes L, Allina A. Women or LARC first? Reproductive autonomy and the promotion of long-acting reversible contraceptive methods. Perspect Sex Reprod Health 2014;46(3):171-5. DOI: 10.1363/46e1614; Long-term reversible contraception. Twelve years of experience with the TCu380A and TCu220C. Contraception 1997;56(6):341–52; Sivin I. Utility and drawbacks of continuous use of a copper T IUD for 20 years. Contraception [Internet] 2007 [cited 2022 Feb 5];75(6 Suppl). Available from: https://pubmed.ncbi.nlm.nih.gov/17531620/; Creinin MD, Schreiber CA, Turok DK, Cwiak C, Chen BA, Olariu AI. Levonorgestrel 52 mg intrauterine system efficacy and safety through 8 years of use. Am J Obstet Gynecol 2022;227(6):871.e1-871.e7; Gemzell-Danielsson K, Apter D, Dermout S, et al. Evaluation of a new, low-dose levonorgestrel intrauterine contraceptive system over 5 years of use. Eur J Obstet Gynecol Reprod Biol [Internet] 2017 [cited 2022 Feb 27];210:22–8. Available from: https://pubmed.ncbi.nlm.nih.gov/27930941/; Mirena package insert [Internet]. 2021 [cited 2022 Mar 12]. Available from: https://labeling.bayerhealthcare.com/html/products/pi/Mirena_PI.pdf; Mejia M, McNicholas C, Madden T, Peipert JF. Association of baseline bleeding pattern on amenorrhea with levonorgestrel intrauterine system use. Contraception [Internet] 2016 [cited 2022 Feb 5];94(5):556–60. Available from: https://pubmed.ncbi.nlm.nih.gov/27364099/; Rowe P, Farley T, Peregoudov A, et al. Safety and efficacy in parous women of a 52-mg levonorgestrel-medicated intrauterine device: A 7-year randomized comparative study with the TCu380A. Contraception [Internet] 2016 [cited 2022 Feb 5];93(6):498–506. Available from: http://www.contraceptionjournal.org/article/S0010782416000718/fulltext; Fan G, Kang S, Ren M, et al. A single-arm phase III study exploring the efficacy and safety of LNG-IUS 8, a low-dose levonorgestrel intrauterine contraceptive system (total content 13.5 mg), in an Asia-Pacific population. Contraception [Internet] 2017 [cited 2022 Feb 5];95(4):371–7. Available from: https://pubmed.ncbi.nlm.nih.gov/27913229/; Liletta Package Insert [Internet]. 2020 [cited 2022 Mar 12]. Available from: https://media.allergan.com/actavis/actavis/media/allergan-pdf-documents/product-prescribing/liletta_pi.pdf; Kyleena Levonorgestrel-releasing intrauterine system (19.5 mg) [Internet]. 2021 [cited 2022 Mar 12]. Available from: https://www.bayer.com/sites/default/files/2020-11/kyleena-pm-en.pdf; Sivin I, Schmidt F, Waldman S. The Copper T 380 intrauterine device: a summary of scientific data. In: The Population Council. New York: 1992; Application Number 21-225: Medical Review of Mirena. In: Center for Drug Research and Evaluation. 2000; Eisenberg DL, Schreiber CA, Turok DK, Teal SB, Westhoff CL, Creinin MD. Three-year efficacy and safety of a new 52-mg levonorgestrel-releasing intrauterine system. Contraception 2015;92(1):10–6; Heinemann K, Reed S, Moehner S, do Minh T. Comparative contraceptive effectiveness of levonorgestrel-releasing and copper intrauterine devices: the European Active Surveillance Study for Intrauterine Devices. Contraception [Internet] 2015 [cited 2022 Feb 27];91(4):280–3. Available from: https://pubmed.ncbi.nlm.nih.gov/25601350/; Turok DK, Gero A, Simmons RG, et al. Levonorgestrel vs. Copper intrauterine devices for emergency contraception. N Engl J Med [Internet] 2021 [cited 2021 Oct 12];384(4):335–44. Available from: https://www.nejm.org/doi/full/10.1056/NEJMoa2022141

ultrasound and thus relatively easy to locate within the uterus. LNG IUDs produce an echolucent (dark) sonographic shadow and can be more difficult to identify with ultrasound, although two of the newer IUDs contain a silver ring on the stem to aid in identification.

Copper 380 mm^2 (Paragard) IUD

The copper 380 mm^2 IUD was introduced in the United States in 1988. It (or the functional equivalents TCu380Ag and TCuT380 slimline) is now available in most countries around the world and has been used by tens of millions of people. The copper 380 mm^2 IUD is the only highly effective, reversible contraceptive method that is hormone-free. Fine copper wire is wound around the vertical stem of the T, and each of the two horizontal arms holds a sleeve of copper. The combined copper surface area of the stem and sleeves is 380 ± 23 mm^2. The device is latex-free and clinically relevant allergy to copper is extremely rare.[39] Serum copper levels are higher in copper 380 mm^2 IUD users compared with nonusers and may be above the normal blood copper level range;[40] however, adverse clinical effects of this elevated blood copper level have not been noted among the millions of people who have used copper 380 mm^2 IUDs worldwide. The copper 380 mm^2 IUD is labeled for 10 years of use, although data indicate high effectiveness for 12 years,[24] and no pregnancies were reported among the few who retained the copper 380 mm^2 IUD for 20 years.[25] Cumulative pregnancy rates for the copper 380 mm^2 IUD are 0.5% to 0.8% (first year),[41,42] 1.4% to 2.5% (7 years),[39,43,44] and 2.2% (12 years).[24] Inert IUDs and copper IUDs with less than 380 mm^2 of copper are less effective than those containing 380 mm^2 or more of copper and are no longer available in the United States.[45,46] In 2005, the US Food and Drug Administration (FDA) clarified package labeling for the copper 380 mm^2 IUD, removing any proscription against use by nulliparous individuals or individuals with more than one sexual partner. Copper 380 mm^2 IUD labeling now also supports placement immediately after an abortion or delivery.

Levonorgestrel IUDs

Currently, there are four LNG IUDs available in the United States. All have T-shaped frames with a reservoir containing levonorgestrel dispersed in polydimethylsiloxane molded around the vertical stem. The reservoirs are covered with a silicone membrane that regulates the release of the hormone. The stems have monofilament polyethylene threads attached to the base to assist with removal. Mirena and Liletta have identical frame sizes and contain 52 mg of LNG. Kyleena and Skyla have slightly smaller frames and lower doses of LNG (19.5 mg and 13.5 mg, respectively). In other countries, IUDs are available with LNG doses as low as 8 mg.[27] Small amounts of levonorgestrel are systemically absorbed and some systemic side effects can occur. However, the daily systemic dose of levonorgestrel with use of a 52 mg LNG IUD[47-49] is about 10% that of an oral contraceptive containing 150 mcg LNG,[50] and the systemic dose of lower dose LNG IUDs is even lower.

52 mg LNG IUDs (Liletta, Mirena)

Millions of individuals in 120 countries around the world[1] have used an LNG 52 mg IUD. The first LNG 52 mg IUD (Mirena) was approved for use in Europe in the early

1990s and in the United States in 2000; it was first sold in the United States in 2001. In 2015, the FDA approved the lower-cost Liletta IUD,[48] which has an identical frame size (32 mm in both height and width), levonorgestrel content, and performance characteristics, although a different inserter. These IUDs release LNG into the endometrial cavity at an initial rate of 19–20 mcg per day,[32] declining to 10 mcg per day after 5 years.[28,49] Cumulative pregnancy rates for the LNG 52 mg IUD are 0.1% to 0.2% (first year),[51,52] 0.5% to 1.1% (5 years),[53,54] and 0.5% (7 years).[43,47,55-59] For emergency contraception, the 52 mg LNG IUD is noninferior to the copper IUD within a margin of 2.5%.[38] Like the copper 380 mm^2 IUD, use of the LNG 52 mg IUD for emergency contraception is evidence-based; however, it is not FDA labeled for this indication.

19.5 mg LNG IUD (Kyleena)

FDA-approved in 2016, the newest IUD available in the United States contains 19.5 mg of LNG at initial placement, with an average daily release rate of 9.8 mcg after 1 year and 7.4 at 5 years.[33] This IUD is labeled by the FDA for 5 years of use, and its cumulative 5-year pregnancy rate is 1.1% ± 0.5%.[53] Extended use of this IUD beyond 5 years may be reasonable given the studies of IUDs containing lower doses of LNG,[29,60] described below.

13.5 mg LNG IUD (Skyla)

FDA-approved in 2013, this IUD contains 13.5 mg of LNG at initial placement and has an average daily release rate of 8 mcg in the first year,[60] declining to approximately 5 mcg at 3 years. This IUD is labeled by the FDA for 3 years of use; it has a first year Pearl Index of 0.48 and a lifetime Pearl Index of 0.9.[29]

Mechanism of Action

IUDs work primarily by preventing sperm from fertilizing ova.[61] Pregnancy is prevented by a combination of the “foreign body effect” of the plastic frame and the specific action of the active ingredient (copper or levonorgestrel) that is released. Exposure to a foreign body causes changes in the intrauterine environment that are toxic to sperm and ova and may impair implantation.[62,63] The production of cytotoxic peptides and activation of enzymes lead to inhibition of sperm motility, reduced sperm capacitation and survival, and increased phagocytosis of sperm and likely ova.[64-66] Copper ions released by the copper 380 mm^2 IUD cause an increase in enzymes, prostaglandins, and white blood cells (macrophages) in uterine and tubal fluids; these impair sperm function and prevent fertilization. The progestin in LNG IUDs thickens cervical mucus, suppresses the endometrium by reducing uterine artery blood flow,[67] and impairs sperm function by changing the uterine immune microenvironment.[68,69] In addition, ovulation may be impaired because of systemic absorption of levonorgestrel.[57] Ovulation suppression is greatest in the initial year of use and with higher LNG levels. According to package inserts, among women using a 52 mg LNG IUD for 1 year, 45% of cycles were ovulatory, and at 4 years, 75% were ovulatory, while with the 19.5 mg and 13.5 mg LNG IUDs, almost all cycles are ovulatory.

Three lines of evidence indicate that IUDs primarily work early in the reproductive process to prevent fertilization, rather than implantation.[41] First, human chorionic gonadotropin assays for early pregnancy do not reveal "chemical pregnancies."[70-72] Second, studies in women undergoing tubal sterilization at mid-cycle, in which the fallopian tubes were flushed and the fluid examined with a microscope to identify fertilized eggs, show markedly fewer fertilized, normally dividing eggs were recovered from IUD users than women using no contraception.[66] Third, IUD users have a significantly decreased risk of ectopic pregnancy compared to women using no contraception,[37,73] which implies that IUDs inhibit fertilization.

Effectiveness

All IUDs available in the United States rank in the top tier of contraceptive effectiveness. IUDs are typically over 20 times as effective as oral contraceptives.[74] (See Table 5-2 in Chapter 5.) IUDs with 52 mg LNG are the most effective IUDs,[37,73] with a cumulative 7-year pregnancy rate of 0.5%, compared with 2.5% for the copper 380 mm^2 IUD.[55] The effectiveness of the copper 380 mm^2 IUD is comparable to permanent contraception via tubal ligation (which has pregnancy rates of 1.3% at 5 years and 1.9% at 10 years[75]), while 52 mg LNG IUDs typically are more effective than tubal ligation.[76] The only contraceptive option more effective than the 52 mg LNG IUD is the subdermal contraceptive implant.[77] As an IUD's LNG dose decreases, the efficacy of the IUD decreases; however, the 13.5 mg LNG IUD appears to be at least as effective as the copper 380 mm^2 IUD.[78] The effectiveness of the copper 380 mm^2 IUD remains high over long-term use; at 12 years the cumulative pregnancy rate is only 2.2%.[79] (See Chapter 5, Effectiveness, Safety, and Comparative Side Effects.)

Cost-Effectiveness

One office visit for IUD placement can provide years of highly effective contraception at a low daily cost. Although the initial cost of an IUD can be high, the overall cost decreases with each year of use,[80] and the costs of undesired pregnancy are considerably higher.[81–83] For individuals with obesity, a levonorgestrel IUD is also a cost-effective strategy for prevention of deaths from endometrial cancer.[84,85]

Advantages

Advantages of IUD contraception include the following:

- High user satisfaction
- High effectiveness
- Impressive safety
- Few contraindications to use; no estrogen
- Convenient and private
- Potential for long-term protection
- Rapid reversibility
- Reduce endometrial cancer risk (with obesity, tamoxifen, and postmenopausal estrogen)
- Reduced dysmenorrhea and menstrual blood loss (LNG IUDs)
- Nearly 100% effective as emergency contraception

- Immediate placement after end of pregnancy (post-abortion, miscarriage, or delivery)
- The possibility of self-removal

The possibility of self-removal by the user is an important difference between IUDs and the other highly effective reversible contraceptive, the subdermal implant. Thread length affects ability to self-remove an IUD, as was demonstrated in one study, in which only 20% of patients who attempted self-removal were successful; therefore, clinicians should clarify patients' preferences before trimming IUD threads.[86] For individuals facing reproductive coercion, IUDs can be made undetectable (except by clinical imaging) by using sterile scissors to remove the threads prior to placement.

User Satisfaction and Continuation Rates

Several studies have demonstrated the effectiveness of the copper 380 mm^2 IUD beyond the duration of use noted on product label. As IUD replacement often causes some discomfort and carries a small risk of uterine perforation or ascending infection, continued use is often advantageous. Satisfaction and continuation rates for IUDs are higher than for all other reversible contraceptives at 1 year (ranging from 78%, as shown in Table 5-2, to 90%).[56,87-90] Although satisfaction and continuation rates are a bit higher for 52 mg LNG than copper 380 mm^2 IUD users at 1 year (satisfaction rates 86% versus 80%, respectively),[90] continuation rates for both IUDs are 77% to 79% at 2 years,[91] 70% at 3 years,[92] greater than 60% at 4 years, and 50% at 5 years.[93]

Ectopic Pregnancy Prevention

Individuals with a history of ectopic pregnancy can safely use either a copper or LNG IUD.[94] In fact, people using no contraception are 10 times more likely than IUD users to develop an ectopic pregnancy.[95]

Protection from Pelvic Inflammatory Disease (PID)

Individuals at risk for or with a history of sexually transmitted infection (STI) or history of PID can safely use an IUD.[96] LNG IUDs, like all progestin-containing contraceptives, decrease risk of PID by thickening cervical mucus, which acts as a barrier to ascending infection.[97,98] All individuals at risk of STI should be encouraged to consider condom use. (See Chapter 23, Reproductive Tract Infections, Including HIV and Other Sexually Transmitted Infections.) If screening for STIs is indicated, screening may be done at the time of IUD placement; those found to be infected can be treated with the IUD in place.[99]

Cancer Protection

Copper IUD use has been associated with lower rates of cervical cancer,[100,101] even after controlling for rates of screening for cervical cancer. Both copper and LNG IUDs have been associated with a reduction in the risk of endometrial cancer. Although the specific mechanism of action by which the copper IUD protects against endometrial cancer is unknown, it may relate to alterations in the endometrium.[102,103] Similarly, progestin-releasing intrauterine contraception has also been shown to protect against endometrial cancer[104] by decreasing endometrial proliferation, as do contraceptives that deliver a progestin systemically.[105] LNG IUDs suppress the endometrium by reducing uterine artery blood flow.[67] The 52 mg LNG IUD has been used to prevent development of endometrial hyperplasia in people using perimenopausal estrogen therapy[106-108] or tamoxifen[104,109,110]; other LNG IUDs may also provide this endometrial protection but have not been studied. The 52 mg LNG IUD also has been used for the treatment of nonatypical endometrial hyperplasia, atypical hyperplasia, and grade 1 stage I endometrial cancer.[110-114] LNG IUD use also has been associated with lower rates of ovarian cancer,[115,116] pancreatic cancer, and lung cancer.[116,117]

Emergency Contraception

IUDs are the most effective method of emergency contraception (EC) when placed up to 7 days following unprotected intercourse; limited data support its use through 10 days from unprotected sex.[118] Although most guidelines recommend placing a copper IUD for EC within 5 days of unprotected sex, some evidence suggests that a copper IUD is highly effective if placed at any time in the menstrual cycle. In 42 studies conducted in 6 countries between 1979 and 2011 that included a total of 7,034 participants, the pregnancy rate was 0.09%.[118] Recent evidence from a randomized controlled trial comparing the LNG 52 mg IUD to the copper IUD for use as EC demonstrated noninferiority of the LNG 52 mg IUD for EC (1-month pregnancy rate of 0.3% in LNG IUD group and 0% in copper IUD group).[38] When an LNG IUD is placed at the time LNG EC pills are taken, pregnancy rates within 2 weeks are less than 1%.[119] (See Chapter 18, Emergency Contraception.)

Noncontraceptive Benefits of LNG IUDs

Overall, LNG IUD use is associated with a reduction in menstrual blood loss compared with using no contraception and using copper IUDs.[56] LNG IUDs reduce dysmenorrhea and menstrual blood loss by inducing endometrial decidualization and atrophy,[120] and the proportion of LNG IUD users with amenorrhea increases with duration of use.[42,56,121] Rates of amenorrhea among IUD users differ markedly by LNG dose (see Chapter 5, Effectiveness, Safety, and Comparative Side Effects).[113,122] and lower-dose LNG IUDs have not been as well-studied for the management of heavy menstrual bleeding. With use of a 52 mg LNG IUD, overall blood loss drops about 90%; this translates into clinically important increases in hemoglobin and iron stores.[42,56] The reduction in menstrual blood loss occurs both for patients with normal coagulation parameters and those with bleeding diatheses or using anticoagulant therapy.[123-125] Some evidence supports using a 52 mg LNG IUD to treat heavy bleeding associated with adenomyosis,[126] leiomyomas,[127] and in those with self-reported heavy menstrual bleeding.[128] Trials have compared this approach to medical treatments with an oral progestin, a nonsteroidal anti-inflammatory drug (NSAID), or mefenamic acid[124] and found 52 mg LNG IUDs superior to the other alternatives. In addition, the 52 mg LNG IUD is an acceptable and cost-effective alternative to endometrial ablation or hysterectomy.[129-132]

Disadvantages and Cautions

Common but benign side effects:

- Changes in menstrual patterns
- Cramping and pain

- Expulsion of the IUD
- Concern of weight gain
- *Actinomyces*-like organisms seen on cervical cytology (Pap smear)

Rare but concerning health risks:

- Pelvic infection
- Uterine perforation
- Pregnancy complications

Changes in Menstrual Patterns

Changes in menstrual patterns are the most common side effects of intrauterine contraception. Irregular bleeding and spotting are common in the early months of use and the most frequent cause of discontinuation. Thus, anticipatory counseling about expected menstrual changes is very important. (See Chapter 4, Person-Centered Reproductive Health Conversations and Contraceptive Counseling, regarding conversations about bleeding.)

Copper 380 mm² IUD

Copper IUD users may find that their menses become heavier, longer, or more uncomfortable, particularly in the first several cycles of copper IUD use. Heavy menses and dysmenorrhea are the most frequent reasons for copper IUD removal in the first year of use.[133] Although these side effects may decrease over time,[134] approximately 2 of every 100 users discontinue use in subsequent years due to bleeding and pain.[53,88] Average monthly menstrual blood loss may be increased by up to 55% throughout the duration of copper IUD use, although this rarely leads to anemia.[135] Limited evidence has demonstrated that NSAIDs used prior to or with onset of menses may reduce blood loss and bleeding duration in copper IUD users.[136] Bleeding irregularities may also be prevented with NSAIDs among new copper IUD users; however, this does not appear to reduce discontinuation rates.[136]

LNG IUDs

Irregular but light bleeding or spotting is the norm in the early months of using an LNG IUD, with considerable improvement after the first 3 months. Overall, LNG IUDs are associated with a reduction in menstrual blood loss and may result in amenorrhea. The majority of LNG IUD users have ovulatory cycles and may continue to experience other cyclic symptoms (e.g., acne or mood changes) while amenorrheic.[56,121,137] The lower the LNG dose, the more likely the individual is to ovulate and have ovulatory symptoms. Side effects that may lead to early discontinuation of an LNG IUD include hormonal side effects, such as breast tenderness, mood changes, hair loss, and acne,[56,87,97] although systemic levels of levonorgestrel are far lower than with other hormonal methods.[47,138] Over time, plasma levels of levonorgestrel gradually decline,[41] and cyclic symptoms may increase.

Cramping and Pain

Most people experience discomfort at the time of IUD placement. Immediately following IUD placement, some patients experience 10 to 30 minutes of uterine cramping accompanied by nausea or feeling faint. Use of intravaginal lidocaine gel or cream may reduce discomfort due to tenaculum placement, and possibly with IUD placement, although studies are conflicting.[139,140] Spraying the cervix with lidocaine 10% may also decrease pain with IUD insertion.[141] Some clinicians offer oral NSAIDs, a paracervical block, or both, prior to IUD placement. In nulliparous patients, use of a 1% lidocaine paracervical block can decrease pain with IUD placement, uterine sounding, and 5 minutes after placement.[142,143] Intracervical blocks are also effective in decreasing pain with tenaculum placement and IUD placement in nulliparous patients.

Some NSAIDs may reduce pain with IUD placement; however, in one randomized trial, use of verbal analgesia was as good as use of oral tramadol for pain control.[144,145] Despite hopes that misoprostol might facilitate IUD placement, multiple randomized trials have not found misoprostol to reduce cramping or increase ease of IUD placement in most cases.[146] However, misoprostol may facilitate IUD placement after a previous failed attempt at IUD placement[147] or for those with multiple prior cesarean sections.[148]

Approximately one-third of nulliparous patients report requiring pain medication for at least 3 days after IUD placement.[140] Along with unscheduled bleeding, dysmenorrhea is one of the primary reasons for discontinuation of use of a copper 380 mm^2 IUD[133,134] and may also affect LNG IUD users.[122] When pelvic pain develops weeks after IUD placement, consider whether the IUD may be partially expelled or dislodged into the cervix and evaluate for infection or pregnancy.

IUD Expulsion

IUD expulsions can be complete (i.e., the IUD is completely outside of uterine cavity and cervical canal) or partial (i.e., all or part of the IUD is in the endocervical canal). Expulsions can be asymptomatic or symptomatic (producing cramping, bleeding, pain, dyspareunia, change in thread length, or a palpable IUD at the exocervical os). The risk of IUD expulsion is greatest in the first year of use,[149] when expulsion occurs in 3% to 10% of copper 380 mm^2 IUD users and 3% to 6% of LNG IUD users. The risk of expulsion is higher for individuals who are nulliparous, younger than 20, have menorrhagia or severe dysmenorrhea, or have an IUD placed immediately postpartum or after a second trimester abortion;[133,150,151] however, IUDs can be successfully used in all these clinical scenarios. Placement immediately after first trimester abortion does not increase expulsion risk.[152] An individual who has expelled one IUD is more likely to experience a repeat expulsion; limited data on repeat expulsion place the risk between 14% and 31% within a year of replacement.[151] Because some IUD expulsions are asymptomatic, some clinicians encourage IUD users to routinely check their IUD threads, especially during the first 6 months of use, when the risk of IUD expulsion is greatest. Offer to explain to users how to check the threads of their IUD so that they have the opportunity to learn how to reassure themselves.

Concern of Weight Gain

Although up to 10% of individuals will report concerns that their weight has increased after placement of an LNG IUD,[122] mean weight change at 1 year for LNG IUD users is 1 kg, which is less than seen with use of subdermal or injectable contraception.[153] Refer to Chapter 4 for Person-Centered Reproductive Health Conversations and Contraceptive Counseling.

Pelvic Infection

Flaws in early research led to exaggerations in estimates of the risk of upper genital tract infection associated with use of IUDs.[10] Rigorous studies[154,155] and reviews of the literature[156] have now established that the risk of infection and infertility among modern IUD users is very low. Both epidemiologic[157] and bacteriologic evidence[158] indicates that the placement process, and not the device or its thread, poses a small transient risk of infection. No procedure that requires traversing the cervical canal can be devoid of all pathogenic organisms. Although sterile technique should be used, endocervical bacteria are routinely introduced to the endometrial cavity regardless of technique.[158] However, antibiotic prophylaxis should not be routinely used before IUD placement.[159] A large randomized controlled trial that evaluated the potential benefit of prophylactic azithromycin given before IUD placement[154] found no benefit. More importantly, this study found that salpingitis was rare with or without prophylaxis: only 1 woman out of about 1,000 in each group developed salpingitis in the early months of IUD use. International experience with IUDs has been similarly favorable. In large trials sponsored by the World Health Organization (WHO), the elevated risk of upper genital tract infection was limited to the first 20 days after placement.[155] Afterwards, the risk returned to a low level and remained there for years. More recent studies have found similarly low risk of PID (0.2-0.5%) and no initial increase in infection following IUD placement; as such, routine screening for gonorrhea or chlamydia is not necessary.[99,160] LNG IUDs appear to protect users from PID because progestins thicken cervical mucus, reducing bacterial infiltration of the upper genital tract.[97,99]

Early assessments of the risk of tubal infertility among IUD users exaggerated risks as well.[161,162] IUD users have no significant differences in return to fertility, whether the IUD was removed because of a desire for pregnancy or because of problems with the IUD.[163,164] Indeed, in a case-control study in Mexico,[165] prior use of a copper IUD was not significantly related to tubal pathology, whereas the presence of antibodies to *Chlamydia trachomatis* was, underscoring that STIs, not IUDs, cause salpingitis. IUD placement does not increase risk of PID compared with no IUD placement among individuals with asymptomatic cervical infection or high risk of STI.[11,166] IUDs can be safely used by people with human immunodeficiency virus (HIV)[167] and those requiring treatment with immunosuppressant medications.[168]

Perforation

Perforation of the uterus can rarely occur at the time of IUD placement; no evidence supports the theory that IUDs can migrate outside the uterus thereafter. The most important determinant of the risk of perforation is the skill of the person placing the IUD. In experienced hands, the risk of perforation is 1 per 1,000 placements or fewer.[41,169] Particular care is required when placing IUDs for those who are breastfeeding as perforation is more likely.[169] However, in a large cohort study, no uterine perforations led to serious illness or to injury of intra-abdominal or pelvic structures.[14] The terms "embedment" (a portion of the IUD abnormally located in the myometrium, but not through the uterine serosa) and "translocation" (IUD location outside of the uterus) refer to the position of the IUD relative to the body of the uterus. Bimanual examination of the uterus (to determine size and position) should generally always be done before attempting to place an IUD to guide correct placement in the endometrial cavity.

Pregnancy Complications

Pregnancy is unlikely with an IUD in place. However, when an individual does conceive with an IUD in place, there is an increased risk that the pregnancy is ectopic compared with those who became pregnant without an IUD in place. It is estimated that among those using no contraception, 2% of pregnancies are ectopic; among individuals using an IUD, 6% to 50% of pregnancies are ectopic.[170,171] Nonetheless, a person is much less likely to develop an ectopic pregnancy while using an IUD than while using less effective methods or no contraception.

Providing the IUD

Most individuals, including teens, can safely use intrauterine contraception. IUDs can be used safely by individuals who are nulliparous, have multiple partners, have a history of ectopic pregnancy, or those with a history of PID if they have no symptomatic cervical or upper genital tract infection at the time of IUD placement. All IUDs also can be used by people with contraindications to estrogen. IUDs can be removed whenever desired. It is appropriate to provide an IUD for those who request one even if they desire pregnancy within the next year or two. See Chapter 4 for recommendations on engaging in person-centered conversations about IUD placement, IUD removal, and reproductive desires.

Choosing IUD Type

Most patients can safely use either a copper or LNG IUD. When counseling a patient about choice of IUD, it is helpful to know their menstrual history, medical history, desire for lighter or less painful menses, and feelings about amenorrhea, unscheduled bleeding or spotting, and hormonal contraception. A current history of anemia, heavy menstrual bleeding, or dysmenorrhea may be compounded by use of the copper 380 mm^2 IUD. When choosing among the LNG IUDs, the patient's feelings about amenorrhea and spotting are more important than their anticipated duration of IUD use. (See Chapter 4, Person-Centered Reproductive Health Conversations and Contraceptive Counseling.)

Contraindications to IUD Use

Few absolute contraindications exist to IUD placement or continued use. The medical eligibility criteria for contraceptive use published by the WHO and US Centers for Disease Control and Prevention (CDC)[172,173] offer clinicians guidelines for determining safe candidates for IUD use. The vast majority of individuals worldwide are good candidates for an IUD. However, intrauterine contraception is contraindicated in people with active pelvic infection, including PID, endometritis, mucopurulent cervicitis, and pelvic tuberculosis, because the presence of a foreign body may impede resolution of the infection. Do not place an IUD for those with known or suspected pregnancy. An IUD should not be newly inserted in individuals awaiting treatment for cervical or endometrial cancer, but may be continued in previously treated patients, and may be placed for those with a history of abnormal cervical cancer screening tests. Evaluate abnormal uterine bleeding before placing an IUD to particularly rule out malignancy, pregnancy, or active infection, so the abnormal bleeding will not be erroneously attributed to the IUD rather than to the preexisting pathology. Placement of an IUD may be difficult with severe cervical stenosis. IUD placement may not be possible with severe uterine distortion from anatomic abnormalities such as bicornuate uteri or fibroids severely distorting the uterine cavity. However, nondistorting fibroids are not a contraindication to intrauterine contraception. IUDs should not be placed for patients with gestational trophoblastic neoplasia who have persistently elevated beta hCG levels or malignant disease with evidence or suspicion of intrauterine disease, although continued use of a previously placed IUD may be acceptable. The copper 380 mm^2 IUD should not be used by individuals with Wilson's disease or copper allergy.[172,174]

Special Issues

Adolescents and Nulliparous Individuals

Adolescent and nulliparous individuals who would like to use an IUD can safely do so; the American Academy of Pediatrics states that IUDs and subdermal implants are appropriate methods of contraception for sexually active adolescents.[175] Future fertility is very unlikely to be affected by IUD use[176] and return to fecundity after IUD removal is prompt. The LNG IUD also can be safely used for menstrual management in adolescents with disabilities when menses may be impacting functional status and quality of life.[177,178]

Younger age, which is associated with nulliparity, is associated with IUD expulsion; however, rates of IUD expulsion remain relatively low.[179] Although nulliparity increases the likelihood of discomfort with IUD placement, it is well tolerated by most teens and nulliparous individuals[180] without requiring use of a smaller-framed IUD. When necessary, gentle cervical dilation with a 13 to15 Fr Pratt dilator can facilitate IUD placement.

In nulliparous patients, offer a lidocaine paracervical or intracervical block at time of IUD placement, as this has been shown to decrease pain with tenaculum placement, IUD placement, and uterine sounding while also providing a better overall experience during the procedure.[142,143,181] Prophylaxis with an oral NSAID and cervical anesthesia may help with discomfort during IUD placement.[142,143,182,183] However, multiple trials have found that most NSAIDs are not effective for reducing pain during IUD placement, although naproxen (300 mg to 550 mg) may have some effect.[145] Misoprostol does not reduce pain or facilitate IUD placement for nulliparous patients.[145]

Individuals who are Breastfeeding/Chestfeeding

IUDs can be placed immediately after delivery of the placenta. Providers should be cautious when placing an IUD for a breastfeeding person as uterine perforation is six times more common than those who are not breastfeeding.[184] However, the absolute risk of perforation remains low, and breastfeeding is not a contraindication to IUD placement.[169,185] People who are concerned that they may experience difficulties initiating breastfeeding may choose to delay initiation of hormonal contraception until they are confident in their breastfeeding abilities.[186] However, breastfeeding individuals can be reassured by evidence which has shown only about a 5% difference in breastfeeding rates with immediate compared to delayed LNG IUD placement.[187,188]

Individuals who are Immunocompromised

IUD use appears safe and effective for people who are immunosuppressed due to organ transplantation,[189] autoimmune disease,[190] or HIV infection.[191] For all these individuals, the benefits of IUD use generally outweigh the potential or known risks, including the risks associated with potential pregnancy. Risk of complications, including infection, when IUDs are used by HIV-infected individuals appear to be equivalent to IUD users without HIV.[192,193] Moreover, a randomized controlled trial found that clinical HIV disease progression was slower among copper 380 mm^2 IUD users than among those using hormonal contraception and that HIV-positive patients assigned to intrauterine contraception were half as likely to become pregnant as those assigned to hormonal contraception.[194]

Individuals with Structural Heart Disease

Intrauterine contraception may be used safely by individuals with structural heart disease.[172] The risk of infectious complications, such as bacterial endocarditis, following IUD placement or removal is negligible, even among those with prosthetic valves or shunts. No evidence suggests that antibiotic prophylaxis is warranted. Whether bacteremia may result from removal of an infected IUD is controversial; prophylaxis 1 hour before removal of the infected IUD (with an antibiotic active against enterococci) may therefore be reasonable for those with prosthetic heart valves or a history of cardiac transplantation.[195]

Individuals with Diabetes Mellitus

Intrauterine contraception has significant benefits for individuals with diabetes mellitus who are at increased risk of vascular disease and adverse birth outcomes if they conceive while glycemic control is poor.[172] Good evidence supports IUD use by individuals with either Type 1 or Type 2 diabetes.[196-199] A rigorous trial of 52 mg LNG IUD use by patients with Type 1 diabetes confirmed no adverse effect on glucose metabolism or insulin requirements.[200] Vascular complications are less common among patients with diabetes who use IUDs than injectable contraception or progestin-only pills.[201]

Individuals with a History of Breast Cancer

The copper 380 mm^2 IUD is generally the preferred contraceptive option for patients with a history of breast cancer who desire future fertility or whose male partners are not interested in vasectomy. However, the LNG IUD may be preferable for patients being treated with tamoxifen, because tamoxifen induces endometrial hyperplasia, which LNG reduces.[173,202] Individuals with a history of breast cancer who are considering using an LNG IUD should be counseled that one study reported that patients using an LNG IUD at the time they were diagnosed with breast cancer who did not have their IUD removed had an increased risk of recurrence compared to those who never used an IUD[203] (although arguably, this is not the relevant comparison group[204] and many oncologists consider this an acceptable option for breast cancer patients).[205] In a cohort study of breast cancer patients of reproductive age, risk of recurrence did not differ with use of hormonal contraception.[206] However, more research is needed on any potential effects of an LNG IUD on breast cancer treatment and risk of recurrence.

In the general population, data are mixed on whether LNG IUD use is associated with a breast cancer diagnosis. A Danish study found an age-adjusted risk difference of 16 additional breast cancer diagnoses per 100,000 woman-years of use of an LNG IUD compared to women who had never used hormonal contraception.[207]

Similarly, a Finnish study found a slightly increased standardized incidence ratio for breast cancer among LNG IUD users.[115] However, a case-control study conducted in Germany and Finland found no association between LNG IUD use and breast cancer diagnosis.[117] Importantly, there are no data to suggest that LNG IUD use increases breast cancer mortality.[208]

Individuals at Risk of Sexually Transmitted Infections

Individuals who are at risk of acquiring STIs should be advised to use condoms but are generally still good candidates for IUD use.[172]

Individuals with a History of Venous Thromboembolism

All IUDs may be used safely by patients with a history of deep venous thrombosis and pulmonary embolism.[172] The 52 mg LNG IUD is preferred for individuals currently on chronic anticoagulation therapy to treat or prevent heavy menstrual bleeding.[123,124] LNG IUDs, unlike hormonal contraception containing estrogen, are not associated with an increased risk of venous thrombosis,[209] even when used by patients with other vascular risk factors.[201]

Individuals with Prior Cesarean Delivery

Patients may safely use an IUD after cesarean section. IUDs can be placed easily at the time of cesarean delivery.[210] Misoprostol (despite its known side effects) may facilitate IUD placement for some patients previously delivered only by cesarean section.[148]

Transgender and Gender Nonconforming Individuals

Transmasculine and gender nonconforming individuals with a uterus may benefit from either a copper or LNG IUD for contraception. Testosterone, which causes menstrual suppression, is teratogenic,[211] and does not reliably inhibit ovulation.[212] LNG IUDs, which reduce menstrual bleeding, may be preferred by those who wish to suppress menses. Clinicians should counsel patients carefully about the copper IUD and the possibility for increased bleeding or cramping, which may negatively impact gender dysphoria. If a transmasculine or gender nonconforming individual chooses to have an IUD placed, providers should be highly sensitive to the unique needs of gender diverse patients who are often marginalized or traumatized by interactions with the health care system. Providers can minimize further trauma by ensuring that the environment is welcoming to people who are gender diverse; using inclusive language; providing care that aligns with principles of Trauma-Informed Care; respecting the patient's bodily autonomy by honoring the patient's control over the encounter; and utilizing methods to reduce or eliminate discomfort during the exam and IUD placement.[212]

Counseling About IUDs

Have sample IUDs readily available in the office so that people can be offered the opportunity to handle and examine what an IUD looks and feels like. Many are surprised at how small and flexible IUDs are. Discussing the option of IUD self-removal may increase interest in IUD use among individuals with concerns

Table 10-2 Misconceptions About the IUD

Misconception	Fact
IUDs must be used for the full lifespan of the IUD.	IUDs can be removed whenever the user desires and have been self-removed by many users.
IUDs are abortifacients.	IUDs prevent fertilization.
IUDs increase the risk of ectopic pregnancy.	IUDs significantly reduce the risk of an ectopic pregnancy compared with the risk if not using contraception or using a less effective contraceptive.
IUDs increase the risk of PID.	The risk of PID with IUD placement is very small and prophylactic antibiotics are not warranted.
IUDs should not be used by people who have not had a child.	IUDs can be easily placed for nulliparas, who have a rapid return of fertility after IUD removal.
IUDs increase the risk of sexually transmitted infections.	People who are at risk of acquiring STIs should be advised to use condoms. It is generally safe for them to use an IUD.

that their clinicians may not respect their reproductive autonomy or that they may have poor access to health care in the future.[86] Be aware of common misconceptions about IUDs (e.g., that the IUD can "float off" and lodge in distant parts of the body, such as heart and brain). Address these sensitively but directly. Use a checklist to remember to share important information with each of your patients. Use the Affirm/Share/Ask Cycle, as described in Chapter 4, with "Teach Back" to help patients retain important information and to confirm understanding. Give each new IUD user an identification card with the type of IUD placed, date of placement, and date replacement is recommended if continued use is desired. (See Chapter 4, Person-Centered Reproductive Health Conversations and Contraceptive Counseling.) **Table 10-2** lists misconceptions about the IUD.

Clinician Training

With appropriate training, IUDs can safely be placed by physicians, nurse practitioners, midwives, and physician assistants. IUD packaging, loading techniques, and placement steps vary among different IUDs so clinicians should receive training for each type of IUD they wish to offer patients. IUD placement should first be practiced with a model and then an adequate number of IUDs should be placed under supervision to demonstrate proficiency. Rather than an absolute number of placements, credentialing should be based on a level of proficiency. Time to proficiency is based in part on competence with intrauterine procedures in general and experience performing IUD placement in patients with a variety of uterine positions and clinical situations. Placement steps and technique for placing an IUD immediately postpartum (immediately after delivery of the placenta) is different than interval placements, so specific training is necessary in this context.

Timing of IUD Placement

The copper IUD may be placed at any time during the menstrual cycle, provided a urine pregnancy test is negative.[213] An LNG IUD may be placed at any time during the menstrual cycle, provided reasonable assurance exists that the patient is not pregnant.[214] The US CDC Selected Practice Recommendations state that a clinician can be reasonably sure a patient is not pregnant if they have no signs or symptoms of pregnancy and meet any of the following criteria:[214]

- Patient is ≤ 7 days from the first day of their last normal menses.
- Patient has not had intercourse since their last normal menses.
- Patient is using a reliable method of contraception correctly and consistently.
- Patient is ≤ 7 days from induced or spontaneous abortion.
- Patient is ≤ 4 weeks postpartum.
- Patient is ≤ 6 months postpartum, amenorrheic, and exclusively breastfeeding.

Screening for chlamydia, gonorrhea, and any other STI that may be indicated can be performed at the time of the IUD placement visit but is not required. Clients who wish to use an IUD should not have to make two clinic visits.[215] In the past, IUD placement during menstrual bleeding was suggested,[41,216] but this approach has no benefits and constrains access to IUDs. Copper IUDs are immediately effective; there is evidence that 52 mg levonorgestrel IUDs are non-inferior to copper IUDs as EC. Use of a backup method is likely not needed for 52 mg LNG IUDs, but this should be a discussion with patients.[38] No backup contraception is needed when an LNG IUD is placed immediately after abortion, miscarriage, delivery, or for a patient who had consistently been using another hormonal contraceptive. No published data indicate a need to wait to resume normal activities such as exercise, sexual activity, tampon use, bathing, or swimming following IUD placement.

Extensive clinical experience has shown the safety and feasibility of IUD placement immediately after abortion or delivery. A systematic review of randomized controlled trials of immediate postabortion placement showed low rates of perforation and PID.[217] Immediate placement after first-trimester abortion is not associated with an increased risk of expulsion; however, continuation rates of IUDs at 6 months are significantly higher among patients who had immediate postabortion placement compared with patients who delayed (94% vs. 83%) placement.[152,218] Placement of IUDs after second-trimester abortion was associated with a slightly higher expulsion rate (7%); however, 54% of patients scheduled to return for delayed placement after a second-trimester abortion did not return.[219] Offering immediate placement of IUDs after second-trimester abortion is an effective way to support some patients' reproductive desires.[220,221]

Placement of IUDs immediately after delivery is popular in many countries and is offered in a growing number of US maternity hospitals, as it is a highly cost-effective approach[222] to optimizing interpregnancy intervals. Expulsion rates are lowest when the IUD is placed within 10 minutes of the expulsion of the placenta, often referred to as postplacental placement,[223] although expulsions appear to be higher with postpartum placement than with interval placements (24% versus 4%), whether IUD placement was done by hand or with instruments. Expulsion of an IUD placed immediately postpartum appears more likely when the IUD contains LNG than copper (17% vs. 4%).[224]

Placement Technique

Review the IUD placement procedure with each patient. In general, a uterine cavity length of 6 cm to 10 cm leads to successful IUD use. IUDs may be placed in larger uterine cavities; however, less is known about the risks of IUD expulsion for these patients. Always place the IUD slowly and gently. Read and follow the manufacturer's instructions on placement (available online).

General Preparation

1. Perform a careful bimanual examination to identify the position and size of the uterus.
2. Many clinicians wash the cervix with an antiseptic, such as povidone-iodine or chlorhexidine. However, no evidence supports this practice and its effect on bacterial colony counts in the endocervix is minimal.[225]
3. Some having an IUD placement may not choose to use anesthesia for IUD placement; however, lidocaine applied to the cervix (as a spray, gel, or injection) may increase comfort during tenaculum placement and IUD placement compared to placebo.[139-141,145] A cervical block (paracervical or intracervical) has been shown to decrease discomfort with IUD placement for nulliparous individuals, and it is reasonable to offer a block to all people having an IUD placed.[143,181,226] A cervical block may be particularly useful for those with a history of difficult or painful attempts at IUD placement or who require cervical dilation to facilitate placement.
4. Routine misoprostol use is not recommended prior to IUD placement but may be considered for those with prior unsuccessful attempts at IUD placement and those with a history of cesarean section.[227]
5. Gently place a tenaculum on the cervix. Apply traction to the tenaculum to stabilize the cervix and straighten the axis of the uterus.
6. Sound the uterus prior to placing the IUD. Advance the sound using the muscles in your fingers and wrist, not your elbow or shoulder. Once you have passed through the external os, pause for a second then proceed to the fundus slowly and gently.
7. Place the IUD at the fundus, remove the placement tube, and trim the threads so they extend 3 to 4 cm from the os and are long enough to curl up in the fornix.

Caution

Instrumentation of the cervical os may result in a vasovagal reaction, including fainting. If a patient feels dizzy, nauseated, ringing in their ears, vision changes, or like they may faint, have them isometrically contract the muscles in their arms, hands, feet, and legs to push blood back to the center of their body.[228-230] This can immediately stop the reflex and prevent syncope. Consider offering anticipatory guidance to the patient prior to IUD placement or removal by telling them that it is not uncommon for people having an IUD placed to get dizzy or even faint. You can go over some of the more common prodromal symptoms with them and have them practice tensing their muscles so they know how to stop the reaction if it starts. Also consider wafting an alcohol swab under their nose, or cooling the patient by removing extra blankets or placing a cool cloth on their forehead. Have the patient remain supine after IUD placement until they feel comfortable sitting up.

IUD Removal

When removing an IUD, apply gentle, steady traction to the IUD threads using gloved hands. If this proves difficult, place a speculum and grasp the threads with a ring forceps. Most IUDs can be easily removed this way; if you cannot remove the IUD with gentle traction, a cervical block may make the removal less painful. After placing the block, use a tenaculum to steady the cervix and straighten the anteversion or retroversion of the uterus and try again. If this technique does not work, dilate the cervix a small amount, and try again. If this is not successful, experienced clinicians may attempt removal with an alligator forceps or packing forceps: with transabdominal ultrasound guidance, grasp the IUD, twist and push gently upwards to dislodge the IUD, and then attempt removal.

If the IUD threads are not visible or palpable, confirm the IUD is in the uterus with ultrasound. If it is, then try using an endocervical brush or small cotton swab to tease the threads out of the endocervical canal. If this is not successful, use of alligator forceps, packing forceps, or a manual vacuum aspirator with a size 6 cannula can help remove the IUD or bring the threads through the external cervical os. Administering a cervical block before cervical manipulation can decrease pain before attempting to remove a "stringless IUD." If this is insufficient to control pain, consider using misoprostol 400 mcg buccally, vaginally, or sublingually before the procedure to help dilate the cervix.[230]

People who desire pregnancy may attempt to conceive immediately after IUD removal.

Timing of IUD Removal for Perimenopausal Patients

As the average age of menopause in the US is 51, consider IUD removal for those over 51 years of age, who have had no menses for the last year. Because LNG IUDs can cause amenorrhea, it can be difficult to identify where a patient is in the menopause transition. However, LNG IUDs may be safely left in place after menopause and provide protection from endometrial proliferation for patients using estrogen for menopausal symptoms.[231]

Managing Problems and Follow-Up

Routine follow-up examination after IUD placement is not required; however, some clinicians offer a follow-up visit approximately 1 month after IUD placement to check that the IUD is in place and that no signs of infection are evident. Further routine visits are not required,[232,233] but IUD users should feel comfortable returning at any time that they have problems, questions, or concerns. Counsel IUD users to seek care when they cannot feel IUD threads that were previously palpable, if their threads seem too long, or the IUD (and not just the thread) is palpable in the cervix. It is helpful to use a sample IUD to demonstrate what this would feel like to the touch. Counseling about the expected changes in bleeding patterns before IUD placement may improve the patient's experience of IUD use and prepare them for anticipated side effects. Unexpected changes in bleeding patterns should be evaluated. Any bleeding pattern that is not acceptable to the patient must be addressed and managed if that is the patient's preference or removed if that is the patient's preference. Refer to Chapter 4 for recommendations for patient-centered counseling about side effects and bleeding changes.

Intermenstrual Bleeding, Spotting, or Excessive Menstrual Flow

Copper IUD users should be counseled to expect some changes in their menstrual bleeding patterns; initial difficulties with bleeding and pain improve for many people after their first 2 months of use.[134] Use of NSAIDs, such as naproxen taken twice daily, can reduce excessive menstrual flow as well as dysmenorrhea.[234] Trials have not demonstrated the superiority of one NSAID product over another. Because local prostaglandin production is involved with excessive bleeding, any prostaglandin synthetase inhibitor should help; in contrast, aspirin and acetaminophen do not. If hemoglobin levels drop, consider oral iron supplementation. Patients with persistent unacceptably heavy menses or dysmenorrhea may consider replacing their copper IUD with an LNG IUD.

Individuals initiating use of an LNG IUD also should be counseled to expect changes in their menses. For most users, the number of bleeding and spotting days decreases considerably after the first 3 months of use. For continued bothersome bleeding, use of naproxen sodium (220–440 mg twice daily for the first 5 days of each month) can be helpful.[235] Other therapies that have been used to manage irregular bleeding induced by progestin-only contraceptives include estrogen (or a combined hormonal contraceptive), tamoxifen, tranexamic acid, mifepristone combined with an estrogen, and doxycycline.[236]

New onset of postcoital, unscheduled, or heavy bleeding in an IUD user may indicate IUD expulsion or pregnancy (intrauterine or ectopic), or less likely malignancy or active infection, and so should be promptly evaluated. Persistent abnormal bleeding also requires clinical evaluation because not all bleeding can be attributed to the IUD. Other gynecologic disorders, such as cervicitis, cervical cancer, or endometrial polyps, may be responsible. In addition, bleeding may accompany endometritis. If there is concern of endometrial hyperplasia with use of a copper 380 mm^2 IUD, biopsy the endometrium using a pipelle with the copper 380 mm^2 IUD left in place.

Chlamydia or Gonorrhea Infection Among IUD Users

If an IUD user acquires chlamydia or gonorrhea infection, standard treatment for them and their partner(s) is indicated with the IUD in place. No evidence suggests that an IUD should be removed in this setting.[237]

Pelvic Inflammatory Disease (PID)

Upper genital tract infections need prompt treatment. The CDC has published standard criteria for diagnosing PID, as well as treatment recommendations,[238] and recommends treating PID without IUD removal criteria.[214] (See http://www.cdc.gov/std/treatment.) However, data on the management of PID with an IUD in place are limited.[239] If no clinical improvement is seen within 48–72 hours of antibiotic treatment, consider removal of the IUD and sending the IUD for culture to assess for possible antibiotic-resistant organisms to guide antibiotic regimen. Individuals who wish to have their IUD removed after being diagnosed with PID should initiate antibiotics prior to removal to decrease the possibility of further complications. Those who wish to have an IUD replaced after treatment of PID should wait until complete resolution of the infection.

Abnormal Cervical Cytology

IUD users do not have an increased risk of abnormal cervical cytology. If a patient with an IUD requires a diagnostic assessment with colposcopy, this can be done without removing the IUD. Take care not to catch the IUD strings in the biopsy forceps when obtaining cervical biopsies. During treatment of a cervical abnormality, the IUD may be left in place. To preserve the IUD threads, loop electrosurgical excision procedures (LEEP) may be performed in two segments (for example, the portion superior to the IUD strings first, followed by the inferior portion), or LEEP may be performed after pushing the threads into the cervical canal (and later bringing the threads back down with a cytobrush). Performing cryotherapy with an IUD in place does not require any accommodation.

Actinomyces-like Organisms Seen on Cytology

An asymptomatic IUD user who has "*Actinomyces*-like organisms" reported on cervical cytology should be informed that this is a finding of limited clinical significance. If the patient is asymptomatic, nothing more needs to be done; the IUD may be left safely in place, and subsequent cervical cancer screening can follow standard timelines. *Actinomyces*-like organisms on cervical cytology does not predict clinical illness. *Actinomyces* species are normal inhabitants of the female genital tract; vaginal culture is not helpful in diagnosing pelvic actinomycosis.[240]

If the IUD user is symptomatic (pelvic pain, discharge, or fever), the device should be removed after initiating antibiotics and the IUD should be sent for culture. IUD removal is recommended when individuals are symptomatic because unlike usual gynecologic pathogens, this genus of bacterium preferentially grows on foreign bodies. Pelvic actinomycosis is a very rare, serious, and poorly understood infection. *Actinomyces* species are sensitive to a variety of antibiotics, including penicillin.

Thread Problems

Missing threads may signal an unsuspected perforation or spontaneous expulsion; alternatively, some threads ascend into the endometrial cavity and descend without known explanation. Ultrasound examination can quickly confirm the presence of the IUD within the endometrial cavity. An IUD that is in the endometrial cavity may be left in place even if the threads are not palpable or visible; no additional surveillance or follow-up is required. However, the patient should be informed that, when removal is desired, this should be done by a clinician experienced in "stringless IUD" removal. If the IUD is not visible in the uterus with ultrasound, perform an abdominal X-ray to determine whether the IUD has been expelled or perforated into the peritoneal cavity. When considering potential causes of missing threads, remember the possibility of (1) an IUD in the uterus with coiled or short threads,

(2) expulsion, (3) an intrauterine pregnancy, (4) IUD embedment in the uterine wall, and (5) translocation into the abdominal cavity.

If a male partner complains of penile discomfort from the thread, it is often because the threads were trimmed too short initially with placement. Let the patient know that the threads may soften with time and if there is adequate string length, show the patient how to tuck the threads under the posterior lip of the cervix. Alternatively, cut the threads shorter to the level of the endocervical canal. This may eliminate the barb-like sensation and obviate the need to replace the IUD. When cutting the threads initially, it is helpful to cut them straight across (perpendicular) rather than at an angle to avoid creating a sharp tip, and avoid making the threads too short. If threads are too long after IUD placement, simply trim them.

Expulsion

Some IUD expulsions are asymptomatic. LNG IUD users with previous amenorrhea who experience return to normal menstrual cycles should be evaluated for asymptomatic IUD expulsion. At other times, expulsions present with symptoms. IUD users complaining of cramping, vaginal discharge, intermenstrual or postcoital bleeding or spotting, dyspareunia for either partner, or lengthened or newly absent strings should be evaluated for partial or complete expulsion. The diagnosis of complete expulsion is confirmed by an ultrasound showing that the IUD is not in the uterus, followed by X-ray demonstrating that the IUD is not in the abdomen or pelvis. The concurrent use of menstrual cups may increase the risk of IUD expulsion, but data are very limited and inconsistent.[241-243] Individuals who have expelled an IUD should be offered emergency contraception if needed. A new IUD can be placed at the time expulsion is diagnosed if the pregnancy test is negative.

Malpositioned IUDs

On occasion, an ultrasound done for unrelated purposes will diagnose a displaced or malpositioned IUD. An IUD is considered well-positioned if the top of the device is at the uterine fundus. An IUD is considered malpositioned if any part extends into the cervical canal, if it is positioned within the lower uterine segment, or if it is rotated. Approximately 10% of IUDs are incidentally found to be malpositioned.[244] When a malpositioned IUD is identified on ultrasound, assess for symptoms such as cramping, heavy menstrual bleeding, or new intermenstrual bleeding or spotting. If the patient is asymptomatic and the IUD is in the lower uterus (not the cervix), removal is not necessary. However, if any part of the IUD extends into the cervical canal, the IUD should be replaced. In this situation, it is not acceptable to push the IUD back up into the uterus.

Fractured IUDs

Although uncommon, IUD breakage or fracture presents a clinical conundrum. The frequency of IUD fracture with currently available devices is not known, but is rare.[245] Most often, fracture of an IUD arm is seen during removal, but there have been reports of spontaneous expulsion of only an IUD stem.[245] If IUD fracture is noted at the time of removal and a fragment remains in the uterus, use of an IUD hook, narrow tip forceps (like alligator forceps), or use of a manual vacuum aspirator with a size 6- or 7-mm cannula to remove the fragment can be attempted in an office setting. Use of a manual vacuum aspirator may have a higher chance of success for IUD fragment removal compared to other initial approaches.[245] Ultrasound or an abdominal X-ray may be useful in establishing whether the fragment is retained, as dislodged fragments may be spontaneously expelled.

Hysteroscopy (either in the operating room or office setting when available) is another option for IUD fragment removal. Hysteroscopy is recommended prior to uterine instrumentation or curettage to allow optimal visualization. If sharp curettage is employed for IUD fragment removal, ultrasound guidance is recommended to minimize uterine trauma.[245]

Additionally, the need to remove an IUD fragment is not known, particularly in patients who are asymptomatic. Although the impact of a retained IUD fragment on future fertility is unknown, one case reported a successful pregnancy and delivery with a remnant IUD arm in the rectovaginal septum.[246]

Translocation

If a copper IUD is found outside the endometrial cavity, it should be removed promptly, because copper in the peritoneal cavity induces adhesion formation, which may involve the adnexa, omentum, and bowel. Laparoscopy is the preferred approach for removal. In contrast, nonmedicated and progestin-bearing devices do not evoke similar intraperitoneal adhesions. No clear medical indication exists for removal of translocated IUDs that do not contain copper,[247] although this is commonly done.

Pregnancy with an IUD in Place

If an individual becomes pregnant with an IUD in place, confirm the pregnancy location (intrauterine or ectopic) as soon as possible. If the IUD strings are visible when a patient presents with a positive pregnancy test, the IUD should be removed, even if abortion is planned for a later date. If the pregnancy is not desired, an abortion procedure can be performed concurrently with IUD removal, and an IUD can be replaced (if the patient desires) at the time of procedural abortion. IUD removal is required before medication abortion to avoid unnecessary discomfort. If pregnancy continuation is desired, patients should be advised of the increased risk of adverse pregnancy outcomes, including spontaneous miscarriage or preterm delivery, septic abortion, and chorioamnionitis, even after removal of the IUD.[248] Regardless of an individual's plans for the pregnancy, early removal of the IUD reduces the risk of these adverse outcomes.[41,249] Delaying IUD removal may increase the difficulty of removal as the uterus grows and the threads are drawn upwards.

If the IUD threads are not visible in the first trimester, removal can be attempted under ultrasound guidance using alligator or packing forceps or hysteroscopy by clinicians with experience in this method of removal;[250] consider antibiotic prophylaxis against infection with this approach. If the threads are not visible in the early second trimester, depending on the IUD location relative to the pregnancy, consider attempting removal with forceps under ultrasound guidance or simply leaving the IUD in place.[251] An IUD left in place during pregnancy carries no known risk of teratogenesis, although data are insufficient regarding the risk of fetal levonorgestrel exposure.[248]

USER INSTRUCTIONS FOR INTRAUTERINE CONTRACEPTION†

Chapter 4 offers recommendations for suggested person-centered language to use when discussing IUDs that considers health literacy. Some basic statements you can use to inform patients about what to expect include:

- Many people have cramps for a few days after IUD placement. This is normal. If you want to take something for pain, products that contain ibuprofen or naproxen sodium are best.
- Expect some spotting in the first few weeks after IUD placement. This is normal. You can use pads or tampons.
- When you feel ready, you can start having sex. Use condoms for protection from STIs, as your IUD will not protect you from these infections. You also can return to other activities, such as exercising, taking baths, swimming, and using tampons, as soon as you feel ready.
- If you want, you can check to make sure that you can feel your IUD threads about once a month and whenever you have had a heavy period, or whenever you would like to check them. Contact your clinician if you cannot feel IUD threads that you were previously able to feel and be sure to use another method of birth control until you have a clinician check whether your IUD is still in your uterus.
- Call your clinician right away if you:
    - Can feel part of the IUD, and not just the threads
    - Have pain or bleeding with sex
    - Have unusually heavy bleeding from your vagina
    - Think you are pregnant
    - Have been, or might have been, exposed to an STI
    - Have unusual pelvic pain, cramping, or soreness in your abdomen
    - Have unexplained fever or chills
- If you are not happy with your IUD, talk to your clinician about ways to reduce your symptoms. There are lots of contraceptive options and your clinician can help you find the one that best meets your current needs.

For Patients Receiving a Copper IUD (Paragard)

- Your Paragard IUD works as soon as it is placed; no backup method is needed.
- During the first 1 to 3 months that you use Paragard, you may have some irregular bleeding or spotting, and your next few menstrual periods may be longer, heavier, and you may have more cramping than usual. Consider using ibuprofen or naproxen sodium to prevent your period from being heavy and to reduce cramping.
- Call your health care provider right away if your period is late or you think you might be pregnant.
- Paragard is effective for up to 12 years, but you don't need to use it for that long unless you want to. You can come in at any time to have it removed.

---

† These instructions are intended to guide providers in educating patients in how to use their method.

For Patients Receiving an LNG IUD

- You may have some irregular bleeding or spotting in addition to your monthly period while you use an LNG IUD, especially during the first 3 to 6 months. If you find this bothersome, talk to your clinician about ways to decrease your bleeding.
- Some people stop having periods right after the IUD is placed, while others notice that their periods get lighter with time. Many people eventually stop having their period—this is perfectly safe. It doesn't mean that you are pregnant.
- Side effects are most common during the first 3 months of IUD use and usually subside over time. You may experience any or none of the following: changes to the way your period comes, lower belly pain, back pain, breast tenderness, headache, mood changes, nausea, and acne.
- Discuss with your health care provider the suggested timing for replacing your LNG IUD.
- Your IUD is effective for up to 3 to 5 years, but you don't need to use it for that long unless you want to. You can come in at any time to have it removed.

Author Disclosures—Economou: none, Mengesha: none, Schwarz: none.

Acknowledgements—The authors would like to thank Drs. Gillian Dean and David Grimes for their contributions to prior versions of this chapter.

References

1. Creinin M, Kohn JE, Tang JH, Serna TB. Society of Family Planning Committee statement on IUD nomenclature. Contraception. 2022;106:1-2. Available from: http://www.contraceptionjournal.org/article/S0010782421004157/fulltext
2. Buhling KJ, Zite NB, Lotke P, Black K. Worldwide use of intrauterine contraception: a review. Contraception. 2014;89(3):162-73.
3. Mosher WD, Jones J, Abma JC. Intended and unintended births in the United States: 1982-2010. Natl Health Stat Rep. 2012;(55):1-28.
4. Kavanaugh ML, Pliskin E. Use of contraception among reproductive-aged women in the United States, 2014 and 2016. F&S Rep. 2020;1(2):83-93. Available from: http://www.fertstertreports.org/article/S2666334120300386/fulltext
5. Stern LF, Simons HR, Kohn JE, Debevec EJ, Morfesis JM, Patel AA. Differences in contraceptive use between family planning providers and the U.S. population: results of a nationwide survey. Contraception. 2015;91(6):464-9. Available from: https://pubmed.ncbi.nlm.nih.gov/25722074/
6. Stanwood NL, Garrett JM, Konrad TR. Obstetrician-gynecologists and the intrauterine device: a survey of attitudes and practice. Obstet Gynecol. 2002;99(2):275-80. Available from: https://pubmed.ncbi.nlm.nih.gov/11814509/
7. Hubacher D, Cheng D. Intrauterine devices and reproductive health: American women in feast and famine. Contraception. 2004;69(6):437-46. Available from: https://pubmed.ncbi.nlm.nih.gov/15157788/
8. Sivin I. Another look at the Dalkon Shield: meta-analysis underscores its problems. Contraception. 1993;48(1):1-12. Available from: https://pubmed.ncbi.nlm.nih.gov/8403900/
9. Branum AM, Jones J. Trends in long-acting reversible contraception use among U.S. women aged 15-44. NCHS Data Brief. 2015;(188):1-8.
10. Hubacher D, Grimes DA, Gemzell-Danielsson K. Pitfalls of research linking the intrauterine device to pelvic inflammatory disease. Obstet Gynecol. 2013;121(5):1091-8. Available from: https://pubmed.ncbi.nlm.nih.gov/23635748/

11. Birgisson NE, Zhao Q, Secura GM, Madden T, Peipert JF. Positive testing for *Neisseria gonorrhoeae* and *Chlamydia trachomatis* and the risk of pelvic inflammatory disease in IUD users. J Womens Health. 2015;24(5):354. Available from: https://pubmed.ncbi.nlm.nih.gov/25836384/
12. Farr G, Amatya R, Acosta M, Ekwempu C, Kisninci H. Clinical performance of the TCu 380A and Lippes Loop IUDs in three developing countries. Contraception. 1995;52(1):17-22. Available from: https://pubmed.ncbi.nlm.nih.gov/8521710/
13. Randic L, Haller H, Perovic M, Farr G. The effect of adding copper onto Lippes Loop IUDs: results from a ten-year study in Yugoslavia. Contraception. 1991;43(3):229-39. Available from: https://pubmed.ncbi.nlm.nih.gov/2036794/
14. Newton J, Szontagh F, Lebech P, Rowe P. A collaborative study of the progesterone intrauterine device (Progestasert). The World Health Organization Task Force on Methods for the Regulation of Implantation. Contraception. 1979;19(6):575-89. Available from: https://pubmed.ncbi.nlm.nih.gov/487808/
15. Jatlaoui TC, Riley HEM, Curtis KM. The safety of intrauterine devices among young women: a systematic review. Contraception. 2017;95(1):17-39. Available from: https://pubmed.ncbi.nlm.nih.gov/27771475/
16. Benson Gold R. Guarding against coercion while ensuring access: A delicate balance. Guttmacher Institute 2014;17(3):8-14.
17. Biggs MA, Tome L, Mays A, Kaller S, Harper CC, Freedman L. The fine line between informing and coercing: Community health center clinicians' approaches to counseling young people about IUDs. Perspect Sex Reprod Health. 2020;52(4):245-52.
18. Sawhill I. Reducing poverty by cutting unplanned births. Health Aff. 2015; Available from: https://www.healthaffairs.org/do/10.1377/forefront.20150821.050064/full/
19. Dehlendorf, Christine; Holt K. The dangerous rise of the IUD as poverty cure [Internet]. The New York Times. 2019; Available from: https://www.nytimes.com/2019/01/02/opinion/iud-implants-contraception-poverty.html
20. Dehlendorf C, Ruskin R, Grumbach K, et al. Recommendations for intrauterine contraception: a randomized trial of the effects of patients' race/ethnicity and socioeconomic status. Am J Obstet Gynecol. 2010;203(4):319.e1-8. Available from: https://pubmed.ncbi.nlm.nih.gov/20598282/
21. Gomez AM, Fuentes L, Allina A. Women or LARC first? Reproductive autonomy and the promotion of long-acting reversible contraceptive methods. Perspect Sex Reprod Health. 2014;46(3):171. Available from: https://www.ncbi.nlm.nih.gov/pmc/articles/PMC4167937/
22. Glaser K, Fix M, Karlin J, Schwarz EB. Awareness of the option of IUC self-removal among US adolescents. Contraception. 2021;104(5):567-70. Available from: http://www.contraceptionjournal.org/article/S0010782421002171/fulltext
23. Ciet P, Litmanovich DE. MR safety issues particular to women. Magn Reson Imaging Clin N Am. 2015;23(1):59-67. Available from: https://pubmed.ncbi.nlm.nih.gov/25476674/
24. Long-term reversible contraception. Twelve years of experience with the TCu380A and TCu220C. Contraception. 1997;56(6):341–52.
25. Sivin I. Utility and drawbacks of continuous use of a copper T IUD for 20 years. Contraception. 2007;75(6 Suppl). Available from: https://pubmed.ncbi.nlm.nih.gov/17531620/
26. Creinin MD, Schreiber CA, Turok DK, Cwiak C, Chen BA, Olariu AI. Levonorgestrel 52 mg intrauterine system efficacy and safety through 8 years of use. Am J Obstet Gynecol. 2022;227(6):871.e1-7.
27. Gemzell-Danielsson K, Apter D, Dermout S, et al. Evaluation of a new, low-dose levonorgestrel intrauterine contraceptive system over 5 years of use. Eur J Obstet Gynecol Reprod Biol. 2017;210:22-8. Available from: https://pubmed.ncbi.nlm.nih.gov/27930941/
28. Mirena package insert [Internet]. 2021; Available from: https://labeling.bayerhealthcare.com/html/products/pi/Mirena_PI.pdf
29. Mejia M, McNicholas C, Madden T, Peipert JF. Association of baseline bleeding pattern on amenorrhea with levonorgestrel intrauterine system use. Contraception. 2016;94(5):556-60. Available from: https://pubmed.ncbi.nlm.nih.gov/27364099/
30. Rowe P, Farley T, Peregoudov A, et al. Safety and efficacy in parous women of a 52-mg levonorgestrel-medicated intrauterine device: A 7-year randomized comparative study with the TCu380A. Contraception. 2016;93(6):498-506. Available from: http://www.contraceptionjournal.org/article/S0010782416000718/fulltext

31. Fan G, Kang S, Ren M, et al. A single-arm phase III study exploring the efficacy and safety of LNG-IUS 8, a low-dose levonorgestrel intrauterine contraceptive system (total content 13.5 mg), in an Asia-Pacific population. Contraception. 2017;95(4):371–7. Available from: https://pubmed.ncbi.nlm.nih.gov/27913229/
32. Liletta Package Insert [Internet]. 2020; Available from: https://media.allergan.com/actavis/actavis/media/allergan-pdf-documents/product-prescribing/liletta_pi.pdf
33. Kyleena levonorgestrel-releasing intrauterine system (19.5 mg) [Internet]. 2021; Available from: https://www.bayer.com/sites/default/files/2020-11/kyleena-pm-en.pdf
34. Sivin I, Schmidt F, Waldman S. The Copper T 380 intrauterine device: a summary of scientific data. New York: The Population Council, 1992.
35. US Food and Drug Administration Center for Drug Research and Evaluation. Application Number 21-225: Medical Review of Mirena; 2000. Available from: https://www.accessdata.fda.gov/drugsatfda_docs/nda/2000/21-225.pdf_Mirena_Medr.pdf
36. Eisenberg DL, Schreiber CA, Turok DK, Teal SB, Westhoff CL, Creinin MD. Three-year efficacy and safety of a new 52-mg levonorgestrel-releasing intrauterine system. Contraception. 2015;92(1):10-6.
37. Heinemann K, Reed S, Moehner S, do Minh T. Comparative contraceptive effectiveness of levonorgestrel-releasing and copper intrauterine devices: the European Active Surveillance Study for Intrauterine Devices. Contraception. 2015;91(4):280-3. Available from: https://pubmed.ncbi.nlm.nih.gov/25601350/
38. Turok DK, Gero A, Simmons RG, et al. Levonorgestrel vs. copper intrauterine devices for emergency contraception. N Engl J Med. 2021;384(4):335-44. Available from: https://www.nejm.org/doi/full/10.1056/NEJMoa2022141
39. Fage SW, Faurschou A, Thyssen JP. Copper hypersensitivity. Contact Dermatitis. 2014;71(4):191-201. Available from: https://pubmed.ncbi.nlm.nih.gov/25098945/
40. de La Cruz D, Cruz A, Arteaga M, Castillo L, Tovalin H. Blood copper levels in Mexican users of the T380A IUD. Contraception. 2005;72(2):122-5.
41. World Health Organization. Mechanism of action, safety and efficacy of intrauterine devices: technical report series 753. Geneva: 1987. Available from: https://apps.who.int/iris/bitstream/handle/10665/38182/WHO_TRS_753.pdf
42. Sivin I, Schmidt F. Effectiveness of IUDs: A review. Contraception. 1987;36(1):55-84.
43. Sivin I, Stern J, Coutinho E, et al. Prolonged intrauterine contraception: a seven-year randomized study of the levonorgestrel 20 mcg/day (LNg 20) and the Copper T380 Ag IUDS. Contraception. 1991;44(5):473-80. Available from: https://pubmed.ncbi.nlm.nih.gov/1797462/
44. World Health Organization. Special Programme of Research, Development and Research Training in Human Reproduction: Task Force on the Safety and Efficacy of Fertility Regulating Methods. The TCu380A, TCu220C, multiload 250 and nova T IUDs at 3, 5 and 7 years of use — Results from three randomized multicentre trials. Contraception. 1990;42(2):141-58.
45. O'Brien PA, Kulier R, Helmerhorst FM, Usher-Patel M, d'Arcangues C. Copper-containing, framed intrauterine devices for contraception: a systematic review of randomized controlled trials. Contraception. 2008;77(5):318-27. Available from: https://pubmed.ncbi.nlm.nih.gov/18402846/
46. French R, Sorhaindo AM, van Vliet HAAM, et al. Progestogen-releasing intrauterine systems versus other forms of reversible contraceptives for contraception. Cochrane Database Syst Rev. 2004;2010(2). Available from: https://www.cochranelibrary.com/cdsr/doi/10.1002/14651858.CD001776.pub2/full
47. Nilsson CG, Lahteenmaki PLA, Luukkainen T, Robertson DN. Sustained intrauterine release of levonorgestrel over five years. Fertil Steril. 1986;45(6):805-7.
48. Liletta NDA Number: 206229 Clinical Pharmacology Review [Internet]. 2014; Available from: https://www.fda.gov/downloads/Drugs/DevelopmentApprovalProcess/DevelopmentResources/UCM446653.pdf
49. Creinin MD, Jansen R, Starr RM, Gobburu J, Gopalakrishnan M, Olariu A. Levonorgestrel release rates over 5 years with the Liletta® 52-mg intrauterine system. Contraception. 2016;94(4):353-6.
50. Basaraba CN, Westhoff CL, Pike MC, Nandakumar R, Cremers S. Estimating systemic exposure to levonorgestrel from an oral contraceptive. Contraception. 2017;95(4):398-404.

51. Luukkainen T, Allonen H, Haukkamaa M, et al. Effective contraception with the levonorgestrel-releasing intrauterine device: 12-month report of a European multicenter study. Contraception. 1987;36(2):169-79.
52. Sivin I, Stern J, Diaz J, et al. Two years of intrauterine contraception with levonorgestrel and with copper: A randomized comparison of the TCu 380Ag and levonorgestrel 20 mcg/day device. Contraception. 1987;35(3):245-55.
53. Sivin I, Mahgoub S el, McCarthy T, et al. Long-term contraception with the levonorgestrel 20 mcg/day (LNg 20) and the Copper T 380Ag intrauterine devices: A five-year randomized study. Contraception. 1990;42(4):361-78.
54. Andersson K, Odlind V, Rybo G. Levonorgestrel-releasing and copper-releasing (Nova T) IUDs during five years of use: A randomized comparative trial. Contraception. 1994;49(1):56-72.
55. Rowe P, Farley T, Peregoudov A, et al. Safety and efficacy in parous women of a 52-mg levonorgestrel-medicated intrauterine device: A 7-year randomized comparative study with the TCu380A. Contraception. 2016;93(6):498-506. Available from: http://dx.doi.org/10.1016/j.contraception.2016.02.024
56. Sivin I, Stern J. Health during prolonged use of levonorgestrel 20 μg/d and the Copper TCu 380Ag intrauterine contraceptive devices: a multicenter study. Fertil Steril. 1994;61(1):70-7.
57. Barbosa I, Olsson SE, Odlind V, Goncalves T, Coutinho E. Ovarian function after seven years' use of a levonorgestrel IUD. Adv Contracept. 1995;11(2):85-95. Available from: https://pubmed.ncbi.nlm.nih.gov/7491859/
58. Xiao B, Zeng T, Wu S, Sun H, Xiao N. Effect of levonorgestrel-releasing intrauterine device on hormonal profile and menstrual pattern after long-term use. Contraception. 1995;51(6):359-65.
59. Hidalgo MM, Hidalgo-Regina C, Bahamondes MV, Monteiro I, Petta CA, Bahamondes L. Serum levonorgestrel levels and endometrial thickness during extended use of the levonorgestrel-releasing intrauterine system. Contraception. 2009;80(1):84-9.
60. Gemzell-Danielsson K, Apter D, Hauck B, et al. The effect of age, parity and body mass index on the efficacy, safety, placement and user satisfaction associated with two low-dose levonorgestrel intrauterine contraceptive systems: subgroup analyses of data from a Phase III Trial. PLoS One. 2015;10(9). Available from: https://www.ncbi.nlm.nih.gov/pmc/articles/PMC4574776/
61. Rivera R, Yacobson I, Grimes D. The mechanism of action of hormonal contraceptives and intrauterine contraceptive devices. Am J Obstet Gynecol. 1999;181(5):1263-9.
62. El-Habashi M, El-Sahwi S, Gawish S, Osman M. Effect of Lippes loop on sperm recovery from human fallopian tubes. Contraception. 1980;22(5):549-55. Available from: https://pubmed.ncbi.nlm.nih.gov/7471742/
63. Ortiz ME, Croxatto HB, Bardin CW. Mechanisms of action of intrauterine devices. Obstet Gynecol Surv. 1996;51(12 Suppl). Available from: https://pubmed.ncbi.nlm.nih.gov/8972502/
64. Sağivroğlu N. Phagocytosis of spermatozoa in the uterine cavity of woman using intrauterine device. Int J Fertil. 1971;16(1):1-14.
65. Ammala M, Nyman T, Strengell L, Rutanen EM. Effect of intrauterine contraceptive devices on cytokine messenger ribonucleic acid expression in the human endometrium. Fertil Steril. 1995;63(4):773-8.
66. Alvarez F, Brache V, Fernandez E, et al. New insights on the mode of action of intrauterine contraceptive devices in women. Fertil Steril. 1988;49(5):768-73.
67. Haliloglu B, Celik A, Ilter E, Bozkurt S, Ozekici U. Comparison of uterine artery blood flow with levonorgestrel intrauterine system and copper intrauterine device. Contraception. 2011;83(6):578-81.
68. Shanmugasundaram U, Hilton JF, Critchfield JW, et al. Effects of the levonorgestrel-releasing intrauterine device on the immune microenvironment of the human cervix and endometrium. Am J Reprod Immunol. 2016;76(2):137-48. Available from: https://onlinelibrary.wiley.com/doi/full/10.1111/aji.12535
69. Achilles SL, Creinin MD, Stoner KA, Chen BA, Meyn L, Hillier SL. Changes in genital tract immune cell populations after initiation of intrauterine contraception. Am J Obstet Gynecol. 2014;211(5):489.e1-9.
70. Segal SJ, Alvarez-Sanchez F, Adejuwon CA, Brache de Mejia V, Leon P, Faundes A. Absence of chorionic gonadotropin in sera of women who use intrauterine devices. Fertil Steril. 1985;44(2):214-8.

71. Wilcox AJ, Weinberg CR, Armstrong EG, Canfield RE. Urinary human chorionic gonadotropin among intrauterine device users: detection with a highly specific and sensitive assay. Fertil Steril. 1987;47(2):265-9.
72. Videla-Rivero L, Etchepareborda JJ, Kesseru E. Early chorionic activity in women bearing inert IUD, copper IUD and levonorgestrel-releasing IUD. Contraception. 1987;36(2):217-26.
73. Ganacharya S, Bhattoa HP, Batár I. Ectopic pregnancy among non-medicated and copper-containing intrauterine device users: a 10-year follow-up. Eur J Obstet Gynecol Reprod Biol. 2003;111(1):78-82.
74. Winner B, Peipert JF, Zhao Q, et al. Effectiveness of long-acting reversible contraception. N Engl J Med. 2012;366(21):1998-2007. Available from: https://www.nejm.org/doi/full/10.1056/NEJMoa1110855
75. Peterson HB, Xia Z, Hughes JM, et al. The risk of pregnancy after tubal sterilization: Findings from the U.S. Collaborative Review of Sterilization. Am J Obstet Gynecol. 1996;174(4):1161-70.
76. Schwarz EB, Lewis CA, Dove MS, et al. Comparative effectiveness and safety of intrauterine contraception and tubal ligation. J Gen Intern Med. 2022;37(16):4168-75. Available from: https://link.springer.com/10.1007/s11606-022-07433-4
77. Tocce K, Sheeder J, Python J, Teal SB. Long acting reversible contraception in postpartum adolescents: Early initiation of etonogestrel implant is superior to IUDs in the outpatient setting. J Pediatr Adolesc Gynecol. 2012;25(1):59-63.
78. Nelson A, Apter D, Hauck B, et al. Two low-dose levonorgestrel intrauterine contraceptive systems: A randomized controlled trial. Obstet Gynecol. 2013;122(6):1205-13.
79. Rowe PJ, Boccard S, Farley TMM, et al. Long-term reversible contraception: Twelve years of experience with the TCu380A and TCu220C. Contraception. 1997;56(6):341-52.
80. Foster DG, Rostovtseva DP, Brindis CD, Biggs MA, Hulett D, Darney PD. Cost savings from the provision of specific methods of contraception in a publicly funded program. Am J Public Health. 2009;99(3):446. Available from: https://www.ncbi.nlm.nih.gov/pmc/articles/PMC2661445/
81. Crespi S, Kerrigan M, Sood V. Budget impact analysis of 8 hormonal contraceptive options. Am J Manag Care. 2013;19(7):e249-55.
82. Bellows BK, Tak CR, Sanders JN, Turok DK, Schwarz EB. Cost-effectiveness of emergency contraception options over 1 year. Am J Obstet Gynecol. 2018;218(5):508.e1-9.
83. Trussell J, Hassan F, Henry N, Pocoski J, Law A, Filonenko A. Cost-effectiveness analysis of levonorgestrel-releasing intrauterine system (LNG-IUS) 13.5 mg in contraception. Contraception. 2014;89(5):451-9.
84. Dottino JA, Hasselblad V, Secord AA, Myers ER, Chino J, Havrilesky LJ. Levonorgestrel intrauterine device as an endometrial cancer prevention strategy in obese women: A cost-effectiveness analysis. Obstet Gynecol. 2016;128(4):747-53.
85. Bernard L, Kwon JS, Simpson AN, et al. The levonorgestrel intrauterine system for prevention of endometrial cancer in women with obesity: A cost-effectiveness study. Gynecol Oncol. 2021;161(2):367-73.
86. Foster DG, Grossman D, Turok DK, et al. Interest in and experience with IUD self-removal. Contraception. 2014;90(1):54-9.
87. Backman T, Huhtala S, Blom T, Luoto R, Rauramo I, Koskenvuo M. Length of use and symptoms associated with premature removal of the levonorgestrel intrauterine system: a nation-wide study of 17,360 users. BJOG. 2000;107(3):335-9. Available from: https://onlinelibrary.wiley.com/doi/full/10.1111/j.1471-0528.2000.tb13228.x
88. Hubacher D, Reyes V, Lillo S, et al. Preventing copper intrauterine device removals due to side effects among first-time users: Randomized trial to study the effect of prophylactic ibuprofen. Human Reprod. 2006;21(6):1467-72.
89. Jensen JT, Nelson AL, Costales AC. Subject and clinician experience with the levonorgestrel-releasing intrauterine system. Contraception. 2008;77(1):22-9.
90. Peipert JF, Zhao Q, Allsworth JE, et al. Continuation and satisfaction of reversible contraception. Obstet Gynecol. 2011;117(5):1105-13.
91. O'Neil-Callahan M, Peipert JF, Zhao Q, Madden T, Secura G. Twenty-four-month continuation of reversible contraception. Obstet Gynecol. 2013;122(5):1083-91.

92. Diedrich JT, Zhao Q, Madden T, Secura GM, Peipert JF. Three-year continuation of reversible contraception. Am J Obstet Gynecol. 2015;213(5):662.e1-8.
93. Diedrich JT, Madden T, Zhao Q, Peipert JF. Long-term utilization and continuation of intrauterine devices. Am J Obstet Gynecol. 2015;213(6):822.e1-6.
94. Ory HW. Ectopic pregnancy and intrauterine contraceptive devices: new perspectives. The Women's Health Study. Obstet Gynecol. 1981;57(2):137-44.
95. Sivin I. Dose- and age-dependent ectopic pregnancy risks with intrauterine contraception. Obstet Gynecol. 1991;78(2):291-8.
96. el Ayadi AM, Rocca CH, Averbach SH, et al. Intrauterine devices and sexually transmitted infection among older adolescents and young adults in a cluster randomized trial. J Pediatr Adolesc Gynecol. 2021;34(3):355-61. Available from: https://pubmed.ncbi.nlm.nih.gov/33276125/
97. Toivonen J. Intrauterine contraceptive device and pelvic inflammatory disease. Ann Med. 1993;25(2):171-3.
98. Toivonen J, Luukkainen T, Allonen H. Protective effect of intrauterine release of levonorgestrel on pelvic infection: three years' comparative experience of levonorgestrel- and copper-releasing intrauterine devices. Obstet Gynecol. 1991;77(2):261-4. Available from: https://europepmc.org/article/med/1899136
99. Turok DK, Eisenberg DL, Teal SB, Keder LM, Creinin MD. A prospective assessment of pelvic infection risk following same-day sexually transmitted infection testing and levonorgestrel intrauterine system placement. Am J Obstet Gynecol. 2016;215(5):599.e1-6. Available from: http://www.ajog.org/article/S0002937816302125/fulltext
100. Roura E, Travier N, Waterboer T, et al. The influence of hormonal factors on the risk of developing cervical cancer and pre-cancer: Results from the EPIC cohort. PLoS One. 2016;11(1):e0147029. Available from: https://journals.plos.org/plosone/article?id=10.1371/journal.pone.0147029
101. Castellsagué X, Díaz M, Vaccarella S, et al. Intrauterine device use, cervical infection with human papillomavirus, and risk of cervical cancer: a pooled analysis of 26 epidemiological studies. Lancet Oncol. 2011;12(11):1023-31.
102. Guleria K, Agarwal N, Mishra K, Gulati R, Mehendiratta A. Evaluation of endometrial steroid receptors and cell mitotic activity in women using copper intrauterine device: Can Cu-T prevent endometrial cancer? J Obstet Gynaecol Res. 2004;30(3):181-7. Available from: https://onlinelibrary.wiley.com/doi/full/10.1111/j.1447-0756.2004.00182.x
103. Curtis KM, Marchbanks PA, Peterson HB. Neoplasia with use of intrauterine devices. Contraception. 2007;75(6):S60-9.
104. Gardner FJE, Konje JC, Bell SC, et al. Prevention of tamoxifen induced endometrial polyps using a levonorgestrel releasing intrauterine system. Long-term follow-up of a randomised control trial. Gynecol Oncol. 2009;114(3):452-6. Available from: http://dx.doi.org/10.1016/j.ygyno.2009.06.014
105. Depot-medroxyprogesterone acetate (DMPA) and risk of endometrial cancer. The WHO Collaborative Study of Neoplasia and Steroid Contraceptives. Int J Cancer. 1991;49(2):186-90.
106. Suvanto-Luukkonen E, Kauppila A. The levonorgestrel intrauterine system in menopausal hormone replacement therapy: five-year experience. Fertil Steril. 1999;72(1):161-3.
107. Suhonen S, Holmström T, Lähteenmäki P. Three-year follow-up of the use of a levonorgestrel-releasing intrauterine system in hormone replacement therapy. Acta Obstet Gynecol Scand. 1997;76(2):145-50. Available from: https://onlinelibrary.wiley.com/doi/full/10.3109/00016349709050071
108. Varila E, Wahlström T, Rauramo I. A 5-year follow-up study on the use of a levonorgestrel intrauterine system in women receiving hormone replacement therapy. Fertil Steril. 2001;76(5):969-73.
109. Gardner FJE, Konje JC, Abrams KR, et al. Endometrial protection from tamoxifen-stimulated changes by a levonorgestrel-releasing intrauterine system: a randomised controlled trial. Lancet. 2000;356(9243):1711-7.
110. Buttini MJ, Jordan SJ, Webb PM. The effect of the levonorgestrel releasing intrauterine system on endometrial hyperplasia: An Australian study and systematic review. Aust NZ J Obstet Gynaecol. 2009;49(3):316-22. Available from: https://onlinelibrary.wiley.com/doi/full/10.1111/j.1479-828X.2009.00981.x

111. Dhar KK, NeedhiRajan T, Koslowski M, Woolas RP. Is levonorgestrel intrauterine system effective for treatment of early endometrial cancer? Report of four cases and review of the literature. Gynecol Oncol. 2005;97(3):924-7.
112. Varma R, Soneja H, Bhatia K, et al. The effectiveness of a levonorgestrel-releasing intrauterine system (LNG-IUS) in the treatment of endometrial hyperplasia—A long-term follow-up study. Eur J Obstet Gynecol Reprod Biol. 2008;139(2):169-75.
113. Hidalgo M, Bahamondes L, Perrotti M, Diaz J, Dantas-Monteiro C, Petta C. Bleeding patterns and clinical performance of the levonorgestrel-releasing intrauterine system (Mirena) up to two years. Contraception. 2002;65(2):129-32.
114. Mittermeier T, Farrant C, Wise MR. Levonorgestrel-releasing intrauterine system for endometrial hyperplasia. Cochrane Database Syst Rev. 2020;2020(9). Available from: https://www.ncbi.nlm.nih.gov/pmc/articles/PMC8200645/
115. Soini T, Hurskainen R, Grénman S, Mäenpää J, Paavonen J, Pukkala E. Impact of levonorgestrel-releasing intrauterine system use on the cancer risk of the ovary and fallopian tube. Acta Oncol. 2016;55(11):1281–4. Available from: https://www.tandfonline.com/doi/abs/10.1080/0284186X.2016.1175660
116. Soini T, Hurskainen R, Grénman S, Mäenpää J, Paavonen J, Pukkala E. Cancer risk in women using the levonorgestrel-releasing intrauterine system in Finland. Obstet Gynecol. 2014;124(2 Part 1):292-9.
117. Dinger J, Bardenheuer K, Minh TD. Levonorgestrel-releasing and copper intrauterine devices and the risk of breast cancer. Contraception. 2011;83(3):211-7. Available from: http://www.contraceptionjournal.org/article/S0010782410006554/fulltext
118. Cleland K, Zhu H, Goldstuck N, Cheng L, Trussell J. The efficacy of intrauterine devices for emergency contraception: a systematic review of 35 years of experience. Hum Reprod. 2012;27(7):1994. Available from: https://www.ncbi.nlm.nih.gov/pmc/articles/PMC3619968/
119. Turok DK, Sanders JN, Thompson IS, Royer PA, Eggebroten J, Gawron LM. Preference for and efficacy of oral levonorgestrel for emergency contraception with concomitant placement of a levonorgestrel IUD: a prospective cohort study. Contraception. 2016;93(6):526-32. Available from: http://www.contraceptionjournal.org/article/S001078241530144X/fulltext
120. ACOG Practice Bulletin No. 110: noncontraceptive uses of hormonal contraceptives. Obstet Gynecol. 2010;115(1):206-18.
121. Rönnerdag M, Odlind V. Health effects of long-term use of the intrauterine levonorgestrel -releasing system. A follow-up study over 12 years of continuous use. Acta Obstet Gynecol Scand 1999;78(8):716-21.
122. Gemzell-Danielsson K, Schellschmidt I, Apter D. A randomized, phase II study describing the efficacy, bleeding profile, and safety of two low-dose levonorgestrel-releasing intrauterine contraceptive systems and Mirena. Fertil Steril. 2012;97(3):616-622.e3. Available from: http://www.fertstert.org/article/S001502821102855X/fulltext
123. Kadir RA, Chi C. Levonorgestrel intrauterine system: bleeding disorders and anticoagulant therapy. Contraception. 2007;75(6):S123–9.
124. Kilic S, Yuksel B, Doganay M, et al. The effect of levonorgestrel-releasing intrauterine device on menorrhagia in women taking anticoagulant medication after cardiac valve replacement. Contraception. 2009;80(2):152–7.
125. Lukes AS, Reardon B, Arepally G. Use of the levonorgestrel-releasing intrauterine system in women with hemostatic disorders. Fertil Steril. 2008;90(3):673–7.
126. Fedele L, Portuese A, Bianchi S, Dorta M, Raffaelli R. Treatment of adenomyosis-associated menorrhagia with a levonorgestrel-releasing intrauterine device. Fertil Steril. 1997;68(3):426-9.
127. Grigorieva V, Chen-Mok M, Tarasova M, Mikhailov A. Use of a levonorgestrel-releasing intrauterine system to treat bleeding related to uterine leiomyomas. Fertil Steril. 2003;79(5):1194-8.
128. Chen BA, Eisenberg DL, Schreiber CA, Turok DK, Olariu AI, Creinin MD. Bleeding changes after levonorgestrel 52-mg intrauterine system insertion for contraception in women with self-reported heavy menstrual bleeding. Am J Obstet Gynecol. 2020;222(4S):S888.e1-S888.e6. Available from: https://pubmed.ncbi.nlm.nih.gov/31866516/
129. Brown PM, Farquhar CM, Lethaby A, Sadler LC, Johnson NP. Cost-effectiveness analysis of levonorgestrel intrauterine system and thermal balloon ablation for heavy menstrual

bleeding. BJOG. 2006;113(7):797-803. Available from: https://onlinelibrary.wiley.com/doi/full/10.1111/j.1471-0528.2006.00944.x

130. Busfield RA, Farquhar CM, Sowter MC, et al. A randomised trial comparing the levonorgestrel intrauterine system and thermal balloon ablation for heavy menstrual bleeding. BJOG. 2006;113(3):257-63. Available from: https://onlinelibrary.wiley.com/doi/full/10.1111/j.1471-0528.2006.00863.x
131. Shaw RW, Symonds IM, Tamizian O, Chaplain J, Mukhopadhyay S. Randomised comparative trial of thermal balloon ablation and levonorgestrel intrauterine system in patients with idiopathic menorrhagia. Aust N Z J Obstet Gynaecol. 2007;47(4):335-40. Available from: https://onlinelibrary.wiley.com/doi/full/10.1111/j.1479-828X.2007.00747.x
132. Hurskainen R, Teperi J, Rissanen P, et al. Clinical outcomes and costs with the levonorgestrel-releasing intrauterine system or hysterectomy for treatment of menorrhagia: Randomized trial 5-year follow-up. JAMA. 2004;291(12):1456-63. Available from: https://jamanetwork.com/journals/jama/fullarticle/198436
133. Rivera R, Chen-Mok M, McMullen S. Analysis of client characteristics that may affect early discontinuation of the TCu-380A IUD. Contraception. 1999;60(3):155-60.
134. Hubacher D, Chen PL, Park S. Side effects from the copper IUD: do they decrease over time? Contraception. 2009;79(5):356-62.
135. Milsom I, Andersson K, Jonasson K, Lindstedt G, Rybo G. The influence of the Gyne-T 380S IUD on menstrual blood loss and iron status. Contraception. 1995;52(3):175-9.
136. Godfrey EM, Folger SG, Jeng G, Jamieson DJ, Curtis KM. Treatment of bleeding irregularities in women with copper-containing IUDs: A systematic review. Contraception. 2013;87(5):549-66. Available from: http://www.contraceptionjournal.org/article/S0010782412008165/fulltext
137. Nilsson CG, Lahteenmaki PLA, Luukkainen T. Ovarian function in amenorrheic and menstruating users of a levonorgestrel-releasing intrauterine device. Fertil Steril. 1984;41(1):52–5.
138. Xiao B, Zhou L, Zhang X, Luukkainen T, Allonen H. Pharmacokinetic and pharmacodynamic studies of levonorgestrel-releasing intrauterine device. Contraception. 1990;41(4):353–62. Available from: https://www.sciencedirect.com/science/article/pii/001078249090035T
139. Abbas AM, Abdellah MS, Khalaf M, et al. Effect of cervical lidocaine–prilocaine cream on pain perception during copper T380A intrauterine device insertion among parous women: A randomized double-blind controlled trial. Contraception. 2017;95(3):251-6.
140. Rapkin RB, Achilles SL, Schwarz EB, et al. Self-administered lidocaine gel for intrauterine device insertion in nulliparous women: A randomized controlled trial. In: Obstetrics and Gynecology. Lippincott Williams and Wilkins; 2016:621-8.
141. Aksoy H, Aksoy Ü, Ozyurt S, Açmaz G, Babayigit M. Lidocaine 10% spray to the cervix reduces pain during intrauterine device insertion: a double-blind randomised controlled trial. J Fam Plann Reprod Health Care. 2016;42(2):83–7. Available from: http://europepmc.org/abstract/MED/25759418
142. Mody SK, Farala JP, Jimenez B, Nishikawa M, Ngo LL. Paracervical block for intrauterine device placement among nulliparous women: A randomized controlled trial. Obstet Gynecol. 2018;132(3):575-82.
143. Akers AY, Steinway C, Sonalkar S, et al. Reducing pain during intrauterine device insertion: A randomized controlled trial in adolescents and young women. Obstet Gynecol. 2017;130(4):795-802.
144. Daykan Y, Battino S, Arbib N, et al. Verbal analgesia is as good as oral tramadol prior to intrauterine device (IUD) insertion, among nulliparous women: A randomized controlled trial. Eur J Obstet Gynecol Reprod Biol. 2021;258:443–6.
145. Lopez LM, Bernholc A, Zeng Y, et al. Interventions for pain with intrauterine device insertion. Cochrane Database Syst Rev. 2015;2015(7). Available from: https://www.cochranelibrary.com/cdsr/doi/10.1002/14651858.CD007373.pub3/full
146. Zapata LB, Jatlaoui TC, Marchbanks PA, Curtis KM. Medications to ease intrauterine device insertion: a systematic review. Contraception. 2016;94(6):739-59.
147. Bahamondes MV, Espejo-Arce X, Bahamondes L. Effect of vaginal administration of misoprostol before intrauterine contraceptive insertion following previous insertion failure: a double blind RCT. Human Reprod. 2015;30(8):1861–6. Available from: https://academic.oup.com/humrep/article/30/8/1861/951174

148. Abdellah MS, Abbas AM, Hegazy AM, El-Nashar IM. Vaginal misoprostol prior to intrauterine device insertion in women delivered only by elective cesarean section: a randomized double-blind clinical trial. Contraception. 2017;95(6):538-43.
149. Aoun J, Dines VA, Stovall DW, Mete M, Nelson CB, Gomez-Lobo V. Effects of age, parity, and device type on complications and discontinuation of intrauterine devices. Obstet Gynecol. 2014;123(3):585-92.
150. Zhang J, Feldblum PJ, Chi I cheng, Farr MG. Risk factors for copper T IUD expulsion: An epidemiologic analysis. Contraception. 1992;46(5):427-33.
151. Bahamondes L, Díaz J, Marchi NM, Petta CA, Cristofoletti MDL, Gomez G. Performance of copper intrauterine devices when inserted after an expulsion. Human Reprod. 1995;10(11): 2917-8. Available from: https://academic.oup.com/humrep/article/10/11/2917/674099
152. Goodman S, Hendlish SK, Benedict C, Reeves MF, Pera-Floyd M, Foster-Rosales A. Increasing intrauterine contraception use by reducing barriers to postabortal and interval insertion. Contraception. 2008;78(2):136-42.
153. Vickery Z, Madden T, Zhao Q, Secura GM, Allsworth JE, Peipert JF. Weight change at 12 months in users of three progestin-only contraceptive methods. Contraception. 2013;88(4):503–8.
154. Walsh T, Grimes D, Frezieres R, et al. Randomised controlled trial of prophylactic antibiotics before insertion of intrauterine devices. Lancet. 1998;351(9108):1005-8.
155. Farley TMM, Rowe PJ, Meirik O, Rosenberg MJ, Chen JH. Intrauterine devices and pelvic inflammatory disease: an international perspective. Lancet. 1992;339(8796):785-8.
156. Grimes DA. Intrauterine device and upper-genital-tract infection. Lancet. 2000;356(9234): 1013–9.
157. Lee NC, Rubin GL, Ory HW, Burkman RT. Type of intrauterine device and the risk of pelvic inflammatory disease. Obstet Gynecol. 1983;62(1):1–6.
158. Mishell DR, Bell JH, Good RG, Moyer DL. The intrauterine device: A bacteriologic study of the endometrial cavity. Am J Obstet Gynecol. 1966;96(1):119-26.
159. Grimes DA, Schulz KF. Prophylactic antibiotics for intrauterine device insertion: a metaanalysis of the randomized controlled trials. Contraception. 1999;60(2):57-63.
160. Sufrin CB, Postlethwaite D, Armstrong MA, Merchant M, Wendt JM, Steinauer JE. Neisseria gonorrhea and chlamydia trachomatis screening at intrauterine device insertion and pelvic inflammatory disease. Obstet Gynecol. 2012;120(6):1314-21.
161. Daling JR, Weiss NS, Metch BJ, et al. Primary tubal infertility in relation to the use of an intrauterine device. N Engl J Med. 2010;312(15):937-41. Available from: https://www.nejm.org/doi/10.1056/NEJM198504113121501
162. Cramer DW, Schiff I, Schoenbaum SC, et al. Tubal infertility and the intrauterine device. N Engl J Med. 1985;312(15):941-7. Available from: https://www.nejm.org/doi/10.1056/NEJM198504113121502
163. Wilson JC. A prospective New Zealand study of fertility after removal of copper intrauterine contraceptive devices for conception and because of complications: A four-year study. Am J Obstet Gynecol. 1989;160(2):391-6.
164. Skjeldestad F, Bratt H. Fertility after complicated and non-complicated use of IUDs. A controlled prospective study. Adv Contracept. 1988;4(3):179-84. Available from: https://europepmc.org/article/med/3239478
165. Hubacher D, Lara-Ricalde R, Taylor DJ, et al. Use of copper intrauterine devices and the risk of tubal infertility among nulligravid women. N Engl J Med. 2001;345(8):561-7. Available from: https://doi.org/10.1056/NEJMoa010438
166. Jatlaoui TC, Simmons KB, Curtis KM. The safety of intrauterine contraception initiation among women with current asymptomatic cervical infections or at increased risk of sexually transmitted infections. Contraception. 2016;94(6):701-12.
167. Tepper NK, Curtis KM, Nanda K, Jamieson DJ. Safety of intrauterine devices among women with HIV: a systematic review. Contraception. 2016;94(6):713-24.
168. Kim CR, Martinez-Maza O, Magpantay L, et al. Immunologic evaluation of the endometrium with a levonorgestrel intrauterine device in solid organ transplant women and healthy controls. Contraception. 2016;94(5):534-40.
169. Heinemann K, Reed S, Moehner S, do Minh T. Risk of uterine perforation with levonorgestrel-releasing and copper intrauterine devices in the European Active Surveillance Study

on Intrauterine Devices. Contraception. 2015;91(4):274-9. Available from: https://pubmed.ncbi.nlm.nih.gov/25601352/

170. Furlong L-A. Ectopic pregnancy risk when contraception fails. A review. J Reprod Med. 2002;47(11):881-5.
171. Backman T, Rauramo I, Huhtala S, Koskenvuo M. Pregnancy during the use of levonorgestrel intrauterine system. Am J Obstet Gynecol. 2004;190(1):50-4.
172. Curtis KM, Tepper NK, Jatlaoui TC, et al. U.S. medical eligibility criteria for contraceptive use, 2016. MMWR Recomm Rep. 2020;65(3):1-104.
173. World Health Organization. Medical eligibility criteria for contraceptive use [Internet]. 2015 . Available from: www.who.int
174. Crandell L, Mohler N. A literature review of the effects of copper intrauterine devices on blood copper levels in humans. Nurs Womens Health. 2021;25(1):71–81.
175. Ott MA, Sucato GS, Braverman PK, et al. Contraception for adolescents. Pediatrics. 2014;134(4):e1257-81. Available from: https://publications.aap.org/pediatrics/article/134/4/e1257/33010/Contraception-for-Adolescents
176. Hubacher D, Lara-Ricalde R, Taylor DJ, Guerra-Infante F, Guzmán-Rodríguez R. Use of copper intrauterine devices and the risk of tubal infertility among nulligravid women. N Engl J Med. 2001;345(8):561–7. Available from: https://doi.org/10.1056/NEJMoa010438
177. Schwartz BI, Alexander M, Breech LL. Intrauterine device use in adolescents with disabilities. Pediatrics. 2020;146(2):e20200016. Available from: https://pubmed.ncbi.nlm.nih.gov/32719107/
178. Quint EH, O'Brien RF. Menstrual management for adolescents with disabilities. Pediatrics 2016;138(1):e20160295. Available from: https://pubmed.ncbi.nlm.nih.gov/27325636/
179. Deans EI, Grimes DA. Intrauterine devices for adolescents: a systematic review. Contraception. 2009;79(6):418-23.
180. Brockmeyer A, Kishen M, Webb A. Experience of IUD/IUS insertions and clinical performance in nulliparous women–a pilot study. Eur J Contracept Reprod Health Care. 2009;13(3): 248-54. Available from: https://www.tandfonline.com/doi/abs/10.1080/02699200802253706
181. de Nadai MN, Poli-Neto OB, Franceschini SA, et al. Intracervical block for levonorgestrel-releasing intrauterine system placement among nulligravid women: a randomized double-blind controlled trial. Am J Obstet Gynecol. 2020;222(3):245.e1-10. Available from: http://www.ajog.org/article/S0002937819311202/fulltext
182. Thiery M. Pain relief at insertion and removal of an IUD: a simplified technique for paracervical block. Adv Contracept. 1985;1(2):167-70.
183. Penney G, Brechin S, de Souza A, et al. FFPRHC Guidance (January 2004). The copper intrauterine device as long-term contraception. J Fam Plann Reprod Health Care. 2004;30(1): 29-41; quiz 42. Available from: https://srh.bmj.com/content/30/1/29
184. Andersson K, Ryde-Blomqvist E, Lindell K, Odlind V, Milsom I. Perforations with intrauterine devices: Report from a Swedish survey. Contraception. 1998;57(4):251-5.
185. Ramos-Rivera M, Averbach S, Selvaduray P, Gibson A, Ngo LL. Complications after interval postpartum intrauterine device insertion. Am J Obstet Gynecol. 2022;226(1):95.e1-8.
186. Chen BA, Creinin MD, Reeves MF, Schwarz EB. Breastfeeding continuation among women using the levonorgestrel-releasing intrauterine device after vaginal delivery. Contraception. 2009;80(2): 204-5. Available from: http://www.contraceptionjournal.org/article/S0010782409001966/fulltext
187. Berry-Bibee EN, Tepper NK, Jatlaoui TC, Whiteman MK, Jamieson DJ, Curtis KM. The safety of intrauterine devices in breastfeeding women: a systematic review. Contraception. 2016;94(6):725-38.
188. Turok DK, Leeman L, Sanders JN, et al. Immediate postpartum levonorgestrel intrauterine device insertion and breast-feeding outcomes: a noninferiority randomized controlled trial. Am J Obstet Gynecol. 2017;217(6):665.e1-8. Available from: https://pubmed.ncbi.nlm.nih.gov/28842126/
189. Browne H, Manipalviratn S, Armstrong A. Using an Intrauterine Device in Immunocompromised Women. Obstet Gynecol. 2008;112(3):667. Available from: https://www.ncbi.nlm.nih.gov/pmc/articles/PMC2607525/
190. Culwell KR, Curtis KM, del Carmen Cravioto M. Safety of contraceptive method use among women with systemic lupus erythematosus: A systematic review. Obstet Gynecol. 2009;114(2):341-53.

191. Curtis KM, Nanda K, Kapp N. Safety of hormonal and intrauterine methods of contraception for women with HIV/AIDS: a systematic review. AIDS 2009;23(Suppl. 1). Available from: https://www.ncbi.nlm.nih.gov/books/NBK76860/
192. Sinei SK, Morrison CS, Sekadde-Kigondu C, Allen M, Kokonya D. Complications of use of intrauterine devices among HIV-1-infected women. Lancet. 1998;351(9111):1238-41.
193. Morrison CS, Sekadde-Kigondu C, Sinei SK, Weiner DH, Kwok C, Kokonya D. Is the intrauterine device appropriate contraception for HIV-1-infected women? BJOG. 2001;108(8): 784-90. Available from: https://onlinelibrary.wiley.com/doi/full/10.1111/j.1471-0528.2001.00204.x
194. Stringer EM, Kaseba C, Levy J, et al. A randomized trial of the intrauterine contraceptive device vs hormonal contraception in women who are infected with the human immunodeficiency virus. Am J Obstet Gynecol. 2007;197(2):144.e1-8.
195. Wilson W, Taubert KA, Gewitz M, et al. Prevention of infective endocarditis. Circulation 2007;116(15):1736-54. Available from: https://www.ahajournals.org/doi/abs/10.1161/CIRCULATIONAHA.106.183095
196. Kjos SL, Ballagh SA, la Cour M, Xiang A, Mishell DR. The copper T380A intrauterine device in women with type II diabetes mellitus. Obstet Gynecol. 1994;84(6):1006-9. Available from: http://europepmc.org/abstract/MED/7970454
197. Kimmerle R, Heinemann L, Berger M. Intrauterine devices are safe and effective contraceptives for type I diabetic women: further evidence. Diabetes Care. 1995;18(11):1506-7.
198. Petersen KR, Skouby SO, Jespersen J. Contraception guidance in women with pre-existing disturbances in carbohydrate metabolism. Eur J Contracept Reprod Health Care. 1996;1(1):53-9.
199. Robinson A, Nwolise C, Shawe J. Contraception for women with diabetes: challenges and solutions. Open Access J Contracept. 2016;7:11. Available from: https://www.ncbi.nlm.nih.gov/pmc/articles/PMC5683149/
200. Rogovskaya S, Rivera R, Grimes DA, et al. Effect of a levonorgestrel intrauterine system on women with type 1 diabetes: a randomized trial. Obstet Gynecol. 2005;105(4):811-5.
201. O'Brien SH, Koch T, Vesely SK, Schwarz EB. Hormonal contraception and risk of thromboembolism in women with diabetes. Diabetes Care. 2017;40(2):233-8. Available from: https://diabetesjournals.org/care/article/40/2/233/37022/Hormonal-Contraception-and-Risk-of-Thromboembolism
202. Schwarz EB, Hess R, Trussell J. Contraception for cancer survivors. J Gen Intern Med. 2009;24(Suppl. 2):401-6. Available from: https://link.springer.com/article/10.1007/s11606-009-1023 8
203. Trinh XB, Tjalma WAA, Makar AP, Buytaert G, Weyler J, van Dam PA. Use of the levonorgestrel-releasing intrauterine system in breast cancer patients. Fertil Steril. 2008;90(1):17-22.
204. Neven P, Amant F, Poppe W, van den Broecke R. Levonorgestrel–releasing intra–uterine systems (LNG-IUS) and breast cancer. Fertil Steril. 2009;91(4):e5.
205. Fu Y, Zhuang Z. Long-term effects of levonorgestrel-releasing intrauterine system on tamoxifen-treated breast cancer patients: a meta-analysis. Int J Clin Exp Pathol. 2014;7(10):6419. Available from: https://www.ncbi.nlm.nih.gov/pmc/articles/PMC4230119/
206. Ostroot MK, Heslin K, Kram JJF, Tjoe JA, Dorton B. Breast cancer recurrence risk after hormonal contraceptive use in survivors of reproductive age. Eur J Obstet Gynecol Reprod Biol. 2021;258:174-8. Available from: https://pubmed.ncbi.nlm.nih.gov/33444811/
207. Mørch LS, Skovlund CW, Hannaford PC, Iversen L, Fielding S, Lidegaard Ø. Contemporary hormonal contraception and the risk of breast cancer. N Engl J Med. 2017;377(23):2228-39. Available from: https://www.nejm.org/doi/full/10.1056/nejmoa1700732
208. Dominick S, Hickey M, Chin J, Su HI. Levonorgestrel intrauterine system for endometrial protection in women with breast cancer on adjuvant tamoxifen. Cochrane Database Syst Rev. 2015;2015(12). Available from: https://www.ncbi.nlm.nih.gov/pmc/articles/PMC6823262/
209. Lidegaard Ø, Løkkegaard E, Svendsen AL, Agger C. Hormonal contraception and risk of venous thromboembolism: national follow-up study. BMJ. 2009;339(7720):557-60. Available from: https://www.bmj.com/content/339/bmj.b2890
210. Levi EE, Stuart GS, Zerden ML, Garrett JM, Bryant AG. Intrauterine device placement during cesarean delivery and continued use 6 months postpartum: A randomized controlled trial. Obstet Gynecol. 2015;126(1):5. Available from: https://www.ncbi.nlm.nih.gov/pmc/articles/PMC5354629/

211. Cipres D, Seidman D, Cloniger C, Nova C, O'Shea A, Obedin-Maliver J. Contraceptive use and pregnancy intentions among transgender men presenting to a clinic for sex workers and their families in San Francisco. Contraception. 2017;95(2):186-9.
212. Krempasky C, Harris M, Abern L, Grimstad F. Contraception across the transmasculine spectrum. Am J Obstet Gynecol. 2020;222(2):134-43. Available from: https://doi.org/10.1016/j.ajog.2019.07.043
213. Turok DK, Godfrey EM, Wojdyla D, Dermish A, Torres L, Wu SC. Copper T380 intrauterine device for emergency contraception: highly effective at any time in the menstrual cycle. Human Reprod. 2013;28(10):2672–6. Available from: https://academic.oup.com/humrep/article/28/10/2672/622225
214. Curtis KM, Jatlaoui TC, Tepper NK, et al. U.S. selected practice recommendations for contraceptive use, 2016. MMWR Recomm Rep. 2021;65(4):1-66.
215. Improving access to contraceptive implants and intrauterine devices. Committee Statement No. 5. American College of Obstetricians and Gynecologists. *Obstet Gynecol*. 2023; 141:866–72.
216. White MK, Ory HW, Rooks JB, Rochat RW. Intrauterine device termination rates and the menstrual cycle day of insertion. Obstet Gynecol. 1980;55(2):220-4.
217. Grimes DA, Lopez LM, Schulz KF, Stanwood NL. Immediate postabortal insertion of intrauterine devices. Cochrane Database Syst Rev. 2010;(6). Available from: https://www.cochranelibrary.com/cdsr/doi/10.1002/14651858.CD001777.pub3/full
218. Bednarek PH, Creinin MD, Reeves MF, Cwiak C, Espey E, Jensen JT. Immediate versus Delayed IUD Insertion after Uterine Aspiration. N Engl J Med. 2011;364(23):2208-17. Available from: https://www.nejm.org/doi/10.1056/NEJMoa1011600
219. Hohmann HL, Reeves MF, Chen BA, Perriera LK, Hayes JL, Creinin MD. Immediate versus delayed insertion of the levonorgestrel-releasing intrauterine device following dilation and evacuation: a randomized controlled trial. Contraception. 2012;85(3):240-5.
220. Goodman S, Hendlish SK, Reeves MF, Foster-Rosales A. Impact of immediate postabortal insertion of intrauterine contraception on repeat abortion. Contraception. 2008;78(2):143-8.
221. Reeves MF, Smith KJ, Creinin MD. Contraceptive effectiveness of immediate compared with delayed insertion of intrauterine devices after abortion: A decision analysis. Obstet Gynecol. 2007;109(6):1286-94. Available from: https://journals.lww.com/greenjournal/Fulltext/2007/06000/Contraceptive_Effectiveness_of_Immediate_Compared.7.aspx
222. Washington CI, Jamshidi R, Thung SF, Nayeri UA, Caughey AB, Werner EF. Timing of postpartum intrauterine device placement: a cost-effectiveness analysis. Fertil Steril. 2015; 103(1):131-7.
223. Eroğlu K, Akkuzu G, Vural G, et al. Comparison of efficacy and complications of IUD insertion in immediate postplacental/early postpartum period with interval period: 1 year follow-up. Contraception. 2006;74(5):376-81.
224. Eggebroten JL, Sanders JN, Turok DK. Immediate postpartum intrauterine device and implant program outcomes: a prospective analysis. Am J Obstet Gynecol. 2017;217(1):51.e1-7.
225. Osborne NG, Wright RC. Effect of preoperative scrub on the bacterial flora of the endocervix and vagina. Obstet Gynecol. 1977;50(2):148-51.
226. Mody SK, Farala JP, Jimenez B, Nishikawa M, Ngo LL. Paracervical block for intrauterine device placement among nulliparous women: A randomized controlled trial. Obstet Gynecol. 2018;132(3):575-82.
227. Tassi A, Parisi N, Londero AP. Misoprostol administration prior to intrauterine contraceptive device insertion: a systematic review and meta-analysis of randomised controlled trials. Eur J Contracept Reprod Health Care. 2020;25(1):76-86. Available from: https://www.tandfonline.com/doi/abs/10.1080/13625187.2019.1706079
228. Brignole M, Croci F, Menozzi C, et al. Isometric arm counter-pressure maneuvers to abort impending vasovagal syncope. J Am Coll Cardiol. 2002;40(11):2053-9.
229. Romme JJCM, Reitsma JB, Go-Schön IK, et al. Prospective evaluation of non-pharmacological treatment in vasovagal syncope. EP Europace. 2010;12(4):567-73. Available from: https://academic.oup.com/europace/article/12/4/567/669268
230. Grubb BP. Neurocardiogenic syncope. N Engl J Med. 2005;352(10):1004-10. Available from: https://www.nejm.org/doi/full/10.1056/NEJMcp042601

231. Wildemeersch D. Safety and comfort of long-term continuous combined transdermal estrogen and intrauterine levonorgestrel administration for postmenopausal hormone substitution – a review. Gynecol Endocrinol. 2016;32(8):598-601. Available from: https://www.tandfonline.com/doi/abs/10.1080/09513590.2016.1177014
232. Hubacher D, Fortney J. Follow-up visits after IUD insertion. Are more better? J Reprod Med. 1999;44(9):801–6. Available from: https://europepmc.org/article/med/10509305
233. Janowitz B, Hubacher D, Petrick T, Dighe N. Should the recommended number of IUD revisits be reduced? Stud Fam Plann. 1994;25(6):362-7. Available from: http://www.jstor.org/stable/2137880
234. Ylikorkala O. Prostaglandin synthesis inhibitors in menorrhagia, intrauterine contraceptive device-induced side effects and endometriosis. Pharmacol Toxicol. 1994;75(s2):86-8.
235. Madden T, Proehl S, Allsworth JE, Secura GM, Peipert JF. Naproxen or estradiol for bleeding and spotting with the levonorgestrel intrauterine system: a randomized controlled trial. Am J Obstet Gynecol. 2012;206(2):129.e1-8.
236. Abdel-Aleem H, d'Arcangues C, Vogelsong KM, Gaffield ML, Gülmezoglu AM. Treatment of vaginal bleeding irregularities induced by progestin only contraceptives. Cochrane Database Syst Rev. 2013;2013(7).
237. Söderberg G, Lindgren S. Influence of an intrauterine device on the course of an acute salpingitis. Contraception. 1981;24(2):137-43.
238. Workowski KA, Bachmann LH, Chan PA, et al. Sexually transmitted infections treatment guidelines, 2021. MMWR Recomm Rep. 2021;70(4):1-187.
239. Tepper NK, Steenland MW, Gaffield ME, Marchbanks PA, Curtis KM. Retention of intrauterine devices in women who acquire pelvic inflammatory disease: a systematic review. Contraception. 2013;87(5):655-60. Available from: https://pubmed.ncbi.nlm.nih.gov/23040135/
240. Lippes J. Pelvic actinomycosis: A review and preliminary look at prevalence. Am J Obstet Gynecol. 1999;180(2):265-9.
241. Seale R, Powers L, Guiahi M, Coleman-Minahan K. Unintentional IUD expulsion with concomitant menstrual cup use: a case series. Contraception. 2019;100(1):85-7. Available from: https://pubmed.ncbi.nlm.nih.gov/30981842/
242. Wiebe ER, Trouton KJ. Does using tampons or menstrual cups increase early IUD expulsion rates? Contraception. 2012;86(2):119-21. Available from: https://pubmed.ncbi.nlm.nih.gov/22464406/
243. Schnyer AN, Jensen JT, Edelman A, Han L. Do menstrual cups increase risk of IUD expulsion? A survey of self-reported IUD and menstrual hygiene product use in the United States. Eur J Contracept Reprod Health Care. 2019;24(5):368-72. Available from: https://www.tandfonline.com/doi/abs/10.1080/13625187.2019.1643836
244. Braaten KP, Benson CB, Maurer R, Goldberg AB. Malpositioned intrauterine contraceptive devices: Risk factors, outcomes, and future pregnancies. Obstet Gynecol. 2011;118(5):1014-20.
245. Wilson S, Tan G, Baylson M, Schreiber C. Controversies in family planning: How to manage a fractured IUD. Contraception. 2013;88(5):599-603. Available from: http://dx.doi.org/10.1016/j.contraception.2013.07.007
246. Ramsewak S, Rahaman J, Persad P, Narayansingh G. Missing intrauterine contraceptive device presenting with strings at the anus. West Indian Med J. 1991;40(4):185-6.
247. Adoni A, ben Chetrit A. The management of intrauterine devices following uterine perforation. Contraception. 1991;43(1):77-81.
248. Brahmi D, Steenland MW, Renner RM, Gaffield ME, Curtis KM. Pregnancy outcomes with an IUD in situ: A systematic review. Contraception. 2012;85(2):131-9. Available from: http://dx.doi.org/10.1016/j.contraception.2011.06.010
249. Foreman H, Stadel B v, Schlesselman S. Intrauterine device usage and fetal loss. Obstet Gynecol. 1981;58(6):669-77.
250. Owen C, Sober S, Schreiber CA. Controversies in family planning: desired pregnancy, IUD in situ and no strings visible. Contraception. 2013;88:330-3. Available from: http://dx.doi.org/10.1016/j.contraception.2012.09.027
251. Schiesser M, Lapaire O, Tercanli S, Holzgreve W. Lost intrauterine devices during pregnancy: maternal and fetal outcome after ultrasound-guided extraction. An analysis of 82 cases. Ultrasound Obstet Gynecol. 2004;23(5):486-9. Available from: https://pubmed.ncbi.nlm.nih.gov/15133801/

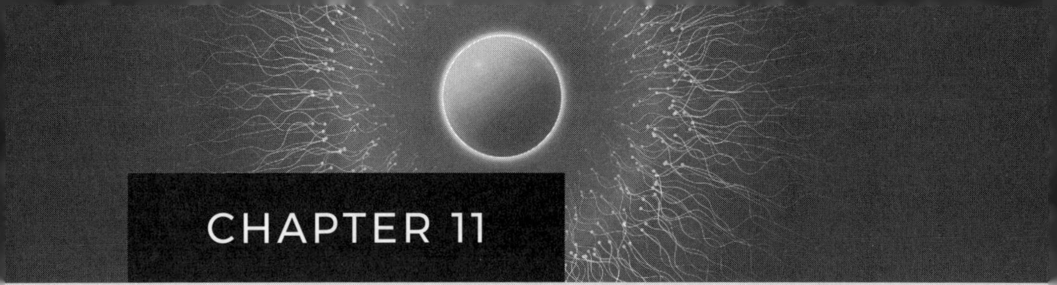

CHAPTER 11

Injectable Contraceptives

Megan Lawley, MD, MPH
Carrie Cwiak MD, MPH

KEY POINTS

- Injectable contraceptives are an effective, convenient method of contraception that may be especially attractive to patients who cannot use or tolerate estrogen or find adherence to shorter-acting methods challenging.
- Use of injectable contraceptives provides the highest possible rate of amenorrhea of all contraceptive methods, thereby providing menstrual suppression and its associated personal and noncontraceptive benefits.
- Adherence to a 3-month schedule for injections is key to effectiveness, and can be increased with the use of regimens for self-injection.
- For patients on a medication that can reduce the serum level of concomitant hormonal contraception, the relatively high progestin dose in depot. medroxyprogesterone acetate (DMPA) alleviates concerns for potential decreased effectiveness due to drug–drug interactions.

The most commonly used injectable contraceptives contain depot medroxyprogesterone acetate (DMPA), marketed as Depo-Provera®. DMPA is a progestin (i.e., synthetic progesterone) that is structurally related to natural progesterone, in contrast to most other progestins utilized in contraceptive products, which are structurally related to testosterone.[1] Depo-Provera is available in two formulations, each administered every 3 months: (1) DMPA-IM, an intramuscular injection containing 150 mg/1 mL (available as a generic), and (2) DMPA-SC, a subcutaneous injection containing 104 mg/0.65 mL. The two formulations are similar in most characteristics (e.g., effectiveness, bleeding profile, side effect profile), so this chapter will only differentiate between DMPA-IM and DMPA-SC when differences exist or studies indicated they included only one formulation. In addition, the term "women" will be used if a cited study identified their participants using that term.

The use of DMPA in the United States (US) has decreased slightly, though it remains a popular method among younger populations. Results from the 2015–2017 National Survey of Family Growth reported that 2.1% of sexually active women not seeking pregnancy used injectable contraception (compared to 3.5%

in 2013–2015).[2,3] The age distribution of users among women at risk remained essentially the same: DMPA use was most common among women at risk aged 15–19 years (12% of women) and 20–24 years (5%), and infrequent among those aged 45–49 years (1%).[4]

Other injectable contraceptives are utilized outside the US and will not be covered in this chapter. These include norethindrone ethanate (NET-EN™), a 2-month progestin-only injectable, as well as monthly estrogen-containing injectables that also contain medroxyprogesterone acetate (Lunelle™), norethindrone ethanate (Mesigyna™), or dihydroxyprogesterone acetophenide.

Mechanism of Action

DMPA is a contraceptive and not a contragestive (which refers to agents that prevent or interrupt implantation in the uterus). The primary contraceptive mechanism of action of DMPA is inhibition of ovulation. Ovulation inhibition occurs through a series of positive and negative feedback loops resulting in the suppression of luteinizing hormone (LH) and follicle-stimulating hormone (FSH) release from the pituitary gland, thus suppressing the mid-cycle LH surge. Ovulation inhibition provided by DMPA is substantial: In a study measuring estradiol and progesterone levels, and follicular development per ultrasound in new DMPA users, no ovulations occurred when DMPA was administered by day 9 of the menstrual cycle.[5] DMPA also has a significant and rapid effect on the cervical mucus, effectively thickening the cervical mucus to prevent sperm transport. In a study measuring cervical mucus scores in new DMPA users, 90% of the participants had a poor cervical mucus score by 24 hours after injection.[6] In addition, DMPA leads to progressively atrophic changes in the endometrium, such that by 12 months of use, endometrial atrophy can be detected by biopsy in 100% of users.[7] Given the profound ovulation suppression caused by DMPA, it is unlikely that the cervical mucus and endometrial effects contribute significantly to its effectiveness.

Effectiveness

DMPA is considered a second-tier contraceptive method in terms of effectiveness—that is, moderately effective. The first-year failure rate with *typical use* is 4%. In contrast, the first-year *perfect use* failure rate of DMPA is only 0.2%. Failure rates reported in clinical trials (i.e., "perfect use") should not be confused with the typical-use failure rate, because participants in clinical trials are highly motivated, monitored closely, and compensated for their time. (See Chapter 5, Safety, Efficacy, and Comparative Risks.) Typical use failure rates, derived from real-world use in which some individuals use DMPA consistently and correctly and others do not, are a better guide for patient counseling. Due to its relatively high progestin dose, the effectiveness of DMPA is not decreased in patients who are overweight or obese.[8] DMPA is metabolized by the liver and avoids the first-pass metabolism that occurs in the gastrointestinal tract. Therefore, the higher progestin dose is not decreased by the concomitant use of medications that induce cytochrome P450 metabolism.[9]

A recent meta-analysis reaffirmed previous studies that demonstrated that patients who self-administered DMPA-SC had no more pregnancies than those who received DMPA-IM. While pregnancy events were rare in all cited studies, meaning the overall effect size was low, this systematic review and meta-analysis confirmed that no significant difference exists in the effectiveness of DMPA-SC and DMPA-IM.[10] In 2021, the Centers for Disease Control and Prevention (CDC) updated its guidance on DMPA-SC, following the World Health Organization (WHO) recommendations published in 2019: Based on moderate-certainty evidence, DMPA-SC is safe, reliable, and has higher continuation rates than its predecessor, DMPA-IM. In a systematic review, six studies demonstrated that at 1 year of use, more participants continued self-administered DMPA-SC than provider-administered DMPA-IM (pooled relative risk [RR] 1.27, 95% confidence interval (CI) 1.16–1.39 for randomized controlled trials (RCTs) and pooled RR = 1.18, 95% CI = 1.10–1.26 for observational studies).[11] This is likely due to several factors, including convenience, increased accessibility and administration, and privacy as demonstrated by the WHO guidance. In addition, patients using DMPA-SC are in control of their experience, which may be important for some, particularly those who want to avoid clinical interactions. Adverse effects and overall side effects from DMPA-SC do not differ from those of DMPA-IM.[11] Two of the cohort studies demonstrated increased skin reactions at the injection sites for DMPA-SC, but this could also be potentially attributable to the type of injection (subcutaneous as opposed to intramuscular) rather than resulting from self-administration.[10]

The manufacturer recommends return for DMPA injections every 13 weeks. The CDC US Selected Practice Recommendations (US SPR) for contraceptive use state that DMPA injections can be provided earlier as needed. In addition, repeat injections can provided up to 15 weeks after the last injection without need for additional contraceptive protection.[12] This recommendation is based on several studies, including a multinational prospective cohort study of 2,290 women initiating DMPA that reported no pregnancies in users who returned from > 13 to < 15 weeks after injection and 1 pregnancy in users who returned from > 15 to < 17 weeks after injection. In this study, 37% of users were breastfeeding at baseline and only a small fraction of users returned more than 13 weeks after injection, which may limit the generalizability of the findings. However, the findings are affirmed by additional studies that found no evidence of pregnancy or ovulation earlier than 15 weeks after injection of DMPA-SC.[13,14]

Decreasing Barriers to Care

Research has shown burgeoning interest in DMPA-SC in adolescents and adults, especially among current and former DMPA-IM users who desired an alternative to repeat clinic visits.[15] A systematic review and meta-analysis included three RCTs comparing self-administration to provider administration of DMPA-SC; it found that self-administered DMPA-SC was associated with a higher continuation rate at 12 months of use (RR 1.35, CI 1.10–1.66), though there was considerable heterogeneity across the studies. Two of the RCTs noted patient satisfaction to be either equal or increased with self-injection.[16] In the third RCT, a single-site trial in the US, 90 of the 91 participants in the self-administered group correctly self-injected and serum DMPA levels were similar between groups.[17] Another RCT included was a multicenter US trial in which, of those who self-administered, 97% reported that self-injection was very or somewhat easy and 87% would recommend self-injection of DMPA-SC to a friend. And among those who received in-clinic administration, 52% reported interest in self-injection in the future.[18]

Health Disparities

Of the roughly 2.3 million DMPA users in the US, 12% are aged 15–19 years old, 12% are Black, and 10% utilize public insurance.[19,20] Given that DMPA-SC has been approved for use by the FDA since 2004, recommended by the WHO for self-administration since 2019, with guidance reaffirmed by the CDC US SPR since May 2021, the question should be asked: why isn't DMPA-SC more available and utilized? Burlando and colleagues[21] proposed several theories as to why ongoing barriers for DMPA-SC exist and disproportionately affect people who already have decreased access to health care. These include unintended and subconscious provider bias related to numerous factors, including racism, limited provider familiarity with DMPA as a contraceptive method, or prioritizing provider concerns about self-administration over the risk of undesired pregnancy.[21] In addition, DMPA-SC may not have comparable coverage by insurance plans to DMPA-IM. While more research on this topic is important, it is also essential for providers to evaluate their own practices and ask themselves why they are not offering DMPA-SC as an option.

Access During Pandemics

Accessing health care safely became essential during the initial stages of the novel coronavirus outbreak in the early months of 2020. Numerous patients were either unable to visit or concerned about coming to health care clinics for their DMPA-IM, which prompted many health care providers and clinics to broaden their considerations of DMPA administration. New approaches included expanding access to DMPA by "curbside administration," whereby people were able to receive their DMPA-IM without having to leave their car, in addition to reevaluating policies regarding self-administration of DMPA-SC.[22]

In a study of current DMPA-IM users conducted during the early months of the COVID-19 pandemic, 37% expressed interest in DMPA-SC and scheduled telehealth appointments to learn self-injection. Of those interested, 58% successfully self-injected DMPA-SC. Of those not interested in DMPA-SC, the most common reasons were fear of self-injection, wanting to stop DMPA, and satisfaction with DMPA-IM.[23] As the COVID-19 pandemic continues or future pandemics emerge, it is evident that self-administration of DMPA-SC increases access for patients and brings greater patient satisfaction than in-clinic administration.[10,11,21]

Advantages

When engaging in shared decision making with a patient, it is important to discuss the relative advantages and disadvantages of each contraceptive method that is safe and available for them to use. Throughout this chapter, we highlight the data that support these important aspects for DMPA. Advantages include:

- Moderately effective, reversible contraception that is not likely to have a decrease in effectiveness when used concurrently with medications that may reduce the effectiveness of other hormonal contraceptives
- Infrequent dosing and the option for self-administration that may be attractive to users who find adherence to shorter-acting methods challenging
- Progestin-only contraception that allows for decreased menstrual bleeding without estrogen-related side effects or contraindications

Menstrual Suppression

Due to the thinning of the endometrium provided by the relatively high progestin dose, DMPA provides the highest rate of amenorrhea among all contraceptive methods. In clinical studies of DMPA-IM, 10% to 30% of users experienced amenorrhea after 1 injection and 40% to 50% of users experienced amenorrhea after 4 injections (i.e., 12 months), indicating increased rates of amenorrhea and decreased days of bleeding over time.[24, 25] Studies of DMPA-SC show the same pattern, with 52% to 64% of users experiencing amenorrhea at 12 months, and 71% of users experiencing amenorrhea at 24 months, with rates of amenorrhea that increased over time.[26] Correspondingly, DMPA users experience a slight increase in hemoglobin levels over time.[24]

DMPA-IM use is also associated with a significant decrease in dysmenorrhea (adjusted OR [aOR] 0.35, 95% CI 0.24–0.51) compared to nonhormonal methods.[27] There have been five RCTs comparing use of DMPA (two with IM, three with SC) to other hormonal therapies (combined oral contraceptives [COCs], leuprolide) in women with a surgical diagnosis of endometriosis; in all, DMPA formulations have been effective in decreasing dysmenorrhea, nonmenstruation-related pelvic pain, and dyspareunia.[28,29] Because progestin levels are sustained with DMPA use and not cyclic, patients may find relief from other menstruation-related symptoms including premenstrual syndrome, premenstrual dysphoric disorder, or menstrual migraines.

Decreased Uterine Leiomyoma Risk

Observational studies suggest a protective effect of DMPA use on uterine leiomyoma development. Most recently, a cohort of 1,693 Black women aged 25–35 years old who did not have a baseline diagnosis of uterine leiomyoma were followed for over 4 years to assess leiomyoma incidence and growth. DMPA use within the previous 2 years was associated with reduced leiomyoma incidence (adjusted hazard ratio [aHR] 0.6, 95% CI 0.4–1.0), and for those who developed leiomyoma, reduced leiomyoma growth (42% mean decrease, 95% CI –51.4 to –30.7), and greater leiomyoma loss (adjusted relative risk [aRR] 1.6, 95% CI 1.1–2.2) compared to never users. Leiomyoma loss was even greater for those who used DMPA within the previous 2–4 years compared to never users (aRR 2.1, 95% CI 1.4–3.1).[30] These findings are consistent with three previous observational studies noting 20% to 60% decreased risk of new or recurrent leiomyoma development with DMPA use, more so with longer durations of use, persisting for years after the last dose.[31]

Treatment for Abnormal Uterine Bleeding

Because of the progestogenic thinning of the endometrium, menstrual blood loss is reduced overall with DMPA use. Therefore, DMPA can provide an effective nonsurgical treatment for heavy menstrual bleeding (HMB) due to a variety of etiologies: anovulation, uterine fibroids, adenomyosis, and coagulopathies. In a pilot study of 48 women with acute HMB, treatment with DMPA-IM followed by oral medroxyprogesterone acetate (Provera) 20 mg three times daily for 3 days resulted in a rapid decrease in bleeding, with a mean time to bleeding cessation of 2.6 days and 100% cessation of bleeding within 5 days.[32] Although there are no RCTs, observational studies have shown that treatment with DMPA-IM significantly decreases leiomyoma-related abnormal uterine bleeding and resulting anemia.[33,34]

Decreased Cancer Risk

Progesterone counteracts the effects of endogenous estrogen in the endometrium, and progestins, including DMPA-IM, have been used to prevent and treat proliferative endometrium, including endometrial hyperplasia and malignancy.[35] A WHO case-control study found ever use of DMPA was associated with an 80% decreased risk of endometrial cancer that persisted up to 8 years after discontinuation.[36] Not surprisingly, data regarding DMPA-IM use and ovarian cancer also suggest a protective effect due to inhibition of ovulation. In a large case-control study, use of DMPA was associated with a 40% decreased risk of epithelial ovarian cancer. This risk was further decreased after at least 3 years of DMPA use.[37] However, earlier studies had demonstrated no statistically significant alteration in ovarian cancer risk.[38]

Disadvantages

Unpredictable Bleeding

The principal complaint associated with DMPA use is unpredictable bleeding, caused by the development of fragile endometrial vessels and local derangement of hemostatic mechanisms due to endometrial atrophy.[39] Less than 10% of DMPA users report regular bleeding at the end of the first year of use. For the remainder of users who experience bleeding at 1 year of use, the pattern is unpredictable and can be infrequent, frequent, or prolonged.[40] Because of the progestogenic thinning of the endometrium, menstrual blood loss is reduced overall; nonetheless, DMPA users may find the unpredictability of their bleeding pattern to be a nuisance. In fact, unpredictable bleeding is the primary reason given for discontinuation of DMPA.[40] Unpredictable bleeding does decrease over time with use and may respond in the interim to temporary administration of therapies such as estrogen or nonsteroidal anti-inflammatory drugs (NSAIDs). Management of bleeding complaints is addressed later in this chapter.

Weight Gain

Aside from unpredictable bleeding, weight gain is the most commonly reported side effect among DMPA users and is a commonly cited reason for discontinuation. However, people gain weight as they age regardless of contraceptive use because their body metabolism changes and therefore weight increases if they make no compensatory changes in nutrition and activity. Key events over the reproductive lifespan, including puberty, pregnancy, and menopause, can have significant effects on metabolism and weight. Early clinical trials of DMPA relied on self-reported weight changes or discontinuation due to the same, which do not necessarily correlate with actual changes in weight with contraceptive use or differential changes among methods.[41]

In a 2016 review of clinical trials that measured weight changes in DMPA users, 15 studies noted no significant differences in mean weight gain or percentage change in body composition associated with DMPA use in comparison to other hormonal or nonhormonal methods. Only three studies found a differential effect. Among them, two retrospective trials compared DMPA to copper intrauterine device (IUD) users: one study found that mean weight gain was higher for DMPA users at 1 year (mean difference 2.28 kg), 2 years (MD 2.71 kg), and 3 years of use (MD 3.17 kg), among normal weight and overweight, but not obese, users; the other study found that mean weight gain was higher for DMPA users at 1 year (1.3 vs 0.2 kg), 4 years

(3.5 vs 1.9 kg), and 10 years of use (6.6 vs 4.9 kg).[41] Bonny et al.[42] compared DMPA use to no hormonal contraceptive use in a small study of 26 adolescents and reported a significant increase in total body fat percentage (11%) and decrease in lean body mass percentage (–4%) at 6 months, though weight gain was not reported. It should be noted that all but one of the 18 trials were considered very low to low in quality.[41] Given that DMPA is the only method that shows an association with weight gain and that weight gain is the most common reason people discontinue it, proactive and informative counseling about weight changes attributable to DMPA use and patient concerns is particularly relevant. (See Chapter 4, Person-Centered Reproductive Health Conversations and Contraceptive Counseling.)

While the mean weight gain attributable to DMPA use may be of negligible or low magnitude for most users, some patients may be more likely to gain significant weight over time with DMPA use. One study of adult DMPA users suggests that a 5% weight change in the first 6 months of use was predictive of more progressive weight gain such that mean weight change was significantly higher (7.03 kg) by 36 months of use in those who experienced early weight gain. Other predictors included nonobese body mass index (BMI) and self-reported increase in appetite.[43] A study of adolescent DMPA users similarly found that DMPA users with a 5% weight change in the first 6 months had a higher mean BMI change (7.6 vs. 2.3) by 18 months of use compared to those that did not have an early weight change.[44] The high loss-to-follow-up rate in both studies limits the generalizability of these findings. Yet, it is reasonable to monitor weight and BMI changes over time in DMPA users to assist in counseling those who are concerned about weight gain. Management of weight gain is addressed later in this chapter.

Delayed Return to Fecundity

Some patients who discontinue DMPA may not experience immediate return to their baseline ovulation, and therefore fecundity or menses, because of the variability in the metabolism of the depot form and variable sensitivity of the hypothalamic gonadotropin-releasing hormone pulse generator to the increased levels of progestin. The mean time to conception after discontinuation has been measured to be 10 months after the last injection, with 90% of conceptions occurring by 17 months after last injection. Since each injection is intended to provide 3 months of contraception, this corresponds to an average delay of 7 months after choosing not to receive the next injection. Time to conception after DMPA discontinuation was not affected by age or by duration of DMPA use but was increased in former users with higher body weight. The return to fertility after DMPA use is longer than for other methods in the short term, but by 18 months after the last injection, conception rates were similar to conception rates after use of nonhormonal contraceptives, suggesting no adverse long-term effect on fertility.[45] Although age did not appear to cause further delay in return to fertility in former DMPA users, the potential delay may be of greater significance to some people of older reproductive age who may want to get pregnant and already experience an age-related decrease in their fecundity.

Health Risks

The US Medical Eligibility Criteria (US MEC) for contraceptive use provides guidelines for providers to follow when assessing health risks associated with the use of various contraceptive methods compared to the risks of unintended pregnancy. The US MEC presents an up-to-date synthesis of the medical literature regarding the risks associated with DMPA use among both healthy patients across the reproductive lifespan and patients with chronic medical conditions. For most patients, the benefits of DMPA far outweigh the risks of DMPA in terms of safety. **In fact, current breast cancer is the only condition for which the health risks associated with DMPA are unacceptable (i.e., US MEC Category 4) and therefore considered a *contraindication* to its use.** However, there are several conditions for which the theoretical or proven risks associated with DMPA use may be greater than the risks associated with an unintended pregnancy (i.e., US MEC Category 3; **Table 11-1**).[9] In comparison, the health risks associated with combined (i.e., estrogen-containing) hormonal contraceptives (CHCs) are unacceptable with most of these conditions, with the exception of severe thrombocytopenia, chronic corticosteroid use, and unexplained vaginal bleeding. Therefore, it may be helpful to think of each of these conditions as a *relative contraindication* to DMPA use, requiring careful clinical thought toward the severity of the condition, the presence of other risk factors, and the patient's access to services. In these clinical circumstances, additional time should be allotted for patient assessment, counseling, and follow up. Relative to other progestin-only and nonhormonal methods, DMPA

Table 11-1 Medical Conditions for which the Risks Typically Outweigh the Advantages of DMPA Use, as Listed in the US Medical Eligibility Criteria for Contraceptive Use

Medical Condition or Characteristic	US MEC Rating
Multiple risk factors for atherosclerotic cardiovascular disease	3
Current or past ischemic heart disease	3
Current or past cerebrovascular accident (stroke)	3
Hypertension with vascular disease or >160 or >100	3
Diabetes mellitus with vascular disease or > 20 years' duration	3
Systemic lupus erythematosus with + antiphospholipid antibodies	3
Systemic lupus erythematosus with severe thrombocytopenia	3(I)
Rheumatoid arthritis on chronic corticosteroid therapy	3(C)
Unexplained vaginal bleeding without evaluation	3
Past breast cancer within 5 years	3
Severe viral hepatitis	3
Hepatocellular adenoma or malignant hepatoma	3

I, initiation; C, continuation

Data from Curtis KM, Tepper NK, Jatlaoui TC, et al. U.S. Medical Eligibility Criteria for contraceptive use, 2016. MMWR Recomm Rep 2016;65(3):1-104.

use may be associated with higher risks in these conditions. Ultimately, the use of DMPA may be reasonable if other methods are not available or acceptable to the patient.

Many medical conditions present no contraindications to use of DMPA; for these conditions, DMPA use neither worsens disease progression nor increases risk of complications. These conditions are assigned "category 1" (use is not restricted) and "category 2" (benefits of use outweigh risks) in the US MEC and include obesity, depression, and venous thromboembolism, among others. In addition, DMPA can help treat abnormal uterine bleeding (AUB) associated with medical conditions like thyroid disorders or anticoagulation. Patients with sickle cell or other preexisting anemias benefit from menstrual suppression. For clinic administrators, protocols can be developed to require additional clinical review to initiate or continue DMPA use in patients with relative contraindications, while allowing for DMPA use without unnecessary barriers with conditions for which little to no risk is observed. For a complete list of the US MEC upon which to make clinical decisions, go to www.cdc.gov, or see Chapter 20, Contraception for People with Medical Conditions for ways to use the guidelines in your everyday practice.

Metabolic Changes

Observational studies measuring serum lipid levels have demonstrated an increase in low-density lipoprotein (LDL) cholesterol and a decrease in HDL cholesterol in DMPA-IM users.[46] A trial by Berenson et al.[47] followed DMPA users for 3 years and found HDL cholesterol levels initially decreased for 6 months but then returned to baseline. Correspondingly, the LDL cholesterol : HDL ratio initially decreased for 6 months but then returned to baseline over the next 24 months of use.[47] No association has been identified between short-term changes in lipid levels during DMPA use and adverse clinical outcomes; accordingly, hyperlipidemia is not a condition currently included in the US MEC.

In a 2003 systematic review of clinical trials that measured insulin and glucose levels in DMPA-IM users, all six studies noted elevated insulin levels at 2–3 hours after an oral glucose challenge, but not with fasting or 1 hour after glucose challenge, in nondiabetic DMPA-IM users compared to baseline. Three of the 6 studies noted elevations in glucose levels in users who were ≥ 68 kg (150 pounds) at baseline or had used DMPA-IM for a longer duration (≥ 4 years).[48] A small 2012 study[49] compared the short-term metabolic effects of DMPA-SC in users of normal weight to users with obesity. At baseline, markers of cardiovascular risk were significantly higher in the users with obesity. Over 18 weeks, there were no differences in BMI, abdominal circumference, HDL cholesterol, or insulin sensitivity in users of normal weight. Among the users with obesity, BMI increased and insulin sensitivity decreased. And like in the Berenson trial previously noted, HDL cholesterol decreased.[49] It is unclear whether these transient changes are clinically significant, especially in users without cardiovascular risk factors. For patients with diabetes of long duration (> 20 years) or with vascular disease (nephropathy, neuropathy, retinopathy), the theoretical or proven risks associated with DMPA use may be greater than the risks associated with pregnancy (i.e., US MEC Category 3).[9]

Cardiovascular Events

In a systematic review, the use of progestin-only contraceptives overall is not associated with an increased risk of venous thromboembolism (VTE), myocardial infarction (MI), or cerebrovascular accident (CVA) in the general population.[50] However, the relatively larger progestin dose in DMPA formulations, the transient adverse effect on lipids, and the potential for weight gain may lead to relatively increased risks for DMPA users. In a WHO multinational case-control study, there was no increased risk of VTE, CVA, or MI with current or recent use (i.e., within the past 3 months) of progestin-only injections, including DMPA-IM, in comparison to nonuse.[51] However, more recent case-control studies have found an increased risk among DMPA users: a 2010 Netherlands study noted an increased risk of VTE in current users (OR 3.0, 95% CI 1.2–7.5), and a 2014 Swedish study noted an increased risk of VTE in current or recent users (OR 2.2, 95% CI 1.3–4).[52,53]

The risk of cardiovascular events associated with DMPA use has also been investigated in populations with preexisting risk factors. The 2014 Swedish study also found an increased risk of VTE in DMPA users with factor V Leiden compared to nonusers without the mutation (OR 16.7, 95% CI 2.4–714), though the confidence interval was quite large and overlapped with other groups that had no increased risk, including those with other thrombophilic mutations.[53] DMPA use was not associated with a significantly increased risk of VTE among smokers or those with personal or family history of VTE.[50] As previously mentioned, the cardiovascular risks associated with pregnancy and CHC use are greater than with DMPA use. Therefore, DMPA remains a viable option for many patients with preexisting cardiovascular risk factors, though there are several conditions for which the theoretical or proven risks associated with DMPA use may be greater than the risks associated with pregnancy (i.e., US MEC Category 3; Table 11-1).[9]

Decreased Bone Mineral Density

In RCTs, current DMPA use has been associated with relative hypoestrogenemia (which increases bone turnover and bone loss) and lower bone mineral density (BMD) in users compared to nonusers.[54] BMD naturally decreases with age. In DMPA users across all ages, BMD declines rapidly during the first year of use and appears to plateau at 2 years of use, mirroring the reversible BMD changes observed during pregnancy and lactation. Adolescents experience a similar decline in BMD during DMPA use, with a rapid return of BMD within 1–2 years of discontinuation, enabling them to attain peak bone mass equal to that of their peers.[55] Decreases in BMD among DMPA-IM users 25–35 years of age are reversible as soon as 2 years after discontinuation.[56] Several studies have demonstrated that even with prolonged DMPA use in perimenopausal women, BMD loss is similarly greatest in the first year of use and then plateaus, with recovery after discontinuation.[57] Finally, postmenopausal women who previously used DMPA do not have lower BMD in comparison to never users, even when DMPA was used up until menopause.[55,58] Although some postulate that decreases in BMD represent a proxy for the more relevant clinical outcome of fracture risk, evidence does not link these two parameters in premenopausal women.

While case-control studies have noted modest increases in fracture risk in both current and past DMPA-IM users versus nonusers, the studies did not adequately control for potential confounders.[59] A Danish case-control study reported an increase in fracture risk with ever use of DMPA (OR 1.44, 95% CI 1.01–2.06), use over 4 years (OR 2.16, 95% CI 1.32–3.53), and users over 50 years old (OR 2.25, 95% CI 1.14–4.42), but without adjusting for potential confounders such as smoking and BMI.[60] A case-control study utilizing the United Kingdom General Practice Research Database reported that longer duration of DMPA use was associated with further increased fracture risk (OR 1.36, 95% CI 1.15–1.6 with 3–9 injections vs. 1.54, 95% CI 1.33–1.78 after 10 injections), but examined fractures typically related to trauma rather than BMD loss and did not adjust for factors related to traumatic fractures. For example, the prevalence of alcohol use disorder (a condition known to be associated with fractures from motor vehicle and other accidents) among the DMPA users was 14%, seven-fold higher than in nonusers, and cases with fractures were three-fold more likely to be classified as having alcohol use disorder than controls.[61] A subsequent retrospective cohort also based on the United Kingdom General Practice Research Database found that DMPA users had higher fracture risk *prior to* the onset of DMPA use versus nonusers (incidence ratio 1.28, 95% CI 1.07–1.58). Furthermore, the risk did not increase further with DMPA use of any duration.[62] People who choose DMPA may have differences from people who choose other methods of contraception, and behavioral dissimilarities reflecting these differences may account for a higher fracture risk among DMPA users compared to those who choose other contraceptives.

Importantly, DMPA use has not been associated with an increase in osteoporotic-related fracture risk.[55,58] The American College of Obstetricians and Gynecologists (ACOG) encourages the use of patient-centered counseling and respect for patient preference. When providers interact with patients who want to start or continue use of DMPA, ACOG discourages avoidance or discontinuation of DMPA use due to concerns of bone health. ACOG also does not recommend routine BMD monitoring in the absence of other risk factors given the lack of evidence to support its use in premenopausal women.[63] For patients with preexisting risk factors for osteoporosis, like chronic steroid therapy, the US MEC recommends considering other contraceptive methods if they are available or acceptable (i.e., US MEC Category 3).[9]

Human Immunodeficiency Virus (HIV) Acquisition

There are several theories for an increased risk of HIV acquisition with DMPA use: decreased systemic level of estrogen that thins the vaginal epithelium, decreased vaginal lactobacilli, or decreased cellular or humoral responses to HIV. In a 2014 systematic review, 3 of 10 observational studies reported an association with DMPA use and increased risk of acquiring HIV.[64] In a more recent systematic review, RCTs found no increased risk of HIV acquisition in DMPA users compared to users of other hormonal and nonhormonal contraceptive methods. For example, the ECHO trial, a RCT of DMPA versus levonorgestrel implant versus copper IUD use in four African countries, found no difference in HIV acquisition among groups. Unique strengths of this trial included a low loss to follow-up rate and adjustments for confounders such as age and herpes infection. Two observational studies have investigated the effect of concurrent bacterial vaginosis (BV) on the risk of HIV acquisition: a cohort study in Mombasa noted an increased risk of HIV (HR 1.72, CI 1.34–2.2) that was not changed by a concurrent BV diagnosis, while a cohort study in Zambia noted an increased risk only in women with concurrent BV. Whether this risk is increased differentially in people with current BV requires further study.[65] Antiretrovirals taken for prevention (i.e., PrEP) or treatment of HIV do not interact with DMPA.[9]

Ten studies have evaluated the vaginal microbiome in DMPA users compared to users of other hormonal or nonhormonal contraceptive methods with mixed results. Of those studies, three have noted a decrease in vaginal lactobacillus and one noted an increase in BV-related bacteria that failed to show a corresponding clinical significance.[66]

Breast Cancer

Breast cancer is responsive to natural progesterone; therefore, current breast cancer is a contraindication to DMPA use (i.e., US MEC Category 4), and a history of breast cancer > 5 years ago is a relative contraindication (i.e., US MEC Category 3).[9] In terms of future risk, a systematic review cited five of six observational studies investigating the association between progestin-only contraceptives use and incidence of breast cancer that found no association. In the remaining case-control study, the risk of breast cancer was increased in current DMPA users aged 35–44 years compared to never users (RR 2.3, 95% CI 1.3–4.1).[67] The more recent Danish Sex Hormone Register Study also found no increase in breast cancer risk associated with DMPA-IM use.[68] These studies were all limited by their observational study design and low numbers of breast cancer cases among participants.

Populations of Interest

The following clinical circumstances or conditions commonly present challenges for clinicians and their patients requesting DMPA despite the benefits DMPA can provide.

Breast/Chestfeeding

Immediate postpartum initiation of DMPA is considered safe whether breast/chestfeeding or not per the US MEC, but this recommendation has been controversial due to hypothetical effects on breast milk production. DMPA provision immediately postpartum is convenient and does not appear to further exacerbate the postpartum risk of VTE that CHC would. There is a potential risk that progestin could interfere with postpartum lactogenesis, milk supply, and duration with potential long-term effects on infant growth. However, in systematic reviews, including 14 nonrandomized clinical trials and observational studies of DMPA initiated in the first 6 weeks postpartum, all but two studies found either no effect on breastfeeding outcomes or improved outcomes among DMPA users.[69,70] Because of the potential risk, the WHO guidance varies from the CDC guidance: the WHO advises against the use of progestin-only injectables in the first six weeks postpartum in breast/chestfeeding people, whereas the CDC concludes that the benefits generally outweigh the risks of use (i.e., US MEC Category 2).[9] One recent study examined the effects of postpartum use of DMPA on milk production, time to onset of secretory activation, lactation duration, and infant consumption in very low birth weight infants and found delayed secondary activation but, overall, no negative effect on milk production or lactation duration.[71] Among these studies, there are few that assessed

DMPA initiation immediately postpartum and no RCTs to date that compare DMPA to nonhormonal or no contraceptive use. If a patient has concerns or preferences about using DMPA while breast/chestfeeding, be respectful of their decision.

Perimenopause

Healthy perimenopausal patients without contraindications can safely use DMPA until they reach menopause. Specifically, for patients in perimenopause, DMPA can reduce AUB and the risk of endometrial hyperplasia associated with anovulatory cycling. DMPA has also been shown to relieve vasomotor symptoms in perimenopausal patients.[72,73] However, as patients get older, additional health issues may evolve that increase the risk of using DMPA. In addition, the unique disadvantages of DMPA (weight gain and delayed return to fecundity) may be disparately concerning to patients in perimenopause. As previously discussed, BMD changes are not exacerbated in users who are in perimenopause, so DMPA need not be discontinued or restricted during perimenopause due to concerns over bone health (i.e., US MEC Category 1).[9] When to stop DMPA is addressed later in this chapter. (See also Chapter 21, Contraception in the Later Reproductive Years.)

Sickle Cell Disease

A systematic review of contraceptive use among women with sickle cell disease cited four studies specifying DMPA use, suggesting that use of DMPA is associated with either a decrease or no change in painful crises, an improvement in hematologic parameters, and no increase in VTE rates. In particular, a small, nonrandomized trial found that DMPA users had a decrease in painful crises at 3 months and 12 months of use compared to baseline, with a greater decrease than in users of either COCs or permanent contraception (30% vs. 45.5% vs. 50% users with crises at 12 months of use, respectively).[74] All studies were small and of fair to poor quality, but since no increase in adverse events was noted, the US MEC concluded that DMPA can be used without restriction in patients with sickle cell disease (i.e., US MEC Category 1).[9]

Providing the Method

Counseling and Assessment for DMPA

Person-centered contraception counseling, as outlined in Chapter 4, is the key to safe and satisfactory DMPA use. DMPA use aligns well with the preferences of patients who seek amenorrhea, find the potential delay in return to fecundity and possible weight gain acceptable, and desire a method that is reversible, with infrequent administration, and no need for an insertion procedure. The benefits of DMPA generally outweigh the risks of DMPA in terms of safety and acceptability. However, some patients have medical conditions or personal characteristics that increase their risk of complications or failure with use. Some patients will not choose DMPA to avoid hormone use or DMPA's potential for weight gain or delayed return to regular menses. And patients seeking the most effective contraception may be better served by using IUDs, implants, or a permanent method.

Explore the patient's medical and menstrual history as well as current medications to ensure there are no conditions that would preclude safe use of DMPA.

A comprehensive history will identify the medical conditions or concomitant medications per the US MEC that are contraindications or cautions to DMPA use. In addition, the previously mentioned US SPR provides guidelines for providers to follow when patients are initiating contraceptive methods, continuing methods, and switching from one method to another. Specifically, although the need for a breast and pelvic examination may be otherwise indicated by the patient's history or symptoms, neither is needed before initiating DMPA in an asymptomatic, healthy patient.[12,75] Two case-control studies compared pelvic examination provided before versus after initiation of DMPA or oral contraceptives and found no differences in incidence of sexually transmitted infections (STIs), abnormal Papanicolaou (pap) tests, or abnormal wet mounts.[76] Wellness exams, including pap and STI testing, may or may not be done at the same time as DMPA initiation or subsequent injections, per patient preference. An assessment of weight and BMI before DMPA initiation and at follow-up visits might be helpful to identify patients who experience weight gain with DMPA use. No other screening or laboratory tests are routinely needed before DMPA initiation unless the patient's medical history or blood pressure indicates a need for further assessment.[12,77] As previously presented, the US MEC provides guidance as to which medical conditions might require further assessment or follow up (https://www.cdc.gov/mmwr/volumes/65/rr/pdfs/rr6503.pdf).

Patients may have misinformation about the health risks posed by DMPA use based on stories from friends and family and from actual or perceived risks presented or exaggerated in media and internet sources. Once your patient expresses a potential interest in using DMPA, it is helpful to explore any misconceptions. Present the potential health and noncontraceptive benefits of DMPA use, not just the possible side effects and risks. Discuss expected bleeding changes, and address how confident they are that they can administer an injection themselves or return for an injection every 3 months. Anticipatory counseling about safety concerns and side effects increases patient satisfaction with their chosen method. (See Chapter 4, Person-Centered Reproductive Health Conversations and Contraceptive Counseling.)

Choosing a Formulation

Although the effectiveness, health benefit: risk ratio, bleeding profile, and side effect profile are similar for DMPA SC and IM formulations, DMPA-SC contains a lower dose than DMPA-IM and therefore each formulation should only be administered as intended. DMPA-SC is prescribed as a single-dose prefilled syringe by Pfizer and can be stored at room temperature. The prefilled syringes have the added benefit of small needle sizes (26-gauge × 3/8-inch needle) and less fluid volume.[78] DMPA-SC is only available as a brand name product can be ordered "Depo-subQ Provera 104." You should explain the relative benefits of DMPA-SC, but the ultimate formulation chosen by your patient may depend on several factors, including self-efficacy and tolerance for self-injection, ability to return to your office or clinic, availability of formulation, or insurance coverage. One of the main reasons DMPA-SC has a higher continuation rate is because it can be self-administered subcutaneously in the anterior thigh or abdomen. Current FDA labeling states DMPA-SC should be administered by a health care provider. Therefore, by prescribing it for self-administration, the provider is prescribing this medication in an "off-label" fashion. Adjusting your prescription instructions and clinical documentation when DMPA-SC is chosen may help ensure insurance coverage. Several national organizations have created standardized tool kits that provide guidance and stepwise instructions regarding prescribing, handling, and billing for DMPA-SC, including National Family Planning & Reproductive Health Administration and National Clinical Training Center for Family Planning.[22]

When to Start DMPA

DMPA can be initiated on any day of the menstrual cycle, as long as it is reasonably certain the patient is not pregnant. Guidelines for how to be reasonably certain a patient is not pregnant can be found in the US SPR and in Box 25-2.[12] This guidance applies to patients who are postabortion, postpartum, breastfeeding, otherwise amenorrheic, or switching from another method of contraception. Initiating DMPA on any day of the menstrual cycle is easy for a patient or your clinic staff to implement and allows a patient to be protected from pregnancy as soon as possible. In a RCT, there were fewer pregnancies (OR 0.36, 95% CI 0.16–0.84) among adolescents and young adults who received same-day DMPA initiation compared to starting a combined hormonal contraceptive as a "bridge" to DMPA initiation 3 weeks later. In addition, twice as many women who received same-day DMPA initiation were very satisfied compared to those who started with a bridge method, even when assessed at 6 months of use.[79]

If the patient is not within the first 7 days of the menstrual cycle, advise use of a back-up method of contraception for the first 7 days of DMPA use. If they need emergency contraception (EC) that day and choose the levonorgestrel (LNG) pill for EC, they can still start DMPA immediately. If they choose ulipristal acetate (UPA) for EC, it is advised to wait 5 days after taking the UPA before initiating hormonal contraception. However, if the patient is choosing DMPA-IM, it is reasonable to provide the DMPA-IM the same day rather than requiring a return visit as the risk of not initiating a regular contraceptive method may be greater than the risk of DMPA-IM reducing the effectiveness of UPA.[12] Regardless of the EC pill chosen, instruct them to repeat a urine pregnancy test in 2-4 weeks. (See Chapter 18, Emergency Contraception.)

If there is a possibility of an undetectable early pregnancy (i.e., less than 10–14 days from unprotected sex), the patient can still receive DMPA that day and take a urine pregnancy test at home (or return to your office or clinic to do so) in 2 weeks. (See Chapter 24, Pregnancy Testing.) Reassure patients that DMPA will not adversely affect an early pregnancy, but that rechecking a urine pregnancy test will detect a pregnancy early enough to allow them to pursue any pregnancy options they choose, especially if they live in a state with laws that restrict reproductive health care. Even if an early pregnancy is missed when DMPA is initiated, data indicate that fetuses inadvertently exposed in utero to DMPA are not at any increased risk for birth defects than are unexposed fetuses.[80,81]

Switching from Other Methods

Patients who switch from other contraceptive methods can start DMPA immediately, using the same guidelines just explained for same-day initiation.[12] For example, if a patient has their contraceptive implant removed, they should start DMPA that same day. If it is not within the first 7 days of scheduled bleeding, advise use of a back-up method of contraception for the first 7 days of DMPA use. The exception is after IUD removal. If the patient has had recent unprotected sex and is ≥ 5 days from the first day of the menstrual cycle, residual sperm in the genital tract may present a risk of pregnancy once the IUD is removed. In which case, there are three options:

- Start DMPA that day and return in 7 days for IUD removal
- Abstain or use a barrier method for the next 7 days and then return for IUD removal and DMPA initiation
- Have the IUD removed that day and take EC. With this option, only the LNG pill is advised. The patient can start DMPA immediately and repeat a urine pregnancy test in 2–4 weeks.[12]

Strategies to Increase Patient Satisfaction

Continuation of DMPA at 12 months is 56%. The most common reason cited for discontinuation of hormonal contraception is side effects. In one study, side effects were more common for DMPA compared to oral contraceptives and transdermal patches (74% vs. 63% vs. 45%). In addition, 31% of the DMPA users also reported not liking the changes in their menstrual cycle.[82] Two RCTs found that structured counseling provided with initiation of DMPA increased continuation (OR 3.78, 95% CI 2.34–6.10). The increase was primarily due to the decrease in discontinuation for menstrual disturbances; discontinuation for other side effects was minimally affected. This demonstrates the value of effective counseling conversations; prior knowledge that menstrual changes are likely allows patients the opportunity to consider whether the bleeding changes would be acceptable to them and avoids distress from an experience of unexpected (and perhaps concerning) bleeding changes.[83] In a prospective study, participants who were told to return to the clinic for side effects or told about the possibility of amenorrhea were more likely (2.7 and 2.5 times, respectively) to continue using DMPA-IM compared to women who did not receive that messaging.[84] It is not clear whether providing reminders to patients, including via text messaging, improves the likelihood of on-time return for repeat injections. One RCT among adolescent DMPA users found that reminders via text message improved on-time return for the first repeat injection only, and only one out of four trials that included adult DMPA users found that patient reminders improve continuation.[83,85]

USER INSTRUCTIONS

Instructions for DMPA use can effectively be provided verbally by a health educator, nurse, or provider or by written instructions, depending on the process that works best in your clinic or office setting. (See Chapter 4, Person-Centered Reproductive Health Conversations and Contraceptive Counseling for recommendations on patient education.)

- Users need to get a DMPA injection every 3 months for it to remain effective. Consider tools that may help users remember, like an app or calendar reminder on a smart phone, or the texting service via www.bedsider.org.
- Patients can start DMPA immediately. Advise them to use a back-up method for the first 7 days if needed and use a condom (internal or external) for dual protection thereafter if they need STI protection.

- Instruct your patient on the warning signs for complications with DMPA use. Even though they are rare, the sequelae of complications can be significant and even life-threatening.

Providing Adequate Supplies

To facilitate access to contraception, the CDC recommends providing up to 1 year's supply (syringes or prescribed refills) when a patient initiates DMPA use.[12] The syringes are packaged as prefilled, single-dose injectable medications and can be stored at room temperature. Ideally, a prescription should include four refills to ensure effective contraception over the course of a year, as each single dose injection should be given every 13 weeks.[22,78] To increase contraceptive access, DMPA injections in the clinic or office can be provided as "nurse-only" visits, decreasing visit time and cost, and increasing flexibility in scheduling. Considering updated cervical cancer screening guidelines, consider reasonable refill protocols for your clinic or office for patients who return less often than annually for a wellness visit. Finally, offer to provide or prescribe condoms and EC pills for all DMPA users.

Follow-Up

Because side effects generally appear in the first few months of DMPA use,[86] encourage patients to return if problems develop, if they have weight concerns, or if they wish to change their method. Although routine follow-up visits are not required, certain populations may benefit from follow-up visits, such as adolescents or adults with chronic medical conditions. At return visits for any reason (i.e., need for a DMPA refill or a wellness visit), responsiveness to patient concerns plays a significant role in patient satisfaction with contraception. Discuss how it has been for them to follow the 3-month injection schedule, whether via return visits or self-administered injections, and remind them adherence is key to DMPA effectiveness. If self-administering their injection, ask what questions or concerns they may have about self-injections.

Managing Issues with DMPA Use

Managing Missed Injections

When initiating DMPA, proactively instruct your patient in what to do after missing an injection:

If it has been more than 13 weeks but less than 15 weeks since the date of your last injection:

- Obtain your DMPA injection as soon as possible via self-injection or return visit.
- No urine pregnancy test, EC, or back-up contraception is needed.

If it has been more than 15 weeks since the date of your last injection:

- Obtain your DMPA injection as soon as possible via self-injection or return visit
- If you had unprotected sex more than 15 weeks after the date of your last injection:
    - Check a urine pregnancy test.

    - Use LNG or UPA pills for EC if you had unprotected sex within the last 5 days.
    - Recheck a urine pregnancy test in 2–4 weeks.
- Use a back-up method of contraception (e.g., condom, abstinence) until your DMPA injection is obtained and for 7 days thereafter.[12]

Managing Bleeding Changes and Side Effects

Active listening, nonjudgmental support, and reassurance with supporting medical evidence may provide support to DMPA users or offer them the opportunity to switch to another method. Listen when a patient expresses distress about side effects and respond with empathy and information. When appropriate, advise the patient that the symptom is usually time limited and offer management. Be clear that side effects are typically not adverse health events and discuss what signs would be concerning. Directly address the patient's concerns about use of DMPA and proactively ask if they are planning to continue DMPA. If the patient decides to switch to a different contraceptive method, offer contraception counseling and facilitate the change. (See Chapter 4, Person-Centered Reproductive Health Conversations and Contraceptive Counseling.)

Bleeding Changes

At 1 year of use, only 10% of DMPA users have regular bleeding episodes. More common bleeding patterns include amenorrhea, or infrequent, irregular, frequent, or prolonged bleeding. Initial DMPA use is associated with the increased likelihood of unpredictable bleeding, with increasing rates of amenorrhea with use over time.[40]

The U.S SPR offers guidance to address complaints of unpredictable bleeding with DMPA:

- Consider whether other clinical causes such as pregnancy, infection, or malignancy are possible and treat them or rule them out accordingly. A change in bleeding pattern that develops after long-term DMPA use may indicate endocrine abnormalities or uterine pathology (e.g., fibroids) that require further assessment.
- If the patient desires treatment, offer the following options for short-term treatment:
    - NSAIDs for 5–7 days
    - COCs or other estrogen supplementation for 10–20 days
- If the bleeding persists and the patient finds it unacceptable, offer counseling and provision of alternative methods.[12]

A Cochrane review evaluated 12 studies of the effectiveness of various treatments for bleeding irregularities with DMPA use. Overall, treatments provided short-term relief from bleeding complaints, though evidence of the long-term effect on DMPA continuation was limited. For example, a RCT of ethinyl estradiol found a profound decrease in bleeding compared to placebo in the first 3 months of use (OR 0.26, 95% CI 0.11–0.6) that tended to wane thereafter, but the loss-to-follow-up rate from the study was high. A RCT of cyclic use of COCs in DMPA users experiencing amenorrhea noted a decrease in amenorrhea (OR 0.38, 95% CI 0.19–0.73) and an increase in DMPA continuation (OR 0.6, 95% CI 0.4–0.88) compared to placebo, but did not follow participants after 6 months. A combined analysis of two RCTs of NSAIDs (mefenamic acid or valdecoxib) versus placebo noted an effect during or just after a bleeding episode (RR 0.42, 95% CI 0.25–0.72). Similarly, tranexamic acid 1,000 mg daily for 5 days decreased bleeding during and for 4 weeks after bleeding episodes (RR 0.13, 95% CI 0.06–0.28). There was no improvement noted with doxycycline.[40]

Weight Gain and Other Side Effects

For many side effects, it is difficult to determine causation versus association—that is, are the side effects caused by the DMPA, or are these symptoms just common among individuals? In a population-based survey of approximately 2,500 Germans, 82% of respondents reported that at least one common symptom (fatigue, headache, muscle pain, etc.) was causing mild impairment, and 22% reported at least one symptom causing severe impairment.[87]

One of the obvious benefits of DMPA is the lack of estrogen-related side effects. Alternatively, some side effects may be more noticeable with the relatively high dose of DMPA in comparison with the other progestin-only methods. Side effects experienced by DMPA users may include headache, bloating, breast tenderness, fatigue, mood changes, and androgenic symptoms such as acne. Systematic reviews of the medical literature have found scant evidence that side effects can be attributed to DMPA use. Specifically, besides bleeding changes, DMPA users in clinical trials were no more likely to report side effects such as menstrual cramping, bloating, or hair loss compared to nonhormonal contraceptive users.[86] Of four observational studies that measured loss of libido, dyspareunia, or adverse effect on arousal or sexual function, only one study noted that DMPA users were more likely to experience loss of libido compared with nonhormonal method users (aOR = 2.24; 95% CI 1.50–3.34).[86] (See Chapter 6, Sexuality and Contraception.)

Three observational studies have evaluated the use of DMPA and found no increased risk of depression, though the studies were of varying quality.[88] Two additional studies have investigated women who initiated DMPA postpartum and found no increased risk of postpartum depression compared to nonhormonal methods.[89] In a systematic review, the results are conflicting regarding DMPA use and any depressive symptoms, finding no increase in mood swings yet an increase in negative mood, though studies did not control for confounders such as relationship satisfaction, life stressors, or socioeconomic instability.[86]

As previously noted, measurement of weight and BMI at initiation and follow-up of DMPA might be helpful in counseling patients regarding weight gain with DMPA use. Early identification of weight gain allows for timely discussion about changes in nutrition, activity, or contraceptive method. Alternatively, lack of significant weight change may be reassuring to patients. A patient's *perception* of their weight change may not correlate with measured changes, or lack thereof, but that does not mean that clinicians should dismiss their perception. Most important, we must listen to a patient's concerns, briefly review the medical evidence about DMPA and weight change, and assist them in weighing the pros and cons of changing methods. (See Chapter 4, Person-Centered Reproductive Health Conversations and Cpntraceptive Counseling.)

When to Stop DMPA

The US SPR, ACOG, and the North American Menopause Society recommend that for patients who wish to avoid pregnancy, use of contraception, including DMPA in eligible patients, should continue until menopause.[90] Patients in perimenopause who are already amenorrheic on DMPA will not be able to use the absence of bleeding to signal the onset of menopause. Reassure patients that they may safely continue DMPA until 55 years of age if they have no contraindications. Alternatively, some users may desire discontinuation as soon as they reach menopause. For these patients, stopping DMPA to allow the resumption of menses may be a reasonable test of menopausal status if a nonhormonal contraceptive method is available and acceptable to them.[91] FSH levels are not substantially suppressed by DMPA use; however, in younger perimenopausal patients, FSH levels can vary widely and should not be relied upon to diagnose menopause. After age 50, DMPA users may be tested on the first day of injection, with menopause confirmed if FSH levels are consistently greater than 30 IU/L at intervals of at least 90 days.[92]

Author Disclosures—Cwiak: None. Lawley: None.

Acknowledgments—Wan-Ju Wu, MD, MPH and Deborah Bartz, MD, MPH, for their work on the previous iteration of this chapter.

References

1. Stanczyk FZ. All progestins are not created equal. Steroids. 2003;68:879-90.
2. Guttmacher Institute. Contraceptive use in the United States by method [fact sheet]. Available from: https://www.guttmacher.org/fact-sheet/contraceptive-method-use-united-states
3. Lessard LN, Karasek D, Ma S, et al. Contraceptive features preferred by women at high risk of unintended pregnancy. Perspect Sex Reprod Health. 2012;44:194-200.
4. Kavanaugh ML, Pliskin E. Use of contraception among reproductive-aged women in the United States, 2014 and 2016. F S Rep. 2020;1(2):83-93.
5. Petta CA, Faundes A, Dunson TR, et al. Timing of onset of contraceptive effectiveness in Depo-Provera users. II. Effects on ovarian function. Fertil Steril. 1998;70:817-20.
6. Petta CA, Faundes A, Dunson TR, et al. Timing of onset of contraceptive effectiveness in Depo-Provera users. I. Changes in cervical mucus. Fertil Steril. 1998;69:252-7.
7. Bastianelli C, Farris M, Bruni V, et al. Effects of progestin-only contraceptives on the endometrium. Expert Rev Clin Pharmacol. 2020;13:1103-23.
8. Lopez LM, Bernholc A, Chen M, et al. Hormonal contraceptives for contraception in overweight or obese women. Cochrane Database Syst Rev. 2016:CD008452.
9. Curtis KM, Tepper NK, Jatlaoui TC, et al. U.S. medical eligibility criteria for contraceptive use, 2016. MMWR Recomm Rep. 2016;65(3):1-103.
10. Kennedy, CE, Yeh, PT, Gaffield, ML, et al. Self-administration of injectable contraception: a systematic review and meta-analysis. BMJ Glob Health. 2019;4:e001350.
11. Curtis KM, Nguyen A, Reeves JA, et al. Update to U.S. selected practice recommendations for contraceptive use: Self-administration of subcutaneous depot medroxyprogesterone acetate. MMWR Morb Mortal Wkly Rep. 2021;70:739-43.
12. Curtis KM, Jatlaoui TC, Tepper NK, et al. U.S. selected practice recommendations for contraceptive use, 2016. MMWR Recomm Rep. 2016;65:1-66.
13. Steiner MJ, Kwok C, Stanback J, et al. Injectable contraception: what should the longest interval be for reinjections? Contraception. 2008;77(6):410-4.
14. Paulen ME, Curtis KM. When can a woman have repeat progestogen-only injectables—depot medroxyprogesterone acetate or norethisterone enantate? Contraception. 2009;80:391–408.
15. Upadhyay UD, Zlidar VM, Foster DG. Interest in self-administration of subcutaneous depot medroxyprogesterone acetate in the United States. Contraception. 2016;94:303-13.
16. Nabhan A, Elshafeey F, Mehrain LM, et al. Self-administered subcutaneous medroxyprogesterone acetate for improving contraceptive outcomes: a systematic review and meta-analysis. BMC Women's Health. 2021;21:359.
17. Beasley A, White KO, Cremers S, Westhoff C. Randomized clinical trial of self versus clinical administration of subcutaneous depot medroxyprogesterone acetate. Contraception. 2014;89:352-6.

18. Kohn JE, Simons HR, Della Badia L, et al. Increased 1-year continuation of DMPA among women randomized to self-administration: results from a randomized controlled trial at Planned Parenthood. Contraception. 2018;97:198-204.
19. Daniels K, Abma JC. Current contraceptive status among women aged 15–49: United States, 2015–2017. NCHS Data Brief, no. 327. National Center for Health Statistics; 2018.
20. Kaiser Family Foundation. DMPA contraceptive injection: use and coverage. Accessed June 15, 2022. Available from: https://www.kff.org/womens-health-policy/fact-sheet/dmpa-contraceptive-injection-use-and-coverage/
21. Burlando AM, Flynn AN, Gutman S, et al. The role of subcutaneous depot medroxyprogesterone acetate in equitable contraceptive care: A lesson from the coronavirus disease 2019 (COVID-19) pandemic. Obstet Gynecol. 2021;138:574-7.
22. National Clinical Training Center for Family Planning. A toolkit for user administration of subcutaneous depot medroxyprogesterone acetate. Kansas City, MO: Author; 2021. Available from: https://ctcfp.org/RiseToolkit1/content/assets/o35EjidVQvCccCfM_I2qdwah5RpxBxx-8-User_Administration_DMPA-SC_Toolkit.pdf
23. Katz M, Newmark RL, Aronstam A, et al. An implementation project to expand access to self-administered depot medroxyprogesterone acetate (DMPA). Contraception. 2020;102:392-5.
24. Schwallie PC, Assenzo JR. Contraceptive use--efficacy study utilizing medroxyprogesterone acetate administered as an intramuscular injection once every 90 days. Fertil Steril. 1973; 24;331-9.
25. Belsey EM. Vaginal bleeding patterns among women using one natural and eight hormonal methods of contraception. Contraception. 1988;38:181-206.
26. Arias RD, Jain JK, Brucker C, et al. Changes in bleeding patterns with depot medroxyprogesterone acetate subcutaneous injection 104 mg. Contraception. 2006;74:234-8.
27. Berenson AB, Odom SD, Breitkopf CR, Rahman M. Physiologic and psychologic symptoms associated with use of injectable contraception and 20 mg oral contraceptive pills. Am J Obstet Gynecol. 2008;199:351.e1-12.
28. Dragoman MV, Gaffield ME. The safety of subcutaneously administered depot medroxyprogesterone acetate (104 mg/0.65 mL): A systematic review. Contraception. 2016;94:202-15.
29. Brown J, Kives S, Akhtar M. Progestagens and anti-progestagens for pain associated with endometriosis. Cochrane Database Syst Rev. 2012;2012(3):CD002122.
30. Harmon QE, Patchel SA, Zhao S, et al. Depot medroxyprogesterone acetate use and the development and progression of uterine leiomyoma. Obstet Gynecol. 2022;139:797-807.
31. Bartels CB, Cayton KC, Chuong FS, et al. An evidence-based approach to the medical management of fibroids: A systematic review. Clin Obstet Gynecol. 2016;59:30-52.
32. Ammerman SR, Nelson AL. A new progestogen-only medical therapy for outpatient management of acute, abnormal uterine bleeding: a pilot study. Am J Obstet Gynecol. 2013;208(6):499 e1-5.
33. Venkatachalam S, Bagratee JS, Moodley J. Medical management of uterine fibroids with medroxyprogesterone acetate (Depo Provera): a pilot study. J Obstet Gynaecol. 2004;24:798-800.
34. Johnson N, Fletcher H, Reid M. Depo medroxyprogesterone acetate (DMPA) therapy for uterine myomata prior to surgery. Int J Gynaecol Obstet. 2004;85:174-6.
35. Kim JJ, Chapman-Davis E. Role of progesterone in endometrial cancer. Semin Reprod Med. 2010;28(1):81-90.
36. World Health Organization. Depot-medroxyprogesterone acetate (DMPA) and risk of endometrial cancer. The WHO Collaborative Study of Neoplasia and Steroid Contraceptives. Int J Cancer. 1991;49(2):186-90.
37. Wilailak S, Vipupinyo C, Suraseranivong V, et al. Depot medroxyprogesterone acetate and epithelial ovarian cancer: a multicentre case-control study. BJOG. 2012;119:672-7.
38. Kaunitz A. Depot medroxyprogesterone acetate contraception and the risk of breast and gynecologic cancer. J Reprod Med. 1996;41:419-27.
39. Andersson K, Odlind V, Rybo G. Levonorgestrel-releasing and copper-releasing (Nova T) IUDs during five years of use: a randomized comparative trial. Contraception. 1994;49:56-72.
40. Abdel-Aleem H, d'Arcangues C, Vogelsong KM, et al. Treatment of vaginal bleeding irregularities induced by progestin only contraceptives. Cochrane Database Syst Rev. 2013 Jul 2;(7):CD003449.

41. Lopez LM, Ramesh S, Chen M, et al. Progestin-only contraceptives: effects on weight. Cochrane Database Syst Rev. 2016:CD008815.
42. Bonny AE, Secic M, Cromer BA. A longitudinal comparison of body composition changes in adolescent girls receiving hormonal contraception. J Adolesc Health. 2009;45:423-5.
43. Le YC, Rahman M, Berenson AB. Early weight gain predicting later weight gain among depot medroxyprogesterone acetate users. Obstet Gynecol. 2009;114:279-84.
44. Bonny AE, Secic M, Cromer B. Early weight gain related to later weight gain in adolescents on depot medroxyprogesterone acetate. Obstet Gynecol. 2011;117:793-7.
45. Schwallie PC, Assenzo JR. The effect of depo-medroxyprogesterone acetate on pituitary and ovarian function, and the return of fertility following its discontinuation: a review. Contraception. 1974;10:181-202.
46. Westhoff C. Depot medroxyprogesterone acetate contraception. Metabolic parameters and mood changes. J Reprod Med. 1996;41(5 Suppl):401-6.
47. Berenson A, Rahman M, Wilkinson G. Effect of injectable and oral contraceptives on serum lipids. Obstet Gynecol. 2009;114:786-794.
48. Kahn HS, Curtis KM, Marchbanks PA. Effects of injectable or implantable progestin-only contraceptives on insulin-glucose metabolism and diabetes risk. Diabetes Care. 2003;26:216-25.
49. Segall-Gutierrez P, Xiang AH, Watanabe RM, et .al. Deterioration in cardiometabolic risk markers in obese women during depot medroxyprogesterone acetate use. Contraception. 2012;85:36-41.
50. Tepper NK, Whiteman MK, Marchbanks PA, et al. Progestin-only contraception and thromboembolism: A systematic review. Contraception. 2016;94:678-700.
51. World Health Organization Collaborative Study of Cardiovascular Disease and Steroid Hormone Contraception. Cardiovascular disease and use of oral and injectable progestogen-only contraceptives and combined injectable contraceptives. Results of an international, multicenter, case-control study. Contraception. 1998;57:315-24.
52. van Hylckama VA, Helmerhorst FM, Rosendaal FR. The risk of deep venous thrombosis associated with injectable depot-medroxyprogesterone acetate contraceptives or a levonorgestrel intrauterine device. Arterioscler Thromb Vasc Biol. 2010;30:2297-2300.
53. Bergendal A, Persson I, Odeberg J, et al. Association of venous thromboembolism with hormonal contraception and thrombophilic genotypes. Obstet Gynecol. 2014;124:600-9.
54. Lopez LM, Grimes DA, Schulz KF, et al. Steroidal contraceptives: effect on bone fractures in women. Cochrane Database Syst Rev. 2014 Jun 24;(6):CD006033.
55. Isley MM, Kaunitz AM. Update on hormonal contraception and bone density. Rev Endocr Metab Disord. 2011;12:93-106.
56. Kaunitz AM, Miller PD, Rice VM, et al. Bone mineral density in women aged 25-35 years receiving depot medroxyprogesterone acetate: recovery following discontinuation. Contraception. 2006;74:90-9.
57. Kaunitz AM, Peipert JF, Grimes DA. Injectable contraception: issues and opportunities. Contraception. 2014;89:331-4.
58. Curtis KM, Martins SL. Progestogen-only contraception and bone mineral density: a systematic review. Contraception. 2006;73:470-87.
59. Lopez LM, Chen M, Long SM, et al. Steroidal contraceptives and bone fractures in women: evidence from observational studies. Cochrane Database Syst Rev. 2015 Jul 21;2015(7):CD009849.
60. Vestergaard P, Rejnmark L, Mosekilde L. The effects of depot medroxyprogesterone acetate and intrauterine device use on fracture risk in Danish women. Contraception. 2008;78:459-64.
61. Meier C, Brauchli YB, Jick SS, et al. Use of depot medroxyprogesterone acetate and fracture risk. J Clin Endocrinol Metab. 2010;95:4909-16.
62. Lanza LL, McQuay LJ, Rothman KJ, et al. Use of depot medroxyprogesterone acetate contraception and incidence of bone fracture. Obstet Gynecol. 2013;121:593-600.
63. American College of Obstetricians and Gynecologists. Committee Opinion No. 602: Depot medroxyprogresterone acetate and bone risk. Obstet Gynecol. 2014;123:1398-1402.
64. Hofmeyr GJ, Singata M, Sneden J. Hormonal contraception for women exposed to HIV infection. Cochrane Database Syst Rev. 2014 May 20;(5):CD009741.
65. Curtis KM, Hannaford PC, Rodriguez MI, et al. Hormonal contraception and HIV acquisition among women: an updated systematic review. Sex Reprod Health. 2020;46:8-16.

66. Ratten LK, Plummer EL, Bradshaw CS. The effect of exogenous sex steroids on the vaginal microbiota: a systematic review. Front Cell Infect Microbiol. 2021;11:732423.
67. Samson M, Porter N, Orekoya O, et al. Progestin and breast cancer risk: a systematic review. Breast Cancer Res Treat. 2016;155:3-12.
68. Morch LS, Skovlund CW, Hannaford PC, et al. Contemporary hormonal contraception and the risk of breast cancer. N Eng J Med. 2017;377:2228-39.
69. Lopez LM, Grey TW, Stuebe AM, et al. Combined hormonal versus nonhormonal versus progestin-only contraception in lactation. Cochrane Database Syst Rev. 2015 Mar 20;(3): CD003988.
70. Phillips SJ, Tepper NK, Kapp N, et al. Progestogen-only contraceptive use among breastfeeding women: a systematic review. Contraception. 2016;94:226-52.
71. Parker LA, Sullivan S, Cacho N, et al. (2021). Effect of postpartum depo medroxyprogesterone acetate on lactation in mothers of very low-birth-weight infants. Breastfeed Med. 2021;16:835-42.
72. Bullock JL, Massey FM, Gambrell RD, Jr. Use of medroxyprogesterone acetate to prevent menopausal symptoms. Obstet Gynecol. 1975;46:165-8.
73. Morrison JC, Martin DC, Blair RA, et al. The use of medroxyprogesterone acetate for relief of climacteric symptoms. Am J Obstet Gynecol. 1980;138:99-104.
74. Haddad LB, Curtis KM, Legardy-Williams JK, et al. Contraception for individuals with sickle cell disease: a systematic review of the literature. Contraception. 2012;85:527-37.
75. Stewart FH, Harper CC, Ellertson CE, et al. Clinical breast and pelvic examination requirements for hormonal contraception: current practice vs evidence. JAMA. 2001;285:2232-9.
76. Tepper NK, Curtis KM, Steenland MW, Marchbanks PA. Physical examination prior to initiating hormonal contraception: a systematic review. Contraception. 2013;87:650-4.
77. Tepper NK, Steenland MW, Marchbanks PA, Curtis KM. Laboratory screening prior to initiating contraception: a systematic review. Contraception. 2013;87:645-9.
78. Pfizer. Depo-SubQ Provera 104 medical information [website]. Available from: https://www.pfizermedicalinformation.com/en-us/patient/depo-subq-provera-104
79. Rickert V, Tiezzi L, Lipshutz J, et al. Depo Now: preventing unintended pregnancies among adolescents and young adults. J Adolesc Health. 2007;40:22-8.
80. Katz Z, Lancet M, Skornik J, et al. Teratogenicity of progestogens given during the first trimester of pregnancy. Obstet Gynecol. 1985;65:775-80.
81. Brent RL. Nongenital malformations following exposure to progestational drugs: the last chapter of an erroneous allegation. Birth Defects Res A Clin Mol Teratol. 2005;73:906-18.
82. Daniels K, Mosher WD. Contraceptive methods women have ever used: United States, 1982-2010. Natl Health Stat Rep. 2013;62:1-15.
83. Mack N, Crawford TJ, Guise J, et al. Strategies to improve adherence and continuation of shorter-term hormonal methods of contraception. Cochrane Database Syst Rev. 2019;4(4):CD004317.
84. Hubacher D, Goco N, Gonzalez B, Taylor D. Factors affecting continuation rates of DMPA. Contraception. 1999;6:345-51.
85. Smith C, Gold J, Ngo TD, et al. Mobile phone-based interventions for improving contraception use. Cochrane Database Syst Rev. 2015;2015(6):CD011159.
86. Dianat S, Fox E, Ahrens KA, et al. Side effects and health benefits of depot medroxyprogesterone acetate: A systematic review. Obstet Gynecol. 2019;133:332-41.
87. Hiller W, Rief W, Brahler E. Somatization in the population: from mild bodily misperceptions to disabling symptoms. Soc Psychiatry Psychiatr Epidemiol. 2006;41:704-12.
88. Worly BL, Gur TL, Schaffir J. The relationship between progestin hormonal contraception and depression: a systematic review. Contraception. 2018;97:478-89.
89. Ti A, Curtis KM. Postpartum hormonal contraception use and incidence of postpartum depression: a systematic review. J Contracept Reprod Health Care. 2019;24:109-16.
90. Shifren JL, Gass ML, Group NRfCCoMWW. The North American Menopause Society recommendations for clinical care of midlife women. Menopause. 2014;21:1038-62.
91. Baldwin MK, Jensen JT. Contraception during the perimenopause. Maturitas. 2013;76:235-42.
92. Juliato CT, Fernandes A, Marchi NM, et al. Usefulness of FSH measurements for determining menopause in long-term users of depot medroxyprogesterone acetate over 40 years of age. Contraception. 2007;76:282-6.

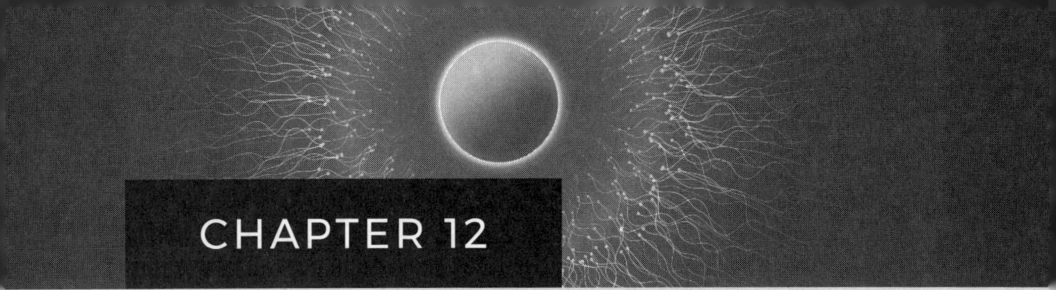

CHAPTER 12

Combined Hormonal Contraceptives (CHCs)

Shaalini Ramanadhan, MD, MCR
Alison Edelman, MD, MPH

KEY POINTS

- Combined hormonal contraceptives (CHCs) are methods that contain both an estrogen and a progestin component.
- CHCs come in a variety of different delivery systems, including oral pills, transdermal patches, and vaginal rings.
- CHCs are not only safe and effective, they also offer many noncontraceptive health benefits.
- Combined oral contraceptives (COCs) are the most commonly used reversible contraceptive method in the United States.
- Adherence to a daily method like COCs can be challenging; studies demonstrate that most patients miss several pills each month.[1]
- Patches and rings do not require daily use and therefore can facilitate consistent and correct use for some users.
- "Quick Start" initiation (e.g., same-day start) and providing a year's worth of CHCs helps improve adherence.[2,3]

Combined oral contraceptives (COCs) have been almost synonymous with contraception in the United States for over half a century. The creation of "the Pill," coupled with the social and legal changes of the 1960s, was a critical step for women in the ongoing struggle for gender equity. Individuals (and couples) could plan and prepare for or prevent pregnancy, thus enabling women to take advantage of educational or professional opportunities. Additionally, by unlinking sexual intercourse and childbearing, the pill enabled women to enjoy sexual activity without the fear of pregnancy.

The first COC approved by the US Food and Drug Administration (FDA) in May 1960 was Enovid-10. Enovid-10 was a monophasic pill with 21 active pills (9.85 mg norethynodrel and 150 mcg mestranol) and 7 placebo pills. The amount of hormones contained in Enovid-10 was significantly higher than today's

COCs. This dose caused nausea and increased the risk of adverse events. Over the years, the doses of the hormones in COCs have dramatically decreased without sacrificing contraceptive efficacy. New synthetic hormones and formulations have since been developed. Initial studies of these higher-dose COCs should be interpreted in this context; health concerns about high-dose pills may not be clinically relevant to current low-dose COCs (i.e., formulations containing < 50 mcg ethinyl estradiol). COC formulations have been continuously evolving, and combined hormonal contraceptive (CHC) options have also been expanding in the last few decades with the approval of contraceptive patches and vaginal rings.

Issues related to eligibility, initiation, side effects, and adverse events are similar for all CHCs regardless of route of administration. In this chapter, we will review these entities together as CHCs. Any pill-, patch-, or ring-specific data or recommendations will be detailed separately.

Clinical Impact of Combined Hormone Contraceptives

Although the widespread public perception is that CHCs are hazardous,[4] recent data about short- and long-term safety of CHC use show minimal health risks.[5] Short-term safety is achieved by appropriate patient selection, and clinicians have better tools now to identify eligible CHC users, as will be explained later in this chapter. Long-term safety data about COCs specifically are reassuring. The Royal College of General Practitioners (RCGP) observed 46,112 women for up to 39 years, accumulating over 819,175 woman-years of experience among ever users and 378,000 woman-years of observational data among never users of COCs.[6] Ever users of COCs had a significant 12% *lower* rate of death from any cause than did never users. The estimated absolute reduction in all causes of mortality for ever users of COCs from that study was 52 per 100,000 women-years. CHCs can reduce the risk of ectopic pregnancy, a leading cause of maternal mortality in early pregnancy, by 90% because they substantially reduce the risk of pregnancy.[7,8] In addition to contraception, other health benefits from CHCs have also been described and will be reviewed in this chapter. The oral contraceptive pill's contributions to women's health have been so enormous that the Centers for Disease Control and Prevention (CDC) recognized family planning (with oral contraceptives and condoms, in particular) as one of the 10 greatest public health achievements of the 20th century, on par with vaccination and control of infectious disease.[9]

Even with advancements made in other methods of contraception and the approval of different forms of CHCs, COCs remain the most commonly used reversible contraceptive method in the United States: 26% of current contraceptors, or 9.7 million reproductive-age women, use COCs.[10] In the most recent National Survey for Family Growth, 82% of US women who have ever been sexually active reported using COCs at some point in their lives.[11] CHCs (including the pill, the patch, and the ring) continue to be an ideal option for those who desire an effective, rapidly reversible method that they control themselves and can stop without input from a clinician, and that provides the many advantages of estrogen. These advantages include the ability for the patient to schedule their bleeding, whether that is monthly or another bleeding pattern, and the option for other noncontraceptive benefits, ranging from the treatment of menstruation-related issues to cancer prevention.

Readers of this chapter will become more effective at providing CHC by understanding how CHCs work, their advantages and disadvantages, and how to manage bleeding changes and side effects. We will review several ways to overcome barriers to using CHCs correctly and consistently; many of these barriers have been historically and arbitrarily created by our health care system. Finally, by providing clinically relevant information, we hope to make patient counseling messages more person-centered and, hopefully, more helpful to the patient. (See Chapter 4, Person-Centered Reproductive Health Conversations and Contraceptive Counseling.)

Mechanism of Action and Formulations

CHCs prevent fertilization. There is no evidence that they work to end or impact pregnancy after fertilization. CHCs are, therefore, contraceptive and not abortifacient or contragestive (which refers to agents that prevent or interrupt implantation in the uterus). The progestin component provides the main contraceptive effect through ovulation suppression. The estrogen component, most often ethinyl estradiol (EE), makes a small contribution to ovulation suppression but primarily helps with cycle control. Ovulation suppression occurs through a series of positive and negative feedback loops resulting in pituitary suppression, thus suppressing the luteinizing hormone (LH) surge (progestin effect) and release of follicle-stimulating hormone (FSH; estrogen effect). (See Chapter 2, Understanding the Physiology of the Menstrual Cycle.) Ovulation suppression provided by even low-dose COC formulations is profound: they suppress 99% to 100% of cyclic ovulations as reported in clinical trials that detected ovulation through serum hormone monitoring.[12]

EE and progestins have other effects on the reproductive system, but it has not been well substantiated that any of these effects contribute significantly to CHC effectiveness:

- Slowing of tubal motility (disruption of ova transport may interfere with fertilization)
- Thickening of cervical mucus (barrier to sperm transport). Blockage of sperm transport has been demonstrated with a levonorgestrel (LNG)-releasing intrauterine system but has not been well studied in terms of CHCs.[13,14]
- Endometrial atrophy, changes in function of endometrial vessels, and alterations in the matrix metalloproteinase content in the endometrium (these are progestin effects that might impede sperm motility and viability or, theoretically, could inhibit implantation)
- Localized edema of the endometrium (an estrogen effect that might affect implantation)

CHC Hormonal Components

CHCs contain both an estrogen and a progestin. In today's CHCs, the estrogen component is most often EE, whereas there are many different types of progestins used.

Estrogen

Estrogen was added to birth control pills to provide better cycle control. Estradiol, the estrogen produced by the ovary, was not initially used in CHCs, specifically

COCs, because it has low bioavailability (percentage of drug that eventually gets into the bloodstream) due to its extensive metabolism in the liver.[15] Instead, the early COCs used mestranol, an estrogenic compound in the first COC, Enovic. Mestranol is a prodrug that converts into EE, an ethinylated estrogen with improved bioavailability compared to estradiol. Over time, the doses of mestranol were reduced from 150 mcg eventually down to 50 mcg; today, the majority of COCs contain less than 35 mcg of EE, with doses as low as 10 mcg. Estradiol and estradiol esters, instead of EE, are currently being developed for use in COCs—two of which, estradiol valerate (E2V, paired with dienogest) and estetrol (E4, paired with drospirenone), are now commercially available in the United States.[16]

E2V is less potent than EE and is thought to have fewer estrogen-related side effects and thus may result in less frequent adverse events. E4 is also thought to have fewer side effects and less metabolic impact. Specifically, E4 is thought to have less metabolism in the liver, less interaction with enzymatic pathways, and more tissue selectivity.[17] In 2021, the first pill containing E4 and drosperinone was released. For both of these new estrogens, large population-level clinical studies are still needed to prove their purported benefits.

Progestins

Because the progestin component provides the main contraceptive effect, therapeutic levels must be maintained for at least 24 hours, with an adequate margin to allow for individual variation in drug absorption and metabolism as well as some allowance for user-adherence variability.[18] Natural progesterone is poorly absorbed from the gastrointestinal tract and is rapidly metabolized, thus it has not been a focus for oral contraceptive development. Synthetic progestins vary in their properties of bioavailability, half-life (the time necessary for the blood level to fall to 50% of its maximum), and clearance. Thus, the progestin dose needed to suppress ovulation varies from type to type.[18] Progestins have often been classified by "generations," a concept developed by the pharmaceutical industry to promote newer compounds. This nomenclature is now considered outdated and inaccurate as it suggests that newer generations are superior to older ones.[19] Instead, current perspectives regard the compound's molecular derivation and the varying levels of in vitro androgenicity and anti-mineralocorticoid activity for each progestin to be most relevant. These in vitro findings may or may not have demonstrable clinical impacts but may be important to some individuals when selecting a progestin.

Combined Oral Contraceptives (COCs)

Formulations

Over decades, COC formulations have changed and the number available has increased. Clinicians and patients now have many options to choose from, which helps to meet individual needs and desires and also addresses cost considerations. COC formulations are either monophasic or multiphasic. Monophasic formulations have the same daily dose of estrogen and progestin in each active pill. Multiphasic formulations have active pills with differing doses of estrogen and progestin; the hormone doses increase as the cycle progresses. Typically, biphasic formulations have two different dose combinations of estrogen and progestin in the active pills, triphasic formulations have three different dose combinations, and quadraphasic formulations have four. COC formulations offering multiphasic combinations of hormones were introduced in an effort to minimize hormonal exposure while maintaining cycle control—although the need for this improvement in regard to safety has not been substantiated given that the doses of modern-day pills are low (i.e., less than 50 mcg EE).

Dosing Regimens

The original COC formulations included hormone-free intervals (when the user takes no pills or placebo pills) to induce a monthly scheduled bleed that patients would interpret as normal menstruation. This scheduled monthly bleeding was thought to be needed for initial acceptance of the pill. Today, it is recognized that this scheduled bleeding is not biologically necessary while using COCs and that it is safe to suppress menstruation.[20] Due to the atrophy caused by the progestin-dominant effect on the endometrial lining, the avoidance of a withdrawal bleed with COC use is safe.

- ***21/7 Formulations.*** The 21-/7-day COC combination came from experience with the early high-dose COCs. Many formulations today still use a 21-/7-day schedule. To prevent breakthrough ovulation using these 21/7 formulations, it is very important that users do not delay starting their next COC pack following a 7 hormone-free interval.
- ***Shortened hormone-free interval.*** Many of the newer COC formulations have increased the number of active pills and decreased the number of placebo pills. Shortening the hormone-free interval appears to improve COC efficacy—likely in its ability to prevent breakthrough ovulation and provide more room for user error.[21] The hormone-free interval can be shortened with any monophasic COC formulation if a 24/4 formulation cannot be obtained or covered by insurance, or if a patient likes their current formulation. A patient can be instructed to adjust the hormone-free interval to be shorter than 7 days, but should be warned not to extend longer than 7 days because that could increase risk of pregnancy.
- ***Extended-cycle use.*** Many patients are afflicted with menstruation-related symptoms that can significantly impact their lives even on 21/7 formulations,[22] and menstrual suppression through COC use is highly effective in alleviating these symptoms.[23] Additionally, many people would prefer to bleed less frequently than once a month.[24] COC users do not need a medical reason to extend the duration of time between scheduled bleeds. The downside of extended cycling is that some users will experience more unscheduled bleeding in the first 3 to 6 months of use, but the unscheduled bleeding will decrease over time in most of these users and is not harmful. Timely ingestion and good adherence likely decrease the frequency of unscheduled bleeding. An occasional 3- to 4-day break[25] (no more frequently than every 30 days) or a pill containing norethindrone acetate[26] may result in more days of amenorrhea.

For some patients, menstrual bleeding reassures them that they are not pregnant. No evidence exists that missing a withdrawal bleed with COC use is indicative of a failure—in fact, many patients experience no bleeding routinely during the hormone-free interval.

Contraceptive Patches

Formulations

The first transdermal contraceptive patch (Ortho Evra®) was approved by the FDA in 2002. Ortho Evra is no longer marketed in the United States, but a generic version of the Ortho Evra patch (Xulane®) was found to be bioequivalent and was approved by the FDA in 2014. It is a thin, flexible patch with three layers: a beige outer protective polyester layer; a middle medicated adhesive layer; and a clear liner. The Ortho Evra patch contained 6 mg of norelgestromin (the primary active metabolite of norgestimate) and 0.75 mg of ethinyl estradiol (EE) in each 20 cm^2 square patch, while Xulane contains 4.86 mg of norelgestromin and 0.53 mg of EE in each 14 cm^2 patch. Both patches release 150 mcg of norelgestromin and 35 mcg of EE daily. In 2020, the FDA approved Twirla®, another transdermal system that releases 30 mcg of EE and 120 mcg of LNG each day in a 28 cm^2 circular patch. These patches can be applied to the buttocks, upper arm, lower abdomen, or upper torso (excluding the breasts). It should be noted that there are differences between the two available patches (Xulane and Twirla) in terms of estradiol exposure. The Xulane patch has been found to have steady state concentrations of EE that are about 60% more than a standard 35-mcg EE-containing oral contraceptive pill.[27] Twirla, on the other hand, has been found to have EE steady state that are 56%–65% less than a standard 35-mcg pill.[28]

Dosing Regimens

The dosing schedule is designed to mimic the 28-day dosing schedule of COCs, with 21 days of active hormones. Each patch provides contraceptive protection for 7 days. A user applies a new patch weekly for 3 weeks, leaves the patch off for a week to allow a scheduled bleed, and then applies a new patch. Extended (84 days) use of the patch resulted in fewer days of bleeding and fewer episodes of bleeding or spotting when compared with cyclic use.[29] Participants in both groups reported more headache days during the patch-off weeks compared with patch-on weeks, but those in the extended group also reported more headache days per week while wearing the patch. Both regimens led to decreased headache frequency over time, and people in both groups were highly satisfied.[29] In one study of 12 weeks of extended patch use, slow accumulation of EE levels was noted over time.[30] No published data evaluate long-term risks of extended patch use; the safety of this practice is unproven and thus extended or continuous patch use is not typically recommended by experts.

Vaginal Rings

Formulations

A vaginal contraceptive ring (NuvaRing®) was approved by the FDA in 2001. NuvaRing is a soft, transparent, flexible ring of ethylene vinyl acetate copolymer, with an outer diameter of 54 mm and a cross-sectional diameter of 4 mm. The ring releases 120 mcg of etonogestrel (3-keto desogestrel; ENG), the major metabolite of desogestrel, and 15 mcg of EE daily. In 2020, an additional vaginal ring (Annovera®) became available in the United States. This year-long contraceptive ring releases 150 mcg of segesterone acetate (SA) and 13 mcg of EE daily. About 6% of American women have ever used NuvaRing.[31] Of those currently using a contraceptive method, 2.6% report using the ring.[10]

Dosing Regimens

The EE/ENG ring is designed to be placed vaginally once every 28 days. Labeling advises that the ring be kept in place for 21 days and removed for a 7-day ring-free period to allow a scheduled bleed. While monthly cycling is the conventional use regimen, data support use of the ring continuously or in extended cycles. Extended use has been used to avoid estrogen-withdrawal side effects during the hormone-free week, to avoid bleeding in individuals who prefer amenorrhea, and to allow ring users to control the timing and frequency of bleeding.

Extended or continuous ring cycles are safe and practical for many users. Individuals can choose the duration of extended use that they prefer; regimens of 84 or 91 days of consecutive use are best studied, but options ranging from 49 to 364 days (changing the ring every 21–31 days) are well tolerated and acceptable. It should be noted that there continues to be active hormone eluted by each ring for 5–6 weeks and studies have shown that levels of hormones remain high enough to suppress ovulation and prevent substantial follicle development.[32,33] Extended use is associated with fewer episodes of scheduled bleeding but may be associated with more unscheduled bleeding. Unscheduled bleeding tends to be more common in the first months and then decreases significantly over the first year of use.[34-36]

One strategy that can help users with adherence is for them to place a new ring on the first day of each calendar month. This can help users remember to switch the ring. Patients choosing continuous use would simply switch the current ring for a new one on the first day of the month. Alternately, users can schedule a bleed by removing the ring for the last 4 days of the calendar month and putting in the subsequent ring on the first day of the next month.

Those who experience persistent or prolonged breakthrough bleeding/spotting with extended ring cycling may benefit from a 4-day hormone-free interval.[37] One recommendation is to follow a flexible "bleeding-signaled" regimen. That is, individuals use the ring continuously until they experience 4 days or more of consecutive bleeding or spotting, at which point they remove the ring for 4 days, and then insert a new ring on the fifth day. A recent study demonstrated that this approach stopped the bleeding episode within 4 days in about 50% of ring users, and within 7 days in over 90%.[36]

The SA/EE ring can be prescribed once for multiple cycles. The ring is placed in the vagina for 21 days and then can be washed and stored in its case for the 7-day hormone free interval. It can then be reinserted and used for up to 13 cycles. Shortening the hormone-free interval and continuous use for this ring has not yet been studied.

Effectiveness

All CHCs are considered "second-tier" contraceptive methods in terms of effectiveness—moderately but not highly effective.

COCs

With COCs, their first-year failure rate with typical use is 9% (see Table 5-2 in Chapter 5, Effectiveness, Safety, and Comparative Side Effects). However, the first-year perfect use failure rate of most COCs is less than 1%. The failure rates reported in clinical trials (i.e., perfect-use) should not be confused with the typical-use failure rate, because participants in clinical trials are highly motivated, monitored closely, and compensated for their time. Typical-use failure rates, derived from real-world use in which some individuals use COCs correctly and others do not, are a better guide for patient counseling. Adolescents and young adults experience even higher typical-use failure rates than adults when using short-acting methods like COCs, the ring, and the patch—almost twice as high.[38]

The gap that exists between perfect-use failure rates and typical-use failure rates is due to human behavior and systems issues that negatively affect users' adherence. Substantial barriers may prevent a patient from gaining timely access to contraceptive supplies and prevent consistent use. A study demonstrated that after 1 month of use, only 72% of COC users returned to the pharmacy on a timely basis for refill.[39] Dispensing a 1-year supply as compared with only one to three pill packs was associated with a 30% reduction in the odds of an unintended pregnancy. Other routine medications are allowed a 90-day supply, so there is precedent for dispensing multiple months at a time.[2] Requiring patients to return each month for refills constitutes a major barrier to successful COC use.[2]

Possession of the COC pack, however, does not guarantee correct daily use. One study, in which a computer chip was placed in the COC pack to record the date and time a pill was removed from the pack, found that although most COC users thought that they took the pills on a daily basis, during the third cycle, 54% of users actually missed three or more pills.[1,40] Taking a daily pill for an asymptomatic condition, such as fecundity, is challenging. Plus, many patients have nuanced attitudes about pregnancy desires and may not be highly motivated to prevent pregnancy.[41,42] Unfortunately, using a smart phone app, signing up for a text messaging service, or setting the alarm on cell phones to remind the patient does not appear to improve adherence, though it did not make it worse.[43] Another strategy for patients who have difficulty with adherence, especially those who forget to start a new pill pack, is to skip the hormone-free interval or placebo week (continuous use) or shorten it to 3 or 4 days (extended use). As previously mentioned, using formulations with fewer placebo pills (e.g., 24/4) has demonstrated lower pregnancy rates,[21] and it is expected that extended use would have lower pregnancy rates as well.

COC users should be advised that fecundity returns quickly with discontinuation,[44] so if pregnancy is not desired, another method should be started immediately. Studies show that 11% of COC users discontinue their COCs in the first month of use, and 19% of those who discontinue fail to adopt a new method.[40]

Contraceptive Patches

In clinical trials and as reported in a Cochrane review,[45] failure rates for patches were similar to those for COCs.[46,47] (For more detailed information about failure rates, see Chapter 5, Effectiveness, Safety, and Comparative Side Effects.) In a pooled analysis of the three pivotal clinical trials of the Ortho Evra patch, 15 pregnancies occurred in 22,160 treatment cycles, with an overall life-table failure rate of 0.8% (95% CI 0.3%–1.3%).[48] For the newer EE/LNG patch, the overall Pearl Index or PI, which represents the number of contraceptive failures per 100 person-years of exposure, was 5.8 (95% CI 4.5–7.2).[49] (For more details on efficacy of patches, see Chapter 5, Effectiveness, Safety, and Comparative Side Effects.) In the Cochrane analysis of patches, and in the EE/LNG patch's key clinical studies, there was lower efficacy seen for individuals of obese body mass index (BMI).[45,49] This will be discussed further in the Special Considerations section of this chapter (p. 388).

Continuation of a method can be an important consideration for providers as users who discontinue a pill, patch, or ring without replacement are at almost immediate risk of pregnancy. In addition, continuation of a method can often be used as a proxy for user satisfaction. Despite its convenience, the contraceptive patch does not have higher continuation rates or lower failure rates than COCs.[50-52] In comparative studies, continuation rates with the patch in typical-use populations were lower than with the vaginal ring (88% vs. 95% over three cycles, $P = 0.03$)[53] or with COCs (67% vs. 89% over three cycles, $P < .001$; and 57% vs. 76% at 1 year, $P = .004$).[52] Another large cohort of young women showed very low continuation rates for the patch; the 12-month continuation rate was 10.9 per 100 person-years compared with 32.7 per 100 person-years for COCs; reported side effects were the most common reasons for discontinuation.[54] In contrast, the contraceptive CHOICE study found continuation rates for the patch were low, but similar to those with COCs and rings, with 1-, 2-, and 3-year patch continuation rates of 49%, 40%, and 28%.[55-57]

In one observational study of teen mothers during the first year postpartum, repeat pregnancy rates were similar for patch users (32%) and COC users (30%) and higher than those of depot medroxyprogesterone acetate (DMPA) users (14%).[50] In another cohort study of women aged 15 to 24, self-reported pregnancy rates were 30.1 per 100 person-years among patch users, compared with 15.6 per 100 person-years among COC users.[54] However, in the contraceptive CHOICE study, participants using COCs, patch, or ring experienced similar failure rates and so were combined: 4.8%, 7.8%, and 9.4% in years 1, 2, and 3.[38]

Although continuation rates among adolescent patch users in one study were higher at 3 months than for COCs (71% vs. 51%), approximately half of both patch and COC users stopped the method by 1 year.[50] Another observational study found that only 38% of adolescent patch users (compared with 60% of COC users) were still using their method after nine cycles, even though no differences were noted in reported side effects or quality of life.[58] In the study of young women reported above, 1-year continuation rates were lowest for patch and DMPA initiators, 10.9 and 12.1 per 100 person-years, compared with 29.4 and 32.7 per 100 person-years for ring and pill users.[54]

Vaginal Rings

Comprehensive data regarding vaginal rings are predominantly from the EE/ENG ring. Failure rates with this vaginal contraceptive ring in clinical trials are low and similar to the patch and COCs.[59] PIs range from 0.25 to 0.96 per 100 person-years with perfect use, to 0.65 to 1.23 overall.[59,60] In one study, more pregnancies occurred in North American sites than in European sites; the overall PI was 1.75 in North America and 0.65 in Europe. Reasons for this difference are unclear but likely reflect differences in participant characteristics among different study settings.[61,62] Typical-use pregnancy rates among those using the ring are about 7% in the first year.

Theoretically, improved ease of adherence to ring regimens could lead to typical-use pregnancy rates lower than those with COCs, which require daily attention. However, this has not been conclusively demonstrated. One recent systematic review noted that, among eight clinical trials, pregnancy rates were similar between the vaginal ring and oral contraceptives.[45] Another systematic review found a trend toward lower pregnancy rates with the ring compared to COCs, though the trend did not meet statistical significance (OR 0.52, 95% CI 0.26–1.04).[63]

Findings about whether adherence is improved with the ring compared with the pill are mixed. Although a noncomparative trial showed high rates of correct and consistent ring use (91%),[63] randomized comparative trials generally have demonstrated similar adherence rates for both methods.[45,59,60] Recently, a systematic review found that the number of study participants able to adhere correctly to ring and pill regimens was similar (63.4% vs. 61.2%), but the number of "compliant cycles" was slightly higher for the ring than COCs (88.3% vs. 86.4%).[64] In trials, 86% to 91% of ring users report perfect adherence,[60,61,63,65-67] although clinical trial settings likely represent a best-case scenario. Studies of typical use find lower adherence rates than seen in clinical efficacy trials.[68]

A randomized crossover study found higher 3-month continuation rates with the ring (94.6%) compared with the patch (88.2%) among those switching from COC,[53] but this short-term study may not reflect real-world experience for those choosing the ring. Twelve-month continuation rates of the ring are in the range of 40% to 55%, generally similar to those of the pill.[57,67,68]

The evidence base for Annovera, the newly released SA/EE ring, is continuing to grow, but initial studies found the ring to have a PI of 2.98 (95% CI 2.13–4.06).[69]

Effectiveness in Patients with Higher Body Weight

COCs

Given the growing number of reproductive-aged individuals with a BMI $\geq$ 30 kg/m^2, the impact that weight might have on COC efficacy is important for public health as well as for personal health. Although it does appear that obesity adversely affects contraceptive steroid hormone pharmacokinetics (e.g., drug levels and how drugs are metabolized),[70,71] the literature has been conflicting regarding the impact on COC effectiveness.[72] Generally, there are few appropriately designed studies for any contraceptive method that explore the relationship between contraceptive efficacy and obesity. The majority of studies are not large enough to investigate the main outcome of interest: pregnancy. However, a study of 10,000 participants with obesity demonstrated that there may be a slight increased risk of pregnancy[73] as did a meta-analysis performed by the FDA of individual study participant data.[74] Likely, obesity plays a small role in decreasing effectiveness, but the small impact is masked by the overwhelming issues of adherence.

Both extended-cycle use of a 20-mcg EE COC and 21/7 use of a 35-mcg EE COC have been to found to provide better suppression of ovarian activity than 21/7 use of a 20-mcg EE COC in people with obesity.[23] For healthy individuals with obesity, COCs are identified as category 2 by the CDC Medical Eligibility Criteria (MEC),[75] and thus safe to use. For patients of any weight or BMI, COCs are still considered second-tier in terms of effectiveness, so if a highly effective method is desired, then an intrauterine device (IUD) or implant or a permanent method should be offered.

Surgical interventions for obesity are an important consideration for prescribers of COCs. After bariatric surgery, fecundity and ovulation rates increase, and the CDC advises against pregnancy in the first 2 years post-surgery as pregnancy outcomes are worse.[76] No clinical trials have assessed the effectiveness of COCs used after bariatric surgery. A case series noted two COC failures in patients after surgery for malabsorptive procedures (biliopancreatic diversion, Roux-en-Y bypass).

Nutritional deficiencies have been noted in patients after these surgeries, suggesting that COC efficacy may be adversely impacted by decreased gastrointestinal absorption. These patients can use COCs with caution (Category 3) if no other method is available or acceptable to the patient. Patients choosing to use COCs should be advised and encouraged to use a second (back-up) method. Concerns about COC effectiveness after bariatric surgery do not apply to other combined hormonal methods such as the transdermal patch and the vaginal ring. Decreased effectiveness of COCs is also not a concern for patients who have had restrictive procedures (banding, gastrectomy), for whom COCs are Category 1.

Contraceptive Patches

Body weight is associated with lower serum levels of EE and norelgestromin in contraceptive patch users.[48] Furthermore, limited evidence suggests that persons weighing more than 90 kg (198 lbs) may be at higher risk of pregnancy when using the contraceptive patch, but evidence is inconsistent. In a pooled analysis of the three pivotal trials for the Ortho Evra patch, 5 of the 15 pregnancies that occurred in patch users were in people weighing more than 90 kg, though such individuals comprised only 3% of the study population.[48] In contrast, another recent observational study found no increased risk of contraceptive failure among those contraceptive patch users with an overweight, or Category 1, 2, or 3 obese BMI, though data were combined with pill and ring user data.[77] The newly approved EE/LNG patch (Twirla) has also been found to have decreased efficacy for higher-BMI patients. For individuals with BMI between 25 and 30, the PI was found to be 5.7 (95% CI 3.0–8.4), and for ≥ 30 the PI was 8.6 (95% CI 5.8–11.5), compared to 3.5 (95% CI 1.8–5.2) for those with BMI < 25.[49]

Vaginal Rings

There are no trials that compare efficacy of the ring between contraceptive users with and without obesity.[32,78] Two studies found similar etonogestrel levels and similar suppression of ovarian follicular development between those with and those without obesity using the ring. These therapeutic levels of hormones and the suppression of follicular development persisted for up to 6 weeks of continuous use.[32,33]

Medication Interactions and the Impact on CHC Effectiveness

One medication can alter the effectiveness of another medication in many ways. The most important way a medication can interact with CHCs is through the liver's cytochrome P450 enzyme activation.[15,18] This is most relevant for COCs and most studies looking at these drug–drug interactions involve COCs. Similar principles apply, however, to rings and patches as metabolism still occurs in the liver after systemic absorption via transdermal or vaginal routes.

Induction of cytochrome P450 will cause more rapid clearance of medications, including contraceptives, that are metabolized by this pathway. Medication development is ongoing, thus the knowledge regarding whether a new medication interacts with a CHC often lags. However, most medication labeling will contain information on its metabolism pathway—if it is a cytochrome P450 inducer, then it is possible that it could decrease COC effectiveness.

The major class of medications that often decrease COC's effectiveness is anticonvulsants such as carbamazepine, phenytoin, and topiramate. Lamotrigine (Lamictal®) is a special case, as the COC is not affected by concurrent use but the lamotrigine level is. Lamotrigine levels drop by almost half when COCs are started because increases in cytochrome P450 start rapidly after COC initiation, and they are slow to normalize after COC cessation.[79] Involving the provider who prescribes lamotrigine in the decision about COC use is critical. For the most up-to-date list, please refer to the CDC MEC (https://www.cdc.gov/reproductivehealth/contraception/mmwr/mec/appendixD.html#drug_interactions).[75]

Antiretrovirals (ARVs) and COCs appear to have varying impacts: they may have no impact on each other, or the COCs may impact the ARVs, or the ARVs may impact the COC. Medication development and treatment regimens for human immunodefciency virus (HIV) are rapidly changing; for the most up-to-date list of potential interactions, please refer to the CDC MEC (https://www.cdc.gov/reproductivehealth/contraception/mmwr/mec/appendixm.html).[75]

Most antibiotics have no impact on the effectiveness of COCs. A systematic review of nearly 200 articles found that only rifampin impaired the effectiveness of COCs.[80] Specific studies of tetracycline, doxycycline, ampicillin, metronidazole, and quinolones demonstrated no impact on medication levels.[81-85]

St. John's Wort is an over-the-counter herbal product that is used to treat depression; evidence is limited, but it may decrease the effectiveness of COCs.[86] Other psychotropic medications do not appear to be of concern.[87]

Advantages

All the items listed below in the COC section below are relevant to all CHCs. Specific additional advantages of the patch and ring follow.

CHCs/COCs

The general benefits of all CHC/COC formulations, regardless of delivery method, are as follows:

- **Rapid reversibility.** A comprehensive review of the literature concluded that the return to fecundity in patients who stop COCs in order to conceive occurs within the first few months after cessation and is comparable to that observed following discontinuation of other contraceptive methods, even with extended use of COCs.[44] Baseline cycling resumes within the first few months of discontinuing COCs. With long-term use, up to 10 years or more, there is similarly no clinically significant delay in return to fecundity.[88]
- **Regulation of bleeding**. Taken cyclically, COCs produce predictable scheduled bleeding. In a randomized controlled trial of patients with abnormal uterine bleeding (AUB), use of COCs was associated with an 80% improvement in bleeding pattern compared with less than 50% with placebo.[89] This includes AUB related to anovulation, which is commonly associated with adolescence, perimenopause, obesity, or polycystic ovary syndrome (PCOS). Predictability in bleeding episodes allows patients to plan their scheduled bleeding to fit their lives, rather than scheduling their lives to fit their bleeding. Patients who use extended-cycle COCs similarly gain control over their scheduled bleeding

and, with time, over unscheduled bleeding.[23] Scheduling bleeding can be done merely for personal preference or convenience. In addition, developmentally or physically disabled adolescents and adults whose menstrual bleeding presents a hygiene challenge to them and their caregivers can benefit.

Benefits of Modified Menstruation

- **Decreased menstrual blood loss.** COCs decrease the number of days of bleeding and the amount of blood loss with each menstruation. In a randomized trial of 45 women with heavy menstrual bleeding (HMB), use of a 30-mcg EE COC was associated with a 43% decrease in menstrual blood loss as compared to placebo.[90] Observational studies have shown that use of COCs can reduce menstrual blood loss and increase hemoglobin levels, and this use is supported in clinical practice guidelines.[91,92] Patients who use extended-cycle regimens reduce their numbers of scheduled bleeding episodes compared with patients who use COCs cyclically. The resulting total blood loss is decreased, though the total number of days of bleeding or spotting is the same.[23] This benefit is particularly important for patients with preexisting anemia from idiopathic HMB, adenomyosis, iron-deficiency anemia, or coagulation defects. COCs may also be effective medical therapy for HMB due to uterine leiomyomas, especially for patients who wish to preserve their fecundity.[91]
- **Decreased dysmenorrhea.** COCs significantly decrease menstruation-related cramping. In a randomized clinical trial of treatment for dysmenorrhea, low-dose COC users reported significantly lower pain scores, fewer absences from school and work, and less need for analgesics than did placebo users.[93] A recent review of the existing literature concluded that for those who wish to use contraception, compared to nonsteroidal anti-inflammatory drugs (NSAIDs), low-dose COCs are the preferred therapy for pain relief from dysmenorrhea; because there are risks associated with taking NSAIDs, COC use is a more suitable long-term option.[94] Extended-cycle COC use, which eliminates scheduled bleeding episodes, may provide even more relief from dysmenorrhea. (See Chapter 2, Understanding the Physiology of the Menstrual Cycle.)
- **Decreased symptoms of endometriosis.** Current COC use is associated with a 50% lower incidence of symptomatic endometriosis among parous patients.[95] The risk of developing endometriomas has been found to be significantly lower in current and past COC users over the age of 25.[96] Long-term cyclic or extended use of COCs following laparoscopic excision of ovarian endometriomas has been found to significantly reduce or delay their recurrence.[97] In addition, COCs decrease menstrual pain with endometriosis.[98] This benefit is enhanced by use of extended-cycle COCs, which reduce the number of painful scheduled bleeding episodes. Also, with extended use of COCs, the progestins induce pseudodecidualization of the endometriotic implants, which makes them inactive and less likely to induce painful inflammation reactions during menstruation.[99] However, such treatment is not curative; the endometriotic implants undergo atrophy during treatment but remain ready for reactivation whenever COCs are stopped.[100]
- **Decreased menstruation-related migraines.** Menstrual migraines are caused by estrogen withdrawal before menstruation, prostaglandin release during menstruation, or both. It is unclear whether use of COCs is associated with

increased frequency of migraine or other headaches as most studies did not control for baseline frequency of headaches or compare COCs with placebo.[101] On the other hand, menstrual migraines can be prevented with the use of extended cycle regimens.[102,103] (See the section on Headaches, in Managing Side Effects, p. 402.)

- **Decreased endometrial cancer risk.** COC (pills containing > 35 mcg of EE) use for at least 12 months reduces the risk of developing endometrial cancer by approximately 40%.[104] A meta-analysis found that longer durations of use were associated with greater decreases in risk, up to a 72% decrease in patients who used COCs for at least 12 years compared with nonusers, and the protection against endometrial cancer endures for up to 20 years after COC discontinuation.[105] Studies suggest that the protection against endometrial cancer is also conferred with lower dose COCs as well.[91] For patients who currently have endometrial hyperplasia (a precursor to endometrial carcinoma), COCs can be used as a treatment to prevent endometrial carcinoma.[75]

Benefits of Suppression of Ovulation

- **Decreased premenstrual symptoms.** There is limited evidence that cyclic use of COCs containing some progestins decrease the symptoms of premenstrual syndrome (PMS) such as breast pain, bloating, and negative affect compared with placebo. In a nonplacebo controlled trial, drospirenone-containing COCs reduced PMS symptoms more than did levonorgestrel-containing COCs.[106] A comparative trial of extended versus cyclic use of a low-dose drospirenone-containing COC noted that extended use was associated with a significant decrease in premenstrual symptoms, including negative mood. The greatest improvement was noted after 6 months of use.[107] A greater clinical benefit may be seen for premenstrual dysphoric disorder (PMDD). As many as 18% of women of reproductive age may have PMDD, which by definition means that their symptoms are severe enough to cause distress.[108] A Cochrane review of randomized clinical trials concluded that use of low-dose drospirenone-containing COCs reduced the severity of symptoms of PMDD. Participants' ability to function and to interact socially during menses also improved.[109] Based on these studies, drospirenone-containing COCs gained approval from the FDA as treatment for the symptoms of PMDD. Extended use of levonorgestrel-containing COCs may also be effective treatment for PMS or PMDD, though studies are not consistent in this finding.[110]
- **Decreased functional ovarian cysts.** The use of low-dose COCs is associated with a reduced prevalence of functional (i.e., postovulatory or luteal) cysts.[111] [111-113] The clinical significance of this benefit is unclear, as most functional cysts regress without needing therapy, although hemorrhagic corpus luteal cysts can rarely pose a surgical emergency. Low-dose COCs taken cyclically (21/7) do not protect as well against ovarian follicle formation, because they do not sufficiently suppress FSH levels.[114-117] Extended cycle use of low-dose COCs more effectively reduces ovarian follicle formation. COCs do not treat existing ovarian cysts because their use does not accelerate regression of cysts,[118] but COCs may prevent the formation of a new cyst, which might be mistaken for the original cyst on repeat exam, and COCs may eliminate the midcycle pain associated with ovarian follicle extrusion.

- **Decreased ovarian cancer risk.** A collaborative reanalysis of data from 45 studies showed that ever users of COCs had a 27% reduced risk of ovarian cancer that persisted for 30 years.[119] The longer the duration of use, the greater the protection: the relative risk decreased by 20% for every 5 years of COC use. Low-dose COC formulations were associated with a similar decrease in risk as older, high-dose formulations containing 50 mcg or more of EE.[120] The Royal College of General Practitioners (RCGP) observational study with up to 39 years of follow-up found that ever users were 47% less likely to die from ovarian cancer than were nonusers (RR 0.53 (0.38–0.72)).[6] A meta-analysis of three observational studies found a similar protective effect among those with *BRCA1* and *BRCA2* mutations who are at higher risk of developing ovarian and breast cancer. Again, the longer the duration of use, the greater the effect. A compelling argument can be made that COCs should be offered to otherwise healthy patients who are at high risk for developing ovarian cancer, even if they do not need contraception.[121]
- **Decreased risk of benign breast conditions.** COC users are less likely to develop fibrocystic breast changes, cysts, or fibroadenoma, especially with longer durations of COC use.[122,123] In one case-control study with over 500 participants, the risk of benign breast conditions was lower in the COC users, regardless of dose of EE, and markedly lower in participants who started COC use before their first full-term pregnancy.[124] COC use does not reduce nor does it elevate the risk of developing ductal hyperplasia with atypia.[123]

Benefits Related to the Estrogen Component

- **Improvement of acne.** Three brand name COC formulations have received formal FDA approval for treatment of mild to moderate acne, but all COC formulations are effective.[125,126] A recent Cochrane review concluded that in nine randomized clinical trials, all COCs were significantly more effective than placebo in reducing the number, severity, and self-assessment of facial acne lesions. In comparative trials of COCs containing varied progestins, few differences were found in effectiveness against acne. [127]COCs reduce acne by suppressing ovarian production of androgens and by inducing hepatic production of sex hormone binding globulin (SHBG). SHBG binds circulating testosterone and, thereby, reduces serum concentrations of free (biologically active) testosterone by up to 50%. In addition, conversion of testosterone to dihydrotestosterone in skin and hair follicles is decreased. Extended-cycle regimens suppress endogenous androgen production more than 21/7 regimens.[128] COCs do not have an immediate impact on acne; patients need to be advised that maximal effect may not be seen for up to 6 months.[129,130] SHBG levels may remain elevated for several months after discontinuation of COCs.[131]
- **Improvement of hirsutism.** Just as estrogen in COCs helps reduce androgen levels and activation of sebum production, it also helps reduce androgenic stimulation of hair growth. With COC use, patients with hirsutism have a reduction in the hair shaft diameter.[132,133] It generally takes 6 months to see the beneficial effect of COCs on hirsutism, and continued use of COCs is necessary to prevent recurrence. In patients with significant androgenic symptoms, as often seen with PCOS, drospirenone-containing COCs may be more effective than other COC formulations in decreasing testosterone levels and

symptomatology.[134,135] In addition, extended-cycle regimens suppress androgen production more than do cyclic 21/7 regimens.[128]

- **Treatment for hot flashes and other perimenopausal symptoms.** One 3-year observational study found that 90% of those with vasomotor symptoms during the perimenopause period had relief with COC therapy compared with 40% with placebo.[136] Extended use of COCs may be more effective as users would not experience a drop in EE during the placebo week. (See Chapter 21, Contraception in the Later Reproductive Years, for more discussion.)
- **Favorable impact on bone for high-risk patients.** Patients who have hypothalamic amenorrhea have low levels of circulating estrogens and are at higher risk for osteoporosis and, later in life, for fractures. COC use increases bone mineral density (BMD) in adolescents with hypothalamic amenorrhea.[137] COC use by patients with osteopenia due to anorexia nervosa is not sufficient to completely protect bone, but when added to anabolic agents such as insulin growth factor, COC use significantly improved that agent's effectiveness.[138] A systematic review concluded there is a possible benefit of COC use in preserving BMD in perimenopausal patients.[139] For patients with normal estrogen levels, the effect of low-dose COCs on BMD is less clear. A review of all observational studies found use of low-dose COCs in healthy people had no effect on bone health overall or fracture risk.[140]

Contraceptive Patches

COCs delivered transdermally (patches) have the following additional benefits:

- **Patches offer an easier and more convenient delivery regimen than pills.** Some users find the weekly patch regimen more convenient than a daily pill regimen. In study populations, the weekly regimen appears to enhance consistent and correct use when compared with daily COC use, particularly among younger users.[46,47,141,142] Adolescents using the contraceptive patch are more likely to use them consistently and correctly than those using COCs.[141,142] Ease of use, the lack of need for daily adherence, and the ease of concealment are among the reported advantages reported by adolescents. However, adolescents are more likely than older users to experience challenges with adherence and use.[142,143]
- **Patches are more forgiving of user error than pills.** Hormone levels remain therapeutic for at least 9 days of use, suggesting that ovulation inhibition would be maintained even if a scheduled patch change was missed for as long as 2 days.[144] Additionally, missed patches (either forgetting to start a new patch or forgetting to change a patch) are less likely to lead to follicular growth or ovulation than are missed COCs.[1] Hormone levels and ovulation are surrogate markers, however, and no studies have evaluated pregnancy rates with missed patches.
- **Patches adhere well under a variety of conditions.** In clinical trials for both Xulane and Twirla, very few patches needed replacement because of complete or partial detachment. Heat, humidity, and exercise do not affect patch adhesion or pharmacokinetics.[144-146] In typical use, however, patch adhesion may be lower. In one three-cycle study of Xulane, almost half of the participants reported that the patch fell off at least once.[53] Adolescents are more likely to

experience application site reactions and patch detachment, so they should receive anticipatory counseling.[142,143]

- **Patches are verifiable**. The user can easily verify the presence of the patch. This reassurance about continued protection may reduce the anxiety some individuals report with COCs—questioning whether they remembered to take their daily pill and worrying that they might forget to take it.
- **Patches provide rapidly reversible contraception.** Fecundity returns rapidly when users discontinue the patch; FSH and LH levels return to nearly baseline levels, and 86% of women ovulate in the month following patch discontinuation.[147]
- **Patches have no significant impact on weight gain.** In a randomized placebo-controlled trial, the contraceptive patch was not associated with weight gain. In a pooled analysis of the clinical trials, the mean change in body weight from baseline to the end of treatment was an increase of 0.3 kg, and 79% of participants remained within 5% of their baseline weight.[148]
- **Patches have no clinically significant metabolic effects.** Although the patch has not been studied in individuals with cardiovascular or other diseases, studies in healthy users have shown no clinically meaningful changes in hematology, blood chemistry, or bone turnover.[149-152] However, the lack impact of the patch on surrogate markers, such as cholesterol or coagulation tests, may not reflect the impact on outcomes of clinical interest such as myocardial infarction or stroke.[153]
- **Patches bypass oral administration and gastrointestinal absorption.** Patches can be used by individuals who cannot take a pill orally or who have abnormal intestinal drug absorption.

Vaginal Rings

COCs delivered transvaginally (rings) have the following additional benefits:

- **Rings are convenient.** Participants in clinical trials report that the ring is easy to insert, comfortable to use, and easy to remove.[61,63,67] Users may easily verify that the device is in place. The ring's effectiveness does not depend on its position, because hormonal absorption occurs through the vaginal walls. The ring rests against the vaginal wall, near or around the cervix;[67] walking and usual movement do not lead to expulsion.[67,154] Although some ring users and their partners report feeling the ring during intercourse, this did not affect acceptability or continuation for most individuals in clinical trials.[63,65] Because the ring does not require daily action and is not coitally dependent, it may be more convenient than other methods such as the diaphragm or COCs.
- **Rings are more forgiving of user error than pills or patches.** Hormone levels remain therapeutic for at least 35 days after placement of the vaginal ring. This suggests that ovulation inhibition would be maintained even if a person forgets to remove the ring for up to 2 weeks beyond schedule. A study demonstrated that contraceptive hormone levels are sustained for up to 6 weeks of use of the same ring, although the incidence of breakthrough bleeding began to increase after 21 days.[32] Ring use for as few as 3 days has been shown to suppress ovarian follicular growth (compared with 7 days for COCs).[155] Removal after 3 days is not recommended, however, as follicular size and ovulation are

only surrogate markers; no studies have evaluated the risk of pregnancy due to shortened dosing timelines or dosing errors during ring use.

- **Vaginal route of delivery allows lower doses of hormones.** The vaginal route of delivery increases the bioavailability of hormones, thus enabling the use of a lower total hormone dose. The ring can be used by individuals who cannot swallow a pill and by individuals with abnormal intestinal absorption. The steady release of hormones via vaginal route also has the potential to decrease side effects that may be associated with oral dosing.
- **Rings are rapidly effective and rapidly reversible.** Hormone levels needed to suppress ovulation are achieved within the first day of vaginal ring use,[156] and as few as 3 consecutive days of vaginal ring use interfere with follicular growth. Return to ovulation after ring removal is rapid, occurring in a median of 17 to 19 days.[157] Return to fecundity can be extrapolated from what we know about COC discontinuation, for which the median time to pregnancy is 3 cycles, with 74% to 95% of those seeking fecundity becoming pregnant within a year of discontinuation.[158]
- **Rings have no adverse effects on cervico-vaginal epithelium.** Ring use does not appear to have adverse effects on the cervico-vaginal epithelium or on cervical cytology.[61,159]
- **Rings have no adverse endometrial effects.** Ring use for up to 2 years did not lead to endometrial hyperplasia or other adverse effects on endometrial histology.[160] Extrapolating from COC data, there is likely in fact a reduction in endometrial hyperplasia risk.
- **Rings can be used concurrently with tampons.** Occasionally, a user may need to insert a ring while still having scheduled bleeding. A pharmacokinetic study showed that tampons can be used concurrently with the ring without any effects on hormone absorption.[161] Ring users need to ensure that the ring is not inadvertently withdrawn at the time of tampon removal.
- **Ring can be removed for up to 2–3 hours without compromising effectiveness.** Although most individuals and their partners do not report discomfort due to the ring during vaginal intercourse, the NuvaRing can be removed or left out for up to 3 hours in any 24-hour period without requiring a backup method. The same ring can then be reinserted.[162] Those who choose to remove and reinsert the ring for this reason should make sure to reinsert within the 3 hours, or it is possible that ring effectiveness could be compromised. The year-long SA/EE ring, Annovera, has a slightly shorter window and needs to be reinserted within 2 hours. If a patient has this ring out for more than 2 hours at once or for a total of more than 2 hours across the 21-day period, the ring can be reinserted, but a backup method should be used for 7 days, as efficacy may be compromised.[69]
- **Rings offer excellent cycle control.** Compared with COCs, the ring may be less likely to produce irregular bleeding, especially in the first few cycles.[64] Most vaginal ring users experience bleeding at the time scheduled.[61,163-165] Extended or continuous use may be associated with an increase in unscheduled bleeding, as can prolonged (> 21 days) use of a single ring.[32,37,166] The frequency and duration of unscheduled bleeding episodes tend to be highest in the first few months of use and decrease over time.
- **Rings have no significant impact on weight gain.** In clinical studies, women are as likely to lose weight as to gain it when using the ring for a year.[59,167]

A recent randomized review noted no large effect on weight among ring users, though the authors noted that available data were limited.[168]

- **Rings are safe in individuals with latex allergies.** Because the ring is made from vinyl acetate, individuals with latex allergies can use it safely.
- **Rings have no clinically significant metabolic effects.** In healthy individuals, the vaginal ring has had no clinically important adverse effects on surrogate markers of disease such as heart rate, blood pressure, blood chemistries, lipids, adrenal and thyroid function, carbohydrate metabolism, or hematology.[61,63,169,170] In a study of patients with type 1 diabetes, ring use did not adversely affect glycemic control or other metabolic measures.[171] These surrogate markers may not reflect the actual risk of adverse outcomes, and no studies have examined long-term metabolic outcomes.
- **Rings do not affect bone density.** In one study, bone mineral density showed no change from baseline after as long as 24 months of contraceptive ring use.[172] The study did not include adolescents or perimenopausal individuals. One study of adolescents and young women found no decrease in bone density at the spine after 12 months of use.[152] No study has looked at risk of fractures.

Disadvantages and Cautions

Before patients decide to use CHCs, they should balance the benefits they would get with CHC use against the possible risks they pose in the context of their individual medical status.

Contraceptive Disadvantages

The disadvantages of CHCs in their various delivery methods are as follows:

- **Scheduled administration.** Pills, patches, and rings all require consistent use by patients on a daily, weekly or monthly basis. Inconsistent use of these methods reduces the effectiveness of protection from pregnancy and increases the incidence of some side effects, especially unscheduled bleeding and spotting. Remembering to start a new pack, patch, or ring can be challenging for some patients. Studies demonstrate that most patients miss several pills each month.[1]
- **Expense and access challenges.** If insurance companies do not provide contraceptive coverage as a benefit, many patients, whether insured or uninsured, must pay out of pocket for their contraception.[173] So for short-acting methods like CHCs, out-of-pocket costs may be required every 1 to 3 months. The cost of branded COCs may easily exceed $80 per pack. Generic formulations are typically less expensive but often cost $30 or more per month. Pharmacies that have generic prescription programs sell a limited number of generic COC formulations for $9 a pack. For users who do have contraceptive coverage, there may be a high copayment, especially for the more expensive formulations. For methods such as Annovera, which is not consistently covered by insurers, out-of-pocket costs can be up to $2,400 but coupons and savings programs can significantly reduce costs. [174] Find out about patients' coverage and their financial constraints when you help them choose CHCs. Often, the number of packs dispensed at pharmacies is severely restricted, so patients are required to return to pharmacies each month or every few months. The mismatch between

calendar months with 30 to 31 days and COC packs with only 28 pills can present additional challenges in COC use. Patients who desire to use extended cycles are faced with even more difficulties in obtaining adequate supplies.

- **Need for privacy as well as ready access.** Adolescents and adults whose parents or partners do not want them to use contraception may not have a secure place to store their CHCs. Practitioners may need to guide them to more private contraceptive methods, if needed.

Health Risks

- **Venous thromboembolism (VTE).** The best evidence suggests the increased risk of **VTE in CHC users is from the estrogen component dependent on dose and duration**, and independent of the progestin used.[175] Higher doses of estrogen are associated with a greater risk of VTE, which is one reason why use of 50 mcg EE COCs is discouraged. Clinically significant VTE occurs when there is an imbalance between two sets of factors that control blood clot formation. Estrogen increases hepatic production of elements that promote clot formation by the extrinsic clotting system (factor VII, factor VIII, factor X) and decreases the production of elements that promote clot lysis (tissue plasminogen activator, antiplasmin). CHC users also develop an increased resistance to anticoagulant effect of activated protein C. The net result is a prothrombotic effect.
    - Progestins alone have virtually no impact on the clotting system, but when combined with estrogen, some progestins can modulate the strength of estrogen's production of extrinsic clotting factors, antithrombin,[176] fibrinolytics, and other steps in blood clot formation. In the mid-1990s, international studies indicated that COCs containing the progestins such as desogestrel and gestodene (not available in the United States) were associated with higher rates of thrombosis (up to a two-fold increase) compared with formulations containing levonorgestrel and norgestrel.[177-179] Because these progestins were designed to reduce the androgenicity of progestin to allow fuller expression of the COC's estrogen component, such concerns were biologically plausible. Reanalyses of those early studies showed no increase in VTE risk with these progestins once corrections were made for biases related to duration of COC use and patient selection.[180] Although more recent observational studies also found as much as a two-fold increased risk of VTE associated with these progestins, the overall incidence of VTEs was expectedly rare (i.e., 6.3 per 10,000).[181,182] Furthermore, for drospirenone-containing COCs, two large cohort studies found no increased VTE risk associated with their use compared with other COC formulations.[183,184] Overall, there is no strong evidence to suggest clinicians need to change their prescribing patterns of COCs containing newer progestins. Discussing the potential benefits versus risks of these newer COC formulations with patients who may be good candidates for them is key to patient informed consent before use.
    - Though the *relative risk* of thrombosis is increased with CHC use, most CHC users face a low *absolute risk* of thrombosis because VTE is a rare event in the healthy young user. A systematic review of the literature estimated the incidence of VTE in reproductive-aged women to be 5 to 10 per 10,000 women-years, which is higher than previous estimates.[185] The most

recent meta-analysis concluded that the risk of VTE was increased three to four times in COC users compared with nonusers, and peaks in the first 12 months of use before declining with further use.[186] In comparison, a population-based cohort found the VTE risk during pregnancy is increased at least four times, and during the postpartum period at least 20 times.[187]

- The risk of VTE increases with age, with nearly a five-fold increase from age 25 to age 50.[188] Another risk factor for VTE is obesity: obese COC users have as much as a three-fold increased risk of VTE when compared with COC users of normal weight.[184] The American College of Obstetricians and Gynecologists (ACOG) recommends caution in prescribing estrogen-containing contraception to patients over age 35 with a BMI > 30,[189] although the US MEC rates obesity as a category 2 condition. Tobacco use also increases the risk of VTE. In one study, smokers aged 18–39 who did not use COCs had double the risk of VTE compared with nonsmokers of the same age who did not use COCs. At even greater risk were smokers who did use COCs: their risk was 8.8 times higher than nonsmokers who did not use COCs.[190] The risks showed a dose response among young smokers, with higher doses of estrogen associated with greater risks of VTE.[191]
- Serum ethinyl estradiol levels of patch users appear to be higher than those of women using a COC containing 35 mcg EE.[192] However, pharmacokinetic measures are surrogate markers and do not necessarily correlate with the magnitude of risk of VTE, stroke, or myocardial infarction. Epidemiologic data are also inconsistent. Several studies have been published, with some studies finding risks similar to those associated with COC use, while others note higher risks with the patch.[178,193-199] The FDA conducted its own review of several databases and found an increased risk of VTE with the contraceptive patch compared with certain COCs, leading to a change in the warning label. In any event, any risk of VTE with patch use is still far below the risk of VTE during pregnancy and the postpartum period. In the Cochrane review, the risk of VTE with patch use was estimated to be 53 per 100,000 women (95% CI 1–294).[45]
- Although ring users have progestin levels similar to those of COC users, their EE levels are two-fold lower than in individuals taking COCs with 35 mg EE and three-fold lower than in individuals wearing the patch.[192] Again, pharmacokinetic measures may not necessarily reflect a decreased risk of estrogen-related side effects or long-term risks. Studies of the ring based on analyses of large databases have also reported somewhat inconsistent results, with some showing a small increased risk of thrombosis among ring users compared with users of levonorgestrel-containing oral contraceptives, and others showing no increase in risk.[39-41] In a Cochrane review of several randomized studies, the risk of VTE with ring use was estimated to be 149 per 100,000 women (95% CI 18–538).[45]
- In general, the CDC MEC does not distinguish between the different combined hormonal methods when categorizing conditions associated with risk of VTE.[200] Furthermore, patients need to know the increase in VTE risk that they experience during CHC use is a completely reversible risk upon discontinuation.

- **Myocardial Infarction (MI).** In healthy, nonsmoking US pill users, it is unlikely that the use of low-dose CHCs (< 50 mcg EE) alone is associated with any significant risk of MI. One pooled analysis showed that the relative risk for MI with low-dose COC use was 1.0.[201] Although a meta-analysis of studies including high-dose COCs showed an overall risk of 2.48 for current users, there was no increased risk for those using 20 mcg formulations.[202] The American College of Cardiology concluded that low-dose COC formulations pose no increased MI risk for current users.[203] Similarly, in a more recent cohort study by Lidegaard et al., the risk of MI doubled in users of COCs containing 30 to 40 mcg of EE, but did not increase in users of COCs containing 20 mcg of EE.[204] In looking at various progestins contained in COCs, the EURAS study (with over 58,000 participants) found no difference in MI rates.[184] Duration of CHC use likewise appears to cause no difference in MI risk.[205] Past CHC users have no increased risk due to their prior CHC use.

- The risks for MI increase with age, but are greatly magnified by the combination of age, smoking, and hypertension.[202,206] In one meta-analysis of COC users, smoking, hypertension, and dyslipidemia each were associated with a nine-fold increased risk for MI.[202] The attributable risk of death from MI in absolute terms with CHC use itself is very low. Estimates are that among women ages 20–24 who do not smoke and do not use COCs, 4 per 1 million die from MI; that risk rises to 10 per million among smokers who use COCs (**Table 12-1**).[176,207]

- **Stroke**. Cerebrovascular disease is rare in young reproductive-age women but becomes more common in women in their 40s. The risk of stroke attributable to current CHC use is likely low with low-dose COCs. One meta-analysis concluded that use of low-dose COCs was associated with a significantly increased risk of ischemic stroke among nonsmoking, nonhypertensive women (RR = 1.9, 95% CI 1.35–2.74).[208] A second meta-analysis concluded that the risk declines with decreasing doses of estrogen.[209] However, little evidence exists assessing the risk of stroke associated with use of COCs with less than 20 mcg EE.[210] There is no apparent increase in the risk of either type of stroke with increasing duration of CHC use[211] or with past use of CHCs.[212] Data are insufficient to

Table 12-1 Age-Specific Estimates of Attributable MI Deaths Due To Low-Dose COC Use per 1 million Users in International Studies: The Effect of Smoking and Hypertension

	Risk of Myocardial Infarction/1 Million Users		
	Age Range (years)		
Risk Category	**20–24**	**30–34**	**40–44**
Healthy nonsmokers	4	6	20
With smoking	10	20	200
With hypertension	100	120	450

Data from Farley TM, Collins J, Schlesselman JJ. Hormonal contraception and risk of cardiovascular disease. An international perspective. Contraception 1998;57:211-30.

make conclusions about how the type or dose of progestin might influence the risk of stroke.[213] CHC use does not affect the risk of *subarachnoid* hemorrhage.[214]

- Risk factors for *ischemic* stroke include smoking, hypertension, diabetes, overweight or obesity, and migraine headaches with aura. The risk factors for *hemorrhagic* stroke include age, hypertension, smoking, obesity, and heavy alcohol use. A recent systematic review found a significant increase in the risk of ischemic stroke among COC users who experienced migraine with aura but no significant increase overall among COC users who reported migraine without aura.[210] (See Chronic Medical Conditions: Migraine Headaches, p. 385.) Most studies suggest there is no synergistic effect between CHC use and hypertension or smoking on risk of ischemic stroke. However, increased risk of ischemic stroke was noted in one study among COC users who did not have blood pressure screening prior to use compared with those who did.[215] And one case-control study found that the risk of hemorrhagic stroke was further increased for COC users who were older than 35 years of age, hypertensive, or smokers.[216] Therefore, it is advisable to avoid estrogen-containing contraceptives if possible in individuals with significant risk factors for stroke.

- **Hyperlipidemia.** Estrogen, specifically EE, is known to decrease low-density lipoprotein (LDL), and to increase high-density lipoprotein (HDL), triglycerides, and total cholesterol. COC users are two to four times more likely to develop abnormal lipid levels compared with COC nonusers.[217] Hypertriglyceridemia is an independent risk factor for early cardiovascular disease. However, CHC-induced lipid changes may not increase a patient's risk for atherosclerosis.[218] Although most modern CHC formulations increase triglycerides by about 30%, these estrogen-induced triglycerides are different in size than endogenously produced triglycerides, and the alterations in lipids nevertheless result in a net decrease in the LDL : HDL ratio, which is a more accurate marker for risk than are absolute levels.[217] The androgen-derived progestins in CHCs may be neutral or may reverse some of estrogen's stimulatory effects on HDL and triglycerides and may increase LDL. The net effect depends upon the dose, potency, and estrogen/androgen balance of each formulation. If LDL levels rise or HDL levels drop significantly with CHC use, change to a formulation with more estrogenic activity and less androgenic activity. Routine screening of lipid levels is not necessary before prescribing or continuing CHCs unless a patient has preexisting hyperlipidemia or a very strong family history of premature cardiovascular disease.[219]
- **Cervical cancer**. Cervical dysplasia and cervical carcinoma are caused by oncogenic (high-risk) types of human papillomavirus (HPV), especially types HPV-16 and -18. A review of cross-sectional studies found no strong evidence for an association between ever using CHCs and having HPV infection.[220] However, a large meta-analysis of 28 studies including 12,531 women with squamous cell and adenocarcinoma found a relative risk (RR) of 1.1 (95% CI 1.1–1.2) for having HPV infection in COC users compared to nonusers after 5 years of COC use, but the RR increased to 1.6 (95% CI 1.4–1.7) after 5 to 10 years, and to 2.2 (95% CI 1.9-2.4) after more than 10 years.[221] However, this CHC-associated risk is lower than the risk that is associated with high parity; women with HPV infection who had seven or more pregnancies had higher RR (8.29) for cervical cancer.[222] Increasing HPV vaccination rates will likely decrease the clinical significance of this associated risk over time.[223]

Despite this slight increase in risk, even long-term CHC users can follow standard guidelines for cervical cancer screening.

- **Breast cancer.** A population-based case-control study investigated the incidence of breast cancer among US women aged 35–64 years and found no increased risk of breast cancer among ever users of COCs compared to never users (RR = 0.9, 95% CI 0.8–1.0) regardless of EE dose, duration of use,[224] or COC formulation.[225] In a prospective cohort of 1.8 million Danish women aged 15–49 years, current and recent users of any hormonal contraception (with the vast majority using low-dose COCs) had an RR of 1.20 (95% CI 1.14–1.26) for breast cancer compared to never users.[226] This translates to an attributable risk of 13 diagnosed cases of breast cancer per 100,000 women using low-dose COCs per year. However, the cohort was limited to women no older than 49 even though the vast majority of breast cancer cases occur above this age. Furthermore, such a small RR in an observational study should be interpreted with caution and not used to suggest causation.[227] Patients should ultimately be counseled on the data and be able to weigh the risks and benefits that meet their contraceptive goals. In regard to high-risk groups, women who carry mutations for *BRCA1* or *BRCA2* and use COCs do not experience any increase in their already high risk of developing breast cancer.[228] Women with a family history of breast cancer (unknown *BRCA* status) do not increase their risk of disease by using CHCs.[229]

Providing the Method

Medical Eligibility

The US MEC for Contraceptive Use provides guidelines for practitioners to follow when assessing risks associated with the use of various contraceptive methods versus the risks of unintended pregnancy.[75] In summary, patients are candidates for CHCs when their health risks from CHC use are less than the health risks they would face with pregnancy. Although the FDA-approved prescribing information also lists medical conditions that are not compatible with CHC use, which may conflict with MEC recommendations, FDA package labeling for many drugs has been shown to be at least 20 years obsolete.[230] The US MEC represents an up-to-date synthesis of the medical literature on the risks associated with CHC use. **Table 12-2** shows a list of medical conditions in which CHC use is contraindicated. For a complete list of the US MEC upon which to make your clinical decisions, go to www.cdc.gov, and see Chapter 20, Contraception for Those with Medical Conditions, for ways in which you can use the guidelines in your everyday practice.

Chronic Medical Conditions

Many medical conditions present no contraindications to use of CHCs; for these conditions, CHC use neither worsens disease progression nor increases risk of complications. These conditions are assigned "category 1" (use is not restricted) and "category 2" (benefits of use outweigh risks) in the US MEC and include thyroid disorders and cystic fibrosis, among others. CHCs can help treat AUB associated with medical conditions like thyroid disorders or anticoagulation. In addition, patients with sickle cell or other preexisting anemias benefit from decreased menstrual

Table 12-2 Medical Conditions Precluding COC Use, As Listed in the US Medical Eligibility Criteria for Contraceptive Use

Medical Conditions Precluding COC Use	US MEC Rating
Current venous thromboembolism	4
History of venous thromboembolism with high risk of recurrence	4
Cerebrovascular or coronary artery disease	4
Valvular heart disease with complications	4
Severe hypertension or with vascular disease	4
Diabetes mellitus with vascular disease or > 20 years' duration	4
Migraine headaches with aura	4
Major surgery with prolonged immobilization	4
Current breast cancer	4
Thrombogenic mutations	4
Systemic lupus erythematosus with + antiphospholipid antibodies	4
Solid organ transplant with complications	4
Peripartum cardiomyopathy with impaired cardiac function	4
Heavy smokers > 35 years of age	4
Hepatic adenoma or carcinoma	4
Severe cirrhosis or acute hepatitis	4
< 21 days postpartum	4
Multiple risk factors for atherosclerotic cardiovascular disease	3/4*

* Category 3 or 4 depending on number of major risk factors for cardiovascular disease.
Data from Curtis KM, Tepper NK, Jatlaoui TC, et al. U.S. Medical Eligibility Criteria for Contraceptive Use, 2016. MMWR Recomm Rep 2016;65(3):1-104.

blood loss. However, sometimes the medications used to treat medical conditions, such as depression and epilepsy, may interact with and decrease the efficacy of CHCs (see Medication Interactions, p. 369). Use of an additional contraceptive method, or substitution with a locally acting method like an IUD, is therefore recommended. (See Chapter 4, Person-Centered Reproductive Health Conversations and Contraceptive Counseling.)

The following are some of the more common medical conditions that present challenges for clinicians and their patients requesting CHCs.

Hypertension

Patients with elevated blood pressure have an increased risk of MI and stroke, and CHC use further increases this risk.[215] However, it is not as clear if well-controlled hypertension is equivalent to normotension. The estrogen component in CHCs increases circulating levels of angiotensinogen. Some patients are sensitive to angiotensinogen metabolites (angiotensin) and experience increases in both systolic and diastolic blood pressures with CHCs. Finally, estrogen, and to some extent progestin, enhance aldosterone activity, which may result in fluid retention and, in turn, an increase in blood pressure. The US MEC recommends that CHC use be avoided in patients with hypertension with uncontrolled elevated blood pressure (systolic blood pressure [SBP] ≥160, diastolic blood pressure [DBP] ≥100) or advanced vascular disease such as retinopathy or nephropathy (category 4), and recommends caution with use of CHCs in individuals with lower elevations of blood pressure (SBP 140–159, DBP 90–99) or those with well-controlled blood pressure, unless no other contraceptive method is available or acceptable (category 3). If you do prescribe CHCs to a patient with treated hypertension, monitor blood pressure carefully. If it rises due to CHC use or due to nonadherence with antihypertensives, the patient may become ineligible for CHC use.[231] In these cases, effective progestin-only or nonhormonal methods are typically available. Patients with a history of gestational hypertension or elevated blood pressures in the 120–139 systolic or 80–89 diastolic range have no restrictions to CHC use. It is important to note that hypertension definitions based on blood pressure ranges as established by the American Heart Association and the American College of Cardiology are slightly different than the ranges used in the US MEC recommendations.

Most studies find no increase in the incidence of hypertension with low-dose COCs, although a 3–5 mmHg rise in blood pressure during COC use is not uncommon.[232,233] One study found that elevated blood pressure occurred in only 41.5 cases per 10,000 COC users.[232] For patients who do experience increases in blood pressures consistent with new onset hypertension during CHC use, stop the CHC and switch to a nonestrogenic contraceptive. Patients with hypertension attributable to CHC use will normalize their blood pressures within 3–6 months of stopping estrogen-containing contraceptives.[203] Patients whose readings do not return to normal after stopping should undergo a standard workup; most will be found to have essential hypertension.

Diabetes

Diabetes increases a patient's risk for microvascular (retinopathy, nephropathy, neuropathy) and macrovascular (coronary artery disease, peripheral artery disease) complications. However, the use of low-dose CHCs by patients with diabetes mellitus does not appear to significantly alter glucose levels or increase risk of vascular complications.[234] CHCs can also provide a diabetic patient the chance to achieve tight glucose control before conception and thereby decrease the risk for maternal and fetal complications, including fetal malformation. Therefore, the US MEC concluded that CHCs may be used by patients with diabetes who do not have vascular disease because the benefits outweigh the risks (category 2). However, the US MEC recommends against the initiation of CHCs in patients with diabetes who have coexisting vascular disease or who have had diabetes for over 20 years, unless no other contraceptive method is available or acceptable (category 3). CHC continuation is contraindicated in diabetic patients who develop micro- or macrovascular complications during CHC use (category 4).[75] In each of these cases, the patient is still eligible for effective progestin-only or nonhormonal methods. Patients with a history of gestational diabetes have no restrictions to CHC use. In these patients, more frequent screening may be needed because they are at higher risk of developing diabetes over time, but CHC use does not appear to increase this risk.[235]

Thrombogenic Mutations

The increase in VTE risk seen with CHC use is greatly magnified in the face of genetic thrombogenic mutation disorders, such as factor V Leiden mutation. The factor V Leiden mutation alone explains 30% of all cases of deep venous thromboses. In the United States, it is estimated that 5.3% of Caucasians, 2.2% of Hispanics, 1.2% of Blacks and Native Americans, and 0.5% of Asians carry this mutation. A World Health Organization (WHO) literature review reported that COC users with factor V Leiden mutations were 6.4–99.0 times more likely to form blood clots than nonusers without the mutation. When an individual who is homozygous for the mutations uses COCs, VTE risk rises 100 times higher than noncarriers who do not use COCs.[236] Genetic mutations in prothrombin also increase VTE risks. For patients with deficiencies in antithrombin, protein C, or protein S, the RRs for VTE are 8–10, with an absolute risk of 120 to 150/100,000 a year. Despite the impact that these mutations may have on a patient's risk for thrombosis, routine laboratory screening of patients prior to initiating CHCs is not recommended.[237]

Migraine Headaches

Before providing hormonal contraception to a patient with preexisting headaches, characterize the type of headache they experience. What a patient calls a "migraine" may actually be a severe nonmigrainous headache. The International Headache Society[238] established guidelines for headache type, including tension, cluster, and migraine headaches. *Tension* headaches are the most common; they are bilateral in location, throbbing in nature, and mild to moderate in intensity. They may be associated with mild or no nausea, and either photo- or phonophobia. *Cluster* headaches are unilateral, severe in intensity, and occur in "clusters" over several days. They may be associated with sympathetic symptoms like eye tearing, nasal congestion, or a feeling of restlessness. There is no contraindication to the use of CHCs with tension or cluster headaches because there is no evidence to suggest that CHC use causes any increased risk of complications.[103]

Migraine headaches are typically unilateral, throbbing in nature, moderate to severe in intensity, and last at least several hours in duration. They are exacerbated by physical activity and associated with nausea and vomiting or both photophobia and phonophobia. Migraines may be preceded by *aura,* which are reversible focal neurologic symptoms that develop gradually, usually prior to onset of headache, and last no more than 60 minutes. Symptoms can include scotoma or flashing lights, loss of vision, numbness, tingling, or trouble speaking. A personal history of migraines is a risk factor for ischemic stroke, and the presence of aura further increases that risk. CHC use increases stroke risk in users with migraines by two- to four-fold. The only study that evaluated COC use and stroke risk by migraine type (aura vs. no aura) found an elevated stroke risk only in users with migraine with aura.[210] Furthermore, the absolute risk of stroke in young women is very low (5 to

10 per 100,000 women-years), but is a catastrophic event.[103] So while CHCs may be prescribed to patients with migraines without aura (category 2), CHCs are contraindicated in patients who experience migraines with aura (category 4).[239] These patients are still eligible for effective progestin-only or nonhormonal methods.

It is important to ask *when* in a menstrual cycle a patient experiences headaches. Headaches due to estrogen withdrawal, whether related to menses or cyclic COC use, are called *menstrual migraines*. By definition, menstrual migraines are not migraine with aura, though they may co-occur in patients with migraine with aura. For menstrual migraines, extended-cycle CHC use could provide relief. Although there is no evidence that a patient's stroke risk decreases if the migraines improve with extended CHC use, the therapeutic relief in symptoms may provide enough benefit to outweigh the minimal risk of stroke.[103,239] If a patient develops new headaches while on CHCs or has worsening of preexisting headaches, provide prompt evaluation and possible discontinuation of estrogen-containing contraceptives. (See Managing Side Effects: Headaches, p. 402.)

Tobacco Use

Although not a medical condition per se, smoking increases CHC users' risk of MI at least 32-fold compared with users with neither risk factor. The risk attributable to smoking alone is greater than the risk attributable to CHCs alone.[240] Indeed, women who smoke as few as three or four cigarettes a day have a 2.5-fold increased risk of coronary heart disease.[241] But 3 to 12 months after stopping smoking, past smokers have the same CHC-related cardiovascular risks as nonsmokers. So, the foremost clinical goal should be to help your patient stop smoking, though this can be challenging. Moderate and heavy smoking (i.e., at least 15 cigarettes a day) by patients over age 35 precludes the use of CHCs (category 4). Light smoking by patients older than 35 merits caution (category 3). The older the smoker, the more cigarettes smoked, and the more comorbid cardiovascular risk factors present, the less likely the patient is to be a candidate for CHCs. In otherwise healthy young patients, the absolute risk of cardiovascular disease is low, so use of CHCs by young adults who smoke is still safer than pregnancy (category 2).

It is not clear which CHC formulation is the best for smokers. On one hand, the ideal CHC would have the lowest EE content (to reduce arterial thrombosis) and the lowest androgenic activity (to minimize any adverse impacts on lipids). On the other hand, the carcinogens in tobacco smoke induce the cytochrome P450 metabolism of EE (see Medication Interactions, p. 369) so that smokers are 47% more likely to have spotting or bleeding than nonsmokers using the same formulation. It is not clear whether this indicates a decrease in contraceptive effectiveness for smokers, but it likely contributes to increased CHC discontinuation.[242] It may be prudent to start smokers and patients who use a nicotine replacement product on a 20-mcg EE COC formulation with an extended cycle. Vaginal rings are another option for smokers who want good cycle control. Effective progestin-only and nonhormonal methods are still viable options.

HIV and AIDS

Worldwide, over 29 million adults are infected with HIV. New infections are concentrated among young adults (15–24 years) and are more likely in women in this age group.[243] With the increased use of antiretroviral therapy (ART) that is highly effective at suppressing the virus, and concomitant improvement in quality of life and pregnancy outcomes, more HIV-infected persons are seeking reversible contraceptive methods. The most recent systematic review concluded that there is no association between COC use and disease progression or death among HIV-positive women.[244] Therefore, CHCs may be safely used (category 1) by HIV-positive patients per the US MEC, whether or not they are taking ARVs or are diagnosed with acquired immunodeficiency syndrome (AIDS).[75] Furthermore, CHC use is not associated with an increased risk of HIV acquisition. A 2016 systematic review included 11 studies of COC use and HIV risk and found either no or only marginally increased risk of HIV acquisition, even among HIV-serodiscordant couples.[245] While correct and consistent use of condoms is effective in preventing sexual transmission, sexual transmission during unprotected sex when the infected partner is fully suppressed (no detectable HIV in the blood by PCR assay), sometimes called "treatment as prevention," is equally effective, such that the CDC states that there is no risk of transmission with oral, anal, or vaginal sex.[246] In addition, some ARVs can interact with CHCs, resulting in a change in the serum level of either the ARV or the CHC. This is another possible reason for HIV-positive individuals to consider condoms in addition to CHCs. (See Medication Interactions, p. 369.)

Rheumatologic Disease

Four studies have shown that the incidence of disease flares does not increase in CHC users with systemic lupus erythematosus (SLE), although patients with severe disease were not studied. Antiphospholipid antibodies in SLE patients are a known risk factor for thromboembolism, so CHC use is contraindicated (category 4). However, patients with mild SLE may use CHCs if they have no antiphospholipid antibodies, even if they are using immunosuppressive therapy (category 2).[247] Effective progestin-only and nonhormonal methods are still a reasonable and safe alternative for all patients with SLE. A review of six studies of COC use in patients with rheumatoid arthritis found no improvement or worsening of disease progression, whether or not they were using immunosuppressive therapy (category 2).[248]

Liver Disease

A systematic review found that COC use did not increase liver transaminase levels, hepatic inflammation, or fibrosis in patients with chronic hepatitis, though studies were all limited by short duration of follow-up. Only one small trial investigated COC use in patients with acute hepatitis and noted no increase in severity of disease. Patients with chronic hepatitis and mild cirrhosis may use COCs. In hepatitis carriers, COC use does not appear to precipitate liver failure or severe dysfunction.[249] US MEC rates CHC use as category 1 for both chronic viral hepatitis and carriers.[75] However, it is recommended that patients with acute hepatitis or with a severe flare or cirrhosis avoid CHC use (category 4).[249]

Low-dose COCs do not appear to be associated with an increased risk of hepatocellular adenoma or other benign liver lesions, though this was noted in the past with high-dose COCs. Preexisting benign hepatic lesions do not appear to be affected by CHC use: in patients who have focal nodular hyperplasia, a type of benign liver tumor, studies of CHC use are limited but nonetheless show no effect on tumor size or number of lesions (category 2). Hepatocellular carcinoma risk is not increased with low-dose COC use,[250] even among high-risk patients (chronic hepatitis B or C, cirrhosis). Although use of CHCs is not associated with a de novo increased risk of benign or malignant liver tumors, the hepatic metabolism of CHCs is significant. Therefore, use of CHCs in patients with hepatocellular adenoma or carcinoma is contraindicated (category 4).[251]

Gallbladder Disease

Low-dose COCs have not been associated with an increased risk of cholelithiasis or cholecystitis, as had been seen earlier with high-dose COCs. However, it may still be possible that low-dose COCs accelerate the course or development of symptomatic gallbladder disease in patients with preexisting gallstones or sludge. The EE in high-dose COCs was found to impair active transport of bile, resulting in cholestatic jaundice with pruritus. Patients who either have current gallbladder disease or a personal history but still have their gallbladder are at higher risk for recurrence and so should not be given CHCs unless other methods are not available (category 3).[75] Patients who have a history of cholestasis treated with cholecystectomy are likely at lower risk, so the US MEC rates their use as a category 2. CHCs do not increase the risk of gallbladder cancer.[252]

Special Considerations for Different Life Stages

Adolescence

Many states guarantee adolescents confidential access to reproductive health care, including contraception, so providing adolescent-friendly services in your office or clinic will increase access for this vulnerable population. If a parent is present, ensure that you are directing your person-centered counseling toward your adolescent patient, and that you also spend some time during the visit speaking to them confidentially. Targeted counseling is important. Adolescents may be more likely to stop using CHCs because of side effects such as nausea or spotting, so actively listen to all their concerns about side effects by using ASA Cycles as described in Chapter 4.[253] Provide concrete counseling; studies show that adolescents anticipate having side effects at much higher rates than actually occur, and they expect to have no difficulty with consistent pill taking.[254] Anticipate that they may find it more challenging to use CHCs correctly and consistently than do older patients. Practitioners and health educators may need to take more time instructing adolescents in what to do for missed pills, including use of condoms and emergency contraception for back-up. Studies have shown that for users of all ages, adherence is improved with once-a-week or once-a-month methods as opposed to taking a pill once a day; however, teens benefit the most from less frequent dosing.[255] For this reason, be sure to also offer the full range of contraceptive methods that are consistent with their preferences. (See Chapter 4, Person-Centered Reproductive Health Conversations and Contraceptive Counseling.)

Many adolescents can also benefit from taking CHCs to treat anovulatory cycling, HMB, primary dysmenorrhea, or acne. If your patient is not sexually active or is contemplating CHC use for noncontraceptive benefits, reassure them that it is common among their peers to use hormonal contraception for noncontraceptive benefits. In particular, the cause for an adolescent's irregular or heavy menstrual bleeding is often anovulation from an immature hypothalamic-pituitary-ovarian axis. CHCs can be used effectively and safely in this circumstance.

Low-dose COCs will not interfere with maturation of the hypothalamic-pituitary-ovarian axis nor stunt growth in height by prematurely closing the epiphyseal plates. Although adolescent CHC users do not accumulate increases in bone mineral density as rapidly as nonusers, this relative decrease is rapidly reversible after CHC cessation.[256,257] Equally important, adolescent patients with AUB should be evaluated to rule out PCOS thyroid disorders, etc., when CHC use is initiated. Clarify that when they stop taking CHCs, menses may return to being abnormal, unless the primary cause of the menstrual disruption has resolved or been treated.

Perimenopause

Healthy patients without contraindications to estrogen can safely use CHCs until they reach menopause. Specifically for perimenopausal patients, CHCs can reduce irregular menstrual bleeding and the risk of endometrial hyperplasia associated with anovulatory cycling. However, as patients get older, additional health issues may evolve that increase the risk of using an estrogen-containing contraceptive method.

CHC users in their 40s or early 50s may not experience symptoms of menopause while taking CHCs. They would not be expected to experience menstrual irregularities or vasomotor symptoms such as hot flashes, especially if CHCs are used on an extended basis. In this context, it may be difficult to detect when menopause occurs. (See Chapter 21, Contraception in the Later Reproductive Years.)

Postpartum

Pregnancy itself is a hypercoagulable state, and the postpartum period is the time that the risk of VTE is greatest.[185] As a result, it is recommended that postpartum patients delay use of estrogen-containing contraception that could further increase VTE risk until at least 21 days after delivery, when those pregnancy-induced changes in the coagulation system start to resolve. For patients with other risk factors for VTE (i.e., age over 35, obesity, cesarean delivery, postpartum hemorrhage, blood transfusion at delivery, preeclampsia, peripartum cardiomyopathy, smoking, immobility), it is advised to wait 42 days before initiating combined hormonal contraception.[75] (See Chapter 19, Contraception After Pregnancy.)

CHCs can be safely initiated immediately after first or second trimester abortion or early pregnancy loss (category 1).[75]

Lactation

High-dose estrogen was once given to postpartum patients to inhibit breast milk formation. From this outdated practice, theoretical concerns persisted for years that CHCs would adversely affect the quality or quantity of breast milk production at any time during breast/chest feeding. As reassuring evidence emerged, the American Academy of Pediatrics approved of estrogen-containing methods once some other source of nutrition (e.g., solid food) was added to the baby's diet. A thorough review of the world literature found that existing trials are insufficient to establish any effect of hormonal contraception on milk quality or its nutrients.[258] (See Chapter 19, Contraception After Pregnancy.) It is important to be respectful of patient's attitudes towards using hormonal contraception during breast/chest feeding as some may prefer not to expose their infant to exogenous hormones. You can share scientific information with a patient while respecting their preference. (See Chapter 4, Person-Centered Reproductive Health Conversations and Contraceptive Counseling.) The US MEC concluded that the benefits of CHC use outweigh the risks (i.e., category 2) in breast/chest feeding patients after 30 days postpartum when no other risk factors for VTE are present, when hypercoagulability is decreased, and when the milk flow is established.[75]

How to Prescribe CHCs

Patients who desire a short-acting reversible method or seek the noncontraceptive benefits of combined hormonal contraception often choose CHCs. The benefits of CHCs generally far outweigh the risks of CHCs. However, some patients have medical conditions or personal characteristics that increase their risk of complications or failure with use. Some patients will not choose CHCs based on their preferences or beliefs about the health or physical effects of hormones in contraceptives.[259] Patients seeking the most effective contraception should be offered IUDs, implants, or a permanent method. Those who have difficulty with daily pill administration should be offered long-acting methods as well as the intermediate-acting hormonal methods: the injection, transdermal patch, or the vaginal ring. (See Chapter 4, Person-Centered Reproductive Health Conversations and Contraceptive Counseling.)

Explore the patient's medical and reproductive health history and family history to ensure there are no conditions that would preclude safe use of CHCs. A comprehensive history will identify the vast majority of medical conditions in the US MEC that are contraindications or cautions to CHC use. In addition, the US Selected Practice Recommendations for Contraceptive Use (US SPR) (https://www.cdc.gov/reproductivehealth/contraception/mmwr/spr/summary.html) provides guidelines for practitioners to follow when initiating contraceptive methods or switching from one method to another, including outlining when screening tests are required before prescribing each method. Specifically, a blood pressure measurement is recommended before CHC initiation.[219] This can be a blood pressure obtained at a prior visit or at a pharmacy, which may be helpful in the setting of telemedicine or other scenarios where a patient is not physically present. An assessment of BMI before CHC initiation might be helpful to inform counseling of patients who subsequently perceive that their CHC use is causing weight gain. Otherwise, no other examinations or laboratory tests are required before initiating CHCs in healthy patients.[260]

Although not absolute contraindications, generalized skin conditions such as psoriasis, eczema, or sunburn may prevent successful patch use. Advise potential patch users weighing more than 90 kg (198 lbs.) that they may want to consider using a second method of contraception or another more effective method, particularly if they think they may forget to change patches on time. However, any potential decrease in effectiveness should be weighed against the risk of adverse outcomes of pregnancy (i.e., individuals with obesity are still candidates for the patch). Similar advice is not needed for individuals with higher BMIs who wish to use the ring. However, individuals may not be suitable candidates for the vaginal ring if they have significant pelvic relaxation, vaginal stenosis or obstruction (if it prevents placement or retention of the ring), conditions that make the vagina more susceptible to irritation or ulceration, or if they experience a discomfort with or an inability or unwillingness to touch their genitals.

Although the need for a breast and pelvic examination may be indicated by the patient's history or symptoms, neither is needed before initiating CHCs in an asymptomatic, healthy patient.[219,261] Wellness exams, including cervical cancer screening and sexually transmitted infection screening, may or may not be done at the same time as CHC initiation, per patient preference. No other screening tests are routinely needed unless the patient's medical history or blood pressure indicates a need for further assessment. The US MEC (https://www.cdc.gov/mmwr/volumes/65/rr/pdfs/rr6503.pdf) provides guidance as to which medical conditions might require further assessment or follow up.[75] In particular, routine screening for thrombotic mutations is not recommended prior to prescribing CHCs.[262]

Once your patient expresses a potential interest in using CHCs, realize that despite the wide range of health *benefits*, attention in the public eye has been focused on possible health *risks* associated with CHC use. Patients may have an inflated estimate of the health risks posed by CHC use. Help them understand that their risks associated with pregnancy are greater than the risk with using CHCs. Discuss noncontraceptive benefits, as well as lifestyle issues, to ensure they feel confident that they can take a pill each day. Anticipatory counseling about safety concerns or side effects may reduce later discontinuation. (See Chapter 4, Person-Centered Reproductive Health Conversations and Contraceptive Counseling.)

When to Start CHCs

CHCs can be initiated on any day of the menstrual cycle, as long as it reasonably certain the patient is not pregnant. Guidelines for how to be reasonably certain a patient is not pregnant can be found in the US SPR. (See Box 25-2 in Chapter 25 on how to be reasonably certain that a woman is not pregnant.) Initiating CHCs on any day of the menstrual cycle is an easy instruction and allows a patient to be protected from pregnancy as soon as possible. If the day the patient would like to start using the CHC is not within the first 5 days of the menstrual cycle, advise them to use a back-up method of contraception for the first 7 days of CHC use. If they need emergency contraception (EC) that day and are using the levonorgestrel (LNG) emergency contraceptive pill, they can still start the CHC immediately. However, if the patient is using ulipristal acetate (UPA; sold under the trade name ella®) for EC, then they should start the CHC 5 days after taking the UPA.[260] The one exception is the E2V/dienogest COC, which should be taken 9 days after UPA use. (See Chapter 18, Emergency Contraception.)

This method of same-day contraceptive initiation was first studied as the "Quick Start" method. A systematic review found that pregnancy rates, unscheduled bleeding, and side effects were not increased when COCs were started after day 5 of the menstrual cycle.[263] It is also the easiest way to teach contraceptive initiation to patients, trainees, and staff. Quick Start is an off-label practice supported by good clinical research, so it's important to reassure your patient that CHCs can be started right away despite how the package may instruct users. As many as 25% of patients given prescriptions for COCs that used outdated Sunday or first menstrual day start protocols did not begin taking the COCs as instructed because they conceived in the interim, forgot the pill-taking instructions, or did not fill the prescription.[3,264] The Quick Start method improved continuation from the first pack of COCs to the second pack when compared with different-day starts, although continuation rates were the same at 3 and 6 months.[265]

For COC users planning to take their pills on a 21/7 or 24/4 schedule, the next scheduled bleeding episode will likely not occur until the patient completes the active pills in the pack and starts the placebo pills. The same applies for 3 weeks of the patch and 3 weeks of ring use. If there is a possibility of an undetectable early pregnancy (i.e., less than 14 days), the patient can still start the CHC and take a urine pregnancy test at home (or return to your office or clinic to do so) in 2 weeks. Reassure patients that the hormones in the pills will not adversely affect an early pregnancy, and that rechecking a urine pregnancy test will detect a pregnancy early enough to allow them to pursue any pregnancy options they choose. Even if an early pregnancy is missed when CHCs are initiated, fetuses inadvertently exposed in utero to CHCs have not been found to have an increased risk for birth defects compared to unexposed fetuses.[266]

Switching from Other Methods

Patients who switch from other contraceptive methods can start CHCs immediately, using the same guidelines just explained for same-day initiation.[260] For example, if a patient is switching from a contraceptive implant to a CHC, advise the patient they can start their CHC the same day the implant is removed and to use a back-up method of contraception for the first 7 days of CHC use. Alternately, they can start the CHC 7 days before having the implant removed.

The exception is after IUD removal. If the patient has had recent intercourse and is more than 5 days from the first day of the menstrual cycle, residual sperm in the genital tract may cause pregnancy once the IUD is removed. In which case, the patient has three options:

- Start the CHC that day and return in 7 days for IUD removal.
- Abstain or use a barrier method for the next 7 days, then return for IUD removal and CHC initiation, and then use a back-up method or abstain for 7 days.
- Have the IUD removed that day and take EC. If the patient is using the LNG emergency contraception pill, a CHC can be started immediately and then a back-up method used for 7 days. If using UPA, then the CHC can be started 5 days after taking the UPA and then a back-up method used for 7 days.

Choosing a Formulation

Clinicians and patients in the United States have more than 70 COC formulations from which to choose, along with two types of patches and two types of rings. Select a CHC based on the hormonal dose and on your patient's clinical context, preferences, past experiences with CHCs, availability, insurance coverage, and cost. Both WHO and the FDA recommend using the lowest-dose CHC to reduce potential side effects, especially in patients who have hormone sensitivity. Although studies have shown that several COCs containing 20 mcg EE (and generally seven placebo pills) were associated with higher rates of unscheduled bleeding and discontinuation than COCs containing more than 20 mcg EE, the progestin components often differed among the COCs compared.[267] Whether the EE dose or the progestin type is responsible for the bleeding differences among COC formulations has yet to be answered.

USER INSTRUCTIONS FOR CHCS

The following bullet points summarize the essential information to include in patient education about each CHC. Instructions for use can effectively be provided by the clinician, nurse, health educator, or written instructions, depending on the process that works best in your clinic or office setting. Health literacy is paramount so adapt these instructions to the educational level of your patients, using plain language and terms that are readily understandable. See Chapter 4, Person-Centered Reproductive Health Conversations and Contraceptive Counseling.

There are some general recommendations for users for all CHCs:

- Start the method immediately, use a back-up method for the first 7 days if needed, and use a barrier method for dual protection if you are at risk for STIs.
- Ask your clinician to provide you with a package of or a prescription for EC. If you forget, you may also get these pills over the counter. You can use these pills if you have had sex that you believe was not fully protected (with or without a method).
- Look out for the warning signs for complications with combined hormonal methods. Even though they are rare, theses complications can be significant and life-threatening. Using the mnemonic "ACHES" with the accompanying graphic can help you remember which signs to look out for (see **Figure 12-1**).

USER INSTRUCTIONS FOR COCS

- It is important to take the pill daily in order for them to remain effective. Although taking a pill at the same time every day is not required to maintain effectiveness, maintaining a daily routine will likely help you remember to take the COC consistently. Pill "apps" and text services or alarms can be helpful.
- Start the pill immediately, use a back-up method for the first 7 days if needed, and use a barrier method for dual protection if you are at risk for STIs.
- Decide with your provider if you want monthly scheduled bleeding or less frequent scheduled bleeding episodes. If you choose extended pill use, your provider can prescribe pills packaged for this purpose. Alternatively, you can use other pill types for extended use by using the active pills, discarding the placebo pills, and starting a new packet right away.
    - If you plan to have scheduled bleeding, remember to start the next pack on the correct day even if you are still having bleeding.
    - If you skip the placebo pills and start the next pack, you may not be able to get another pack of pills until the usual refill time due to insurance issues. Your provider can change the way they order the pill to make sure you do not run out.

USER INSTRUCTIONS FOR CONTRACEPTIVE PATCHES

- Store patches at room temperature (25°C or 77°F) in their protective pouches, and do not put them in the refrigerator or freezer. Use one patch for 7 days.

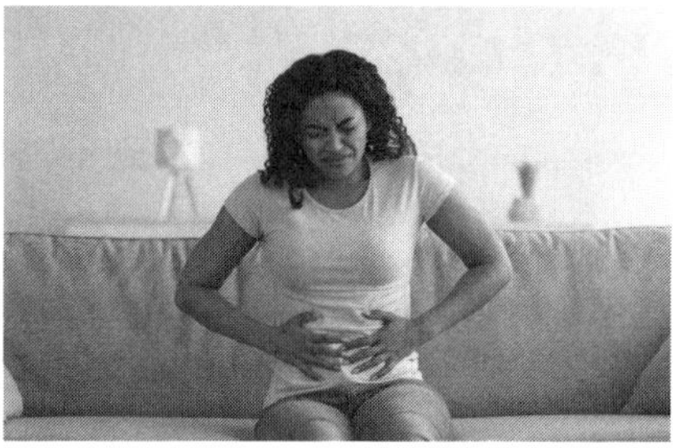

ABDOMINAL PAIN

- Blood clot in the pelvis or liver [mesenteric or pelvic vein thrombosis]
- Vomiting
- Cramping
- Weakness

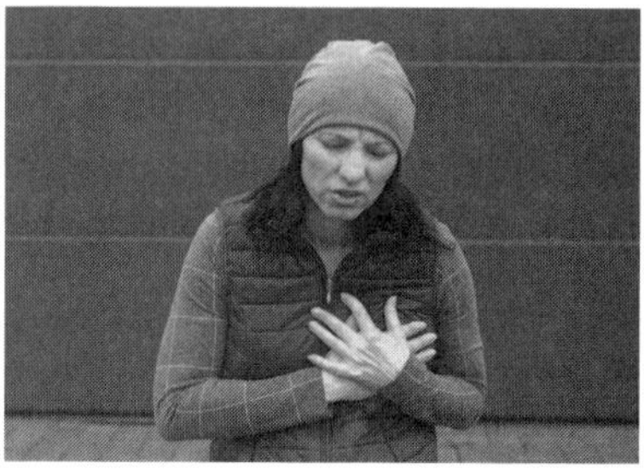

CHEST PAIN

- Blood clot in the lung or heart vessels [pulmonary embolism or myocardial infarction]
- Heart attack, angina
- Chest or heart pain, left arm and shoulder pain
- Coughing and shortness of breath

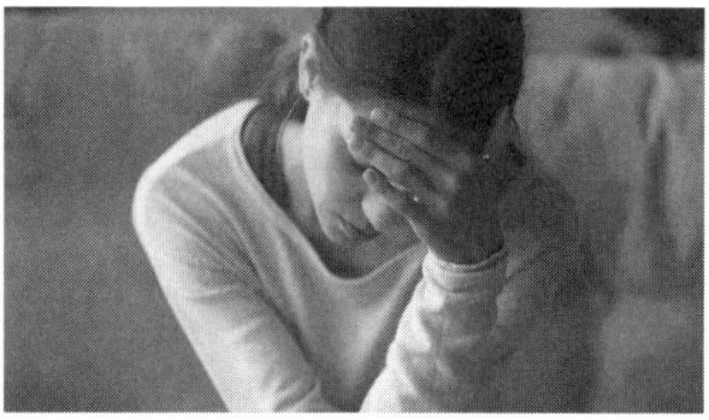

HEADACHES

- Stroke
- Blurred vision, spots, zigzag lines, weakness, difficulty speaking
- Sudden intellectual impairment

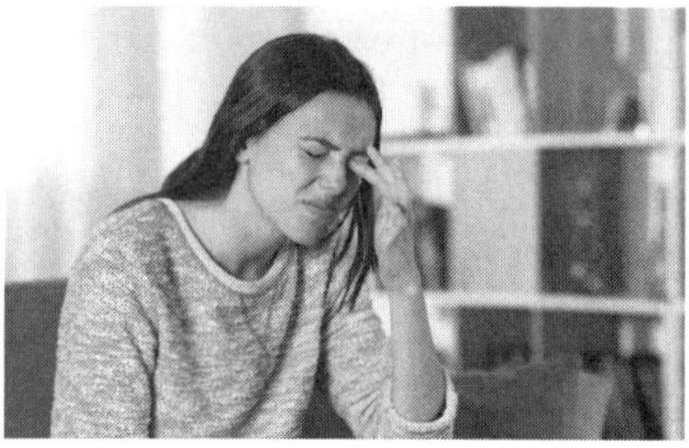

EYE PROBLEMS

- Stroke or retinal vein thrombosis
- Complete or partial loss of vision

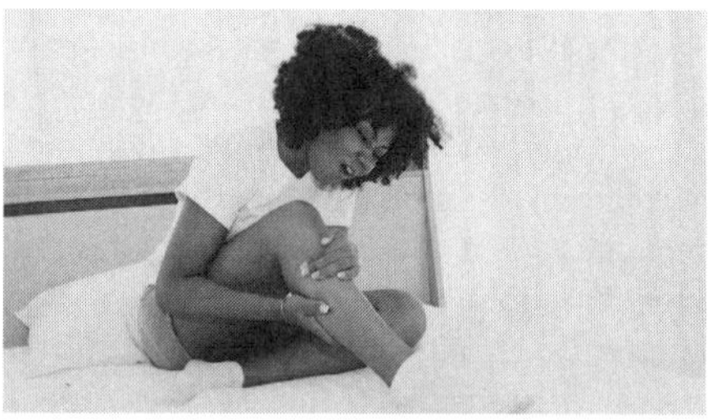

SEVERE LEG PAIN

- Inflammation and blood clots of a leg in the leg [thrombophlebitis]
- Swelling, heat or redness, tenderness in leg

You should also return to the office if you develop severe mood swings or depression, become jaundiced (yellow-colored skin), miss 2 periods or have signs of pregnancy.

Figure 12-1 Warning signs of CHC complications: ACHES mnemonic.

Modified from Hatcher RA 2003, Used with permission

Apply a new patch once a week on the same day for 3 weeks in a row. During the fourth week, do not wear a patch. At the end of the week, start another cycle of patches.

- Each patch is packaged in an individual foil packet. Open the pouch by tearing along the top edge and one side edge. Peel the foil pouch apart and open it. Using a fingernail to peel the unit off the foil pouch, lift out the patch along with its clear plastic cover—take care not to remove the clear liner as you remove the patch.
- Fold the patch open. While holding onto one half, peel the plastic off the other half. Avoid touching the sticky surface after you remove the liner.
- Apply the sticky side of the opened patch to your skin, and then remove the other half of the clear liner. You can put the patch on your buttocks, abdomen (belly), upper torso (except the breasts), or on the outer upper arm. Avoid placing patches in areas that rub together, such as under bra straps or underwear bands. Only apply the patch to clean, dry skin, and never put it over skin that is irritated, sunburned, red, or infected. Make sure there are no creams, oils, powder, sunscreen, or sweat on the skin, as these prevent the patch from sticking well. Press firmly on the patch for 10 seconds. Run your finger around the patch to make sure that all parts of the patch are sticking and to smooth out wrinkles.
- Keep the patch in place for 7 days, and then remove it. Check the patch every day to make sure it is sticking to your skin. You can wear the patch while bathing, showering, swimming, and exercising.
- To remove the patch, grasp it by an edge and pull it off. Fold it closed on itself on the sticky side to seal in the medication.
- Discard the patch in the garbage; do not flush it into the toilet.
- If any stickiness or adhesive remains on your skin, remove it using baby oil or lotions.
- At the beginning of the second week, remove the first patch and apply a new patch on a different spot on your body. Every new patch should be applied on the same day of the week, called the "patch change day." There is enough hormone in each patch to prevent pregnancy for up to 9 days, so you do not need to apply a new patch at the same time of the day. Wear the new patch for 7 days. Repeat this for a third week.
- During the fourth week, do not wear a patch. You will begin your menstrual period.
- After a week without wearing a patch, apply a new "first week" patch on the same day of the week you applied your other patches, even if you are still having bleeding.

USER INSTRUCTIONS FOR VAGINAL RINGS

NuvaRing

- If you have multiple rings or are going to store a ring for more than 4 months, refrigerate the rings at 2° to 8°C (36° to 46°F) to extend the shelf-life beyond 4 months. Rings may be stored for up to 4 months at room temperature, 25°C (77°F).
- Each ring comes in a resealable foil pouch. After washing and drying your hands, remove the ring and keep the foil pouch for ring disposal.

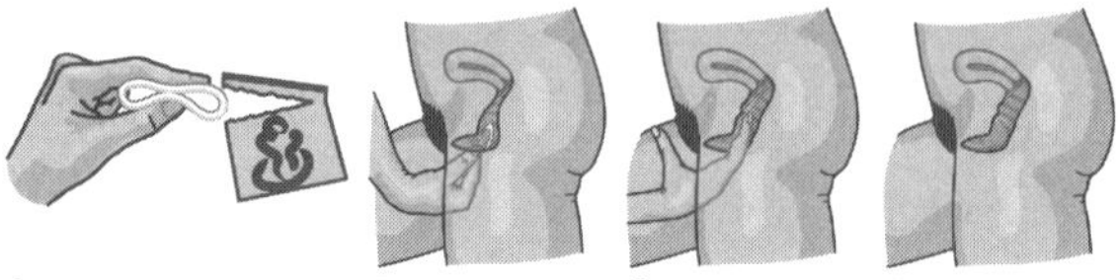

Figure 12-2 Inserting the ring.
Reproduced from Organon USA I. NuvaRing prescribing information. Roseland, NJ: Organon group of companies; 2005.

- To insert the ring into your vagina, use any position you find most comfortable: standing with one leg up, squatting, or lying down (see **Figure 12-2**). Hold the ring between your thumb and index finger and press the sides of the ring together so that it makes a long loop. Insert the folded ring into your vagina and using your index finger, gently push the ring into your vagina until it is comfortable; the muscles of your vagina should keep it in place. The does not need to be in any particular position in your vagina in order to prevent pregnancy.
- Leave the ring in place for 3 weeks. You do not need to remove the ring for intercourse. If you do remove the ring for intercourse, do not leave it out of the vagina for more than 3 hours in any 24-hour period.
- After 3 weeks of use, remove the ring for 4–7 days. During this break, you will experience bleeding, like a light period.
- Before removing the ring, wash and dry your hands. Insert your index finger into your vagina until you feel the rim of the ring. Remove the ring by hooking your index finger under whatever part of the ring you can feel or by grasping the rim between your index and middle finger and pulling it out. Place the used ring in the foil pouch and throw it away in a trash container out of the reach of children and pets (do not flush it down the toilet).
- After the 4- to 7-day break, insert a new vaginal ring to begin the cycle again. Insert the new ring even if you have not finished bleeding.
- If the ring is out of your vagina for more than 3 hours during the 21-day period, reinsert it and use additional contraception for the next 7 days. If you have had unprotected intercourse, consider using EC.

Annovera

- Wash your hands with mild soap and water. Dry them well. Take the ring out of its package. Wash the ring with mild soap and water, rinse, and pat dry with a clean cloth towel or paper towel.
- Hold the ring between your thumb and first (index) finger. Press the sides of the ring together to make it narrow.
- Choose a position that is comfortable for you. For example, lying down, squatting, or standing with one leg up.
- Gently insert the folded ring into your vagina. Push the ring further up into your vagina using your index finger. Push it in as far as you can. It sometimes helps to push down with the muscles in your vagina while you are inserting the ring. When you insert the ring, it may be in different positions in your vagina, but it does not have to be in an exact position for it to work. Mark your vaginal ring "in day" on your calendar.

    - If you feel the ring in your vagina or if it feels uncomfortable, you may not have pushed it into your vagina far enough. Use your index finger to gently push the ring as far as you can into your vagina. There is no danger of the ring being pushed too far up in the vagina or getting lost. You should not feel the ring after you have placed it into your vagina. Some individuals and their partners may be aware of the ring in the vagina during sexual intercourse.
    - You do not need to remove the ring for intercourse. If you do remove the ring for intercourse, do not leave it out of the vagina for more than 2 hours in any 21-day period.
- To remove the ring, first wash and dry your hands. Choose the position that is most comfortable for you. Put your index finger into your vagina and hook it through the ring. Gently pull downward and forward to remove and pull it out. It sometimes helps to push down with the muscles in your vagina while you are removing the ring. Wash the ring with mild soap and lukewarm water, pat it dry, and store in the case provided. Mark your ring "out day" on your calendar.

Providing Adequate Supplies

To facilitate access to contraception, the CDC recommends providing up to 1 year's supply (dispensing or prescribing 3–12 months) of CHCs when a patient initiates use.[260] For patients who obtain their CHCs from a pharmacy, many commercial and Medicaid insurance plans will provide a 90-day supply at a time if the prescription is written as such. In light of updated cervical cancer screening guidelines, consider reasonable refill protocols for your office or clinic for patients who return less often than annually for a wellness visit. A systematic review of the literature found that COC continuation rates are greater when more pill packs are given at one time.[268] Finally, offer to prescribe or provide condoms and EC for all CHC users.

Follow-Up

Because side effects that may lead to CHC discontinuation generally appear in the first few months of CHC use,[253] encourage patients to return if problems develop or if they wish to change their method. Many patients discontinue CHCs without consulting their clinicians. Although routine follow-up visits are not required, certain populations may benefit from follow-up visits, such as adolescents and adults with chronic medical conditions. At return visits for any reason (i.e., need for a CHC refill or a wellness visit), be responsive to patient concerns about their CHC. Acknowledge how difficult it is for many people to remember to take pills daily,[269] and remind them that such daily pill-taking is critical for CHC effectiveness. Support them in assessing how well they are able to take their daily pill.

Managing Problems Associated with use of Combined Hormonal Contraceptives

Users of CHCs may encounter issues with their chosen method; for instance, they may have a delayed or missed dose. Providing clear directions to the patient can help manage these challenges. Below are some common situations that arise with CHCs and example instructions you can provide.

Combined Oral Contraceptives

COC users commonly miss taking their pill daily.[1] After having taken at least 7 COCs at the correct time, patients are at little risk for ovulation until they subsequently miss 7 consecutive pills. Breakthrough ovulation and unintended pregnancy are more likely to occur if the patient missing pills is using a 21/7 formulation.[21] COCs containing 20 mcg or less of EE are associated with more breakthrough ovulation with missed pills.[270] When initiating COCs, proactively instruct your patient in what to do after missing one or more pills:

For one late or missed active (hormonal) pill:

- Take one active pill as soon as possible.
- Continue taking your pills daily on time, which may mean taking two pills in one day.
- No back-up contraception is needed.
- Emergency contraception is not typically needed unless pills were also missed earlier in the packet or at the end of the previous packet.

For two or more late or missed active (hormonal) pills:

- Take one active pill as soon as possible.
- Continue taking your pills daily on time, which may mean taking two pills in one day.
- Use condoms or abstain from vaginal sex until you have taken active pills for 7 days in a row.
- If pills were missed during the last week of active pills (days 15 through 21 of a packet), finish the active pills in the current packet and start a new packet the next day without using any placebo pills, OR use condoms or abstain from vaginal sex until you have taken active pills in the new packet for 7 days in a row.
- Use LNG EC pills if you missed COCs during the first week of a packet and you had any unprotected intercourse. If you have vomiting or severe diarrhea within 24 hours of taking your pill, treat this as a missed pill.

Contraceptive Patches

Dislodged or detached patches:

- If the patch is partially or completely detached for less than 24 hours:
    - Put the patch back on the skin and press it firmly, applying pressure for 10 seconds, and make sure that the edges are sticking well. If it does not stick well, remove the patch and apply a new patch.
    - Do not use other adhesives or wraps to hold the patch in place. No additional contraception is needed, and the patch change day will be the same. If the edges stick well, you can continue to use the patch for the full 7 days.
- If the patch has been partially or completely detached for more than 24 hours or you do not know how long it has been unstuck:
    - Start a new patch cycle immediately and use additional contraceptive protection for 7 days.
    - You will now have a new patch-change day; if unprotected intercourse has occurred, EC may be needed.

Table 12-3 **Management of Missed or Forgotten Patches**

When Patch Forgotten/Missed	Management
Week 1	■ If a patch is forgotten or is applied late during the first week, and you have had unprotected intercourse, you can use EC. ■ You should place a patch immediately. ■ You should use an additional contraceptive method or abstain for 7 days. ■ Remember to change the patch each week, from now on, on the day of the week the new patch was applied.
Weeks 2 or 3	■ *1–2 days late*: If you forget to remove and replace a patch, remove the old patch and replace it with a new patch immediately. You do not need an additional contraceptive method or emergency contraception, and your patch change day does not change. ■ *More than 2 days late*: Remove the old patch and place a new one immediately. Use EC if you have had unprotected intercourse (especially if you are 4 or more days late in applying the patch). Use additional contraception or abstinence for 7 days; the next patch will be applied 7 days later on the same day of the week that the new patch was applied.
Week 4	■ If you forget to remove the third patch, just remove the patch. ■ You do not need an additional contraceptive method or EC; a new patch is placed on your usual change day.

Missed or forgotten patches: Missed or forgotten patches may mean that a user has forgotten to place a patch at all in the first week of the cycle, or forgotten to remove and replace a patch during the second or third weeks. Management of forgotten patches depends upon which patch is missed and for how long (**Table 12-3**).

Application-site reactions:

- To decrease the risk of skin irritation, change where on your body you put the patch each time you put on a new one.
- Do not apply the patch to areas of skin that are irritated or cut.
- If you have a skin reaction at a place where you put a patch, you can remove the patch and apply a new patch in a different place.

Vaginal Rings

Expelled or removed rings:

- You may accidentally remove the ring, or it may get pushed out of your body (e.g., while removing a tampon, while you are having intercourse, while you are having a bowel movement, or if you do strenuous physical activity such as marathon running).

- Rinse the ring with lukewarm water (for comfort) and reinsert it as soon as possible. If ring is lost, the user should insert a new ring and continue using the ring the same way you were before the ring came out.
- If the EE/ENG ring has been *out for more than 3 hours, but less than 48 hours*, reinsert it as soon as possible, and continue wearing it until the scheduled removal day.[260] No additional contraceptive is needed. Consider EC if unprotected intercourse occurred in the first week of a cycle.
- If the EE/ENG ring has been *out for more than 48 hours*, instructions may vary depending on week of the cycle.
  - Generally, reinsert the ring as soon as possible, and continue it until the scheduled removal day.
  - Use additional contraception or avoid intercourse until the ring has been in for 7 days.
  - If you leave the ring out of your vagina for more than 7 days during the *third week of the cycle or later*:
    - Skip your patch-free week by finishing the third week of ring use and starting a new ring immediately.
    - If you are unable to start a new ring immediately, use back-up contraception (e.g., condoms) or avoid sexual intercourse until a new ring has been worn for 7 consecutive days.
- If the SA/EE ring is out for a total of more than 2 hours during 21 days of use, use additional contraception or avoid intercourse until the ring has been in for 7 days.

Forgotten or late ring:

- If you leave the ring in the vagina for more than 3 weeks (but less than 5 weeks), it is still effective in preventing pregnancy.
- Remove the ring and insert a new one or reinsert (if the SA/EE ring is used) after a 1-week interval if following a monthly regimen, or immediately if extended or continuous use is preferred.
- If the NuvaRing was left in place for more than 5 weeks, the ring may not protect you against pregnancy. (A recent study is reassuring that serum ENG levels persist up to 6 weeks,[32] but more data are needed to confirm contraceptive effectiveness for the EE/ENG ring.)
- Consider taking EC and use an additional contraceptive method until a new ring has been in place for at least 7 days.

Disconnected (broken) ring:

- If your contraceptive ring has broken, discard the ring and replace it with a new ring.
- You do not need additional contraception as long as you can insert a new ring quickly.

Vaginal symptoms:

- You may feel that you have more vaginal discharge or wetness while using the ring, but this does not always mean you have an infection.
- There is no increased risk of vaginal infection with ring use. If you have vaginal itching or a foul odor, you may need to be evaluated and treated.
- Even if you do not have an infection, if the discharge is bothersome to you, you may want to change methods.

Managing Side Effects

Side effects are the most common reason for CHC discontinuation. In one large study, 34% of women reported that side effects were the main reason for discontinuation of their COC.[253] Many of these side effects have been determined not to be caused by CHCs while others remain difficult to determine causation or association—meaning, is it the CHC, or are these symptoms just common among individuals? In a population-based survey of approximately 2,500 Germans, 82% of respondents reported that at least one common symptom (fatigue, headache, muscle pain, etc.) was causing mild impairment and 22% reported at least one symptom causing severe impairment.[271] Reported side effects may occur more commonly in women than men when the patient is preconditioned to expect them, such as by warning them that they might experience symptoms.[272]

However, perception is often everything. Active listening to and being supportive of patients in a nonjudgmental manner while still providing them the evidence about an issue may satisfy the patient or provide the opportunity to switch to another method. Be clear that side effects are not adverse events and discuss what signs would be concerning. Advise patients that side effects are usually time-limited. Address the patient's main concerns about use of CHCs directly. Support them in their decision if they decide to switch to a different CHCs or different formulation or a completely different contraceptive method.

Amenorrhea or Unscheduled Bleeding

Initial CHC use is associated with unscheduled bleeding and the timing of initiation (i.e., Quick Start versus Sunday start) does not change the amount or duration of this bleeding.[273] Over time, bleeding should become more scheduled when using a CHC that has a scheduled nonhormonal pill break. Advise patients that the overall amount of bleeding they experience during a scheduled bleed is typically less than during natural menstruation. Likely the most common reason for unscheduled spotting or bleeding is missed or late pills.

As mentioned previously, extended-cycling formulations with skipped or delayed withdrawal can have a longer duration of unscheduled bleeding, but for most users that bleeding will improve over time.[23] If unscheduled bleeding becomes a nuisance with extended cycling, a 3- to 4-day break in CHC use[25] or supplementing with a pill containing norethindrone acetate[26] may result in more days of amenorrhea.

Before changing CHC type for complaints of unscheduled bleeding, rule out more serious causes, such as pregnancy, infection (vaginitis and cervicitis), or medications or compounds that interfere with CHC metabolism (certain anticonvulsants, cigarette smoking, St. John's Wort, rifampin). Consider changing the patient's CHC formulation if unscheduled spotting or bleeding persists after the first several months of use. Switch earlier if a patient is planning to discontinue due to the bleeding pattern. No research indicates that any specific CHC or formulation is best at eliminating unscheduled spotting or bleeding.

Experiencing amenorrhea during the time a scheduled withdrawal bleed should occur could be completely normal. The incidence likely varies for different individuals. COCs containing estradiol valerate combined with dienogest, as compared with an EE-levonorgestrel COC, appear to have shorter and less intense scheduled withdrawal bleeds as well as more likelihood of amenorrhea during the scheduled withdrawal week.[274] If there is cause for concern, the most obvious cause of amenorrhea—pregnancy—should be ruled out. Thyroid problems, prolactinoma, hypothalamic amenorrhea due to stress or excessive exercise, or anovulatory states (such as PCOS or obesity) are often masked by CHCs. Other specific conditions, such as cervical stenosis, need to be evaluated if the patient has recently had cervical surgery (e.g., D&C, cone biopsy, LEEP, etc.). In general, reassurance can be given that they are not pregnant and, given the progestin-dominant effect on the endometrium, the lining of the uterus is not "building up." Additionally, the patient could consider intermittently using a home pregnancy test if that might be helpful to reduce anxiety around concerns about pregnancy. If the patient desires cyclic bleeding, consider switching to a different pill, triphasic formulation, or other method.

Weight Changes

Randomized clinical trials have demonstrated that, on average, patients do *not* experience more weight gain with low-dose COCs than with placebo or no intervention.[168,275,276] In a prospective trial of women using triphasic COCs with daily weight measurements for 4 months, no changes in mean weight fluctuations were noted during the cycle.[277] A 9-year study showed that COC use by adolescents was *not* associated with either weight gain or increased body fat.[278] In clinical trials, women who use CHCs do not typically gain more weight than they normally do in the same time interval without CHCs. A Cochrane review confirmed that available evidence is insufficient to determine the effect of combination contraceptives on weight, but concluded that no large effect was evident.[168] However, it is important for clinicians to understand that what troubles a patient is their experience and *perception* of weight changes and that often a patient's opinions about weight change in clinical trials may not correlate with measured changes on a scale.

The most common reason for weight gain in adults is simply age—as adults age, their metabolism changes and weight increases if no changes to diet or exercise are made. In addition, women have several events over their lifetime that can significantly act upon their metabolism and thus their weight, including puberty, each successive pregnancy, and menopause.[279-282] The hypothesized mechanisms for CHC-related weight gain include changes to the renin-angiotensin-aldosterone system causing fluid retention and hypertrophy of adipose tissue. But as no clear clinical evidence has been found, it is unlikely that any of these mechanisms cause significant problems. Nonetheless, individual weight changes related to CHC may exist, and given that weight changes are an incredibly sensitive topic for many people, the most important thing is listen to a patient's concerns, briefly review what we know about CHCs and weight changes, and balance the pros/cons of changing methods.

Headaches

Headaches are common,[283] but if a patient develops new headaches while on a CHC or has worsening of preexisting headaches, evaluate promptly and consider possible discontinuation of estrogen-containing contraceptives (see Chronic Medical Conditions: Headaches earlier in this chapter or Chapter 20, Contraception for Those with Medical Conditions). Women report experiencing fewer headaches with extended regimens as compared with cyclic COCs.[23] For menstrual migraines, extended-cycle CHC use could also provide relief.[103,239]

Headache complaints decrease with continued use of CHCs. Patients experiencing headaches during the first cycle have only a 1 in 3 chance of having those headaches the second month of use. The risk drops to 1 in 10 by the third cycle.

A systematic review of the literature found that there is no scientific evidence to support the common clinical practice of switching formulations to treat headache. However, the authors suggested that manipulation of the extent or duration of estrogen withdrawal might be beneficial, especially if the headaches worsen during bleeding.[284] Stepwise evaluation of the headache is necessary. For discussion on headache classification, see Chapter 20, Contraception for Those with Medical Conditions.

- **Confirm whether the headaches started or worsened in frequency or severity with the onset of CHC use.** New or worsening symptoms prompt medical evaluation. Stop CHCs during evaluation, especially if the headaches are severe or if the patient develops any aura with the headaches. Progestin-only pills may be used. If the headaches are not serious, consider lowering estrogen doses.
- **Rule out other causes**. Measure the patient's blood pressure. Obtain a personal history of medication use, caffeine intake, and other prescription, nonprescription, and recreational drug use. Inquire about recent trauma. Note if there are other associated problems with vision, sensation, or other functions. Evaluate for signs and symptoms of transient ischemic attacks, cerebrovascular accidents, temporal arteritis, sinusitis, viremia, sepsis, allergy, temporomandibular joint (TMJ) disorders, dental problems, drug use, alcohol or caffeine withdrawal, or central nervous system tumor.
- **Characterize the type of headache.** The consequences are different for different types of headaches. If a patient develops new-onset migraine or a worsening in the severity or frequency of migraine headaches during the active pill days, they may no longer be a candidate for CHCs. *If associated neurologic aura develops, stop the CHC immediately* and provide contraception without estrogen. On the other hand, if the symptoms develop or worsen only during the hormone-free interval (when the estrogen levels drop), it may be possible to offer extended use, low-dose COCs to reduce menstrual migraines.

Mood Swings and Depression

There is a common belief that CHCs adversely impact mood, but the published evidence is significantly flawed,[285] and recent publications have been conflicting, either demonstrating a protective effect[286] or not.[287] It is important to note that the study reporting an increased risk of depression in COC users had a risk estimate well below 2, which is considered by epidemiologists to be not significant. In those with existing depression, CHC use does not appear to worsen the condition.[288]

If patients do report an increase in depressive symptoms, moodiness, and other emotional states when on CHCs, respond with empathy. Discuss options with the patient like considering an empiric change to a lower dose formulation or CHC cessation. However, it is also important to identify when in a patient's cycle these symptoms develop. If the symptoms appear just before the menses, then extended use of active pills may help to suppress or prevent cycle-related mood changes.[24] For those who suffer from PMDD, all CHCs likely have the ability to suppress or reduce symptoms, and consideration should be given to extended dosing (eliminating the scheduled withdrawal week). The COC containing drospirenone/EE has an FDA indication for treatment of PMDD. A systematic review of drospirenone-containing pills for PMDD demonstrates that in the first 3 months of use, participants experienced less severe symptoms, but data were insufficient to determine a longer impact.[109] In addition, the use of placebo had a significant beneficial impact on symptoms. (See Chapter 2, Understanding the Physiology of the Menstrual Cycle.)

If you have any concern about your patient suffering from an underlying depressive or anxiety disorder, perform or refer for an explicit evaluation and treatment. Stopping CHC use is not adequate therapy and may not even be indicated. Suicidal patients need emergency treatment by specialists.

Sexual Changes

Studies have failed to find a clear association between libido and CHC use.[289-291] However, sexual desire and libido are not linear processes and can be influenced by a variety of internal and external factors (see Chapter 6, Sexuality and Contraception). A subset of individuals may be adversely affected by changes in the amount and consistency of vaginal lubrication. In addition to recommending a sexual lubricant, it may be useful to switch to a lower dose formulation; however, no clear guidance exists regarding what to do when patients experience these symptoms. A study comparing a 30 mcg EE/LNG versus a 20 mcg EE/LNG pill demonstrated an increase in sexual desire.[292] Given this evidence, it is conceivable that other lower-dose hormonal methods might also provide improvement.

Skin Changes

Estrogen stimulates the production and activity of melanocytes, which can cause darkening of pigmented areas (for example, the linea nigra on the abdomen) or a dark patch on the face (melasma or chloasma). Patients with darker skin pigment are more susceptible. After discontinuation of estrogen, the melasma can fade over time but often incompletely. Progestin-only methods may be preferable for at-risk patients. In vitro studies have demonstrated that progesterone reduces the proliferation rate of melanocytes as compared with 17B-estradiol.[293] Recommend consistent use of sunscreen and hats in those at risk or if melasma has already occurred. If a patient is particularly bothered by these skin changes, refer to a dermatology specialist.

Estrogen can also stimulate the formation of telangiectasias, which are fine, dilated intracutaneous capillaries and small terminal arteries. Telangiectasias are not clinically significant but may be cosmetically disturbing to a patient. Avoid the use of estrogen-containing hormonal methods in patients troubled by telangiectasia.

As mentioned earlier, CHCs are used as treatment for acne.[127] If using CHCs in the treatment of acne, the effect is not immediate and may take several months before benefits become apparent to the patient. Although certain CHCs have received FDA approval for the treatment of acne, all CHCs should have a similar effect given their ability to decrease free testosterone by increasing SHBG. If it appears the patient's CHC may be contributing to acne, consider extended-use cycling or switch to a CHC with a progestin component with low androgenicity formulation, such as a drospirenone-containing formulation.[294]

Mastalgia

Breast tissue is dynamic and responsive to hormone exposure. For example, breast volume varies greatly during the menstrual cycle. An imaging study found that overall volume of the breast varies by 76 mL during the menstrual cycle![295] Mastalgia, or breast tenderness, is not an uncommon complaint, especially with initiation of CHCs.

A properly fitting bra with adequate support is the first recommendation. A Cochrane review of COCs with different progestin types found that desogestrel-containing pill users complained less of breast tenderness than did those using a drospirenone-containing pill.[296] COC users with a lower EE component (20 mcg) also report less breast pain than do those using higher EE pills.[270] If the symptoms develop just before or during withdrawal bleeding, extended-cycle CHCs should also be helpful.

Gastrointestinal Complaints

Working at the level of the central nervous system, estrogen can induce nausea or vomiting. Progesterone slows gastric peristalsis and can increase constipation and sensations of bloating and distention. Most affected patients acclimate to the hormones, and nausea resolves within 1 to 3 months of use. If a patient complains of nausea, they can try taking the pills with food or at night. Patients with onset of severe gastrointestinal symptoms should be promptly evaluated for other causes, as this is likely unrelated to CHC use.

If vomiting or diarrhea is related to taking the pill, try the following approaches:

- Switch to a progestin-only formulation.
- Decrease the dose of the estrogen-component.

Author Disclosures—Ramanadhan: none; Edelman: consultant for World Health Organization, CDC, Gynuity Health Projects, Genzyme, Agile Therapeutics, HRA Pharma and FHI360; Nexplanon trainer for Merck; author for UptoDate (royalties received); research funding from Merck and National Institutes of Health (received NIH grant funding for several of the studies referenced in the chapter specific to obesity and contraceptive effectiveness)

Acknowledgements—Thank you to Carrie Cwiak, MD, MPH, Anne Burke, MD, MPH, and Kavita Nanda, MD, MHS, who were all contributing authors to the prior edition of the CHC chapters. Thank you to Abigail Liberty, MD, MSPH and Megan A. Cohen, MD, MPH for editorial review.

Appendix—Many high-quality resources now exist for providers in creating their own COC user instructions or in referring patients to use. One such site is Planned Parenthood's online resources: www.plannedparenthood.org/learn/birth-control/birth-control-pill. For additional resources, see Chapter 27.

References

1. Potter L, Oakley D, de Leon-Wong E, Canamar R. Measuring compliance among oral contraceptive users. Fam Plann Perspect. 1996;28:154-8.
2. Foster DG, Hulett D, Bradsberry M, Darney P, Policar M. Number of oral contraceptive pill packages dispensed and subsequent unintended pregnancies. Obstet Gynecol. 2011;117:566-72.
3. Westhoff C, Kerns J, Morroni C, Cushman LF, Tiezzi L, Murphy PA. Quick start: novel oral contraceptive initiation method. Contraception. 2002;66:141-5.
4. Tessler SL, Peipert JF. Perceptions of contraceptive effectiveness and health effects of oral contraception. Womens Health Iss. 1997;7:400-6.
5. Brabaharan S, Veettil SK, Kaiser JE, et al. Association of Hormonal contraceptive use with adverse health outcomes: An umbrella review of meta-analyses of randomized clinical trials and cohort studies. JAMA Netw Open. 2022;5:e2143730.
6. Hannaford PC, Iversen L, Macfarlane TV, Elliott AM, Angus V, Lee AJ. Mortality among contraceptive pill users: cohort evidence from Royal College of General Practitioners' Oral Contraception Study. BMJ. 2010;340:c927.
7. Franks AL, Beral V, Cates W, Jr., Hogue CJ. Contraception and ectopic pregnancy risk. Am J Obstet Gynecol. 1990;163:1120-3.

8. Marchbanks PA, Annegers JF, Coulam CB, Strathy JH, Kurland LT. Risk factors for ectopic pregnancy. A population-based study. JAMA. 1988;259:1823-7.
9. Centers for Disease Control and Prevention. Ten great public health achievements--United States, 1900-1999. MMWR Morb Mortal Wkly Rep. 1999;48:241-3.
10. Daniels K, Daugherty J, Jones J, Mosher W. Current contraceptive use and variation by selected characteristics among women aged 15-44: United States, 2011-2013. Natl Health Stat Rep. 2015:1-14.
11. Daniels K, Mosher WD. Contraceptive methods women have ever used: United States, 1982-2010. Natl Health Stat Rep. 2013:1-15.
12. Seidman L, Kroll R, Howard B, Ricciotti N, Hsieh J, Weiss H. Ovulatory effects of three oral contraceptive regimens: a randomized, open-label, descriptive trial. Contraception. 2015;91: 495-502.
13. Lewis RA, Taylor D, Natavio MF, Melamed A, Felix J, Mishell D, Jr. Effects of the levonorgestrel-releasing intrauterine system on cervical mucus quality and sperm penetrability. Contraception. 2010;82:491-6.
14. Natavio MF, Taylor D, Lewis RA, et al. Temporal changes in cervical mucus after insertion of the levonorgestrel-releasing intrauterine system. Contraception. 2013;87:426-31.
15. Stanczyk FZ, Archer DF, Bhavnani BR. Ethinyl estradiol and 17beta-estradiol in combined oral contraceptives: pharmacokinetics, pharmacodynamics and risk assessment. Contraception. 2013;87:706-27.
16. Nelson A, Parke S, Mellinger U, Zampaglione E, Schmidt A. Efficacy and safety of a combined oral contraceptive containing estradiol valerate/dienogest: results from a clinical study conducted in North America. J Womens Health (Larchmt). 2014;23:204-10.
17. Coelingh Bennink HJ, Holinka CF, Diczfalusy E. Estetrol review: profile and potential clinical applications. Climacteric. 2008;11 Suppl 1:47-58.
18. Stanczyk FZ. All progestins are not created equal. Steroids. 2003;68:879-90.
19. Creinin MD, Jensen JT. Oral contraceptive generations - Time to stop using a marketing myth to define nomenclature. Contraception. 2020;102:143-4.
20. Edelman A. Menstrual nirvana: amenorrhea through the use of continuous oral contraceptives. Curr Womens Health Rep. 2002;2:434-8.
21. Dinger J, Minh TD, Buttmann N, Bardenheuer K. Effectiveness of oral contraceptive pills in a large US cohort comparing progestogen and regimen. Obstet Gynecol. 2011;117:33-40.
22. Sulak PJ, Scow RD, Preece C, Riggs MW, Kuehl TJ. Hormone withdrawal symptoms in oral contraceptive users. Obstet Gynecol. 2000;95:261-6.
23. Edelman A, Micks E, Gallo MF, Jensen JT, Grimes DA. Continuous or extended cycle vs. cyclic use of combined hormonal contraceptives for contraception. Cochrane Database Syst Rev. 2014 Jul 29;2014(7):CD004695. Available from: https://www.ncbi.nlm.nih.gov/pmc/articles/PMC6837850/.
24. Sulak PJ, Kuehl TJ, Ortiz M, Shull BL. Acceptance of altering the standard 21-day/7-day oral contraceptive regimen to delay menses and reduce hormone withdrawal symptoms. Am J Obstet Gynecol. 2002;186:1142-9.
25. Sulak PJ, Kuehl TJ, Coffee A, Willis S. Prospective analysis of occurrence and management of breakthrough bleeding during an extended oral contraceptive regimen. Am J Obstet Gynecol. 2006;195:935-41.
26. Edelman AB, Koontz SL, Nichols MD, Jensen JT. Continuous oral contraceptives: are bleeding patterns dependent on the hormones given? Obstet Gynecol. 2006;107:657-65.
27. Mylan Pharmaceuticals. Xulane prescribing information. 2022. Available from: https://dailymed.nlm.nih.gov/dailymed/fda/fdaDrugXsl.cfm?type=display&setid=f7848550-086a-43d8-8ae5-047f4b9e4382.
28. Archer DF, Stanczyk FZ, Rubin A, Foegh M. Ethinyl estradiol and levonorgestrel pharmacokinetics with a low-dose transdermal contraceptive delivery system, AG200-15: a randomized controlled trial. Contraception. 2012;85:595-601.
29. Stewart FH, Kaunitz AM, Laguardia KD, Karvois DL, Fisher AC, Friedman AJ. Extended use of transdermal norelgestromin/ethinyl estradiol: a randomized trial. Obstet Gynecol. 2005;105:1389-96.
30. Lavelanet AF, Rybin D, White KoC. The pharmacokinetics of 12-week continuous contraceptive patch use. Contraception. 2017;95 6:578-85.

31. Benson LS, Micks EA. Why stop now? Extended and continuous regimens of combined hormonal contraceptive methods. Obstet Gynecol Clin North Am. 2015;42 4:669-81.
32. Dragoman M, Petrie K, Torgal A, Thomas T, Cremers S, Westhoff CL. Contraceptive vaginal ring effectiveness is maintained during 6 weeks of use: a prospective study of normal BMI and obese women. Contraception. 2013;87:432-6.
33. Westhoff CL, Torgal AH, Mayeda ER, et al. Pharmacokinetics and ovarian suppression during use of a contraceptive vaginal ring in normal-weight and obese women. Am J Obstet Gynecol. 2012;207:39.e1-6.
34. Miller L, Verhoeven CH. Extended regimens of the contraceptive vaginal ring: a randomized trial. Obstet Gynecol. 2005;106:473-82.
35. Guazzelli CAF, Barreiros FA, Barbosa R, de Araújo FF, Moron AF. Extended regimens of the vaginal contraceptive ring: cycle control. Contraception. 2009;80:430-5.
36. Weisberg E, Merki-Feld GS, McGeechan K, Fraser IS. Randomized comparison of bleeding patterns in women using a combined contraceptive vaginal ring or a low-dose combined oral contraceptive on a menstrually signaled regimen. Contraception. 2015;91:121-6.
37. Sulak PJ, Smith V, Coffee A, Witt I, Kuehl AL, Kuehl TJ. Frequency and management of breakthrough bleeding with continuous use of the transvaginal contraceptive ring: a randomized controlled trial. Obstet Gynecol. 2008;112:563-71.
38. Winner B, Peipert JF, Zhao Q, et al. Effectiveness of long-acting reversible contraception. N Engl J Med. 2012;366:1998-2007.
39. Foster DG, Parvataneni R, de Bocanegra HT, Lewis C, Bradsberry M, Darney P. Number of oral contraceptive pill packages dispensed, method continuation, and costs. Obstet Gynecol. 2006;108:1107-14.
40. Potter L. Oral contraceptive compliance and its role in the effectiveness of the method. In: Cramer J, Spilker B, eds. Patient compliance in medical practice and clinical trials. New York: Raven Press; 1991:195-207.
41. Nettleman MD, Chung H, Brewer J, Ayoola A, Reed PL. Reasons for unprotected intercourse: analysis of the PRAMS survey. Contraception. 2007;75:361-6.
42. Jones RK. Change and consistency in US women's pregnancy attitudes and associations with contraceptive use. Contraception. 2017;95:485-90.
43. Hou MY, Hurwitz S, Kavanagh E, Fortin J, Goldberg AB. Using daily text-message reminders to improve adherence with oral contraceptives: a randomized controlled trial. Obstet Gynecol. 2010;116:633-40.
44. Barnhart KT, Schreiber CA. Return to fertility following discontinuation of oral contraceptives. Fertil Steril. 2009;91:659-63.
45. Lopez LM, Grimes DA, Gallo MF, Stockton LL, Schulz KF. Skin patch and vaginal ring versus combined oral contraceptives for contraception. Cochrane Database Syst Rev. 2013 Apr 30;2013(4):CD003552. Available from: https://www.ncbi.nlm.nih.gov/pmc/articles/PMC7154336/.)
46. Audet M-C, Moreau M, Koltun WD, et al. Evaluation of contraceptive efficacy and cycle control of a transdermal contraceptive patch vs an oral contraceptive: a randomized controlled trial. JAMA. 2001;285:2347-54.
47. Urdl W, Apter D, Alperstein A, et al. Contraceptive efficacy, compliance and beyond: factors related to satisfaction with once-weekly transdermal compared with oral contraception. Eur J Obstet Gynecol Reprod Biol. 2005;121:202-10.
48. Zieman M, Guillebaud J, Weisberg E, Shangold GA, Fisher AC, Creasy GW. Contraceptive efficacy and cycle control with the Ortho Evra™/Evra™ transdermal system: the analysis of pooled data. Fertil Steril. 2002;77:13-8.
49. Nelson AL, Kaunitz AM, Kroll R, et al. Efficacy, safety, and tolerability of a levonorgestrel/ethinyl estradiol transdermal delivery system: Phase 3 clinical trial results. Contraception. 2021;103:137-43.
50. Thurman AR, Hammond N, Brown HE, Roddy ME. Preventing repeat teen pregnancy: postpartum depot medroxyprogesterone acetate, oral contraceptive pills, or the patch? J Pediatr Adolesc Gynecol. 2007;20:61-5.
51. Jick SS, Hagberg KW, Kaye JA, Jick H. The risk of unintended pregnancies in users of the contraceptive patch compared to users of oral contraceptives in the UK General Practice Research Database. Contraception. 2009;80:142-51.

52. Bakhru A, Stanwood N. Performance of contraceptive patch compared with oral contraceptive pill in a high-risk population. Obstet Gynecol. 2006;108:378-86.
53. Creinin MD, Meyn LA, Borgatta L, et al. Multicenter comparison of the contraceptive ring and patch: a randomized controlled trial. Obstet Gynecol. 2008;111:267-77.
54. Raine TR, Foster-Rosales A, Upadhyay UD, et al. One-year contraceptive continuation and pregnancy in adolescent girls and women initiating hormonal contraceptives. Obstet Gynecol. 2011;117:363.
55. Peipert JF, Zhao Q, Allsworth JE, et al. Continuation and satisfaction of reversible contraception. Obstet Gynecol. 2011;117:1105-13.
56. O'Neil ME, Peipert JF, Zhao Q, Madden T, Secura G. Twenty-four–month continuation of reversible contraception. Obstet Gynecol. 2013;122:1083.
57. Diedrich JT, Zhao Q, Madden T, Secura GM, Peipert JF. Three-year continuation of reversible contraception. Am J Obstet Gynecol. 2015;213:662.e1-8.
58. Sucato GS, Land SR, Murray PJ, Cecchini R, Gold MA. Adolescents' experiences using the contraceptive patch versus pills. J Pediatr Adolesc Gynecol. 2011;24:197-203.
59. Oddsson K, Leifels-Fischer B, de Melo NR, et al. Efficacy and safety of a contraceptive vaginal ring (NuvaRing) compared with a combined oral contraceptive: a 1-year randomized trial. Contraception. 2005;71:176-82.
60. Ahrendt H-J, Nisand I, Bastianelli C, et al. Efficacy, acceptability and tolerability of the combined contraceptive ring, NuvaRing, compared with an oral contraceptive containing 30 μg of ethinyl estradiol and 3 mg of drospirenone. Contraception. 2006;74:451-7.
61. Dieben TO, Roumen FJ, Apter D. Efficacy, cycle control, and user acceptability of a novel combined contraceptive vaginal ring. Obstet Gynecol. 2002;100:585-93.
62. Gerlinger C, Trussell J, Mellinger U, et al. Different Pearl Indices in studies of hormonal contraceptives in the United States: impact of study population. Contraception. 2014;90:142-6.
63. Roumen F. Contraceptive efficacy and tolerability with a novel combined contraceptive vaginal ring, NuvaRing. Eur J Contracept Reprod Health Care. 2002;7:19-24.
64. Lopez-Picado A, Lapuente O, Lete I. Efficacy and side-effects profile of the ethinylestradiol and etonogestrel contraceptive vaginal ring: a systematic review and meta-analysis. Eur J Contracept Reprod Health Care. 2017;22:131-46.
65. Roumen FJ, op ten Berg MM, Hoomans EH. The combined contraceptive vaginal ring (NuvaRing®): first experience in daily clinical practice in The Netherlands. Eur J Contracept Reprod Health Care. 2006;11:14-22.
66. Merki-Feld GS, Hund M. Clinical experience with the combined contraceptive vaginal ring in Switzerland, including a subgroup analysis of previous hormonal contraceptive use. Eur J Contracept Reprod Health Care. 2010;15:413-22.
67. Roumen FJ, Mishell Jr DR. The contraceptive vaginal ring, NuvaRing®, a decade after its introduction. Eur J Contracept Reprod Health Care. 2012;17:415-27.
68. Lete I, Doval JL, Pérez-Campos E, et al. Self-described impact of noncompliance among users of a combined hormonal contraceptive method. Contraception. 2008;77:276-82.
69. TherapeuticsMD. Highlights of prescribing information for ANNOVERA. 2020. (Available at https://www.annovera.com/pi.pdf.)
70. Edelman AB, Carlson NE, Cherala G, et al. Impact of obesity on oral contraceptive pharmacokinetics and hypothalamic-pituitary-ovarian activity. Contraception. 2009;80:119-27.
71. Westhoff CL, Torgal AH, Mayeda ER, Pike MC, Stanczyk FZ. Pharmacokinetics of a combined oral contraceptive in obese and normal-weight women. Contraception. 2010;81:474-80.
72. Lopez LM, Bernholc A, Chen M, et al. Hormonal contraceptives for contraception in overweight or obese women. Cochrane Database Syst Rev. 2016 Aug; 2016(8):CD008452. Available from: https://www.ncbi.nlm.nih.gov/pmc/articles/PMC9063995/.
73. Dinger JC, Cronin M, Mohner S, Schellschmidt I, Minh TD, Westhoff C. Oral contraceptive effectiveness according to body mass index, weight, age, and other factors. Am J Obstet Gynecol. 2009;201:263.e1-9.
74. Yamazaki M, Dwyer K, Sobhan M, et al. Effect of obesity on the effectiveness of hormonal contraceptives: an individual participant data meta-analysis. Contraception. 2015;92:445-52.

75. Centers for Disease Control and Prevention. U.S. medical eligibility criteria for contraceptive use, 2010. MMWR Recomm Rep. 2016;65.
76. American College of Obstetricians and Gynecologists. ACOG practice bulletin no. 105: bariatric surgery and pregnancy. Obstet Gynecol. 2009;113:1405-13.
77. McNicholas C, Zhao Q, Secura G, Allsworth JE, Madden T, Peipert JF. Contraceptive failures in overweight and obese combined hormonal contraceptive users. Obstet Gynecol. 2013;121:585.
78. Dragoman MV, Simmons KB, Paulen ME, Curtis KM. Combined hormonal contraceptive (CHC) use among obese women and contraceptive effectiveness: a systematic review. Contraception. 2017;95:117-29.
79. Sabers A, Buchholt JM, Uldall P, Hansen EL. Lamotrigine plasma levels reduced by oral contraceptives. Epilepsy Res. 2001;47:151-4.
80. Dickinson BD, Altman RD, Nielsen NH, Sterling ML. Drug interactions between oral contraceptives and antibiotics. Obstet Gynecol. 2001;98:853-60.
81. Murphy AA, Zacur HA, Charache P, Burkman RT. The effect of tetracycline on levels of oral contraceptives. Am J Obstet Gynecol. 1991;164:28-33.
82. Neely JL, Abate M, Swinker M, D'Angio R. The effect of doxycycline on serum levels of ethinyl estradiol, norethindrone, and endogenous progesterone. Obstet Gynecol. 1991;77:416-20.
83. Joshi JV, Joshi UM, Sankholi GM, et al. A study of interaction of low-dose combination oral contraceptive with ampicillin and metronidazole. Contraception. 1980;22:643-52.
84. Maggiolo F, Puricelli G, Dottorini M, Caprioli S, Bianchi W, Suter F. The effect of ciprofloxacin on oral contraceptive steroid treatments. Drugs Exp Clin Res. 1991;17:451-4.
85. Friedman CI, Huneke AL, Kim MH, Powell J. The effect of ampicillin on oral contraceptive effectiveness. Obstet Gynecol. 1980;55:33-7.
86. Berry-Bibee EN, Kim MJ, Tepper NK, Riley HE, Curtis KM. Co-administration of St. John's wort and hormonal contraceptives: a systematic review. Contraception. 2016;94:668-77.
87. Berry-Bibee EN, Kim MJ, Simmons KB, et al. Drug interactions between hormonal contraceptives and psychotropic drugs: a systematic review. Contraception. 2016;94:650-67.
88. Mikkelsen EM, Riis AH, Wise LA, Hatch EE, Rothman KJ, Sorensen HT. Pre-gravid oral contraceptive use and time to pregnancy: a Danish prospective cohort study. Hum Reprod. 2013;28:1398-405.
89. Davis A, Godwin A, Lippman J, Olson W, Kafrissen M. Triphasic norgestimate-ethinyl estradiol for treating dysfunctional uterine bleeding. Obstet Gynecol. 2000;96:913-20.
90. Farquhar C, Brown J. Oral contraceptive pill for heavy menstrual bleeding. Cochrane Database Syst Rev. 2009 Oct 7;(4):CD000154.
91. ACOG Practice Bulletin No. 110: noncontraceptive uses of hormonal contraceptives. Obstet Gynecol. 2010;115:206-18.
92. National Collaborating Centre for Women's and Children's Health. Heavy menstrual bleeding: Clinical guideline. London: RCOG Press; 2007. Available from: https://www.nice.org.uk/guidance/ng88/evidence/full-guideline-pdf-4782291810)
93. Davis AR, Westhoff C, O'Connell K, Gallagher N. Oral contraceptives for dysmenorrhea in adolescent girls: a randomized trial. Obstet Gynecol. 2005;106:97-104.
94. Zahradnik HP, Hanjalic-Beck A, Groth K. Nonsteroidal anti-inflammatory drugs and hormonal contraceptives for pain relief from dysmenorrhea: a review. Contraception. 2010;81:185-96.
95. Sangi-Haghpeykar H, Poindexter AN, 3rd. Epidemiology of endometriosis among parous women. Obstet Gynecol. 1995;85:983-92.
96. Westhoff C, Britton JA, Gammon MD, Wright T, Kelsey JL. Oral contraceptive and benign ovarian tumors. Am J Epidemiol. 2000;152:242-6.
97. Seracchioli R, Mabrouk M, Frasca C, et al. Long-term cyclic and continuous oral contraceptive therapy and endometrioma recurrence: a randomized controlled trial. Fertil Steril. 2010;93:52-6.
98. Harada T, Momoeda M, Taketani Y, Hoshiai H, Terakawa N. Low-dose oral contraceptive pill for dysmenorrhea associated with endometriosis: a placebo-controlled, double-blind, randomized trial. Fertil Steril. 2008;90:1583-8.
99. Parazzini F, Ferraroni M, Bocciolone L, Tozzi L, Rubessa S, La Vecchia C. Contraceptive methods and risk of pelvic endometriosis. Contraception. 1994;49:47-55.

100. Nisolle-Pochet M, Casanas-Roux F, Donnez J. Histologic study of ovarian endometriosis after hormonal therapy. Fertil Steril. 1988;49:423-6.
101. Edlow AG, Bartz D. Hormonal contraceptive options for women with headache: a review of the evidence. Rev Obstet Gynecol. 2010;3:55-65.
102. Martin VT. Menstrual migraine: a review of prophylactic therapies. Curr Pain Headache Rep. 2004;8:229-37.
103. Harris M, Kaneshiro B. An evidence-based approach to hormonal contraception and headaches. Contraception. 2009;80:417-21.
104. Combination oral contraceptive use and the risk of endometrial cancer. The Cancer and Steroid Hormone Study of the Centers for Disease Control and the National Institute of Child Health and Human Development. JAMA. 1987;257:796-800.
105. Schlesselman JJ. Risk of endometrial cancer in relation to use of combined oral contraceptives. A practitioner's guide to meta-analysis. Hum Reprod. 1997;12:1851-63.
106. Sangthawan M, Taneepanichskul S. A comparative study of monophasic oral contraceptives containing either drospirenone 3 mg or levonorgestrel 150 microg on premenstrual symptoms. Contraception. 2005;71:1-7.
107. Coffee AL, Kuehl TJ, Willis S, Sulak PJ. Oral contraceptives and premenstrual symptoms: comparison of a 21/7 and extended regimen. Am J Obstet Gynecol. 2006;195:1311-9.
108. Halbreich U, Borenstein J, Pearlstein T, Kahn LS. The prevalence, impairment, impact, and burden of premenstrual dysphoric disorder (PMS/PMDD). Psychoneuroendocrinology. 2003;28 Suppl 3:1-23.
109. Lopez LM, Kaptein AA, Helmerhorst FM. Oral contraceptives containing drospirenone for premenstrual syndrome. Cochrane Database Syst Rev. 2012 Feb 15;(2):CD006586.
110. Freeman EW, Halbreich U, Grubb GS, et al. An overview of four studies of a continuous oral contraceptive (levonorgestrel 90 mcg/ethinyl estradiol 20 mcg) on premenstrual dysphoric disorder and premenstrual syndrome. Contraception. 2012;85:437-45.
111. Lanes SF, Birmann B, Walker AM, Singer S. Oral contraceptive type and functional ovarian cysts. Am J Obstet Gynecol. 1992;166:956-61.
112. Vessey M, Metcalfe A, Wells C, McPherson K, Westhoff C, Yeates D. Ovarian neoplasms, functional ovarian cysts, and oral contraceptives. Br Med J (Clin Res Ed). 1987;294: 1518-20.
113. Christensen JT, Boldsen JL, Westergaard JG. Functional ovarian cysts in premenopausal and gynecologically healthy women. Contraception. 2002;66:153-7.
114. Holt VL, Cushing-Haugen KL, Daling JR. Oral contraceptives, tubal sterilization, and functional ovarian cyst risk. Obstet Gynecol. 2003;102:252-8.
115. Young RL, Snabes MC, Frank ML, Reilly M. A randomized, double-blind, placebo-controlled comparison of the impact of low-dose and triphasic oral contraceptives on follicular development. Am J Obstet Gynecol. 1992;167:678-82.
116. Chiaffarino F, Parazzini F, La Vecchia C, Ricci E, Crosignani PG. Oral contraceptive use and benign gynecologic conditions. A review. Contraception. 1998;57:11-8.
117. Grimes DA, Godwin AJ, Rubin A, Smith JA, Lacarra M. Ovulation and follicular development associated with three low-dose oral contraceptives: a randomized controlled trial. Obstet Gynecol. 1994;83:29-34.
118. MacKenna A, Fabres C, Alam V, Morales V. Clinical management of functional ovarian cysts: a prospective and randomized study. Hum Reprod. 2000;15:2567-9.
119. Collaborative Group on Epidemiological Studies of Ovarian Cancer, Beral V, Doll R, Hermon C, Peto R, Reeves G. Ovarian cancer and oral contraceptives: collaborative reanalysis of data from 45 epidemiological studies including 23,257 women with ovarian cancer and 87,303 controls. Lancet. 2008;371:303-14.
120. Ness RB, Grisso JA, Klapper J, et al. Risk of ovarian cancer in relation to estrogen and progestin dose and use characteristics of oral contraceptives. SHARE Study Group. Steroid Hormones and Reproductions. Am J Epidemiol. 2000;152:233-41.
121. Jensen JT, Speroff L. Health benefits of oral contraceptives. Obstet Gynecol Clin North Am. 2000;27:705-21.
122. Brinton LA, Vessey MP, Flavel R, Yeates D. Risk factors for benign breast disease. Am J Epidemiol. 1981;113:203-14.

123. Rohan TE, Miller AB. A cohort study of oral contraceptive use and risk of benign breast disease. Int J Cancer. 1999;82:191-6.
124. Charreau I, Plu-Bureau G, Bachelot A, Contesso G, Guinebretiere JM, Le MG. Oral contraceptive use and risk of benign breast disease in a French case-control study of young women. Eur J Cancer Prev. 1993;2:147-54.
125. Palatsi R, Hirvensalo E, Liukko P, et al. Serum total and unbound testosterone and sex hormone binding globulin (SHBG) in female acne patients treated with two different oral contraceptives. Acta Derm Venereol. 1984;64:517-23.
126. Wishart JM. An open study of Triphasil and Diane 50 in the treatment of acne. Australas J Dermatol. 1991;32:51-4.
127. Arowojolu AO, Gallo MF, Lopez LM, Grimes DA. Combined oral contraceptive pills for treatment of acne. Cochrane Database Syst Rev. 2012 Jul 11;(7):CD004425.
128. Sullivan H, Furniss H, Spona J, Elstein M. Effect of 21-day and 24-day oral contraceptive regimens containing gestodene (60 microg) and ethinyl estradiol (15 microg) on ovarian activity. Fertil Steril. 1999;72:115-20.
129. Redmond GP, Olson WH, Lippman JS, Kafrissen ME, Jones TM, Jorizzo JL. Norgestimate and ethinyl estradiol in the treatment of acne vulgaris: a randomized, placebo-controlled trial. Obstet Gynecol. 1997;89:615-22.
130. Lucky AW, Henderson TA, Olson WH, Robisch DM, Lebwohl M, Swinyer LJ. Effectiveness of norgestimate and ethinyl estradiol in treating moderate acne vulgaris. J Am Acad Dermatol. 1997;37:746-54.
131. Panzer C, Wise S, Fantini G, et al. Impact of oral contraceptives on sex hormone-binding globulin and androgen levels: a retrospective study in women with sexual dysfunction. J Sex Med. 2006;3:104-13.
132. Dewis P, Petsos P, Newman M, Anderson DC. The treatment of hirsutism with a combination of desogestrel and ethinyl oestradiol. Clin Endocrinol (Oxf). 1985;22:29-36.
133. Lobo RA. The androgenicity of progestational agents. Int J Fertil. 1988;33 Suppl:6-12.
134. De Leo V, Di Sabatino A, Musacchio MC, et al. Effect of oral contraceptives on markers of hyperandrogenism and SHBG in women with polycystic ovary syndrome. Contraception. 2010;82:276-80.
135. Kriplani A, Periyasamy AJ, Agarwal N, Kulshrestha V, Kumar A, Ammini AC. Effect of oral contraceptive containing ethinyl estradiol combined with drospirenone vs. desogestrel on clinical and biochemical parameters in patients with polycystic ovary syndrome. Contraception. 2010;82:139-46.
136. Shargil AA. Hormone replacement therapy in perimenopausal women with a triphasic contraceptive compound: a three-year prospective study. Int J Fertil. 1985;30(1):15, 18-28.
137. Hergenroeder AC, Smith EO, Shypailo R, Jones LA, Klish WJ, Ellis K. Bone mineral changes in young women with hypothalamic amenorrhea treated with oral contraceptives, medroxyprogesterone, or placebo over 12 months. Am J Obstet Gynecol. 1997;176:1017-25.
138. Grinspoon S, Thomas L, Miller K, Herzog D, Klibanski A. Effects of recombinant human IGF-I and oral contraceptive administration on bone density in anorexia nervosa. J Clin Endocrinol Metab. 2002;87:2883-91.
139. Nappi C, Bifulco G, Tommaselli GA, Gargano V, Di Carlo C. Hormonal contraception and bone metabolism: a systematic review. Contraception. 2012;86:606-21.
140. Lopez LM, Chen M, Mullins S, Curtis KM, Helmerhorst FM. Steroidal contraceptives and bone fractures in women: evidence from observational studies. Cochrane Database Syst Rev. 2015 Jul 21;2015(7):CD009849. Available from: https://www.ncbi.nlm.nih.gov/pmc/articles/PMC8917344/.
141. Archer DF, Bigrigg A, Smallwood GH, Shangold GA, Creasy GW, Fisher AC. Assessment of compliance with a weekly contraceptive patch (Ortho Evra™/Evra™) among North American women. Fertil Steril. 2002;77:27-31.
142. Rubinstein ML, Halpern-Felsher BL, Irwin Jr CE. An evaluation of the use of the transdermal contraceptive patch in adolescents. J Adolesc Health 2004;34:395-401.
143. Bodner K, Bodner-Adler B, Grünberger W. Evaluation of the contraceptive efficacy, compliance, and satisfaction with the transdermal contraceptive patch system Evra: a comparison between adolescent and adult users. Arch Gynecol Obstet. 2011;283:525-30.

144. Abrams LS, Skee D, Natarajan J, Wong FA. Pharmacokinetic overview of Ortho Evra™/Evra™. Fertil Steril. 2002;77:3-12.
145. Zacur HA, Hedon B, Mansour D, Shangold GA, Fisher AC, Creasy GW. Integrated summary of Ortho Evra™/Evra™ contraceptive patch adhesion in varied climates and conditions. Fertil Steril. 2002;77:32-5.
146. Ocheltree T, Wittes J, Case J, et al. Adhesion evaluation of AG200-15: An investigational transdermal contraceptive delivery system. Adv Ther. 2019;36:3381-9.
147. Pierson RA, Archer DF, Moreau M, et al. Ortho Evra™/Evra™ versus oral contraceptives: follicular development and ovulation in normal cycles and after an intentional dosing error. Fertil Steril. 2003;80:34-42.
148. Sibai BM, Odlind V, Meador ML, Shangold GA, Fisher AC, Creasy GW. A comparative and pooled analysis of the safety and tolerability of the contraceptive patch (Ortho Evra™/Evra™). Fertil Steril. 2002;77:19-26.
149. Creasy GW, Fisher AC, Hall N, Shangold GA. Transdermal contraceptive patch delivering norelgestromin and ethinyl estradiol. Effects on the lipid profile. J Reprod Med. 2003; 48:179-86.
150. Graziottin A. A review of transdermal hormonal contraception: focus on the ethinylestradiol/norelgestromin contraceptive patch. Treat Endocrinol. 2006;5:359-65.
151. Kiriwat O, Petyim S. The effects of transdermal contraception on lipid profiles, carbohydrate metabolism and coagulogram in Thai women. Gynecol Endocrinol. 2010;26:361-5.
152. Massaro M, Di Carlo C, Gargano V, Formisano C, Bifulco G, Nappi C. Effects of the contraceptive patch and the vaginal ring on bone metabolism and bone mineral density: a prospective, controlled, randomized study. Contraception. 2010;81:209-14.
153. Grimes DA, Schulz KF. Surrogate end points in clinical research: hazardous to your health. Obstet Gynecol. 2005;105:1114-8.
154. Barnhart KT, Timbers K, Pretorius ES, Lin K, Shaunik A. In vivo assessment of NuvaRing® placement. Contraception. 2005;72:196-9.
155. Killick S. Complete and robust ovulation inhibition with NuvaRing. Eur J Contracept Reprod Health Care. 2002;7:13-8.
156. Timmer CJ, Mulders TM. Pharmacokinetics of etonogestrel and ethinylestradiol released from a combined contraceptive vaginal ring. Clin Pharmacokinet. 2000;39:233-42.
157. Mulders TM, Dieben TO, Bennink HJC. Ovarian function with a novel combined contraceptive vaginal ring. Hum Reprod. 2002;17:2594-9.
158. Mansour D, Gemzell-Danielsson K, Inki P, Jensen JT. Fertility after discontinuation of contraception: a comprehensive review of the literature. Contraception. 2011;84:465-77.
159. Roumen FJ, Boon ME, van Velzen D, Dieben TO, Coelingh Bennink HJ. The cervico-vaginal epithelium during 20 cycles' use of a combined contraceptive vaginal ring. Hum Reprod. 1996;11:2443-8.
160. Bulten J, Grefte J, Siebers B, Dieben T. The combined contraceptive vaginal ring (NuvaRing) and endometrial histology. Contraception. 2005;72:362-5.
161. Verhoeven CH, Dieben TO. The combined contraceptive vaginal ring, NuvaRing®, and tampon co-usage. Contraception. 2004;69:197-9.
162. Organon & Co. NuvaRing® prescribing information. 2023. Available from: https://www.organon.com/product/usa/pi_circulars/n/nuvaring/nuvaring_pi.pdf.
163. Bjarnadóttir RI, Tuppurainen M, Killick SR. Comparison of cycle control with a combined contraceptive vaginal ring and oral levonorgestrel/ethinyl estradiol. Am J Obstet Gynecol. 2002;186:389-95.
164. Oddsson K, Leifels-Fischer B, Wiel-Masson D, et al. Superior cycle control with a contraceptive vaginal ring compared with an oral contraceptive containing 30 microg ethinylestradiol and 150 microg levonorgestrel: a randomized trial. Hum Reprod. 2005;20:557-62.
165. Milsom I, Lete I, Bjertnaes A, et al. Effects on cycle control and bodyweight of the combined contraceptive ring, NuvaRing, versus an oral contraceptive containing 30 microg ethinyl estradiol and 3 mg drospirenone. Hum Reprod. 2006;21:2304-11.
166. Weisberg E, Merki-Feld GS, McGeechan K, Fraser IS. Randomized comparison of bleeding patterns in women using a combined contraceptive vaginal ring or a low-dose combined oral contraceptive on a menstrually signaled regimen. Contraception. 2015;91:121-6.

167. O'Connell KJ, Osborne LM, Westhoff C. Measured and reported weight change for women using a vaginal contraceptive ring vs. a low-dose oral contraceptive. Contraception. 2005;72:323-7.
168. Gallo MF, Lopez LM, Grimes DA, Carayon F, Schulz KF, Helmerhorst FM. Combination contraceptives: effects on weight. Cochrane Database Syst Rev. 2014 Jan 29;(1):CD003987.
169. Tuppurainen M, Klimscheffskij R, Venhola M, Dieben TO. The combined contraceptive vaginal ring (NuvaRing) and lipid metabolism: a comparative study. Contraception. 2004;69:389-94.
170. Barreiros FA, Guazzelli CAF, Barbosa R, Torloni MR, Barbieri M, Araujo FF. Extended regimens of the combined contraceptive vaginal ring containing etonogestrel and ethinyl estradiol: effects on lipid metabolism. Contraception. 2011;84:155-9.
171. Grigoryan OR, Grodnitskaya EE, Andreeva EN, Chebotnikova TV, Melnichenko GA. Use of the NuvaRing hormone-releasing system in late reproductive-age women with type 1 diabetes mellitus. Gynecol Endocrinol. 2008;24:99-104.
172. Massai R, Mäkäräinen L, Kuukankorpi A, Klipping C, Duijkers I, Dieben T. The combined contraceptive vaginal ring and bone mineral density in healthy pre-menopausal women. Hum Reprod. 2005;20:2764-8.
173. Sonfield A, Gold RB, Frost JJ, Darroch JE. U.S. insurance coverage of contraceptives and the impact of contraceptive coverage mandates, 2002. Perspect Sex Reprod Health. 2004;36:72-9.
174. Bedsider.org. Birth control ring. 2021. Available from: https://www.bedsider.org/birth-control/the_ring#costs_tab.
175. Shapiro S, Dinger J. Risk of venous thromboembolism among users of oral contraceptives: a review of two recently published studies. J Fam Plann Reprod Health Care. 2010;36:33-8.
176. Cardiovascular disease and steroid hormone contraception. Report of a WHO Scientific Group. World Health Organ Tech Rep Ser. 1998;877:i-vii, 1-89.
177. Effect of different progestagens in low oestrogen oral contraceptives on venous thromboembolic disease. World Health Organization Collaborative Study of Cardiovascular Disease and Steroid Hormone Contraception. Lancet. 1995;346:1582-8.
178. Jick SS, Kaye JA, Russmann S, Jick H. Risk of nonfatal venous thromboembolism with oral contraceptives containing norgestimate or desogestrel compared with oral contraceptives containing levonorgestrel. Contraception. 2006;73:566-70.
179. Romero A, Alonso C, Rincon M, et al. Risk of venous thromboembolic disease in women A qualitative systematic review. Eur J Obstet Gynecol Reprod Biol. 2005;121:8-17.
180. Spitzer WO, Lewis MA, Heinemann LA, Thorogood M, MacRae KD. Third generation oral contraceptives and risk of venous thromboembolic disorders: an international case-control study. Transnational Research Group on Oral Contraceptives and the Health of Young Women. BMJ. 1996;312:83-8.
181. van Hylckama Vlieg A, Helmerhorst FM, Vandenbroucke JP, Doggen CJ, Rosendaal FR. The venous thrombotic risk of oral contraceptives, effects of oestrogen dose and progestogen type: results of the MEGA case-control study. BMJ. 2009;339:b2921.
182. Lidegaard O, Lokkegaard E, Svendsen AL, Agger C. Hormonal contraception and risk of venous thromboembolism: national follow-up study. BMJ. 2009;339:b2890.
183. Seeger JD, Loughlin J, Eng PM, Clifford CR, Cutone J, Walker AM. Risk of thromboembolism in women taking ethinylestradiol/drospirenone and other oral contraceptives. Obstet Gynecol. 2007;110:587-93.
184. Dinger JC, Heinemann LA, Kuhl-Habich D. The safety of a drospirenone-containing oral contraceptive: final results from the European Active Surveillance Study on oral contraceptives based on 142,475 women-years of observation. Contraception. 2007;75:344-54.
185. Heinemann LA, Dinger JC. Range of published estimates of venous thromboembolism incidence in young women. Contraception. 2007;75:328-36.
186. Manzoli L, De Vito C, Marzuillo C, Boccia A, Villari P. Oral contraceptives and venous thromboembolism: a systematic review and meta-analysis. Drug Saf. 2012;35:191-205.
187. Heit JA, Kobbervig CE, James AH, Petterson TM, Bailey KR, Melton LJ, 3rd. Trends in the incidence of venous thromboembolism during pregnancy or postpartum: a 30-year population-based study. Ann Intern Med. 2005;143:697-706.
188. Naess IA, Christiansen SC, Romundstad P, Cannegieter SC, Rosendaal FR, Hammerstrom J. Incidence and mortality of venous thrombosis: a population-based study. J Thromb Haemost. 2007;5:692-9.

189. American College of Obstetricians and Gynecologists. ACOG practice bulletin No. 73: Use of hormonal contraception in women with coexisting medical conditions. Obstet Gynecol. 2006;107:1453-72.
190. Pomp ER, Rosendaal FR, Doggen CJ. Smoking increases the risk of venous thrombosis and acts synergistically with oral contraceptive use. Am J Hematol. 2008;83:97-102.
191. Sidney S, Cheetham TC, Connell FA, et al. Recent combined hormonal contraceptives (CHCs) and the risk of thromboembolism and other cardiovascular events in new users. Contraception. 2013;87:93-100.
192. van den Heuvel MW, van Bragt AJ, Alnabawy AK, Kaptein MC. Comparison of ethinylestradiol pharmacokinetics in three hormonal contraceptive formulations: the vaginal ring, the transdermal patch and an oral contraceptive. Contraception. 2005;72:168-74.
193. Jick S, Kaye JA, Li L, Jick H. Further results on the risk of nonfatal venous thromboembolism in users of the contraceptive transdermal patch compared to users of oral contraceptives containing norgestimate and 35 microg of ethinyl estradiol. Contraception. 2007;76:4-7.
194. Jick SS, Hagberg KW, Kaye JA. ORTHO EVRA and venous thromboembolism: an update. Contraception. 2010;81:452-3.
195. Cole JA, Norman H, Doherty M, Walker AM. Venous thromboembolism, myocardial infarction, and stroke among transdermal contraceptive system users. Obstet Gynecol. 2007; 109:339-46.
196. Dore DD, Norman H, Loughlin J, Seeger JD. Extended case-control study results on thromboembolic outcomes among transdermal contraceptive users. Contraception. 2010;81:408-13.
197. Jick SS, Hagberg KW, Hernandez RK, Kaye JA. Postmarketing study of ORTHO EVRA and levonorgestrel oral contraceptives containing hormonal contraceptives with 30 mcg of ethinyl estradiol in relation to nonfatal venous thromboembolism. Contraception. 2010;81:16-21.
198. Lidegaard Ø, Nielsen LH, Skovlund CW, Løkkegaard E. Venous thrombosis in users of nonoral hormonal contraception: follow-up study, Denmark 2001-10. BMJ. 2012;344:e2990.
199. Tepper NK, Dragoman MV, Gaffield ME, Curtis KM. Nonoral combined hormonal contraceptives and thromboembolism: a systematic review. Contraception. 2017;95:130-9.
200. Curtis KM, Tepper NK, Jatlaoui TC, et al. U.S. medical eligibility criteria for contraceptive use, 2016. MMWR Recomm Rep. 2016;65:1-103.
201. Petitti DB. Clinical practice. Combination estrogen-progestin oral contraceptives. N Engl J Med. 2003;349:1443-50.
202. Khader YS, Rice J, John L, Abueita O. Oral contraceptives use and the risk of myocardial infarction: a meta-analysis. Contraception. 2003;68:11-7.
203. Shufelt CL, Bairey Merz CN. Contraceptive hormone use and cardiovascular disease. J Am Coll Cardiol. 2009;53:221-31.
204. Margolis KL, Adami HO, Luo J, Ye W, Weiderpass E. A prospective study of oral contraceptive use and risk of myocardial infarction among Swedish women. Fertil Steril. 2007;88:310-6.
205. Acute myocardial infarction and combined oral contraceptives: results of an international multicentre case-control study. WHO Collaborative Study of Cardiovascular Disease and Steroid Hormone Contraception. Lancet. 1997;349:1202-9.
206. Schwingl PJ, Ory HW, Visness CM. Estimates of the risk of cardiovascular death attributable to low-dose oral contraceptives in the United States. Am J Obstet Gynecol. 1999;180:241-9.
207. Farley TM, Collins J, Schlesselman JJ. Hormonal contraception and risk of cardiovascular disease. An international perspective. Contraception. 1998;57:211-30.
208. Gillum LA, Mamidipudi SK, Johnston SC. Ischemic stroke risk with oral contraceptives: A meta-analysis. JAMA 2000;284:72-8.
209. Xu Z, Li Y, Tang S, Huang X, Chen T. Current use of oral contraceptives and the risk of first-ever ischemic stroke: A meta-analysis of observational studies. Thromb Res. 2015;136:52-60.
210. Tepper NK, Whiteman MK, Zapata LB, Marchbanks PA, Curtis KM. Safety of hormonal contraceptives among women with migraine: A systematic review. Contraception. 2016; 94:630-40.
211. Hannaford PC, Croft PR, Kay CR. Oral contraception and stroke. Evidence from the Royal College of General Practitioners' Oral Contraception Study. Stroke. 1994;25:935-42.
212. Curtis KM, Chrisman CE, Peterson HB, WHO Programme for Mapping Best Practices in Reproductive Health. Contraception for women in selected circumstances. Obstet Gynecol. 2002;99:1100-12.

213. Kemmeren JM, Tanis BC, van den Bosch MA, et al. Risk of Arterial Thrombosis in Relation to Oral Contraceptives (RATIO) study: oral contraceptives and the risk of ischemic stroke. Stroke. 2002;33:1202-8.
214. Feigin VL, Rinkel GJ, Lawes CM, et al. Risk factors for subarachnoid hemorrhage: an updated systematic review of epidemiological studies. Stroke. 2005;36:2773-80.
215. Curtis KM, Mohllajee AP, Martins SL, Peterson HB. Combined oral contraceptive use among women with hypertension: a systematic review. Contraception. 2006;73:179-88.
216. Haemorrhagic stroke, overall stroke risk, and combined oral contraceptives: results of an international, multicentre, case-control study. WHO Collaborative Study of Cardiovascular Disease and Steroid Hormone Contraception. Lancet. 1996;348:505-10.
217. Berenson AB, Rahman M, Wilkinson G. Effect of injectable and oral contraceptives on serum lipids. Obstet Gynecol. 2009;114:786-94.
218. Walsh BW, Sacks FM. Effects of low dose oral contraceptives on very low density and low density lipoprotein metabolism. J Clin Invest. 1993;91:2126-32.
219. Tepper NK, Steenland MW, Marchbanks PA, Curtis KM. Laboratory screening prior to initiating contraception: a systematic review. Contraception. 2013;87:645-9.
220. Green J, Berrington de Gonzalez A, Smith JS, et al. Human papillomavirus infection and use of oral contraceptives. Br J Cancer. 2003;88:1713-20.
221. Smith JS, Green J, Berrington de Gonzalez A, et al. Cervical cancer and use of hormonal contraceptives: a systematic review. Lancet. 2003;361:1159-67.
222. Munoz N, Franceschi S, Bosetti C, et al. Role of parity and human papillomavirus in cervical cancer: the IARC multicentric case-control study. Lancet. 2002;359:1093-101.
223. Ursin G, Peters RK, Henderson BE, d'Ablaing G, 3rd, Monroe KR, Pike MC. Oral contraceptive use and adenocarcinoma of cervix. Lancet. 1994;344:1390-4.
224. Marchbanks PA, McDonald JA, Wilson HG, et al. Oral contraceptives and the risk of breast cancer. N Engl J Med. 2002;346:2025-32.
225. Marchbanks PA, Curtis KM, Mandel MG, et al. Oral contraceptive formulation and risk of breast cancer. Contraception. 2012;85:342-50.
226. Morch LS, Skovlund CW, Hannaford PC, Iversen L, Fielding S, Lidegaard O. Contemporary Hormonal Contraception and the Risk of Breast Cancer. N Engl J Med. 2017;377:2228-39.
227. Grimes DA, Schulz KF. False alarms and pseudo-epidemics: the limitations of observational epidemiology. Obstet Gynecol. 2012;120:920-7.
228. Figueiredo JC, Haile RW, Bernstein L, et al. Oral contraceptives and postmenopausal hormones and risk of contralateral breast cancer among BRCA1 and BRCA2 mutation carriers and noncarriers: the WECARE Study. Breast Cancer Res Treat. 2010;120:175-83.
229. Gaffield ME, Culwell KR, Ravi A. Oral contraceptives and family history of breast cancer. Contraception. 2009;80:372-80.
230. Mullen WH, Anderson IB, Kim SY, Blanc PD, Olson KR. Incorrect overdose management advice in the Physicians' Desk Reference. Ann Emerg Med 1997;29:255-61.
231. Lubianca JN, Faccin CS, Fuchs FD. Oral contraceptives: a risk factor for uncontrolled blood pressure among hypertensive women. Contraception. 2003;67:19-24.
232. Chasan-Taber L, Willett WC, Manson JE, et al. Prospective study of oral contraceptives and hypertension among women in the United States. Circulation. 1996;94:483-9.
233. Darney P. Safety and efficacy of a triphasic oral contraceptive containing desogestrel: results of three multicenter trials. Contraception. 1993;48:323-37.
234. Visser J, Snel M, Van Vliet HA. Hormonal versus non-hormonal contraceptives in women with diabetes mellitus type 1 and 2. Cochrane Database Syst Rev. 2013 Mar 28;2013(3):CD003990. Available from: https://www.ncbi.nlm.nih.gov/pmc/articles/PMC6485821/.
235. Nelson AL, Le MH, Musherraf Z, Vanberckelaer A. Intermediate-term glucose tolerance in women with a history of gestational diabetes: natural history and potential associations with breastfeeding and contraception. Am J Obstet Gynecol. 2008;198:699.e1-7; discussion e7-8.
236. Vandenbroucke JP, Koster T, Briet E, Reitsma PH, Bertina RM, Rosendaal FR. Increased risk of venous thrombosis in oral-contraceptive users who are carriers of factor V Leiden mutation. Lancet. 1994;344:1453-7.
237. Vandenbroucke JP, van der Meer FJ, Helmerhorst FM, Rosendaal FR. Factor V Leiden: should we screen oral contraceptive users and pregnant women? BMJ. 1996;313:1127-30.

238. Headache Classification Subcommittee of the International Headache Society. The International Classification of Headache Disorders: 2nd edition. Cephalalgia. 2004;24 Suppl 1:9-160.
239. Curtis KM, Mohllajee AP, Peterson HB. Use of combined oral contraceptives among women with migraine and nonmigrainous headaches: a systematic review. Contraception. 2006;73:189-94.
240. Chasan-Taber L, Stampfer M. Oral contraceptives and myocardial infarction--the search for the smoking gun. N Engl J Med. 2001;345:1841-2.
241. Willett WC, Green A, Stampfer MJ, et al. Relative and absolute excess risks of coronary heart disease among women who smoke cigarettes. N Engl J Med 1987;317:1303-9.
242. Kroon LA. Drug interactions with smoking. Am J Health Syst Pharm. 2007;64:1917-21.
243. Murray CJ, Ortblad KF, Guinovart C, et al. Global, regional, and national incidence and mortality for HIV, tuberculosis, and malaria during 1990-2013: a systematic analysis for the Global Burden of Disease Study 2013. Lancet. 2014;384:1005-70.
244. Phillips SJ, Polis CB, Curtis KM. The safety of hormonal contraceptives for women living with HIV and their sexual partners. Contraception. 2016;93:11-6.
245. Polis CB, Curtis KM, Hannaford PC, et al. An updated systematic review of epidemiological evidence on hormonal contraceptive methods and HIV acquisition in women. AIDS. 2016;30:2665-83.
246. Centers for Disease Control and Prevention. HIV Treatment as Prevention. 2022. Available from: https://www.cdc.gov/hiv/risk/art/index.html.
247. Culwell KR, Curtis KM, del Carmen Cravioto M. Safety of contraceptive method use among women with systemic lupus erythematosus: a systematic review. Obstet Gynecol. 2009;114:341-53.
248. Farr SL, Folger SG, Paulen ME, Curtis KM. Safety of contraceptive methods for women with rheumatoid arthritis: a systematic review. Contraception. 2010;82:64-71.
249. Kapp N, Tilley IB, Curtis KM. The effects of hormonal contraceptive use among women with viral hepatitis or cirrhosis of the liver: a systematic review. Contraception. 2009;80:381-6.
250. Combined oral contraceptives and liver cancer. The WHO Collaborative Study of Neoplasia and Steroid Contraceptives. Int J Cancer. 1989;43:254-9.
251. Kapp N, Curtis KM. Hormonal contraceptive use among women with liver tumors: a systematic review. Contraception. 2009;80:387-90.
252. Milne R, Vessey M. The association of oral contraception with kidney cancer, colon cancer, gallbladder cancer (including extrahepatic bile duct cancer) and pituitary tumours. Contraception. 1991;43:667-93.
253. Westhoff CL, Heartwell S, Edwards S, et al. Oral contraceptive discontinuation: do side effects matter? Am J Obstet Gynecol. 2007;196:412.e1-6; discussion e6-7.
254. Rosenthal SL, Cotton S, Ready JN, Potter LS, Succop PA. Adolescents' attitudes and experiences regarding levonorgestrel 100 mcg/ethinyl estradiol 20 mcg. J Pediatr Adolesc Gynecol. 2002;15:301-5.
255. Archer DF, Cullins V, Creasy GW, Fisher AC. The impact of improved compliance with a weekly contraceptive transdermal system (Ortho Evra) on contraceptive efficacy. Contraception. 2004;69:189-95.
256. Lopez LM, Grimes DA, Schulz KF, Curtis KM. Steroidal contraceptives: effect on bone fractures in women. Cochrane Database Syst Rev. 2009 Apr 15;(2):CD006033.
257. d'Arcangues C. WHO statement on hormonal contraception and bone health. Contraception. 2006;73:443-4.
258. Lopez LM, Grey TW, Stuebe AM, Chen M, Truitt ST, Gallo MF. Combined hormonal versus nonhormonal versus progestin-only contraception in lactation. Cochrane Database Syst Rev. 2015:CD003988.
259. Cheung E, Free C. Factors influencing young women's decision making regarding hormonal contraceptives: a qualitative study. Contraception. 2005;71:426-31.
260. Curtis KM, Jatlaoui TC, Tepper NK, et al. U.S. Selected Practice Recommendations for Contraceptive Use, 2016. MMWR Recomm Rep. 2016;65:1-66.
261. Stewart FH, Harper CC, Ellertson CE, Grimes DA, Sawaya GF, Trussell J. Clinical breast and pelvic examination requirements for hormonal contraception: Current practice vs evidence. JAMA. 2001;285:2232-9.

262. Comp PC. Should coagulation tests be used to determine which oral contraceptive users have an increased risk of thrombophlebitis? Contraception. 2006;73:4-5.
263. Brahmi D, Curtis KM. When can a woman start combined hormonal contraceptives (CHCs)? A systematic review. Contraception. 2013;87:524-38.
264. Oakley D, Sereika S, Bogue EL. Oral contraceptive pill use after an initial visit to a family planning clinic. Fam Plann Perspect. 1991;23:150-4.
265. Westhoff C, Heartwell S, Edwards S, et al. Initiation of oral contraceptives using a quick start compared with a conventional start: a randomized controlled trial. Obstet Gynecol. 2007;109:1270-6.
266. Brent RL. Nongenital malformations following exposure to progestational drugs: the last chapter of an erroneous allegation. Birth Defects Res A Clin Mol Teratol. 2005;73:906-18.
267. Gallo MF, Nanda K, Grimes DA, Lopez LM, Schulz KF. 20 microg versus >20 microg estrogen combined oral contraceptives for contraception. Cochrane Database Syst Rev. 2008 Oct 8;(4):CD003989.
268. Steenland MW, Rodriguez MI, Marchbanks PA, Curtis KM. How does the number of oral contraceptive pill packs dispensed or prescribed affect continuation and other measures of consistent and correct use? A systematic review. Contraception. 2013;87:605-10.
269. Osterberg L, Blaschke T. Adherence to medication. N Engl J Med. 2005;353:487-97.
270. Gallo MF, Nanda K, Grimes DA, Lopez LM, Schulz KF. 20 microg versus >20 microg estrogen combined oral contraceptives for contraception. Cochrane Database Syst Rev. 2013 Aug 1;2013(8):CD003989. Available from: https://www.ncbi.nlm.nih.gov/pmc/articles/PMC7173696/.
271. Hiller W, Rief W, Brahler E. Somatization in the population: from mild bodily misperceptions to disabling symptoms. Soc Psychiatry Psychiatr Epidemiol. 2006;41:704-12.
272. Klosterhalfen S, Kellermann S, Braun S, et al. Gender and the nocebo response following conditioning and expectancy. Journal of psychosomatic research 2009;66:323-8.
273. Westhoff C, Morroni C, Kerns J, Murphy PA. Bleeding patterns after immediate vs. conventional oral contraceptive initiation: a randomized, controlled trial. Fertil Steril. 2003;79:322-9.
274. Ahrendt HJ, Makalova D, Parke S, Mellinger U, Mansour D. Bleeding pattern and cycle control with an estradiol-based oral contraceptive: a seven-cycle, randomized comparative trial of estradiol valerate/dienogest and ethinyl estradiol/levonorgestrel. Contraception. 2009;80:436-44.
275. Coney P, Washenik K, Langley RG, DiGiovanna JJ, Harrison DD. Weight change and adverse event incidence with a low-dose oral contraceptive: two randomized, placebo-controlled trials. Contraception. 2001;63:297-302.
276. Goldzieher JW, Moses LE, Averkin E, Scheel C, Taber BZ. A placebo-controlled double-blind crossover investigation of the side effects attributed to oral contraceptives. Fertil Steril. 1971;22:609-23.
277. Rosenberg M. Weight change with oral contraceptive use and during the menstrual cycle. Results of daily measurements. Contraception. 1998;58:345-9.
278. Lloyd T, Lin HM, Matthews AE, Bentley CM, Legro RS. Oral contraceptive use by teenage women does not affect body composition. Obstet Gynecol. 2002;100:235-9.
279. Flegal KM, Kruszon-Moran D, Carroll MD, Fryar CD, Ogden CL. Trends in Obesity Among Adults in the United States, 2005 to 2014. JAMA. 2016;315:2284-91.
280. Panotopoulos G, Raison J, Ruiz JC, Guy-Grand B, Basdevant A. Weight gain at the time of menopause. Hum Reprod. 1997;12 Suppl 1:126-33.
281. Abraham S, Boyd C, Lal M, Luscombe G, Taylor A. Time since menarche, weight gain and body image awareness among adolescent girls: onset of eating disorders? J Psychosom Obstet Gynaecol. 2009;30:89-94.
282. Phelan S. Pregnancy: a "teachable moment" for weight control and obesity prevention. Am J Obstet Gynecol. 2010;202:135.e1-8.
283. Scher AI, Stewart WF, Liberman J, Lipton RB. Prevalence of frequent headache in a population sample. Headache. 1998;38:497-506.
284. Loder EW, Buse DC, Golub JR. Headache as a side effect of combination estrogen-progestin oral contraceptives: a systematic review. Am J Obstet Gynecol. 2005;193:636-49.

285. Schaffir J, Worly BL, Gur TL. Combined hormonal contraception and its effects on mood: a critical review. Eur J Contracept Reprod Health Care. 2016;21:347-55.
286. Keyes KM, Cheslack-Postava K, Westhoff C, et al. Association of hormonal contraceptive use with reduced levels of depressive symptoms: a national study of sexually active women in the United States. Am J Epidemiol. 2013;178:1378-88.
287. Skovlund CW, Morch LS, Kessing LV, Lidegaard O. Association of hormonal contraception with depression. JAMA Psychiatry. 2016;73:1154-62.
288. Pagano HP, Zapata LB, Berry-Bibee EN, Nanda K, Curtis KM. Safety of hormonal contraception and intrauterine devices among women with depressive and bipolar disorders: a systematic review. Contraception. 2016;94:641-9.
289. Pastor Z, Holla K, Chmel R. The influence of combined oral contraceptives on female sexual desire: a systematic review. Eur J Contracept Reprod Health Care. 2013;18:27-43.
290. Davis AR, Castano PM. Oral contraceptives and libido in women. Annu Rev Sex Res. 2004;15:297-320.
291. Burrows LJ, Basha M, Goldstein AT. The effects of hormonal contraceptives on female sexuality: a review. J Sex Med. 2012;9:2213-23.
292. Strufaldi R, Pompei LM, Steiner ML, et al. Effects of two combined hormonal contraceptives with the same composition and different doses on female sexual function and plasma androgen levels. Contraception. 2010;82:147-54.
293. Wiedemann C, Nagele U, Schramm G, Berking C. Inhibitory effects of progestogens on the estrogen stimulation of melanocytes in vitro. Contraception. 2009;80:292-8.
294. Thorneycroft l H, Gollnick H, Schellschmidt I. Superiority of a combined contraceptive containing drospirenone to a triphasic preparation containing norgestimate in acne treatment. Cutis. 2004;74:123-30.
295. Hussain Z, Roberts N, Whitehouse GH, Garcia-Finana M, Percy D. Estimation of breast volume and its variation during the menstrual cycle using MRI and stereology. Br J Radiol. 1999;72:236-45.
296. Lawrie TA, Helmerhorst FM, Maitra NK, Kulier R, Bloemenkamp K, Gulmezoglu AM. Types of progestogens in combined oral contraception: effectiveness and side-effects. Cochrane Database Syst Rev. 2011 May 11;(5):CD004861.

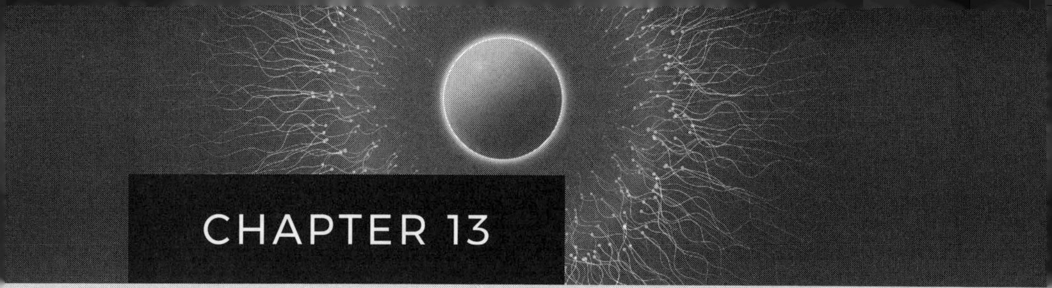

CHAPTER 13

Progestin-only Pills

Charita L. Roque, MD, MPH
Anne E. Burke, MD, MPH

KEY POINTS

- Progestin-only pills contain a progestin hormone and no estrogen.
- Progestin-only pills are highly effective if taken as directed.
- Progestin-only pills are safe for almost all people, including many with contraindications to combined oral contraceptive pills.
- The most common side effect of progestin-only pill users is irregular bleeding.
- Distribution of progestin-only pills over the counter without a prescription could increase access to effective contraception without compromising safety.

Progestin-only pills (POPs), sometimes called *minipills*, contain only a progestin hormone. There are two types of progestin-only pills currently available by prescription in the United States. These are norethindrone, which consists of active pills that users take once every day without hormone-free breaks, and, as of 2019, drospirenone, which consists of 24 daily pills with 4 hormone-free days.[1] (See **Table 13-1**.) In July 2023, the Food and Drug Administration approved a norgestrel-containing progestin only pill for over-the-counter use.[2]

Mechanism of Action

POPs may prevent pregnancy by the following mechanisms:

- Thickens cervical mucus, which impairs sperm penetration
- Alters luteinizing hormone (LH) and follicle-stimulating hormone (FSH) secretion, resulting in inhibition of ovulation in some proportion of cycles
- Decreases tubal motility by reducing activity of the cilia in the fallopian tube, which prevents the sperm and the egg from meeting

Table 13-1 Progestin-Only Oral Contraceptives Currently Available in the United States[3]

	Norethindrone	Drospirenone
Brand Names	Micronor®, Camila®, others	Slynd®
Strength	0.35 mg (28 active tablets)	4 mg (24 active/4 inactive tablets)
Half-life	About 9 hours	About 30 hours
Dosage	1 tablet daily × 28 days	1 active tablet daily × 24 days + hormone-free tablets for 4 days
Missed Doses	If dose is > 3 hours late, backup contraception recommended × 48 hours	If ≥ 2 active doses missed, backup contraception recommended × 7 days
Cost*	$25 for 28 days	$194 for 28 days

* Wholesale acquisition cost

Reprinted with special permission from The Medical Letter on Drugs and Therapeutics, February 10, 2020; Vol. 62 (1591):18-19.

The specific mechanism active in a particular cycle may vary among users and, in any single user, between cycles.[4] Studies found drospirenone 4 mg inhibits ovulation as effectively as desogestrel, which has ovulation rates similar to combined hormonal contraceptives.[5] This contrasts with norethindrone-containing pills, which do not suppress ovulation consistently due to lower doses of norethindrone compared to combined oral contraceptive (COC) pills.[4,6]

Effectiveness

POPs can be a highly effective contraceptive method when taken as directed. They are included in the second tier of effectiveness, along with COC pills, injectable contraceptives, and hormonal patches and rings (see Figure 5-2 in Chapter 5, Effectiveness, Safety, and Comparative Side Effects). In clinical studies for the norethindrone POP, all of which were conducted at least 20 years ago, the first-year failure rate ranged from 0.2%–13.2% (see Appendix B: Method Efficacy Tables, which is included in the eBook).[7] The quality of many of these studies was poor. Effectiveness and pregnancy failure rates for POPs are often reported in conjunction with rates for COCs. Of 100 users of POPs and COCs, seven will experience a pregnancy with typical use and 0.3 of 100 will become pregnant with perfect use (see Table 5-2).

In typical use, factors such as age, coital frequency, lactation, and compliance with pill-taking may influence pregnancy rates more than relatively minor differences in inherent method efficacy.[8] Guidelines on use of POPs emphasize that for maximum efficacy, the pills must be taken within several hours of the same time every day. This recommendation is based primarily on data about serum progestin levels after ingestion of the norethindrone POP, which peak shortly after pill ingestion and then decline to nearly undetectable levels 24 hours later.[6] However, no clinical data are available that correlate pregnancy rates with timeliness in taking

POPs. Phase II studies found that drospirenone-containing pills inhibited ovulation in nearly all participants despite intentional 24-hour delays in pill intake and a planned 4-day hormone hiatus. The ovulation rate for norethindrone POPs is 30% to 40%, whereas among participants who consistently took drospirenone daily, the ovulation rate was 0.8%, which is similar to that of COCs (1.1% to 2%).[9]

Scant data are available comparing efficacy of different POP products. The package insert for norethindrone, the POP most commonly available in the United States, reports a typical-use failure rate of 5% per year.[10] A large clinical trial for drospirenone reported a confirmed pregnancy rate of 1.2%, with a Pearl Index of 2.9 (95% confidence interval [CI] 1.5–5.1).[11] The package insert for this pill reports a pregnancy rate of 1.8%.[11] One randomized trial found no significant difference in efficacy between POPs containing norethindrone and POPs containing levonorgestrel (not available in the United States).[6] Pregnancy rates in both POP groups in this trial were greater than 9% at 1 year, higher than in many other studies.

A Cochrane review of randomized controlled trials of POPs from 1972 to 2007 found too little evidence to compare the effectiveness of different formulations, including desogestrel, levonorgestrel, norethindrone, ethynodiol diacetate plus mestranol, and norethindrone plus mestranol, of POPs either to each other or to COCs.[6] There have been two prospective, multicenter studies examining the effectiveness of drospirenone with a total of 1,571 participants. One study followed the safety of drospirenone, while in the other, participants were randomized to either drospirenone 4 mg or desogestrel 75 mg, a formulation available in Europe. They reported Pearl Indices of 0.7052 and 1.4, respectively.[5,13] The 41-site European trial of drospirenone 4 mg with 713 participants found a pregnancy rate of 0.5% (95% CI, 0%–1.07%) for all participants and 0.64% (95% CI, 1%–1.37%) for participants under 35 years of age over 13 cycles.[1]

POPs are widely believed to be less effective than COCs, but this belief is not supported by rigorous evidence.[6] One randomized trial comparing two COC and two POP preparations found that the pregnancy rate was significantly lower in one group of COC users than the rates in the other three groups. Losses from the study for reasons other than pregnancy were very high in all the groups, which seriously compromised the comparisons.[14] Another small study comparing a POP to a COC (neither of which is currently marketed) found no pregnancies in either group, although the study contained only 43 women in each group who used the assigned method for only 6.7 and 9.2 cycles on average.[15]

Advantages

POPs have numerous beneficial features, as described here.

1. **Safety.** Since POPs do not contain estrogen, they are even safer than COCs. Data suggest that neither norethindrone nor drospirenone POPs appear to be associated with an increase in risk of hypertension, cardiovascular disease and stroke, breast cancer, or blood clots.[1,16–20] However, rigorous data on safety of POPs as distinct from or in comparison to COCs are relatively scant.
2. **Few contraindications.** According to the US Medical Eligibility Criteria for Contraceptive Use (US MEC), POPs can safely be used by almost all patients.[21–23] These criteria list many fewer contraindications to POPs than to COCs. Progestin-only methods are contraindicated (US MEC category 4) for

those with current breast cancer. They are to be used with caution (US MEC category 3) in patients with severe cirrhosis, malignant liver tumors or hepatocellular adenoma, prior stroke, or systemic lupus erythematosus. POPs are also MEC category 3 for patients more than 5 years out from breast cancer; patients taking medications that alter progestin metabolism, such as anti-epileptics (e.g., phenytoin, carbamazepine) and rifampin; and those with a history of malabsorptive procedures.[24] A database study examining reproductive-age women seeking preventive care between 2009 and 2015 found only 4.36% had US MEC category 3 or 4 conditions.[25]

3. **Acceptable efficacy,** especially if the pills are taken as directed. As mentioned previously, depending on formulation, efficacy may be less vulnerable to user error for some POPs compared to others.
4. **Improved menstrual symptoms.** POPs cause menstrual cycle changes that some users perceive as favorable (for another perspective, see also Disadvantages in the following section). They may also reduce the severity of menstrual cramps.[25] Drospirenone demonstrates antimineralocorticoid and antiandrogenic effects, which may result in decreased water retention, weight gain, and breast tenderness before menses.[26]
5. **Simple, fixed daily regimen.** Users of norethindrone POPs take the same type of pill every day (same color and hormone content, no placebo days). This straightforward regimen is easy for clinicians to explain and for patients to understand. With drospirenone POPs, users follow a 24 + 4 regimen, which may be familiar from COC pills.
6. **Immediate reversibility.** Limited data suggest that fertility is normal immediately after stopping use of POPs, regardless of the duration of POP use.[27]
7. **Noncontraceptive health benefits.** POPs may reduce the incidence of painful crises in people with sickle cell disease through stabilization of red blood cell membranes and may relieve pelvic pain associated with endometriosis and reduce frequency and severity of migraines.[28–30] Daily use of progestin has also been associated with reduced risk of endometrial cancer, though there are no data specific to POPs.[31]

Disadvantages and Cautions

POPs also have disadvantages, as described here.

1. **Menstrual cycle disturbances.** POPs often cause bleeding changes. These changes are unpredictable and may include short cycles, irregular periods, bleeding episodes, and spotting, and less commonly, prolonged bleeding or amenorrhea. Analysis of bleeding patterns of participants in six clinical trials studying various methods of contraception showed that norethindrone POP users typically had less regular bleeding patterns and more total bleeding or spotting days over time than users of COCs, likely due to decreased ovulation suppression with POPs.[32]

   On the other hand, a multicenter trial of drospirenone found decreases in unscheduled bleeding, duration of bleeding, prolonged bleeding, and spotting over the course of several cycles.[1] Whether or not bleeding patterns tend to become more regular with increased duration of POP use is unknown. Bleeding irregularities caused by POPs are not inherently dangerous, but they can complicate the detection of pregnancy or mask underlying pathologies and thus cause patients to delay seeking care. They are also a common reason for discontinuing POPs, although some people consider the altered bleeding pattern to be a benefit, particularly if they experience a decrease in total bleeding.

2. **Other side effects.** Potential POP side effects include headache, nausea, breast tenderness, fatigue, and androgenic symptoms such as hirsutism and acne. The precise extent to which these common symptoms are actually caused by the pills cannot be determined from available data.[27] Of note, desogestrel has less androgenic activity while drospirenone-containing pills demonstrate antiandrogenic activity.[33,34] Studies give conflicting results regarding progestin effects on mood and mood disorders, but the US MEC designate POP as category 1 for those with depressive disorders and those using selective serotonin reuptake inhibitors (SSRIs).[35]
3. **Possibly vulnerable efficacy**. To maximize contraceptive efficacy, norethindrone POP users are advised to take pills at the same time each day and to use a backup method if pills are taken more than 3 hours late. In contrast, drospirenone-containing POPs more consistently inhibit ovulation, allowing missed-pill forgiveness similar to COCs[36]. (See Chapter 12, Combined Hormonal Contraceptives [CHCs].)
4. **Lower efficacy than some other methods in preventing ectopic pregnancy.** Rigorous data are not available about the effect of POPs on the absolute risk of ectopic pregnancy. One early report suggested that POP users may be at higher risk of an ectopic pregnancy than users of no method or of other methods, but other data refute that contention. However, up to 10% of pregnancies that occur among POP users may be ectopic, a proportion higher than is seen in users of COCs.[27] Given the contraceptive effectiveness of POP, the absolute risk of ectopic pregnancy is low, and substantially lower than that experienced by those using no contraception.
5. **Ovarian cysts.** Unlike COCs, which substantially inhibit ovarian activity and reduce the risk of functional ovarian cysts, norethindrone POPs do not prevent development of functional ovarian cysts or persistent follicles.[37] Most ovarian cysts cause minor or no symptoms and resolve without treatment.
6. **Lack of protection against sexually transmitted infections (STIs).** Progestin-only contraceptives provide no known substantial protection against STIs, including human immunodeficiency virus (HIV).

Special Issues

Breastfeeding

Given the elevated risk of venous thromboembolism in the postpartum period and previously held concerns regarding the effects of combined hormonal contraception on breastfeeding and breastmilk, norethindrone-containing POPs have long been recommended for postpartum contraception. A small amount of the progestin in pills passes into breast milk, which exposes a breastfeeding baby to the hormone. A meta-analysis examining 47 studies regarding duration and initiation of breastfeeding along with infant outcomes for people using progestin-only methods found no negative impact on breastfeeding duration, composition of breast milk, or infant development. Participants had either longer breastfeeding rates or no difference from historical controls.[38–40] No strong or consistent evidence exists suggesting harm for either norethindrone or drospirenone.[41,42] Both the World Health Organization (WHO) and US MECs recommend that the benefits of initiating and using POPs at any point after delivery postpartum generally outweigh the risks. Because of their safety, tolerability, and short list of contraindications, providers have increasingly recognized that POPs are also appropriate choices for nonlactating people, and outside of the immediate postpartum period. (See Chapter 19, Contraception After Pregnancy.)

Drug Interactions

Interactions between POPs and other drugs have not been well studied, but it is reasonable to suspect that they may be similar to interactions with COCs. Since POPs produce relatively low progestin levels even in the absence of other drugs, POPs may not be a good contraceptive option for people who are taking certain drugs on a chronic basis. These drugs include rifampicin, certain anticonvulsants, and some antiretroviral drugs, which affect the metabolism of ingested steroid hormones and lower serum levels of the contraceptive hormone.[25] People on these drugs can increase the effectiveness of their contraceptive use by adding a second contraceptive that is nonhormonal like a barrier method, spermicide, or withdrawal. Advise POP users who want to maintain effectiveness while temporarily taking a potentially interacting drug to use a backup method while on the medication, and possibly for some period of time after stopping it. Although some providers have proposed that POP users should increase the dose of POPs while taking a potentially interacting drug, no data are available on the efficacy or advisability of this idea.

Weight

A Cochrane review identified two comparative trials of POP effects on weight. One trial showed no significant weight change after 6 months of use of either a norethisterone or levonorgestrel POP. Another study of perimenopausal women that compared desogestrel POP to control showed no change in weight or body mass index after 12 months, with the desogestrel group showing a greater increase in fat mass.[43] No significant weight, heart rate, or blood pressure changes were observed with drospirenone POP in Phase III clinical trials.[5]

Renal Impairment

Drospirenone has not been demonstrated to affect renal function but does pose a theoretical risk of hyperkalemia. The concentration of serum potassium remained constant across study participants with normal to moderate renal impairment.[44,45]

Providing the Method

Almost all people can safely use POPs, including most people who are not eligible to take COCs. The US MEC does not restrict the use of POPs based on conditions such as age, smoking status, or medical conditions such as hypertension or migraine with aura.[21,24] No examination or laboratory test is needed to determine whether a person is eligible to receive POPs.

The WHO MEC and the US MEC list few category 3 or 4 contraindications to POPs (**Table 13-2**). Only one condition, current breast cancer, is classified as category 4, indicating that POPs pose an unacceptable health risk to those with this condition.

Table 13-2 Contraindications To Use of Progestin-Only Pills

Condition	US MEC
Current breast cancer	4
Past breast cancer and no evidence of current disease for 5 years	3
Severe cirrhosis, malignant liver tumors, or hepatocellular adenoma	3
History of bariatric surgery (malabsorptive procedure)	3
History of/current ischemic heart disease or stroke while on POPs	3*
Systemic lupus erythematosus with positive or unknown antiphospholipid antibodies	3
Enzyme-inducing anticonvulsants, (phenytoin, carbamazepine, barbiturates, primidone, topiramate, oxcarbazepine), rifampicin, or rifabutin	3

* Continuation only, not initiation. ± WHO MEC Category 3, including benign hepatocellular adenoma

Data from US Medical Eligibility Criteria (US MEC) for contraceptive use, 2016. CDC. Published November 19, 2020. Accessed May 16, 2021. https://www.cdc.gov/reproductivehealth/contraception/mmwr/mec/summary.html; Serfaty D. Update on the contraceptive contraindications. J Gynecol Obstet Hum Reprod. 2019;48(5):297-307. DOI:10.1016/j.jogoh.2019.02.006

Immediate start of certain kinds of POPs following use of ulipristal acetate (UPA) emergency contraceptive pills may counteract the ability of UPA to suppress ovulation, putting the user at risk of pregnancy from the act of intercourse that has already occurred.[46] Whether UPA counteracts the efficacy of POPs is not known, although one study showed that UPA did not interfere with the ability of COC pills to induce ovarian quiescence.[47] Until more is known, POPs should not be initiated within 5 days after taking UPA and people using POPs who need oral emergency contraception should be advised to use regimens that do not contain UPA. If a user of POPs takes UPA, they would need a backup contraceptive if they have sex within the following 5 days and then for the first 7 days after restarting the POP (See Chapter 18, Emergency Contraception.).

People who want to avoid irregular bleeding or amenorrhea may not desire norethindrone POPs. As norethindrone pills should be taken at close to the same hour each day, they may not be as effective for people whose schedules do not allow such consistency. People taking drospirenone POPs may have a more predictable bleeding pattern than those on norethindrone pills.

Counseling

Patients considering POPs should be advised about their advantages and disadvantages, described above. (See Chapter 4, Person-Centered Reproductive Health Conversations and Contraceptive Counseling.)

Timing of Initiation

A person may start taking POPs at any time when it is reasonably certain that they are not pregnant and if they have not used UPA emergency contraception within the last 5 days. (See Box 25-2 on how to be reasonably certain that a woman is not pregnant.)

The 2016 US Selected Practice Recommendations for Contraceptive Use indicate that no backup method is needed if a person starts POPs within the first 5 days after onset of menses. They would need a backup method if they had vaginal intercourse within the first 2 days after starting norethindrone POPs or within the first 7 days after starting drosprinenone POPs.[48,49]

Distribution of Commodities

Currently in the United States, POPs are available only by prescription. However, the recent approval of Opill for over-the-counter access should increase availability. Pharmacists can also prescribe contraception in 17 states and the District of Columbia.[50] Provide or prescribe as many packs of POPs as the patient wants. Advise the patient to check with their insurance carrier about any limits on the number of packs that may be dispensed at one time under their policy.

Managing Problems and Follow-Up

Abnormal bleeding in people using POPs can be managed through number of approaches, including reassurance, prostaglandin inhibitors, estrogen supplementation, or a method switch. (See Chapter 2, Understanding the Physiology of the Menstrual Cycle.)

If a patient becomes pregnant while using POPs, be vigilant for the possibility of ectopic pregnancy.

USER INSTRUCTIONS FOR PROGESTIN-ONLY PILLS*

To use POPs, follow these instructions:

1. Start taking the pills during the first 5 days of your normal menstrual period or on any day you are reasonably sure that you are not pregnant. If you are switching from estrogen-containing oral contraceptive pills (regular birth control pills), skip the inactive pills at the end of the pack, and instead start the POPs the day after the last active pill. If you are switching from a longer-acting progestin-only method (such as Depo-Provera or a levonorgestrel intrauterine device [IUD]), you may start the pills the same day the prior method is discontinued, or earlier, to minimize the time a backup method is needed.
2. Use a backup method, such as condoms, every time you have vaginal sex within 2 days after starting POPs. A backup method is not needed if drospirenone pills are started on the first day of a menstrual period.
3. Take one pill every day. Choose a time and take the pill at that time (or within 3 hours after that time if using a norethindrone POP).
4. Start the next pack the day after the last pack is finished. Do not take any break or days off between packs. Always have your next pack ready *before* you finish each pack.

---

* These instructions are intended to guide providers in educating patients in how to use their method.

5. If, while taking a norethindrone POP, you miss a pill during the 3-hour window, take it as soon as you remember and continue taking one pill each day at the usual time, even if that means you will take two pills in one day. Use a backup method such as condoms or abstain from vaginal sex during the next 48 hours. Take further pills at the usual time. If you miss taking a drospirenone POP, take the next pill as soon as you remember and use a nonhormonal backup method for 7 days after the missing pill(s).
6. If you vomit or have severe diarrhea within 4 hours after taking a pill, your body might not properly absorb the medicine in the POPs. Keep taking the pills on schedule, but use a backup method such as condoms every time you have sex, until 48 hours after the vomiting or diarrhea are over.
7. Get a pregnancy test if:
   - Your menstrual period is late, you have not taken all your pills on time, and you had sex without a condom or other backup method.
   - You have not had any periods for 2 months.
   - You are concerned about pregnancy for any reason.

   Keep taking the pills daily until you know the pregnancy test result. If the result is positive, then stop taking the pills and consult your clinician about your options. If the result is negative, then the late or missed periods are probably due to the pills and are not dangerous. Consult your clinician about other possible causes and your options.
8. Certain medicines and some over-the-counter preparations can reduce the effectiveness of POPs. If you take any other drug while using POPs, ask your clinician whether it might interact with POPs. If so, you should use a backup method (such as condoms) during the entire time you are taking the other drug and possibly for some time (up to a month) after you stop taking it. If you are planning to take the other drug for a long period of time, consult with your clinician about whether a contraceptive method other than POPs might be appropriate for you.
9. Changes in your menstrual periods (frequency and length and bleeding between periods) are common in people taking POPs. These changes are usually not dangerous. If you have unusual bleeding, keep taking the POPs. If the bleeding lasts for more than 8 days, is particularly heavy, occurs after intercourse, or if you want to switch to another contraceptive method that is less likely to cause bleeding irregularities, consult your clinician.
10. If you have other problems or questions while taking POPs, if you want to avoid pregnancy you can keep taking the pills according to schedule while you figure out what to do.
11. If you stop taking POPs and do not want to become pregnant, start using another contraceptive immediately, or abstain from vaginal sex. Your ability to become pregnant returns right away after you stop POPs.
12. If you have had sex that was not properly protected by POPs or another contraceptive method, consider using emergency contraception (EC). Choose a copper IUD, a levonorgestrel IUD (52 mg only), or morning-after pills that contain levonorgestrel. Emergency contraceptives containing UPA could interact with the hormone in POPs, meaning they might not work as well to prevent pregnancy, resulting in decreased effectiveness.

Box 13-1 Emergency Contraceptives (EC)

Emergency contraceptive pills or placement of a copper or a 52 mg levonorgestrel IUD after unprotected intercourse substantially reduces the risk of pregnancy. POP users should take EC regimens other than UPA. If a POP user does choose UPA as an EC method, they should not restart the POP until 5 days after taking the UPA. They would need to abstain from intercourse or use a backup contraceptive for those 5 days plus an additional 7 days after restarting the POPs.

Methods in Development

The characteristics of POPs make them eminently suitable for distribution over the counter: they are safe, contraindications are rare and readily recognizable by users themselves, and the regimen is very simple.[25,51] Further, overdose is not a concern. In a recent survey, a substantial proportion of US adults and teens indicated interest in using a POP if one was available over the counter.[52] The characteristics of POPs make them eminently suitable for distribution over the counter: they are safe, contraindications are rare and readily recognizable by users themselves, and the regimen is very simple.[25,51] Further, overdose is not a concern. In a recent survey, a substantial proportion of US adults and teens indicated interest in using a POP if one was available over the counter.[52] The effort to make POPs available without a prescription has been ongoing for several years. On July 13, 2023, years of advocacy and research culminated with the US Food and Drug Administration's authorization of Opill, a POP containing norgestrel 0.075 mg, for over the counter use. Opill's properties are similar to the norethindrone POP.[53,54,55]

While recent changes in some states, such as the prescription of contraceptives by pharmacists and greater provision of telehealth services, have increased access to oral contraceptives, the ultimate availability of over-the-counter POPs is an important step.[56,57]

Author Disclosures—Roque: none. Burke: research funding from Chemo and Merck, mediated through Johns Hopkins University.

Acknowledgments—Elizabeth Raymond, MD, and Daniel Grossman, MD, for their work on the previous iteration of this chapter.

References

1. Archer DF, Ahrendt HJ, Drouin D. Drospirenone-only oral contraceptive: results from a multicenter noncomparative trial of efficacy, safety and tolerability. Contraception. 2015;92(5): 439-44. DOI:10.1016/j.contraception.2015.07.017.
2. FDA Approves First Nonprescription Daily Oral Contraceptive. FDA. Published July 13, 2023. Accessed July 25, 2023. (https://www.fda.gov/news-events/press-announcements/fda-approves-first-nonprescription-daily-oral-contraceptive)
3. Drospirenone (Slynd) - a new progestin-only oral contraceptive. Med Lett Drugs Ther. 2020; 62(1591):18-9.
4. Teal S, Edelman A. Contraception selection, effectiveness, and adverse effects: A review. JAMA. 2021;326(24):2507-18. DOI:10.1001/jama.2021.21392.

5. Palacios S, Colli E, Regidor P. Multicenter, phase III trials on the contraceptive efficacy, tolerability and safety of a new drospirenone-only pill. Acta Obstet Gynecol Scand. 2019;98(12): 1549-57. DOI:10.1111/aogs.13688.
6. Grimes DA, Lopez LM, O'Brien PA, Raymond EG. Progestin-only pills for contraception. Cochrane Database Syst Rev. 2013;(11):CD007541. DOI:10.1002/14651858.CD007541.pub3.
7. Sales Vieira C, Celis C, Galán G, Hernández L, Díaz I, López J. Drospirenone: a Latin American perspective for oestrogen-free oral contraception. Eur J Contracept Reprod Health Care. 2021;26(1):73-8. DOI:10.1080/13625187.2020.1837364.
8. Steiner M, Dominik R, Trussell J, Hertz-Picciott I. Measuring contraceptive effectiveness: a conceptual framework. Obstet Gynecol. 1996;88(3 Suppl):24S-30S. DOI:10.1016/0029-7844(96)00251-7.
9. Duijkers IJM, Heger-Mahn D, Drouin D, Colli E, Skouby S. Maintenance of ovulation inhibition with a new progestogen-only pill containing drospirenone after scheduled 24-h delays in pill intake. Contraception. 2016;93(4):303-9. DOI:10.1016/j.contraception.2015.12.007.
10. U.S. National Library of Medicine. CAMILA norethindrone tablet. DailyMed database. Accessed February 28, 2022. (https://dailymed.nlm.nih.gov/dailymed/lookup.cfm?setid=a786be85-49ba-4369-b510-7dccc10f7f18)
11. Kimble T, Burke AE, Barnhart KT, Archer DF, Colli E, Westhoff CL. A 1-year prospective, open-label, single-arm, multicenter, phase 3 trial of the contraceptive efficacy and safety of the oral progestin-only pill drospirenone 4 mg using a 24/4-day regimen. Contracept X. 2020; 2:100020. DOI:10.1016/j.conx.2020.100020.
12. Exeltis USA. Slynd (drospirenone tablets): US FDA approved product information. Published online May 2019. Accessed February 27, 2022. (www.accessdata.fda.gov/drugsatfda_docs/label/2019/211367s000lbl.pdf)
13. Cahill EP, Kaur S. Advances in contraception research and development. Curr Opin Obstet Gynecol. 2020;32(6):393-8. DOI:10.1097/GCO.0000000000000666.
14. Sheth A, Jain U, Sharma S, et al. A randomized, double-blind study of two combined and two progestogen-only oral contraceptives. Contraception. 1982;25(3):243-52. DOI:10.1016/0010-7824(82)90047-6.
15. Paulsen ML, Varaday A, Brown BW, Kalman SM. A randomized contraceptive trial comparing a daily progestogen with a combined oral contraceptive steroid. Contraception. 1974;9(5): 497-506. DOI:10.1016/0010-7824(74)90061-4.
16. Sitruk-Ware R. Hormonal contraception and thrombosis. Fertil Steril. 2016;106(6):1289-94. DOI:10.1016/j.fertnstert.2016.08.039.
17. Mantha S, Karp R, Raghavan V, Terrin N, Bauer KA, Zwicker JI. Assessing the risk of venous thromboembolic events in women taking progestin-only contraception: a meta-analysis. BMJ. 2012;345:e4944. DOI:10.1136/bmj.e4944.
18. Chakhtoura Z, Canonico M, Gompel A, Scarabin PY, Plu-Bureau G. Progestogen-only contraceptives and the risk of acute myocardial infarction: a meta-analysis. J Clin Endocrinol Metab. 2011;96(4):1169-74. DOI:10.1210/jc.2010-2065.
19. Samson M, Porter N, Orekoya O, et al. Progestin and breast cancer risk: a systematic review. Breast Cancer Res Treat. 2016;155(1):3-12. DOI:10.1007/s10549-015-3663-1.
20. Blanco-Molina MA, Lozano M, Cano A, Cristobal I, Pallardo LP, Lete I. Progestin-only contraception and venous thromboembolism. Thromb Res. 2012;129(5):e257-62. DOI:10.1016/j.thromres.2012.02.042.
21. Medical eligibility criteria for contraceptive use. 5th ed. World Health Organization; 2015. Accessed February 21, 2022. (http://www.ncbi.nlm.nih.gov/books/NBK321151/)
22. Curtis KM, Tepper NK, Jatlaoui TC, et al. U.S. medical eligibility criteria for contraceptive use, 2016. MMWR Recomm Rep. 2016;65(3):1-103. DOI:10.15585/mmwr.rr6503a1.
23. Curtis KM, Zapata LB, Pagano HP, Nguyen A, Reeves J, Whiteman MK. Removing unnecessary medical barriers to contraception: Celebrating a decade of the U.S. Medical Eligibility Criteria for Contraceptive Use. J Womens Health. 2021;30(3):293-300. DOI:10.1089/jwh.2020.8910.

24. Centers for Disease Control and Prevention. US Medical Eligibility Criteria (US MEC) for Contraceptive Use, 2016. Published November 19, 2020. Accessed May 16, 2021. (https://www.cdc.gov/reproductivehealth/contraception/mmwr/mec/summary.html)
25. Dutton C, Kim R, Janiak E. Prevalence of contraindications to progestin-only contraceptive pills in a multi-institution patient database. Contraception. 2021;103(5):367-70. DOI:10.1016/j.contraception.2021.01.010.
26. Kubba A, Guillebaud J, Anderson RA, MacGregor EA. Contraception. Lancet. 2000;356(9245):1913-9. DOI:10.1016/S0140-6736(00)03269-4.
27. Horvath S, Schreiber CA, Sonalkar S. Contraception. In: Feingold KR, Anawalt B, Boyce A, et al., eds. Endotext. MDText.com, Inc.; 2000. Accessed February 21, 2022. (http://www.ncbi.nlm.nih.gov/books/NBK279148/)
28. Haddad LB, Curtis KM, Legardy-Williams JK, Cwiak C, Jamieson DJ. Contraception for individuals with sickle cell disease: a systematic review of the literature. Contraception. 2012;85(6):527-37. DOI:10.1016/j.contraception.2011.10.008.
29. Casper RF. Progestin-only pills may be a better first-line treatment for endometriosis than combined estrogen-progestin contraceptive pills. Fertil Steril. 2017;107(3):533-6. DOI:10.1016/j.fertnstert.2017.01.003.
30. Grandi G, Barra F, Ferrero S, et al. Hormonal contraception in women with endometriosis: a systematic review. Eur J Contracept Reprod Health Care. 2019;24(1):61-70. DOI:10.1080/13625187.2018.1550576.
31. Weiderpass E, Adami HO, Baron JA, et al. Risk of endometrial cancer following estrogen replacement with and without progestins. J Natl Cancer Inst. 1999;91(13):1131-7. DOI:10.1093/jnci/91.13.1131.
32. Zigler RE, McNicholas C. Unscheduled vaginal bleeding with progestin-only contraceptive use. Am J Obstet Gynecol. 2017;216(5):443-50. DOI:10.1016/j.ajog.2016.12.008
33. Bosanac SS, Trivedi M, Clark AK, Sivamani RK, Larsen LN. Progestins and acne vulgaris: a review. Dermatol Online J. 2018;24(5):13030/qt6wm945xf.
34. Muhn P, Krattenmacher R, Beier S, Elger W, Schillinger E. Drospirenone: A novel progestogen with antimineralocorticoid and antiandrogenic activity: Pharmacological characterization in animal models. Contraception. 1995;51(2):99-110. DOI:10.1016/0010-7824(94)00015-O.
35. Centers for Disease Control and Prevention. Summary chart of U.S. medical eligibility criteria for contraceptive use. (https://www.cdc.gov/reproductivehealth/contraception/pdf/summary-chart-us-medical-eligibility-criteria_508tagged.pdf)
36. HRA Pharma. Opill (norgestrel, 0.075 mg tablets) for Rx-to-OTC switch. Meeting May 9-10, 2023. Accessed May 18, 2023. (https://www.fda.gov/media/167893/download)
37. Tayob Y, Adams J, Jacobs HS, Guillebaud J. Ultrasound demonstration of increased frequency of functional ovarian cysts in women using progestogen-only oral contraception. Br J Obstet Gynaecol. 1985;92(10):1003-9. DOI:10.1111/j.1471-0528.1985.tb02994.x.
38. Glasier A, Bhattacharya S, Evers H, et al. Contraception after pregnancy. Acta Obstet Gynecol Scand. 2019;98(11):1378-85. DOI:10.1111/aogs.13627.
39. Phillips SJ, Tepper NK, Kapp N, Nanda K, Temmerman M, Curtis KM. Progestogen-only contraceptive use among breastfeeding women: a systematic review. Contraception. 2016;94(3):226-52. DOI:10.1016/j.contraception.2015.09.010.
40. Baird DC. The impact of contraception on lactation. Am Fam Physician. 2016;93(5):356-7.
41. National Library of Medicine (US). Drospirenone. In: Drugs and lactation database (LactMed); 2006. Accessed February 21, 2022. (http://www.ncbi.nlm.nih.gov/books/NBK501356/)
42. Bhardwaj NR, Espey E. Lactation and contraception. Curr Opin Obstet Gynecol. 2015;27(6):496-503. DOI:10.1097/GCO.0000000000000216.
43. Lopez LM, Edelman A, Chen M, Otterness C, Trussell J, Helmerhorst FM. Progestin-only contraceptives: effects on weight. Cochrane Database Syst Rev. 2013;(7):CD008815. DOI:10.1002/14651858.CD008815.pub3.
44. Rapkin AJ, Winer SA. Drospirenone: a novel progestin. Expert Opin Pharmacother. 2007;8(7):989-99. DOI:10.1517/14656566.8.7.989
45. Schürmann R, Blode H, Benda N, Cronin M, Küfner A. Effect of drospirenone on serum potassium and drospirenone pharmacokinetics in women with normal or impaired renal function. *J Clin Pharmacol.* 2006;46(8):867-75. DOI:10.1177/0091270006289973.

46. Brache V, Cochon L, Duijkers IJM, et al. A prospective, randomized, pharmacodynamic study of quick-starting a desogestrel progestin-only pill following ulipristal acetate for emergency contraception. Hum Reprod (Oxf). 2015;30(12):2785-93. DOI:10.1093/humrep/dev241.
47. Cameron ST, Berger C, Michie L, Klipping C, Gemzell-Danielsson K. The effects on ovarian activity of ulipristal acetate when "quickstarting" a combined oral contraceptive pill: a prospective, randomized, double-blind parallel-arm, placebo-controlled study. Hum Reprod (Oxf). 2015;30(7):1566-72. DOI:10.1093/humrep/dev115.
48. Exeltis USA. Slynd: What you need to know about starting birth control pills. Published July 27, 2021. Accessed February 26, 2022. (https://slynd.com/what-you-need-to-know-about-starting-birth-control-pills/)
49. Curtis KM. U.S. Selected practice recommendations for contraceptive use, 2016. MMWR Recomm Rep. 2016;65. DOI:10.15585/mmwr.rr6504a1.
50. Guttmacher Institute. Pharmacist-prescribed contraceptives. Published December 7, 2020. Accessed August 26, 2022. (https://www.guttmacher.org/state-policy/explore/pharmacist-prescribed-contraceptives)
51. White K, Potter JE, Hopkins K, Fernández L, Amastae J, Grossman D. Contraindications to progestin-only oral contraceptive pills among reproductive-aged women. Contraception. 2012; 86(3):199-203. DOI:10.1016/j.contraception.2012.01.008.
52. Grindlay K, Grossman D. Interest in Over-the-Counter Access to a Progestin-Only Pill among Women in the United States. Womens Health Iss. 2018;28(2):144-51. DOI:10.1016/j.whi.2017.11.006.
53. Commissioner of the FDA Approves First Nonprescription Daily Oral Contraceptive. Published July 13, 2023. Accessed July 25, 2023. (https://www.fda.gov/news-events/press-announcements/fda-approves-first-nonprescription-daily-oral-contraceptive)
54. Ibis Reproductive Health. Ibis announces groundbreaking partnership with HRA Pharma to move a birth control pill over the counter [press release]. Published December 30, 2016. Accessed February 28, 2022. (https://www.ibisreproductivehealth.org/news/ibis-announces-groundbreaking-partnership-hra-pharma-move-birth-control-pill-over-counter)
55. HRA Pharma. Perrigo's HRA Pharma submits application to FDA for first-ever OTC birth control pill [press release]. Published July 11, 2022. Accessed August 26, 2022. (https://www.hra-pharma.com/articles/perrigos-hra-pharma-submits-application-to-fda-for-first-ever-otc-birth-control-pill-66)
56. Williams RL, Meredith AH, Ott MA. Expanding adolescent access to hormonal contraception: an update on over-the-counter, pharmacist prescribing, and web-based telehealth approaches. Curr Opin Obstet Gynecol. 2018;30(6):458-64. DOI:10.1097/GCO.0000000000000497.
57. Upadhya KK, Santelli JS, Raine-Bennett TR, Kottke MJ, Grossman D. Over-the-counter access to oral contraceptives for adolescents. *J Adolesc Health.* 2017;60(6):634-40. DOI:10.1016/j.jadohealth.2016.12.024.

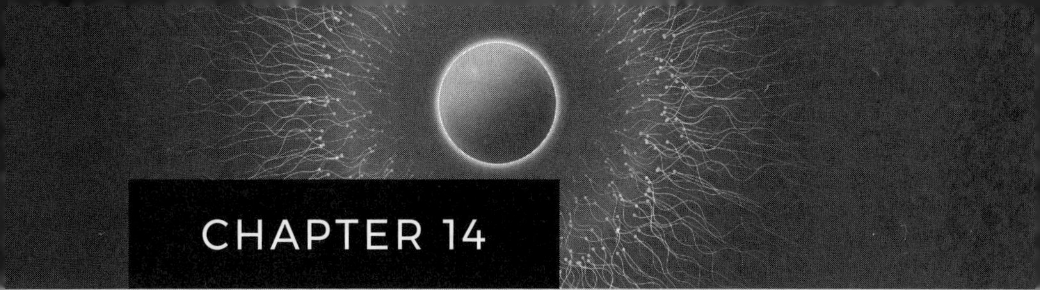

CHAPTER 14

External (Male) Condoms

Lee Warner, PhD, MPH
Markus J. Steiner, PhD, MSPH
Riley J. Steiner, PhD, MPH

KEY POINTS

- When used consistently and correctly, external (male) latex condoms can reduce the risk of pregnancy *and* sexually transmitted infections (STIs), including human immunodeficiency virus (HIV).
- Condoms are inexpensive, available without a prescription, and easy to use.
- Individuals potentially at risk for STIs, including adolescents, should be counseled to use condoms even if they already rely on more effective methods of contraception.

External condoms, also known as male condoms and hereafter referred to as condoms, remain among the most widely available and commonly used contraceptive methods in the United States. (For information on internal [female] condoms, see Chapter 16, On-Demand, Internal Methods.) When used consistently and correctly, condoms reduce the risk of both pregnancy and sexually transmitted infections (STIs), including human immunodeficiency virus (HIV). This multipurpose prevention role is widely recognized by national and international health organizations as a unique benefit of condoms.[1,2]

Although condom use increased markedly in the United States during the late 1990s and early 2000s, largely in response to the HIV and STI epidemics, use has since stabilized or declined according to multiple national surveys of adolescents and adults.[3] For example, data from the National Youth Risk Behavior Survey (YRBS) indicate the prevalence of condom use at last intercourse among sexually active high school students increased by one-third from 46% in 1991 to a peak of 63% in 2003.[4] However, condom use has since gradually declined to 52% in 2021.[5]

Use of condoms for contraception among reproductive-age women appears to have declined as well, according to the National Survey of Family Growth (NSFG).

In 1995, 20% of women reported using condoms as their most effective contraceptive method, compared with 16% in 2006–2010, and 8.4% in 2017–2019.[6,7] Estimates from 2017–2019 indicate that condoms are the fourth-most-popular method among women using contraception behind female sterilization, male sterilization, and oral contraceptive pills.[7] Among men aged 15–44, NSFG data from 2011–2015 indicate that one-third of sexually active men used a condom at last sexual intercourse in the past 12 months.[8] Condom use thus continues to be an important part of public health efforts to prevent undesired pregnancies as well as new cases of infection with HIV and other STIs.

Mechanism of Action

The condom acts as a physical barrier by covering the penile glans and shaft. The condom prevents pregnancy by blocking the passage of semen; it prevents infections by covering the major portals of entry and exit for many STI pathogens. Because of their coitally dependent nature, condoms must be used consistently and correctly with each act of intercourse to be effective. Among contraceptive methods that are physical barriers, condoms provide the most protection of the genital tract and effective protection against many STIs (see section on Special Issues).

A sheath worn over the penis can be traced as far back as 1350 B.C., when Egyptian men wore decorative covers for their penises. In 1564 A.D., Fallopius first described linen sheaths used to protect against syphilis.[9] Protective sheaths were made from dried animal intestines in the 18th century, when according to some sources, they were first given the name "condom," presumably after inventor Colonel Cundum. The advent of vulcanized rubber in 1843 led to the mass production of condoms made from natural rubber latex.[10] During the past three decades, manufacturers have used synthetic materials (e.g., polyurethane and polyisoprene) to develop new condom options.

Condom Options

Condoms are available in a variety of shapes, sizes, colors, and thicknesses, as well as with or without lubricants or spermicides, and with or without reservoir-tip or nipple-ends. Condoms can be straight-sided or tapered toward the closed end, textured (e.g., ribbed) or smooth, solid-colored or nearly transparent, odorless or scented, and flavored. Most condoms commercially available in the United States are about 7 inches (180 mm) long, 2 inches (52 mm) wide, and approximately 0.003 inches (0.08 mm) thick.

Condoms are made from three types of material—latex, natural membrane, and synthetic (**Table 14-1**). More than 80% of condoms commercially available in the United States are manufactured from natural rubber latex ("rubber" condoms).[11] A small proportion (<5%) are made from the intestinal cecum of lambs and are better known as "natural skin," "natural membrane," or (incorrectly) "lambskin" condoms. Natural membrane condoms contain small pores that do not allow the passage of sperm but may permit the passage of viruses, including hepatitis B virus, herpes simplex virus, and HIV.[12,13] Because of this porosity, natural membrane condoms may not provide the same level of protection against STIs as latex condoms and are thus not recommended for this purpose. No clinical data

Table 14-1 Characteristics of latex, natural membrane, and synthetic male condoms.

	Material		
Characteristic	**Latex**	**Natural Membrane**	**Synthetic**
Material	Natural rubber	Lamb cecum	Polyurethane or polyisoprene*
Lubricant use	Water-based or silicone-based†	Any	Any
Cost	Low	Moderate	Moderate/high
Recommended for prevention of pregnancy	Yes	Yes	Yes‡
Recommended for prevention of STIs, including HIV	Yes	No	Yes‡

* Most synthetic condoms currently available are made from polyurethane or polyisoprene.

† Users should consult package labeling to ensure compatibility of silicone-based lubricants with latex condoms.

‡ For latex sensitive or allergic persons.

are available on the effectiveness of natural membrane condoms for STI prevention, however. The remaining 15% or so of condoms are manufactured from synthetic materials, such as polyurethane and polyisoprene.[11] Synthetic condoms are generally more resistant to deterioration, have a longer shelf-life, and are compatible with use of both oil-based and water-based lubricants. For pregnancy prevention, synthetic condoms have rates of clinical failure that are comparable to their latex counterparts.[14] The effectiveness of synthetic condoms to prevent STIs, including HIV, has not been extensively studied, and US Food and Drug Administration (FDA) labeling restricts their recommended use to persons who are sensitive or allergic to latex;[15] however, based on their physical properties and laboratory testing, synthetic condoms likely provide contraception and STI protection similar to that of latex condoms. Finally, although still commercially available in the United States, use of condoms lubricated with the spermicide nonoxynol-9 (N-9), which is a surfactant, is not recommended. Condoms with N-9 lack additive benefit compared with other lubricated condoms and are associated with increased risk for HIV infection and among women, bacterial urinary tract infections and adverse effects on the vaginal epithelium.

Condom Testing

Condoms are regulated as Class II medical devices and subject to random sampling and testing by the FDA. Every condom is tested electronically for holes and weak spots before it is packaged and released for sale. Samples of condoms also undergo a series of additional laboratory tests for leakage, strength, dimensional requirements, and package integrity.[16] If the sample condoms fail any of these tests, the entire lot is rejected and destroyed. Imported condoms are required to comply with the same performance requirements as condoms produced domestically.

Effectiveness Against Pregnancy

Method failure of the condom is uncommon. Of 100 couples using condoms consistently and correctly (i.e., perfectly), 2 are estimated to become pregnant during the first 12 months of use. However, couples vary widely in how consistently or correctly they use condoms. Among couples using condoms for contraception, about 13 of every 100 will become pregnant during the first year of typical use. (A summary of studies of contraceptive failure for condoms, as well as a detailed discussion of the estimates used to derive these rates, can be found in Chapter 5 on safety, efficacy, and comparative risks.)

Condom effectiveness depends heavily on the skill level and experience of the user. The marked difference between the probabilities of pregnancy during typical use versus perfect use of condoms generally reflects problems with use. Examples of problems leading to reduced effectiveness of condoms against pregnancy, as well as STIs, include the following:

1. **Not using condoms with every act of sexual intercourse.** Nonuse of condoms, rather than poor condom quality or other condom-related problems, is the most common problem.[17,18] A leading priority for any prevention program should be to address factors that lead to nonuse of condoms, including lack of device acceptability, poor skills for negotiating use with partners, and latex allergy or sensitivity.
2. **Not using condoms throughout sexual intercourse.** Studies have documented that users put condoms on after starting intercourse or remove condoms prior to ejaculation.[19-24] These behaviors represent product misuse and could expose partners to risk of pregnancy or STIs despite condom use.
3. **Breakage and slippage.** Although users may express concern that the condom will break or fall off during use, these events are rare with proper use, tend to be concentrated among a small proportion of users,[25] and occur infrequently with properly fitting condoms.[26,27] Most studies show that during vaginal sex, condoms break approximately 2% of the time during intercourse or withdrawal and a similar proportion slip off completely.[21,28-32] Relevant to STI/HIV prevention, some studies have found that rates of breakage and slippage during anal intercourse may be slightly higher than during vaginal intercourse, yet one recent study found that breakage and slippage was lower for anal intercourse than vaginal intercourse.[33]
4. **Using improper lubricants with latex condoms.** Unlike water-based and most silicone-based lubricants, oil-based lubricants (e.g., petroleum jelly, baby oil, and hand lotions) reduce latex condom integrity[34] and may facilitate breakage (see **Table 14-2**). People may mistakenly believe oil-based products that readily wash off with water to be water-based lubricants. Note that oil-based products in general can be safely used as lubricants with currently available polyurethane and polyisoprene condoms.

Detailed instructions for condom use, as well as considerations for counseling, are provided at the end of this chapter.

Table 14-2 Examples of types of lubricant products that should and should not be used with latex condoms.

Safe	Not Safe
Saliva	Baby oil
Silicone	Cold creams
Water	Edible oils (e.g., olive, peanut, corn, sunflower)
Water-based or silicone-based lubricants	Hand and body lotions
	Massage oil
	Petroleum jelly
	Rubbing alcohol or silicone-based lubricants
	Suntan oil and lotions
	Vaginal infection medications in cream or suppository form
	Vegetable or mineral oil

Advantages

When used consistently and correctly, condoms provide an effective, nonhormonal option for preventing pregnancy, which some users may prefer. Importantly, condoms are the only available method known to reduce the risk of pregnancy *and* STIs, including HIV. By preventing STIs and their long-term sequelae, condoms protect future fertility.

Whether used for pregnancy or STI prevention, other benefits of condoms include:

1. **Accessibility.** Condoms are widely available and typically over the counter. Usage does not require medical examination, prescription, or fitting.
2. **Low cost.** Condoms are among the most inexpensive and cost-effective contraceptives, especially considering the added protection offered against STIs. Condoms are often available at low cost in both the private and public sectors and often for free from publicly funded programs.
3. **Portability.** Condoms can be easily and discreetly carried, for example, in wallets or purses.
4. **Minimal side effects.** Condoms rarely cause medical problems among users. The most frequent side effect is typically latex sensitivity or allergy; individuals with this condition can be directed to use synthetic condoms, particularly if STIs are of concern (see the section on Managing Problems and Follow-up on p. 442 in this chapter, as well as Chapter 23).
5. **Delayed ejaculation.** For some individuals, condom use may help prolong intercourse and also prevent premature ejaculation.

Disadvantages and Cautions

Condoms also have disadvantages that may result in inconsistent or nonuse of the method.

1. **Reduced sensation.** Many users and their partners report that condoms reduce sensitivity. Individuals can experiment with different types of condoms (and lubricants) to find ones that are most suitable.
2. **Problems with erection.** Individuals who cannot consistently maintain an erection when using condoms may find the method unacceptable. In these cases, where culturally acceptable, involving the partner in putting the condom on as part of foreplay may be helpful. While occasional erectile difficulties are a normal (yet nonetheless challenging) occurrence, frequent difficulties may be an early warning sign of underlying medical problems, such as coronary heart disease or diabetes, and should be evaluated by a clinician.[35,36]
3. **Lack of spontaneity.** Many individuals dislike interrupting sexual activity to put on the condom and may find the coitally dependent nature of condom use to be inconvenient. For some users, involving their partner in putting on the condom may help facilitate use.
4. **Challenges with partner negotiation.** Some individuals may be embarrassed to obtain condoms or to suggest or initiate condom use because they perceive condom use implies a lack of trust or intimacy. In some instances, individuals may be unwilling to use condoms for other reasons. Offer to teach individuals (and partners, when appropriate) about condoms and how to successfully negotiate their use. (See section on Providing Condoms—Counseling, p. 440).
5. **Latex allergy or sensitivity**. A small proportion of individuals and their partners, especially health care workers repeatedly exposed to latex, may be allergic or sensitive to latex and thus unable to use latex condoms. Synthetic condoms are excellent alternatives. (See section on Managing Problems and Follow-up.)

Special Issues

Effectiveness Against STIs, Including HIV

The primary noncontraceptive benefit of condom use is the protection conferred against STIs, including HIV. When placed on the penis before any genital contact and used throughout intercourse, condoms prevent direct contact with semen; genital lesions and subclinical viral shedding on the glans and shaft of the penis; and penile, vaginal, or anal discharges or infectious fluids. Condoms thus greatly reduce the risk of STIs that are transmitted primarily to or from the penile urethra (such as gonorrhea, chlamydia, trichomoniasis, hepatitis B infection, and HIV). Condoms also provide protection against STIs that are transmitted primarily through skin-to-skin contact or contact with mucosal surfaces (such as genital herpes, human papillomavirus [HPV] and HPV-associated diseases, syphilis, and chancroid) to the extent that these areas are covered by the condom.[15] Protection may be less when these STIs involve areas not covered by the condom.[37] In vitro laboratory studies indicate that latex condoms provide an effective physical barrier against passage of even the smallest sexually transmitted pathogen, hepatitis B.[38-43] Latex and synthetic condoms also can be used during anal and oral intercourse to reduce the risk of STIs, including HIV,[15] and in 2022, FDA authorized the first condom specifically indicated for anal intercourse, i.e., One Male Condom. This natural latex condom, which is available in a variety of sizes and fits, also can be used during vaginal intercourse.[44]

The level of protection condoms provide is likely to vary for different STIs because STIs differ in their routes of transmission, as well as in their infectivity and prevalence.[45-47] Well-designed clinical studies of discordant couples (where one partner is infected and the other is not) have shown consistent use of latex condoms to be highly effective against penile-vaginal transmission of HIV infection.[48] Two meta-analyses of these studies place the estimated effectiveness of consistent (though not necessarily correct) condom use for HIV prevention between approximately 80% and 95%.[49,50] A well-designed study of HIV-discordant men who have sex with men estimated the protective effect of consistent condom use to be in the same range.[51] Studies and systematic reviews have also found condom use to be associated with reduced risk of many other STIs, including gonorrhea, chlamydia, trichomoniasis, syphilis, genital herpes, HPV infection and HPV-associated conditions, and sexually transmitted Zika virus infection.[47,52-74] Although clinical studies of effectiveness against most STIs other than HIV have generated varying estimates of the protective effect,[54] much of this inconsistency can be attributed to limitations in study design (e.g., incomplete assessment of condom use and whether individuals were exposed to infected partners). We refer readers elsewhere for more extensive discussion of condom effectiveness for STI prevention.[47,54,72,75]

Condom Use and Sexual Behaviors

Concern been raised about whether condom use may result, paradoxically, in greater sexual risk due to changes in other sexual behaviors (i.e., risk compensation), such as earlier onset of sexual activity or increased number of sexual partners.[76] Studies that have evaluated whether such an effect exists or whether it outweighs the protective effects of condom use suggest that condom promotion is not associated with increases in sexual activity. A review of 174 condom-related prevention approaches concluded that interventions designed to reduce the risk of HIV infection do not increase unsafe sexual behavior.[77] Since that review was published, reviews of school-based condom availability programs have reached similar conclusions specifically for adolescent populations.[78-80]

Condom Use with Other Prevention Strategies

General consensus holds that condoms must play a central role in any STI/HIV prevention program.[81] However, the appropriate mix of condom use versus other prevention strategies (e.g., abstinence, mutual monogamy, preexposure prophylaxis [PrEP] for HIV prevention) remains a challenge. For one, condoms may not be used sufficiently for effective STI/HIV prevention. As examples, even among study populations where a known or suspected risk for infection is present (e.g., couples discordant for HIV or genital herpes simplex virus [HSV], pregnant women residing in areas with a Zika virus outbreak), fewer than half of couples report regular use of condoms.[49,50,59,82]

Additionally, as the availability of biomedical strategies for HIV prevention has increased (e.g., PrEP, circumcision, treatment as prevention), concerns have been raised that such strategies may result in decreased condom use and increased risk for other STIs. This may be less of a concern for circumcision—a meta-analysis found no association between circumcision and decreased condom use[83]—than for PrEP, where the evidence is less clear.[84,85]

The use of condoms with contraceptive methods that are more effective (i.e., permanent contraception [male and female sterilization], intrauterine devices [IUDs], implants, injectables, patches, rings, oral contraception) is recommended for sexually active individuals seeking to prevent pregnancy who are also at risk of STIs.[2,86] Although use of a condom plus another contraceptive method could dramatically reduce the risk of both pregnancy and STIs,[87] this strategy is not commonly practiced,[8,88] including among adolescents who are at disproportionate risk for STIs.[5,89] Moreover, evidence from studies of women of reproductive age,[90,91] including adolescents,[92-94] suggests that condom use is lower among users of implants and IUDs compared with users of injectables, patches, rings, and oral contraception.[95] While the explanation for these differences warrants further research,[95-97] such findings underscore the value of integrating pregnancy and STI prevention in health education and clinical practice.[98]

Providing Condoms

Counseling

Provider counseling about condoms has been associated with increased reports of condom use in multiple studies.[82,99] As with counseling about other contraceptive methods, it is important to address risks and benefits and ensure that condom use counseling is client-centered and tailored to an individual's needs, preferences, and ability to use condoms effectively. (See Chapter 4, Person-Centered Reproductive Health Conversations and Contraceptive Counseling.) Because condoms, when used consistently and correctly, also confer protection against STIs, clients' risk for infection and prevention motivations (e.g., protecting future fertility associated with untreated infections) should also be used to tailor counseling messages.[86]

Depending on the client, providers may emphasize messages related to condom use for pregnancy prevention, STI prevention, or both. It is important that, regardless of the purpose, any counseling addresses how to use condoms most effectively (i.e., consistently and correctly). For counseling messages related to general advantages and potential disadvantages (including how to address them), see sections on Advantages and Disadvantages and Cautions.

Pregnancy Prevention

- Advise clients that in order to be effective, condoms should be used with every act of intercourse because it is challenging to predict when ovulation may occur.
- Although preventing pregnancy is often cited as the most important reason for using condoms,[100-103] clients may find it difficult to understand contraceptive failure rates.[104] Consider showing them a scale of the relative effectiveness of contraceptives when communicating condom failure rates (see Chapter 5, Effectiveness, Safety, and Comparative Side Effects and Chapter 4, Person-Centered Reproductive Health Conversations and Contraceptive Counseling).
- Emergency contraception can be used as a backup method for pregnancy prevention in case a condom breaks, falls off, or is not used (see Chapter 18, Emergency Contraception).

STI Prevention

- Work with the client interactively to prioritize their understanding of the benefit of consistent and correct condom use during sexual activities that can transmit STIs, including HIV. Recommend that clients use a new condom for each act of anal, vaginal, or oral intercourse that involves penile contact when any risk of infection exists. (See Chapter 4, Person-Centered Reproductive Health Conversations and Contraceptive Counseling.)
- Strongly recommend that clients use condoms during pregnancy when there is a risk for STIs to protect their fetus, their partner(s), and themselves.
- If recommending condom use for STI prevention with a highly effective method of contraception, emphasize this reason to clients who may assume that condom use is for additional protection against pregnancy. This message may be especially important for promoting condom use with IUDs and implants since backup contraception is unnecessary with these methods.
- Because simultaneous use of condoms for STI prevention with a more effective method of contraception may be challenging for some clients, suggest a brief trial period. If using two methods proves difficult, work with clients to overcome barriers or identify more feasible strategies for adequate protection against both pregnancy and STIs.
- If a condom breaks, falls off, or is not used, offer clients STI testing. If HIV is a possibility, offer postexposure prophylaxis for HIV prevention.

Effective Use

- Emphasize that condoms are most effective when used correctly during every act of intercourse.
- Routinely assess consistency and correctness of condom use using a two-step process.
    - First, ask clients how often they are using condoms, whether they use condoms that fit properly, when they choose to use or not use condoms, and, if not using consistently, address barriers to use.
    - Second, to identify potential misuse, ask clients to explain (and perhaps demonstrate on an appropriate model of a penis) how they use condoms. If needed, review user instructions with the client (see User Instructions for Condoms, p. 442).
- Advise client to have several condoms available in case a condom is torn or put on incorrectly, or repeated intercourse is desired.
- Assess the likelihood of a partner's negative reaction to the suggestion of condom use, and help clients develop responses they feel comfortable using if a partner objects to using condoms. Counsel or refer as appropriate if you are concerned about intimate partner violence.
- Encourage clients to practice putting on a condom, including in the dark. When providing instruction on how to use condoms, have the client unroll a condom onto a model of a penis.
- Advise clients taking vaginal medications (e.g., for yeast infections) to use synthetic condoms or remain abstinent until the medication is finished and the infection is cured. These medications often contain oil-based ingredients that can damage latex condoms.

Condom Availability

It is important that providers have condoms readily available and accessible for clients, ideally at no cost. Clients should also be able to obtain a large number of condoms each visit, in case accessing health care is a challenge or obtaining condoms from other settings is difficult. Consider providing a variety of types of condoms, including latex and synthetic options (as well as internal [female] condoms). Because simply making condoms available may not result in sufficient use,[18] incorporating condom use counseling as part of condom availability efforts is important.

Managing Problems and Follow-Up

Persons sensitive or allergic to natural rubber latex may experience irritation, allergic contact dermatitis, or systemic anaphylactic symptoms when exposed to latex-containing products.[105,106] While 1% to 6% of the US population are estimated to be allergic to latex, the prevalence of latex sensitivity is thought to be much higher (8% to 12%) among health care and laboratory workers who have repeated exposure to latex-containing medical devices (e.g., surgical and examination gloves, catheters, intubation tubes, anesthesia masks, and dental dams).[107,108] Proteins in the latex appear to be the primary source of allergic reactions. All clients should be questioned for potential latex allergy. Ask whether the client experiences itching, rash, or wheezing after wearing latex gloves or inflating a balloon. If you suspect a client has generalized latex sensitivity, consider recommending synthetic condoms and refer the client for allergy skin testing.[109] While latex condom use is contraindicated for clients with general latex sensitivity, both synthetic and natural membrane condoms can be recommended for prevention of pregnancy, while only synthetic condoms should be recommended for prevention of STIs, including HIV.

Allergic reactions that occur only after exposure to latex condoms and not after exposure to other latex-containing products may be attributable to brand-specific condom attributes such as spermicides, lubricants, perfumes, local anesthetics, or other chemical agents added during the manufacturing process.[110] Advise clients to try different brands of latex and synthetic condoms. In any case, clients should immediately contact their health care provider for follow-up if they or their partner(s) experience a severe allergic reaction while using latex condems. Additional comprehensive information on latex allergy can also be obtained from the Asthma and Allergy Foundation of America (see www.aafa.org/latex-allergy).

USER INSTRUCTIONS FOR CONDOMS

During a World Health Organization Experts Meeting (Geneva, June 22–24, 2005) to develop a Global Handbook for Family Planning Providers, consensus was reached on five key condom instructions.

More detailed instructions for using condoms (including **Box 14-1**) are included as follows and can be found elsewhere https://www.cdc.gov/condomeffectiveness/external-condom-use.html):

Box 14-1 Five Key Instructions for Condom Use

1. Use a new condom for each act of intercourse if any risk of pregnancy or STIs exists.
2. Before any genital contact, place the condom on the tip of the erect penis with the rolled side out.
3. Unroll the condom all the way to the base of the erect penis.
4. Immediately after ejaculation, hold the rim of the condom and withdraw the penis while it is still erect.
5. Throw away the used condom safely.

Before Intercourse

1. Have on hand an adequate supply of latex or synthetic condoms and lubricant if a condom may be needed, even if using another contraceptive. Have extra condoms available in case the first is damaged, torn before use, put on incorrectly, or repeated intercourse is desired.
2. Discuss condom use with your partner before having intercourse.

At Time of Intercourse

1. Open the condom package carefully to avoid damaging it with fingernails, teeth, or other sharp objects.
2. Before any genital contact between partners, put the condom on the erect penis.
3. Unroll the condom a short distance to make sure the condom is being unrolled in the correct direction. Then hold the tip of the condom and unroll it down to the base of the erect penis. If the condom does not unroll easily, it has probably been put on inside-out. Discard the condom and begin with a new one, because flipping it over and using it could expose your partner to infectious organisms contained in the pre-ejaculate.
4. Adequate lubrication is important. For latex condoms, use only water-based lubricants like water or saliva, or lubricating jellies (like silicone-based lubricants, or spermicidal lubricants, jellies, foam, or suppositories). Avoid oil-based lubricants (like cold cream, mineral oil, cooking oil, petroleum jelly, body lotions, massage oil, or baby oil), which can damage latex condoms (see Table 14-2).
5. Keep the condom on the penis until after intercourse. If the condom breaks or falls off during intercourse but before ejaculation, stop and put on a new condom. Use a new condom when you have different types of intercourse within a single session (e.g., after anal sex, change the condom before having vaginal sex to decrease the risk of urinary tract infection).

After Intercourse

1. Soon after ejaculation, withdraw the penis while it is still erect. Hold the condom firmly against the base of the penis to prevent slippage and leakage of semen.
2. Check the condom for visible damage such as holes, then wrap it in tissue and discard. Do not flush condoms down the toilet.

3. If the condom breaks, falls off, leaks, is damaged, or is not used, the following may help:
   - Discuss the possibility of pregnancy or infection with your partner and contact your health care provider as soon as you can. Do not douche. Emergency contraception may be used to prevent pregnancy if it is started within 5 days (120 hours) of having unprotected intercourse. (See Chapter 18, Emergency Contraception.)
   - Consider getting tested for STIs. If HIV is a possibility, postexposure prophylaxis for HIV prevention is available.

Repeated Intercourse

Use a new condom from "beginning to end" with each act of anal, vaginal, or oral intercourse. Do not reuse condoms.

Taking Care of Supplies

1. Store condoms in a cool, dry place out of direct sunlight (excessive heat will weaken latex).
2. Check the expiration or manufacture date on the box or individual package of condoms. Expiration dates are marked as "Exp"; otherwise, the date is the manufacture date (MFG). Latex condoms should not be used beyond their expiration date or more than 5 years after the manufacturing date. Condoms in damaged packages or that show obvious signs of deterioration (e.g., brittleness, stickiness, or discoloration) should not be used regardless of their expiration date.

Author Disclosures—Warner: none; Steiner MJ: none; Steiner RJ: none

References

1. UNFPA, WHO, UNAIDS. Position statement on condoms and the prevention of HIV, other sexually transmitted infections and unintended pregnancy. (www.unaids.org/en/resources/presscentre/featurestories/2015/july/20150702_condoms_prevention).
2. Grubb LK, Committee on Adolescence. Barrier protection use by adolescents during sexual activity. Pediatrics. 2020;146(2). DOI: 10.1542/peds.2020-007237.
3. Anderson JE, Warner L, Macaluso M. Condom use among US adults at last sexual intercourse, 1996-2008: an update from national survey data. Sex Transm Dis. 2011;38(10):919-21. DOI: 10.1097/OLQ.0b013e31822545d9.
4. Kann L, McManus T, Harris WA, et al. Youth Risk Behavior Surveillance - United States, 2017. MMWR Surveill Summ. 2018;67(8):1-114. DOI: 10.15585/mmwr.ss6708a1.
5. Szucs LE, Pampati S, Li J. MD1;Role of the COVID-19 Pandemic on Sexual Behaviors and Receipt of Sexual and Reproductive Health Services Among U.S. High School Students — Youth Risk Behavior Survey, United States, 2019–2021. MMWR Suppl 2023;72(Suppl-#1):55-65.
6. Jones J, Mosher W, Daniels K. Current contraceptive use in the United States, 2006-2010, and changes in patterns of use since 1995. Natl Health Stat Rep. 2012(60):1-25. (https://www.ncbi.nlm.nih.gov/pubmed/24988814).
7. Daniels K, Abma JC. Current contraceptive status among women aged 15-49: United States, 2017-2019. NCHS Data Brief. 2020(388):1-8. (https://www.ncbi.nlm.nih.gov/pubmed/33151146).
8. Copen CE. Condom use during sexual intercourse among women and men aged 15-44 in the United States: 2011-2015 National Survey of Family Growth. Natl Health Stat Rep. 2017(105):1-18. (https://www.ncbi.nlm.nih.gov/pubmed/29155683).

9. Valdiserri RO. Cum hastis sic clypeatis: the turbulent history of the condom. Bull N Y Acad Med. 1988;64(3):237-45. (https://www.ncbi.nlm.nih.gov/pubmed/3069159).
10. Murphy JS. The condom industry in the United States, 1990. Jefferson NC: McFarland & Company, Inc., 1990.
11. Global Industry Analysts Inc. Condoms: A global business strategic report. San Jose, CA, 2008.
12. Carey RF, Lytle CD, Cyr WH. Implications of laboratory tests of condom integrity. Sex Transm Dis. 1999;26(4):216-20. DOI: 10.1097/00007435-199904000-00006.
13. Lytle CD, Routson LB, Seaborn GB, Dixon LG, Bushar HF, Cyr WH. An in vitro evaluation of condoms as barriers to a small virus. Sex Transm Dis. 1997;24(3):161-4. DOI: 10.1097/00007435-199703000-00007.
14. Gallo MF, Grimes DA, Lopez LM, Schulz KF. Non-latex versus latex male condoms for contraception. Cochrane Database Syst Rev. 2006(1):CD003550. DOI: 10.1002/14651858.CD003550.pub2.
15. Workowski KA, Bachmann LH, Chan PA, et al. Sexually transmitted infections treatment guidelines, 2021. MMWR Recomm Rep. 2021;70(4):1-187. DOI: 10.15585/mmwr.rr7004a1.
16. American Society for Testing Materials. Annual book of ASTM standards. Rubber products: standard specifications for rubber contraceptives (male condoms-D3492). West Conshohocken, PA: American Society for Testing Materials, 2016.
17. Steiner MJ, Cates W, Jr., Warner L. The real problem with male condoms is nonuse. Sex Transm Dis. 1999;26(8):459-62. DOI: 10.1097/00007435-199909000-00007.
18. Warner L, Steiner MJ. Condom access does not ensure condom use: you've got to be putting me on. Sex Transm Infect. 2002;78(3):225. DOI: 10.1136/sti.78.3.225.
19. Calzavara L, Burchell AN, Remis RS, et al. Delayed application of condoms is a risk factor for human immunodeficiency virus infection among homosexual and bisexual men. Am J Epidemiol. 2003;157(3):210-7. DOI: 10.1093/aje/kwf195.
20. Sanders SA, Yarber WL, Kaufman EL, Crosby RA, Graham CA, Milhausen RR. Condom use errors and problems: a global view. Sex Health. 2012;9(1):81-95. DOI: 10.1071/SH11095.
21. Warner L, Newman DR, Kamb ML, et al. Problems with condom use among patients attending sexually transmitted disease clinics: prevalence, predictors, and relation to incident gonorrhea and chlamydia. Am J Epidemiol. 2008;167(3):341-9. DOI: 10.1093/aje/kwm300.
22. Warner L, Clay-Warner J, Boles J, Williamson J. Assessing condom use practices. Implications for evaluating method and user effectiveness. Sex Transm Dis. 1998;25(6):273-7. DOI: 10.1097/00007435-199807000-00001.
23. Paz-Bailey G, Koumans EH, Sternberg M, et al. The effect of correct and consistent condom use on chlamydial and gonococcal infection among urban adolescents. Arch Pediatr Adolesc Med. 2005;159(6):536-42. DOI: 10.1001/archpedi.159.6.536.
24. Hensel DJ, Stupiansky NW, Herbenick D, Dodge B, Reece M. When condom use is not condom use: an event-level analysis of condom use behaviors during vaginal intercourse. J Sex Med. 2011;8(1):28-34. DOI: 10.1111/j.1743-6109.2010.02031.x.
25. Steiner M, Piedrahita C, Glover L, Joanis C. Can condom users likely to experience condom failure be identified? Fam Plann Perspect. 1993;25(5):220-3, 226. (https://www.ncbi.nlm.nih.gov/pubmed/8262171).
26. Reece M, Herbenick D, Sanders SA, Monahan P, Temkit M, Yarber WL. Breakage, slippage and acceptability outcomes of a condom fitted to penile dimensions. Sex Transm Infect. 2008;84(2):143-9. DOI: 10.1136/sti.2007.028316.
27. Crosby RA, Yarber WL, Graham CA, Sanders SA. Does it fit okay? Problems with condom use as a function of self-reported poor fit. Sex Transm Infect. 2010;86(1):36-8. DOI: 10.1136/sti.2009.036665.
28. Albert AE, Warner DL, Hatcher RA, Trussell J, Bennett C. Condom use among female commercial sex workers in Nevada's legal brothels. Am J Public Health. 1995;85(11):1514-20. DOI: 10.2105/ajph.85.11.1514.
29. Cook L, Nanda K, Taylor D. Randomized crossover trial comparing the eZ.on plastic condom and a latex condom. Contraception. 2001;63(1):25-31. DOI: 10.1016/s0010-7824(00)00193-1.
30. Valappil T, Kelaghan J, Macaluso M, et al. Female condom and male condom failure among women at high risk of sexually transmitted diseases. Sex Transm Dis. 2005;32(1):35-43. DOI: 10.1097/01.olq.0000148295.60514.0b.

31. Macaluso M, Kelaghan J, Artz L, et al. Mechanical failure of the latex condom in a cohort of women at high STD risk. Sex Transm Dis. 1999;26(8):450-8. DOI: 10.1097/00007435-199909000-00006.
32. Walsh TL, Frezieres RG, Peacock K, et al. Effectiveness of the male latex condom: combined results for three popular condom brands used as controls in randomized clinical trials. Contraception. 2004;70(5):407-13. DOI: 10.1016/j.contraception.2004.05.008.
33. Siegler AJ, Rosenthal EM, Sullivan PS, et al. Levels of clinical condom failure for anal sex: A randomized cross-over trial. EClinicalMedicine 2019;17:100199. DOI: 10.1016/j.eclinm.2019.10.012.
34. Voeller B, Coulson AH, Bernstein GS, Nakamura RM. Mineral oil lubricants cause rapid deterioration of latex condoms. Contraception. 1989;39(1):95-102. DOI: 10.1016/0010-7824(89)90018-8.
35. Weinberg AE, Eisenberg M, Patel CJ, Chertow GM, Leppert JT. Diabetes severity, metabolic syndrome, and the risk of erectile dysfunction. J Sex Med. 2013;10(12):3102-9. DOI: 10.1111/jsm.12318.
36. Katsiki N, Wierzbicki AS, Mikhailidis DP. Erectile dysfunction and coronary heart disease. Curr Opin Cardiol. 2015;30(4):416-21. DOI: 10.1097/HCO.0000000000000174.
37. Steiner M, Warner L, Stone KM, Cates W. Condoms and other barrier methods for prevention of STD/HIV infection, and pregnancy. In: Holmes KK, Sparling PF, Mardh PA, eds. Sexually transmitted diseases. 4th ed. New York, NY: McGraw-Hill; 2008.
38. Carey RF, Herman WA, Retta SM, Rinaldi JE, Herman BA, Athey TW. Effectiveness of latex condoms as a barrier to human immunodeficiency virus-sized particles under conditions of simulated use. Sex Transm Dis. 1992;19(4):230-4. DOI: 10.1097/00007435-199207000-00009.
39. Conant MA, Spicer DW, Smith CD. Herpes simplex virus transmission: condom studies. Sex Transm Dis. 1984;11(2):94-5. DOI: 10.1097/00007435-198404000-00009.
40. Katznelson S, Drew WL, Mintz L. Efficacy of the condom as a barrier to the transmission of cytomegalovirus. J Infect Dis. 1984;150(1):155-7. DOI: 10.1093/infdis/150.1.155.
41. Rietmeijer CA, Krebs JW, Feorino PM, Judson FN. Condoms as physical and chemical barriers against human immunodeficiency virus. JAMA. 1988;259(12):1851-3. (https://www.ncbi.nlm.nih.gov/pubmed/2830416).
42. Van de Perre P, Jacobs D, Sprecher-Goldberger S. The latex condom, an efficient barrier against sexual transmission of AIDS-related viruses. AIDS. 1987;1(1):49-52. (https://www.ncbi.nlm.nih.gov/pubmed/3122790).
43. Judson FN, Ehret JM, Bodin GF, Levin MJ, Rietmeijer CA. In vitro evaluations of condoms with and without nonoxynol 9 as physical and chemical barriers against Chlamydia trachomatis, herpes simplex virus type 2, and human immunodeficiency virus. Sex Transm Dis. 1989;16(2):51-6. DOI: 10.1097/00007435-198904000-00001.
44. Food and Drug Administration. FDA permits marketing of first condom specifically indicated for anal intercourse. (https://www.fda.gov/news-events/press-announcements/fda-permits-marketing-first-condom-specifically-indicated-anal-intercourse).
45. Cates W, Jr. The condom forgiveness factor: the positive spin. Sex Transm Dis. 2002;29(6):350-2. DOI: 10.1097/00007435-200206000-00007.
46. Mann JR, Stine CC, Vessey J. The role of disease-specific infectivity and number of disease exposures on long-term effectiveness of the latex condom. Sex Transm Dis. 2002;29(6):344-9. DOI: 10.1097/00007435-200206000-00006.
47. Warner L, Stone KM, Macaluso M, Buehler JW, Austin HD. Condom use and risk of gonorrhea and chlamydia: a systematic review of design and measurement factors assessed in epidemiologic studies. Sex Transm Dis. 2006;33(1):36-51. DOI: 10.1097/01.olq.0000187908.42622.fd.
48. Cates W, Jr. The NIH condom report: the glass is 90% full. Fam Plann Perspect. 2001;33(5):231-3. (https://www.ncbi.nlm.nih.gov/pubmed/11589545).
49. Weller S, Davis K. Condom effectiveness in reducing heterosexual HIV transmission. Cochrane Database Syst Rev. 2002(1):CD003255. DOI: 10.1002/14651858.CD003255.
50. Pinkerton SD, Abramson PR. Effectiveness of condoms in preventing HIV transmission. Soc Sci Med. 1997;44(9):1303-12. DOI: 10.1016/s0277-9536(96)00258-4.

51. Smith DK, Herbst JH, Zhang X, Rose CE. Condom effectiveness for HIV prevention by consistency of use among men who have sex with men in the United States. J Acquir Immune Defic Syndr. 2015;68(3):337-44. DOI: 10.1097/QAI.0000000000000461.
52. d'Oro LC, Parazzini F, Naldi L, La Vecchia C. Barrier methods of contraception, spermicides, and sexually transmitted diseases: a review. Genitourin Med. 1994;70(6):410-7. DOI: 10.1136/sti.70.6.410.
53. Manhart LE, Koutsky LA. Do condoms prevent genital HPV infection, external genital warts, or cervical neoplasia? A meta-analysis. Sex Transm Dis. 2002;29(11):725-35. DOI: 10.1097/00007435-200211000-00018.
54. Holmes KK, Levine R, Weaver M. Effectiveness of condoms in preventing sexually transmitted infections. Bull World Health Org. 2004;82(6):454-61. (https://www.ncbi.nlm.nih.gov/pubmed/15356939).
55. Koss CA, Dunne EF, Warner L. A systematic review of epidemiologic studies assessing condom use and risk of syphilis. Sex Transm Dis. 2009;36(7):401-5. DOI: 10.1097/OLQ.0b013e3181a396eb.
56. Winer RL, Hughes JP, Feng Q, et al. Condom use and the risk of genital human papillomavirus infection in young women. N Engl J Med. 2006;354(25):2645-54. DOI: 10.1056/NEJMoa053284.
57. Casper C, Wald A. Condom use and the prevention of genital herpes acquisition. Herpes. 2002;9(1):10-4. (https://www.ncbi.nlm.nih.gov/pubmed/11916494).
58. Wald A, Langenberg AG, Krantz E, et al. The relationship between condom use and herpes simplex virus acquisition. Ann Intern Med. 2005;143(10):707-13. DOI: 10.7326/0003-4819-143-10-200511150-00007.
59. Wald A, Langenberg AG, Link K, et al. Effect of condoms on reducing the transmission of herpes simplex virus type 2 from men to women. JAMA. 2001;285(24):3100-6. DOI: 10.1001/jama.285.24.3100.
60. Barlow D. The condom and gonorrhoea. Lancet. 1977;2(8042):811-3. DOI: 10.1016/s0140-6736(77)90737-1.
61. Ramstedt K, Forssman L, Giesecke J, Granath F. Risk factors for Chlamydia trachomatis infection in 6810 young women attending family planning clinics. Int J STD AIDS. 1992;3(2):117-22. DOI: 10.1177/095646249200300208.
62. Upchurch DM, Brady WE, Reichart CA, Hook EW, 3rd. Behavioral contributions to acquisition of gonorrhea in patients attending an inner city sexually transmitted disease clinic. J Infect Dis. 1990;161(5):938-41. DOI: 10.1093/infdis/161.5.938.
63. Fennema JS, van Ameijden EJ, Coutinho RA, Van den Hoek A. Clinical sexually transmitted diseases among human immunodeficiency virus-infected and noninfected drug-using prostitutes. Associated factors and interpretation of trends, 1986 to 1994. Sex Transm Dis. 1997;24(6):363-71. DOI: 10.1097/00007435-199707000-00010.
64. Levine WC, Revollo R, Kaune V, et al. Decline in sexually transmitted disease prevalence in female Bolivian sex workers: impact of an HIV prevention project. AIDS. 1998;12(14):1899-906. DOI: 10.1097/00002030-199814000-00022.
65. Hooper RR, Reynolds GH, Jones OG, et al. Cohort study of venereal disease. I: the risk of gonorrhea transmission from infected women to men. Am J Epidemiol. 1978;108(2):136-44. DOI: 10.1093/oxfordjournals.aje.a112597.
66. Baeten JM, Nyange PM, Richardson BA, et al. Hormonal contraception and risk of sexually transmitted disease acquisition: results from a prospective study. Am J Obstet Gynecol. 2001;185(2):380-5. DOI: 10.1067/mob.2001.115862.
67. Cates WC, Jr., Holmes KK. Re: Condom efficacy against gonorrhea and nongonococcal urethritis. Am J Epidemiol. 1996;143(8):843-4. DOI: 10.1093/oxfordjournals.aje.a008826.
68. Sanchez J, Gotuzzo E, Escamilla J, et al. Sexually transmitted infections in female sex workers: reduced by condom use but not by a limited periodic examination program. Sex Transm Dis. 1998;25(2):82-9. DOI: 10.1097/00007435-199802000-00005.
69. Schwartz MA, Lafferty WE, Hughes JP, Handsfield HH. Risk factors for urethritis in heterosexual men. The role of fellatio and other sexual practices. Sex Transm Dis. 1997;24(8):449-55. DOI: 10.1097/00007435-199709000-00002.

70. Hogewoning CJ, Bleeker MC, van den Brule AJ, et al. Condom use promotes regression of cervical intraepithelial neoplasia and clearance of human papillomavirus: a randomized clinical trial. Int J Cancer. 2003;107(5):811-6. DOI: 10.1002/ijc.11474.
71. Bleeker MC, Hogewoning CJ, Voorhorst FJ, et al. Condom use promotes regression of human papillomavirus-associated penile lesions in male sexual partners of women with cervical intraepithelial neoplasia. Int J Cancer. 2003;107(5):804-10. DOI: 10.1002/ijc.11473.
72. Alfonsi GA, Shlay J. The effectiveness of condoms for the prevention of sexually transmitted diseases. Curr Womens Health Rev. 2005;1:151-9.
73. Nielson CM, Harris RB, Nyitray AG, Dunne EF, Stone KM, Giuliano AR. Consistent condom use is associated with lower prevalence of human papillomavirus infection in men. J Infect Dis. 2010;202(3):445-51. DOI: 10.1086/653708.
74. World Health Organization. Annex B2. Evidence review, key question (2): Does consistent and correct condom use reduce transmission of Zika virus? WHO guidelines for the prevention of sexual transmission of Zika virus. Geneva: World Health Organization; 2020.
75. Crosby R, DiClemente RJ, Holtgrave DR, Wingood GM. Design, measurement, and analytical considerations for testing hypotheses relative to condom effectiveness against non-viral STIs. Sex Transm Infect. 2002;78(4):228-31. DOI: 10.1136/sti.78.4.228.
76. Richens J, Imrie J, Copas A. Condoms and seat belts: the parallels and the lessons. Lancet. 2000;355(9201):400-3. DOI: 10.1016/S0140-6736(99)09109-6.
77. Smoak ND, Scott-Sheldon LA, Johnson BT, Carey MP. Sexual risk reduction interventions do not inadvertently increase the overall frequency of sexual behavior: a meta-analysis of 174 studies with 116,735 participants. J Acquir Immune Defic Syndr. 2006;41(3):374-84. DOI: 10.1097/01.qai.0000185575.36591.fc.
78. Wang T, Lurie M, Govindasamy D, Mathews C. The effects of school-based condom availability programs (CAPs) on condom acquisition, use and sexual behavior: A systematic review. AIDS Behav. 2018;22(1):308-20. DOI: 10.1007/s10461-017-1787-5.
79. Andrzejewski J, Liddon N, Leonard S. Condom availability programs in schools: A review of the literature. Am J Health Promot. 2019;33(3):457-67. DOI: 10.1177/0890117118791118.
80. Algur E, Wang E, Friedman HS, Deperthes B. A systematic global review of condom availability programs in high schools. J Adolesc Health. 2019;64(3):292-304. DOI: 10.1016/j.jadohealth.2018.11.013.
81. Halperin DT, Steiner MJ, Cassell MM, et al. The time has come for common ground on preventing sexual transmission of HIV. Lancet. 2004;364(9449):1913-5. DOI: 10.1016/S0140-6736(04)17487-4.
82. Salvesen von Essen B, Kortsmit K, Warner L, et al. Preventing sexual transmission of Zika virus infection during pregnancy, Puerto Rico, USA, 2016(1). Emerg Infect Dis. 2019;25(11):2115-9. DOI: 10.3201/eid2511.190915.
83. Gao Y, Yuan T, Zhan Y, et al. Association between medical male circumcision and HIV risk compensation among heterosexual men: a systematic review and meta-analysis. Lancet Glob Health. 2021;9(7):e932-41. DOI: 10.1016/S2214-109X(21)00102-9.
84. Kumar S, Haderxhanaj LT, Spicknall IH. Reviewing PrEP's effect on STI incidence among men who have sex with men-balancing increased STI screening and potential behavioral sexual risk compensation. AIDS Behav. 2021;25(6):1810-8. DOI: 10.1007/s10461-020-03110-x.
85. Traeger MW, Schroeder SE, Wright EJ, et al. Effects of pre-exposure prophylaxis for the prevention of Human Immunodeficiency Virus infection on sexual risk behavior in men who have sex with men: A systematic review and meta-analysis. Clin Infect Dis. 2018;67(5):676-686. DOI: 10.1093/cid/ciy182.
86. Gavin L, Moskosky S, Carter M, et al. Providing quality family planning services: Recommendations of CDC and the U.S. Office of Population Affairs. MMWR Recomm Rep. 2014; 63(RR-04):1-54. (https://www.ncbi.nlm.nih.gov/pubmed/24759690).
87. Cates W, Jr., Steiner MJ. Dual protection against unintended pregnancy and sexually transmitted infections: what is the best contraceptive approach? Sex Transm Dis. 2002;29(3):168-74. DOI: 10.1097/00007435-200203000-00007.
88. Higgins JA, Smith NK, Sanders SA, et al. Dual method use at last sexual encounter: a nationally representative, episode-level analysis of US men and women. Contraception. 2014;90(4): 399-406. DOI: 10.1016/j.contraception.2014.06.003.

89. Kottke M, Whiteman MK, Kraft JM, et al. Use of dual methods for protection from unintended pregnancy and sexually transmitted diseases in adolescent African American women. J Pediatr Adolesc Gynecol. 2015;28(6):543-8. DOI: 10.1016/j.jpag.2015.04.008.
90. Pazol K, Kramer MR, Hogue CJ. Condoms for dual protection: patterns of use with highly effective contraceptive methods. Public Health Rep. 2010;125(2):208-17. DOI: 10.1177/003335491012500209.
91. Eisenberg DL, Allsworth JE, Zhao Q, Peipert JF. Correlates of dual-method contraceptive use: an analysis of the National Survey of Family Growth (2006-2008). Infect Dis Obstet Gynecol. 2012;2012:717163. DOI: 10.1155/2012/717163.
92. Kortsmit K, Williams L, Pazol K, et al. Condom use with long-acting reversible contraception vs non-long-acting reversible contraception hormonal methods among postpartum adolescents. JAMA Pediatr. 2019;173(7):663-670. DOI: 10.1001/jamapediatrics.2019.1136.
93. Steiner RJ, Liddon N, Swartzendruber AL, Rasberry CN, Sales JM. Long-acting reversible contraception and condom use among female US high school students: Implications for sexually transmitted infection prevention. JAMA Pediatr. 2016;170(5):428-34. DOI: 10.1001/jamapediatrics.2016.0007.
94. Walsh-Buhi ER, Helmy HL. Trends in long-acting reversible contraceptive (LARC) use, LARC use predictors, and dual-method use among a national sample of college women. J Am Coll Health. 2018;66(4):225-36. DOI: 10.1080/07448481.2017.1399397.
95. Steiner RJ, Pampati S, Kortsmit KM, Liddon N, Swartzendruber A, Pazol K. Long-Acting reversible contraception, condom use, and sexually transmitted infections: A systematic review and meta-analysis. Am J Prev Med. 2021;61(5):750-60. DOI: 10.1016/j.amepre.2021.04.032.
96. Steiner RJ, Swartzendruber A, Cushing K, et al. Being on the safe side: A qualitative study of condom use motivations according to contraceptive type among adolescents in Atlanta, Georgia. J Pediatr Adolesc Gynecol. 2019;32(4):388-94. DOI: 10.1016/j.jpag.2019.02.122.
97. Raidoo S, Tschann M, Elia J, Kaneshiro B, Soon R. Dual-method contraception among adolescents and young people: Are long-acting reversible contraception users different? A qualitative study. J Pediatr Adolesc Gynecol. 2020;33(1):45-52. DOI: 10.1016/j.jpag.2019.09.008.
98. Steiner RJ, Liddon N, Swartzendruber AL, Pazol K, Sales JM. Moving the message beyond the methods: Toward integration of unintended pregnancy and sexually transmitted infection/HIV prevention. Am J Prev Med. 2018;54(3):440-3. DOI: 10.1016/j.amepre.2017.10.022.
99. Morroni C, Heartwell S, Edwards S, Zieman M, Westhoff C. The impact of oral contraceptive initiation on young women's condom use in 3 American cities: missed opportunities for intervention. PLoS One. 2014;9(7):e101804. DOI: 10.1371/journal.pone.0101804.
100. Cooper ML, Agocha VB, Powers AM. Motivations for condom use: do pregnancy prevention goals undermine disease prevention among heterosexual young adults? Health Psychol. 1999;18(5):464-74. DOI: 10.1037//0278-6133.18.5.464.
101. Harvey SM, Washburn I, Oakley L, Warren J, Sanchez D. Competing priorities: Partner-specific relationship characteristics and motives for condom use among at-risk young adults. J Sex Res. 2017;54(4-5):665-76. DOI: 10.1080/00224499.2016.1182961.
102. Crosby RA, Milhausen RR, Graham CA, et al. Condom use motivations and selected behaviours with new versus established sex partners. Sex Health. 2014;11(3):252-7. DOI: 10.1071/SH13159.
103. O'Sullivan LF, Udell W, Montrose VA, Antoniello P, Hoffman S. A cognitive analysis of college students' explanations for engaging in unprotected sexual intercourse. Arch Sex Behav. 2010;39(5):1121-31. DOI: 10.1007/s10508-009-9493-7.
104. Steiner MJ, Dalebout S, Condon S, Dominik R, Trussell J. Understanding risk: a randomized controlled trial of communicating contraceptive effectiveness. Obstet Gynecol. 2003;102(4):709-17. DOI: 10.1016/s0029-7844(03)00662-8.
105. Zaza S, Reeder JM, Charles LE, Jarvis WR. Latex sensitivity among perioperative nurses. AORN J. 1994;60(5):806-12. DOI: 10.1016/s0001-2092(07)63329-8.
106. National Institute for Occupational Safety and Health. Preventing allergic reactions to natural rubber latex in the workplace DHHS (NIOSH) Publication Number 97-135, 1997.
107. Food and Drug Administration. Don't be misled by "Latex Free" claims. (https://www.fda.gov/consumers/consumer-updates/dont-be-misled-latex-free-claims).

108. Food and Drug Administration. Allergic reactions to latex-containing medical devices Rockville, MD: Food and Drug Administration; 1991.
109. Yassin MS, Lierl MB, Fischer TJ, O'Brien K, Cross J, Steinmetz C. Latex allergy in hospital employees. Ann Allergy. 1994;72(3):245-9. (https://www.ncbi.nlm.nih.gov/pubmed/8129217).
110. Hamann CP, Kick SA. Update: immediate and delayed hypersensitivity to natural rubber latex. Cutis 1993;52(5):307-11. (https://www.ncbi.nlm.nih.gov/pubmed/8299394).

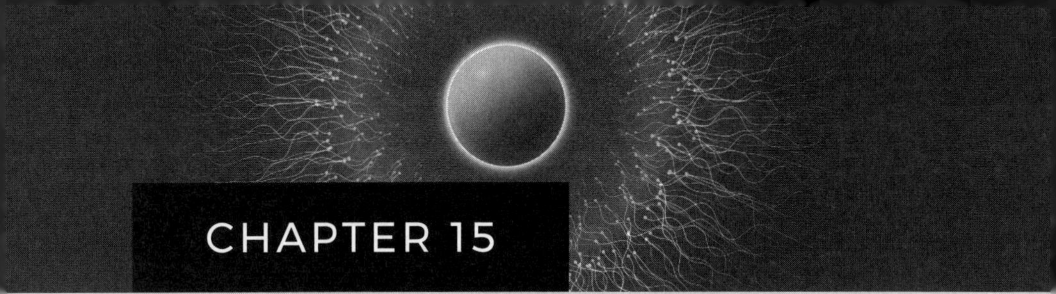

CHAPTER 15

Fertility Awareness-Based Methods

Rachel Peragallo Urrutia, MD
Chelsea B. Polis, PhD

KEY POINTS

- Fertility awareness-based methods (FABMs) teach users to try to identify days of high and low fecundity; that information can be used to avoid pregnancy by avoiding vaginal-penile intercourse without backup contraception on highly fecund days.
- Regardless of whether they choose to use an FABM to avoid pregnancy, most people can find value in learning fertility awareness.
- There are several different kinds of FABMs; each uses one or more biomarkers and a unique set of rules or algorithms to try to identify days of high and low fecundity.
- FABMs can address preferences of some people to use a method that has no side effects, can be used together with their partner(s), and can be used to achieve or avoid pregnancy.

Fertility awareness–based methods (FABMs) of family planning depend on trying to identify the days in each menstrual cycle when intercourse is most likely to result in a pregnancy. Some FABMs simply involve keeping track of cycle days to help identify which days of the menstrual cycle are most likely to be fecund. Other FABMs involve observing, recording, and interpreting the body's fertility signs.[1]

FABMs rely on five biological facts:[2-5]

- A period of fecundity occurs during each menstrual cycle.
- There is a single ovulatory event each cycle.
- The ovum has a limited life span (it can be fertilized only in the short time span of 12–24 hours after release).
- Sperm have a longer but still limited life span of 3 to 5 days in cervical mucus and the upper genital tract.
- People using FABMs can monitor menstrual cycle length and/or cycle-related signs to attempt to estimate the period of potential fecundity (often called "the fertile window").

To avoid pregnancy, users must either use an additional method or avoid vaginal-penile intercourse completely during the fertile window. Although terminology varies, those who use an additional method on fertile days are often described as using a "fertility awareness–based method (FABM)" while those who abstain are often described as using "natural family planning (NFP)."[1] This chapter uses the term "FABM" to indicate that the client can choose to abstain or use an alternative method on fertile days. Studies suggest that many people seeking family planning services would be interested in FABMs if they were explained to them appropriately, regardless of their intention to abstain or use an additional method on fertile days.[6] Data from the US National Survey of Family Growth between 2013 and 2017 suggest recent increases in FABM use, with 3.4% of contracepting women currently using FABMs.[7]

Mechanism of Action

The mechanism of action of FABMs is to avoid having viable sperm in the female reproductive tract at the time the oocyte can be fertilized. FABMs use one or more indicators to try to identify the beginning and end of the span of potentially fertile days during each menstrual cycle. Users then can then modify their sexual behavior during this time by either abstaining or using an additional method in order to avoid pregnancy.

Different FABMs rely on different indicators. FABMs discussed throughout this chapter include:

- Methods based on tracking of days of the menstrual cycle (e.g., the Standard Days Method)
- Methods based on observation of cervical secretions (e.g., the TwoDay Method, the Billings Ovulation Method)
- Methods based primarily on tracking changes in basal body temperature (e.g., Natural Cycles)
- Methods based on tracking of multiple indicators of fertility (e.g., sympto-thermal methods) and urinary hormone-based methods (e.g., the Marquette Model).
- Methods that rely upon mini-computers (which use predictive algorithms to try to identify the fertile time) as well as smartphone applications (apps) and devices discussed where relevant.

FABMs can be effective for preventing pregnancy when used correctly.[1] While perfect use of each individual FABM may be differently defined, it generally includes consistently avoiding vaginal-penile intercourse or using an additional contraceptive method on days of the menstrual cycle that are more likely to lead to pregnancy. Therefore, by definition, incorrect use of FABMs involves intercourse without other contraception, including withdrawal, precisely on the days more likely to lead to pregnancy.

In most cycles, ovulation occurs at or very near the middle of the cycle.[8] It is commonly believed that there are only about 6 days during each cycle when intercourse without contraception can actually result in pregnancy (the day of ovulation plus the 5 days preceding ovulation, given that sperm can survive in the female genital tract for this long).[2,3] However, as ovulation does not occur on the same day each cycle, the actual number of potentially fertile days identified by each FABM is greater. In some cases, this may be 12 days or longer, given the variability in biomarker changes relative to the actual day of ovulation.[9,10]

Methods Based on Tracking Days of the Menstrual Cycle

FABMs such as the Standard Days Method and the Rhythm Method (sometimes called calendar rhythm) involve counting the days in the menstrual cycle to identify the days of high fecundity. In cycles that range between 26 and 32 days long (approximately 78% of cycles), the fertile window is highly likely to fall within cycle days 8 to 19, though the actual timing of the ovulation and days of fecundity likely varies a bit from cycle to cycle.[11] In shorter or longer cycles, the fertile window shifts accordingly (sooner in shorter cycles and later in longer cycles).[12]

The Standard Days Method requires that menstrual cycles are between 26 and 32 days long. The fertile window is defined as days 8 through 19. Users of the Standard Days Method can keep track of the fertile window using a paper calendar, a physical ring of cycle beads, or a smartphone application.[13] For Rhythm Method users, it is important to have a record of the length of the previous 6 to 12 menstrual cycles prior to starting use, in order to try to identify the longest and shortest of these cycles. Once these are noted, calculations are performed to identify the probable days of fertility during the current cycle.[14] Although many people report using the rhythm method, survey results from many countries show that among users who state they are using "rhythm" or "calendar rhythm" method, as many as half do not know and/or are not adhering to the rules of the formal Rhythm Method. Rather, they are using the term "rhythm method" to refer to abstaining from intercourse on a few days of the menstrual cycle when they believe, often erroneously, that pregnancy is most likely to occur.[15] As such, it is likely that "rhythm" has simply become a generic term for occasional abstinence related to cycle timing.

Newer menstrual cycle length–based FABMs employ algorithms to try to identify the fertile window, based on user-provided information on menstrual cycle lengths. Clue Birth Control (FDA approved but not yet marketed in the United States) uses a Bayesian computer algorithm that was developed using a database of cycles from users with known fertile windows. This algorithm makes individualized fertile window predictions based on each user's cycle lengths compared with those from that database.[16]

Methods Based on Observation of Cervical Secretions

FABMs such as the TwoDay Method and the Billings Ovulation Method (and variants such as the Creighton Model) involve observing the presence of, absence of, and changes in cervical mucus secretions at the vulva to try to identify the beginning and end of the fertile window. The day of ovulation is typically within ± 3 days of the last day of highest-quality mucus ("peak day").[17] Penile-vaginal intercourse without backup contraception is typically avoided during days with the presence of any cervical mucus, and for a set number of days after the cervical mucus disappears.

Methods Based Primarily on Tracking Changes in Basal Body Temperature

FABMs based primarily on basal body temperature, such as Natural Cycles, typically also include a menstrual cycle length calculation to try to identify the beginning of the fertile window. Penile-vaginal intercourse without backup contraception is typically avoided starting a set number of days prior to the predicted ovulation and until a set number of days after the increase in basal body temperature. When compared to using luteinizing hormone (LH) surge or ultrasonography, the increase in basal body temperature typically occurs within ± 2 days of the actual day of ovulation.[18-20] Natural Cycles, an app that requires a subscription fee, uses a statistical algorithm that accounts for the start of menstruation and the date that basal body temperature increases from previous cycles to try to identify the fertile window in the current cycle. Over time, the algorithm enables more days of vaginal-penile intercourse without backup contraception ("green days").

Methods Based on Tracking Multiple Indicators of Fertility

Symptothermal methods involve observation of at least two fertility indicators, typically cervical secretions and basal body temperature. Some symptothermal method protocols also involve observation of changes in cervical position, a menstrual length calculation, or both. Changes in all these signs are caused by fluctuations in circulating hormone levels during the cycle. A set of rules is then applied by the user to try to identify the fertile window. Single-check symptothermal methods typically instruct the user to define the beginning of fertile window as the first appearance of cervical mucus and the end of the fertile window as the increase in basal body temperature.[21] Double-check methods (e.g., Thyma, Sensiplan) typically rely on two markers of fertility to both begin and end the fertile window.[22–24] For Sensiplan, for example, the beginning of the fertile window is typically determined by the user based either on menstrual cycle dates and/or days of temperature increase from previous cycles, or appearance of first cervical mucus, **whichever comes first.** The fertile window ends on the third day of the basal body temperature increase or the third day after the peak mucus day, **whichever comes last.**[22]

Methods Based on Urinary Hormone Monitoring

The Marquette Model, a symptohormonal method, utilizes a self-test device (the Clearblue® Fertility Monitor) to measure urinary hormones. Rising estradiol levels in the early portion of the cycle are used to determine the beginning of the fertile window, and the LH surge determines the end of the fertile window. The LH surge is typically detected one day before or after ovulation. Clearblue is FDA approved in the US as a LH test. Marquette users can opt to use the monitor alone or can also track changes in cervical mucus and/or basal body temperature.

FABM Apps and Devices

Over 1,000 smartphone applications are currently available to help people track their menstrual cycles. Most are not appropriate for pregnancy prevention because they lack data on whether the application can be used effectively as a contraceptive and do not provide transparent information about their accuracy at identifying the fertile days,[25] although the millions of people who have downloaded them do not necessarily know this. Furthermore, some apps with contraceptive effectiveness evidence have conducted direct-to-consumer advertising that may not be fully transparent.[26] Thus, providers should be prepared to be an informed resource for patients in identifying and selecting which apps provide accurate information and are appropriate for their particular needs. There are two main categories of apps for which some evidence exists to support use with (or as) FABMs to avoid pregnancy: apps that facilitate the use of an existing FABM and apps that use a predictive algorithm and are themselves a contraceptive method.

Apps that Facilitate Use of an Existing FABM

In theory, apps that replace pencil and paper charts (or other tools) for tracking various biomarkers are intended to maintain fidelity with the underlying FABM, including that the user (not the app) remains responsible for interpreting fertility signs to try to identify the fertile window. If an app accurately represents the FABM on which it is based, effectiveness for pregnancy avoidance could be the same as that for the underlying method, though to our knowledge, studies confirming this do not yet exist. Internet and/or smartphone apps exist for the Billings Ovulation Method, Standard Days Method,[13] TwoDay Method, and the Marquette Method.

Apps Based Upon Predictive, Embedded Algorithms

Many apps exist that purportedly employ predictive modeling to try to identify the fertile window for the user. Few have been empirically tested to determine their effectiveness for avoiding pregnancy, and most share no information about how their predictive modeling was developed, given intellectual property concerns. Only two such apps are currently FDA-cleared for use as contraception: Natural Cycles and Clue Birth Control (Clue is not yet available in the United States as of this printing).

In addition, some FABM users may use devices (often linked to basal body temperature thermometers), wearables, or other direct-to-consumer products that aim to help detect changes in biomarkers of fertility (some of which may also include predictive algorithms). For example, basal body temperature mini-computers such as LadyComp® or Daysy® have not at the time of this writing been assessed through standard prospective effectiveness studies (though some manufacturers have made claims about effectiveness).[27] Numerous wearables in existence or development aim to help track changes in biomarkers of fertility including cervical mucus, mean resting temperature, and quantitative urinary metabolites. Other direct-to-consumer devices include those that quantitatively measure urinary hormones and metabolites including LH, progesterone, and estrogen. None of these products has been assessed for use for pregnancy prevention through standard prospective effectiveness studies, although a few have been studied for ovulation detection.[28-30] Natural Cycles received FDA clearance to pull temperature data from the Oura ring for use within its algorithm.[31] The Oura ring collects temperature trend data, which automatically syncs to the Natural Cycles app. The FDA clearance to use the Oura ring with the Natural Cycles algorithm was based on validation studies using basal body temperature devices. Effectiveness data for this device/app combination for use in pregnancy prevention is not available.

Effectiveness

Successful use of FABMs for avoiding pregnancy depends on (1) the accuracy of the method in identifying the fertile window, (2) the ability of the person using the method (or the algorithm upon which the method is based) to correctly interpret the information to identify the fertile window, and (3) the ability of the user and their partner(s) to follow the instructions of the method—that is, to use a backup contraceptive method and/or avoid penile-vaginal intercourse on the days the method identifies as fertile. Motivation to avoid pregnancy by both members of the couple is a factor in successful use.[32] As noted above, while perfect use of each FABM may be defined differently, it includes consistently avoiding vaginal-penile intercourse or using an additional method on days of the menstrual cycle that are more likely to lead to pregnancy.

Among women in the United States who self-report use of either "rhythm or safe period by calendar" or a "safe period by temperature or cervical mucus test, natural family planning" as their contraceptive method, about 15 out of 100 will become pregnant in the first year of typical use,* based upon an unpublished estimate from an analysis of the 2006–2010 National Survey of Family Growth (NSFG) (which is adjusted for underreporting of abortion).[34,35]

Use of this estimate—which "lumps together" a range of FABMs—has been controversial, and warrants additional explanation. National surveys in the United States can theoretically be used to estimate typical-use effectiveness of individual FABMs, but this is challenging in practice, given the low utilization of FABMs broadly. Small numbers of users can lead to instability in estimates. For this reason, estimation of typical effectiveness for *individual* FABMs has not been possible in US surveys to date. To overcome this statistical limitation, analyses of NSFG data have "lumped" various FABM methods together to enable generation of an overall typical use estimate across all women who self-report using an FABM. However, greater than 80% of FABM use in recent NSFG surveys consists of self-reported calendar rhythm method use. Given colloquial use of terms such as "rhythm" (as described previously), individuals self-reporting use of these methods may include women not following formal rules for the Rhythm Method, but instead those who are attempting to time intercourse based on their own (correct or incorrect) understanding of the fertile period. Thus, such "lumped" estimates may not be applicable to individual FABMs but are provided to shed light on the typical experience of users in the United States who report using these methods.

Population-based survey data from the NSFG or other surveys have been used by experts to estimate typical-use failure rates for most other contraceptive methods. These surveys allow experts to monitor the actual experience across a range of contraceptive users with differing demographic characteristics. Typical- and perfect-use rates derived from clinical trials can also be considered, but they should be interpreted differently. Participants in clinical trials are more highly selected (and thus, less generalizable) than those in population-based surveys. In addition, their behaviors may be influenced by frequent contact with investigators and study staff, which may be particularly important for methods that are highly user-dependent, such as FABMs. Furthermore, many FABM clinical trials have used inappropriate

---

* This specific estimate was not published as part of the most recent NSFG effectiveness manuscript because the number of segments of use (257) did not meet the prespecified minimum of observations (50) per month for the first 12 months and should be interpreted with caution. This estimate is substantially lower than the estimate derived from the previous (2002) NSFG33 (24%); it is unclear if this change relates to instability in the estimates given the small number of women reporting use of these methods, to improved use of these methods between the two survey periods, or to other factors.

methodological approaches,[36,37] and estimates vary substantially by FABM studied, study quality, and country context.[37,38]

A systematic review published in 2018 comprehensively summarized the best available evidence on FABM effectiveness derived from clinical trials.[37] Of the 53 included studies, none were considered high quality, 21 were considered moderate quality, and 32 were considered low quality for the question of interest. Estimated perfect- and typical-use pregnancy probabilities for individual FABMs from the moderate-quality, prospective studies in the 2018 review are summarized later, along with some subsequently published estimates. As described previously, these are largely derived from clinical trials, and should thus be interpreted as "best-case scenarios." FABMs that have not yet been tested in standard contraceptive effectiveness studies are not described.

Methods Based on Tracking Days of the Menstrual Cycle

Standard Days Method

According to moderate-quality prospective studies, among 100 users, 11–14 will become pregnant during the first year of typical use[39–41] and five will become pregnant during the first year of perfect use.[40]

The Rhythm Method

No moderate- or higher-quality prospective studies estimating typical or perfect use rates for the rhythm method have been identified.

Clue Birth Control

Clue opts to use the upper bound of the confidence interval from their study, suggesting that 8 of 100 users will become pregnant during the first year of typical use and 3 will become pregnant during the first year of perfect use. The study was published in 2018 and has not been formally assessed for quality in a systematic review.[42] Although FDA-approved, Clue is not available in the United States at the time of this printing.

Methods Based on Observation of Cervical Secretions

TwoDay Method

According to a moderate-quality prospective study, among 100 new users, 14 will become pregnant during the first year of typical use and 4 will become pregnant during the first year of perfect use.[43]

Billings Ovulation Method

According to moderate-quality prospective studies, among 100 new users, 11–34 will become pregnant during the first year of typical use[23,24,44,45] and 1–3 will become pregnant during the first year of perfect use.[44,45]

Marquette Method (Mucus Only)

According to moderate-quality prospective studies, among 100 new users, 4–19 will become pregnant during the first year of typical use,[46-48] and 3 will become pregnant during the first year of perfect use.[46]

Creighton Model Fertility Care System

No moderate- or higher-quality prospective studies estimating typical or perfect use rates for this method have been identified; to date, analyses of this method have been conducted in a manner distinct from other contraceptive effectiveness calculations.

Methods Based Primarily on Tracking Changes in Basal Body Temperature

Natural Cycles

According to a moderate-quality prospective study, among 100 new users of Natural Cycles, 10 will become pregnant during the first year of typical use.[49] Estimates from several recently published studies, which have not undergone formal quality assessment in a systematic review, suggest that among 100 new users, 6–7 will become pregnant during typical use.[50-52] The newer studies also suggest that among 100 new users, 1–2 will become pregnant during the first year of perfect use.

Methods Based on Tracking Multiple Indicators of Fertility

Symptothermal Methods

According to a moderate-quality prospective study, among 100 new users of Sensiplan (one type of symptothermal method), 2 will become pregnant during 1 year of typical use and <1 will become pregnant during 1 year of perfect correct use.[22] However, according to moderate-quality prospective studies of other symptothermal methods (e.g., symptothermal single check, Thyma method), among 100 new users, 11–33 will become pregnant during 1 year of typical use,[21,23,24] and perfect use estimates are unavailable.

Methods Based on Urinary Hormone Monitoring

Marquette Method (Urinary Hormone-Based, or Urinary Hormone Plus Mucus-Based)

According to moderate-quality prospective studies, among 100 new users, 2–7 will become pregnant during 1 year of typical use.[46–48] In one study (197 users) of the monitor-only method, there were zero perfect-use pregnancies.[46]

Advantages

Characteristics of FABMs perceived by some to be advantages may be perceived by others as disadvantages.[1] For example, the importance of the partner's participation in method use is positive for some sexual partners, but the ability to negotiate the timing and circumstances of sexual activity is difficult to achieve for others. Some people choose FABMs precisely because of the opportunity for daily awareness of fertility signs or cycle day, while others may find this burdensome. For some, the lack of side effects and the ability to prevent pregnancy without the need of a device or medication offsets the fact that FABMs can be less forgiving of incorrect use as compared to some other methods of family planning.[53] In a recent survey of 1,400 users of the digital FABM Natural Cycles, 71% of users stated they began using the method to avoid hormone use.[54]

A subset of FABMs, often referred to as natural family planning (NFP), are used only in conjunction with abstinence during the fertile window due to religious reasons, such as religious prohibitions on using alternative methods (such as condoms) or engaging in nonpenile-vaginal sexual practices.[55] For some users, this link between NFP methods and religious teachings is desirable, while for others this is unacceptable.

Being knowledgeable about cyclic fertility may be beneficial, regardless of which family planning method a person uses or whether they choose to use family planning at all, in part because the method is adaptable to other purpose if fertility intentions change. FABMs and fertility awareness information in general can be used for a number of purposes:

1. ***To avoid pregnancy.*** For maximum effectiveness, users should abstain from penile-vaginal intercourse or use an additional method during days of higher fertility.
2. ***To become pregnant.*** Users have intercourse on the days that are most likely to lead to pregnancy. Depending on the method used, these may include certain days of the cycle, the days certain types of cervical secretions are observed, and/or the days when urinary estradiol metabolites and LH are highest. The day in which intercourse is most likely to lead to pregnancy appears to be the day prior to the actual day of ovulation.[2,3,56] A 2015 Cochrane review concluded that insufficient data are available to draw conclusions on the effectiveness of timed intercourse for the outcomes of live birth, adverse events, and clinical pregnancy.[57] However, none of the studies involved in this review included cervical mucus monitoring or urinary estrogen metabolite monitoring. Additionally, several subsequent studies have shown that use of apps with biomarkers of fertility may shorten time to pregnancy.[58,59] Also, many people trying to conceive are interested in and have positive feelings towards using an app,[60] despite a specific gender, income, and race normalization by some apps, which could contribute to social inequities.[61,62] In the specific situation of HIV, among serodiscordant couples who desire pregnancy, FABMs could be used to maximize the chances of pregnancy using timed intercourse, while minimizing exposure of the HIV-uninfected partner to the virus,[63] though other HIV prevention strategies remain important to minimize HIV transmission risk.[64]
3. ***To detect pregnancy.*** A postovulatory temperature rise sustained for 18 or more days is an excellent early indicator that pregnancy is underway.[65]
4. ***To detect impaired fertility.*** Charting fertility signs costs relatively little and can aid in diagnosing and treating fertility problems due to infrequent or absent ovulation. People who menstruate but do not ovulate tend to have meandering basal body temperature and cervical mucus patterns throughout the cycle, rather than the typical cyclic patterns.
5. ***To detect a need for medical attention.*** Changes in cervical and vaginal secretions, abdominal pain, prolonged menstrual bleeding, intermenstrual bleeding, and other signs or symptoms may indicate the need for further medical evaluation. This potential use of FABMs has not been well studied.

6. *To help contribute to medical knowledge.* In the era of FABM apps, some patients may appreciate being able to more easily contribute to updated and expanded information on normal and abnormal gynecologic function.[58,62,66] Some users may appreciate contributing in this way, but this desire would need to be counterbalanced with a understanding and an agreement about how their data would be protected and used.

Disadvantages and Cautions

FABMs are unforgiving of incorrect or inconsistent use, leading many to report higher typical-use pregnancy rates than most other methods, such as provider-dependent methods. While FABMs produce no physical side effects, they offer no protection against sexually transmitted infections (STIs), including infection with the human immunodeficiency virus (HIV). Some methods may also require an investment of time working with an experienced instructor.

Certain conditions and life stages that increase the likelihood of irregular/less predictable cycles may make FABMs more difficult to use, and those patients require more extensive counseling and follow-up:

- Recent childbirth
- Current breast/chestfeeding
- Recent menarche
- Anovulatory cycling as with polycystic ovary syndrome (PCOS)
- Recent discontinuation of hormonal contraceptive methods
- Approaching menopause

FABMs are also not recommended for persons who are unable to abstain or use other contraceptive methods during the fertile days or who are unable to negotiate the timing of intercourse. **Table 15-1** provides contraindications for particular FABM categories.

Special Issues and Populations

Acceptability

Family planning providers are less likely to routinely include information about FABMs than about other contraceptive methods.[67-69] A recent study of Title X providers revealed that 43% believed FABMs were not a viable option for most patients, 44% were neutral, and only 11% felt that FABMs were a viable option for most patients. Those who had more training on FABMs were more likely to offer them as an option.[67] A 2009 study in Canada demonstrated that most primary care physicians underestimate efficacy of FABMs and only a small proportion provide information about them.[69] (See Chapter 4, Person-Centered Reproductive Health Conversations and Contraceptive Counseling.)

Recent development of FABMs that are easy to use without detailed instructions or time with instructors may make FABMs more accessible for users and increase interest of providers in recommending these methods. It is relatively easy to incorporate a discussion of simpler methods such as Standard Days Method and TwoDay Method into the context of regular clinical or community-based services, thus potentially making these methods more widely available.[70] Also, newer algorithm-based FABM apps can be downloaded and used right away by patients with minimal instruction.

Table 15-1 Reasons Why Particular FABMs Could Be Contraindicated

Reasons	Calendar-Based Methods	Cervical Mucus Methods	Basal Body Temperature–Based Methods	Sympto-thermal Methods	Urinary Hormone–Based Methods
Irregular cycles	⊘				
Postpartum amenorrhea	⊘		⊘		
Reluctance or inability to interpret cervical mucus		⊘		⊘	
Reluctance or inability to measure basal body temperature			⊘	⊘	
Cycles with reproductive tract infections or individuals with chronic vaginitis that affect cervical mucus		⊘		⊘	
Intermenstrual bleeding not distinguishable from menstruation or that masks secretions	⊘	⊘		⊘	
Clinical detection of female genital cutting		⊘		⊘	

Data from Urrutia RP, Polis CB, Jensen ET, Greene ME, Kennedy E, Stanford JB. Effectiveness of fertility awareness-based methods for pregnancy prevention: a systematic review. Obstet Gynecol. 2018 Sep;132(3):591-604.

Some individuals, providers, and program managers worry that using FABMs will hamper one's sexual life, making the method less acceptable and leading to discontinuation. Analysis of intercourse patterns of users of the Sensiplan Method, Standard Days Method, and the TwoDay Method show that people who use these methods have intercourse as frequently as those who use other methods (average 4–6 coital acts per month).[70-72] The pattern of intercourse differs, however, as those who use FABMs tend to have sex more frequently during the infertile days and avoid intercourse during their fertile days.[70]

Safety

Unintended pregnancies among those who use FABMs usually result from having intercourse at the beginning or end of the fertile window, as users try to avoid intercourse on what they perceive to be the highest-risk days. Thus, concerns have been raised about a potential increased risk of birth defects or poor pregnancy outcomes in these pregnancies due to aged ovum or sperm. Research suggests that no such increased risks exist, with the possible exception of women who have had a prior spontaneous abortion.[73,74]

Sex Selection

A study of about 1,000 births showed no association between the timing of intercourse during the fertile window and the sex ratio at birth.[75] These results do not substantiate claims that it is possible to select the sex of the child by timing intercourse further from or closer to the time of ovulation.

Providing Fertility Awareness-Based Methods

Counseling

A critical component of providing FABMs is helping individuals and couples decide how they want to handle their fertile days (i.e., by abstaining or using another method) to avoid pregnancy. Those who choose to use an alternative method (such as a barrier method) on those days should be instructed on correct use of the alternative method and counseled accordingly.

A second critical component for providers is understanding that each FABM is unique and being conversant in how different FABMs may best serve different types of users. Providers should (1) be aware of published effectiveness data for individual FABMs, (2) be able to provide information to access the two FDA-cleared FABM apps, (3) consider learning how to instruct patients in simpler FABMs (e.g., Standard Days Method and TwoDay Method), and (4) consider building relationships with FABM instructors in their area, enabling them to refer patients for instruction in how to use the FABM of their choice. In a study of Title X providers, those who knew an FABM instructor in their area were more likely to recommend use of FABMs.[67]

Regarding learning time, it takes less than 20 minutes to learn that fertility should be considered likely on days 8 to 19 of the cycle and to keep track of cycle days (i.e., to use the Standard Days Method) or to learn how to notice the presence or absence of secretions (i.e., to use the TwoDay Method).[76] Additional counseling may improve correct use. Those using other FABMs typically need an instructor's teaching to observe, record, and interpret the fertility signs and patterns. However, this type of instruction is increasingly becoming available online. Based on general medical practice within the National Health Service in Great Britain, it takes approximately 4 to 6 hours over three cycles to teach symptothermal fertility awareness skills, including charting fertility signs (cervical secretions and basal body temperature) and identifying the fertile time.[77] The Billings Ovulation Method is typically taught in three 30- to 60-minute sessions over 3 months. The Marquette Symptohormonal Method is typically taught in two to three 30-minute sessions over several cycles (see **Figure 15-1**).

An interactive infographic to assist with counseling including effectiveness and features of the different FABMS is available at https://www.bmj.com/content/366/bmj.l4245.

Provider Training

Providers with an interest could certainly be trained as FABM instructors for individual methods (e.g., Billings Ovulation, Marquette, Symptothermal). The Reproductive Health National Training Center has several continuing medical education (CME) lectures available around FABM effectiveness and counseling (https://rhntc.org/search?keys=fabm) and has developed an e-learning module for providers around FABMs (https://www.ctcfp.org/fertility-awareness-based-methods-of-contraception/) (see **Figure 15-2**).

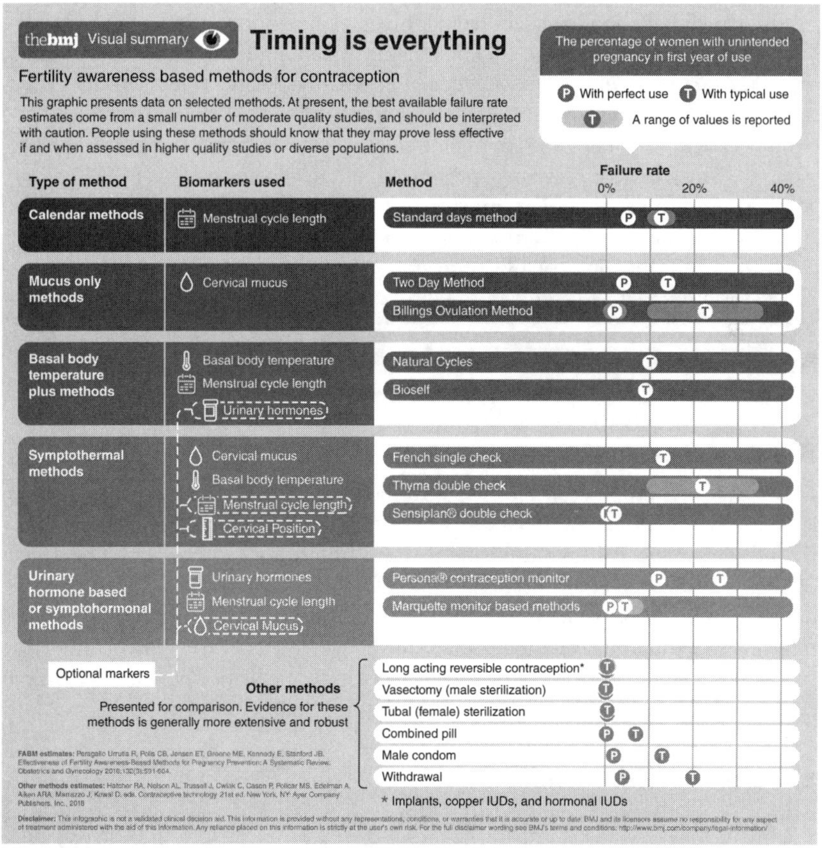

Figure 15-1 Fertility awareness-based methods for pregnancy prevention infographic.

Reproduced from Urrutia RP, Polis CB. Fertility awareness based methods for pregnancy prevention. BMJ 2019 Jul 11;366:l4245. doi: 10.1136/bmj.l4245

FABM Training Resources for Clinicians

- Standard Days Method: online, free, 1- to 2-hour training module (CME). https://www.fptraining.org/projects/standard-days-method-sdm
- TwoDay Method: online, free toolkit. https://toolkits.knowledgesuccess.org/toolkits/twoday/twoday-method-quick-start-approach
- Sensiplan™ teacher training (available at cost). https://www.sensiplan-im-netz.de/?page_id=910.
- Sensiplan™ handbook and workbook for learners of the method (available at cost). https://replyobgyn.com/store/product/sensiplan-the-handbook/.
- Billings Ovulation Method: religious components, teacher training, and online instruction for learners (available at cost). https://www.woombinternational.org/global-outreach.
- Marquette Symptohormonal Method: religious components, teacher training (available at cost). https://www.marquettemethod.com/

FABM Overview Documents

- World Health Organization's medical eligibility criteria for contraceptive use, Fifth Edition. https://www.who.int/publications/i/item/9789241549158
- Family Planning Handbook: A Global Handbook for Providers, Ch. 18, 2018. http://fphandbook.org/sites/default/files/global-handbook-2018-full-web.pdf
- Free webinars from the National Clinical Training Center for Family Planning, supported by the US Office of Population Affairs Title X Family Planning Program
    - Understanding and counseling potential users on fertility awareness-based methods for pregnancy prevention. https://vimeo.com/264114233
    - Effectiveness of fertility awareness-based methods for pregnancy prevention. https://vimeo.com/284453322
    - Fertility apps: a new approach for fertility awareness-based methods. https://vimeo.com/277724852

Figure 15-2 Resources on FABM for family planning providers.

Reproduced from Urrutia RP, Polis CB. Fertility awareness based methods for pregnancy prevention. BMJ 2019 Jul 11;366:l4245. DOI: 10.1136/bmj.l4245.

Starting the Method

Each FABM has unique rules for when to start using the method as contraception. Most can be used right away but users may need to consider themselves potentially fecund for a period of time until the patterns of fertility can be clearly identified. Billings Ovulation Method users are asked to avoid intercourse for the first cycle of use in order to better identify their basic infertile and fertile patterns of cervical mucus. Symptothermal method users must consider themselves potentially fertile and avoid intercourse until the first ovulation can be confirmed by both a change in cervical secretions and a basal body temperature shift.

Special Considerations

Users of hormonal birth control who want to transition to an FABM may have specific considerations for FABM use. For example, Standard Days Method and TwoDay Method have not been tested for use until at least 3 months after the hormonal method was discontinued. The symptothermal methods can be used right away but typically have special instructions for those discontinuing hormonal contraceptive methods.[22] Persons who use emergency contraception (EC) while using an FABM should be advised that EC could result in changes in cycle length and timing of ovulation in the forthcoming cycle.[78]

Persons who desire to use FABMs during postpartum amenorrhea and/or lactational amenorrhea will have unique challenges as they identify their first period of fecundity, which may occur before their first menstrual bleed. Some methods including the Billings Ovulation Method, Sensiplan, and the Marquette Method provide instructions for this category of users, but there has been little published data on method use among breastfeeding and postpartum individuals.[47,79-82]

The Billings Ovulation Method, Standard Days Method, and TwoDay Method have undergone effectiveness testing among populations with lower literacy and may be better options for those who have literacy or other learning challenges. Any of the FABMs should be able to be used in accordance with the teachings of most religions.[1]

For some FABM studies, particularly those done in the United States, populations evaluated tend to be higher income, White, monogamous, higher in religiosity, heterosexual, and cis-gendered.[37,61] Studies on the Billings Ovulation Method, Standard Days Method, and TwoDay Method have been conducted in African, Latin American, and Southeast Asian populations.[45] Additional research is needed to understand use of these methods among more diverse populations.

Managing Problems and Follow-Up

Some FABM users have difficulty interpreting their biomarkers of fertility. This is particularly common for the methods that require user interpretation (e.g., the Billings Ovulation Method and symptothermal methods). In this case, users should be encouraged to work with an experienced instructor to help with their interpretation and/or to determine if they will be able to use the method successfully going forward. Providers should also take this opportunity to review the users' fertility tracking. They may be able to identify a medical problem that needs treatment. In addition to promoting health, treatment of that problem may help users better interpret their signs of fertility in the future. For example, a user who perceives having copious cervical mucus on every day of the cycle who is unable to identify any mucus pattern may have an untreated vaginal infection. A user with no clear basal body temperature shift may be having regular bleeding without ovulation caused by undiagnosed PCOS or thyroid dysfunction.

Providers should consider offering new users of an FABM follow-up in 2–3 months to be sure that the method they have chosen is a good fit for them. This would allow the opportunity to partner with patients to choose a different FABM or a different contraceptive method. It may also offer providers who are less familiar with FABMs an opportunity to learn more about these methods through their patients' experiences and fertility tracking.

If a user has an unintended pregnancy, it may be helpful for them to have an FABM instructor review their FABM use to determine the cause; this may inform the patient's decision about whether to use the same method in the future. For example, if the assumptions the user made about fertility were incorrect, further instruction may help them have a lower chance of unintended pregnancy during future use.

USER INFORMATION

Instructions are presented here for a sample of FABMs which do not require working with a trained instructor: Standard Days Method, Clue Birth Control, TwoDay Method, and Natural Cycles. Other methods (e.g., Billings Ovulation Method, Symptothermal Methods, the Marquette Method) require working with a trained instructor; brief information is provided for how to access more information on the use of these methods.

Methods Based on Tracking Days of the Menstrual Cycle

Standard Days Method

The Standard Days Method can be used by people whose menstrual cycles are between 26 and 32 days long. Cycle length is the number of days from the first day of menstrual bleeding until the last day before your next menstrual bleeding starts. About 78% of menstruating people have cycles in the 26- to 32-day range.[26] If you choose this method, you will need to monitor your cycle lengths over time to be sure they stay in this range. Some people have longer or shorter cycles as they get older. If over the course of 1 year you have more than one cycle that is shorter than 26 days or longer than 32 days, you should use a different method. You may also need to wait a few months after stopping hormonal birth control to start using this method. To use the Standard Days Method, you will need keep track of the days of your menstrual cycle, starting with the first day of your menstrual bleeding in your next cycle.

1. Count the first day of your menstrual bleeding as day 1.
2. Continue counting every day.
3. **To prevent pregnancy.** On days 1 to 7, you can have penile-vaginal intercourse without backup contraception. (You may be bleeding on these days.) On days 8 to 19, you will have to use a different method, like a condom, or not have penile-vaginal intercourse. You can have penile-vaginal intercourse without backup contraception again starting on day 20 and for the rest of the cycle and until day 8 of the following cycle.
4. **To try to become pregnant.** You should try to have penile-vaginal intercourse without contraception frequently, as often as every day, between days 8 and 19 of your cycle.

Many people who use the Standard Days Method use CycleBeads to help them keep track of their cycle days. This color-coded string of beads with a ring you move daily helps to identify whether it is a fertile or infertile day and whether your cycle length is appropriate for using this method. Other users write the days down on a paper calendar. More recently, people are using the CycleBeads app (https://www.cyclebeads.com) on their smartphones (see **Figure 15-3**). To do this, enter the period start date (first day of bleeding) into the app, and the app tells you your daily fertility status and cycle length appropriateness.

Clue Birth Control

Clue Birth Control was developed for 18- to 45-year-old users who have had at least 12 months of predictable 20- to 40-day cycles. The length of your shortest and

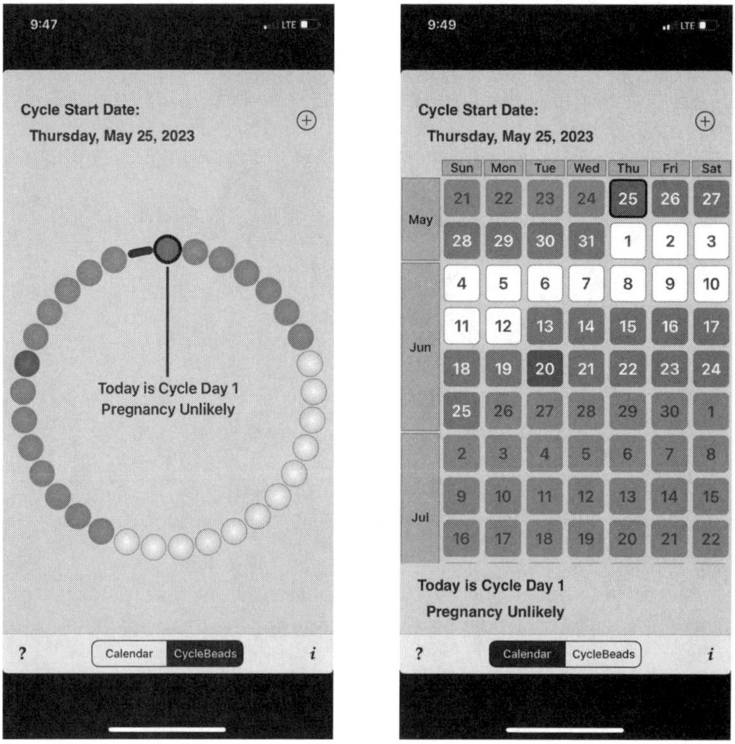

Figure 15-3 CycleBeads app for Standard Days Method.

Reproduced from Vasiliu A. 7 Fertility apps you can use to get pregnant or as birth control; 2015. https://www.bytesin.com/7-fertility-period-tracker-apps-can-use-get-pregnant-birth-control/

longest cycle should not vary by more than 9 days. At this time, the approved Clue Birth Control Internet app is not available for use. Please visit https://helloclue.com/ for information about future availability. If the app can be downloaded, you will be asked to input the date of the start of your most recent menstrual cycle. If you have kept track of prior menstrual cycle dates, you can also input those into the app. You will need to tell the app if you are trying to conceive or trying to avoid pregnancy. The app will then try to identify the days when you should either plan or avoid penile-vaginal sex (without backup contraception), depending on your goals. When each new menstrual cycle starts, you will enter the first day of menstrual bleeding into the app and keep track of which days are predicted to be high and low fertility. These days may change over time as the app gets used to your cycles and the variation in your cycles.

Methods Based on Observation of Cervical Secretions

TwoDay Method

The TwoDay Method (see **Figure 15-4**) is based on whether or not you have any cervical secretions present. You can track this when you go to the bathroom. If you notice any type of secretions "today" or "yesterday," you should consider yourself fertile "today." If you did not notice any secretions "today" or "yesterday," consider

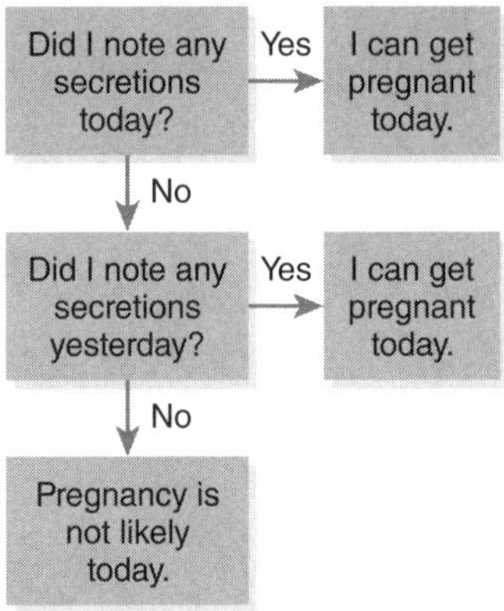
Did I note any secretions today?
Yes
I can get pregnant today.
No
Did I note any secretions yesterday?
Yes
I can get pregnant today.
No
Pregnancy is not likely today.

Figure 15-4 TwoDay Method Algorithm

Reproduced from the Institute for Reproductive Health. TwoDay method; n.d. https://www.irh.org/twoday-method/

yourself not fertile "today." There are lots of different ways to keep track of cervical secretions, like a paper calendar or a smartphone app. You should choose whatever works best for you.

To use the TwoDay Method:

1. Check for secretions every time before you urinate. You can:
   - Look at the secretions in your underwear or in toilet paper,
   - Touch the secretions on your vulva (the outside of your vagina), or
   - Feel the sensation of wetness at your vulva.
2. Determine whether you are fertile or not TODAY based on the presence or absence of secretions. You can ask yourself these two questions:
   - Did I notice ANY secretions of any type TODAY?
   - Did I notice ANY secretions of any type YESTERDAY?

   If you noticed ANY secretions TODAY or YESTERDAY, you can become pregnant if you have sex today. If you did not notice secretions of any type today or yesterday, you are not likely to get pregnant if you have sex today.
3. **To prevent pregnancy.** Avoid penile-vaginal intercourse without backup contraception if you noticed any secretions of any type either today or yesterday.
4. **To become pregnant.** Penile-vaginal intercourse is suggested as frequently as every day on days with secretions.
5. If you have continuous secretions for more than 2 weeks, or if your secretions are malodorous or irritating, you may have an infection that requires medical attention and should contact your health care provider.

Billings Ovulation Method

The Billings Ovulation Method teaches users to notice changes in their cervical mucus throughout the cycle. The Billings Ovulation Method was designed and has been studied with users relying on an experienced instructor to teach this method.

People who are interested in using this method can learn more here: https://billings.life/en/.

Methods Based Primarily on Tracking Changes in Basal Body Temperature

Natural Cycles

Natural Cycles can be used by anybody over the age of 18 who menstruates. You will have to purchase access to the Natural Cycles app (see **Figure 15-5**) and a basal body thermometer. The basal body thermometer must be accurate to two decimal places. You will then be asked to input the date of the start of your most recent menstrual cycle in the app. If you have kept track of prior menstrual period dates, you can also input those into the app. You will need to tell the app if you are trying to conceive or trying to avoid pregnancy. Then, you need to take your temperature first thing in the morning before getting out of bed and record it in the app. It is recommended to take your temperature at least 5 days out of the week (and ideally every day); if a user measures temperature less frequently, there will be a larger number of days identified as potentially fertile ("red days"). The app will predict when you can have or avoid penile-vaginal intercourse without backup contraception, depending on your goals. Be sure to check the app every day for the prediction about fertility; sometimes the fertile days predicted by the app can change after input of new information.

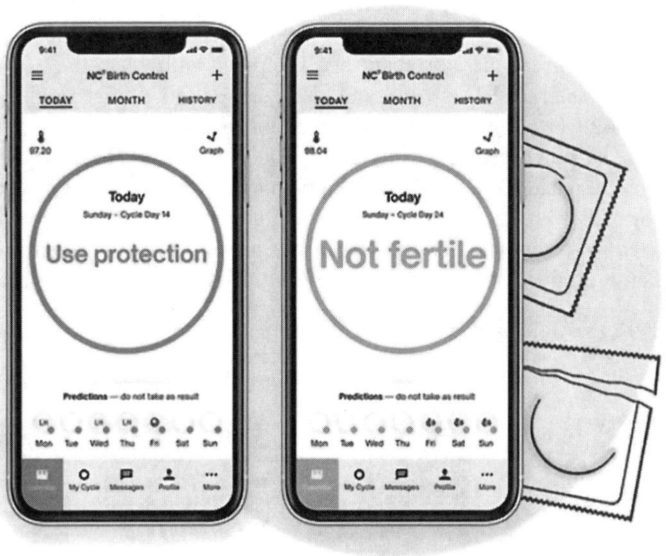

Image: Natural Cycles

Figure 15-5 Natural Cycles App

Courtesy of Natural Cycles.

Methods Based on Tracking Multiple Indicators of Fertility

Some people who are using an FABM prefer to observe more than one indicator of fertility. Most who use a symptothermal approach use both cervical secretions and basal body temperature (BBT) to try to identify the fertile time; some people additionally track cervical position, and some include monitoring cycle length (see **Figure 15-6**). There are several variants of the symptothermal method (e.g., Sensiplan™, or others taught by provider groups). Traditionally, people using a symptothermal method recorded their observations for various biomarkers with a paper-and-pencil chart. More recently, apps such as Kindara, Sympto, and Lady Cycle serve this purpose; patients record their observations, including their temperature, directly into the app, which stores this information so fertility status can be assessed according to the instructions of the method. However, there are no studies on the effectiveness of these apps, so it is not recommended to depend on their predictions. Instead, you can use the app to keep track of your observations and make your own predictions about fertility based on what you have learned with an experienced teacher. SensiplanTM is a symptothermal method that has been studied for effectiveness (see **Figure 15-7**). Users who are interested in this method can find instructors and written materials at the following websites: https://replyobgyn.com/store/and https://www.sensiplan.de/en.

Methods Based on Urinary Hormone Monitoring

Marquette Method users may observe multiple biomarkers of fertility including cervical mucus changes, basal body temperature changes, and urinary hormones (see **Figure 15-8**). However, the urinary hormone changes appear to be used with equal or better effectiveness on their own compared with when they are combined with other biomarkers. The Marquette Method is designed to be used together with the ClearBlue Fertility Monitor and compatible test sticks. The monitor and test sticks must be purchased and are readily available online. The Marquette Method has been designed to be used with the help of a trained instructor who can be found with this website: https://www.marquettemethod.com/. Protocols for use are targeted to specific user groups depending on their experience with the method and their reproductive category (e.g., regular cycles, postpartum, breastfeeding).

Author Disclosures—Urrutia: part of salary was paid for clinical work done July 2014 through March 2022 at Reply OB/Gyn& Fertility, a clinic focused on offering access to FABMs and FABM education. Polis: none.

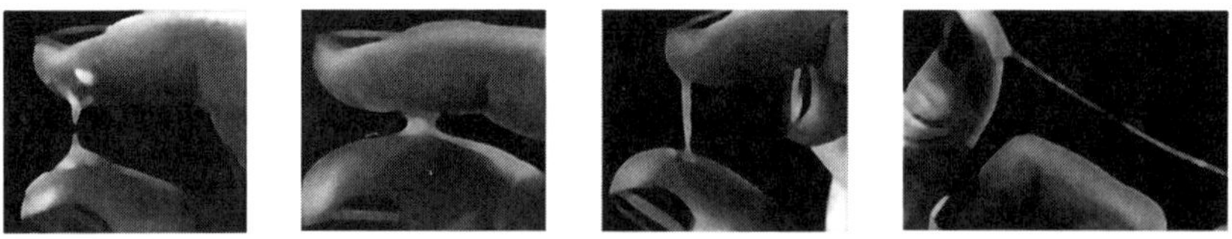

Whitish, creamy (S) | Milky or cloudy, tough elastic (S) | Whitish or yellowish, some tough elastic (S) | Translucent, stretchy (S+)

Figure 15-6 Cervical Mucus Secretions

Reproduced from Malteser Arbeitsgruppe NFP. Natural and safe: the handbook: family planning with Sensiplan™. CycleForth LLC; May 2019

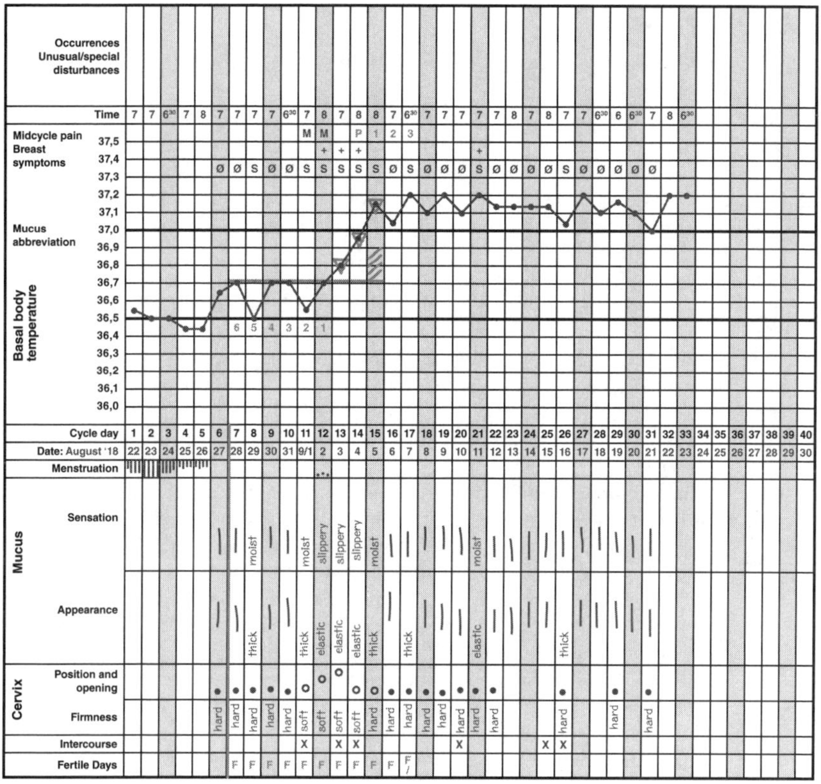

Figure 15-7 Symptothermal variations during a model menstrual cycle.

Reproduced from Malteser Arbeitsgruppe NFP. Natural and safe: the workbook: family planning with Sensiplan™. CycleForth LLC; May 2019. p. 12

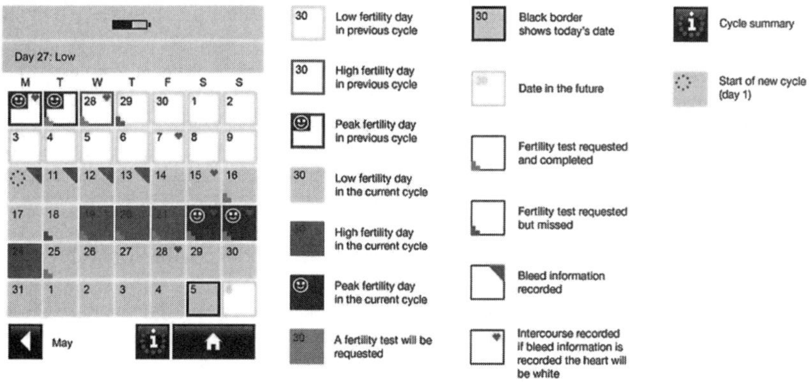

Example monthly summary screen and explanation of symbols

Figure 15-8 Marquette Model Chart

Courtesy of Marquette University.

References

1. Urrutia RP, Polis CB. Fertility awareness based methods for pregnancy prevention. BMJ. 2019;366:l4245.
2. Lynch CD, Jackson LW, Buck Louis GM. Estimation of the day-specific probabilities of conception: current state of the knowledge and the relevance for epidemiological research. Paediatr Perinat Epidemiol. 2006;20 Suppl 1:3-12.
3. Wilcox AJ, Weinberg CR, Baird DD. Timing of sexual intercourse in relation to ovulation. Effects on the probability of conception, survival of the pregnancy, and sex of the baby. N Engl J Med. 1995;333(23):1517-21.
4. Zinaman M, Drobnis EZ, Morales P, et al. The physiology of sperm recovered from the human cervix: acrosomal status and response to inducers of the acrosome reaction. Biol Reprod. 1989;41(5):790-7.
5. Faust L, Bradley D, Landau E, et al. Findings from a mobile application-based cohort are consistent with established knowledge of the menstrual cycle, fertile window, and conception. Fertil Steril. 2019;112(3):450-7.e3.
6. Stanford JB, Lemaire JC, Thurman PB. Women's interest in natural family planning. J Fam Pract. 1998;46(1):65-71.
7. Brewer M, Stevens L. Use of fertility awareness-based methods of contraception: Evidence from the National Survey of Family Growth, 2013-2017. Contraception. 2021;104(2):183-7.
8. Lamprecht VM, Grummer-Strawn L. Development of new formulas to identify the fertile time of the menstrual cycle. Contraception. 1996;54(6):339-43.
9. Kleinschmidt TK, Bull JR, Lavorini V, et al. Advantages of determining the fertile window with the individualised Natural Cycles algorithm over calendar-based methods. Eur J Contracept Reprod Health Care. 2019;24(6):457-63.
10. Najmabadi S, Schliep KC, Simonsen SE, Porucznik CA, Egger MJ, Stanford JB. Cervical mucus patterns and the fertile window in women without known subfertility: a pooled analysis of three cohorts. Hum Reprod. 2021;36(7):1784-95.
11. Arévalo M, Sinai I, Jennings V. A fixed formula to define the fertile window of the menstrual cycle as the basis of a simple method of natural family planning. Contraception. 1999;60(6): 357-60.
12. Bull JR, Rowland SP, Scherwitzl EB, Scherwitzl R, Danielsson KG, Harper J. Real-world menstrual cycle characteristics of more than 600,000 menstrual cycles. NPJ Digital Med. 2019;2:83.
13. Özçelik E, Uzuner A, Karahan Ö, Atici E, Özendi Y. Standard days method: comparison of CycleBeads and Smartphone app. Int Med. 2020;2(5):294.
14. Kambic RT, Lamprecht V. Calendar rhythm efficacy: a review. Adv Contracept. 1996;12(2):123-8.
15. Che Y, Cleland JG, Ali MM. Periodic abstinence in developing countries: an assessment of failure rates and consequences. Contraception. 2004;69(1):15-21.
16. Li D, Heyer L, Jennings VH, Smith CA, Dunson DB. Personalised estimation of a woman's most fertile days. Eur J Contracept Reprod Health Care. 2016;21(4):323-8.
17. Porucznik CA, Cox KJ, Schliep KC, Stanford JB. Pilot test and validation of the peak day method of prospective determination of ovulation against a handheld urine hormone monitor. BMC Womens Health. 2014;14:4.
18. Morris N, Underwood L, Easterling W. Temporal relationship between basal body temperature nadir and luteinizing hormone surge in normal women. Fertil Steril. 1976;27(7):780-3.
19. Guida M, Tommaselli GA, Palomba S, et al. Efficacy of methods for determining ovulation in a natural family planning program. Fertil Steril. 1999;72(5):900-4.
20. Martinez AR, van Hooff MH, Schoute E, van der Meer M, Broekmans FJ, Hompes PG. The reliability, acceptability and applications of basal body temperature (BBT) records in the diagnosis and treatment of infertility. Eur J Obstet Gynecol Reprod Biol. 1992;47(2):121-7.
21. Weeks JR. An evaluation of the use-effectiveness of fertility awareness methods of family planning. J Biosoc Sci. 1982;14(1):25-32.
22. Frank-Herrmann P, Heil J, Gnoth C, et al. The effectiveness of a fertility awareness based method to avoid pregnancy in relation to a couple's sexual behaviour during the fertile time: a prospective longitudinal study. Hum Reprod. 2007;22(5):1310-9.

23. Medina JE, Cifuentes A, Abernathy JR, Spieler JM, Wade ME. Comparative evaluation of two methods of natural family planning in Colombia. Am J Obstet Gynecol. 1980;138(8):1142-7.
24. Wade ME, McCarthy P, Braunstein GD, et al. A randomized prospective study of the use-effectiveness of two methods of natural family planning. Am J Obstet Gynecol. 1981;141(4): 368-76.
25. Johnson S, Marriott L, Zinaman M. Can apps and calendar methods predict ovulation with accuracy? Curr Med Res Opin. 2018;34(9):1587-94.
26. Hough A, Bryce M. Exaggerating contraceptive efficacy: the implications of the Advertising Standards Authority action against Natural Cycles. BMJ Sex Reprod Health. 2019;45(1):71-2.
27. Polis CB. Published analysis of contraceptive effectiveness of Daysy and DaysyView app is fatally flawed. Reprod Health. 2018;15(1):113.
28. Maijala A, Kinnunen H, Koskimäki H, Jämsä T, Kangas M. Nocturnal finger skin temperature in menstrual cycle tracking: ambulatory pilot study using a wearable Oura ring. BMC Womens Health. 2019;19(1):150.
29. Shilaih M, Clerck V de, Falco L, Kübler F, Leeners B. Pulse rate measurement during sleep using wearable sensors, and its correlation with the menstrual cycle phases, a prospective observational study. Sci Rep. 2017;7(1):1294.
30. Bouchard TP, Fehring RJ, Mu Q. Quantitative versus qualitative estrogen and luteinizing hormone testing for personal fertility monitoring. Expert Rev Mol Diagn. 2021;21(12):1349-60.
31. Natural Cycles Fertility App Wins FDA Clearance For Oura Ring Integration :: Medtech Insight [Internet]. (https://medtech.pharmaintelligence.informa.com/MT145673/Natural-Cycles-Fertility-App-Wins-FDA-Clearance-For-Oura-Ring-Integration)
32. Fehring RJ, Schneider M, Barron ML, Pruszynski J. Influence of motivation on the efficacy of natural family planning. MCN Am J Matern Child Nurs. 2013;38(6):352-8.
33. Kost K, Singh S, Vaughan B, Trussell J, Bankole A. Estimates of contraceptive failure from the 2002 National Survey of Family Growth. Contraception. 2008;77(1):10-21.
34. Sundaram A, Vaughan B, Kost K, et al. Contraceptive failure in the United States: Estimates from the 2006-2010 National Survey of Family Growth. Perspect Sex Reprod Health. 2017;49(1):7-16.
35. Sundaram A. FABM effectiveness in 2006-2010 NSFG data. 2017; In: Polis CB, ed. Personal Communication, 2017
36. Trussell J, Kost K. Contraceptive failure in the United States: a critical review of the literature. Stud Fam Plann. 1987;18(5):237-83.
37. Peragallo Urrutia R, Polis CB, Jensen ET, Greene ME, Kennedy E, Stanford JB. Effectiveness of Fertility awareness-based methods for pregnancy prevention: A systematic review. Obstet Gynecol. 2018;132(3):591-604.
38. Freundl G, Sivin I, Batár I. State-of-the-art of non-hormonal methods of contraception: IV. Natural family planning. Eur J Contracept Reprod Health Care. 2010;15(2):113-23.
39. Gribble JN, Lundgren RI, Velasquez C, Anastasi EE. Being strategic about contraceptive introduction: the experience of the Standard Days Method. Contraception. 2008;77(3):147-54.
40. Arévalo M, Jennings V, Sinai I. Efficacy of a new method of family planning: the Standard Days Method. Contraception. 2002;65(5):333-8.
41. Burkhart MC, de Mazariegos L, Salazar S, Lamprecht VM. Effectiveness of a standard-rule method of calendar rhythm among Mayan couples in Guatemala. Int Fam Plann Perspect. 2000;26(3):131.
42. Jennings V, Haile LT, Simmons RG, Spieler J, Shattuck D. Perfect- and typical-use effectiveness of the Dot fertility app over 13 cycles: results from a prospective contraceptive effectiveness trial. Eur J Contracept Reprod Health Care. 2019;24(2):148-53.
43. Arévalo M, Jennings V, Nikula M, Sinai I. Efficacy of the new TwoDay Method of family planning. Fertil Steril. 2004;82(4):885-92.
44. Bhargava H, Bhatia JC, Ramachandran L, Rohatgi P, Sinha A. Field trial of Billings ovulation method of natural family planning. Contraception. 1996;53(2):69-74.
45. Trussell J, Grummer-Strawn L. Further analysis of contraceptive failure of the ovulation method. Am J Obstet Gynecol. 1991;165(6 Pt 2):2054-9.
46. Fehring RJ, Schneider M, Raviele K, Rodriguez D, Pruszynski J. Randomized comparison of two Internet-supported fertility-awareness-based methods of family planning. Contraception. 2013;88(1):24-30.

47. Fehring RJ, Mu Q. Cohort efficacy study of natural family planning among perimenopause age women. J Obstet Gynecol Neonatal Nurs. 2014;43(3):351-8.
48. Fehring RJ, Schneider M. Effectiveness of a natural family planning service program. MCN Am J Matern Child Nurs. 2017;42(1):43-9.
49. Berglund Scherwitzl E, Gemzell Danielsson K, Sellberg JA, Scherwitzl R. Fertility awareness-based mobile application for contraception. Eur J Contracept Reprod Health Care. 2016;21(3): 234-41.
50. Berglund Scherwitzl E, Lundberg O, Kopp Kallner H, Gemzell Danielsson K, Trussell J, Scherwitzl R. Perfect-use and typical-use Pearl Index of a contraceptive mobile app. Contraception. 2017;96(6):420-5.
51. Pearson JT, Chelstowska M, Rowland SP, et al. Natural Cycles app: contraceptive outcomes and demographic analysis of UK users. Eur J Contracept Reprod Health Care. 2021;26(2):105-10.
52. Pearson JT, Chelstowska M, Rowland SP, et al. Contraceptive effectiveness of an FDA-cleared birth control app: Results from the Natural Cycles U.S. Cohort. J Womens Health (Larchmt). 2021;30(6):782-8.
53. Coombe J, Wigginton B, Loxton D, Lucke J, Harris ML. How young Australian women explain their use of condoms, withdrawal and fertility awareness: a qualitative analysis of free-text comments from the CUPID study. Cult Health Sex. 2021;24(11):1563-74.
54. Pearson JT, Rowland SP, Scherwitzl EB, Danielsson KG, Scherwitzl R. Adoption of a digital app-based fertility awareness based method of birth control in the US [04I]. Obstet Gynecol. 2020;135:92S-3S.
55. Obelenienė B, Narbekovas A, Juškevičius J. Anthropological and methodical differences of natural family planning and fertility awareness-based methods. Linacre Q. 2021;88(1):14-23.
56. Mu Q, Fehring RJ. Efficacy of achieving pregnancy with fertility-focused intercourse. MCN Am J Matern Child Nurs. 2014;39(1):35-40.
57. Manders M, McLindon L, Schulze B, Beckmann MM, Kremer JAM, Farquhar C. Timed intercourse for couples trying to conceive. Cochrane Database Syst Rev. 2015;(3):CD011345.
58. Stanford JB, Willis SK, Hatch EE, Rothman KJ, Wise LA. Fecundability in relation to use of mobile computing apps to track the menstrual cycle. Hum Reprod. 2020;35(10):2245-52.
59. Johnson S, Stanford JB, Warren G, Bond S, Bench-Capon S, Zinaman MJ. Increased likelihood of pregnancy using an app-connected ovulation test system: A randomized controlled trial. J Womens Health (Larchmt). 2020;29(1):84-90.
60. Blair D-L, Morgan HM, McLernon DJ. Women's perspectives on smartphone apps for fertility tracking and predicting conception: a mixed methods study. Eur J Contracept Reprod Health Care. 2021;26(2):119-27.
61. Grenfell P, Tilouche N, Shawe J, French RS. Fertility and digital technology: narratives of using smartphone app "Natural Cycles" while trying to conceive. Sociol Health Illn. 2021;43(1):116-32.
62. Favaro C, Pearson JT, Rowland SP, et al. Time to pregnancy for women using a fertility awareness based mobile application to plan a pregnancy. J Womens Health (Larchmt). 2021;30(11):1538-45.
63. Liao C, Wahab M, Anderson J, Coleman JS. Reclaiming fertility awareness methods to inform timed intercourse for HIV serodiscordant couples attempting to conceive. J Int AIDS Soc. 2015;18:19447.
64. Zia Y, Velloza J, Oluoch L, et al. Use of fertility awareness methods as a component of safer conception for women in HIV-serodifferent relationships in Kenya. Reprod Health. 2021;18(1):73.
65. Kotz HL. Basal body temperature record: a multipurpose diagnostic tool. JOGN Nurs. 1973;2(4):43-8.
66. Tatsumi T, Sampei M, Saito K, et al. Age-dependent and seasonal changes in menstrual cycle length and body temperature based on big data. Obstet Gynecol. 2020;136(4):666-74.
67. Webb S, Cheng A-L, Simmons R, Peragallo Urrutia R, Jennings V, Witt J. A mixed-methods assessment of health care providers' knowledge, attitudes, and practices around fertility awareness-based methods in Title X clinics in the United States. Womens Health Rep (New Rochelle). 2020;1(1):354-65.
68. Stanford JB, Thurman PB, Lemaire JC. Physicians' knowledge and practices regarding natural family planning. Obstet Gynecol. 1999;94(5 Pt 1):672-8.

69. Choi J, Chan S, Wiebe E. Natural family planning: physicians' knowledge, attitudes, and practice. J Obstet Gynaecol Can. 2010;32(7):673-8.
70. Sinai I, Arévalo M. It's all in the timing: coital frequency and fertility awareness-based methods of family planning. J Biosoc Sci. 2006;38(6):763-77.
71. Gnoth C, Frank-Herrmann P, Freundl G, Kunert J, Godehardt E. Sexual behavior of natural family planning users in Germany and its changes over time. Adv Contracept. 1995;11(2):173-85.
72. Lehmiller JJ, Garcia JR, Gesselman AN, Mark KP. Less sex, but more sexual diversity: changes in sexual behavior during the COVID-19 coronavirus pandemic. Leis Sci. 2020;:1-10.
73. Gray RH, Simpson JL, Kambic RT, et al. Timing of conception and the risk of spontaneous abortion among pregnancies occurring during the use of natural family planning. Am J Obstet Gynecol. 1995;172(5):1567-72.
74. Simpson JL, Gray R, Perez A, et al. Fertilisation involving ageing gametes, major birth defects, and Down's syndrome. Lancet. 2002;359(9318):1670-1.
75. Gray RH, Simpson JL, Bitto AC, et al. Sex ratio associated with timing of insemination and length of the follicular phase in planned and unplanned pregnancies during use of natural family planning. Hum Reprod. 1998;13(5):1397-400.
76. Germano E, Jennings V. New approaches to fertility awareness-based methods: incorporating the Standard Days and TwoDay Methods into practice. J Midwifery Womens Health. 2006;51(6):471-7.
77. Knight J. The complete guide to fertility awareness. Routledge; 2016.
78. Gainer E, Kenfack B, Mboudou E, Doh AS, Bouyer J. Menstrual bleeding patterns following levonorgestrel emergency contraception. Contraception. 2006;74(2):118-24.
79. Bouchard T, Fehring RJ, Schneider M. Efficacy of a new postpartum transition protocol for avoiding pregnancy. J Am Board Fam Med. 2013;26(1):35-44.
80. Perez A, Labbok M, Barker D, Gray R. Use-effectiveness of the ovulation method initiated during postpartum breastfeeding. Contraception. 1988;38(5):499-508.
81. Labbok MH, Stallings RY, Shah F, et al. Ovulation method use during breastfeeding: is there increased risk of unplanned pregnancy? Am J Obstet Gynecol. 1991;165(6 Pt 2):2031-6.
82. Redmond JJ, Jensen ET, Stanford JB, Greene ME, Kennedy E, Urrutia RP. Effectiveness of fertility awareness-based methods for pregnancy prevention during the postpartum period. Contraception. 2022;114:32-40.

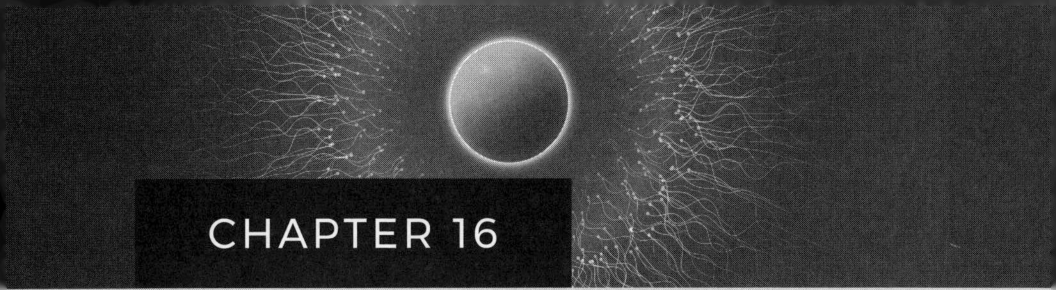

CHAPTER 16

On-Demand, Internal Methods

Kelly Culwell, MD, MPH
Joely Pritzker, MS, FNP-C

KEY POINTS

- These are nonhormonal, "on-demand" methods. They were previously referred to as vaginal barrier methods.
- Only spermicides are available over the counter or online without clinician consultation.
- Many can be combined with each other or other methods to increase contraceptive efficacy or to provide noncontraceptive benefits.
- Typical-use failure rates for these methods are generally higher than for other methods, but they still significantly reduce the user's risk for pregnancy compared to unprotected intercourse.
- All are rapidly reversible.
- Consider offering a prescription for emergency contraception in advance for users of these methods.

On-demand, internal contraceptive methods have features that appeal to many potential users in the United States. Encompassing a wide range of formulations and styles, including gels, foams, films, diaphragms, and cervical caps, these methods are controlled by the person who could potentially become pregnant and/or who is seeking sexually transmitted infection (STI) protection. Sometimes referred to as pericoital methods, these contraceptive options are used at the time of coitus, without ongoing contraceptive use outside of acts of intercourse. They are all nonhormonal and thus can be used by patients with a wide range of medical conditions or other health risks. Some are available over the counter, eliminating the need to get a prescription. For methods requiring a prescription, most can be obtained via telehealth visit, removing the barrier of an in-clinic office visit. Many are modestly priced and do not need to be purchased until the need arises, although being prepared by having the chosen method available in advance promotes consistent use.

All on-demand methods are rapidly reversible. Additionally, most reduce transmission of at least some STIs. Should a person become pregnant while using these methods, exposure in early pregnancy is not associated with nor is expected to cause increased risk of birth defects in the fetus.[1,2]

These methods were previously referred to as vaginal barrier methods. Newer language—on-demand, internal, and/or pericoital—has emerged to more fully capture the diversity of individuals who opt to use these options. Transgender and nonbinary individuals may use different terminology to refer to the anatomical vagina. (See Chapter 4, Person-Centered Reproductive Health Conversations and Contraceptive Counseling and Chapter 22, Contraception for Lesbian, Gay, Bisexual, Transgender, Gender Diverse, Queer/Questioning, Intersex, Asexual, and Other Individuals.) In addition to its contraceptive purpose and vaginal STI protection, the internal condom (FC2) is commonly used for anal sex for STI protection.

While the language used to describe these methods continues to evolve, internal contraceptive agents are among some of the oldest recorded methods of contraception. Egyptian papyri described vaginal plugs of honey, gum, acacia, and crocodile dung, as well as sponges. Different societies used local products such as bamboo paper, seaweed, and willow leaves. In early second-century Rome, soft wool balls combined with acidic fruit and nuts were described.

Contraceptive methods in this category continue to attract growing interest. In May 2020, the US Food and Drug Administration (FDA) approved a new method in this group. Phexxi, a novel, nonhormonal pH modulator gel, joins the list of existing options individuals can choose from. Older on-demand, internal methods have been retooled and reintroduced: the original female condom (Reality) returned as FC2, and the Caya diaphragm has effectively replaced the older, more specifically sized diaphragms. The FemCap was redesigned slightly and is the only cervical cap available in the United States. See **Table 16-1** for summary of characteristics of internal, on-demand methods available in the United States.

On-demand, internal barriers, spermicides, and gels may be used alone or in combination with each other to enhance efficacy. The cervical cap and diaphragm must be used together with a contraceptive gel or spermicide. Most of these methods can be combined with other hormonal and nonhormonal methods, from intrauterine devices (IUDs) to coitus interruptus, to enhance pregnancy and/or STI protection. Some exceptions exist. For example, the internal and external condoms should never be used together; diaphragms and cervical caps should not be used with IUDs.

Because of the large gap between failure rates with perfect and typical use, providers should engage in shared decision-making conversations with patients who opt to use these methods. (See Chapter 4, Person-Centered Reproductive Health Conversations and Contraceptive Counseling.) These conversations can help troubleshoot potential challenges, encourage precoital practice, and offer patients who select these methods a prescription (with refills) for emergency contraception, if desired. (See Chapter 18, Emergency Contraception.)

Mechanism of Action

All internal barriers, spermicides, and gels prevent fertilization by blocking sperm transport into the upper genital tract. The internal condom provides a physical barrier that lines the vagina and partially shields the perineum and does not require use of a

Table 16-1 Summary of Characteristics of Internal, On-Demand Contraceptive Methods

			First-Year Failure Rates With			
Device	**Description**	**Mechanism**	**Correct and Consistent Use**	**Typical Use**	**Availability**	**Special Features**
FC2 (female condom) Scented Unscented	Nitrile sheath with an unattached flexible ring at top to aid in placing and stabilizing ring in vaginal vault and a second ring attached at bottom remaining outside the introitus	Barrier	5%	21%	Requires prescription from clinician or online provider	■ Single use protection ■ Can be placed in advance ■ One size ■ No need for spermicide
Caya (contraceptive diaphragm)	Silicone rubber molded device with circular nylon spring to stabilize against vaginal walls; spermicide-filled cup fits over cervix	Barrier & spermicide	6% to 12.5%	12% to 18%	Requires prescription Clinician may need to check size and placement	■ Reusable ■ Can be used for up to 2 years ■ Single-size can accommodate 65- to 80-mm vaginal measurement ■ Used with spermicidal gel ■ May be used for multiple acts of intercourse by adding more spermicide vaginally

(continues)

Table 16-1 Summary of Characteristics of Internal, On-Demand Contraceptive Methods *(continued)*

			First-Year Failure Rates With			
Device	**Description**	**Mechanism**	**Correct and Consistent Use**	**Typical Use**	**Availability**	**Special Features**
FemCap (cervical cap)	■ Silicone rubber "brimmed hat" ■ Spermicide placed inside and outside dome, which covers cervix ■ Brim stabilizes the cap against vaginal walls	Barrier & spermicide	13.5% at 6 months		Requires prescription from clinician or online provider	■ Reusable for up to 1 year ■ Sized by obstetric history with clinician confirmation ■ Used with spermicidal gel ■ May be used for up to 48 hours for multiple acts without adding more spermicide
Phexxi	■ pH modulating vaginal gel	Inhibits sperm motility through acid buffering of seminal fluid	6.6% to 9.9% at 7 cycles	13.6% at 7 cycles	Requires prescription from clinician or online provider	■ Single-use prefilled applicator ■ Can be used immediately before or up to 1 hour before intercourse ■ Additional application needed for each act of vaginal intercourse ■ Has lubricating properties
Spermicides*	■ Foams, films, gels, creams, and suppositories releasing nonoxynoyl-9	Spermicide	18%	28%	Over-the-counter	Different formulations may need different lead times to activate within the vagina, but all are active as single agents for 1 hour of use

*For more details on different types of spermicides, see Table 16-2

spermicidal agent. Other barriers combine both a physical barrier, to prevent sperm entry into the cervical canal, and a spermicide agent, to kill sperm. The diaphragm and the cervical cap hold the spermicide in place in front of the cervix. Phexxi, the pH modulator gel, maintains an acidic vaginal environment, inhibiting sperm motility.

Advantages

For Internal, On-Demand Contraceptives as a Group

1. **User-controlled.** These methods are primarily controlled by the person who can potentially become pregnant, including initiation and discontinuation. No partner action is needed, especially for those methods that can be applied in advance of coitus. However, negotiation with a partner/partners may be required for the visible methods, as well as for those that need to be placed at the time of coitus.
2. **Available if external condom not an option.** Internal barriers may be used when the external condom cannot or will not be used.
3. **Nonhormonal.** Options in this contraceptive group do not affect endogenous hormone production or menstrual cycles. May be used by people who desire to avoid the use of hormonal contraception or who have medical contraindications to its use.
4. **On-demand contraception.** These methods are used only at the time of coitus. For individuals or couples with infrequent intercourse, this may significantly reduce costs and the burden of maintaining ongoing contraceptive methods.
5. **Immediately reversible.** All these methods are immediately reversible simply by discontinuing their use. There is no delayed return to fecundity.
6. **Portable.** Generally, these methods are portable. They can fit into a bag to be carried with the user.
7. **May be combined.** Many of these methods can be combined to enhance efficacy or to provide other noncontraceptive benefits. They may also be used during potential fertile days identified by fertility awareness methods.

Disadvantages

For Internal, On-Demand Contraceptives as a Group

1. **Must be used with every act of intercourse without exception to achieve maximum effectiveness.** Intermittent or inconsistent use greatly increases failure rates.
2. **Requires comfort and proficiency with vaginal or rectal placement.** The user must be comfortable placing the method in the vagina or rectum (for STI protection) or having a partner place it. Comfort with touching one's own genitals or placing materials into the vagina or rectum varies greatly among individuals.[3]
3. **Coitally dependent use.** The user needs time to place the method prior to genital-to-genital contact. This may diminish spontaneity in some sexual encounters.
4. **Higher failure rates.** As a group, these methods can significantly reduce the chance of pregnancy, particularly in comparison with nonuse of contraception. In typical use, however, they have higher failure rates than other contraceptive methods, similar to the behavioral methods, such as coitus interruptus or fertility awareness methods.

Internal Condom (FC2)

The internal condom currently available in the United States is called FC2. It is a single-use, soft, flexible, tapered nitrile sheath that measures 180 mm in length. The sheath is shaped to fit the anatomy of the vagina. The outer ring is oval with a diameter of 72 mm. The mid-body diameter of the sheath is 66 cm, while the inner ring that ultimately rests at the vault has a 58-mm diameter. This inner ring, made of polyurethane, helps introduce the sheath through the introitus and guide the condom to the top of the vagina. The inner ring is not affixed to the rest of the device. The inner ring should be placed as far into the vault as it can go, above the pubic bone; it may cover the cervix or it may be positioned above the cervix in the vault. The outer polyurethane ring is attached to the edge of the condom and folds over on itself slightly to cover the user's external genitalia partially or completely. The nitrile sheath is coated internally and externally with a silicone-based lubricant to ease placement and to reduce friction during coitus. This lubricant does not have any spermicidal activity. Nitrile is a synthetic rubber latex and can be used by those with allergies to natural latex. Nitrile is an impermeable material that effectively transmits body heat but blocks passage of microbes. Petroleum- and silicone-based products can be used as lubricants without threatening the integrity of the condom. FC2 can be stored anywhere at a wide range of temperatures. The FC2 is available by prescription, but can be readily obtained via telehealth visits.

As a dual protection method, FC2 offers both pregnancy and STI prevention. In October 2018, FC2 was reclassified by the FDA as a "single use internal condom," a change from its previous classification as a "single use female condom."[4] This reclassification acknowledges the well-established practice of using internal condoms for anal sex. Public health groups and community organizations support internal condoms for anal sex, though this use is still technically off-label. For this STI prevention purpose, it is recommended that the inner ring be removed after placement and before beginning anal intercourse.

Effectiveness

The FDA quotes FC2 first-year failure rates as being the same as its predecessor—the Reality female condom. Those rates are 5% with perfect use and 21% with typical use. Clinical experience shows that users may experience an early learning curve. Rates of functional failures, such as breakage, slippage, invagination, and misdirection, were highest in the first five uses of internal condoms (7.7% with the first condom, decreasing to 1.2% with the fifth one).[5] For this reason, some experts advise not relying exclusively on the internal condom for the first several uses of the method. It is recommended that emergency contraception prescriptions be offered in advance for FC2 users in case of method failure. (See Chapter 18, Emergency Contraception.)

Advantages

In addition to the general advantages for the methods listed previously, the internal condom has specific features that many users can appreciate.

1. **STI protection.** The nitrile material is a synthetic rubber latex that blocks passage of even the smallest sexually transmitted pathogens, either into or out

of the condom, thus providing protection to both the user and the partner. The FDA-approved labeling states that FC2 is indicated for the prevention of human immunodeficiency virus (HIV)/acquired immunodeficiency syndrome (AIDS) and other STIs with vaginal use. It can be used off-label for protection during anal sex. In some studies, focus groups have found that users perceive the internal condom as an improvement over the male condom for STD protection, because it is in the user's control.[6] Also, it provides some amount of vulvar coverage, theoretically providing additional protection against STIs passed through skin-to-skin transmission, such as herpes simplex virus, though additional research is needed.[7]

2. **Can be used when external condoms cannot be used**—either due to issues of erectile dysfunction or because the penis cannot be fitted with any of the currently available external condoms.[8] Studies show that placement of the external condom is associated with softening or complete loss of erection in nearly one-third of condom users.[9] This is not an issue with the internal condom.
3. **Can be used during menses.** The internal condom does not interfere with menstrual flow, but it also does not control it.
4. **May be used in the postpartum period.** Sizing is not needed.
5. **Pleasure-positive features.** Nitrile warms to body temperature and avoids the cold shock that can be associated with latex condoms. The internal condom can be placed up to 8 hours before coitus, avoiding disruption during the arousal/excitement phase. If the silicone lubricant on the internal condom does not provide satisfactory lubrication, the user can add more silicone-based, petroleum-based, or water-soluble lubricants. There is a potential for the internal condom to increase sexual pleasure at several points. The pressure of the inner ring along the vaginal wall, the stimulation of the outer ring against the clitoris, and the pressure of the inner ring against the head of the penis have all been reported as sources of heightened sexual pleasure with use.

Disadvantages

1. **Proper placement required for efficacy.** Comfort and accuracy with the placement procedure requires practice. Users in focus groups described the placement procedure as "too complicated" with the two rings,[10] though a more recent study demonstrated more ease of use.[11] Even those experienced with diaphragm use have commented that the ring is slippery. The relatively high rates of early functional failures can be discouraging, but those errors diminish rapidly and after continuous uses, technical problems are very rare. The penis must be guided (usually manually) into the condom to prevent misdirection, avoiding entering the space between the vaginal wall or anus and the outer surface of the condom. For some couples, guiding the penis can be enjoyable, but for others it might be less appealing.
2. **Vaginal placement.** The internal condom requires users to be willing and able to place the condom vaginally. Many patients are unfamiliar with the anatomy of the vagina. They do not know that the vagina is a flexible, expandable space that is between 6.5 cm to 12.5 cm in length.[12] It is also finite, with items placed inside unable to migrate to other areas of the body. This unfamiliarity raises several concerns that affect acceptance of the female condom:

- Some potential users surveyed were very concerned about the size and shape of the female condom. In one study, a participant was quoted as saying, "By (just) looking at it, (FC2) it was scary and even the shape looks horrible." Another said, "The ring looked scary, in fact, the entire structure of FC2 is very scary."[10]
- Many of the potential users thought they needed to advance the condom to the level of the cervix to cover it, like a diaphragm. They did not appreciate that coverage of the cervix is automatic. The inner ring just needs to rest in an area that will not apply pressure to internal structures.
- It cannot be used with other vaginal methods such as a diaphragm, cervical cap, sponge, or NuvaRing® because the inner ring of FC2 fits into the same place at the cervix.

Appropriate counseling, including the use of visual aids, can help address anatomical misconceptions as it relates to internal condom use.

3. **Visible.** The female condom is quite visible to the partner. Use without the partner's knowledge may not be successful or realistic.[6]
4. **Potential discomfort with use.** Incorrect introduction or misplacement introduces the possibly of discomfort or pain with its use.[10]
5. **Prescription only.** Though FC2 was originally approved by FDA for over-the-counter provision, it is not currently available without a prescription. However, it can be easily prescribed via telemedicine, as it does not require an examination or device placement and has very few medical limitations to use.
6. **Local irritation.** Some users have reported a burning sensation, rash, or pruritus during use of the FC2 or for hours following its removal.
7. **May interrupt sex.** If it has not been placed in advance, placement may interrupt sex.
8. **Relatively expensive.** The cost of this single-use condom may present challenges for users who must pay out-of-pocket for the condoms and who may have frequent acts of intercourse.

USER INSTRUCTIONS FOR FC2*

Users should be reminded to place the FC2 with every act of intercourse. The FC2 can be placed up to 8 hours before intercourse. These are intended as single-use devices. One study did find that, in monogamous relationships, carefully washing and disinfecting the device enabled reuse of a single internal condom for up to 10 times—however, this practice is not recommended at this time.[13,14] After removal, the outer ring of the sheath should be twisted closed to contain the ejaculate. The used condom should be disposed of in the solid waste garbage. Providers should caution users not to combine internal condoms with external condoms.

* These instructions are intended to guide providers in educating patients in how to use their method.

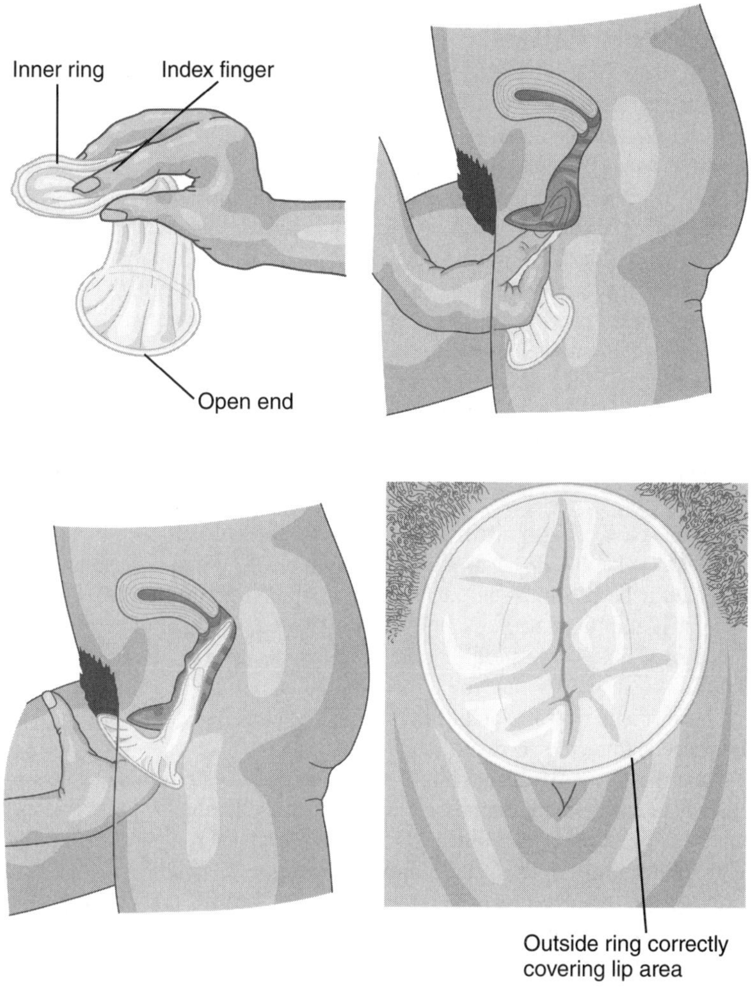

Figure 16-1 FC2 step-by-step detailed instructions.

Figure 16-1 displays step-by-step instructions for use of FC2 that are included in the packaging. Additional information, including video demonstrations, is available at https://fc2.us.com/how-to-use/.

The most important points are:

1. Place the inner ring of the condom as high in the vagina as comfortably possible.
2. Ensure that the penis enters into the condom and stays within the condom during intercourse.
3. After the penis has exited the condom, grasp the outer ring of FC2 and twist it once to seal the fluids inside the condom before removing it.
4. Use a new condom with each act of intercourse.

Caya Diaphragm

The Caya diaphragm has essentially replaced earlier dome-shaped, fitted diaphragms in the United States. Caya (previously known as the SILCS diaphragm) is a lightweight, reusable silicone rubber device molded with a circular nylon spring. It measures 75 mm in length and 67 mm in maximum width. Its spring enables Caya to be used for a variety of vaginal and cervical sizes and in users who have different degrees of vaginal support. Caya can be used by patients who would have been fitted with older diaphragms ranging in size from 65–80 mm. About 80% of potential users meet that criterion. The Caya has two cuplike structures. The large, oval, dome-shaped cervical cup fits over cervix and holds spermicide in place over the cervical os. The smaller, everted removal dome tucks behind the symphysis and facilitates removal of the device. The rim is flexible and eases placement through the introitus. Textured dimples on the sides of the rim help the user identify the best position to grasp the unit during placement. Caya has a notch in the anterior edge of the rim to reduce pressure against the urethra. (See **Figure 16-2**.) Caya fits people with varying body types. The user must be willing and able to place and remove the device or be able to enlist partner help to perform those tasks.

The Caya diaphragm is used with spermicide.[15] About 1 teaspoon of spermicide should be put into the larger cup and spread around the rim just before placement. If additional acts of coitus are anticipated, Caya should be left in place and additional spermicide should be added into the vagina. Caya should be kept in place for at least 6 hours after the last act of coitus, but it should not be left in the vagina for more than a total of 24 hours. One Caya can be reused for up to 2 years before it needs to be replaced.

While the Caya is available in only one size and does not need to be sized as specifically as earlier diaphragms were, it is still available only by prescription. Professional examination is recommended to ensure proper fitting and to support the patient's ability to use, place, and remove it correctly. The clinician needs to have clean models in the office available to verify the fit. "Test fit" units are available online for clinicians to use for this function.

Studies show that 75% of interested patients easily placed Caya correctly following instructions. With additional instruction, 94% were able to place, position, and remove this diaphragm.[16] After the patient has placed Caya, perform a bimanual exam to confirm correct fit and correct placement. Check to see that:

- The larger dome completely covers the cervix.
- The back rim of Caya is past the cervix and pressed comfortably against the posterior fornix.
- There is no buckling of the rim. Such buckling would suggest that the Caya is too large.
- There is no spinning of Caya when you attempt to rotate it in place. Such spinning would demonstrate that Caya is too small for this user.
- The front rim tucks behind the symphysis pubis.

Also verify that the patient is able to place and remove Caya while in the office.

Effectiveness

In the Caya clinical trial with 450 diaphragm users, in which 150 used Caya with N-9 spermicide, the total 6-month Kaplan-Meier cumulative pregnancy

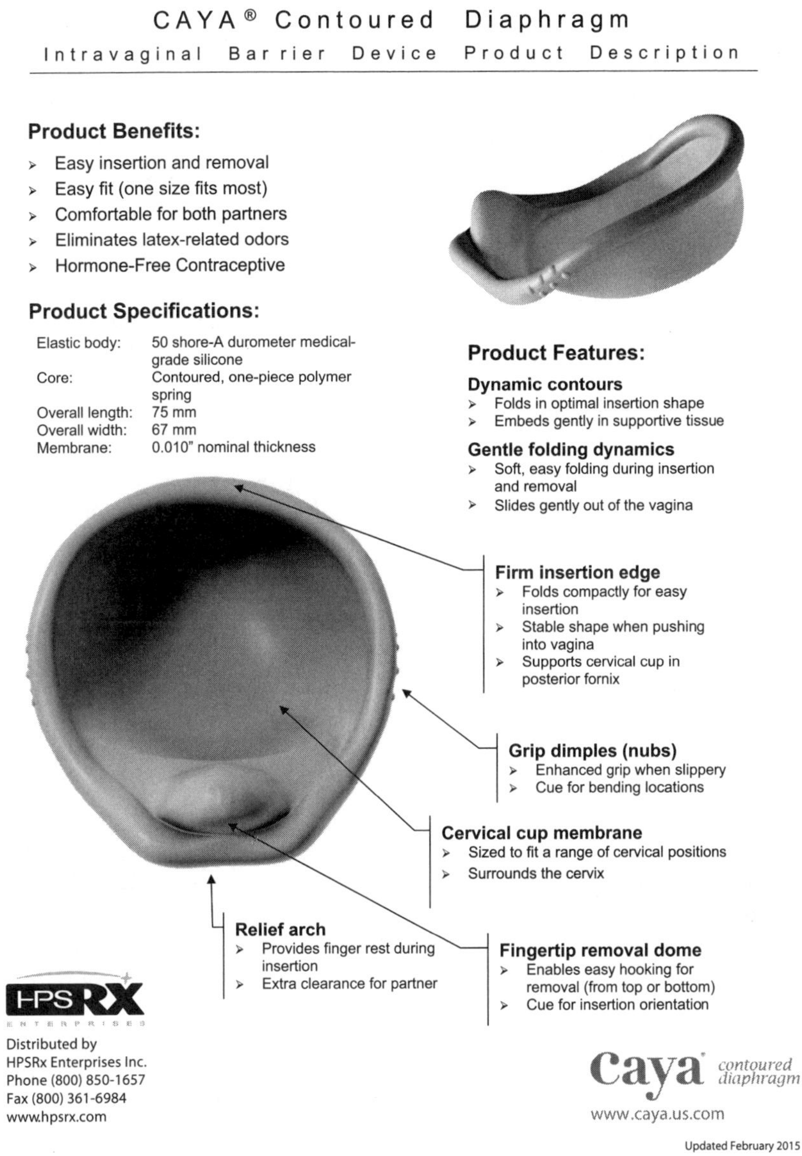

Figure 16-2 Caya Diaphragm

Reproduced from Caya contoured diaphragm. Intravaginal barrier device product description. 2015.

rate for Caya was 12.5% (95% CI, 5.4%–19.5%). This rate was annualized to 14% with correct and consistent use and 17.8% total failure rate with use seen in that trial (not equivalent to typical-use failure rates quoted for other methods). This compared to the 6-month pregnancy rate of 10.7% with the older, standard, fitted round-domed diaphragms.[16] Reanalysis of these data for this book yielded estimates that varied slightly from published estimates—failure rates with perfect use of 16.3% and total failure rate of 17.4%. It is

It is still possible to order a silicone Milex wide-seal diaphragm in either an arching or omniflex style from the manufacturer. These silicone diaphragms are available in eight sizes ranging from 60–95 mm in 5-mm increments. The use of these more traditional dome-shaped diaphragms has diminished in part because very few practitioners have fitting rings to enable formal sizing (fitting) of diaphragms. However, it is feasible to size someone reasonably well on bimanual exam by measuring the distance between the tip of your middle finger of your examining hand when it is placed against the posterior vaginal fornix and the mark on the upper edge of your index finger where it touches the inferior edge of the pubic arch. This is much like measuring the conjugate angle in obstetrics. The number of millimeters in length to the nearest 5 mm gives you the size of diaphragm needed. After the patient purchases the diaphragm, you would test it in place using all the same maneuvers you used to check Caya to confirm correct sizing prior to having the patient use it for contraception.

generally recommended that a prescription for emergency contraception be offered to users of Caya to be used if case difficulties are encountered with its use. (See Chapter 18, Emergency Contraception.)

Advantages

In addition to the general advantages offered by barrier methods, Caya offers the following advantages:

1. **Reusable.** The diaphragm is reusable for up to 2 years. The only element that needs to be periodically resupplied is the spermicide, which is available over the counter.
2. **Some STI risk reduction.** Diaphragms traditionally have been associated with lower risks for transmitting cervical infection, such as gonorrhea and chlamydia.[17] However, no confirmation of that protection with the newer diaphragms has been published.
3. **Can be used with other methods.** The Caya diaphragm can be combined with methods except IUDs, FC2 (internal condoms), and cervical caps to enhance pregnancy protection.
4. **Diaphragm is not often detected** by the partner during coitus and usually does not bother the partner.
5. **Multiple acts of intercourse possible.** More spermicide must be added in the vagina in front of device before each act.
6. **Easy to clean.** The material does not absorb odors.
7. **Pleasure-positive features.** The spermicide may provide vaginal lubrication. The diaphragm can be placed in advance of coitus, so sex is not interrupted.

Disadvantages

1. **Proper placement required for efficacy.** Users need practice to learn correct placement and removal. Placement of the Caya diaphragm is generally quickly mastered, but over 5% of potential users are not able to learn how to place the device, even with extra instruction and extensive encouragement. The product instructions suggest that the user practice placement a few times before relying on it for pregnancy protection.

2. **Clinician visit suggested and prescription required.** For patients who have never used a diaphragm before, a clinician visit is highly recommended to confirm appropriate fit. For patients who know their previous diaphragm size, an exam may not be necessary. Caya is available only by prescription.
3. **May interrupt sex.** If the Caya is not placed in advance, the need to do so before intercourse may disrupt sexual pleasure.
4. **Postcoital delays.** Caya must be left in place for 6 hours following last act of coitus.
5. **Twenty-four-hour limit**. Caya must be removed within 24 hours of placement.
6. **Not for immediate postpartum use.** Caya should not be used in the immediate (6 week) postpartum period until the cervix and vagina normalize and correct sizing can be reconfirmed.

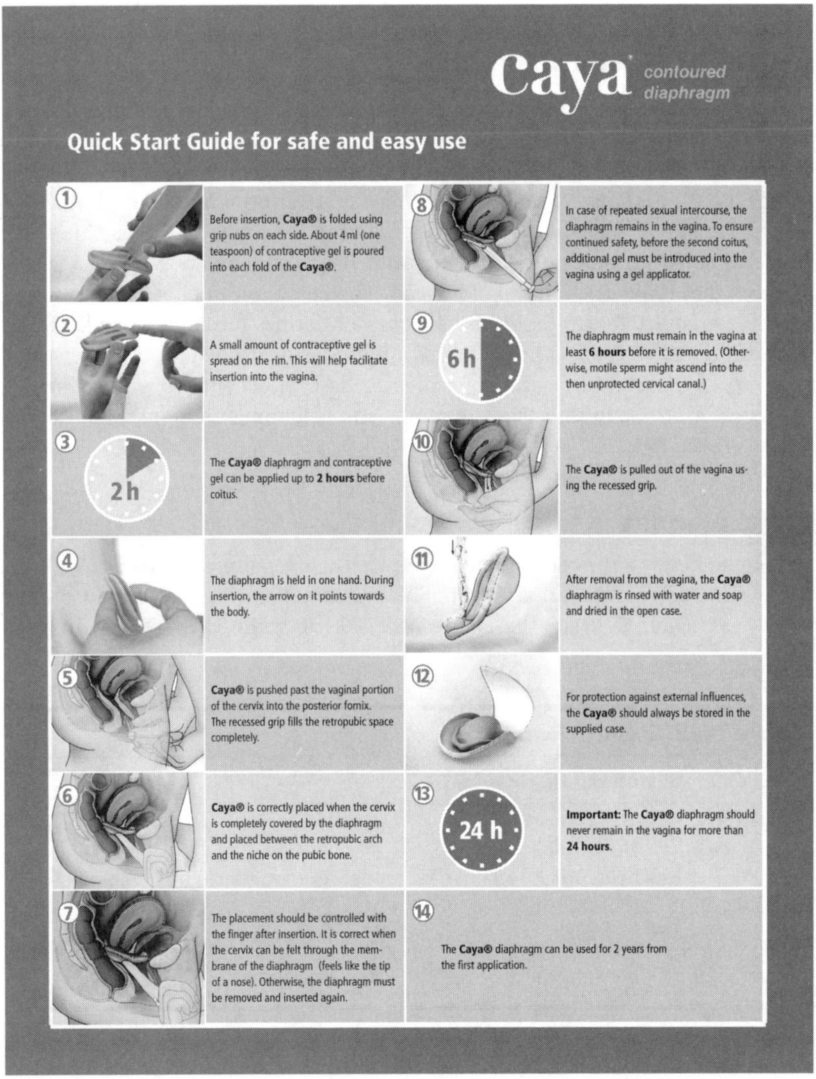

Figure 16-3 Detailed instructions on placement and removal of Caya diaphragm.

Reproduced from Caya contoured diaphragm. Quick start guide for safe and easy use. n.d. https://www.medintim.de/assets/downloads/caya-quick-start-guide-en.pdf

USER INSTRUCTIONS FOR CAYA DIAPHRAGM*

Instructions for use of Caya diaphragm are clearly outlined in English and Spanish in the manufacturer's 10-step illustrated guidelines. We have reprinted the English language instructions in **Figure 16-3**. The website https://www.caya.us.com/how-to-use-caya/ has a video that also helps instruct patients in detail, in English and Spanish, on how to use this device.

After removal, the diaphragm should be rinsed clean, dried, and stored in a clean, dry container.

FemCap Cervical Cap

FemCap is a reusable, surgical-grade silicone device shaped like a brimmed hat. It has a bowl that fits over the cervix, a rim that fits high into the vaginal vault, and a variable-size brim that stabilizes the unit against the vaginal walls. The wider brim fits against the posterior vaginal wall and the narrower brim fits anteriorly. Spermicide is placed into the bowl, in the space between the brim, on the outside of the bowl and along the outer surface of the brim. There is a thin loop of silicone over the bowl that facilitates removal of the cap. The FemCap can be used for multiple acts of intercourse for up to 48 hours. Some authorities recommend adding extra spermicide into the vagina prior to repeat episodes of intercourse, but that is not necessary. The user must wait 6 hours after the last act of coitus to remove the cap. The cap is available in three sizes generally corresponding to the user's obstetrical history (**Table 16-2**).

Effectiveness

FemCap's efficacy varies depending on parity. The overall pregnancy rate with use is 23% in a 12-month period. For nulliparous users and parous users without a history of vaginal delivery, the failure rate is 14%, while for parous individuals

Table 16-2 Sizing of FemCap

Size	Obstetrical History
22 mm	Nulligravida
26 mm	Has been pregnant, but has not delivered full term baby vaginally
30 mm	Has delivered a term baby vaginally

Data from FemCap. n.d. How to determine which FemCap™ is right for you. https://femcap.com/new/size-matters/

* These instructions are intended to guide providers in educating patients in how to use their method.

with a history of vaginal delivery, the failure rate is 29%.[18] In a small randomized 6-month trial, the pregnancy rate with FemCap was nearly twice that of the All-flex diaphragm (13.5% vs. 7.9%).[19] (Because of small number of users in the United States, the FemCap was not included among the methods assessed in Chapter 5, Efficacy, Safety, and Comparative Side Effect.) It is generally recommended that the user be offered a prescription for emergency contraception to have available in case any difficulties are encountered with FemCap use. (See Chapter 18, Emergency Contraception.)

Advantages

1. **Easy to fit (clinician benefit).** Size is determined by obstetric history. It does not require an in-clinic pelvic exam, though one may be recommended to confirm appropriate fit.
2. **Well tolerated.** The FemCap has fewer side effects than seen with older cervical caps or diaphragms: fewer urinary tract infections and no increase in cervical dysplasia.
3. **Multiple acts possible with one use.** Users can participate in multiple acts of intercourse for up to 48 hours with no additional spermicide needed, but some users report unpleasant odor with such prolonged use.
4. **Reusable.** One FemCap can be used for 1 year. Annual replacement is encouraged to reduce risk of recurrent vaginal infection.
5. **Easy to clean.** The silicone does not absorb odors.

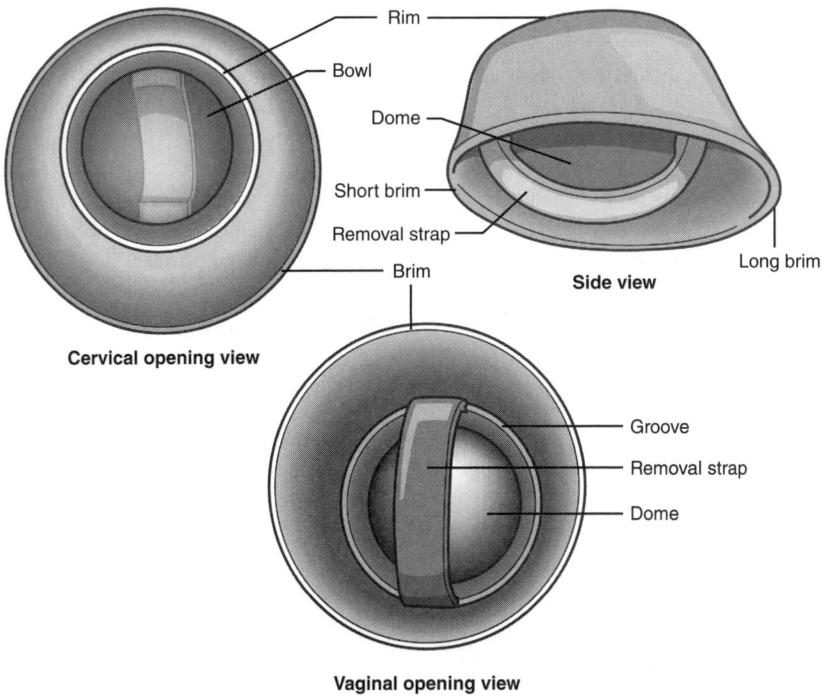

Figure 16-4 FemCap

6. **May be combined with other methods.** FemCap can be used together with other methods except IUDs, diaphragms, or sponges.
7. **Pleasure-positive features.** The user may place the device in advance of coitus, so sex is not interrupted. It is compatible with lubricants and petroleum-based, water-based, or silicone lubricants can be used.

Disadvantages

1. **Prescription required and clinician exam suggested.** FemCap requires a prescription, and a pelvic exam is recommended after obtaining the cervical cap to confirm appropriate cervical coverage.
2. **Will not fit all interested potential users.** Only 80% of potential users can be fit. The device will not work if the cervix is adherent to or flat against the vaginal wall.
3. **Vaginal placement.** Users need to be willing and able to place device vaginally. New users need to practice correct placement.
4. **May interrupt sex.** If it has not been placed in the vagina in advance, placement may interrupt sex.
5. **Postcoital delays.** Users must leave the cap in place for 6 hours after last coitus.
6. **Resizing needed.** The cap needs to be resized after the user gives birth or has a miscarriage or abortion.
7. **Potential discomfort or problems with use.** Users and their partners may feel discomfort or pain, especially if the cap is placed incorrectly.[20]
8. **Potential for cervical trauma.** Some users have reported blood on the cap, indicating some degree of cervical trauma—usually with removal. However, there have been no reports of increased infection or dysplasia with FemCap use.
9. **May be difficult to remove.** The addition of a removal strap did not increase ease of removal.[20] Some patients need directed counselling to apply pressure directly against the dome to break suction before trying to remove the cap.
10. **Limitations on use.** FemCap should not be used during menses; in the immediate (6 week) postpartum period until cervix normalizes; or with cervicitis, pelvic inflammatory disease, or history of toxic shock syndrome.

USER INSTRUCTIONS FOR FEMCAP*

1. Place the FemCap at least 15 minutes in advance of coitus.
2. Wash your hands and genitalia.
3. Place ¼ teaspoon of spermicide into the inside of the bowl and ½ teaspoon in the groove between the brim and outside of the bowl. Spread spermicide over brim.
4. Find a comfortable position, like when placing a tampon or menstrual cup (standing with one leg elevated, lying on back, or squatting). Feel for your cervix.

---

* These instructions are intended to guide providers in educating patients in how to use their method.

5. Squeeze the sides of the cap together to make it thin for introduction into your vagina.
6. Separate the lips of the vulva and slide the FemCap through the opening to your vagina with the longer brim placed against the lower side of your vagina (the side closer to your anus).
7. Advance the cap inside your vagina in a downward angle toward your anus and deeper into your vagina, until it reaches your cervix.
8. Rotate the cap to cover your cervix. Tug on strap to make sure it will stay in place during intercourse.
9. Leave the cap in place for 6 hours after last intercourse. Do not use the cap for longer than 48 hours for any one use.

Removal

1. Wait 6 hours after last act of sex to remove FemCap.
2. Assume a position that allows you to feel your cervix. Squatting works well for many users.
3. Introduce one or two fingers into your vagina.
4. Slip your finger under the strap and press against dome of the cap to break the suction (make a dimple in it).
5. Hook the strap with your finger, rotate it slightly, and gently pull the cap down toward the opening of your vagina.
6. Check for blood. Rinse the cap with soap and water. Dry. Store in clean, dry container.

Spermicides

Spermicides are available over the counter without a prescription in a variety of formulations—as gels and creams (usually for use with other barrier methods), foams (used as single agents or as the agent used before additional acts of intercourse with diaphragms), sponges (need to add liquid to activate spermicide), foaming suppositories, and films (which need 15 minutes to melt within vagina). See **Table 16-3**.

All spermicides currently available in the United States use N-9 as their active ingredient. N-9 acts as a detergent to disrupt the membranes of the sperm's flagella

Table 16-3 Spermicides Used As a Single Agent

Base or Carrier	Onset of Action	Duration of Action
Foam ■ Aerosol container	Immediate	≤ 60 min.
Creams and gels ■ Single-use packets ■ Reusable applicator	Immediate	≤ 60 min.
Suppositories	10-15 min.	≤ 60 min.
Film	15 min.	≤ 60 min.

and body to immobilize or destroy it. However, N-9 can have the same disruptive effect on the epithelial cells of the vagina, cervix, and rectum, which can increase the transmission of HIV. Therefore, patients at high risk for HIV should not use spermicides alone or in combination with other methods.[21] That would include those who have higher-risk partners as well as couples who are HIV-serodiscordant. Even in patients with low risk for STIs, the detergent action of N-9 can cause vaginal or penile irritation that can preclude its use.

Spermicidal gels, creams, and foam are commonly marketed for use with a diaphragm, but they can also be used alone for contraception. One application delivers 52.5 mg to 150 mg of N-9, depending on the product: the spermicide concentration ranges from 8% to 12.5% in foams, and from 2% to 4% in gels and creams. Foams are useful for immediate application in case another method malfunctions (condom slipped off, etc.).

Spermicidal suppositories can be used alone for contraception or with an external or internal condom. Suppositories have a spermicide concentration of 3% to 5% and provide 100 mg to 125 mg of N-9. Adequate time between placement and intercourse (10 to 15 minutes depending on the product) is essential for the spermicide to dissolve and disburse.

Spermicidal film containing N-9 can be used alone for contraception or with condoms, or, more rarely, with diaphragms or cervical caps. Each paper-thin sheet of film has a spermicide concentration of 28% and contains 72 mg to 100 mg of N-9.

The *contraceptive sponge* is a single-use spermicide. This small, pillow-shaped polyurethane sponge contains 1 gram of N-9 spermicide. The concave dimple on one side is designed to fit over the cervix and decrease the chance of dislodgement during intercourse. The other side of the sponge is covered with a woven polyester loop to facilitate removal.

The sponge protects for up to 24 hours, no matter how many times intercourse occurs. After the last act of intercourse, the sponge must be left in place for at least 6 hours before it is removed and discarded. Wearing the sponge for longer than 24 hours is not recommended because of the rare risk of toxic shock syndrome. **Beginning in 2020, the only contraceptive sponge marketed in the United States was unavailable due to manufacturing issues. At the time of this writing, it is unknown when or if the product will be available again in the future.**

Mechanisms of Action

Spermicidal preparations consist of two components: (1) a carrier/base (gel, foam, sponge, cream, film, suppository, or tablet) and (2) a chemical available in different doses and concentrations to kill the sperm. The carrier/base helps disperse the spermicide in the vagina. In the case of viscous gel and foam, the formulation itself may provide both lubrication and an additional barrier effect. Most formulations provide protection if sperm is released within 60 minutes of use. Later acts of intercourse require that additional spermicide be added to the vagina before intromission.

When combined with other barriers (cervical cap, diaphragm, or condoms), spermicide boosts the effectiveness of those methods.[22]

Effectiveness

Spermicides are among the least effective of all modern methods of family planning.[23] With correct and consistent use, spermicides as a single agent have a

16% first-year failure rate. With typical use, that rate rises to 21%, again demonstrating that methods requiring initiation at or around the time of coitus can have larger gaps between potential protection offered and actual protection achieved. Formulations with higher concentrations of N-9 are more effective.[24] There do not appear to be any differences in efficacy by delivery system for the same dose of spermicide.[23] It is recommended that a prescription for emergency contraceptives be offered to users to have on hand if they have a problem with correctly using spermicide with any act of coitus. (See Chapter 18, Emergency Contraception.)

Some researchers have attributed the relatively higher rates of pregnancy with spermicides to the user instructions that are provided in these over-the-counter methods. In one analysis, the "how to use" sections were found to be hard to understand, with reading levels that ranged from 8th to 12th grade and with line drawing illustrations that were fairly small. Overall, none of the products had instructions that scored high on all the features that make instructions user-friendly.[25]

Researchers have developed models that can predict patients who will have < 5% pregnancy risk with spermicides. For example, users aged over 35 who engage infrequently in intercourse and have low parity are more likely to use spermicides with greater success.[26] In general, it has been difficult to develop meaningful estimates of efficacy for these methods because of the widely varying failure rates in different studies.[24]

Sponge Effectiveness

The efficacy of the contraceptive sponge has been analyzed separately from the other types of spermicides. The failure rates for the sponge are similar to those seen with other spermicides—12% with correct and consistent use and 17% with typical use. However, some studies seem to indicate higher failure rates with parous users (20% perfect use and 27% typical use) compared to nulliparous users (9% perfect use and 14% typical use). A Cochrane systematic review found two studies to compare the efficacy of the contraceptive sponge to the traditional fitted, domed diaphragms. A US study found 12-month pregnancy rates for the sponge versus diaphragm were 17.4% versus 12.8%. In a UK study, those rates were 24.5% versus 10.9%.[27]

Advantages

1. **Readily available.** Spermicidal products are available over the counter without prescription and can be purchased online or in stores.
2. **Pleasure-positive features.** Spermicidal gel, creams, and foams can provide additional lubrication with intercourse.
3. **Flexible timing of placement.** Users can insert spermicide immediately before or up to one hour prior to intercourse so the sex act does not need to be interrupted.
4. **Postpartum use allowed.** Spermicidal products can be used postpartum, but only after lochia has stopped.
5. ***For sponge only.*** The sponge material absorbs ejaculate and may be less messy.

Disadvantages

1. **May require negotiation with partner.** The limited 1-hour duration of action may prevent opportunities for advance placement and may interrupt sex.
2. **Delayed onset of activity.** Spermicidal suppository and film require 15 minutes to melt and activate, which may interrupt coitus.
3. **May be messy.** Some forms (foams, gel) may be messy during and after coitus. Douching and perhaps bathing is to be discouraged for at least 6 hours following coitus. (Douching is discouraged in virtually all situations because it disrupts the vaginal defense system. Here it could also diminish the effectiveness of the spermicide.)
4. **Can cause local reaction or urinary tract infections.** Spermicide ingredients can cause irritation, allergic-type reactions, or dermatitis affecting the vagina, vulva, penis, anus, or oral cavity.
5. **Limited candidates.** Spermicidal products should not be used by those at high risk for HIV. Also, those with allergies to the ingredients cannot use the products.
6. **Taste may be unpleasant.**

USER INSTRUCTIONS FOR SPERMICIDES*

The product packaging for each product provides directions for use. Foams and gels are placed by an applicator into the vagina as close to the cervix as possible and are immediately active. Suppositories and films also need to be placed as close to the cervix as possible and must be put in the vagina 10–15 minutes prior to intercourse to allow time for the suppository or film to melt and disperse. Incomplete dissolution of a suppository may reduce its contraceptive efficacy and may cause an uncomfortable gritty sensation or friction for one or both partners. Placing film on the tip of the penis for insertion is not recommended; the film will not have adequate time to dissolve, and it may not be properly placed to adequately cover the cervical os.

The sponge should be removed from the packaging and wet thoroughly until visibly sudsy. The sponge is folded upward, with dimple side up and placed deep in the vagina. The loop will be on the bottom for easier removal. After placement, the sponge is immediately effective. There is no need to delay intercourse. The sponge must be left in place for at least 6 hours after sex, but not longer than 30 hours in total.

Vaginal pH Modulator

The vaginal pH modulator, Phexxi, is a vaginally administered gel that was approved by the US FDA in May 2020 for use as an on-demand method of contraception.[28] It comes in a box of 12 prefilled, individually wrapped, single-use

---

* These instructions are intended to guide providers in educating patients in how to use their method.

disposable applicators and is only available by prescription. Phexxi is immediately active upon vaginal application or can be applied up to an hour before vaginal intercourse.

Phexxi, originally studied under the name ACIDFORM, is an acid-buffering gel that modulates vaginal pH to the range of 3.5–4.5, even in the presence of alkaline semen.[29] The active ingredients are L-lactic acid, citric acid, and potassium bitatrate, which are all either naturally occurring in the human body or naturally found in food or as food additives.[30] The applicator is similar to many other vaginally administered products with a cap and plunger and is made of high-density polyethylene.

While Phexxi is approved as a standalone contraceptive method, it has been shown to be compatible with all other barrier forms of contraception including internal and external condoms and diaphragms.[2] Phexxi also has lubricating properties based on the inactive ingredients forming the gel base and was cleared by the FDA as a personal lubricant in 2004, but never marketed for this purpose.

A Phase 2B study found that Phexxi decreased acquisition of chlamydia and gonorrhea by 50% and 78%, respectively, in women with a history of recently treated infection with either chlamydia or gonorrhea.[31] Unfortunately, results of a larger Phase 3 trial failed to confirm these findings making the future development of Phexxi for STI protection uncertain.[32]

Effectiveness

In an initial Phase 3 study conducted in the United States and Russia, Phexxi was found to be noninferior to a commercially available N-9–containing spermicidal gel.[33] In a follow-up study conducted in the United States only, the seven-cycle cumulative typical use pregnancy rate (the primary endpoint used for FDA approval) was 13.7% (95%, CI 10.0–17.5)[34] and the seven-cycle rate with perfect use ranged from 6.7% to 9.9%, depending on the method used to calculate evaluable perfect-use cycles and the definition of per-protocol, on-treatment pregnancies.[35]

Mechanism of Action

Phexxi's contraceptive properties are primarily related to its acid buffering capacity.[2] The average pH of the vagina is between 3.5 and 4.5. At pH levels less than 5, sperm are immobilized. Semen has a pH of 7.2–8.0 and helps protect sperm by raising the vaginal pH to 6 or above. Phexxi counters this rise in pH that would occur during and after ejaculation and has been shown to be able to keep pH below 5 even when diluted with semen up to a 3:1 ratio and completely immobilized sperm at a 2:1 ratio of semen to gel.[29] The volume of Phexxi (5 g) should therefore be sufficient to maintain the pH of the vagina below 5 with typical volumes of ejaculate, which range between 2 and 5 mL.[30]

Though only labeled for administration up to 1 hour before intercourse due to the design of the pivotal clinical trials, the bioadhesive properties of Phexxi and maintenance of viscosity even with seminal dilution should allow for a greater time window for application. Phase 1 studies demonstrated a maintenance of sperm immobilization when vaginal intercourse occurred up to 8–10 hours after application and a layer of product could be seen on cervical and vaginal surfaces with colposcopic examination up to 12 hours after administration.[36,37] Phexxi's persistent ability to keep the pH below 5 is important because in vitro studies have demonstrated that about one-third of sperm that are initially immobilized by a low pH are able to regain motility when pH is raised above 5.5.[30]

The concerns of epithelial disruption and increased risk of HIV and STIs seen with spermicides containing N-9 have not been seen with use of Phexxi and would not be expected due to the differing mechanisms of action and lack of surfactants in Phexxi's formulation.[37]

Advantages

1. **Easy to administer.** Product comes in individually wrapped prefilled single-use applicators that are similar to other commonly used vaginal preparations and tampons. No device or fitting is required.
2. **Flexible timing of placement.** Users can administer the gel immediately before or up to 1 hour prior to intercourse so the sex act does not need to be interrupted.
3. **Pleasure-positive features.** The gel provides additional lubrication with intercourse and was cleared by the FDA as a personal lubricant prior to the studies demonstrating contraceptive benefit.
4. **Rapid onset of activity.** The gel is immediately active upon placement.
5. **Can be used with all other methods**, including all barrier methods. The prescribing information for Phexxi recommends avoiding use with the vaginal ring due to theoretical concerns regarding impact of the gel on the integrity or drug-release properties of the ring.
6. **Less messy.** The viscosity and bioadhesive nature of gel was designed to ensure less leakage of product than other vaginal medications. This contributes to the effectiveness of Phexxi and may make the product less messy and thus more acceptable to users and their partners.
7. **Can be initiated postpartum as soon as it is safe to resume vaginal intercourse.** No studies have been conducted on the impact of Phexxi on breastfeeding, but any maternal systemic exposure of the active ingredients is not expected to lead to safety concerns.
8. **Does not contain N-9,** the active ingredient in all other commercially available vaginal contraceptive gels, and therefore does not have the restrictions on use by people at risk for HIV or STIs or who may have an allergy or sensitivity to N-9.
9. **Can be used at any time during menstrual cycle.**

Disadvantages

1. **Prescription only.** Phexxi is not available over the counter and requires a prescription. However, Phexxi can be easily prescribed via telemedicine as it does not require an examination or device placement and has very few medical limitations to use.
2. **Vaginal placement.** Users need to be comfortable inserting an applicator into the vagina, similar to placing a tampon.
3. **May require negotiation with partner.** The limited 1-hour duration of action may prevent opportunities for advance placement.

4. **Single-use only.** An additional application of gel is required for each additional act of intercourse, even if within the initial 1-hour window.
5. **Can cause local reaction.** Up to 18% of users in clinical studies reported at least one episode of local genital irritation. These genitourinary symptoms were generally mild and improved over time. There was no difference in reported genitourinary side effects in users of Phexxi versus placebo in the Phase 2B study evaluating the prevention of chlamydia and gonorrhea.
6. **Limitations on use.** Phexxi is not effective if administered after vaginal intercourse. Use in people with a history of recurrent urinary tract infections (UTIs, >3 in the past year) is not recommended because of the theoretical risk of UTI with vaginally administered gels in this population. Studies did not show an increased risk of UTI with use of Phexxi compared with placebo or the expected baseline population risk, but potential subjects with a history of recurrent UTI were excluded from participation.

USER INSTRUCTIONS FOR PHEXXI*

Phexxi is available in individually wrapped, prefilled single use applicators. The applicator is very similar to other that used in other vaginally administered preparations or to standard tampon applicators. Phexxi can be administered in whatever position the user prefers—standing with one foot elevated, seated, or lying down. Users remove the prefilled applicator and plunger rod from the individual foil pouch and place the plunger rod just inside the applicator until the tip of the plunger rod connects to the inside of the applicator. Care should be taken not to push the plunger too far into the applicator, as this could cause the gel to be expressed into the cap. After the plunger rod is connected, the cap is removed. The applicator has a grooved area toward the bottom to indicate the best position to hold the applicator for insertion. The applicator is inserted into the vagina as far as is comfortable and the plunger rod is pushed into the applicator with the index finger until it stops at the base of the applicator. The plunger is then removed and disposed.

Once administered, a single application will be sufficient to cover one act of intercourse occurring within 1 hour. If more than 1 hour passes before intercourse or if an additional act of intercourse occurs (even within 1 hour), an additional application of gel is necessary.

Author Disclosures—Culwell: Former Employee of Evofem Biosciences (Phexxi); Pritzker: Trainer for Organon

References

1. Gallaway MS, Waller DK, Canfield MA, Scheuerle A. The association between use of spermicides or male condoms and major structural birth defects. Contraception. 2009;80(5):422-9. DOI: 10.1016/j.contraception.2009.03.007.
2. Evofem Biosciences. Phexxi prescribing information. (https://www.accessdata.fda.gov/drugsatfda_docs/label/2022/208352s002lbl.pdf).

* These instructions are intended to guide providers in educating patients in how to use their method.

3. van der Straten A, Sahin-Hodoglugil N, Clouse K, Mtetwa S, Chirenje MZ. Feasibility and potential acceptability of three cervical barriers among vulnerable young women in Zimbabwe. J Fam Plann Reprod Health Care. 2010;36(1):13-9. DOI: 10.1783/147118910790290966.
4. US Food and Drug Administration. Obstetrical and gynecological devices; reclassification of single-use female condom, to be renamed single-use internal condom. Final order. Fed Regist. 2018 Sep 27;83(188):48711-3.
5. Beksinska M, Smit J, Greener R, Piaggio G, Joanis C. The female condom learning curve: patterns of female condom failure over 20 uses. Contraception. 2015;91(1):85-90. DOI: 10.1016/j.contraception.2014.09.011.
6. Hart GJ, Pool R, Green G, Harrison S, Nyanzi S, Whitworth JA. Women's attitudes to condoms and female-controlled means of protection against HIV and STDs in south-western Uganda. AIDS Care. 1999;11(6):687-98. DOI: 10.1080/09540129947596.
7. Langenberg A. Interrupting herpes simplex virus type 2 transmission: the role of condoms and microbicides. Herpes. 2004;11 Suppl 3:147A-54A. (http://europepmc.org/abstract/MED/15319084).
8. Cecil M, Nelson AL, Trussell J, Hatcher R. If the condom doesn't fit, you must resize it. Contraception. 2010;82(6):489-90. DOI: 10.1016/j.contraception.2010.06.007.
9. Crosby RA, Sanders SA, Yarber WL, Graham CA, Dodge B. Condom use errors and problems among college men. Sex Transm Dis. 2002;29(9):552-7. DOI: 10.1097/00007435-200209000-00010.
10. Mogale R, Mulaudzi FM, Peu MD, Mataboge MS, Ngunyulu R, Phiri SS. The constraints and concerns regarding the size and/or shape of the second generation female condom: The narratives from the healthcare providers. Afr J Prim Health Care Fam Med. 2016;8(2):e1-7. DOI: 10.4102/phcfm.v8i2.1146.
11. Chen BA, Blithe, D. L., Muraguri, G. R., et al. Acceptability of the woman's condom in a phase III multicenter open-label study. Contraception. 2019;99(6):357-62. DOI: https://doi.org/10.1016/j.contraception.2019.02.006.
12. Soo MJ, Bharwani N, Rockall AG. Vagina and vulva: Imaging techniques, normal anatomy and anatomical variants. In: Hamm B, Ros PR, eds. Abdominal imaging. Berlin, Heidelberg: Springer Berlin Heidelberg; 2013:2201-10.
13. Philpott A. Re-use of the female condom: now for the practical realities. Reprod Health Matters. 2003;11(22):185-6. DOI: 10.1016/s0968-8080(03)02296-1.
14. Potter B, Gerofi J, Pope M, Farley T. Structural integrity of the polyurethane female condom after multiple cycles of disinfection, washing, drying and relubrication. Contraception. 2003;67(1):65-72. DOI: 10.1016/s0010-7824(02)00418-3.
15. Mauck CK, Brache V, Kimble T, et al. A phase I randomized postcoital testing and safety study of the Caya diaphragm used with 3% Nonoxynol-9 gel, ContraGel or no gel. Contraception. 2017;96(2):124-30. DOI: 10.1016/j.contraception.2017.05.016.
16. Schwartz JL, Weiner DH, Lai JJ, et al. Contraceptive efficacy, safety, fit, and acceptability of a single-size diaphragm developed with end-user input. Obstet Gynecol. 2015;125(4):895-903. DOI: 10.1097/aog.0000000000000721.
17. d'Oro LC, Parazzini F, Naldi L, La Vecchia C. Barrier methods of contraception, spermicides, and sexually transmitted diseases: a review. Genitourin Med. 1994;70(6):410-7. DOI: 10.1136/sti.70.6.410.
18. US Food and Drug Administation. FemCap Summary of Safety and Effectiveness Data. 2003. (https://www.accessdata.fda.gov/cdrh_docs/pdf/P010043b.pdf.)
19. Mauck C, Callahan M, Weiner DH, Dominik R. A comparative study of the safety and efficacy of FemCap, a new vaginal barrier contraceptive, and the Ortho All-Flex diaphragm. The FemCap Investigators' Group. Contraception. 1999;60(2):71-80. DOI: 10.1016/s0010-7824(99)00068-2.
20. Mauck CK, Weiner DH, Creinin MD, et al. FemCap with removal strap: ease of removal, safety and acceptability. Contraception. 2006;73(1):59-64. DOI: 10.1016/j.contraception.2005.06.074.
21. Tepper NK, Curtis KM, Cox S, Whiteman MK. Update to U.S. medical eligibility criteria for contraceptive use, 2016: Updated recommendations for the use of contraception among women at high risk for HIV infection. MMWR Morb Mortal Wkly Rep. 2020;69(14):405-10. DOI: 10.15585/mmwr.mm6914a3.

22. Bounds W, Guillebaud J, Dominik R, Dalberth BT. The diaphragm with and without spermicide. A randomized, comparative efficacy trial. J Reprod Med. 1995;40(11):764-74.
23. Raymond EG, Trussell J, Weaver MA, Reeves MF. Estimating contraceptive efficacy: the case of spermicides. Contraception. 2013;87(2):134-7. DOI: 10.1016/j.contraception.2012.06.014.
24. Grimes DA, Lopez LM, Raymond EG, Halpern V, Nanda K, Schulz KF. Spermicide used alone for contraception. Cochrane Database Syst Rev 2013(12):Cd005218. DOI: 10.1002/14651858.CD005218.pub4.
25. Zite NB, Wallace LS. Do instructions for over-the-counter pre-coital female contraceptives promote "perfect use"? Contraception. 2009;79(3):211-5. DOI: 10.1016/j.contraception.2008.10.002.
26. Schreiber CA, Ratcliffe SJ, Sammel MD, Whittaker PG. A self-assessment efficacy tool for spermicide contraceptive users. Am J Obstet Gynecol. 2016;214(2):264.e1-7. DOI: 10.1016/j.ajog.2015.10.018.
27. Kuyoh MA, Toroitich-Ruto C, Grimes DA, Schulz KF, Gallo MG. Sponge versus diaphragm for contraception. Cochrane Database Syst Rev. 2002(3):CD003172. DOI: 10.1002/14651858.Cd003172.
28. US Food and Drug Administration. Drug approval package: PHEXXI. (https://www.accessdata.fda.gov/drugsatfda_docs/nda/2020/208352Orig1s000TOC.cfm.)
29. Garg S, Anderson RA, Chany CJ, 2nd, et al. Properties of a new acid-buffering bioadhesive vaginal formulation (ACIDFORM). Contraception. 2001;64(1):67-75. DOI: 10.1016/s0010-7824(01)00217-7.
30. Nelson AL. An overview of properties of Amphora (Acidform) contraceptive vaginal gel. Expert Opin Drug Saf. 2018;17(9):935-43. DOI: 10.1080/14740338.2018.1515197.
31. Chappell BT, Mena LA, Maximos B, Mollan S, Culwell K, Howard B. EVO100 prevents chlamydia and gonorrhea in women at high risk of infection. Am J Obstet Gynecol. 2021;225(2):162.e1-14. DOI: 10.1016/j.ajog.2021.03.005.
32. https://www.prnewswire.com/news-releases/evofem-reports-top-line-results-from-phase-3-evoguard-clinical-trial-evaluating-evo100-for-prevention-of-chlamydia-and-gonorrhea-infection-in-women-301646667.html
33. Barnhart K, Dart C, Culwell K. Efficacy, safety and acceptability of aciform (Amphora) and nonoxynol-9 containing vaginal gels [16N]. Poster presentation. American College of Obstetricians and Gynecologists (ACOG) annual clinical meeting. Washington, D.C.; May 14–15, 2016.
34. Thomas MA, Chappell BT, Maximos B, Culwell KR, Dart C, Howard B. A novel vaginal pH regulator: results from the phase 3 AMPOWER contraception clinical trial. Contracept X. 2020;2:100031. DOI: 10.1016/j.conx.2020.100031.
35. Chappell BT, Culwell K, Dart C. Perfect-use pregnancy rates with vaginal pH regulatory: efficacy results from AMPOWER. Poster presentation at the Virtual Annual Clinical and Scientific Meeting of the American College of Obstetricians and Gynecology (ACOG); April 24-27, 2020. (https://www.evofem.com/wp-content/uploads/2021/08/Chappell-et-al.-Perfect-use-pregnancy-rates-with-vaginal-pH-regulator_Efficacy-results-from-AMPOWER.-Poster-Presentation.-ACOG-2020..pdf.)
36. Amaral E, Perdigão A, Souza MH, et al. Postcoital testing after the use of a bio-adhesive acid buffering gel (ACIDFORM) and a 2% nonoxynol-9 product. Contraception. 2004;70(6):492-7. DOI: 10.1016/j.contraception.2004.06.007.
37. Amaral E, Faúndes A, Zaneveld L, Waller D, Garg S. Study of the vaginal tolerance to Acidform, an acid-buffering, bioadhesive gel. Contraception. 1999;60(6):361-6. DOI: 10.1016/s0010-7824(99)00102-x.

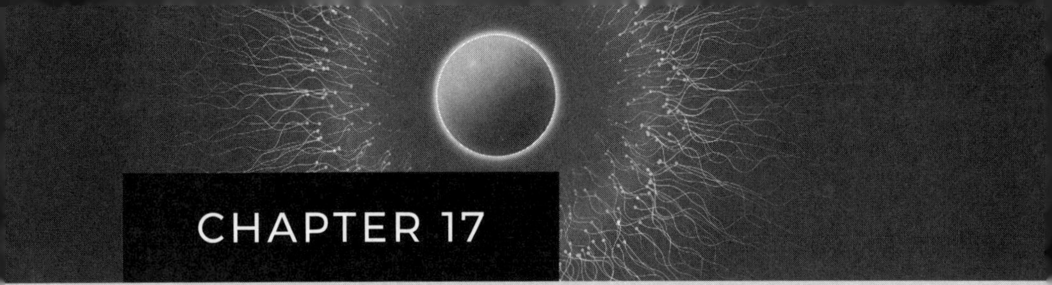

CHAPTER 17

Coitus Interruptus (Withdrawal, the Pull-Out Method)

Rachel K. Jones, PhD

KEY POINTS

- Sixty-six percent of all sexually active women report having used withdrawal at some point in their lives, and for 7% of women it is the most effective method they are currently using.
- Withdrawal can be used alone, at the same time as other methods (dual use), or alternating with other methods (rotating use).
- Withdrawal's perfect-use failure rate is estimated to be 4%. Typical-use failure rates are as high as 20%.
- Spermatozoa appear in the pre-ejaculatory fluid of some individuals, and there is a small chance this could cause pregnancy even if withdrawal occurs prior to ejaculation.

Coitus interruptus, more commonly referred to as withdrawal or the pull-out method, is the practice of an individual withdrawing the penis from the vagina and away from the external genital organs of their partner before ejaculation, with the intention of reducing the risk of pregnancy. Coitus interruptus was a natural response to the discovery that ejaculation into the vagina caused pregnancy. The method was probably widely practiced throughout history, playing a role in the European fertility transitions—when the continent transformed from a rural, agrarian society to an urban, industrial one—that occurred prior to the advent of modern contraceptive methods.[1,2]

Over the last four decades, couples have increasingly relied on coitus interruptus. Some 66% of heterosexually experienced women report having *ever* practiced withdrawal according to the 2017–2019 National Survey of Family Growth (NSFG)[3]; comparable figures were 60% in 2006–2010, 41% in 1995, and 25% in 1982.[4] Only pills and condoms were more often reported as methods ever used.

Among women using contraception in 2016, 7% were relying on coitus interruptus as their most effective method, a slight increase from 5% in 2008.[5] But the pull-out method is likely used more frequently, due to both multiple method use and underreporting. Most studies evaluate contraception based on the most effective method used. Estimate of reliance on withdrawal in the last month doubled when use of multiple methods were taken into account, from 8% to 16% among all women using contraception in the 2013–2015 NSFG.[6] Because it is often used as a secondary method, and because some individuals perceive withdrawal to be ineffective at preventing pregnancy,[7–9] many individuals may not report use unless they are specifically asked about it.

Mechanism of Action

Withdrawal inhibits fertilization by preventing contact between spermatozoa and the ovum. The couple may have penile-vaginal intercourse until ejaculation is impending, at which time the penis is withdrawn from the vagina and away from the external genitalia of the partner. The individual responsible for withdrawing must rely on their own sensations to determine when ejaculation is about to occur. The pre-ejaculate, which is usually released just prior to full ejaculation, generally goes unnoticed by both the partners during their course of sexual activity and so cannot be relied upon as a sign that ejaculation is about to occur.

Effectiveness

The method has not been examined in clinical trials, but the perfect-use failure rate is estimated to be 4%. Data from the 2006–2010 NSFG suggest that the typical-use failure rate is 20%.[10] The difference between the typical-use and perfect-use failure rates speak to the difficulty couples have in using withdrawal consistently and correctly.

When the penis becomes erect, pre-ejaculate, a lubricating secretion produced by the Littre or Cowper's glands, is emitted. Although two studies examining the pre-ejaculate for the presence of spermatozoa found none,[11,12] two other studies found spermatozoa, though in small numbers. In one of these studies, 8 of 23 samples contained clumps of a few hundred sperm, which could theoretically have posed a risk of fertilization.[13] In a study designed specifically to determine whether pre-ejaculate contained sperm potentially capable of fertilizing an egg, researchers examined pre-ejaculate samples from 27 men within 2 hours of production.[14] The pre-ejaculate of 37% of men contained motile sperm, though the number of sperm in each sample was very low. The study also found that subjects either consistently had sperm in their pre-ejaculate or consistently did not. The best available evidence suggests that the risk of pregnancy posed by pre-ejaculate is low, though not zero.

As with other contraceptive methods, withdrawal's effectiveness in preventing pregnancy is associated not only with characteristics of the method (whether the pre-ejaculate contains sperm) but also with characteristics of the users. Individuals who are less experienced with using the method or who have difficulty in telling when ejaculation will occur could have a greater risk of causing pregnancy. Research also suggests that women reporting lower motivation to avoid pregnancy are more likely to use withdrawal,[15,16] which may result in inconsistent use of the method.

Advantages

As a method of contraception, withdrawal has several distinct advantages. It costs nothing, requires no devices, involves no chemicals, and is available in most situations. Some couples may select withdrawal as their method because it requires no physical examination or contact with a clinic or pharmacy.[17] Practicing coitus interruptus causes no medical side effects. It also enables both partners to take a responsible and active role in fertility regulation and may foster a dialogue on contraception and sexuality between the partners. It is a backup contraceptive that is almost always available and can enhance the effectiveness of other methods.

Disadvantages and Cautions

Because the method must be used with each coital act, and complete withdrawal is required for it to be effective, the probability of pregnancy with typical use (20%) is substantially higher than that for hormonal methods or long-acting contraception. One reason for contraceptive failure may be that the partner with the penis is not motivated or is not able to withdraw completely in time for every act of intercourse.[18] For some, interruption of the excitement or plateau phase of the sexual response cycle may diminish pleasure.[19] In addition, some people with a vagina may feel anxiety in relinquishing control over pregnancy prevention to their partners. One qualitative study of young men found that reproductive coercion involving withdrawal was reported to have been committed by both partners.[19] Some men reported intentionally not pulling out prior to ejaculation even though they had told their partner they would, and there were also instances when women attempted to prevent their male partner from withdrawing (e.g., by holding them).

Special Issues

Sexually Transmitted Infections

Because not all pathogens are transmitted solely by seminal fluid, withdrawal does not completely protect from exposure to sexually transmitted infections (STIs), notably those STIs that infect epithelium, including genital herpes and human papillomavirus.

The seminal fluid that emerges from the penis prior to ejaculation may contain some human immunodeficiency virus (HIV),[13] if the ejaculating partner is not virally suppressed with effective antiretroviral therapy (ART).[20] However, coitus interruptus may decrease HIV exposure by reducing the amount of semen that enters the vagina. In stable discordant couples (the man was infected with HIV and the woman was not), coitus interruptus reduced the rate of HIV acquisition in women by more than half in one study.[21] Because these studies examined only stable heterosexual couples, the findings may not hold true in other circumstances or for those with more than one HIV-infected partner.

Although coitus interruptus may be less likely than intercourse with ejaculation to transmit HIV, individuals have become infected while their partners consistently practiced withdrawal. Coitus interruptus has not been studied as a way to reduce HIV transmission from vagina to penis. Viral suppression with ART of the infected partner ("treatment as prevention") is the most effective way to prevent sexual transmission of HIV.

Use Patterns

Among US women using contraception, reliance on withdrawal as the primary method of contraception has shown slight fluctuations, from 5% in 2008 to 8% in 2014[22] and 7% in 2016.[5]

Among US women using a contraceptive method, reliance on withdrawal as the most effective method was most common among individuals in their 20s (9% to 11%) compared to 5% among adolescents 15–19 and 5% to 7% among those in their 30s.[5] The same study also found reports of withdrawal to be higher among women who reported not receiving any sexual and reproductive health care in the last year compared to those who did (13% and 7%, respectively). This latter pattern suggests that lack of access to health care, which is more common among disadvantaged groups, might contribute to reliance on withdrawal. However, use of the method was higher among non-poor women compared to those with poverty-level incomes (8% and 3%) and among those with a high school degree (or higher) compared to those without one (7% to 8% vs. 3%). One study using the 2013–2017 NSFG found that, among women at risk of unintended pregnancy (including nonusers, who were not included in the above statistics), reliance on withdrawal was higher among those residing in urban than rural areas (8% compared to 4%).[23] These patterns indicate that many demographic groups use withdrawal; therefore, information about the method should be included in sexual health educational and counseling materials.

Individuals and couples who use withdrawal adopt a variety of use patterns. In 2015, nearly one in five (18%) women using contraception reported using more than one method at last sex, and withdrawal accounted for three of the four top contraceptive combinations.[24] One national study found that a majority of adult women using withdrawal in the last month also used another contraceptive, and only 35% of withdrawal users reported using this method alone.[16] Users of withdrawal were as likely to report that they used it with condoms as they were to report that they used it with a highly effective method such as the pill or the IUD.[16,25]

Research suggests that adolescents who use withdrawal typically do so in combination with other methods, and this practice has increased over time. Among sexually active female adolescents 15–19 any use of withdrawal at last penile-vaginal intercourse increased from 17% to 23% between 2006–2019 and comparable figures for males were 19% and 27%.[26] For both genders, the rise in withdrawal was due to increases in dual (or more) method use. In 2006–2010, 9% of adolescent females reported using withdrawal with another method, and 8% reported it to be the most effective method. By 2015–2019 use of withdrawal with other methods increased to 17%, and the proportion using it as the most effective method declined slightly, to 6%. Similar patterns were seen among males. Use of withdrawal with another method increased from 16% to 22%, and only 3% to 4% reported it as most effective method in either time period.

Qualitative and quantitative studies provide further insights into the ways that individuals and couples use withdrawal: at the same time as other methods (dual use), switching between methods (rotating use), and alternating between the two strategies (dual and rotating use) over a 1-month period.[16] Studies also suggest that individuals and couples use withdrawal for a variety of reasons, including having no other method on hand, as "extra insurance" against pregnancy, concerns about side effects of hormonal methods, as well as other reasons.[9,25,27]

One study suggests that US couples may rely on withdrawal for reasons other than pregnancy prevention. Among a national sample of adolescent and adults, 60% reported that in the last year ejaculation occurred "somewhere other than in [your/partner's] vagina, such as on [your/their] back or belly, [your/their] face, or into a sheet/towel."[28] One in five of all respondents indicated it occurred most of the time. Pregnancy prevention was the most common reason for extra-vaginal ejaculation, cited by 39% of respondents, and similar proportions, 17%, indicated it was used because it was sexy or arousing and/or to avoid mess on clothes or underwear. When respondents were asked about their most recent act of penile-vaginal intercourse, 12% reported use of "withdrawal (pulling out; removing penis before ejaculation)" when it was included in a randomized list of 10 contraceptive methods. However, on a subsequent question, 21% of respondents reported that ejaculation had occurred somewhere other than the vagina.

The above results have several potential implications. Even if withdrawal is being used for reasons other than pregnancy prevention, extra-vaginal ejaculation is likely to reduce the possibility of pregnancy if it is used regularly. The Lu et al.[28] study did not report the frequency with which other methods were being used when extra-vaginal ejaculation occurred. However, if individuals and couples are using extra-vaginal ejaculation on a regular basis along with methods such as condoms or the pill, typical-use failure rates for these methods might be lower since two methods are actually being used. Thus, future surveys might consider asking where ejaculation occurs and not limit reporting to types of contraception used. Similarly, research efforts to estimate typical use failure rates should work to better identify whether and how dual use of withdrawal or extra-vaginal ejaculation with other methods impact method effectiveness.

Providing the Method

Some individuals who rely on withdrawal may not consider it to be a "real" or effective method[7,8] and may not report that they use it when contraception is being discussed with a health care provider. One study found that withdrawal was brought up only in 15% of women's contraceptive visits, and discussions were typically brief and initiated by the patient.[29] Thus, health care providers may need to ask specifically about use of the method, including the context in which it is used. Moreover, given that withdrawal can be part of several contraceptive strategies, providers should determine if dual, rotating, or both strategies are being used. Given that reliance on the method is seen among almost all groups, discussions of withdrawal are relevant for all patient populations. Health care professionals should refrain from framing use of withdrawal as negative or ineffective.[29] (See Chapter 4, Person-Centered Reproductive Health Conversations and Contraceptive Counseling.) It is possible that typical-use failure rates for the method would improve if couples had more information about how to use it most effectively. Some users or potential users may have questions related to the fertile period, pre-ejaculate fluid, and the risk of any negative health effects, including exposure to STIs. Finally, inform the individual or couple about emergency contraception, including intrauterine contraception, and provide a supply of emergency contraceptive pills and instruct them on their use to help decrease the risk of pregnancy. (See Chapter 18, Emergency Contraception.)

USER INSTRUCTIONS FOR COITUS INTERRUPTUS*

Note that when creating written instructions for patients, a general rule is to aim for a fifth- to sixth-grade reading level due to health literacy considerations.

1. To practice withdrawal, the individual should remove their penis from the partner's vagina when they feel they are about to ejaculate, making sure that ejaculation occurs away from the partner's genitalia.
2. Withdrawal will not prevent pregnancy if an individual cannot predictably withdraw their penis prior to ejaculation.
3. Pre-ejaculate fluid can be released as soon as the penis becomes erect to or just before ejaculation. In some individuals, this pre-ejaculate fluid may contain small numbers of sperm, which could possibly cause a pregnancy. Individuals may not be aware when pre-ejaculate fluid has been released.
4. If more than one act of intercourse takes place within a relatively short period of time, the tip of the penis should be wiped off before intercourse to remove any sperm remaining from a previous ejaculation.
5. There is postcoital protection that can be used should any ejaculate come in contact with the vagina. If you think you or your partner may have been exposed to pregnancy, you can obtain emergency contraception through a pharmacy or at a health care center.

Author Disclosure—Jones: none

References

1. Santow G. Coitus interruptus and the control of natural fertility. Pop Stud. 1995;49:19-43.
2. Knodel J, van de Walle E. Lessons from the past: policy implications of historical fertility studies. In Watkins SC, ed., The decline of fertility in Europe. Princeton University Press; 2017: 390-419.
3. Centers for Disease Control and Prevention. Key statistics from the National Survey of Family Growth – C listing. [Internet]. (https://www.cdc.gov/nchs/nsfg/key_statistics/c-keystat.htm)
4. Daniels K, Mosher WD. Contraceptive methods women have ever used: United States, 1982-2010. Natl Health Stat Rep. 2013;(62):1-15.
5. Kavanaugh ML, Pliskin E. Use of contraception among reproductive-aged women in the United States, 2014 and 2016. F&S Rep. 2020;1:83-93. (http://www.sciencedirect.com/science/article/pii/S2666334120300386).
6. Polis CB, Jones RK. Multiple contraceptive method use and prevalence of fertility awareness based method use in the United States, 2013–2015. Contraception. 2018;98:188-92. doi.org/10.1016/j.contraception.2018.04.013.
7. Jones RK, Fennell J, Higgins JA, Blanchard K. Better than nothing or savvy risk-reduction practice? The importance of withdrawal. Contraception. 2009;79(6):407-10.
8. Arteaga S, Gomez AM. "Is that a method of birth control?" a qualitative exploration of young women's use of withdrawal. J Sex Res. 2016;53:626-32.

* These instructions are intended to guide providers in educating patients in how to use their method.

9. Frohwirth L, Blades N, Moore AM, Wurtz H. The complexity of multiple contraceptive method use and the anxiety that informs it: implications for theory and practice. Arch Sex Behav. 2016;45(8):2123-35.
10. Sundaram A, Vaughan B, Kost K, et al. Contraceptive failure in the United States: estimates from the 2006–2010 National Survey of Family Growth. Perspect Sex Reprod Health. 2017;49:7-16.
11. Ilaria G, Jacobs J, Polsky B, et al. Detection of HIV-1 DNA sequences in pre-ejaculatory fluid. Lancet. 1992;340:1469.
12. Zukerman Z, Weiss DB, Orvieto R. Does preejaculatory penile secretion originating from Cowper's Gland contain sperm? J Assist Reprod Genet. 2003;20:157-9.
13. Pudney J, Oneta M, Mayer K, Seage G, Anderson D. Pre-ejaculatory fluid as potential vector for sexual transmission of HIV-1. Lancet. 1992;340:1470.
14. Killick SR, Leary C, Trussell J, Guthrie KA. Sperm content of pre-ejaculatory fluid. Hum Fertil. 2011;14(1):48-52.
15. Higgins JA, Wang Y. Which young adults are most likely to use withdrawal? The importance of pregnancy attitudes and sexual pleasure. Contraception. 2015;91:320-7.
16. Jones RK, Lindberg LD, Higgins JA. Pull and pray or extra protection? Contraceptive strategies involving withdrawal among US adult women. Contraception. 2014;90:416-21.
17. Rogow D, Horowitz S. Withdrawal: a review of the literature and an agenda for research. Stud Fam Plann. 1995;26:140-53.
18. Latack KR, Patel J, Moog D, Spencer D, Nguyen BT. Withdrawal method inquiries and user experiences: an analysis of content posted on 4 gendered forums on Reddit. Contraception. 2021;104:170-5.
19. Hamm M, Evans M, Miller E, Browne M, Bell D, Borrero S. "It's her body": low-income men's perceptions of limited reproductive agency. Contraception. 2019;99:111-7.
20. Politch JA, Mayer KH, Anderson DJ. HIV-1 is undetectable in preejaculatory secretions from HIV-1-infected men on suppressive HAART. AIDS. 2016;30:1899-903.
21. De Vincenzi I. A longitudinal study of human immunodeficiency virus transmission by heterosexual partners. N Engl J Med. 1994;331:341-6.
22. Kavanaugh ML, Jerman J. Contraceptive method use in the United States: trends and characteristics between 2008, 2012 and 2014. Contraception. 2018;97:14–21.
23. Janis JA, Ahrens KA, Kozhimannil KB, Ziller EC. Contraceptive method use by rural–urban residence among women and men in the United States, 2006 to 2017. Womens Health Iss. 2021;31:277-85.
24. Kavanaugh ML, Pliskin E, Jerman J. Use of concurrent multiple methods of contraception in the United States, 2008 to 2015. Contracept X. 2021;3:100060. DOI: 10.1016/j.conx.2021.100060.
25. Harris ML, Coombe J, Forder PM, Lucke JC, Bateson D, Loxton D. Young women's complex patterns of contraceptive use: Findings from an Australian cohort study. Perspect Sex Reprod Health. 2020;52:181-90.
26. Lindberg LD, Firestein L, Beavin C. Trends in U.S. adolescent sexual behavior and contraceptive use, 2006-2019. Contracept X. 2021;3:100064. DOI: 10.1016/j.conx.2021.100064.
27. Berglas NF, Kimport K, Mays A, Kaller S, Biggs MA. "It's worked well for me": young women's reasons for choosing lower-efficacy contraceptive methods. J Pediatr Adolesc Gynecol. 2021;34:341-7.
28. Fu T, Hensel DJ, Beckmeyer JJ, Dodge B, Herbenick D. Considerations in the measurement and reporting of withdrawal: findings from the 2018 National Survey of Sexual Health and Behavior. J Sex Med. 2019;16:1170-77.
29. Kimport K. Talking about male body-based contraceptives: the counseling visit and the feminization of contraception. Soc Sci Med. 2018;201:44-50.

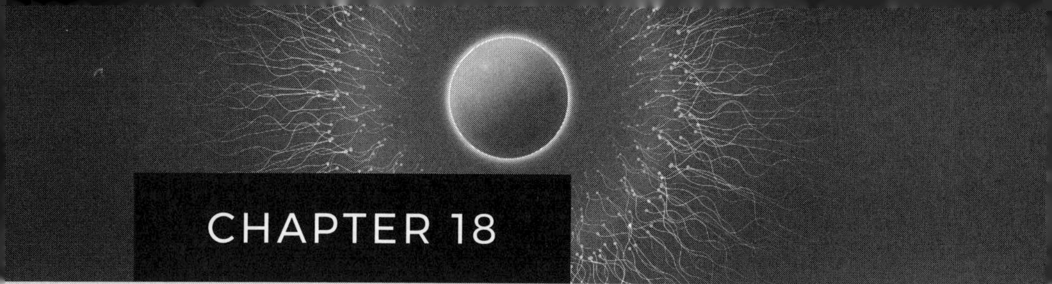

CHAPTER 18

Emergency Contraception

Eleanor Bimla Schwarz, MD, MS
Kelly Cleland, MPA, MPH
David Turok, MD, MPH

KEY POINTS

- Emergency contraception (EC) substantially reduces the chance of pregnancy after an episode of unprotected intercourse.
- Placement of a copper intrauterine device (IUD) after unprotected intercourse reduces the risk of pregnancy within the month to <0.1%.
- A single randomized controlled trial supports placement of the levonorgestrel 52 mg IUD for emergency contraception with a pregnancy risk of 0.3%.
- Emergency contraceptive pills (ECPs) taken within 5 days of unprotected intercourse are effective but less effective than IUD placement. From most to least effective, these pills contain:
    - Ulipristal acetate 30 mg (*UPA*)
    - Levonorgestrel (LNG) 1.5 mg (*Plan B One-Step and several generic versions*)
    - Higher-than-usual doses of routine oral contraceptives containing ethinyl estradiol and either levonorgestrel or norgestrel (*Preven* is no longer marketed)
- ECPs are safe for everyone; if someone is already pregnant, EC pills are ineffective but have not been shown to be harmful to pregnancy.

Overview

Emergency contraception can be safely used after intercourse to prevent pregnancy.

In addition to postcoital IUD placement,[1,2] two types of dedicated emergency contraceptive pills (ECPs) are currently available for use in the United States:

- *ella*, a single 30-mg ulipristal acetate (UPA) pill, was approved by the US Food and Drug Administration (FDA) in 2010. In the United States, people must obtain a prescription for UPA; as of January 2015, the European Medicines Agency allows pharmacist dispensing of UPA ECPs without a prescription.
- *Plan B One-Step* and its generic forms (e.g., *My Way, Take Action, EContra One-Step,* and *Aftera*) that consist of a single 1.5-mg levonorgestrel (LNG) pill are available without a prescription to anyone who wishes to purchase them in the United States.

Although until February 2014, a prescription was required for women under age 17 to obtain generic levonorgestrel ECPs, this restriction has been removed. The two-dose version of LNG ECPs (Plan B and its generic forms) is no longer sold in the United States.

Less-effective ECPs include use of combined oral contraceptives (COCs) containing ethinyl estradiol and either norgestrel or LNG, sometimes called the Yuzpe regimen. (**Table 18-1** provides examples of how to create doses of at least 100 mcg of ethinyl estradiol and 50 mcg levonorgestrel by taking up to six COC pills at once, and then again 12 hours later). Preven, a dedicated product containing two doses of 0.1 mg ethinyl estradiol and 0.5 mg LNG, was approved for use in 1998 but withdrawn from the market in 2004, as more effective ECPs with fewer side effects were available. Emergency use of combined pills containing norethindrone was found in one study to have an efficacy slightly lower than that for combined pills containing LNG.[3] No published studies are available for EC use of combined pills containing gestodene, etonorgestrel, or other progestogens; such pills should therefore not be used for EC. There are no contraindications for the use of any ECP by anyone of any age except in pregnancy, and that contraindication is only because the EC will not prevent or halt pregnancy once it is already established.

In the United States, access to mifepristone remains constrained by individuals who seek to limit access to abortion services. However, in a handful of countries including Armenia, China, Russia, Moldova, Ukraine, and Vietnam, mifepristone in doses of 10–25 mg is available as an ECP. Mifepristone prevents ovulation by blocking the effects of progesterone by binding to its receptors. Depending on whether the drug is administered before or after ovulation, it can also disrupt luteal-phase events and endometrial development.[4] Mifepristone is more effective and causes less nausea and vomiting and fewer side effects than does the Yuzpe regimen[3,5-7] and LNG EC[3]; it has not been directly compared to UPA.

Meloxicam (a COX-2 inhibitor) given for five consecutive days in the late follicular phase at a dose of 30 mg may also be an effective option for EC. This regimen does not alter the endocrine profile of the cycle and causes no menstrual disturbance.[8,9] (In contrast, celecoxib, another COX-2 inhibitor, appears to have no potential for EC.[10]) However, the effectiveness of meloxicam has yet to be compared to other EC options in a randomized controlled fashion, and it is not sold as an emergency contraceptive.

Barriers to Use

The major barriers to use of EC are awareness, access, and cost. Many potential users still may not know that EC is available, effective, and safe. In addition, many health care providers have limited knowledge of EC.[11] Nevertheless, among US women aged 15–44 who have ever had intercourse, the proportion that had ever used ECPs increased from 2% in 2002 to 18% in 2011–2013[12] and 23% in 2015.[13]

Even in cases of rape, many hospital emergency departments do not provide EC services,[14-18] despite the fact that legal precedent indicates that failure to provide EC constitutes inadequate care and provides grounds to sue the hospital.[19] It is estimated that thousands of pregnancies resulting from rape each year could be prevented by use of EC.[20] Since 2013, the Department of Justice *National Protocol for Sexual Assault Medical Forensic Examinations*,[21,22] has noted the importance of timely provision of EC.

Table 18-1 **The Yuzpe Regimen: Examples of combined hormonal, levonorgestrel-containing regimens for use when more effective EC options are not available.**

Brand	Company	Two Doses 12 hours Apart	Ethinyl Estradiol per Dose (μg)	Levonorgestrel per Dose (mg)
Afirmelle	Aurobindo	5 white pills	100	0.50
Altavera	Sandoz	4 peach pills	120	0.60
Amethia	Actavis	4 white pills	120	0.60
Amethia Lo	Actavis	5 white pills	100	0.50
Amethyst	Actavis	6 white pills	120	0.54
Aubra	Afaxys	5 white pills	100	0.50
Aviane	Teva	5 orange pills	100	0.50
Ayuna	Aurobindo	4 orange pills	100	0.50
Camrese	Teva	4 light blue-green pills	120	0.60
CamreseLo	Teva	5 orange pills	100	0.50
Chateal	Afaxys	4 white pills	120	0.60
Cryselle[a]	Teva	4 white pills	120	0.60
Elinest[a]	Novast	4 orange pills	120	0.60
Enpresse	Teva	4 orange pills	120	0.50
Falmina	Novast	5 orange pills	100	0.50
Introvale	Sandoz	4 peach pills	120	0.60
Jolessa	Teva	4 pink pills	120	0.60
Kurvelo	Lupin	4 peach pills	120	0.60
Larissia	Ammeal	4 white pills	120	0.60
Lessina	Teva	5 pink pills	100	0.50
Levlen	Bayer	4 light brown pills	120	0.50
Levonest	Novast	4 light brown pills	120	0.50
Levora	Actavis	4 white pills	120	0.60
Lillow	Amneal	4 white pills	120	0.60

(continues)

Table 18-1 The Yuzpe Regimen: Examples of combined hormonal, levonorgestrel-containing regimens for use when more effective EC options are not available. *(continued)*

Brand	Company	Two Doses 12 hours Apart	Ethinyl Estradiol per Dose (μg)	Levonorgestrel per Dose (mg)
LoSeasonique	Teva	5 orange pills	100	0.50
Low-Ogestrel[a]	Actavis	4 white pills	120	0.60
Lutera	Actavis	5 white pills	100	0.50
Lybrel	Wyeth	6 yellow pills	120	0.54
Marlissa	Glenmark	4 peach pills	120	0.60
Myzilra	Novast	4 yellow pills	120	0.50
Nordette	Teva	4 light-orange pills	120	0.60
Orsythia	Vintage	5 pink pills	100	0.50
Portia	Teva	4 pink pills	120	0.60
Seasonale	Teva	4 pink pills	120	0.60
Seasonique	Teva	4 light-blue-green pills	120	0.60
Setlakin	Novast	4 pink pills	120	0.60
Sronyx	Actavis	5 white pills	100	0.50
Triphasil	Wyeth	4 yellow pills	120	0.50
Trivora	Actavis	4 pink pills	120	0.50
Vienva	Sandoz	5 white pills	100	0.50

Notes: [a]The progestogen in Cryselle, Elinest, and Low-Ogestrel is norgestrel, which contains two isomers, only one of which (LNG) is bioactive; the amount of norgestrel in each tablet is twice the amount of LNG.

Promoting Awareness and Use

Multiple initiatives have encouraged greater awareness and use of EC (see Additional Information and Materials). These include advance prescription and dispensing of EC, pharmacist EC prescribing and dispensing, EC availability in vending machines, online sales, and use of telemedicine. Advance prescription of ulipristal acetate for anyone beginning a new contraceptive method and any heterosexually active person of reproductive capability who desires it is a worthwhile consideration, though not supported by evidence. The majority of new contraceptive method users will not be using their selected method within the year, and the expiration date for oral EC will likely be several years in the future.

Some have voiced concern that making ECPs more widely available will cause individuals who know they can use ECPs to become less diligent with other contraception and prevention of sexually transmitted infections (STIs). However, many studies have now demonstrated that making ECPs more widely available did not increase sexual risk-taking.[23-40] Also, working to increase access to EC supports patient autonomy and person-centered care. In the four studies that examined the impact of easier access to ECPs on rates of STIs, access to ECPs did not affect incidence of STIs.[27,35,38,40] Another study demonstrated that educating teens about ECPs did not increase their level of sexual activity or use of EC but did increase their knowledge about proper administration of ECPs.[41]

Over-the-Counter (OTC) Availability

There are no medical reasons for ECPs to require a prescription.[42,43] However, changing oral LNG from prescription to OTC status in the United States was a long and politically charged process; although ulipristal acetate is available without a prescription in Europe, in the United States it remains only available with a prescription. In most pharmacies, oral LNG ECPs are now located on the shelf in the family planning aisle and can be purchased regardless of age. Stating concerns about potential shoplifting, some pharmacies choose to keep ECPs and other relatively expensive medications in a locked cabinet.

Two unintended, negative outcomes of OTC access to oral levonorgestrel EC in the United States included significant price increases and loss of insurance coverage for ECPs for most Americans whose health insurance covers only prescription drugs. Some states have sought to require insurance coverage of OTC contraceptives. However, OTC access may still reduce opportunities for health care providers to counsel patients about use of more effective, longer-term contraceptive methods when they present for EC,[44] such as the copper or levonorgestrel IUD.

Cost-Effectiveness

Studies based on economic models have shown that EC has the potential to be cost-effective by preventing unintended pregnancies.[45] In the United States, placement of a copper T IUD is cost saving within a 1-year horizon, even if some patients opt to have their IUD removed within a few months of placement,[46] as a copper T380A IUD remains highly effective for at least 12 years when desired.[47] ECPs have also been shown to be cost-effective, regardless of whether they are provided when needed or provided in advance of need.[48-55] However, all of the above studies have assumed that ECPs would actually be used after unprotected intercourse. Unfortunately, randomized controlled trials have not demonstrated that increasing access to ECPs reduces pregnancy or abortion rates at the population level. Although an ecological study from Chile reported an association between access to EC pills and lower rates of pregnancy,[56] and a study from Utah noted that increased uptake of oral levonorgestrel EC was associated with a decrease in birth and abortion rates,[57] neither study was able to control for use of other contraceptives, which may have also varied over time. Therefore, while ECPs have been shown to be cost-effective when used by those seeking EC, at the population level, advance provision of ECPs has not been shown to be cost-effective, because individuals provided ECPs in advance of need have used the ECPs so rarely. However, cost-effectiveness and population-level effects should not drive decision-making about patient care or about availability of ECPs; ECPs are an important strategy for individuals seeking to prevent pregnancy, regardless of larger-scale public health effects. (See Chapter 4, Person-Centered Reproductive Health Conversations and Contraceptive Counseling.)

Mechanism of Action

Copper IUDs

When used as a regular method of contraception, copper IUDs act to prevent fertilization. Emergency placement of a copper IUD is significantly more effective than use of ECPs, reducing the risk of pregnancy following unprotected intercourse to less than 0.1%.[58] This very high level of effectiveness implies that emergency placement of a copper IUD likely prevents sperm–egg union as well as having some postfertilization effect. The important point is that effectiveness and mechanism of action are not independent;[59] a regimen without a postfertilization effect could not be 100% effective in typical populations, which inevitably include some users who take ECPs after ovulation, and potentially fertilization, have already occurred. (See Chapter 10, Intrauterine Devices [IUDs].)

Levonorgestrel 52 mg IUDs

For ongoing contraceptive use, LNG IUDs prevent sperm–egg union by thickening the cervical mucus in a way that makes it impenetrable to sperm. The EC mechanism for levonorgestrel IUDs is not specifically known. A progestin burst does occur with placement, but that may not be similar enough to an LNC-ECP to cause ovulation delay or inhibition. Inert IUDs do generate an inflammatory response that likely prevents fertilization,[60,61] and the presence of the plastic frame for a levonorgestrel IUD could do the same. Levonorgestrel in the genital tract interferes with sperm transport,[62] sperm capacitation, penetration of the zona pellucida,[63] and oviduct transport,[64,65] though it is not known if the amount and intrauterine delivery of LNG released with LNG IUD placement could create these effects.

Emergency Contraceptive Pills (ECPs)

ECPs prevent pregnancy without any postfertilization effects, though the data supporting this for LNG ECPs exceeds the strength of that for UPA ECPs.[66,67] As with the birth control pill, patch, ring, shot, and implant,[68] and even lactation,[69] ECPs prevent pregnancy primarily by delaying or inhibiting ovulation, thereby preventing fertilization. As there is no scientific method to test for fertilization, it is not possible to definitively rule out the possibility that any contraceptive methods, including lactational amenorrhea, inhibit implantation of a fertilized egg in the endometrium.

ECPs do not cause abortion[70] or harm an established pregnancy, which begins with implantation, according to medical authorities such as the FDA, the National Institutes of Health[71] and the American College of Obstetricians and Gynecologists (ACOG).[72]

Ulipristal Acetate

A number of studies have demonstrated that UPA can delay ovulation.[73-75] Timing of treatment can make a difference. In one study, 34 women were treated when the size of the leading follicle was 18 to 22 mm.[76] Each woman contributed one cycle treated with placebo and another with UPA. Follicular rupture failed to occur within 5 days following UPA treatment in 20 (59%) subjects while normal ovulation was observed in all women within 5 days after placebo intake. Follicular rupture failed to occur within 5 days after treatment with UPA in all women treated before onset of the luteinizing hormone (LH) surge, in 79% of women treated after the onset of the LH surge but before the LH peak, and in 8% of women treated after the LH peak. Another study was designed to assess whether UPA EC has similar efficacy when used before and after ovulation. The researchers measured pregnancy rates in 700 women who took UPA within 120 hours of unprotected sex. The women were classified as preovulatory or postovulatory based on several parameters, including serum LH, estradiol and progesterone levels, presence and size of a lead ovarian follicle >10 mm in mean diameter, and self-reported cycle length. Among women in the preovulatory group, 77.6% of expected pregnancies were prevented, while in women who took UPA EC on the day of ovulation or after, 36.4% of pregnancies were prevented. The pregnancy rate in the preovulatory group was significantly lower than would be expected without the use of EC, while the rate in the postovulatory group was not different than would have been expected without any use of EC.[77] This result builds on earlier work suggesting that the primary mechanism of action of UPA EC is interference with ovulation. Other studies have focused on potential effects of UPA on the endometrium: one found that UPA altered the endometrium, but whether this change would inhibit implantation is unknown.[78] An in vitro study found that UPA, at the dosage used for EC, does not affect human embryo implantation.[79] However, data from mouse models suggest that a single dose of UPA may affect embryo-endometrial interaction.[80,81] UPA does not impair sperm function.[82,83]

Levonorgestrel ECPs

LNG EC does not interfere with implantation. A systematic review of 33 studies assessing the effect of LNG EC on implantation and fertility found no evidence that LNG EC affects fetal development or causes miscarriage or stillbirth.[65] Although this lack of impact on implantation is clear on European labels, US drug labels continue to be a source of confusion. Early treatment with ECPs containing only the progestogen LNG has been shown to impair the ovulatory process and luteal function.[84-88] The above-mentioned systematic review included a subset of 10 studies that demonstrated LNG EC does not alter endometrial receptivity for implantation relative to controls. Seven of the eight in vivo studies in the review assessing endometrial receptivity markers demonstrated no change with LNG compared to controls. One study showed LNG taken before the LH surge altered the luteal phase secretory pattern of glycodelin in serum and the endometrium.[89] Glycodelin is a protein that the endometrium produces that reduces sperm capacitation and inhibits sperm–egg binding.[90] However, two later studies explicitly designed to assess endometrial glycodelin expression found no alteration in the secretory pattern.[91,92] The second of these studies also found no effect on other endometrial receptivity biomarkers or progesterone receptors. In another study, LNG taken before the LH surge increased serum and intrauterine concentrations of glycodelin at the time of ovulation, implying the possibility of an additional mechanism of action of LNG in inhibiting sperm-egg binding.[93] This included two in vitro studies showing that LNG does not impair the attachment of human blastocysts to endometrial tissue models and has no effect on the expression of endometrial receptivity markers.[94,95] LNG interference with sperm migration and function is less clear. One study showed LNG negatively impacting sperm function at all levels of the genital tract;[96] however, another study designed to assess this issue found that LNG 1.5 mg had no effect on the quality of cervical mucus or on the passage of spermatozoa into the uterine cavity,[91] and more recently, a study found an effect on sperm function only with much higher levels of LNG than are used for emergency contraception.[97] Despite the strong evidence supporting the prevention of ovulation as the main mechanism of action and a lack of evidence of a postfertilization/implantation effect, for years the package labeling for Plan B One Step still included the language "It may also prevent fertilization of a released egg or attachment of a fertilized egg to the uterus." In December 2022, following a thorough review of the evidence, the language suggesting an anti-implantation effect was finally removed, and the updated label states that "Plan B One-Step® works before release of an egg from the ovary."[98]

Croxatto and colleagues[99] have argued that most, if not all, of the contraceptive effect of LNG ECPs can be explained by inhibited or dysfunctional ovulation, based on the existing animal and human studies, including two human studies comparing observed and expected pregnancies when LNG ECPs were administered before and after ovulation. In the first study, 0 pregnancies were observed when LNG ECPs were taken on or before the day of ovulation (in contrast to the 4 pregnancies that would have been expected without use of ECPs), whereas 3 pregnancies occurred when ECPs were taken after the day of ovulation (versus 3.5 expected pregnancies).[100] In a follow-up study, 0 pregnancies were observed when LNG ECPs were taken before the day of ovulation (in contrast to the 16 pregnancies that would have been expected without use of ECPs,) whereas when ECPs were taken on or after the day of ovulation, 8 pregnancies occurred (versus 8.7 expected pregnancies).[101] While some find the existing human and animal studies adequate to conclude that ECPs have no post-fertilization effect,[98,102,103] others may feel that this question has not been answered until it is scientifically possible to determine whether fertilization has occurred prior to implantation.

Combined ECPs

Several clinical studies have shown that combined ECPs containing ethinyl estradiol and LNG can inhibit or delay ovulation.[104-107] This mechanism of action may explain the effectiveness of combined ECPs when used during the first half of the menstrual cycle, before ovulation has occurred. Some studies have shown histologic or biochemical alterations in the endometrium after treatment with the regimen, leading to the conclusion that combined ECPs may act by impairing endometrial receptivity to subsequent implantation of a fertilized egg.[102,108-110] However, other, more recent studies have found no such effects on the endometrium.[101,111,112] Additional possible mechanisms include interference with corpus luteum function; thickening of the cervical mucus resulting in trapping of sperm; alterations in the tubal transport of sperm, egg, or embryo; and direct inhibition of fertilization.[96,98,113,114] No clinical data exist that support direct inhibition of fertilization.

Effectiveness

Intrauterine Devices

More than 7,000 postcoital placements of copper IUDs have been reported in the literature since the practice was introduced in 1976. With only 10 known failures, this approach has a pregnancy rate of less than 0.1%.[58] In a review of this literature, IUDs were placed up to 7 days after unprotected intercourse (UPI) in three studies, up to 10 days after UPI in one study, and up to 10+ days after UPI in one study; there were 0 pregnancies. There was one pregnancy (0.1%) in one study in which IUDs were placed up to 5+ days after UPI. A reanalysis of Chinese data found 0 pregnancies in 52 women when the IUD was placed >5 days after UPI.[115]

Efficacy data for use of a levonorgestrel IUD for emergency contraception has been a longstanding question. In a recent randomized noninferiority trial, the levonorgestrel 52 mg IUD was noninferior to the copper 380 mm^2 IUD for emergency contraception.[116] In this study, one pregnancy occurred among 317 levonorgestrel 52 mg IUD EC users. These data are miniscule in comparison to the large, accumulated data supporting the copper IUD as the most effective form of EC. An ongoing study assessing reproducibility of the LNG 52 mg IUD EC findings (ClinicalTrials.gov Identifier: NCT05444582) will provide a more accurate EC pregnancy risk point estimate. The study leverages the 2022 change in the Planned Parenthood Federation of America's Standards and Guidelines, which now include provision of the LNG 52 mg IUD alone for EC. However, US Centers for Disease Control and Prevention and World Health Organization (WHO) clinical guidelines still support use of oral LNG along with LNG IUD placement for EC users. This practice would be most appropriate for those reporting mid-cycle unprotected intercourse, thus at the highest risk of pregnancy.

ECPs

Studies clearly show that both LNG and UPA ECPs are more effective than doing nothing to prevent pregnancy after unprotected intercourse.[117]

Ulipristal Acetate

The antiprogestin UPA (30 mg in a single dose) is the most effective ECP available in the United States, with reported estimates of effectiveness ranging from 62% to 85% risk reduction.[76,118-120] Two randomized trials compared the efficacy of LNG and UPA, one up to 72 hours after unprotected intercourse[117] and the second up to 120 hours after intercourse.[116] When these two studies were combined in a meta-analysis, the odds of pregnancy were 42% lower for UPA taken within 72 hours and 65% lower when taken within the first 24 hours.[116] In the second randomized study, UPA prevented significantly more pregnancies than did LNG in the 72- to 120-hour subgroup. The reason seems to be that UPA is more effective than LNG in postponing imminent ovulation. LNG is no more effective than a placebo in preventing ovulation when the leading follicle reaches 15–17 mm.[87] In contrast, by the time the follicle reaches 18–20 mm (which indicates that ovulation should occur within the next 48 hours) and the probability of conception without medication is >30%, UPA delayed ovulation for at least 5 days in 59% of cycles (versus 0% for the placebo).[72]

Mifepristone

Three randomized trials compared the efficacy of LNG 1.5 mg and 10 mg mifepristone for use as EC. Two trials found no significant difference in efficacy of the two-dose LNG (0.75 mg each) regimen and mifepristone; pregnancy rates for the two regimens were respectively 1.8% and 1.5% in the first trial,[121] and 2.0% and 1.3% in the second.[122] The first trial also included a one-dose LNG (1.5 mg) regimen, which yielded a pregnancy rate of 1.5%. A meta-analysis of 20 Chinese randomized trials found that a mid-dose (25 mg or 50 mg) of mifepristone had a lower failure rate than LNG; for the 13 trials that reported side effects, mifepristone was more tolerable but the delay in menses was greater for mifepristone.[2] A meta-analysis of 11 randomized trials (9 Chinese, 1 United Kingdom,[120] and one multinational[119]) found that low-dose (<25 mg) mifepristone was more effective than LNG, but when only the four high-quality studies were included, mifepristone was not superior.[2] Another Chinese trial found that the antiprogestin gestrinone was as effective as 10 mg mifepristone.[123] As yet, mifepristone has not been directly compared to UPA for EC.

Progestogen-Only (LNG) and Combined Regimens

Twelve studies of the LNG regimen, which together included a total of more than 13,500 women, reported estimates of effectiveness between 52% and 100%; that is, this regimen reduced the chance of pregnancy by that amount.[98,116,117,119,120,124-129] A meta-analysis of eight studies of the combined regimen, which in total included more than 3,800 women, concluded that the regimen prevents about 74% of expected pregnancies; the proportion ranged from 56% to 89% in the different studies.[130] A more recent analysis using possibly improved methodology found an effectiveness of 53% and 47% in two of the largest trials of the combined regimen.[131] Combined data from two randomized trials that directly compared the LNG and combined regimens showed a relative risk of pregnancy of 0.51 (95% confidence limits 0.31–0.83), indicating that the chance of pregnancy among women who received the LNG regimen was about half the chance among those who received the combined regimen.[115,124,125] This estimate makes *no* assumption about the number of pregnancies that would have been observed in the absence of treatment. The results imply that (1) if the Yuzpe regimen is completely inefficacious, then the LNG regimen has an efficacy of 49% and (2) for every additional 2 percentage points of efficacy of the Yuzpe regimen, 1 percentage point of efficacy is added to the LNG regimen.

A pilot study of 41 women found that adding a COX-2 inhibitor (meloxicam 15 mg) to 1.5 mg LNG significantly increased the proportion of cycles with no follicular rupture or with ovulatory dysfunction (88% vs. 66%, P=.012), and that COX-2 inhibitors can disturb the ovulatory process after the onset of the LH surge.[132]

Treatment Delay

Several studies have indicated that both the combined and LNG regimens are more effective the sooner after sex the pills are taken.[7,119,122,125,126,131,136] Other studies have not found that delays in use have this effect,[3,117,120,121,123,124,128,132,133] although sample sizes were often small. The initial studies showed that these regimens are effective when used up to 72 hours after intercourse.[125,133] Consequently,

US product package instructions for LNG ECPs advise use only within that time frame. Subsequent studies indicate that the regimens continue to be moderately effective if started between 72 and 120 hours.[119,123,126,133,134] However, a pooled analysis of four WHO trials of the LNG regimen shows no decline in efficacy until day 5, when it may offer no protection at all.[134] Analysis of the pooled data from the two Phase III trials of UPA showed no statistically significant effect of treatment delay (0–24 hours, 25–48 hours, 49–72 hours, 73–96 hours, and 97–120 hours) on pregnancy rates ($P = .91$).[135] No data are available establishing efficacy if ECPs are taken more than 120 hours after intercourse, when sperm are unlikely to be viable.

Body Mass Index

Analysis of data from the two randomized trials of the UPA and LNG regimens found that women with higher BMI taking ECP had a significantly higher risk of pregnancy than did women of lower weight. In fact, women with a BMI of ≥30 who took LNG EC were as likely to experience a pregnancy as those who had taken no ECP.[136] The label for NorLevo (LNG 1.5 mg) in Europe was changed in November 2013 to reflect additional analyses of these data; the label stated: "In clinical trials, contraceptive efficacy was reduced in women weighing 75 kg or more and LNG was not effective in women who weighed more than 80 kg."[137] However, the European Medicines Agency, after reviewing additional data from three WHO trials[119,125,126] that did not find reduced efficacy with increasing weight or BMI, removed that statement from the Norlevo label in July 2014.[138] In May 2016, the US FDA similarly announced that the evidence was too limited to merit a label change, and encouraged EC manufacturers to further study the relationship between obesity and the effectiveness of ECP. The WHO then published a report with data from four studies (the three above plus one more) that did find a higher failure rate for women with higher BMI, but only after controlling for other factors in a regression model. It is notable that there was no effect of weight in contrast to BMI; the rate was not higher among women weighing >80 kg.[139]

However, a pharmacokinetic study found that the serum concentration of LNG 1.5 mg was about 50% lower in women with BMI >35 compared with those whose BMI was <25.[140] The same study found that doubling the dose of LNG EC (from 1.5 mg to 3.0 mg) appeared to produce serum concentration levels similar to those in women with BMI <25 who had taken the regular dose (1.5 mg). This small study did not measure endpoints more directly related to effectiveness (ovulation or pregnancy), but it suggests that obesity does affect the bioavailability of LNG EC. However, a newer pharmacodynamic study powered to detect a 30% difference in follicle rupture delay >5 days, compared single versus double dosing of LNG among individuals with BMI higher than 30. The study found no significant difference in follicular rupture among those who used a double dose of LNG (3.0 mg) and those who used a single dose (1.5 mg).[141] Another pharmacokinetic study (involving 32 women) similarly found that 24 hours after the women ingested LNG ECPs, serum concentration levels were 50% lower among women with BMI of 30–40 compared to those less than 25.[142] Following use of UPA, however, blood levels were similar among women with BMI >30 and those with BMI <25. The effect of weight on the efficacy of combined ECPs has not been studied. When acceptable, an IUD is always the most effective option for EC, especially for patients who are obese. The American Society for Emergency Contraception recommends placing special emphasis on the IUD or UPA for those with higher body weights. In addition, they recommend that advocates disseminate information about all EC options and encourage heavier EC users desiring oral treatment to consult a clinician or an online service to obtain UPA after unprotected intercourse.[143] For heavier people unable to obtain UPA or an IUD, there is no harm in taking oral LNG for EC, though it has likely low efficacy in pregnancy prevention.

Repeated Use

Repeated use of ECPs is far less effective than most other contraceptive methods. For a typical individual who repeatedly used LNG ECPs, the chance of pregnancy after 1 year would be 20%.[144] In a recent study of women with infrequent intercourse (up to six times a month) using LNG ECPs, the pregnancy rate was 11 per 100 women-years.[145] While repeated use of EC is less effective, aside from pregnancy, there are not additional safety concerns with this approach.

Population Impact of ECPs

Only two[146,147] of 16 published studies have demonstrated that increasing access to ECPs reduces pregnancy or abortion rates,[148,149] although one demonstration project[150] and five clinical trials[37-40] were specifically designed to address this issue. One explanation for this result is that even when provided with ECPs in advance of need, most individuals use ECPs too rarely after unprotected sex to result in a substantial population impact. In the San Francisco trial, 45% of the women in the advance provision group who had unprotected intercourse during the study period did not use ECPs.[38] In the Nevada/North Carolina trial, 33% of women in the advance provision group had unprotected intercourse at least once without using ECPs.[40] In the Nevada/North Carolina trial, increased access to EC increased use of ECPs most among women who were at lower baseline risk of pregnancy.[151] This may explain in part why increased access to EC has increased use of EC without measurable effect on pregnancy rates in clinical trials. The two exceptions come from the same study, which occurred among women initiating the lactational amenorrhea method in Egypt. Participants were randomized to either receive a single dose of oral levonorgestrel EC or not.[37] In the final analysis of 2,708 participants, those in the advance provision group had a lower pregnancy rate (0.4% versus 5.3%, $P = .0001$) in the first 6 months postpartum, but the reason is that these women were far more likely to start using an ongoing contraceptive; the authors argue that using ECPs allowed the women time to get to a clinic for ongoing contraception. All of these studies used the LNG EC regimen, which is less effective than UPA, so it is possible that similar studies using UPA would find a greater population-level effect. EC will be increasingly important for individuals in places where abortion is severely restricted or entirely unavailable, but it will never be able to prevent all need for abortion.

Reproductive Coercion and Emergency Contraception

For some individuals, such as those facing reproductive coercion, repeated use of ECPs may be the best pregnancy prevention strategy they are aware of, or the one they feel best suits their needs.[152] Patients identified as repeatedly using ECPs should not be condemned, but rather compassionately engaged in a discussion to explore potential contraceptive challenges. (See Chapter 4, Person-Centered Reproductive Health Conversations and Contraceptive Counseling.) For those facing reproductive coercion, an IUD with the strings trimmed so they don't exit the cervix is often an ideal option, as it offers long-term, highly effective, unobtrusive contraception, without the need to store contraceptive supplies at home. For those desiring continuation of a normal menstrual pattern a copper IUD would be ideal. For those able to accommodate a period of heavier or irregular bleeding followed by long-term lighter or no bleeding, a levonorgestrel IUD could also be an option.

Advantages and Indications

Emergency contraceptives can prevent pregnancy after unprotected sexual intercourse or after a contraceptive "accident." This makes EC an essential part of treatment following sexual assault.[153] EC may also be appropriate in the following circumstances:[69,154]

- No contraceptive was used at the time of intercourse.
- An external (male) condom slipped, broke, or leaked.
- An internal (female) condom, diaphragm, or cervical cap was placed incorrectly, dislodged during intercourse, removed too early, or found to be torn.
- A patient missed two or more active COC pills during the first week of a pill pack and had any unprotected intercourse. A patient was late or missed one or more active pills in addition to also having missed taking a pill earlier in the packet or at the end of the previous packet. (Vomiting and severe diarrhea within 24 hours of taking a pill should be treated as a missed pill.)
- A person who is lactating is incompletely protected by lactational amenorrhea (because menses have returned, or baby has received feedings other than breast milk).
- Contraceptive use was delayed:
    - 3 or more hours late for a norethindrone-containing progestogen-only pill
    - More than 14 days late for a Depo-Provera (DMPA) injection
    - 2 or more days late placing a new vaginal ring after a hormone-free interval.
    - 2 or more days late starting a new patch cycle
- An internal condom was placed or removed incorrectly, leading to spillage of semen, or the penis was inserted mistakenly between the internal condom and the vaginal wall, resulting in the potential presence of intravaginal semen.
- An attempt at coitus interruptus resulted in ejaculation in the vagina or on external genitalia.
- Someone practicing a fertility awareness–based method (FABM) or periodic abstinence inadvertently had intercourse on a fertile day of the cycle.
- An IUD user cannot feel the IUD string, or the IUD was removed less than 7 days after the last act of intercourse.
- Someone was exposed to a possible teratogen such as Zika virus or isotretinoin when not protected by effective contraception.

The copper IUD may be an especially useful option for people who present 4 or 5 days after unprotected intercourse, because it provides highly effective emergency contraception and ongoing contraception. Early data suggest the same for the levonorgestrel 52 mg IUD.

Side Effects

Copper-Releasing or Levonorgestrel 52 mg IUD

Side effects after emergency placement of an IUD are similar to those seen after routine placement and may include abdominal discomfort and vaginal bleeding or spotting. (See Chapter 10, Intrauterine Devices [IUDs].)

ECPs

Nausea and Vomiting. These side effects impact about 13% to 29% of patients treated with either LNG or UPA ECPs;[116,117] the incidence of nausea was significantly higher with UPA than LNG in one randomized trial[117] but not in the other.[116] This is a significant improvement over the initial oral EC option of combined estrogen-progestogen ECPs, which produced nausea in about 50% of users, and vomiting in about 20%. Other reported complaints include fatigue, breast tenderness, headache, lower abdominal pain, dizziness, and diarrhea. Side effects are similar for the LNG and UPA regimens.[116,117] Side effects subside within a day or two after treatment is completed.

There is no research to indicate whether it is necessary to repeat the ECP dose if vomiting occurs within 2 hours after taking ECPs. Some practitioners take the view that a replacement dose should be given orally, or vaginally to prevent the tablets from being vomited a second time. Other providers, believing that nausea and vomiting are evidence of hormonal effects on the central nervous system and thus of absorption of the drugs, conclude that a replacement dose is not necessary unless an ECP tablet is visible in the vomitus.

Effects on Future Fertility and Inadvertently Exposed Pregnancies. There is no evidence that ECPs have any long-term or adverse effects on fertility. One study of 332 pregnant women who had used LNG ECPs in the conception cycle found no increased risk of birth defects.[155] Combined data from postmarketing surveillance and clinical trials of UPA found no teratogenic effects among 232 pregnancies with a known outcome in which the woman and conceptus were exposed to UPA.[156] Data on ulipristal from the German Federal Institute for Drugs and Medical Devices has also been reassuring.[157] Moreover, two observations provide reassurance for any concern about birth defects.[110] First, in the event of treatment failure, ECPs are taken long before organogenesis starts so, they should not have a teratogenic effect. Second, studies that have examined births to individuals who inadvertently continued to take COCs (including high-dose formulations) without knowing they were pregnant have found no increased risk of birth defects.[158-160] For this reason, the FDA removed warnings about adverse effects of combined oral contraceptives on the fetus from contraceptive package inserts years ago.[161]

Available evidence suggests that ECPs do not increase the chance that a pregnancy following ECP use will be ectopic; moreover, like all contraceptive methods, ECPs reduce the absolute risk of ectopic pregnancy by preventing ovulation, and thus pregnancy. Ectopic pregnancies represent 0.6% to 1% of oral ECP failures,[162,163] demonstrating no increased risk of ectopic pregnancy compared to overall ectopic pregnancy risk. So, just like in all early pregnancy evaluations, it is important to keep this possibility in mind whenever an ECP treatment failure occurs.

Menstrual Changes. Two studies have been specifically designed to assess the effects of LNG ECPs on bleeding patterns. Outcomes examined included length of the treatment and posttreatment cycles (where the first day of bleeding is cycle day 1), duration of bleeding during the menstrual period, and unscheduled bleeding. All three found that the length of the menstrual cycle can be shortened when treatment occurs early in the cycle.

The first study found that when taken in the first 3 weeks of the cycle, LNG 1.5 mg in a single dose significantly shortened that cycle as compared both to the usual cycle length and to the cycle length in a comparison group of similar women who had not taken ECPs. The magnitude of this effect was greater the earlier the pills were taken. However, when this regimen was taken later in women's cycles, it had no effect on cycle length, but it did cause prolongation of bleeding during the next menstrual period. Unscheduled bleeding was uncommon after ECP use, although more common than among women who had not taken ECPs.[164]

The second study compared the baseline cycle with the treatment and posttreatment cycles when LNG 1.5 mg was administered in a single dose. Cycle length was significantly shortened by 1 day when ECPs were taken in the preovulatory phase of the cycle and was significantly lengthened by 2 days when ECPs were taken in the postovulatory phase. No difference in cycle length was observed for women who took ECPs during the periovulatory phase of the cycle (from 2 days before to 2 days after the expected day of ovulation). In both the treatment and posttreatment cycles, the duration of bleeding during the menstrual period increased significantly when ECPs were taken in the periovulatory or postovulatory phase. The length of the posttreatment cycle remained significantly longer when ECPs were taken in the postovulatory phase. During the treatment cycle, 15% of women experienced unscheduled bleeding; this was significantly more common when ECPs were taken in the preovulatory phase.[165] Per the Cochrane review assessing interventions for EC, EC users taking ulipristal acetate are more likely than levonorgestrel EC users to have their menses return after the expected date (RR 1.65, 95% CI 1.42 to 1.92, 2 RCTs, n = 3,593).

Cautions

There are no true contraindications to the use of any ECPs.[166] However, in the United States, the labeling for LNG and UPA ECPs identifies known or suspected pregnancy as a contraindication. When ECPs are used during pregnancy they are not harmful, but they are ineffective.[167] All FDA-approved ECPs are estrogen-free, and thus safe even with vascular disease or migraine with aura. In all cases, use of UPA or LNG ECPs is preferable to use of combined estrogen-progestogen ECPs, as in addition to being safer, they are more effective.

Few adverse events have been reported for individuals using EC. Both UPA and oral LNG have an excellent safety profile. Without estrogen, they avoid elevating the risk of thrombosis, the most worrisome, though rare, major complications of estrogen-containing contraception. Common side effects of ulipristal acetate (all occurring in less than one in five EC users) include headache, abdominal pain, nausea, dysmenorrhea, fatigue, and dizziness.[168] For levonorgestrel EC users, common side effects include those above as well as, dizziness, breast pain, and vomiting.[169]

Lactation

During the first 6 months postpartum, individuals who are exclusively nursing and amenorrheic have little risk of pregnancy. There are no restrictions on use of any ECPs based on lactation status.[169] One study that examined LNG pharmacokinetics in plasma and milk of lactating women who take 1.5 mg for EC concluded that to limit infant exposure to the period of maximum LNG excretion in milk, mothers may consider avoiding nursing for 8 hours after they take ECPs;[170] however, the US Medical Eligibility Criteria for Contraceptive Use (US MEC) recommends no change in breast/chest feeding patterns. In a study of the effects of levonorgestrel ECPs on infant health and development, no adverse effects were noted.[171] In another study that compared outcomes among women who took LNG ECPs (after nursing) and among women who used progestogen-only oral contraceptives, no adverse effects were noted on maternal or infant health or continued lactation among the women who took ECPs.[172] The label for ella states, "It is not known if UPA is excreted in human milk. However, UPA is detected in milk of lactating rats. Because many drugs are excreted in human milk, risk to the breast-fed child cannot be excluded. Use of UPA by breastfeeding women is not recommended."[173] The US MEC states that there is no restriction on use of UPA by those who are lactating but recommends that they refrain from breast/chest feeding and discard pumped milk for 24 hours.[169] There are no contraindications to use of either copper or levonorgestrel 52 mg IUDs by lactating individuals.

Drug Interactions

Although medications that induce hepatic enzymes (such as phenytoin, rifampin, or efavirenz) could theoretically reduce the effectiveness of ECPs[174] by impacting pharmacokinetic profiles,[175] whether they actually reduce ECP effectiveness has not been directly studied. Nonetheless, caution is warranted, and patients taking such medications should be offered prompt access to placement of a copper or levonorgestrel 52 mg IUD as an alternative to ECPs. The UK's EC Guidelines have suggested "consider double-dose (3 mg) LNG if taking an enzyme inducer," but studies have not been conducted to inform this recommendation. Similarly, no clear guidance is available regarding adjustment of UPA dosing for those taking hepatic enzyme–inducing agents.[172] No significant interactions have been found with concurrent use of ECP and most antibiotics.

UPA is an antiprogestin. Therefore, there are implications for immediately starting progestogen-containing contraceptives after taking UPA (or using UPA after recently taking a progestogen). One randomized, double-blind, placebo-controlled study found no difference in the time (14 days) to achieve ovarian quiescence after taking UPA and starting a daily pill between the placebo group and the group who took a combined oral contraceptive starting the day after taking UPA.[176] A second randomized cross-over study examined women who quick-started a desogestrel progestogen-only oral contraceptive (75 μg desogestrel, not available in the United States) after taking UPA or a placebo.[177] The findings showed that initiating desogestrel the day after UPA significantly reduced UPA's ability to delay ovulation, from 97% to 55%. However, no significant differences were found in time to ovarian quiescence or cervical mucus penetrability with continued use of desogestrel. The FDA updated the ella package label to include warnings regarding the coadministration of ella and hormonal contraception. The label now states that if a patient wishes to use hormonal contraception after using ella, the ongoing method should be initiated no sooner than 5 days after taking ella, and that a reliable barrier method should be used until the next menstrual period. The label also now states that because ella and the progestogen component of hormonal contraceptives both bind to the progesterone receptor, using them together may impair the ability of ella to delay ovulation.

For people using COCs who miss pills and wish to use UPA as EC, one study indicates that for consistent pill users who miss three pills on days 5–7 of the cycle, it may be reasonable to immediately continue taking a daily combined pill,[178] although another study indicated that this may decrease the effectiveness of both contraceptives.[179]

Eligibility criteria and contraindications for placement of an IUD as EC are the same as for all IUD placements. (See Chapter 10, Intrauterine Devices [IUDs].) If concern exists about STIs (e.g., after unprotected intercourse with a new sexual partner or sexual assault), testing for STIs can occur at the time of IUD placement; if clinical suspicion of STI based on history is high, empiric antibiotics may be given. Patients who are found to harbor an STI after an IUD has been placed can be effectively treated with antibiotics with the IUD in place.

Providing Emergency Contraception

Although pregnancy can result from intercourse only during the fertile phase of the menstrual cycle, anyone requesting EC within 120 hours of unprotected intercourse should be offered treatment.[116,119,123,133,134]

It is important to remember that determining pregnancy risk is rarely straightforward. Although the probability of conception is low except for the 5 days just before ovulation and on the day of ovulation (see Figure 18-1, graph 1),[180] neither the patient nor the clinician is likely to actually know on which day ovulation occurs. What may be known are prior menstrual period dates. Plotting the probability of pregnancy based on menstrual period dates (see **Figure 18-1**, graph 2) shows that late (or early) ovulation is common enough that pregnancy risk is above 1% beginning as early as cycle day 7 and continuing until at least day 39.[181]

Counseling

In counseling patients who seek EC treatment, remember that those in need of EC are often facing a difficult and stressful situation. Be respectful of patients and responsive to their needs. (See Chapter 4, Person-Centered Reproductive Health Conversations and Contraceptive Counseling.)

Patients may feel embarrassed about not using an ongoing method of contraception or they may feel like a failure if they think they did not use their method correctly or if their contraceptive method failed, such as when a condom slips or breaks. Rape survivors will feel traumatized. Patients may be very concerned about possible infection, especially in cases of rape. Counsel patients and provide STI diagnostic services (or referrals) and information about preventive measures. If appropriate, explain reporting requirements regarding statutory rape. Be supportive of the patient's choices and refrain from making judgmental comments or indicating disapproval through body language or facial expressions. A supportive attitude is person-centered. Centering the individual will

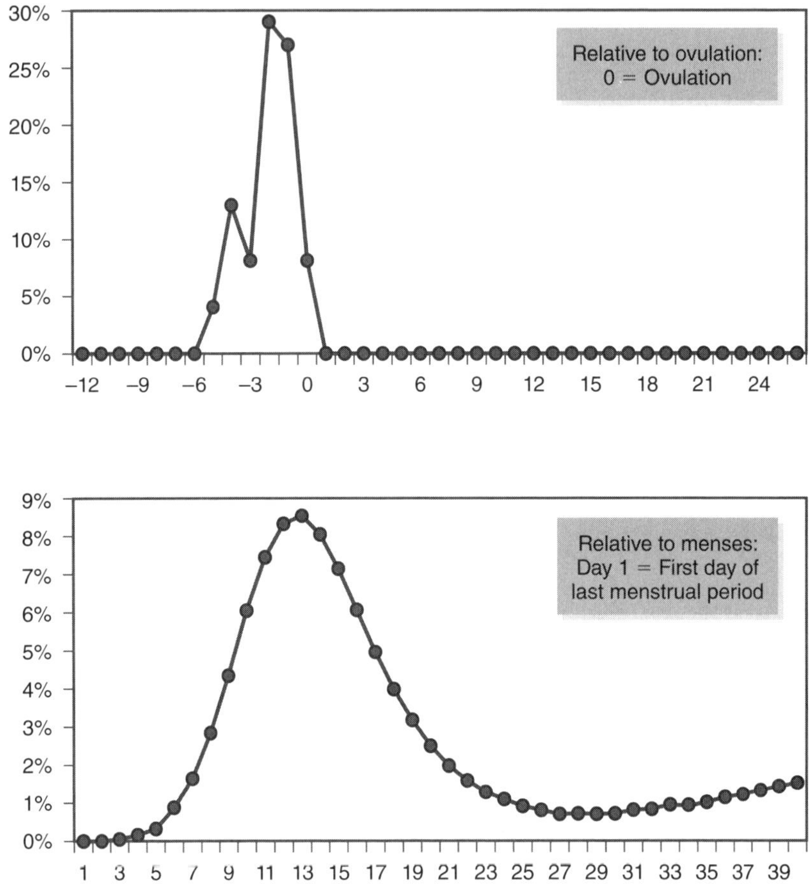

Figure 18-1 Pregnancy probability by cycle day.

Data from Wilcox AJ, Dunson DB, Weinberg CR, Trussell J, Baird DD. Likelihood of conception with a single act of intercourse: providing benchmark rates for assessment of post-coital contraceptives. Contraception 2001;63:211-5.

help with adherence to contraceptive plans and contribute to making the patient feel comfortable following up with counseling about regular contraceptive use and STI prevention. Patients should be advised that EC offers no protection against STIs, including infection with the human immunodeficiency virus (HIV). Therefore, postexposure HIV prophylaxis and emergency treatment of other infections may also be needed. (See Chapter 23, Reproductive Tract Infections, Including HIV and Other Sexually Transmitted Infections.)

Patients who would not have an abortion if EC treatment fails can be reassured that pregnancies occurring despite EC treatment do not have an increased risk of birth defects or other adverse outcomes.

Frequent Use

Advise the patient that ECPs are less effective than other contraceptives. However, repeated use of combined or LNG ECPs is not known to pose health risks to users other than pregnancy. The label for ella states that "Repeated use of ella within the same menstrual cycle is not recommended, as safety and efficacy of repeat use within the same cycle has not been evaluated."[172] However, a pharmacodynamic study of repeated use of UPA EC (every 7 days for 8 weeks) showed no safety concerns, indicating that UPA can be safely used more than once per cycle. However, the same study found that the majority of women in a smaller subgroup ovulated at least once during this period, suggesting that this may not be an effective longer-term method.[181]

Use After 72 Hours

Although most studies of ECP treatment have specified that treatment be administered within 72 hours, more recent studies have demonstrated the efficacy of ECPs up to 120 hours after unprotected intercourse.[119,123,133,134] However, a reanalysis of WHO studies concluded that LNG may not be effective at all after 96 hours.[136] Nonetheless, UPA is labeled for use up to 120 hours after intercourse.[116,118,175]

A number of studies demonstrate low pregnancy rates even when IUDs are placed 6–14 days after unprotected intercourse. For 134 copper IUD users reporting intercourse 6–14 days prior to IUD placement, there were 0 pregnancies (97.5% CI 0%–2.7%).[182] In a similar study of levonorgestrel 52 mg IUD users, there was 1 pregnancy among 187 participants (0.5%, 95% CI 0.01%–2.9%).[183] These findings suggest that, beyond their use for EC, either of these IUDs can be placed at any time in the menstrual cycle (when there is a negative pregnancy test) with low risk of pregnancy regardless of recent unprotected intercourse.

Use After Multiple Acts of Unprotected Intercourse

If more than 120 hours have elapsed since the time of the first unprotected act of intercourse, ECPs may be less effective in preventing pregnancy that resulted from that first exposure. Providing ECPs, however, would not be expected to disrupt or harm subsequent pregnancy development and would reduce the risk that pregnancy would result from later acts of intercourse that occurred within the preceding 120 hours. For IUDs, multiple episodes of unprotected intercourse in the same menstrual cycle of EC use does not appear to decrease EC efficacy.[184]

Ongoing Contraception

Patients requesting EC should be offered information and services for regular contraception (see Chapter 4, Person-Centered Reproductive Health Conversations and Contraceptive Counseling). However, not everyone will want contraceptive counseling or want to use other contraceptives. Thus, while it is recommended that providers offer contraception counseling, adoption of an ongoing regular method of contraception should never be a prerequisite for providing EC. It is coercive to withhold EC (or other services) unless a patient agrees to contraceptive counseling or starts ongoing contraception. If the reason for requesting EC is that the regular contraceptive method failed, offer to discuss reasons for failure and how this might be prevented in the future. Note that there are specific protocols to follow for initiating hormonal contraception after taking UPA for EC given the potential interaction between UPA and progestogen-containing contraceptives.

Before Providing Emergency Contraceptive Treatment

Although many people now obtain EC over the counter, when a clinician is consulted it is important to make certain the patient does not want to become pregnant, is aware of the range of available EC options, and understands there is still a chance of pregnancy after treatment. Describe common side effects; advance counseling about possible side effects helps patients know what to expect and may lead to greater satisfaction. A pregnancy test may be helpful if there is some doubt about whether the patient may have become pregnant after previous episodes of unprotected sex, earlier in the month. If this is not the case, pregnancy testing is unnecessary. If the patient is pregnant, ECP treatment will not be effective. Those with negative pregnancy tests can use ECPs to reduce their risk of becoming pregnant. Patients who do not have a period within 3 weeks of taking ECPs should be instructed to take a pregnancy test to see if they have become pregnant.[185] Pregnancy testing has been performed prior to IUD EC placement in the trials of this treatment.

Make sure patients understand that ECPs will not protect them from pregnancy if they engage in unprotected intercourse in the days or weeks following treatment. Because ECPs, especially UPA, can delay ovulation, a patient could be at risk of pregnancy if unprotected intercourse occurs within the first few days after ECP treatment. Individuals using LNG ECPs can start an ongoing hormonal method immediately, but those who use UPA should wait to start an ongoing method for 5 days after the last episode of unprotected sex before starting or resuming a hormonal method (unless they missed their pills on days 5, 6, and 7—in this case, there is evidence that they can immediately restart their pill after taking UPA). Anyone who needs EC because of missed or late pills, patch, or ring should be advised to resume their method if desired. For LNG ECP and UPA ECP users who have missed 3 days or fewer of their regular hormonal contraception, this can occur immediately. Other UPA ECP users should wait 5 days to resume their method. Patients who would like to start ongoing contraception should be counseled to determine the most appropriate EC method, taking into consideration which ongoing method they would like to use, and whether they are at greater risk of pregnancy from the previous act of intercourse or future acts of intercourse. EC users should abstain from intercourse or use a barrier method of contraception for 7 days after taking LNG or UPA.

EC Treatment Regimens

ECPs. For maximum effectiveness, ECP treatment should be started as soon as possible after unprotected intercourse, and within 120 hours. Treatment with UPA (one 30 mg tablet) is the most effective ECP option. LNG ECP treatment (LNG 1.5 mg tablet) is more effective and causes significantly less nausea and vomiting than treatment with combined estrogen-progestogen ECP options (e.g., ethinyl estradiol 0.1 to 0.2 mg and LNG 0.5 to 0.6 mg in each dose).

Combined estrogen-progestogen treatment involves two doses taken 12 hours apart. If necessary, adjust the timing for the second dose by a few hours to avoid a middle-of-the-night dose. Drugs and doses are shown in Table 18-1.

Intrauterine Devices. Placement of an IUD up to 2 weeks after unprotected sex may provide effective postcoital contraception.[182,183] If emergency IUD placement is planned, but cannot be carried out immediately, some patients may wish to take an ECP until their IUD is placed.

After Providing EC Treatment

Offer contraception counseling (see Chapter 4, Person-Centered Reproductive Health Conversations and Contraceptive Counseling). Oral LNG EC users wishing to continue use of a previously selected method of routine contraception can begin immediately. For UPA EC users, delay initiation of progestogen-containing contraception for 5 days, unless they have been using COCs and only missed 3 days or less. In that case, they should resume their COC immediately.[184] No follow-up is needed unless a normal menstrual period does not occur within 3 weeks, the patient suspects pregnancy, or if other reasons for concern arise. If there is any concern of pregnancy, perform a pregnancy test.

If EC has failed and the patient is pregnant, provide appropriate services or referrals. Recent use of UPA does not preclude subsequent use of mifepristone as needed to end an undesired pregnancy. For patients who decide to continue the pregnancy, reassure them that there is no evidence of any teratogenic effect following the use of ECPs. Pregnancy following emergency placement of an IUD should be managed with prompt counseling and a discussion of the rationale for recommending immediate removal of the IUD (see Chapter 10, Intrauterine Devices [IUDs]).

Advance Prescription of UPA

Provide a prescription in advance of need to interested patients for use when needed in the coming year. Alternatively, those who need EC can order UPA online (with overnight delivery in the United States) from Nurx (https://www.nurx.com/emergency contraception/) or Simple Health (https://www.simplehealth.com/birth-control/ella).

Additional Information and Materials

Additional information and materials are available from the following sources:

- The American Society for Emergency Contraception (www.americansocietyforec.org) offers clinical guidance about EC and information about EC access in the United States.
- ACOG Practice Bulletin No. 152: Emergency Contraception. *Obstet Gynecol* 2015;126:e1-e11.
- UK Faculty of Sexual and Reproductive Health Clinical Guideline: Emergency Contraception, amended December 2020 (https://www.fsrh.org/documents/ceu-clinical-guidance-emergency-contraception-march-2017/)

USER INSTRUCTIONS FOR EMERGENCY CONTRACEPTION*

Note that when creating patient education materials, health literacy and cultural considerations should be prioritized. (See Chapter 4, Person-Centered Reproductive Health Conversations and Contraceptive Counseling.)

* These instructions are intended to guide providers in educating patients in how to use their method.

ECP users should receive medication labeling that identifies the specific product prescribed and the number of tablets needed for each dose (see Table 18-1). Give the following instructions to ensure correct use.

1. **Take your ECP as directed:**
   a. **Ulipristal acetate (*ella*).** Swallow one tablet as soon as possible within 120 hours after unprotected sex. Taking more pills will not make you less likely to become pregnant.
   b. **LNG ECPs (*Plan B One-Step [or generic equivalent such as My Way, Take Action, or Aftera]*).** Swallow one tablet as soon as possible within 120 hours after unprotected sex. Taking more pills will not make you less likely to become pregnant.
   c. **Combined estrogen-progestogen ECPs.** Swallow the first dose as soon as possible within 120 hours after unprotected sex. Do not take any extra pills. Taking more pills will not make you less likely to become pregnant but may make you more nauseated and cause vomiting. Swallow the second dose 12 hours after taking the first dose. If necessary, you can delay the second dose by a few hours to avoid having to take your second dose in the middle of the night.

   Consider taking anti-nausea medication (two 25 mg tablets of meclizine) 1 hour before the first dose. About one-half of those who use combined ECPs have temporary nausea. It is usually mild and should stop in a day or so. If you vomit within 2 hours after taking a dose, call your clinician. You may need to repeat a dose of ECP.
2. **If your period does not start within 3 weeks, take a pregnancy test and/or see your clinician.** Your next period may start a few days earlier or later than usual. If you think you may be pregnant, see your clinician as soon as possible, whether or not you plan to continue the pregnancy.
3. **After you have taken your ECP, if you have unprotected intercourse the ECP will not give you protection from pregnancy. You will not be protected unless you are using condoms or another method of birth control.**
4. **If you discuss options for ongoing birth control with your clinician, they can let you know when you can start using your method and when it will start working.**

Instructions for patients who have placement of an IUD for EC are the same as for anyone who has an IUD placed (see Chapter 10, Intrauterine Devices [IUDs].)

Author Disclosures—Schwarz and Cleland, none; Turok: serves as a consultant for Sebela Pharmaceuticals and the national principal investigator for FDA trials of a copper and levonorgestrel IUD. The University of Utah's Division of Family Planning receives research funding from Bayer Women's Health Care, Organon (previously Merck & Co. Inc.), Cooper Surgical, Sebela Pharmaceuticals, Femasys, and Medicines360.

References

1. Trussell J, Ellertson C. Efficacy of emergency contraception. Fertility Control Reviews. 1995;4:8–11.
2. Shen J, Che Y, Showell E, Chen K, Cheng L. Interventions for emergency contraception. Cochrane Database Syst Rev. 2019;1(1):CD001324.

3. Ellertson C, Webb A, Blanchard K, et al. Modifying the Yuzpe regimen of emergency contraception: a multi-center randomized, controlled trial. Obstet Gynecol. 2003;101:1160-7.
4. Van Look PF, von Hertzen H. Clinical uses of antiprogestogens. Hum Reprod Update. 1995;1:19-34.
5. Glasier A, Thong KJ, Dewar M, Mackie M, Baird DT. Mifepristone (RU 486) compared with high-dose estrogen and progestogen for emergency postcoital contraception. N Engl J Med. 1992;327:1041-4.
6. Webb AM, Russell J, Elstein M. Comparison of Yuzpe regimen, danazol, and mifepristone (RU486) in oral postcoital contraception. BMJ. 1992;305:927-31.
7. Ashok PW, Stalder C, Wagaarachchi PT, Flett GM, Melvin L, Templeton A. A randomised study comparing a low dose of mifepristone and the Yuzpe regimen for emergency contraception. BJOG. 2002;109:553-60.
8. Hester KE, Harper MJK, Duffy DM. Oral administration of the cyclooxygenase-2 (COX-2) inhibitor meloxicam blocks ovulation in non-human primates when administered to simulate emergency contraception. Hum Reprod. 2010;25:360-7.
9. Jesam C, Salvatierra AM, Schwartz JL, Croxatto HB. Suppression of follicular rupture with meloxicam, a cyclooxygenase-2 inhibitor: potential for emergency contraception. Hum Reprod. 2010;25:368-73.
10. Edelman AB, Jensen JT, Doom C, Hennebold JD. Impact of the prostaglandin synthase-2 inhibitor celecoxib on ovulation and luteal events in women. Contraception. 2013;87:352-7.
11. Batur P, Cleland K, McNamara M, Wu J, Pickle S, EC Survey Group. Emergency contraception: A multispecialty survey of clinician knowledge and practices. Contraception. 2016;93:145-52.
12. National Center for Health Statistics. Special tabulation. (https://www.cdc.gov/nchs/nsfg/key_statistics/e.htm)
13. Hussain R, Kavanaugh ML. Changes in use of emergency contraceptive pills in the United States from 2008 to 2015. Contracept X. 2021;3:100065.
14. Patel A, Tilmon S, Bhogireddy V, Chor J, Patel D, Keith L. Emergency contraception after sexual assault: changes in provision from 2004 to 2009. J Reprod Med. 2012;57:98-104.
15. Patel A, Panchal H, Piotrowski ZH, Patel D. Comprehensive medical care for victims of sexual assault: a survey of Illinois hospital emergency departments. Contraception. 2008;77:426-30.
16. Kavanaugh ML, Saladino RA, Gold MA. Emergency contraception services for adolescents: a National Survey of Children's Hospital Emergency Department Directors. J Pediatr Adolesc Gynecol. 2009;22:111-9.
17. Goyal M, Zhao H, Mollen C. Exploring emergency contraception knowledge, prescription practices, and barriers to prescription for adolescents in the emergency department. Pediatrics. 2009;123:765-70.
18. Gilmore AK, McKee G, Flanagan JC, et al. Medications at the Emergency Department After Recent Rape. J Interpers Violence. 2021 Mar 18:886260521997434.
19. Goldenring JM, Allred G. Post-rape care in hospital emergency rooms. Am J Public Health. 2001;91:1169-70.
20. Stewart FH, Trussell J. Prevention of pregnancy resulting from rape: a neglected preventive health measure. Am J Prevent Med 2000;19:228-9.
21. US Dept of Justice, Office on Violence Against Women. National protocol for sexual assault medical forensic examinations: adults/adolescents. Washington DC: US Dept of Justice; 2004.
22. US Dept of Justice, Office on Violence Against Women. National protocol for sexual assault medical forensic examinations: adults/adolescents, 2nd ed. Washington DC: US Dept of Justice; 2013. (https://www.ojp.gov/pdffiles1/ovw/228119.pdf)
23. Glasier A, Baird D. The effects of self-administering emergency contraception. N Engl J Med 1998;339:1-4.
24. Raine T, Harper C, Leon K, Darney P. Emergency contraception: advance provision in a young, high-risk clinic population. Obstet Gynecol 2000;96:1-7.
25. Hazari K. Use of emergency contraception by women as a back-up method. Health Popul 2000;23:115-122.
26. Jackson RA, Schwarz EB, Freedman L, Darney P. Advance supply of emergency contraception: effect on use and usual contraception—a randomized trial. Obstet Gynecol 2003;102:8-16.

27. Gold MA, Wolford JE, Smith KA, Parker AM. The effects of advance provision of emergency contraception on adolescent women's sexual and contraceptive behaviors. J Pediatr Adolesc Gynecol 2004;17:87-96.
28. Lo SS, Fan SYS, Ho PC, Glasier AF. Effect of advanced provision of emergency contraception on women's contraceptive behavior: a randomized controlled trial. Hum Reprod. 2004;19:2404-10.
29. Belzer M, Sanchez K, Olson J, Jacobs AM, Tucker D. Advance supply of emergency contraception: a randomized trial in adolescent mothers. J Pediatr Adolesc Gynecol 2005;18:347-54.
30. Trussell J, Raymond E, Stewart FH. Letter to the editor. Comment on: Advance supply of emergency contraception [J Pediatr Adolesc Gynecol 2005 Oct;18(5):347-54]. J Pediatr Adolesc Gynecol 2006;19:251.
31. Walsh TL, Frezieres RG. Patterns of emergency contraception use by age and ethnicity from a randomized trial comparing advance provision and information only. Contraception 2006;74:110-7.
32. Marston C, Meltzer H, Majeed A. Impact on contraceptive practice of making emergency hormonal contraception available over the counter in Great Britain: repeated cross sectional surveys. BMJ 2005;331(7511):271-3.
33. Moreau C, Bajos N, Trussell J. The impact of pharmacy access to emergency contraceptive pills in France. Contraception 2006;73:602-8.
34. Schwarz EB, Gerbert B, Gonzales R. Computer-assisted provision of emergency contraception: a randomized controlled trial. J Gen Intern Med 2008;23:794-9.
35. Ekstrand M, Larsson M, Darj E, Tydén T. Advance provision of emergency contraceptive pills reduces treatment delay: a randomised controlled trial among Swedish teenage girls. Acta Obstet Gynecol Scand 2008;87:354-9.
36. Ekstrand M, Tydén T, Darj E, Larsson M. Twelve-month follow-up of advance provision of emergency contraception among teenage girls in Sweden-a randomized controlled trial. Ups J Med Sci 2013;118:271-5.
37. Shaaban OM, Hassen SG, Nour SA, Kames MA, Yones EM. Emergency contraceptive pills as a backup for lactational amenorrhea method (LAM) of contraception: a randomized controlled trial. Contraception 2013;87:363-369.
38. Raine TR, Harper CC, Rocca CH, et al. Direct access to emergency contraception through pharmacies and effect on unintended pregnancy and STIs: a randomized controlled trial. JAMA 2005;293:54-62.
39. Hu X, Cheng L, Hua X, Glasier A. Advanced provision of emergency contraception to postnatal women in China makes no difference in abortion rates: a randomized controlled trial. Contraception 2005;72:111-6.
40. Raymond EG, Stewart F, Weaver M, Monteith C, Van Der Pol B. Randomized trial to evaluate the impact of increased access to emergency contraceptive pills. Obstet Gynecol 2006;108:1098-106.
41. Graham A, Moore L, Sharp D, Diamond I. Improving teenagers' knowledge of emergency contraception: cluster randomized controlled trial of a teacher led intervention. BMJ 2002;234(7347):1179-84.
42. Ellertson C, Trussell J, Stewart F, Winikoff B. Should emergency contraceptive pills be available without prescription? J Am Med Wom Assoc. 1998;53 Suppl 2:S226-9, 232.
43. Grimes DA, Raymond EG, Scott Jones B. Emergency contraception over-the-counter: the medical and legal imperatives. Obstet Gynecol 2001;98:151-5.
44. Trussell J, Guthrie KA. Talking straight about emergency contraception. J Fam Plan Reprod Health Care. 2007;33:139-42.
45. Bellows BK, Tak CR, Sanders JN, Turok DK, Schwarz EB. Cost-effectiveness of emergency contraception options over 1 year. Am J Obstet Gynecol. 2018;218(5):508.e1-508.e9.
46. Trussell J, Leveque JA, Koenig JD, et al. The economic value of contraception: a comparison of 15 methods. Am J Public Health. 1995;85:494-503.
47. Sivin I. Utility and drawbacks of continuous use of a copper T IUD for 20 years. Contraception. 2007;75:Suppl S70-5.
48. Trussell J, Koenig J, Ellertson C, Stewart F. Preventing unintended pregnancy: the cost-effectiveness of three methods of emergency contraception. Am J Public Health. 1997;87:932-7.

49. Trussell J, Koenig J, Stewart F, Darroch JE. Medical care cost savings from adolescent contraceptive use. Fam Plann Perspect. 1997;29:248-55, 295.
50. Trussell J, Wiebe E, Shochet T, Guilbert É. Cost savings from emergency contraceptive pills in Canada. Obstet Gynecol. 2001;97:789-93.
51. Trussell J, Shochet T. Cost-effectiveness of emergency contraceptive pills in the public sector in the USA. Expert Rev Pharmacoeconomics Outcomes Res. 2003;3:433-40.
52. Trussell J, Calabretto H. Cost savings from use of emergency contraceptive pills in Australia. Aust N Z J Obstet Gynaecol. 2005;45:308-11.
53. Foster DG, Rostovtseva DP, Brindis CD, Biggs MA, Hulett D, Darney PD. Cost savings from the provision of specific methods of contraception in a publicly funded program. Am J Public Health. 2009;99:446-51.
54. Foster DG, Raine TR, Brindis C, Rostovtseva DP, Darney PD. Should providers give women advance provision of emergency contraceptive pills? A cost-effectiveness analysis. Womens Health Iss. 2010;20:242-7.
55. Bayer LL, Edelman AB, Caughey AB, Rodriguez MI. The price of emergency contraception in the United States: what is the cost-effectiveness of ulipristal acetate versus single-dose levonorgestrel? Contraception. 2013;87:385-90.
56. Bentancor A, Clarke D. Assessing Plan B: the effect of the morning-after pill on children and women. Econ J. 2017;127:2525-52.
57. Turok DK, Simonsen SE, Marshall N. Trends in levonorgestrel emergency contraception use, births, and abortions: the Utah experience. Medscape J Med. 2009;11(1):30.
58. Cleland K, Zhu H, Goldstruck N, Cheng L, Trussell J. The efficacy of IUDs for emergency contraception: a systematic review of 35 years of experience. Hum Reprod. 2012;27:1994-2000.
59. Mikolajczyk RT, Stanford JB. Levonorgestrel emergency contraception: a joint analysis of effectiveness and mechanism of action. Fertil Steril. 2007;88:565-71.
60. Black TR, Goldstuck ND, Spence A. Post-coital intrauterine device insertion - a further evaluation. Contraception. 1980; 22:653.
61. Guillebaud J, Kubba A, Rowlands S, et al. Post-coital contraception with Danazol, compared with an ethinyloestradiol—norgestrel combination or insertion of an intra-uterine device. J Obstet Gynaecol. 1983; 3:S64.
62. Bylander A, Nutu M, Wellander R, et al. Rapid effects of progesterone on ciliary beat frequency in the mouse fallopian tube. Reprod Biol Endocrinol. 2010;8:48.
63. Tamburrino L, Marchiani S, Minetti F, et al. The CatSper calcium channel in human sperm: relation with motility and involvement in progesterone-induced acrosome reaction. Hum Reprod. 2014;29:418.
64. Mahmood T, Saridogan E, Smutna S, et al. The effect of ovarian steroids on epithelial ciliary beat frequency in the human Fallopian tube. Hum Reprod. 1998;13:2991.
65. Nutu M, Weijdegård B, Thomas P, et al. Distribution and hormonal regulation of membrane progesterone receptors beta and gamma in ciliated epithelial cells of mouse and human fallopian tubes. Reprod Biol Endocrinol. 2009;7:89.
66. Endler M, Li RHW, Genzell Danielsson K. Effect of levonorgestrel emergency contraception on implantation and fertility: A review. Contraception 2022;109:8-18.
67. Li RHW, Resche-Rigon M, Bagchi IC, Gemzell-Danielsson K, Glasier A. Does ulipristal acetate emergency contraception (ella®) interfere with implantation? Contraception 2019;100(5):386-90.
68. American College of Obstetricians and Gynecologists. Statement on contraceptive methods. Washington DC: American College of Obstetricians and Gynecologists; July 1998.
69. Díaz S, Cárdenas H, Brandeis A, Miranda P, Salvatierra AM, Croxatto HB. Relative contributions of anovulation and luteal phase defect to the reduced pregnancy rate of breastfeeding women. Fertil Steril. 1992;58:498-503.
70. World Health Organization. Levonorgestrel for emergency contraception [Fact sheet]. Geneva (Switzerland): World Health Organization; 2005.
71. Protection of Human Subjects, 45 C.F.R. Sect. 46.202 (2009).
72. Hughes EC (ed). Committee on Terminology, The American College of Obstetricians and Gynecologists, Obstetric-Gynecologic Terminology. Philadelphia (PA): F.A. Davis Company; 1972.

73. Brache V, Cochon L, Deniaud M, Croxatto HB. Ulipristal acetate prevents ovulation more effectively than levonorgestrel: analysis of pooled data from three randomized trials of emergency contraception regimens. Contraception. 2013;88:611-8.
74. Stratton P, Hartog B, Hajizadeh N, et al. A single mid-follicular dose of CDB-2914, a new antiprogestin, inhibits folliculogenesis and endometrial differentiation in normally cycling women. Hum Reprod. 2000;15:1092-9.
75. Nallasamy S, Kim J, Sitruk-Ware R, Bagchi M, Bagchi I. Ulipristal blocks ovulation by inhibiting progesterone receptor-dependent pathways intrinsic to the ovary. Reprod Sci. 2013;20:371-81.
76. Brache V, Cochon L, Jesam C, et al. Immediate preovulatory administration of 30 mg ulipristal acetate significantly delays follicular rupture. Hum Reprod. 2010;25:2256-63.
77. Li HWR, Lo SST, Ng EHY, Ho PC. Efficacy of ulipristal acetate for emergency contraception and its effect on the subsequent bleeding pattern when administered before or after ovulation. Hum Reprod. 2016;31:1200-7.
78. Stratton P, Levens ED, Hartog B, Piquion J, Wei Q, Merino M, Nieman LK. Endometrial effects of a single early luteal dose of the selective progesterone receptor modulator CDB-2914. Fertil Steril. 2010;93:2035-41.
79. Berger C, Boggavarapu NR, Menezes J, Lalitkumar PG, Gemzell-Danielsson K. Effects of ulipristal acetate on human embryo attachment and endometrial cell gene expression in an in vitro co-culture system. Hum Reprod. 2015;30:800-11.
80. Munuce MJ, Gómez-Elías MD, Caille AM, Bahamondes L, Cuasnicú PS, Cohen DJ. Mechanisms involved in the contraceptive effects of ulipristal acetate. Reproduction. 2020 Mar;159(3):R139-R149. DOI: 10.1530/REP-19-0355.
81. Gómez-Elías MD, May M, Munuce MJ, Bahamondes L, Cuasnicú PS, Cohen DJ. A single post-ovulatory dose of ulipristal acetate impairs post-fertilization events in mice. Mol Hum Reprod. 2019;25(5):257-64.
82. Zumoffen C, Gómez-Elías MD, Caille AM, et al. Study of the effect of ulipristal acetate on human sperm ability to interact with tubal tissue and cumulus-oocyte-complexes. Contraception. 2017;95(6):586-91.
83. Li HWR, Gemzell-Danielsson K. Mechanisms of action of emergency contraception pills. Eur J Contracept Reprod Health Care. 2019;24(1):11-2.
84. Hapangama D, Glasier AF, Baird DT. The effects of peri-ovulatory administration of levonorgestrel on the menstrual cycle. Contraception. 2001;63:123-9.
85. Durand M, del Carmen Cravioto M, Raymond EG, et al. On the mechanisms of action of short-term levonorgestrel administration in emergency contraception. Contraception. 2001;64:227-34.
86. Marions L, Hultenby K, Lindell I, Sun X, Ståbi B, Gemzell Danielsson K. Emergency contraception with mifepristone and levonorgestrel: mechanism of action. Obstet Gynecol 2002;100:65-71.
87. Marions L, Cekan SZ, Bygdeman M, Gemzell-Danielsson K. Effect of emergency contraception with levonorgestrel or mifepristone on ovarian function. Contraception. 2004;69:373-7.
88. Croxatto HB, Brache V, Pavez M, Cochon L, et al. Pituitary-ovarian function following the standard levonorgestrel emergency contraceptive dose or a single 0.75-mg dose given on the days preceding ovulation. Contraception. 2004;70:442-50.
89. Durand M, Séppala M, del Carmen Cravioto M, et al. Late follicular phase administration of levonorgestrel as an emergency contraceptive changes the secretory pattern of glycodelin in serum and endometrium during the luteal phase of the menstrual cycle. Contraception. 2005;71:451-7.
90. Seppälä M, Taylor RN, Koistinen H, Koistinen R, Milgrom E. Glycodelin: a major lipocalin protein of the reproductive axis with diverse actions in cell recognition and differentiation. Endocr Rev. 2002;23:401-30.
91. do Nascimento JA, Seppala M, Perdigao A, et al. In vivo assessment of the human sperm acrosome reaction and the expression of glycodelin-A in human endometrium after levonorgestrel-emergency contraceptive pill administration. Hum Reprod. 2007;22:2190-5.
92. Palomino WA, Kohen P, Devoto L. A single midcycle dose of levonorgestrel similar to emergency contraceptive does not alter the expression of the L-selectin ligand or molecular markers of endometrial receptivity. Fertil Steril. 2010;94:1589-94.

93. Durand M, Koistinen R, Chirinos M, Rodríguez JL, Zambrano E, Seppälä M, Larrea F. Hormonal evaluation and midcycle detection of intrauterine glycodelin in women treated with levonorgestrel as in emergency contraception. Contraception. 2010;82:526-33.
94. Lalitkumar PG, Lalitkumar S, Meng CX, et al. Mifepristone, but not levonorgestrel, inhibits human blastocyst attachment to an in vitro endometrial three-dimensional cell culture model. Human Reprod. 2007;22:3031-7.
95. Meng CX, Andersson KL, Bentin-Ley U, Gemzell-Danielsson K, Lalitkumar PG. Effect of levonorgestrel and mifepristone on endometrial receptivity markers in a three-dimensional human endometrial cell culture model. Fertil Steril. 2009;91:256-64.
96. Kesserü E, Garmendia F, Westphal N, Parada J. The hormonal and peripheral effects of d-norgestrel in postcoital contraception. Contraception. 1974;10:411-24.
97. Yeung WS, Chiu PC, Wang CH, Yao YQ, Ho PC. The effects of levonorgestrel on various sperm functions. Contraception 2002;66:453-7.
98. Food and Drug Administration. Levonorgestrel 1.5 mg tablet emergency contraceptive labeling supplement for update to mechanism of action. December 23, 2022. (https://www.accessdata.fda.gov/drugsatfda_docs/label/2022/021998Orig1s005SumR.pdf)
99. Croxatto HB, Ortiz ME, Müller AL. Mechanisms of action of emergency contraception. Steroids. 2003;68:1095-8.
100. Novikova N, Weisberg E, Stanczyk FZ, Croxatto HB, Fraser, IS. Effectiveness of levonorgestrel emergency contraception given before or after ovulation—a pilot study. Contraception. 2006;74:349-50.
101. Noé G, Croxatto HB, Salvatierra AM, Reyes V, Villarroel C, Muñoz C, Morales G, Retamales A. Contraceptive efficacy of emergency contraception with levonorgestrel given before or after ovulation. Contraception. 2011;84:486-92.
102. Emergency contraception's mode of action clarified. Popul Briefs 2005;11:2. (http://www.popcouncil.org/uploads/pdfs/pbmay05.pdf).
103. Gemzell-Danielsson K, Berger C, Lalitkumar PGL. Emergency contraception - mechanisms of action. Contraception. 2013;87:300-8.
104. Swahn ML, Westlund P, Johannisson E, Bygdeman M. Effect of post-coital contraceptive methods on the endometrium and the menstrual cycle. Acta Obstet Gynecol Scand. 1996;75:738-44.
105. Ling WY, Robichaud A, Zayid I, Wrixon W, MacLeod SC. Mode of action of dl-norgestrel and ethinylestradiol combination in postcoital contraception. Fertil Steril. 1979;32:297-302.
106. Rowlands S, Kubba AA, Guillebaud J, Bounds W. A possible mechanism of action of danazol and an ethinylestradiol/norgestrel combination used as postcoital contraceptive agents. Contraception. 1986;33:539-45.
107. Croxatto HB, Fuentalba B, Brache V, et al. Effects of the Yuzpe regimen, given during the follicular phase, on ovarian function. Contraception. 2002;65:121-8.
108. Kubba AA, White JO, Guillebaud J, Elder MG. The biochemistry of human endometrium after two regimens of postcoital contraception: a dl-norgestrel/ethinylestradiol combination or danazol. Fertil Steril. 1986;45:512-6.
109. Ling WY, Wrixon W, Zayid I, Acorn T, Popat R, Wilson E. Mode of action of dl-norgestrel and ethinylestradiol combination in postcoital contraception. II. Effect of postovulatory administration on ovarian function and endometrium. Fertil Steril. 1983;39:292-7.
110. Yuzpe AA, Thurlow HJ, Ramzy I, Leyshon JI. Post coital contraception—a pilot study. J Reprod Med. 1974;13:53-8.
111. Taskin O, Brown RW, Young DC, Poindexter AN, Wiehle RD. High doses of oral contraceptives do not alter endometrial a1 and anb3 integrins in the late implantation window. Fertil Steril. 1994;61:850-5.
112. Raymond EG, Lovely LP, Chen-Mok M, Seppälä M, Kurman RJ, Lessey BA. Effect of the Yuzpe regimen of emergency contraception on markers of endometrial receptivity. Hum Reprod. 2000;15:2351-5.
113. Glasier A. Emergency postcoital contraception. N Engl J Med. 1997;337:1058-64.
114. Ling WY, Wrixon W, Acorn T, Wilson E, Collins J. Mode of action of dl-norgestrel and ethinylestradiol combination in postcoital contraception. III. Effect of preovulatory administration following the luteinizing hormone surge on ovarian steroidogenesis. Fertil Steril. 1983;40:631-6.

115. Turok DK, Godfrey EM, Wojdyla D, Dermish A, Torres L, Wu SC. Copper T380 intrauterine device for emergency contraception: highly effective at any time in the menstrual cycle. Hum Reprod. 2013;28:2672-6.
116. Turok DK, Gero A, Simmons RG, Kaiser JE, Stoddard GJ, Sexsmith CD, Gawron LM, Sanders JN. Levonorgestrel vs. copper intrauterine devices for emergency contraception. N Engl J Med. 2021;384(4):335-44.
117. Raymond E, Taylor D, Trussell J, Steiner MJ. Minimum effectiveness of the levonorgestrel regimen of emergency contraception. Contraception. 2004;69:79-81.
118. Glasier AF, Cameron ST, Fine PM, et al. Ulipristal acetate versus levonorgestrel for emergency contraception: a randomised non-inferiority trial and meta-analysis. Lancet. 2010;375:555-62.
119. Creinin MD, Schlaff W, Archer DF, et al. Progesterone receptor modulator for emergency contraception: a randomized controlled trial. Obstet Gynecol. 2006;108:1089-97.
120. Fine P, Mathé H, Ginde S, Cullins V, Morfesis J, Gainer E. Ulipristal acetate taken 48-120 hours after intercourse for emergency contraception. Obstet Gynecol. 2010;115:257-63.
121. von Hertzen H, Piaggio G, Ding J, et al. Low dose mifepristone and two regimens of levonorgestrel for emergency contraception: a WHO multicentre randomised trial. Lancet. 2002;360:1803-10.
122. Hamoda H, Ashok PW, Stalder C, Flett GM, Kennedy E, Templeton A. A randomized trial of mifepristone (10 mg) and levonorgestrel for emergency contraception. Obstet Gynecol. 2004;104:1307-13.
123. Wu S, Dong J, Cong J, Wang C, VonHertzen H, Godfrey EM. Gestrinone compared with mifepristone for emergency contraception: a randomized controlled trial. Obstet Gynecol. 2010;115:740-4.
124. Arowojolu AO, Okewole IA, Adekunle AO. Comparative evaluation of the effectiveness and safety of two regimens of levonorgestrel for emergency contraception in Nigerians. Contraception. 2002;66:269-73.
125. Ngai SW, Fan S, Li S, et al. A randomized trial to compare 24h versus 12h double dose regimen of levonorgestrel for emergency contraception. Hum Reprod. 2004;20:307-11.
126. Ho PC, Kwan MS. A prospective randomized comparison of levonorgestrel with the Yuzpe regimen in post-coital contraception. Hum Reprod. 1993;8:389-92.
127. Task Force on Postovulatory Methods of Fertility Regulation. Randomised controlled trial of levonorgestrel versus the Yuzpe regimen of combined oral contraceptives for emergency contraception. Lancet. 1998;352:428-33.
128. Dada OA, Godfrey EM, Gilda Piaggio G, von Hertzen H. A randomized, double-blind, noninferiority study to compare two regimens of levonorgestrel for emergency contraception in Nigeria. Contraception. 2010;82:373-8.
129. Farajkhoda T, Khoshbin A, Enjezab B, Bokaei M, Karimi Zarchi M. Assessment of two emergency contraceptive regimens in Iran: levonorgestrel versus the Yuzpe.Niger J Clin Pract. 2009;12:450-2.
130. Trussell J, Rodríguez G, Ellertson C. Updated estimates of the effectiveness of the Yuzpe regimen of emergency contraception. Contraception. 1999;59:147-51.
131. Trussell J, Ellertson C, von Hertzen H, Bigrigg A, Webb A, Evans M, Ferden S. Leadbetter C. Estimating the effectiveness of emergency contraceptive pills. Contraception. 2003;67:259-65.
132. Massai MR, Forcelledo ML, Brache V, et al. Does meloxicam increase the incidence of an ovulation induced by single administration of levonorgestrel in emergency contraception? A pilot study. Hum Reprod. 2007;22:434-9.
133. Yuzpe AA, Lancee WJ. Ethinylestradiol and dl-norgestrel as a postcoital contraceptive. Fertil Steril. 1977;28:932-6.
134. Piaggio G, Kapp N, von Hertzen H. Effect on pregnancy rates of the delay in the administration of levonorgestrel for emergency contraception: a combined analysis of four WHO trials. Contraception. 2011;84:35-39.
135. Moreau C, Trussell J. Results from pooled phase III studies of ulipristal acetate for emergency contraception. Contraception. 2012;86:673-680.
136. Glasier A, Cameron ST, Blithe D, et al. Can we identify women at risk of pregnancy despite using emergency contraception? Data from randomized trials of ulipristal acetate and levonorgestrel. Contraception. 2011;84:363-7.

137. European Medicines Agency. Annex III: Amendments to relevant sections of the summary of product characteristics and package leaflet for Levonorgestrel-containing emergency contraceptive medicinal products. (http://www.ema.europa.eu/docs/en_GB/document_library/Referrals_document/Emergency_contraceptives_31/WC500176384.pdf)
138. European Medicines Agency. Levonorgestrel and ulipristal remain suitable emergency contraceptives for all women, regardless of bodyweight [press release]. July 7, 2014. (http://www.ema.europa.eu/ema/index.jsp?curl=pages/news_and_events/news/2014/07/news_detail_002145.jsp&mid=WC0b01ac058004d5c1)
139. Festin MP, Peregoudov A, Seuc A, Kiarie J, Temmerman M. Effect of BMI and body weight on pregnancy rates with LNG as emergency contraception: analysis of four WHO HRP studies. Contraception. 2017;95:50-54.
140. Edelman A, Cherala G, Blue S, Erikson D, Jensen J. Impact of obesity on the pharmacokinetics of levonorgestrel-based emergency contraception: single and double dosing. Contraception. 2016;94:52-57.
141. Edelman AB, Hennebold JD, Bond K, et al. Double dosing levonorgestrel-based emergency contraception for individuals with obesity: a randomize controlled trial. Obstetr Gynecol. 2022;140(1):48-54.
142. Praditpan P, Hamouie A, Basaraba CN, Nandakumar R, Cremers S, Davis AR, Westhoff CL. Pharmacokinetics of levonorgestrel and ulipristal acetate emergency contraception in women with normal and obese body mass index. Contraception. 2017;95:464-9.
143. American Society for Emergency Contraception. Efficacy of emergency contraception and body weight: Current understanding and recommendations. 2022. (https://www.americansocietyforec.org/_files/ugd/0cdab4_12f4b1c5cdf64feab998bc561692137c.pdf)
144. Trussell J, Ellertson C, Stewart F, Raymond EG, Shochet T. The role of emergency contraception. Am J Obstet Gynecol. 2004;190:S30-8.
145. Festin MP, Bahamondes L, Nguyen TM, et al. A prospective, open-label, single arm, multicentre study to evaluate efficacy, safety and acceptability of pericoital oral contraception using levonorgestrel 1.5 mg. Hum Reprod. 2016;31:530-40.
146. Shaaban OM, Hassen SG, Nour SA, Kames MA, Yones EM. Emergency contraceptive pills as a backup for lactational amenorrhea method (LAM) of contraception: a randomized controlled trial. Contraception. 2013;87:363-9.
147. Shaaban OM, Abbas AM, Mahmoud HR, Yones EM, Hassen SG, Zakherah MS. Counseling and in-advance provision of levonorgestrel emergency contraceptive pills decrease the rate of unplanned pregnancy during breastfeeding: a randomized controlled trial. J Matern Fetal Neonatal Med. 2019;32(8):1250-5.
148. Raymond EG, Trussell J, Polis C. Population effect of increased access to emergency contraceptive pills: a systematic review. Obstet Gynecol. 2007;109:181-8.
149. Polis CB, Grimes DA, Schaffer K, Blanchard K, Glasier A, Harper C. Advance provision of emergency contraception for pregnancy prevention. Cochrane Database Syst Rev. 2007 Apr18;(2):CD005497.
150. Glasier A, Fairhurst K, Wyke S, Ziebland S, Seaman P, Walker J, Lakha F. Advanced provision of emergency contraception does not reduce abortion rates. Contraception. 2004;69:361-6.
151. Baecher L, Weaver MA, Raymond EG. Increased access to emergency contraception: why it may fail. Hum Reprod. 2009;24:815-9.
152. Raymond EG, Shochet T, Drake JK, Westley E. What some women want? On-demand oral contraception. Contraception. 2014;90:105-10.
153. Feldhaus KM. A 21st-century challenge: improving the care of the sexual assault victim. Ann Emerg Med. 2002;39:653-5.
154. World Health Organization. Selected practice recommendations for contraceptive use. 2nd ed. Geneva (Switzerland); 2005.
155. Zhang L, Chen J, Wang Y, Ren F, Yu W, Cheng L. Pregnancy outcome after levonorgestrel-only emergency contraception failure: a prospective cohort study. Hum Reprod. 2009;24:1605-11.
156. Levy DP, Jager M, Kapp N, Abitbol JL. Ulipristal acetate for emergency contraception: postmarketing experience after use by more than 1 million women. Contraception. 2014;89:431-3.

157. Wagner JK, Dathe K, Schaefer C, Hoeltzenbein M. Ulipristal acetate and pregnancy outcome-an observational study. Hum Reprod. 2020;35(4):751-8. DOI: 10.1093/humrep/deaa024.
158. Raman-Wilms L, Tseng AL, Wighardt S, Einarson TR, Koren G. Fetal genital effects of first-trimester sex hormone exposure: a meta-analysis. Obstet Gynecol. 1995;85:141-9.
159. Bracken MB. Oral contraception and congenital malformations in offspring: a review and meta-analysis of the prospective studies. Obstet Gynecol. 1990;76:552-7.
160. Simpson JL, Phillips OP. Spermicides, hormonal contraception and congenital malformations. Adv Contraception. 1990;6:141-67.
161. US Food and Drug Administration. Prescription drug products; certain combined oral contraceptives for use as postcoital emergency contraception. Fed Regist. 1997;62:8610-2.
162. Trussell J, Hedley A, Raymond E. Ectopic pregnancy following use of progestin-only ECPs [letter]. J Fam Plann Reprod Health Care. 2003;29:249.
163. Cleland K, Raymond E, Trussell J, Cheng L, Zhu H. Ectopic pregnancy and emergency contraception: a systematic review. Obstet Gynecol. 2010;115:1263-6.
164. Raymond EG, Goldberg A, Trussell J, Hays M, Roach E, Taylor D. Bleeding patterns after use of levonorgestrel emergency contraceptive pills. Contraception. 2006;73:376-81. Erratum in: Contraception. 2006;74:349-50. Erratum in: Contraception. 2007;75:476-7.
165. Gainer E, Kenfack B, Mboudou E, Doh AS, Bouyer J. Menstrual bleeding patterns following levonorgestrel emergency contraception. Contraception. 2006;74:118-24.
166. Centers for Disease Control and Prevention. U.S. Medical Eligibility Criteria for Contraceptive Use, 2016. MMWR Recomm Rep. 2016;65(3):1-108.
167. Wagner JK, Dathe K, Schaefer C, Hoeltzenbein M. Ulipristal acetate and pregnancy outcome-an observational study. Hum Reprod. 2020 Apr 28;35(4):751-758. DOI: 10.1093/humrep/deaa024. PMID: 32322890.
168. Ulipristal acetate. US FDA approved product information. National Library of Medicine. (https://www.dailymed.nlm.nih.gov/dailymed/drugInfo.cfm?setid=2bf93d23-cddd-4613-9066-5b5fa090404b)
169. Teva Women's Health, Inc. Plan B (levonorgestrel). Highlights of prescribing information. 2017. (https://www.accessdata.fda.gov/drugsatfda_docs/label/2017/021045s016lbl.pdf)
170. Gainer E, Massai R, Lillo S, et al. Levonorgestrel pharmacokinetics in plasma and milk of lactating women who take 1.5 mg for emergency contraception. Hum Reprod. 2007;22:1578-84.
171. Shaaban OM, Abbas AM, Mahmoud HR, Yones EM, Mahmoud A, Zakherah MS. Levonorgestrel emergency contraceptive pills use during breastfeeding; effect on infants' health and development. J Matern Fetal Neonatal Med. 2019;32(15):2524-8. DOI: 10.1080/14767058.2018.1439470.
172. Polakow-Farkash S, Gilad O, Merlob P, Stahl B, Yogev Y, Klinger G. Levonorgestrel used for emergency contraception during lactation-A prospective observational cohort study on maternal and infant safety. J Matern Fetal Neonatal Med 2013;26:219-21.
173. Afaxys, Inc. ella: Highlights of prescribing information. 2015. (http://www.accessdata.fda.gov/drugsatfda_docs/label/2015/022474s007lbl.pdf)
174. Le Corvaisier C, Capelle A, France M, Bourguignon L, Tod M, Goutelle S. Drug interactions between emergency contraceptive drugs and cytochrome inducers: literature review and quantitative prediction. Fundam Clin Pharmacol. 2021;35(2):208-16. DOI: 10.1111/fcp.12601.
175. Carten ML, Kiser JJ, Kwara A, Mawhinney S, Cu-Uvin S. Pharmacokinetic interactions between the hormonal emergency contraception, levonorgestrel (Plan B), and Efavirenz. Infect Dis Obstet Gynecol. 2012;2012:137192. DOI: 10.1155/2012/137192.
176. Cameron ST, Berger C, Michie L, Klipping C, Gemzell-Danielsson K. The effects on ovarian activity of ulipristal acetate when 'quickstarting' a combined oral contraceptive pill: a prospective, randomized, double-blind parallel-arm, placebo-controlled study. Hum Reprod. 2015;30:1566-72.
177. Brache V, Cochon L, Duijkers IJM, et al. A prospective, randomised pharmacodynamic study of quick-starting desogestrel progestin-only pill following ulipristal acetate for emergency contraception. Hum Reprod. 2015;30:2785-93.

178. Banh C, Rautenberg T, Duijkers I, et al. The effects on ovarian activity of delaying versus immediately restarting combined oral contraception after missing three pills and taking ulipristal acetate 30 mg. Contraception. 2020;102(3):145-151.
179. Edelman AB, Jensen JT, McCrimmon S, Messerle-Forbes M, O'Donnell A, Hennebold JD. Combined oral contraceptive interference with the ability of ulipristal acetate to delay ovulation: A prospective cohort study. Contraception. 2018;98(6):463-466.
180. Wilcox AJ, Dunson DB, Weinberg CR, Trussell J, Baird DD. Likelihood of conception with a single act of intercourse: providing benchmark rates for assessment of post-coital contraceptives. Contraception. 2001;63:211-5.
181. Jesam C, Cochon L, Salvatierra AM, et al. A prospective, open-label, multicenter study to assess the pharmacodynamics and safety of repeated use of 30 mg ulipristal acetate. Contraception. 2016;93:310-6.
182. Thompson I, Sanders JN, Schwarz EB, Boraas C, Turok DK. Copper intrauterine device placement 6-14 days after unprotected sex. Contraception. 2019;100(3):219-21.
183. Boraas CM, Sanders JN, Schwarz EB, Thompson I, Turok DK. Risk of pregnancy with levonorgestrel-releasing intrauterine system placement 6-14 days after unprotected sexual intercourse. Obstet Gynecol. 2021 Apr 1;137(4):623-625.
184. BakenRa A, Gero A, Sanders J, Simmons R, Fay K, Turok DK. Pregnancy risk by frequency and timing of unprotected intercourse before intrauterine device placement for emergency contraception. Obstet Gynecol. 2021;138(1):79-84.
185. Grimes DA, Raymond EG. Bundling a pregnancy test with the Yuzpe regimen of emergency contraception. Obstet Gynecol. 1999;94:471-3.

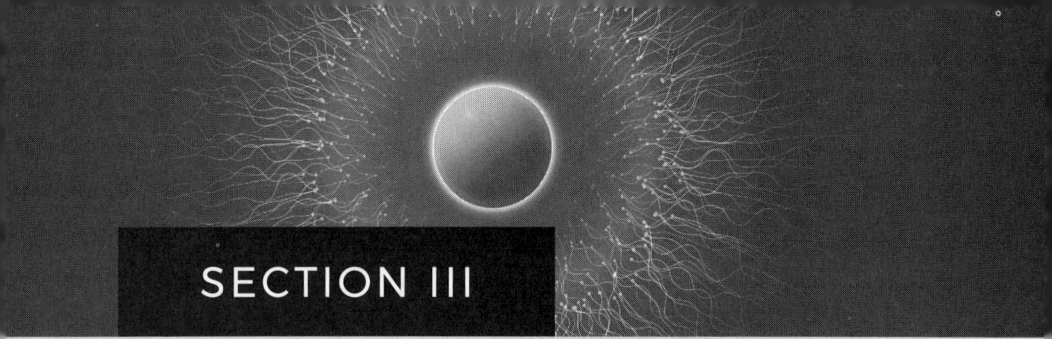

SECTION III

Contraception During Life Stages and Medical Conditions

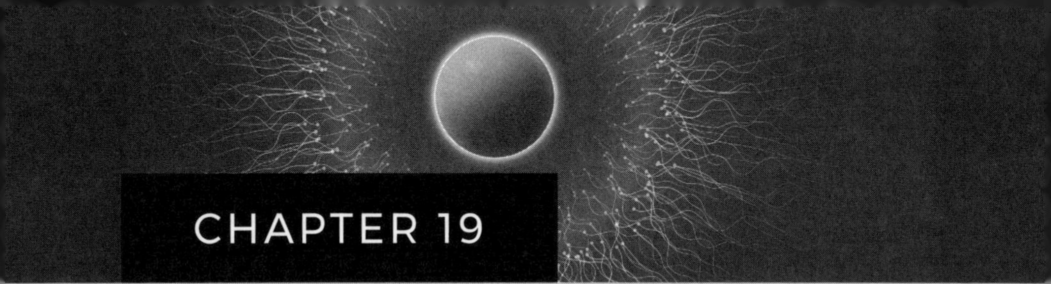

CHAPTER 19

Contraception After Pregnancy

Crystal Goldsmith, MD, MS
Melissa Kottke, MD, MPH, MBA

KEY POINTS

- Postpartum is a unique and dynamic time requiring a personalized and iterative approach to contraceptive counseling.
- The postpartum period is one of unmet contraceptive need.
- Lactational amenorrhea is a highly effective, temporary method of birth control that is available immediately postpartum.
- Progestin-only and nonhormonal contraceptive methods may be initiated immediately postpartum.
- Estrogen-containing contraceptives should be avoided for 3–6 weeks postpartum depending upon individual characteristics.
- All methods are considered compatible with breastfeeding at some point.

Postpartum is a unique time in a person's life. Individuals may experience a variety of health, physiological, emotional, and relational changes. Postpartum people may have different goals for their family size after delivery. Further, they may have different priorities for their contraception postpartum compared to prior to delivery, such as compatibility with breastfeeding, child-spacing, efficacy, ease of use, or noncontraceptive benefits. Importantly, the postpartum time-period is one of unmet contraceptive need; therefore, person-centered contraceptive counseling and conscious connection to an individual's preferred contraceptive can help support reproductive autonomy during this time.

A note on language: postpartum individuals may have diverse gender identities, future needs for pregnancy prevention, and preferences for infant feeding. Furthermore, robust empirical data on postpartum contraceptive needs and human milk feeding for people who use gender-affirming therapies in the postpartum period are lacking. Throughout this chapter, when possible, we will use gender-neutral terms for the postpartum individual unless citing specific studies' terminology. We will also use the term breastfeeding, as much of the empirical literature pertaining to contraception does, but we acknowledge that the terms chest feeding and human milk feeding are more inclusive terms and may be preferred by some.

Counseling about Contraception After Pregnancy

As with contraceptive counseling during other times in an individual's life, patient-centered counseling and shared decision-making should be employed. (See Chapter 4, Person-Centered Reproductive Health Conversations and Contraceptive Counseling.) Pregnancy and the postpartum period are incredibly dynamic, and many factors may change during this time that influence a person's contraceptive needs and goals. Counseling about postpartum contraception should begin during prenatal care and should be readdressed periodically. Several factors that are unique for postpartum individuals may be relevant to discuss, including (but not limited to) return of fecundity, birth spacing, medical conditions, anticipated system barriers, and individual preferences and goals, including desire for breastfeeding.

Postpartum Infertility

During pregnancy, cyclic ovarian function is suspended. The corpus luteum, which arises from the ovulated follicle, secretes steroids, including estrogen and progesterone, that are essential in maintaining the early weeks of pregnancy. Later, these steroids are secreted by the placenta and play a more dominant role in the hormonal support of the pregnancy. Luteal and placental steroids suppress the circulating levels of follicle-stimulating hormone (FSH) and luteinizing hormone (LH) and disrupt their pulsatile release from the pituitary.[1] When the placenta is delivered, the levels of estrogen and progesterone drop significantly, the levels of FSH and LH gradually recover, and the pituitary resumes the pulsatile release of FSH and LH.[2]

After delivery, there is a natural period of infertility due to changing hormonal milieu, but the duration is variable and unpredictable. Most nonlactating postpartum individuals resume menses within 4 to 6 weeks of delivery. On average, the first ovulation occurs 45 days postpartum, although not all first menses are preceded by normal luteal phases. About one-third of first cycles are anovulatory, and a proportion of first ovulatory cycles have a deficient corpus luteum that secretes subnormal amounts of steroids. In the second and third menstrual cycles, 15% are anovulatory and 25% of ovulatory cycles have luteal-phase defects.[3] Breastfeeding suppresses ovarian function and extends the period of infertility.[4] This is discussed further later in the section on lactational amenorrhea.[5]

Postpartum Sexual Activity

Ovulation alone does not create risk for pregnancy; ovulation with exposure to sperm, however, does. A review of the return to sexual activity and intercourse postpartum indicates that many people resume sexual intercourse within several weeks of delivery.[6] In small samples of people who were breastfeeding, monthly coital frequency in the second month postpartum averaged 2.4, increasing to 3.2 to 4.9 in the third postpartum month.[7] There is no medically necessary waiting period before resuming sexual activity after delivery. Each person must make that decision for themselves. Clinicians can use these data to provide anticipatory guidance to patients and to ensure that they have what they need to prevent pregnancy. Importantly, delaying discussion of contraception to some arbitrary point in the future may not meet the patient's needs and could create risk for unwanted pregnancy.

Birth Spacing Recommendations

Discussion of an individual's reproductive desires during the prenatal period can include recommendations about birth spacing. Short interpregnancy intervals (IPIs: the intervals between a live birth and conception of another pregnancy) have been associated with adverse maternal and infant outcomes. These include preterm birth, small for gestational age, infant mortality, and uterine rupture in those with a previous cesarean.[8–11] Systematic reviews have suggested that these outcomes have stronger associations in low-resource settings. As a result, the World Health Organization (WHO) advises an IPI of at least 24 months.[11] The American College of Obstetricians and Gynecologists (ACOG) advises that people should be counseled to avoid IPIs shorter than 6 months and be counseled about the risks and benefits of repeat pregnancy sooner than 18 months.[9] Not surprisingly, the choice to use contraception and the type of contraception selected are related to IPI. Balancing the patient's individual goals with the risk of adverse health outcomes is critical.

System Factors

Unfortunately, system factors may present barriers between postpartum individuals and their desired contraceptive method. For example, as many as 40% of postpartum individuals do not attend their postpartum visit.[12] This is influenced by several factors, but is higher in people with limited resources.[13] Further, some individuals lose insurance coverage weeks after delivery or never have coverage beyond emergency coverage of the delivery. Finally, some religiously affiliated hospitals do not allow any contraceptive service delivery, and others have policies that do not support immediate provision of injections, intrauterine devices (IUDs), implants, or permanent contraception.[9] While not completely predictable, clinicians can help patients navigate the known barriers and plan around them accordingly. This may include advocating for permanent, or long-acting and reversible, contraception in the hospital setting and/or providing prescriptions in advance of need, arranging for early follow-up postpartum, and increasing awareness of local resources for contraception, like Title X and other publicly funded sources. Likewise, it is important to ensure that patients who have implant or IUD placement in the immediate or early postpartum period have information regarding and access to services for removal when desired, especially for those who lose insurance coverage after delivery.

Patient Preferences and Goals

As with any other time in a person's life, an individual's preferences and goals for seeking and preventing pregnancy, as well as characteristics for contraception if desired, should be prioritized during contraceptive counseling. (See Chapter 4, Person-Centered Reproductive Health Conversations and Contraceptive Counseling.) A postpartum individual may have different contraceptive priorities than they had before pregnancy and may differentially prioritize safety, ease of use, noncontraceptive benefits, or long-term or permanent protection. Unique to the postpartum time, a person may also want assurance that contraception is compatible with breastfeeding.

The practice of breastfeeding is supported by most leading public health and professional societies around the world. Breastfeeding facilitates attachment and bonding. Human milk has both nutritional and anti-infective advantages for the infant. The infant ingests substances that provide host-protection, humoral factors, and allergy prophylaxis. These are particularly concentrated in the colostrum, the high-protein, high-antioxidant fluid secreted in the first few days postpartum. The mixtures of protein, fat, carbohydrate, and trace elements in breastmilk change to meet the infant's evolving needs as breastfeeding proceeds from month to month.[14,15] There are both short-term and long-term health benefits of breastfeeding to the infant. Breastfeeding reduces the risk of acute otitis media, nonspecific diarrheal disease, respiratory tract infections, atopic dermatitis, asthma, type 1 diabetes, childhood leukemia, sudden infant death syndrome, and necrotizing enterocolitis.[16] Later in life, having been breastfed is associated with significant positive effects in blood pressure, serum cholesterol, overweight and obesity, and risk of type 2 diabetes.[17] In the United States, there are few absolute contraindications to breastfeeding; individuals living with HIV infection should talk with their doctors about the risk of transmission of HIV in breastmilk.[18]

Breastfeeding also has protective effects for the postpartum individual against premenopausal cancers of the ovary, endometrium, and breast; type 2 diabetes; hypertension; cardiovascular disease; and stroke.[19–24] Breastfeeding increases caloric expenditure, and as such, breastfeeding may facilitate return to prepregnancy weight. Finally, breastfeeding supports a rapid return of uterine tone. Oxytocin, which induces uterine contractions, is released from the posterior pituitary when the nipple is stimulated by suckling. During lactation, the body's estrogen levels are very low, and vaginal lubrication may be less than usual and begin later during sexual activity. Vaginal lubrication improves when cycling resumes or when the frequency of breastfeeding declines.[25]

Most medications taken by the breastfeeding individual are safe for the infant, and excellent references are available that list and describe those medications that may require an interruption of breastfeeding.[26] Breastfeeding requires additional protein, calcium, iron, and several vitamins and other micronutrients. The increased needs for specific nutrients can be provided by a well-balanced diet, although many are encouraged to continue their prenatal vitamins during breastfeeding. Supplements are generally unnecessary unless the diet is deficient in one or more of these nutrients.[27]

Despite the wide endorsement for breastfeeding, the United States falls short in the breastfeeding goals of Healthy People 2030: 42.4% of infants exclusively breastfed through 6 months and 54.1% breastfed at 1 year.[28] According to the US Breastfeeding Report Card,[29] among infants born in 2019, most (83.2%) received some breast milk, but 19.2% also received formula before 2 days of age. At 6 months, 55.8% of infants received any breast milk and 24.9% received breast milk exclusively. Support for breastfeeding is wide and multilevel factors (i.e., individual, financial, cultural, workplace, insurance, education, and family leave) can influence breastfeeding. When it comes to individual patient counseling and contraception, it is prudent to seek to understand an individual's priorities with breastfeeding as well as pregnancy prevention and work collaboratively to outline a plan that supports all of the patient's goals.

While data show that use of hormonal contraception during breastfeeding is safe for the infant, some people prefer not to expose their infant to hormones of any kind. Providers can respectfully query patients about what is concerning to them about hormones and offer to share data that are relevant to their specific concern. Providers can offer reassurance that there are no harmful effects of using hormonal contraception while breastfeeding for the infant, but providers should respect this preference and work with the patient to find a method that is aligned with their preferences and values. (See Chapter 4, Person-Centered Reproductive Health Conversations and Contraceptive Counseling.)

Individualized Recommendations and Timing of Initiation

While delivery is an event, the postpartum period, including contraceptive care, is a continuum. In 2018, ACOG released its new approach and guidance for "Optimizing Postpartum Care." In it, they outline that postpartum care should be "an ongoing process rather than a single encounter, and that services and support [be] tailored to…individual needs." The document encourages initial contact with the postpartum individual within 3 weeks of delivery as well as a comprehensive postpartum visit within 12 weeks of delivery. Importantly, during this dynamic time, an individual's goal and health can change and influence the contraception that is most appropriate for them at the time. An iterative, personalized approach is necessary.[9] The clinician must consider timing of initiation and take into account breastfeeding goals. The US Medical Eligibility Criteria for Contraceptive Use (US MEC) outlines the initiation of breastfeeding status.[30] These recommendations are outlined in **Table 19-1**.

There are a couple of key themes identified from the US MEC recommendations. First, most methods are safe for use immediately after birth in most people, including IUDs, implants, and progestin-only contraceptive methods. Second, all contraceptive methods are considered safe with breastfeeding (potentially at different time points). Finally, combined hormonal contraception (CHC) should not be used in the first 3 weeks postpartum. There is no risk of pregnancy during this time, and the risk of venous thromboembolism (VTE) is increased. As such, there is no added benefit and an increase in potential for harm. The increased risk of VTE decreases over time from delivery, and individuals who are not breastfeeding and who do not have other VTE risk factors can safely begin to use CHC after 3 weeks, accordingly. The postpartum period, itself, increases risk of VTE substantially, but it is important to recognize the other factors that can increase this risk. Some of these are commonly encountered in postpartum individuals and may not have been a part of prenatal discussions about postpartum contraceptive planning. Factors that increase VTE risk postpartum include age ≥35 years, previous VTE, thrombophilia, immobility, transfusion at delivery, peripartum cardiomyopathy, BMI ≥30 kg/m^2, postpartum hemorrhage, postcesarean delivery, preeclampsia, and smoking.[30] Some of these factors would independently discourage CHC use (e.g., previous VTE or thrombophilia); however, some generally are not associated with increased risk outside of the immediate postpartum period (e.g., postcesarean delivery or postpartum hemorrhage). Clinicians need to take into account these factors and potentially new medical conditions when counseling about safety of contraceptive methods postpartum.

Table 19-1 **US Medical Eligibility Criteria for Postpartum and Breastfeeding Individuals**

Postpartum Initiation of Contraception	Etonogestrel Implant or Progestin Only Pills	Depo-medroxyprogesterone Acetate	Combined Hormonal Contraception
Less than 21 days after delivery	2/1*	2/1*	4
21–29 days w/VTE risk factors**	2/1*	2/1*	3
21–29 days w/o VTE risk factors**	2/1*	2	3/2*
30–42 days w/ VTE risk factors**	1	1	3
30–42 days w/o VTE risk factors**	1	1	2
More than 42 days	1	1	2/1*
Postplacental Placement		**Levonorgestrel IUD**	**Copper 380-A IUD**
Less than 10 minutes after placental delivery		2/1*	1
More than 10 minutes and less than 4 weeks		2	2
4 weeks or later		1	1
Postpartum sepsis		4	4

*Breastfeeding/nonbreastfeeding

**Postpartum venous thromboembolism (VTE) risk factors: age ≥35 years, previous VTE, thrombophilia, immobility, transfusion at delivery, peripartum cardiomyopathy, BMI ≥30 kg/m^2, postpartum hemorrhage, postcesarean delivery, preeclampsia, smoking

Data from Curtis KM, Tepper NK, Jatlaoui TC, et al. U.S. Medical Eligibility Criteria for Contraceptive Use, 2016. MMWR Recomm Rep 2016;65(3):1-104.

Postpartum Considerations for Contraceptive Methods

Lactational Amenorrhea Method (LAM)

Breastfeeding is a natural, temporary contraceptive method uniquely available to postpartum individuals. The sensitivity of the nipple and areola increases at birth.[31] Infant suckling stimulates the nerve endings in the nipple and areola. Nerve impulses are passed to the hypothalamus, stimulating the release of various hormones, including those that regulate prolactin. Prolactin controls the rate of milk production but is not believed to play a major role in suppressing ovarian function.[32] Instead, suckling appears to disrupt the pulsatile release of gonadotropin-releasing hormone (GnRH) by the hypothalamus,[33] perhaps by increasing hypothalamic b-endorphin production.[34] The disruption of GnRH release in turn averts the normal pulsatility of LH, which is required for follicle development and some steroid synthesis in the ovary. Plasma levels of FSH return to normal follicular phase values by 4–8 weeks postpartum in breastfeeding individuals.[33] In contrast, LH pulsation is disorganized in terms of the frequency or the amplitude of the LH pulse in most lactating individuals throughout much of the period of lactational amenorrhea.[35] Small amounts of secreted estrogen at this time are insufficient to trigger an LH surge necessary to induce ovulation.[36]

Full or nearly full breastfeeding is necessary to rely on LAM for contraception and is associated with longer periods of lactational amenorrhea and infertility than is combination feeding (formula and human milk). Frequent stimulation of the breast by suckling day and night helps maintain the cascade of neuroendocrine events that produces the contraceptive effect.[37] The breastfeeding characteristics that contribute significantly to delay the return of ovulation include a high frequency of breastfeeds, a long total duration of feedings, a short interval between breastfeeds, and the presence of night feeds.[3,38] If introduction of solid/supplemental foods does not decrease this optimal amount of suckling, small amounts of supplementation should have little or no effect on the return of ovulation. However, if LAM is to be relied upon for contraception, supplements should be given only infrequently, in small amounts, and not by bottle. **Table 19-2** describes different infant feeding patterns and can be helpful in determining whether the person is fully or nearly fully

Table 19-2 Breastfeeding Patterns and Impact on Fertility Inhibition

Breastfeeding practice	Criteria	Fertility inhibition
Exclusive	Breastfeeds only: ■ < 4 hours daytime intervals ■ < 6 hours nighttime intervals	Significant
Almost exclusive	Breastfeeds with *infrequent* supplementation: ■ < 4 hours daytime intervals ■ < 6 hours nighttime intervals Only 5-15% of feeds supplemented, the fewer the better. Supplementation may include vitamins, mineral water, juice, or ritualistic feeds	Significant
High partial	Breastfeeds are great preponderance of feeds: ■ < 4 hours daytime intervals ■ < 6 hours nighttime intervals Only 5-15% of feeds supplemented, the fewer the better.	Significant, but any supplementation or interruption of the breastfeeding pattern can restore fertility

(continues)

Table 19-2 Breastfeeding Patterns and Impact on Fertility Inhibition *(continued)*

Breastfeeding practice	Criteria	Fertility inhibition
Medium partial	About half of all feeds are breastfeeds	Little
Low partial	Great preponderance of feeds are NOT breastfeeds	Little

Milk expression, such as by hand or pump, may not fully substitute for breastfeeding in terms of its fertility-inhibiting effect.

breastfeeding.[39,40] *Milk expression, such as by hand or pump, may not fully substitute for breastfeeding in terms of its fertility-inhibiting effect.* Individuals relying on LAM after returning to work and using milk expression during working hours demonstrated an elevated 6-month probability of pregnancy (5.2% compared to 2%).[41] This suggests that adequate milk production and full feeding with breastmilk may not suppress fertility as sufficiently as frequent suckling by the infant. Ultimately, the relationship between milk expression, milk volume, and hormonal regulation is complex and warrants additional study, particularly in countries where postpartum individuals have minimal maternity leave. While many parents are highly motivated to breastfeed, those returning to work are half as likely to breastfeed compared to nonworking counterparts.[42–44] While this highlights the importance of paid family leave in supporting breastfeeding families, focus also must turn to supporting breastfeeding individuals within the workplace. Research demonstrates that providing adequate break time and a private location to express breastmilk doubles exclusive breastfeeding rates. Patients receiving verbal support from managers were also more likely to continue to breastfeed.[45] Moreover, insurance coverage of breastfeeding services and supplies are essential.

If a person exclusively breastfeeds and has not experienced any postpartum menses, the risk of pregnancy is 2% in the first 6 months following a birth.[37,39,46] (See **Figure 19-1** and Table 19-2.) Four prospective clinical studies of the contraceptive effect of LAM demonstrated a cumulative 6-month life-table perfect-use probability of pregnancy ranging from 0.5% to 1.5% among those who relied solely on LAM.[5,47–49] While pregnancy rates during the use of LAM compare favorably with those for many other methods of contraception (see Chapter 5, Effectiveness, Safety, and Comparative Side Effects), even greater effectiveness could be achieved by a combination of breastfeeding and use of additional contraception.

Ovulation can occur even if a breastfeeding person has not yet resumed menstruation. The probability that ovulation will precede the first menses increases over time:[38,50]

- 33% to 45% during the first 3 months postpartum
- 64% to 71% during months 4 through 12
- 87% to 100% after 12 months.

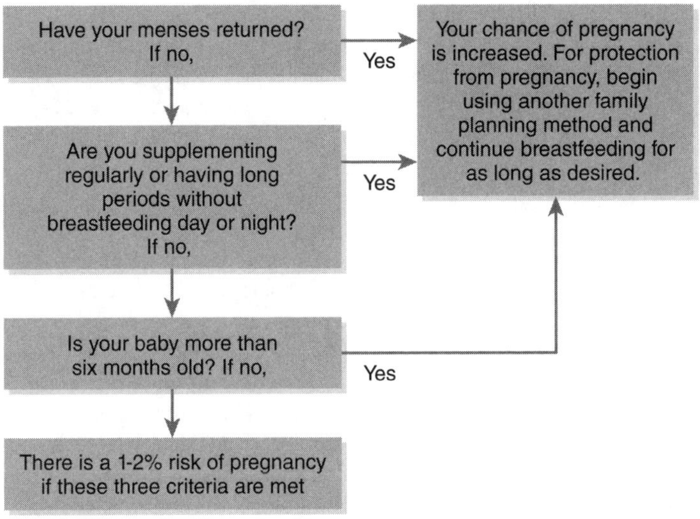

Figure 19-1 LAM: Lactational Amenorrhea Method

Even though about 60% of ovulations preceding first menses have an adequate luteal phase,[50] patients need to be aware that lactational amenorrhea becomes increasingly unreliable as an indicator of infertility beyond 6 months postpartum. Accordingly, additional contraception should be considered for individuals who are breastfeeding but are not able to fully or nearly fully breastfeed, whose menses have resumed, or who rely on nonsuckling milk expression or infant supplementation, and for those who are six months or greater postpartum.

Permanent Contraception

Patients who have achieved their desired family size or are done with childbearing may be interested in permanent contraception options, including vas or tubal surgery. It is essential to discuss immediate postpartum contraceptive surgery well before the delivery to help ensure that consent is fully informed and appropriate paperwork is completed. Studies consistently demonstrate that only half of patients requesting postpartum tubal surgery will be able to get it. Those who do not receive their requested procedure had twice the rate of pregnancy at 12 months compared to those who had not requested the procedure.[51] Barriers exist at all levels, from religiously affiliated hospitals denying procedures, to lack of available operating room (OR) time, to health care provider bias.[52] Nearly two-thirds of those unable to access tubal surgery at time of delivery were denied because of unsigned or invalid Medicaid consent forms.[53]

Permanent contraception via tubal surgery performed during the immediate postpartum period can be a more cost-effective and simpler technique than interval procedures. After a vaginal delivery, tubal surgery should be performed by mini-laparotomy within 48 hours or else delayed for 4 to 6 weeks. After 48 hours, access to the tubes is reduced. Tubal surgery can be performed at the time of cesarean delivery through the abdominal incision. As with mini-laparotomy after vaginal delivery, tubal surgery at the time of cesarean may need to be delayed in the case of severe complications.[54] While tubal surgery is a highly effective method of contraception, a small risk of sterilization failure persists for at least a decade. Partial salpingectomy performed postpartum, however, carries a very low 10-year pregnancy risk.[55] Recently, there has been a shift toward bilateral total rather than partial salpingectomy. This is due to evidence suggesting a tubal origin for some ovarian cancers and a possible decreased risk for ovarian cancers in those undergoing total bilateral salpingectomy compared to traditional methods of tubal surgery. There is conflicting data regarding the impact of total versus partial salpingectomy on OR time and costs in the postpartum setting.[56–58] Differences, if they exist, are minimal and should not be a barrier to offering this procedure.[59]

For patients desiring to breastfeed, skin-to-skin contact and the first suckling episode are recommended within the first hour after birth (known as the "golden hour"). For people who deliver vaginally, permanent contraception procedures should be performed after the golden hour. For patients delivered by cesarean, skin-to-skin contact and suckling may be accomplished in the OR. Use of spinal, epidural, and general anesthesia are not contraindications to breastfeeding. General anesthesia, however, may interfere with breastfeeding given food and fluid restrictions preoperatively and increased operative stress levels. Thus, neuraxial analgesia is preferred for postpartum surgery. Nonetheless, patients need not discard breastmilk and may resume breastfeeding as soon as they are awake and alert and have recovered from the anesthetic effects.[60]

Partner vas surgery is an effective method that can be done in an outpatient setting and allows participation of the partner in the pregnancy prevention. Pregnancy or the postpartum period may be a convenient time for a vas surgery, in that the inherent postpartum infertility plus any lactational infertility can act as a bridge until the vasectomy can be relied upon for contraception (generally about 3 months postprocedure; see Chapter 8, Permanent Contraception). Partner vas surgery does not interfere with breastfeeding.

Intrauterine Devices

Intrauterine devices (IUDs) provide the potential for long-acting birth control and require little effort for new parents. IUDs placed postpartum are best placed either (1) immediately after the expulsion of the placenta, or (2) after 4 weeks postpartum. It is less desirable to place an IUD in between because of the higher expulsion rate that occurs during uterine involution.[61] However, studies have demonstrated the feasibility, safety, and acceptability of IUD insertion less than 4 weeks postpartum.[62,63] An IUD can be inserted during a cesarean delivery through the uterine incision prior to closure. Immediate post-placental-delivery IUD placement should not be performed when chorioamnionitis is present because of the elevated risk of infection.[64] Immediate postpartum placement has not been associated with excessive bleeding or endometritis.[65] Expulsion rates following immediate postpartum placement are higher than those following interval placement 4–6 weeks postpartum or later.[66] One small pilot study has examined expulsion rates in people receiving an immediate postplacental IUD after vaginal compared to cesarean birth and found that risk of expulsion was 4.5 times greater following vaginal birth.[67] Subsequent studies similarly report lower expulsion rates when an IUD is placed after cesarean birth when compared to placement after a vaginal birth.[68,69] One study suggests that the LNG 52 mg

IUD demonstrates a greater risk of expulsion when placed immediately postpartum compared to the copper 380 mm^2 IUD.[70] Despite higher rates of expulsion immediately postpartum, a review by Lopez and colleagues identified that utilization of an IUD at 6 months postpartum is twice as high for those who had an IUD placed immediately postpartum due to access issues with later placement.[71] Individuals who have an IUD placed immediately postpartum are more likely to experience missing IUD strings or malpositioned IUDs and so postpartum care and follow-up remain important.

Perforation risk may be higher among those who are breastfeeding (3.7–6.3/1000 vs. 1/1000 in nonbreastfeeding individuals). The increased risk persists for at least 18 weeks postpartum.[72,73] This modest increase in perforation risk does not suggest that IUDs should not be placed in those who are breastfeeding. However, providers should quote the 3–7:1000 risk of perforation rather than 1:1000 when counseling and obtaining informed consent for those who are postpartum. Clinicians placing IUDs should be aware of this increased risk and take care during placement to approach the fundus slowly and intentionally when sounding and placing the IUD to avoid momentum.

All available IUDs are excellent options for individuals desiring a reversible, highly effective, contraceptive. As a nonhormonal method, the copper on the Cu 380 mm^2 IUD has no plausible impact on the quantity or quality of breastmilk. Similarly, the LNG IUDs are considered safe with breastfeeding.[30,74] (See Table 19-1, MEC for Postpartum Contraception.) A randomized controlled trial has evaluated time to lactogenesis and breastfeeding continuation in women assigned to postplacental placement of an LNG 52 mg IUD versus placement 4–8 weeks postpartum. No differences were noted in time to mature milk or in continuation of breastfeeding at 3 months.[75] (See Chapter 10, Intrauterine Devices [IUDs].)

Progestin-only Contraception

Placement of the progestin-only contraceptive implant in the immediate postpartum period has been evaluated in several studies.[76–78] A randomized controlled trial assigned people to contraceptive implant placement in the immediate postpartum period (within 60 hours) or at the postpartum visit (at 4–8 weeks postpartum). The onset of mature milk was not different between these groups and continuation of breastfeeding (both any and exclusive) did not differ at 6 months. Of note, 20% of participants randomized to delayed placement did not attend their postpartum visit and did not have an implant placed. All women in the immediate postpartum group had the implant placed. This supports prior data demonstrating that immediate use of postpartum implants is associated with a decrease in rapid repeat pregnancies and is highly cost-effective.[79] No comparative study has demonstrated a difference in breastmilk quality or infant growth or development for people utilizing an etonogestrel contraceptive implant during breastfeeding.[80,81] Based on available data, both the US MEC and the WHO MEC[82] find use of postpartum implants safe at all time points among both breastfeeding and nonbreastfeeding patients.

There is theoretical concern about administration of injectable progestin immediately upon delivery and before the onset of mature milk because injectables result in faster, higher circulating levels of hormone than other noninjectable methods.[83] To date, this theoretical concern has not been supported by data. Two small studies have shown that depot medroxyprogesterone acetate (DMPA) injection immediately postpartum has no impact on lactation, though neither study had power to detect small differences.[77,84] WHO's study of DMPA provided at 6 weeks postpartum demonstrated no impact on infant growth or development and small increases in the breastmilk production compared with nonhormonal methods of contraception.[85] The US MEC does not distinguish injectables from any other progestin-only method and describes all progestin-only methods as having benefits that outweigh the risks at any time postpartum.[30]

The use of progestin-only pills is considered safe for use during lactation.[85–87] Frequently, people are started on the progestin-only pill (POP) in the immediate postpartum period, with a plan to switch to CHC when the risk for VTE has declined and lactation is better established. It is essential to counsel fully regarding the differences in combination versus progestin-only pills. Specifically, the most commonly used POP in the United States (norethindrone 0.35 mg) is nearly entirely metabolized within 24 hours, requiring users take the pill at the same time daily.[88] People should be given a clear timeline regarding when they may safely transition to a CHC, if that is their goal.

In 2019, a POP containing drospirenone 4 mg was approved by the FDA. Ovulation inhibition is greater with the drospirenone pill compared to the norethindrone pill, eliminating the requirement to take it at the same time every day.[89] A single study has evaluated the presence of drospirenone in breast milk among 12 pill users and found 0.11% of the maternal daily dose.[90] These findings suggest use of drospirenone pills among breastfeeding patients would be unlikely to impact lactation. However, there have been no studies evaluating clinical breastfeeding outcomes such as breastfeeding continuation. Additionally, phase 3 trials demonstrated no VTE events, suggesting that drosprinenone-only pill use would be safe for use in the immediate postpartum period.[91]

Combined Hormonal Contraception

CHC use (including the combination pill, patch, injectable, and vaginal ring) is contraindicated <21 days postpartum for all patients due to the increased risk for VTE during the immediate postpartum period. The risk of VTE in the postpartum period is five times the risk during pregnancy and remains elevated through at least the sixth postpartum week.[92,93] The CDC MEC concluded the risks of CHC use outweigh the benefits in the first 42 days in the presence of patient characteristics (age, obesity, preeclampsia, postpartum hemorrhage, etc.) that increase VTE risk and in the first 30 days in the absence of those risk factors.[30]

CHC use among breastfeeding patients has been the subject of multiple reviews.[94–96] The evidence is inconsistent regarding the effect of CHC on breastfeeding and insufficient regarding the impact on the infant when CHC was initiated less than 6 weeks postpartum. Older studies demonstrate a decrease in milk volume and breastfeeding, but they may reflect the use of COCs with higher doses of estrogen than are used today. Indeed, higher-dose COCs were prescribed historically to suppress lactation.[85] Newer studies suggest no impact on milk volume[97] or breastfeeding duration[98] but include only short-term data regarding breastfeeding. The WHO MEC considers the evidence regarding decreased breastmilk production to contraindicate the use of COCs in the first 6 weeks of breastfeeding and to relatively contraindicate it in the period from 6 weeks to 6 months.[82] However, the US MEC considers CHC safe for use in postpartum people after 6 weeks regardless of breastfeeding status (See Table 19-1).[30]

Other Methods

Emergency contraceptive pills (ECPs) are considered safe for use in the postpartum period. Use of levonorgestrel ECPs has been studied in breastfeeding individuals, demonstrating no impact on milk quantity or infant growth and development.[99] Therefore the WHO and US MEC indicate that levonorgestrel (LNG) ECP can be used with no restriction by breastfeeding individuals.[30,82] Ulipristal acetate (UPA) has no published data regarding use during breastfeeding. The manufacturer of UPA recommends restricting use during breastfeeding (in the prescribing information)[100]—however, UPA levels rapidly decline over 24 hours. Thus, the US MEC deems it safe for use (Category 1) during lactation but recommends discarding breastmilk for 24 hours after use.[30] The WHO MEC takes a more conservative stand, listing UPA as a Category 2 contraceptive during lactation and recommending breastmilk be discarded for a full week after use.[82] More research should be done to further delineate the presence of UPA in breastmilk. Advanced prescription of LNG ECP to patients planning to use LAM has been shown to decrease short interval pregnancies.[101] Placement of an IUD is the most effective form of emergency contraception, and an IUD may be placed in postpartum and breastfeeding patients as described above. (See Chapter 18, Emergency Contraception.)

Condoms and spermicides are readily available and do not require a prescription. In the United States, barrier methods are the most widely used contraceptive among lactating mothers in the first 6 months postpartum.[6] Both internal and external condoms can offer a readily available, on-demand contraceptive option. Lubricated condoms may be useful in the postpartum period because of increased vaginal dryness. Similarly, spermicides may help offset dryness. However, all spermicides currently available in the United States use nonoxynol 9 (N-9), which acts as a detergent to disrupt the membranes of the sperm's flagella and body to immobilize or destroy it. N-9 can have the same disruptive effect on the epithelial cells of the vagina, cervix, and rectum, which can denude the epithelium and cause vaginal or penile irritation (See Chapter 16, On-Demand Internal Methods). In animal studies, N-9 is absorbed through the skin and secreted in breastmilk.[102] The question of whether N-9 is secreted in breastmilk has not been completely evaluated in humans. (See Chapter 14, External (Male) Condoms.) A new contraceptive vaginal pH modulator that does not contain N-9 is available, and though data on use postpartum and during breastfeeding are limited, the biological plausibility of concern is extremely low as its mechanism of action is to keep the pH of the vagina low even after deposition of high-pH semen.

Diaphragms and cervical cap use needs to be delayed in the postpartum setting. It is recommended to avoid use until 6 weeks postdelivery. The ensures the uterus has involuted and the cervix has returned to a nonpregnant size and shape. Additionally, the risk of toxic shock syndrome is increased when blood, including the postpartum lochia, is present.[103] Finally, the perineum may be tender, causing patients to prefer to delay fitting due to discomfort. Of note, the contraceptive sponge and cervical cap (though not the diaphragm) have higher failure rates among parous individuals *even during perfect use.* (See Chapter 16, On-Demand Internal Methods.) Inform patients about this decrease in efficacy so they can make an informed choice of a contraceptive method.

Fertility awareness–based methods cannot be used before menstrual cycles are reestablished and cyclic signs of fertility return.[104] The return of fertility symptoms after the first postpartum menses may be especially difficult for new users to identify and may lead to an increased risk for pregnancy.[105] Basal body temperature cannot be ascertained before at least 6 hours of uninterrupted sleep. Thus, the person who gets up in the night to care for an infant is precluded from using the temperature symptom to help determine ovulation. (See Chapter 15, Fertility Awareness-Based Methods.)

Withdrawal may be an acceptable method for couples in the postpartum period. Withdrawal can be effective if used correctly and consistently. (See Chapter 17, Coitus Interruptus [Withdrawal, the Pull-Out Method].)

Postpartum abstinence is 100% effective in preventing pregnancy if practiced consistently by those who choose not to have sexual intercourse. However, it can be difficult for some people to maintain. Counsel postpartum individuals about other contraceptive methods if they are going to have intercourse. (See Chapter 7, Abstinence and Sexual Health: What Every Clinician Needs to Know.)

Summary

The postpartum period is dynamic and one of unmet contraceptive need. Estrogen-containing contraception should be avoided for the first 3 to 6 weeks, depending upon individual characteristics. Outside of this time, most contraceptives are safe and effective for both breastfeeding and nonbreastfeeding individuals. Postpartum may be associated with new medical conditions and new childbearing goals, and as such, this can be a time where person-centered care and an individualized iterative process may be particularly valuable.

Resources for Patients

Postpartum Birth Control FAQ from ACOG
https://www.acog.org/womens-health/faqs/postpartum-birth-control
Breastfeeding support
https://breastfeeding.support
https://www.llli.org
Medication safety with breastfeeding from CDC
https://www.cdc.gov/breastfeeding/breastfeeding-special-circumstances/vaccinations-medications-drugs/prescription-medication-use.html
Postpartum Support International
https://www.postpartum.net

Author Disclosures—Goldsmith: none. Kottke: investigator-initiated grant funding from Organon, consultant fee from HRA Pharma.

Acknowledgments—Kathy Irene Kennedy, DrPH, MA, for work on the previous iteration of this chapter.

References

1. Hodgen G, Itskovitz J. Recognition and maintenance of pregnancy. In: The physiology of reproduction. New York: Reaven Press; 1988.
2. Willson J. The puerperium. In Willson JR, Carrington ER, Ledger WJ, Laros RK, Mattox JH (eds). Obstetrics and gynecology. St. Louis, MO: CV Mosby Company; 1987:598-607.
3. Gray RH, Campbell OM, Zacur HA, Labbok MH, MacRae SL. Postpartum return of ovarian activity in nonbreastfeeding women monitored by urinary assays. J Clin Endocrinol Metab. 1987;64(4):645-50.
4. McNeilly AS. Lactational control of reproduction. Reprod Fertil Dev. 2001;13(7–8):583-90.
5. Labbok MH, Hight-Laukaran V, Peterson AE, Fletcher V, von Hertzen H, Van Look PF. Multicenter study of the Lactational Amenorrhea Method (LAM): I. Efficacy, duration, and implications for clinical application. Contraception. 1997;55(6):327-36.

6. Labbok MH. Postpartum sexuality and the Lactational Amenorrhea Method for contraception. Clin Obstet Gynecol. 2015;58(4):915-27.
7. Visness CM, Kennedy KI. The frequency of coitus during breastfeeding. Birth. 1997;24(4):253-7.
8. Conde-Agudelo A, Rosas-Bermúdez A, Kafury-Goeta AC. Birth spacing and risk of adverse perinatal outcomes: a meta-analysis. JAMA. 2006;295(15):1809-23.
9. ACOG Committee Opinion No. 736: Optimizing postpartum care. Obstet Gynecol. 2018; 131(5):e140-50.
10. Ahrens KA, Nelson H, Stidd RL, Moskosky S, Hutcheon JA. Short interpregnancy intervals and adverse perinatal outcomes in high-resource settings: An updated systematic review. Paediatr Perinat Epidemiol. 2019;33(1):O25-47.
11. World Health Organization. Report of a WHO technical consultation on birth spacing: Geneva, Switzerland 13-15 June 2005. World Health Organization; 2007. (https://apps.who.int/iris/handle/10665/69855)
12. Bennett WL, Chang H-Y, Levine DM, et al. Utilization of primary and obstetric care after medically complicated pregnancies: an analysis of medical claims data. J Gen Intern Med. 2014;29(4):636-45.
13. Bryant AS, Haas JS, McElrath TF, McCormick MC. Predictors of compliance with the postpartum visit among women living in healthy start project areas. Matern Child Health J. 2006;10(6):511-6.
14. Heinig MJ, Dewey KG. Health advantages of breast feeding for infants: a critical review. Nutr Res Rev. 1996;9(1):89-110.
15. Riordan J, Wambach K. Breastfeeding and human lactation. Jones & Bartlett Learning; 2010.
16. Ip S, Chung M, Raman G, et al. Breastfeeding and maternal and infant health outcomes in developed countries. Evid Rep Technol Assess (Full Rep). 2007;(153):1-186.
17. Horta BL, Bahl R, Martinés JC, Victora CG. Evidence on the long-term effects of breastfeeding: systematic review and meta-analyses. World Health Organization;2007:52.
18. World Health Organization. Guideline: updates on HIV and infant feeding. (https://www.who.int/publications-detail-redirect/9789241549707)
19. Eidelman AI, Schanler RJ, et al. Breastfeeding and the use of human milk. Pediatrics 2012; 129(3):e827-41.
20. Schwarz EB. Infant feeding in America: enough to break a mother's heart? Breastfeed Med. 2013;8(5):454-7.
21. Rosenblatt KA, Thomas DB. Prolonged lactation and endometrial cancer. WHO collaborative study of neoplasia and steroid contraceptives. Int J Epidemiol. 1995;24(3):499-503.
22. Aune D, Norat T, Romundstad P, Vatten LJ. Breastfeeding and the maternal risk of type 2 diabetes: a systematic review and dose-response meta-analysis of cohort studies. Nutr Metab Cardiovasc Dis. 2014;24(2):107-15.
23. Breast cancer and breastfeeding: collaborative reanalysis of individual data from 47 epidemiological studies in 30 countries, including 50302 women with breast cancer and 96973 women without the disease. Lancet. 2002;360(9328):187-95.
24. Sung HK, Ma SH, Choi J-Y, et al. The effect of breastfeeding duration and parity on the risk of epithelial ovarian cancer: a systematic review and meta-analysis. J Prev Med Pub Health. 2016;49(6):349.
25. Gutzeit O, Levy G, Lowenstein L. Postpartum female sexual function: risk factors for postpartum sexual dysfunction. Sex Med. 2020;8(1):8-13.
26. Sachs HC, Frattarelli DAC, et al. The transfer of drugs and therapeutics into human breast milk: an update on selected topics. Pediatrics. 2013;132(3):e796-809.
27. Institute of Medicine (US) Committee on Nutritional Status During Pregnancy and Lactation. Nutrition during lactation. Washington DC: National Academies Press; 1991.
28. Office of Disease Prevention and Health Promotion. Healthy People 2030. (https://health.gov/healthypeople/search?query=breastfeeding)
29. Centers for Disease Control and Prevention. Breastfeeding report card, United States. 2022. (https://www.cdc.gov/breastfeeding/pdf/2022-Breastfeeding-Report-Card-H.pdf.)
30. Curtis KM, Tepper NK, Jatlaoui TC, et al. U.S. medical eligibility criteria for contraceptive use, 2016. MMWR Recomm Rep. 2016;65(3):1-103.
31. Robinson JE, Short RV. Changes in breast sensitivity at puberty, during the menstrual cycle, and at parturition. Br Med J. 1977;1(6070):1188-91.
32. Diaz S, Seron-Ferre M, Croxatto H, Veldhuis J. Neuroendocrine mechanisms of lactational infertility in women. Biol Res. 1995;10.

33. McNeilly AS. Neuroendocrine changes and fertility in breast-feeding women. Prog Brain Res. 2001;133:207-14.
34. Gordon K, Renfree MB, Short RV, Clarke IJ. Hypothalamo-pituitary portal blood concentrations of beta-endorphin during suckling in the ewe. J Reprod Fertil. 1987;79(2):397-408.
35. Diaz S, Croxatto HB. Contraception in lactating women. Curr Opin Obstet Gynecol. 1993;5(6): 815-22.
36. McNeilly A, Tay C, Glaiser A. Physiological mechanisms underlying lactational amenorrhea. In: Human reproductive ecology: interactions of environment, fertility and behavior. New York: Academy of Sciences, 1994: 145-55.
37. Kennedy KI, Rivera R, McNeilly AS. Consensus statement on the use of breastfeeding as a family planning method. Contraception. 1989;39(5):477-96.
38. Campbell OM, Gray RH. Characteristics and determinants of postpartum ovarian function in women in the United States. Am J Obstet Gynecol. 1993;169(1):55-60.
39. Labbok M, Cooney KA, Coly S. Guidelines: breastfeeding, family planning, and the Lactational Amenorrhea Method-LAM. Washington, DC: Institute for Reproductive Health; 1994.
40. Labbok M, Krasovec K. Toward consistency in breastfeeding definitions. Stud Fam Plann. 1990;21(4):226-30.
41. Valdés V, Labbok MH, Pugin E, Perez A. The efficacy of the Lactational Amenorrhea Method (LAM) among working women. Contraception. 2000;62(5):217-9.
42. Brown CRL, Dodds L, Legge A, Bryanton J, Semenic S. Factors influencing the reasons why mothers stop breastfeeding. Can J Public Health. 2014;105(3):e179-85.
43. Ogbuanu C, Glover S, Probst J, Liu J, Hussey J. The effect of maternity leave length and time of return to work on breastfeeding. Pediatrics. 2011;127(6):e1414-27.
44. Gianni ML, Bettinelli ME, Manfra P, et al. Breastfeeding difficulties and risk for early breastfeeding cessation. Nutrients. 2019;11(10):2266.
45. Dinour LM, Szaro JM. Employer-based programs to support breastfeeding among working mothers: a systematic review. Breastfeed Med. 2017;12:131-41.
46. World Health Organization Task Force on Methods for the Natural Regulation of Fertility. The WHO multinational study of breastfeeding and lactation amenorrhoea. III. Pregnancy during breast-feeding. Fertil Steril. 1999;72(3):431-40.
47. Kazi A, Kennedy KI, Visness CM, Khan T. Effectiveness of the lactational amenorrhea method in Pakistan. Fertil Steril. 1995;64(4):717-23.
48. Perez A, Labbok MH, Queenan JT. Clinical study of the lactational amenorrhoea method for family planning. Lancet. 1992;339(8799):968-70.
49. Ramos R, Kennedy KI, Visness CM. Effectiveness of lactational amenorrhoea in prevention of pregnancy in Manila, the Philippines: non-comparative prospective trail. BMJ 1996;313(7062):909-12.
50. Lewis PR, Brown JB, Renfree MB, Short RV. The resumption of ovulation and menstruation in a well-nourished population of women breastfeeding for an extended period of time. Fertil Steril. 1991;55(3):529-36.
51. American College of Obstetricians and Gynecologists, Committee on Health Care for Underserved Women. Access to postpartum sterilization: ACOG Committee Opinion, Number 827. Obstet Gynecol. 2021;137(6):e169-76.
52. Henkel A, Beshar I, Goldthwaite LM. Postpartum permanent contraception: updates on policy and access. Curr Opin Obstet Gynecol. 2021;33(6):445-52.
53. Morris J, Ascha M, Wilkinson B, et al. Desired sterilization procedure at the time of cesarean delivery according to insurance status. Obstet Gynecol. 2019;134(6):1171-7.
54. Kilpatrick SJ (ed.). Guidelines for perinatal care. American Academy of Pediatrics; 2017.
55. Peterson HB. Sterilization. Obstet Gynecol. 2008;111(1):189-203.
56. Wagar MK, Godecker A, Landeros MV, Williams M. Postpartum salpingectomy compared with standard tubal ligation after vaginal delivery. Obstet Gynecol. 2021;137(3):514-20.
57. Garcia C, Moskowitz OM, Chisholm CA, et al. Salpingectomy compared with tubal ligation at Cesarean delivery: a randomized controlled trial. Obstet Gynecol. 2018;132(1):29-34.
58. Venkatesh KK, Clark LH, Stamilio DM. Cost-effectiveness of opportunistic salpingectomy vs tubal ligation at the time of cesarean delivery. Am J Obstet Gynecol. 2019;220(1):106.e1-10.
59. Mills K, Marchand G, Sainz K, et al. Salpingectomy vs tubal ligation for sterilization: a systematic review and meta-analysis. Am J Obstet Gynecol. 2021;224(3):258-65.e4.
60. Anderson PO. General anesthesia while breastfeeding. Breastfeed Med. 2021;16(4):275-7.

61. Lichtenstein Liljeblad K, Kopp Kallner H, Brynhildsen J. Effectiveness, safety and overall satisfaction of early postpartum placement of hormonal IUD compared with standard procedure: An open-label, randomized, multicenter study. Acta Obstet Gynecol Scand. 2022;101(4):424-30.
62. Zerden ML, Stuart GS, Charm S, Bryant A, Garrett J, Morse J. Two-week postpartum intrauterine contraception insertion: a study of feasibility, patient acceptability and short-term outcomes. Contraception. 2017;95(1):65-70.
63. Baldwin MK, Edelman AB, Lim JY, Nichols MD, Bednarek PH, Jensen JT. Intrauterine device placement at 3 versus 6 weeks postpartum: a randomized trial. Contraception. 2016;93(4):356-63.
64. O'Hanley K, Huber DH. Postpartum IUDS: keys for success. Contraception. 1992;45(4):351-61.
65. Welkovic S, Costa LO, Faúndes A, de Alencar Ximenes R, Costa CF. Post-partum bleeding and infection after post-placental IUD insertion. Contraception. 2001;63(3):155-8.
66. Letti Müller AL, Lopes Ramos JG, Martins-Costa SH, et al. Transvaginal ultrasonographic assessment of the expulsion rate of intrauterine devices inserted in the immediate postpartum period: a pilot study. Contraception. 2005;72(3):192-5.
67. Levi E, Cantillo E, Ades V, Banks E, Murthy A. Immediate postplacental IUD insertion at cesarean delivery: a prospective cohort study. Contraception. 2012;86(2):102-5.
68. Chen BA, Reeves MF, Creinin MD, Schwarz EB. Postplacental or delayed levonorgestrel intrauterine device insertion and breast-feeding duration. Contraception. 2011;84(5):499-504.
69. Lester F, Kakaire O, Byamugisha J, et al. Intracesarean insertion of the Copper T380A versus 6 weeks postcesarean: a randomized clinical trial. Contraception. 2015;91(3):198-203.
70. Goldthwaite LM, Sheeder J, Hyer J, Tocce K, Teal SB. Postplacental intrauterine device expulsion by 12 weeks: a prospective cohort study. Am J Obstet Gynecol. 2017;217(6):674.e1-8.
71. Lopez LM, Bernholc A, Hubacher D, Stuart G, Van Vliet HAAM. Immediate postpartum insertion of intrauterine device for contraception. Cochrane Database Syst Rev. 2015;(6):CD003036.
72. O'Brien PA, Pillai S. Uterine perforation by intrauterine devices: a 16-year review. J Fam Plann Reprod Health Care. 2017;43(4):289-95.
73. Heinemann K, Barnett C, Reed S, Möhner S, Do Minh T. IUD use among parous women and risk of uterine perforation: a secondary analysis. Contraception. 2017;95(6):605-7.
74. Berry-Bibee EN, Tepper NK, Jatlaoui TC, Whiteman MK, Jamieson DJ, Curtis KM. The safety of intrauterine devices in breastfeeding women: a systematic review. Contraception. 2016;94(6):725-38.
75. Turok DK, Leeman L, Sanders JN, et al. Immediate postpartum levonorgestrel intrauterine device insertion and breast-feeding outcomes: a noninferiority randomized controlled trial. Am J Obstet Gynecol. 2017;217(6):665.e1-8.
76. Gurtcheff SE, Turok DK, Stoddard G, Murphy PA, Gibson M, Jones KP. Lactogenesis after early postpartum use of the contraceptive implant: a randomized controlled trial. Obstet Gynecol. 2011;117(5):1114-21.
77. Halderman LD, Nelson AL. Impact of early postpartum administration of progestin-only hormonal contraceptives compared with nonhormonal contraceptives on short-term breast-feeding patterns. Am J Obstet Gynecol. 2002;186(6):1250-6; discussion 1256-8.
78. Braga GC, Ferriolli E, Quintana SM, Ferriani RA, Pfrimer K, Vieira CS. Immediate postpartum initiation of etonogestrel-releasing implant: A randomized controlled trial on breastfeeding impact. Contraception. 2015;92(6):536-42.
79. Han L, Teal SB, Sheeder J, Tocce K. Preventing repeat pregnancy in adolescents: is immediate postpartum insertion of the contraceptive implant cost effective? Am J Obstet Gynecol. 2014;211(1):24.e1-7.
80. Brito MB, Ferriani RA, Quintana SM, Yazlle MEHD, Silva de Sá MF, Vieira CS. Safety of the etonogestrel-releasing implant during the immediate postpartum period: a pilot study. Contraception. 2009;80(6):519-26.
81. Reinprayoon D, Taneepanichskul S, Bunyavejchevin S, et al. Effects of the etonogestrel-releasing contraceptive implant (Implanon) on parameters of breastfeeding compared to those of an intrauterine device. Contraception. 2000;62(5):239-46.
82. World Health Organization. Medical Eligibility Criteria for Contraceptive Use. 5th ed. Geneva, Switzerland: WHO; 2015.
83. Kennedy KI, Short RV, Tully MR. Premature introduction of progestin-only contraceptive methods during lactation. Contraception. 1997;55(6):347-50.
84. Brownell EA, Fernandez ID, Fisher SG, et al. The effect of immediate postpartum depot medroxyprogesterone on early breastfeeding cessation. Contraception. 2013;87(6):836-43.

85. Tankeyoon M, Dusitsin N, Chalapati S, et al. Effects of hormonal contraceptives on milk volume and infant growth. WHO Special Programme of Research, Development and Research Training in Human Reproduction Task Force on Oral Contraceptives. Contraception. 1984;30(6):505-22.
86. Moggia AV, Harris GS, Dunson TR, et al. A comparative study of a progestin-only oral contraceptive versus non-hormonal methods in lactating women in Buenos Aires, Argentina. Contraception. 1991;44(1):31-43.
87. Bjarnadóttir RI, Gottfredsdóttir H, Sigurdardóttir K, Geirsson RT, Dieben TO. Comparative study of the effects of a progestogen-only pill containing desogestrel and an intrauterine contraceptive device in lactating women. BJOG. 2001;108(11):1174-80.
88. Stanczyk FZ, Brenner PF, Mishell DRJ, Ortiz A, Gentzschein EK, Goebelsmann U. A radioimmunoassay for norethindrone (NET): measurement of serum NET concentrations following ingestion of NET-containing oral contraceptive steroids. Contraception. 1978;18(6):615-33.
89. Chiara Del Savio M, De Fata R, Facchinetti F, Grandi G. Drospirenone 4 mg-only pill (DOP) in 24+4 regimen: a new option for oral contraception. Expert Rev Clin Pharmacol. 2020;13(7):685-94.
90. Melka D, Kask K, Colli E, Regidor P-A. A single-arm study to evaluate the transfer of drospirenone to breast milk after reaching steady state, following oral administration of 4-mg drospirenone in healthy lactating female volunteers. Womens Health. 2020;16:1745506520957192.
91. Palacios S, Colli E, Regidor P-A. Multicenter, phase III trials on the contraceptive efficacy, tolerability and safety of a new drospirenone-only pill. Acta Obstet Gynecol Scand. 2019;98(12):1549-57.
92. Heit JA, Kobbervig CE, James AH, Petterson TM, Bailey KR, Melton LJ 3rd. Trends in the incidence of venous thromboembolism during pregnancy or postpartum: a 30-year population-based study. Ann Intern Med. 2005;143(10):697-706.
93. Pomp ER, Lenselink AM, Rosendaal FR, Doggen CJM. Pregnancy, the postpartum period and prothrombotic defects: risk of venous thrombosis in the MEGA study. J Thromb Haemost. 2008;6(4):632-7.
94. Lopez LM, Grey TW, Stuebe AM, Chen M, Truitt ST, Gallo MF. Combined hormonal versus nonhormonal versus progestin-only contraception in lactation. Cochrane Database Syst Rev. 2015;(3):CD003988.
95. Jackson E. Controversies in postpartum contraception: when is it safe to start oral contraceptives after childbirth? Thromb Res. 2011;127 Suppl 3:S35-9.
96. Tepper NK, Phillips SJ, Kapp N, Gaffield ME, Curtis KM. Combined hormonal contraceptive use among breastfeeding women: an updated systematic review. Contraception. 2016;94(3):262-74.
97. Bahamondes L, Bahamondes MV, Modesto W, et al. Effect of hormonal contraceptives during breastfeeding on infant's milk ingestion and growth. Fertil Steril. 2013;100(2):445-50.
98. Espey E, Ogburn T, Leeman L, Singh R, Ostrom K, Schrader R. Effect of progestin compared with combined oral contraceptive pills on lactation: a randomized controlled trial. Obstet Gynecol. 2012;119(1):5-13.
99. Shaaban OM, Abbas AM, Mahmoud HR, Yones EM, Mahmoud A, Zakherah MS. Levonorgestrel emergency contraceptive pills use during breastfeeding; effect on infants' health and development. J Matern Fetal Neonatal Med. 2019;32(15):2524-8.
100. HRA Pharma America, Inc. Ella (ulipristal acetate) prescribing information [Internet]. 2020 (https://dailymed.nlm.nih.gov/dailymed/drugInfo.cfm?setid=2bf93d23-cddd-4613-9066-5b5fa090404b)
101. Shaaban OM, Hassen SG, Nour SA, Kames MA, Yones EM. Emergency contraceptive pills as a backup for lactational amenorrhea method (LAM) of contraception: a randomized controlled trial. Contraception. 2013;87(3):363-9.
102. Chvapil M, Eskelson CD, Stiffel V, Owen JA, Droegemueller W. Studies on Nonoxynol-9. II. Intravaginal absorption, distribution, metabolism and excretion in rats and rabbits. Contraception. 1980;22(3):325-39.
103. Faich G, Pearson K, Fleming D, Sobel S, Anello C. Toxic shock syndrome and the vaginal contraceptive sponge. JAMA. 1986;255(2):216-8.
104. Howise PW. Natural regulation of fertility. Brit Med Bull. 1993;49(1):182-99.
105. Labbok MH, Stallings RY, Shah F, et al. Ovulation method use during breastfeeding: is there increased risk of unplanned pregnancy? Am J Obstet Gynecol. 1991;165(6 Pt 2):2031-6.

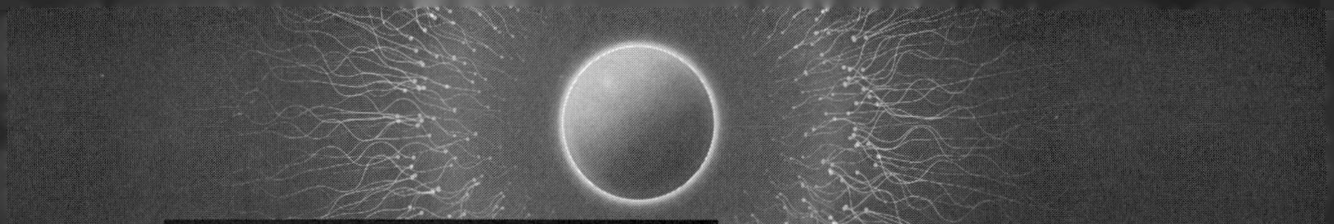

CHAPTER 20

Contraception for People with Medical Conditions

Jennifer Villavicencio, MD, MPP
Rebecca H. Allen, MD, MPH

KEY POINTS

- Individuals with chronic medical problems typically have an increased risk of health complications at baseline as a result of their condition(s).
- For patients with medical concerns, the risks associated with pregnancy are often greater than the risks associated with contraceptive use.
- The US Medical Eligibility Criteria for Contraceptive Use (US MEC) provides evidence-based guidelines that facilitate the important task of helping patients with medical issues choose appropriate contraception.

Most people with chronic medical conditions can safely use a variety of methods of contraception. Health care providers caring for individuals with medical conditions may be concerned about the effects of contraceptives on the medical condition, and therefore may avoid providing contraceptives or addressing family planning needs. However, adverse outcomes and disease progression are often greater during pregnancy than during contraceptive use. Pregnancy itself can pose serious health risks to patients who have particular medical conditions (**Table 20-1**).[1] Given that the increase in maternal morbidity and mortality in the United States is due in part to chronic maternal conditions, providing appropriate contraceptive care is critical.[2] Additionally, the impact of systemic and structural racism on the health and well-being of Black people, Indigenous people, and people of color in the United States, including higher rates of chronic medical conditions, intersects and potentially compounds other racial and ethnic inequities in contraceptive care.[3]

Table 20-1 Conditions Associated with Increased Risk for Adverse Health Events as a Result of Pregnancy

- Breast cancer
- Complicated valvular heart disease
- Cystic fibrosis
- Diabetes: insulin dependent; with nephropathy, retinopathy, or neuropathy or other vascular disease; or of >20 years' duration
- Endometrial or ovarian cancer
- Epilepsy
- Gestational trophoblastic disease
- Hepatocellular adenoma and malignant liver tumors (hepatoma)
- History of bariatric surgery within the past 2 years
- HIV: not clinically well or not receiving antiretroviral therapy
- Hypertension (systolic ≥160 mm Hg or diastolic ≥100 mm Hg)
- Ischemic heart disease
- Peripartum cardiomyopathy
- Schistosomiasis with fibrosis of the liver
- Severe (decompensated) cirrhosis
- Sickle cell disease
- Solid organ transplantation within the past 2 years
- Stroke
- Systemic lupus erythematosus
- Thrombogenic mutations

Modified from Curtis KM, Tepper NK, Jatlaoui TC, et al. U.S. Medical Eligibility Criteria for Contraceptive Use, 2016. MMWR Recomm Rep 2016;65(3):1-104. Available free of charge from https://www.cdc.gov/mmwr/volumes/65/rr/pdfs/rr6503.pdf. Reference to specific commercial products, manufacturers, companies, or trademarks does not constitute its endorsement or recommendation by the U.S. Government, Department of Health and Human Services, or Centers for Disease Control and Prevention.

The Safety of Contraceptive Methods

Understanding Risk Estimates

Understanding the following fundamental statistical concepts will help in understanding the risks reported by studies and in interpreting those risks for our patients.

In contraceptive studies, the *relative risk* (RR) is the probability that an outcome will occur in users of a contraceptive method compared with the probability that that outcome will occur in nonusers of that method. Statistically, this is written as a ratio of users versus nonusers:

$$\text{RR} = \frac{\text{Probability of outcome X in } \textit{users} \text{ of method Y}}{\text{Probability of outcome X in } \textit{nonusers} \text{ of method Y}}$$

A relative risk of 1.0 means that use of a contraceptive method is not associated with the risk of an outcome either way: neither an increase nor a decrease. For example, because combined oral contraceptive (COC) use has no effect on eye color, the relative risk of having brown eyes with COC use compared with (for instance) condom use would be 1.0. However, if an outcome happens more often in users of that method, the relative risk will be greater than 1.0. Alternatively, if an outcome happens less often in users of the method, the relative risk will be less than 1.0. For example, the relative risk of developing ovarian cancer associated with COC use is 0.73, which means that, compared with women who have never used COC, COC users have a 27% reduction in the risk of developing ovarian cancer (1 – 0.73 = 0.27).[4] If there is only a slight increase in risk (RR = 1.10, or a 10% increase), the clinical importance of the increase in risk is generally small—unless the problem is very common or very serious. The "odds ratio" (OR) and the "hazard ratio" (HR) represent similar calculations and should be interpreted as you would a RR in clinical settings. The change in risk with use of a particular contraceptive method may be related to the method itself (causation) or to a common characteristic among users of that method (association).

The *absolute risk* of an outcome happening is also important to know. Even if the relative risk is very high, the absolute risk of an event may still be low, if the background risk in the population is low. For example, the relative risk of developing a benign liver tumor with COC use is 500. This risk appears to be quite high until you understand that this is such a rare occurrence that the chance that a COC user will develop a benign liver tumor (i.e., the absolute risk) is only 1 in 50,000 COC users.[30] A large multiple of a rare event is still a rare event.

The *attributable risk* reflects how much of the RR is associated with the use of the contraceptive method versus the background risk in the population of nonusers. For example, people frequently report having headaches. COC users also report having headaches. The attributable risk is typically what patients truly want to know: how much more or less often they are apt to have headaches because they are using COCs.

Finally, the *confidence interval* (CI) is another statistical principle that is useful. Studies will report both RR and its confidence interval. This is important because the RR calculated in a study is only an estimate. Because studies are based on *samples* of people, no one study ever reflects the experience of all individuals. So when researchers calculate the RR in a study, they also calculate (based on how many subjects were involved in the study and how similar the experiences of those subjects were) the probable limits within which the true answer would fall if all people were studied. The 95% confidence interval (95% CI) means that 95 times out of 100, the real answer lies between the two values quoted. For example, when a study of women with migraine with aura reports an increased risk of stroke with COC use with a RR = 3.0 (95% CI = 1.3, 11.3), the reader would know that the event occurred 3 times more often in COC users than in nonusers. However, the study also calculated with 95% confidence that the real risk lies somewhere between a 30% and an 11-fold increase.[5]

A crucial rule when interpreting the confidence interval is that a relative risk is statistically significant only if *both* confidence interval numbers reflect the same answer: either there is an increase or a decrease in risk. A confidence interval that includes the number 1 suggests that the answer is not clearly either an increased risk or a decreased risk, and therefore the relative risk is *not* statistically significant and should *not* change practice. For example, if a study of contraceptive patch users reports an increase in venous thromboembolism (VTE) with an RR = 2.0 (95% CI = 0.9, 4.1), the researchers are suggesting that patch users are two times more likely to experience the event compared to nonusers of the patch. However, the real answer is that the risk of the event could range widely, from 10% *less* often to 4.1 times *more* often.[6] Because the study could not determine whether the event actually increased or decreased among patch users, the outcome of the study is not statistically significant and should not alter clinical practice.

Permanent Contraception

Fallopian tube and vas deferens surgery are permanent, safe, and highly effective methods of preventing pregnancy.[7] The risks vary according to the type procedure and anesthesia used. Vasectomy can be performed under local anesthesia in the outpatient setting. In contrast, surgery on the fallopian tubes through laparotomy or laparoscopy is typically performed under regional or general anesthesia in a hospital. Both, however, are associated with a low rate of complications.[8] There are few medical conditions that represent a contraindication to the permanent contraceptive method itself. Examples include a known allergy to any required components of the devices used to complete the procedure or extensive scarring due to previous surgeries or endometriosis that obscures the fallopian tubes. However, certain medical conditions place individuals at a higher risk for undergoing surgery, especially under general anesthesia. The risk of surgery must then be balanced against any acceptable alternative contraceptive methods that the person is eligible to use that are safer to administer, still effective at preventing pregnancy, and acceptable to the individual. (See Chapter 4, Person-Centered Reproductive Health Conversations and Contraceptive Counseling and Chapter 8, Permanent Contraception.)

Intrauterine Contraception

Intrauterine contraception can be used by most individuals with medical problems. Regardless of the type of intrauterine device (IUD), the mechanism of action is local, and so intrauterine contraception has the advantage of no known drug–drug interactions. The main contraindications to IUD placement include pregnancy, active uterine or cervical infection, and a distorted uterine cavity unable to accommodate the device.[1] Other concerns include cancer in the genital tract (e.g., cervical cancer, endometrial cancer, and gestational trophoblastic disease with intrauterine involvement), which is a contraindication, and patients with complicated solid organ transplantation (e.g., graft failure, rejection, or cardiac allograft vasculopathy), who can use the IUD with caution. Due to its levonorgestrel (LNG) content, the hormonal IUD is contraindicated in patients with current breast cancer. Anecdotally, the LNG IUD is sometimes used by patients desiring contraception with a history of breast cancer if they also have abnormal uterine bleeding (AUB) and are not appropriate candidates for surgical management.[9,10] While the LNG acts directly on the uterus and cervix, there is a small amount of systemic absorption. A stable serum concentration of 150–200 pg/mL of levonorgestrel occurs after placement of the 52 mg LNG IUD.[11] This concentration is roughly 30 times lower than the 6.2 ng/mL from a 150 mcg LNG-containing oral contraceptive pill.[12] Due to the small amount of systemic absorption, there are theoretical concerns for the LNG IUD in individuals who have hepatocellular adenoma, hepatoma, and severe decompensated cirrhosis. The copper IUD is the only nonhormonal long-acting reversible contraceptive. For individuals with severe thrombocytopenia or severe anemia, there is concern that the copper IUD could increase menstrual blood loss. (See Chapter 10, Intrauterine Devices [IUDs].)

Progestin-Only Contraceptives

Systemic progestin-only contraceptives have very few contraindications and can be used by most individuals with medical problems. These methods include the etonogestrel subdermal implant (Nexplanon), depot medroxyprogesterone acetate (DMPA) injection, and progestin-only oral contraceptives (only available as norethindrone or drospirenone in the United States). Progestin-only contraceptives are effective options for patients who have cardiovascular risk factors or conditions because progestins do not increase the risk of cardiovascular complications: normotensive users of progestin-only methods do not have higher rates of VTE, myocardial infarction (MI), or cerebrovascular accident (CVA) compared to normotensive nonusers.[13,14] Because DMPA is a high-dose contraceptive, there is theoretical concern that use of DMPA may be associated with slightly increased risk of cardiovascular complications compared to lower dose progestin-only methods.[15] It is important to remind patients that their *absolute risk* of cardiovascular complications is not negligible, but that risk is primarily *attributable* to their medical condition, and not to their contraceptive. In addition, progestin-only contraceptives may provide noncontraceptive benefits: inhibition of ovulatory cycling (except for the norethindrone progestin-only pill), decreased menstrual blood loss, and decreased anemia.[16] For patients with heavy menstrual bleeding, menstrual migraines, anticoagulant therapy, or sickle cell anemia, for example, the menstrual suppression provided by their contraceptive may actually improve their medical condition while providing effective protection from undesired pregnancy.

Progestin-only contraceptives are contraindicated in patients with current breast cancer. Progestins are metabolized in the liver via the microsomal P450 system, so they must be used with caution in the setting of hepatocellular adenoma, hepatomas, and severe decompensated cirrhosis. Similarly, medication interactions are possible with low-dose progestin-only contraceptives (implant and progestin-only pills [POPs]).[1] Although most medication interactions do not harm the contraceptive user per se, they may result in reducing the effectiveness of the contraceptive. Therefore, a backup contraceptive may need to be added to preserve effectiveness, but the use of the primary method itself is not contraindicated. (See Chapter 9, Contraceptive Implant; Chapter 11, Injectable Contraceptives; and Chapter 13, Progestin-Only Pills.)

Combined Hormonal Contraceptives

For individuals with chronic medical conditions that increase their baseline risk of cardiovascular complications, the use of combined hormonal contraceptives (CHCs) is contraindicated. These methods include combined oral contraceptives (COCs), the transdermal patch, and the vaginal ring. Although the transdermal patch and vaginal rings are nonoral, their estrogen component—ethinyl estradiol (EE)— nevertheless increases the risk of VTE compared to nonusers of CHCs, and although the risk of arterial thromboembolism (MI and CVA) associated with CHC use may be negligible in healthy users, individuals with hypertension, migraines with aura, or tobacco use at age 35 and older will have further increases in risk that increase the risk of CHC.[5,17,18] In individuals for whom CHCs are not contraindicated but should be used with caution (e.g., those with obesity), using a combined method with the lowest estrogen dose acceptable is still an option. Alternative estrogens to EE available in the United States include estradiol valerate and estetrol. These newer estrogen components in CHCs may ultimately prove to have less cardiovascular risk.[19]

Use of the transdermal patch is associated with a 60% increase in EE exposure compared with a COC containing 30 mcg of EE. In contrast, use of the monthly vaginal ring is associated with EE exposure three times lower than with the patch and two times lower than with COCs.[20] It is unclear whether this means use of the patch is associated with a comparatively increased risk, or use of the monthly ring is associated with a comparatively decreased risk, of cardiovascular complications compared with use of COCs. There are no EE exposure comparative studies including the yearly vaginal ring published yet, but the predicted serum EE concentration after 364 days of continuous use is 43 pmol/L.[21] Nevertheless, the relative EE exposure may be relevant when counseling a patient in choosing the CHC with the lowest EE dose that aligns with the desired noncontraceptive benefits.

Like progestin-only contraceptives, CHCs provide noncontraceptive benefits due to inhibition of ovulation, suppression of menstruation, and decrease in androgen levels.[16] For patients with menstrual-related disorders, AUB, or increased androgen levels, their contraceptive may add the benefit of improving their medical condition in addition to providing effective protection from undesired pregnancy.

As with all hormonal methods, CHCs are contraindicated in patients with current breast cancer. EE is metabolized in the liver to a greater extent than progestins, and so their use is contraindicated in the setting of hepatocellular adenoma, hepatomas, active hepatitis, and severe decompensated cirrhosis. Interactions can occur with medications that induce hepatic cytochrome P450 metabolism.[1] A backup contraceptive may need to be added to preserve effectiveness, but the use of the primary method itself is not contraindicated. Concurrent use of the yearly vaginal ring with specific medication regimens for the treatment of hepatitis C is contraindicated.[22] (See Chapter 12, Combined Hormonal Contraceptives.)

Emergency Contraception

Oral emergency contraception (EC) includes the option of 1.5 mg of LNG or 30 mg of ulipristal acetate (UPA). Because the medications are a one-time dose, there is limited clinical impact and there are no contraindications.[1] All individuals with medical conditions should have access to EC and be offered advance provision.

Individuals taking hepatic enzyme inducers should be warned that the efficacy of EC pills may be reduced, as enzyme inducers may increase metabolism of LNG and UPA. For these patients, the first-line option for EC is the copper IUD or LNG IUD. For patients for whom the IUD is not acceptable or available, a double-dose of LNG (3 mg) may be used. This approach is safe, although the efficacy is not known. UPA is not recommended for patients taking enzyme inducers.[31] Additionally, an individual's weight may impact the efficacy of EC pills, especially LNG pills.

Placement of a copper IUD or LNG IUD is a highly effective form of EC and allows for ongoing contraception in people with medical conditions. (See Chapter 18, Emergency Contraception.)

Risks of Pregnancy

An individual who experiences and continues a pregnancy is exposed to small but real health risks; the risk of VTE is increased at least 22-fold in postpartum women compared to nonpregnant women of reproductive age.[23] For individuals with certain medical conditions, risks of pregnancy complications such as VTE, uncontrolled blood pressure, or stroke are increased. In addition, pregnancy loss and congenital defects are more likely in patients with poorly controlled diabetes. Pregnancy in those taking teratogenic medications (e.g., antiepileptic drugs, isotretinoin) is associated with an elevated risk of birth defects. See Table 20-1 for the list of medical conditions associated with increased risk for adverse health events as a result of pregnancy. For these conditions, the known risks of pregnancy are typically greater than any actual or theoretical risk associated with appropriate contraceptive use. When pregnancy is desired, the risk-benefit ratio may shift for the individual since their goals for health would then include having a healthy pregnancy. Many individuals with medical conditions who desire pregnancy will have better pregnancy outcomes or better health outcomes for themselves if they optimize disease management or make medication adjustments to avoid teratogenic medications prior to pregnancy. They will benefit from person-centered conversations about their reproductive desires. In these conversations, providers can educate about potential risks and explore options for optimizing pregnancy outcomes. In preparation, contraception may be used to postpone pregnancy until therapy is completed (e.g., transplant, bariatric surgery, chemotherapy) or the medical condition is better controlled and therefore risks of pregnancy complications decreased. (See Chapter 4, Person-Centered Reproductive Health Conversations and Contraceptive Counseling.)

CDC Medical Eligibility Criteria for Contraceptive Use

Development of the Guidelines

The Centers for Disease Control and Prevention (CDC) developed the US Medical Eligibility Criteria for Contraceptive Use (US MEC) as guidelines intended to assist health care providers in determining what methods are safe to use in the context of particular medical conditions.[1] (See Appendix A: US MEC Summary Chart on page A-1.) The World Health Organization (WHO) published the first MEC for global use in 1996. These guidelines were developed based on systematic reviews of the medical literature concerning the safety of contraceptive use in patients with chronic medical illnesses or other conditions. After review of the literature, an expert working group was convened to determine the final guidelines based on the literature. Therefore, where the literature was limited, expert opinion prevailed. The WHO MEC was designed as an overarching document as a starting point for countries to adapt their own guidelines for use. The CDC adapted the WHO guidance and published the first US MEC in 2010. The United Kingdom published its MEC shortly before that. It is important to recognize that the CDC provided substantial technical support to the WHO in developing its MEC, and in turn relied on the same process for developing the US MEC. Where the US MEC appears to conflict from the WHO MEC—as in recommendations for breastfeeding individuals, for example—this reflects where the CDC adapted the MEC to be relevant to the US population rather than a differing interpretation of the literature.

Using the Recommendations in Practice

The US MEC will have the greatest benefit for patients if it is used by health care providers in everyday practice in order to decrease unnecessary barriers to contraceptive access. The US MEC app can be downloaded for free from the CDC for use in a smartphone. If a provider does not have access to a smartphone in their clinical setting, the guidelines can be downloaded to a desktop, or laminated charts can be used (apps, guidelines, and charts are available for free from www.cdc.gov/reproductivehealth/contraception/mmwr/mec/summary.html).

The MEC uses a four-tiered category system to denote level of risk associated with the use of a particular contraceptive among individuals with a particular condition, compared to the risk associated with pregnancy.[1] Pregnancy, rather than simply nonuse of the contraceptive, is the comparative condition because the great majority of sexually active people (85%) will become pregnant within 1 year if using no contraceptive. (See Chapter 5, Effectiveness, Safety, and Comparative Side Effects.) Category 1 conveys that the benefits of use of the contraceptive outweigh the risks of use. Category 2 indicates that the benefits of use still outweigh the risks of use, but that additional follow-up after initiation of the contraceptive may be warranted. Using category 1 and 2 contraceptive methods freely can eliminate barriers to contraceptive use that may be based on misperception of risk rather than actual evidence of risk. Use of category 1 and 2 contraceptives may be more easily incorporated into your clinical practice, more easily taught to trainees who may have limited family planning experience, or may provide assurance that additional referral before contraceptive initiation is not needed. Similarly, medical conditions for which all contraceptive methods are category 1 and 2 should be considered as conditions for which there are no significant contraceptive safety concerns due to the condition itself (see **Table 20-2**).

Categories Indicating Risk Potential

Category 3 indicates that the risks of using the contraceptive method outweigh the benefits, although the method may be used if nothing else is available or acceptable to the patient. This category most closely approximates the health care provider asking, "Are the risks from pregnancy greater that the risks from this contraceptive method?" If yes, then clinical judgment guides us to use the contraceptive method. Health care providers may understandably require more family planning experience before they are comfortable prescribing category 3 methods to their patients. Within a group practice or clinic, category 3 methods may signal when referral to a more experienced health care provider is needed. Prescribing a category 3 contraceptive method typically requires more time within a clinical visit to explain to patients the risks and benefits of the method, as well as alternative methods. Follow-up may be needed to assure that continued use is safe.

Category 4 conveys that an unacceptable risk is associated with use of that contraceptive in patients with that condition. Category 4 methods should be used only in rare circumstances and when there is no alternative method that is safe to use; for

Table 20-2 Conditions that Are Generally Not a Contraindication for Contraceptives

Age	Benign breast cysts
Past ectopic pregnancy	Family history of cancer
Obesity	Ovarian cancer
Gestational hypertension	Dysmenorrhea
Gestational diabetes	Uterine fibroids
Varicose veins	Cervical dysplasia
Migraines without aura	HIV
Epilepsy	Thyroid disease
Depression	Cystic fibrosis
Abnormal uterine bleeding	Sickle cell anemia
Endometriosis	Iron deficiency anemia
Benign ovarian cysts	Antibiotic use

Data from: Curtis KM, Tepper NK, Jatlaoui TC, et al. U.S. Medical Eligibility Criteria for Contraceptive Use, 2016. MMWR Recomm Rep 2016;65(3):1-104

example, a patient with breast cancer using tamoxifen may benefit from protection of the endometrium conferred by the LNG IUD (the decision is best made in consultation with the medical oncologist).

The US MEC allows for documentation of clinical decision making to be more standardized, objective, recognizable, and feasible. For example, within an electronic medical record, a smart text or autotext can be used to concisely state, "Use of this contraceptive is category 1 (can use) in the CDC US Medical Eligibility Criteria." Notes can be forwarded to other health care providers, such as the cardiologist caring for your patient with a history of peripartum cardiomyopathy, so that recommendations for care are well understood and communicated among the health care team. Advocating for the highest-quality care for our patients requires conversations with the other health care providers involved in their care. In these circumstances, the expertise of other health care providers should be respected. However, subspecialty providers rarely if ever ask patients about their reproductive desires and might not have expertise in contraception and therefore may be uncomfortable due to their lack of knowledge or misinformation they have heard. Their discomfort is understandable but must be responded to with education and resources that provide accurate information about the risks of various contraceptive methods. The mutual goal is to provide safe care and minimize harm to the patient. (See Chapter 4, Person-Centered Reproductive Health Conversations and Contraceptive Counseling.)

The US MEC lists recommendations for contraceptive use in the presence of over 60 conditions. All contraceptive methods available in the United States are included; recommendations are listed separately for natural family planning, barrier methods, permanent contraception (the US MEC lists this as "sterilization"), and emergency contraception, as they do not involve the prolonged provision of medication.

For Medical Conditions Not Listed in the US MEC

Some medical conditions are not listed because there is not enough medical evidence on contraception use in that population of patients to inform recommendations. So how do health care providers manage the patient with a medical condition that is not listed in the US MEC? In this case, the following should be considered:

- Consider the risks inherent in the condition itself and review the recommendations for conditions that have similar risk. For example, cerebral aneurysm is not listed in the MEC but migraine with aura is, and so following the guidelines for migraine with aura might be prudent in order to avoid an increased risk of stroke with contraceptive use.
- Consider the themes of the US MEC, including that:
  - Estrogen-containing contraceptives increase cardiovascular risk
  - Progestins generally do not
  - Nearly all women are eligible for at least one of the reversible long-acting contraceptive methods (implant or IUD)
- Research other sources, such as UpToDate, PubMed, etc. for guidance.
- Consult with the other health care providers involved in your patient's care.

Assessment of Medical Eligibility for Contraception

Screening for Medical Conditions

A comprehensive patient history, updated annually, will reveal the majority of contraindicating conditions. A pelvic examination will detect the majority of contraindications to IUD placement. The US Selected Practice Recommendations for Contraceptive Use (SPR) provides guidelines to all health care providers as to how to prescribe contraception.[24] The SPR is included in the smart phone app that contains the US MEC and is also available at www.cdc.gov/reproductivehealth/contraception/mmwr/mec/summary.html. Specifically, the US SPR reviews the screening tests that are needed before initiation of contraception. Blood pressure measurement before initiation of CHCs contributes to the safety of their use. COC users with unmeasured blood pressure were more likely to have complications after contraceptive initiation than users with measured blood pressure.[25] Documenting users' weight and body mass index (BMI) at initiation of all contraceptive methods may contribute to the effectiveness of follow-up and future counseling as significant weight gain caused by contraceptive use is a concern for many patients. While patients require a pelvic examination before IUD placement in order to rule out anatomic changes that preclude correct placement and decrease the risk of complications related to placement due to unrecognized infection, pregnancy, or cancer, a pelvic examination is not required prior to initiating other contraceptive methods.[26] Screening for anemia, hyperlipidemia, or diabetes does not contribute to the safety of contraceptive use, so is it not required before initiating or continuing contraceptive use. Screening the general population for thrombogenic mutations before CHC use is not cost-effective, but it may be indicated in patients with a strong family history of thromboembolism.[27] The performance of tests for sexually transmitted infections, human papillomavirus testing, pap testing, and mammograms do not increase the safety of contraceptive use and should not be required before the provision of contraception unless an individual's history indicates the need for the test.[26]

Initiating a Method Using the US MEC

Clinical Scenario 1

> A 32-year-old patient with a known history of high blood pressure presents for contraception. They are not taking any medications because they lost their health insurance. Their blood pressure is measuring consistently 160/100 mm Hg. What method(s) can they safely use?

Based on US MEC recommendations (**Table 20-3**), estrogen-containing methods are considered contraindicated for this patient due to the higher risk of stroke, acute MI, and peripheral arterial disease.[28,29] They can safely use an IUD, implant, progestin-only pill, or any reversible nonhormonal method. There are theoretical concerns about the effect of LNG on lipids and limited evidence suggests that among those with hypertension, users of POPs or DMPA had a small increased risk for cardiovascular events compared with those who did not use these methods.[30] However,

Table 20-3 **The US MEC Categories for Clinical Scenario 1**

Hypertension	Cu-IUD	LNG-IUD	Implants	DMPA	POP	CHC
Adequately controlled hypertension	1	1	1	2	1	3
Elevated blood pressure levels: Systolic 140–159 mm Hg or diastolic 90–99 mm Hg	1	1	1	2	1	3
Elevated blood pressure levels: Systolic ≥160 mm Hg or diastolic ≥100 mm Hg	1	2	2	3	2	4
Vascular disease	1	2	2	3	2	4

Cu-IUD, copper intrauterine device; LNG-IUD, levonorgestrel intrauterine device; DMPA, depot medroxyprogesterone acetate; POP, progestin-only pill; CHC, combined hormonal contraception.

Modified from Curtis KM, Tepper NK, Jatlaoui TC, et al. U.S. Medical Eligibility Criteria for Contraceptive Use, 2016. MMWR Recomm Rep 2016;65(3):1-104. Available free of charge from https://www.cdc.gov/mmwr/volumes/65/rr/pdfs/rr6503.pdf. Reference to specific commercial products, manufacturers, companies, or trademarks does not constitute its endorsement or recommendation by the U.S. Government, Department of Health and Human Services, or Centers for Disease Control and Prevention.

because the absolute risk of cardiovascular events is quite small, the rating is only category 2 for POPs, LNG IUD, and the implant. For DMPA, there is further concern about its hypoestrogenic effects and reduced high-density lipoprotein (HDL) levels, which raises the rating to 3. It is safer for the patient to use one of the methods that is category 1 or 2. Nevertheless, if after explaining the potential risk to the patient, they still choose to use DMPA, this method is an option since it is not a category 4. If the patient would like permanent contraception with tubal surgery, that would also be a safe option once the blood pressure is controlled.

Clinical Scenario 2. When patients present with multiple medical conditions, the condition with the highest category number should determine the safety of the contraceptive choice for the patient. The US MEC does have a category that helpfully provides recommendations for the patient with multiple conditions. The category is entitled *multiple risk factors for atherosclerotic cardiovascular disease*, and it takes into account older age, smoking, diabetes, hypertension, low HDL, high low-density lipoprotein, or high triglyceride levels:

> A 25-year-old patient with obesity recently diagnosed with Type 2 diabetes mellitus presents for contraception (**Table 20-4**). They are currently taking metformin for diabetes. They also have a history of migraines with aura. What method(s) can they safely use?

Based on US MEC recommendations, combined hormonal contraception is contraindicated (i.e., is the condition with the highest category, category 4) in patients with migraine with aura due to the increased risk of stroke.[18] They can safely use a progestin-only or nonhormonal method.

Clinical Scenario 3. Other US MEC recommendations include two ratings for a single condition. In this case, it is the clinical circumstances or severity of the condition that will dictate which rating applies:

> A 40-year-old patient with long-standing Crohn's disease presents for contraception (**Table 20-5**). What method(s) can they safely use?

Table 20-4 The US MEC Categories for Clinical Scenario 2

	Cu-IUD	LNG-IUD	Implants	DMPA	POP	CHC
Migraine with aura	1	1	1	1	1	4
BMI ≥30 kg/m²	1	1	1	1	1	2
Noninsulin-dependent diabetes mellitus	1	2	2	2	2	2

Cu-IUD, copper intrauterine device; LNG-IUD, levonorgestrel intrauterine device; DMPA, depot medroxyprogesterone acetate; POP, progestin-only pill; CHC, combined hormonal contraception.

Modified from Curtis KM, Tepper NK, Jatlaoui TC, et al. U.S. Medical Eligibility Criteria for Contraceptive Use, 2016. MMWR Recomm Rep. 2016;65(3):1-104.

Table 20-5 The US MEC Categories for Clinical Scenario 3

	Cu-IUD	LNG-IUD	Implants	DMPA	POP	CHC
Inflammatory bowel disease (ulcerative colitis or Crohn's disease)	1	1	1	2	2	2/3

Cu-IUD, copper intrauterine device; LNG-IUD, levonorgestrel intrauterine device; DMPA, depot medroxyprogesterone acetate; POP, progestin-only pill; CHC, combined hormonal contraception.
Modified from Curtis KM, Tepper NK, Jatlaoui TC, et al. U.S. Medical Eligibility Criteria for Contraceptive Use, 2016. MMWR Recomm Rep 2016;65(3):1-104. Available free of charge from https://www.cdc.gov/mmwr/volumes/65/rr/pdfs/rr6503.pdf. Reference to specific commercial products, manufacturers, companies, or trademarks does not constitute its endorsement or recommendation by the U.S. Government, Department of Health and Human Services, or Centers for Disease Control and Prevention.

In their case, use of CHC will depend on the severity of their disease. Individuals with inflammatory bowel disease have a higher baseline risk for VTE compared to those who are unaffected.[31] Nevertheless, for patients with mild inflammatory bowel disease and no other risk factors for VTE, the benefits of CHC generally outweigh the risks, so a rating of 2 is given.[32] For individuals with severe inflammatory bowel disease or other risk factors for VTE such as surgery or immobilization, the rating for CHC is increased to a 3 because the risks generally outweigh the benefits. This patient can safely use for progestin-only or nonhormonal methods.

Continuing a Method Based on the MEC

Certain US MEC recommendations are subdivided into two subcategories: Initiation (I) of a new contraceptive method (a method that the patient is not using currently) and continuation (C) of a currently used contraceptive method. If an individual's condition changes or they develop a new medical condition while using a contraceptive, the category rating and risk-benefit profile may change:

Clinical Scenario 4

> A 35-year-old patient with systemic lupus erythematosus presents for contraception (**Table 20-6**). They are negative for anti-phospholipid antibodies and are not taking immunosuppressants. They do have severe thrombocytopenia with platelets measuring 30,000/mcl. What method(s) can they safely use?

Both the copper IUD and DMPA are given a category 3 rating for initiation of the method in this setting. This is due to concerns for preexisting heavy menstrual bleeding with severe thrombocytopenia that may be worsened by the copper IUD, and the potential for irregular bleeding with DMPA, a medication that cannot be reversed rapidly. However, if a patient already has a copper IUD in place or is on DMPA and develops severe thrombocytopenia, the recommendation changes to

Table 20-6 The US MEC Categories for Clinical Scenario 4

	Cu-IUD		LNG-IUD	Implants	DMPA		POP	CHC
	I	C			I	C		
Systemic lupus erythematosus with severe thrombocytopenia	3	2	2	2	3	2	2	2

I, initiation; C, continuation; Cu-IUD, copper intrauterine device; LNG-IUD, levonorgestrel intrauterine device; DMPA, depot medroxyprogesterone acetate; POP, progestin-only pill; CHC, combined hormonal contraception.
Modified from Curtis KM, Tepper NK, Jatlaoui TC, et al. U.S. Medical Eligibility Criteria for Contraceptive Use, 2016. MMWR Recomm Rep. 2016;65(3):1-104.

Table 20-7 The US MEC Categories for Clinical Scenario 5

	Cu-IUD		LNG-IUD		Implants	DMPA	POP	CHC
	I	C	I	C				
Current PID	4	2	4	2	1	1	1	1

I, initiation; C, continuation; Cu-IUD, copper intrauterine device; LNG-IUD, levonorgestrel intrauterine device; DMPA, depot medroxyprogesterone acetate; POP, progestin-only pill; CHC, combined hormonal contraception.
Modified from Curtis KM, Tepper NK, Jatlaoui TC, et al. U.S. Medical Eligibility Criteria for Contraceptive Use, 2016. MMWR Recomm Rep 2016;65(3):1-104. Available free of charge from https://www.cdc.gov/mmwr/volumes/65/rr/pdfs/rr6503.pdf. Reference to specific commercial products, manufacturers, companies, or trademarks does not constitute its endorsement or recommendation by the U.S. Government, Department of Health and Human Services, or Centers for Disease Control and Prevention.

a category 2 rating for either. In this case, if the patient is already tolerating the method, one can consider continuing and observing for any signs of worsening bleeding. They are also a candidate for other progestin-only or nonhormonal methods, with the exception of surgery for permanent contraception, until the thrombocytopenia is improved.

Clinical Scenario 5

> A 21-year-old patient desires an IUD for contraception. They present with fever, pelvic pain, and foul-smelling vaginal discharge. They have cervical motion tenderness and uterine tenderness on exam. You diagnose them with pelvic inflammatory disease and treat them with antibiotics. What method(s) can they safely use that day?

In this case, placement of the IUD is contraindicated due to current pelvic inflammatory disease (**Table 20-7**). The patient is eligible for all the other methods of contraception. However, if they had developed pelvic inflammatory disease with the IUD already in place, the recommendation for continuation is a category 2. The IUD can be continued while the infection is being treated provided the patient is clinically improving.[24]

Counseling Patients with Medical Conditions on Contraceptive Methods

Counseling individuals with complex medical conditions will likely take additional time in order to address the various contributing factors, including social determinants, that may be multifaceted in this population. If possible, allotting additional time for these visits will enable you to address the increased complexity of the medical decision-making that will be required.

While contraception decision making may be more complex for individuals with medical conditions, prioritizing an individual's preferences and lived experiences while engaging in person-centered counseling remains critical to each encounter. Additionally, health care providers should be aware of the intersections that race, ethnicity, gender identity, trauma, and socioeconomic factors have with chronic health condition management, and the resulting inequities in health outcomes as well as access to contraception. (See Chapter 4, Person-Centered Reproductive Health Conversations and Contraceptive Counseling.)

Review All Medically Eligible Effective Methods

Once the patient has been screened for medical eligibility based on a review of the medical history and concomitant medications, review the available options. Individuals may have preconceived ideas regarding different methods of contraception, so dispel any misconceptions about efficacy or safety (see Chapter 5, Effectiveness, Safety, and Comparative Side Effects). The effect of any particular method on the patient's disease process or concomitant medications should be discussed. While you ideally should be able to provide the desired method that same day, the patient may need time to reflect and decide on a personal best option.

Discuss Future Reproductive Desires

Individuals with chronic medical problems should be queried regarding their reproductive goals (see Chapter 4, Person-Centered Reproductive Health Conversations and Contraceptive Counseling.) If an individual is certain that future pregnancy is not desired, permanent contraception should be offered. Individuals with chronic medical problems who do desire future pregnancy may want to time their pregnancy according to disease control or remission. If their medical condition would lead to serious pregnancy-related complications they strongly want to avoid, then they may want to consider higher-efficacy methods such as the implant or IUD.[33,34] Short-term contraception use may benefit individuals desiring pregnancy to allow time to optimize management of their chronic health condition. For example, individuals with diabetes mellitus desiring pregnancy should be informed of ways to minimize risks of birth defects and early pregnancy loss, including working towards normal blood glucose levels prior to conception.[35] Similarly, patients with epilepsy or rheumatologic disorders should be evaluated for the possibility of changing to nonteratogenic medications or tapering to monotherapy with lower risk medication prior to conception to avoid the risk of birth defects.[36]

Consider Impact of Health Conditions and Treatment on Adherence

Medication interactions can directly decrease contraceptive hormonal levels and potentially decrease contraceptive method effectiveness. Patients may face challenges in adhering to their contraceptive method due to factors related to their medical condition. Consider your patient's existing medical regimen, requirements for therapy, or schedule of other health care visits. For example, patients with daily oral medication regimens might find it easy to incorporate a daily COC, but those with weekly dialysis will not be able to maintain adequate serum hormone levels with COCs, and individuals with frequent hospitalizations may not be able to return to your office or clinic on time for DMPA injections.

Physical and mental ability to adhere to a contraceptive method must also be considered: for example, has an individual's history of stroke impaired their memory such that adherence to contraceptives that require them to remember to take a pill daily or change a patch weekly is difficult? Does a physical disability make vaginal ring placement challenging? Ultimately, your patient is the best judge of their ability to adhere to a specific method and their preferences and values should always be prioritized.

Individuals with chronic medical conditions may believe they are not able to conceive; accordingly, even if avoiding pregnancy is of high priority, adherence to contraception may not be a focus for them amid the other challenges of managing a medical condition. Individuals with certain medical conditions have lower fecundity than their counterparts without those medical conditions due to decreased fertility or less frequent sexual activity as a result of their disease. Some of these patients erroneously believe that they are not able to become pregnant at all. It is critical that these patients receive individualized information so they are able to make informed choices about contraception. Providers can engage patients in conversations designed to explore misinformation, give them accurate estimates about their ability to get pregnant, and give them scientifically detailed information about their risk of pregnancy-related complications. (See Chapter 4, Person-Centered Reproductive Health Conversations and Contraceptive Counseling.)

Consider Noncontraceptive Benefits and Bleeding Profiles

Individuals with chronic medical problems, depending on their condition, may benefit from the noncontraceptive effects of various methods. This may be an important part of their contraception decision-making process. For example, a hormonal method that reduces menstrual blood loss and dysmenorrhea may be of particular benefit for patients with severe anemia or for those on anticoagulants. Long-term benefits such as protection against ovarian and endometrial cancer may be important to patients with a family history of ovarian cancer or with chronic anovulation, respectively.

Incorporate Contraceptive Choice

Compared to healthy individuals, those with medically complex conditions may have primary goals for their health that are more closely aligned with their chronic medical condition(s) than contraception itself. Even when the focus is contraception, individuals with medical conditions will want to know (1) how each of their contraceptive options will affect their disease control or progression, (2) how each option might interact with their ongoing medication regimen, and (3) how each option might increase or decrease the symptoms or side effects that currently challenge them or introduce new side effects. Whether healthy or medically complex, engaging in shared decision-making with the patient is critical. As with other medications prescribed for a prolonged time, the process of informed consent before use of any contraceptive will require a review of the benefits and risks that are supported by evidence, with added clinical guidance when the evidence is lacking (see Chapter 4, Person-Centered Reproductive Health Conversations and Contraceptive Counseling). The additional social aspects that govern contraceptive choice cannot be ignored. For example, while an implant or an IUD may be the safest method for your medically complex patient to use, they may feel hesitant choosing a contraceptive that they cannot stop on their own if they changed their mind. This becomes even more challenging when the racial, ethnic, or socioeconomic inequities in access to health care impacts the ability of an individual to immediately discontinue a contraceptive method that requires clinician intervention. Listening to your patients, addressing their concerns, and respecting their preferences, values, and choices will foster provider-patient relationships that are invaluable to successfully helping them optimize their health.

Author Disclosures—Allen: Nexplanon trainer (Organon), research support (Bayer), consultant (Cadence Health and Merck). Villavicencio: None.

Acknowledgments—Kathryn M. Curtis, PhD, Herbert B. Peterson, MD and Carrie Cwiak, MD, MPH, for their work on the previous iteration of this chapter.

References

1. Curtis KM, Tepper NK, Jatlaoui TC, et al. U.S. medical eligibility criteria for contraceptive use, 2016. MMWR Recomm Rep. 2016;65:1-104.
2. Creanga AA, Berg CJ, Syverson C, et al. Pregnancy-related mortality in the United States, 2006-2010. Obstet Gynecol. 2015;125:5-12.
3. Centers for Disease Control and Prevention. Racial and ethnic approaches to community health. (https://www.cdc.gov/nccdphp/dnpao/state-local-programs/reach/)
4. Collaborative Group on Epidemiological Studies of Ovarian Cancer, Beral V, Doll R, et al. Ovarian cancer and oral contraceptives: collaborative reanalysis of data from 45 epidemiological studies including 23,257 women with ovarian cancer and 87,303 controls. Lancet. 2008;371:303-14.
5. Chang CL, Donaghy M, Poulter N. Migraine and stroke in young women: case-control study. The World Health Organisation Collaborative Study of Cardiovascular Disease and Steroid Hormone Contraception. BMJ. 1999;318:13-8.
6. Jick SS, Hagberg KW, Hernandez RK, et al. Postmarketing study of ORTHO EVRA and levonorgestrel oral contraceptives containing hormonal contraceptives with 30 mcg of ethinyl estradiol in relation to nonfatal venous thromboembolism. Contraception. 2010;81:16-21.
7. American College of Obstetricians and Gynecologists. ACOG practice bulletin no. 133: benefits and risks of sterilization. Obstet Gynecol. 2013;121:392-404.
8. Stuart GS, Ramesh SS. Interval female sterilization. Obstet Gynecol. 2018;131:117-24.
9. Chin J, Konje JC, Hickey M. Levonorgestrel intrauterine system for endometrial protection in women with breast cancer on adjuvant tamoxifen. Cochrane Database Syst Rev. 2009:CD007245.
10. Ostroot MK, Heslin K, Kram JJF, et al. Breast cancer recurrence risk after hormonal contraceptive use in survivors of reproductive age. Eur J Obstet Gynecol Reprod Biol. 2021;258:174-8.
11. Bayer Healthcare Pharmaceuticals. Mirena prescribing information. 2008. (https://www.accessdata.fda.gov/drugsatfda_docs/label/2008/021225s019lbl.pdf.)
12. Duramed Pharmaceuticals. Seasonique prescribing information. 2010. (https://www.accessdata.fda.gov/drugsatfda_docs/label/2010/021840s008lbl.pdf.)

13. Chakhtoura Z, Canonico M, Gompel A, et al. Progestogen-only contraceptives and the risk of acute myocardial infarction: a meta-analysis. J Clin Endocrinol Metab. 2011;96:1169-74.
14. Chakhtoura Z, Canonico M, Gompel A, et al. Progestogen-only contraceptives and the risk of stroke: a meta-analysis. Stroke. 2009;40:1059-62.
15. Tepper NK, Whiteman MK, Marchbanks PA, et al. Progestin-only contraception and thromboembolism: A systematic review. Contraception. 2016;94:678-700.
16. American College of Obstetricians and Gynecologists. ACOG Practice Bulletin No. 110: noncontraceptive uses of hormonal contraceptives. Obstet Gynecol. 2010;115:206-18.
17. Ischaemic stroke and combined oral contraceptives: results of an international, multicentre, case-control study. WHO Collaborative Study of Cardiovascular Disease and Steroid Hormone Contraception. Lancet. 1996;348:498-505.
18. Champaloux SW, Tepper NK, Monsour M, et al. Use of combined hormonal contraceptives among women with migraines and risk of ischemic stroke. Am J Obstet Gynecol. 2017;216:489 e1-7.
19. Dinger J, Do Minh T, Heinemann K. Impact of estrogen type on cardiovascular safety of combined oral contraceptives. Contraception. 2016;94:328-39.
20. van den Heuvel MW, van Bragt AJ, Alnabawy AK, et al. Comparison of ethinylestradiol pharmacokinetics in three hormonal contraceptive formulations: the vaginal ring, the transdermal patch and an oral contraceptive. Contraception. 2005;72:168-74.
21. Liu JH, Plagianos M, Archer DF, et al. Segesterone acetate serum levels with a regression model of continuous use of the segesterone acetate/ethinyl estradiol contraceptive vaginal system. Contraception. 2021;104:229-34.
22. Population Council. Annovera prescribing information. (https://www.accessdata.fda.gov/drugsatfda_docs/label/2018/209627s000lbl.pdf.)
23. Jackson E, Curtis KM, Gaffield ME. Risk of venous thromboembolism during the postpartum period: a systematic review. Obstet Gynecol. 2011;117:691-703.
24. Curtis KM, Jatlaoui TC, Tepper NK, et al. U.S. selected practice recommendations for contraceptive use, 2016. MMWR Recomm Rep. 2016;65:1-66.
25. Tepper NK, Curtis KM, Steenland MW, et al. Blood pressure measurement prior to initiating hormonal contraception: a systematic review. Contraception. 2013;87:631-8.
26. Stewart FH, Harper CC, Ellertson CE, et al. Clinical breast and pelvic examination requirements for hormonal contraception: Current practice vs evidence. JAMA. 2001;285:2232-9.
27. Vandenbroucke JP, van der Meer FJ, Helmerhorst FM, et al. Factor V Leiden: should we screen oral contraceptive users and pregnant women? BMJ. 1996;313:1127-30.
28. Khader YS, Rice J, John L, et al. Oral contraceptives use and the risk of myocardial infarction: a meta-analysis (structured abstract). Contraception. 2003;68:11-7.
29. Gillum LA, Mamidipudi SK, Claiborne Johnston S. Ischemic stroke risk with oral contraceptives: a meta-analysis (structured abstract). JAMA. 2000;284:72-8.
30. World Health Organization. Cardiovascular disease and use of oral and injectable progestogen-only contraceptives and combined injectable contraceptives. Results of an international, multicenter, case-control study. World Health Organization Collaborative Study of Cardiovascular Disease and Steroid Hormone Contraception. Contraception. 1998;57:315-24.
31. Sridhar A, Cwiak CA, Kaunitz AM, et al. Contraceptive considerations for women with gastrointestinal disorders. Dig Dis Sci. 2017;62:54-63.
32. Zapata LB, Paulen ME, Cansino C, et al. Contraceptive use among women with inflammatory bowel disease: A systematic review. Contraception. 2010;82:72-85.
33. Mavranezouli I, Larc Guideline Development G. The cost-effectiveness of long-acting reversible contraceptive methods in the UK: analysis based on a decision-analytic model developed for a National Institute for Health and Clinical Excellence (NICE) clinical practice guideline. Human Reprod. 2008;23:1338-45.
34. Lipetz C, Phillips CJ, Fleming CF. The cost-effectiveness of a long-acting reversible contraceptive (Implanon) relative to oral contraception in a community setting. Contraception. 2009;79:304-9.
35. Gabbe SG, Graves CR. Management of diabetes mellitus complicating pregnancy. Obstet Gynecol. 2003;102:857-68.
36. Davis AR, Pack AM, Dennis A. Contraception for women with epilepsy. In: Allen RA, Cwiak C, eds. Contraception for the medically challenging patient. New York: Springer; 2014:135-46.

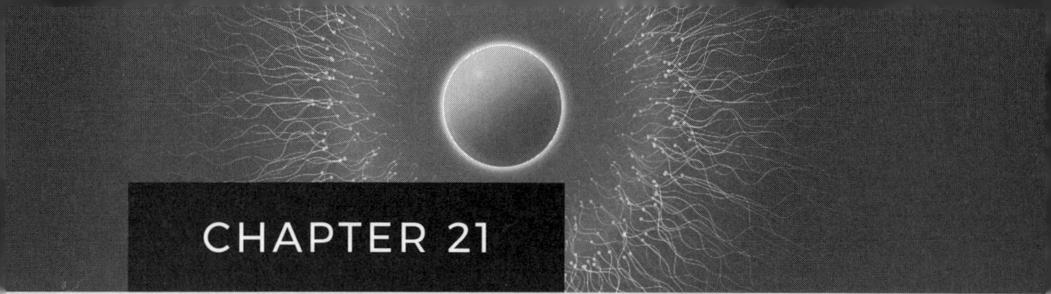

CHAPTER 21

Contraception in the Later Reproductive Years

Amanda Y. Black, MD, MPH
Alexandra Sherman, WHNP-BC, MSCP
Taniqua A. Miller, MD, MSCP

KEY POINTS

- Although fertility declines with increasing age, individuals still need contraception if they wish to avoid pregnancy.
- There are no contraceptive methods that are contraindicated on the basis of age alone. However, medical conditions become more prevalent with increasing age and should be considered when choosing a contraceptive method.
- For most healthy, nonsmoking individuals, the benefits of contraception use during the perimenopause outweigh potential risks associated with the method. Noncontraceptive benefits of some methods may help to improve quality of life during the perimenopause and decrease cancer risks.
- The LNG-IUD provides an effective method of perimenopausal contraception, and can readily transition into the progestin component of post-menopausal hormone therapy (HT)

Menopause is a normal physiologic event, indicating the cessation of ovarian follicular function and ovulation. It is defined as the final menstrual period and is a retrospective diagnosis. Individuals are considered postmenopausal 1 year after their last natural menses. Perimenopause is a transitional period characterized by fluctuating hormone levels, irregular menstrual cycles, and the onset of vasomotor symptoms (flashes and flushes) that may increase in severity as menopause approaches.[1] Perimenopause starts with altered ovarian hormone production. The onset of menopause-related symptoms continues for an indefinite amount of time after the last natural menstrual period.[2] The mean age of menopause is 51 years, the average age of onset of perimenopause is 46 (range 39–51), and the average duration is 5 years (range 2–8).[3] During this time, shortening of the follicular phase leads to a decrease in cycle length. Menstrual cycles may become increasingly irregular and unpredictable; more than 75% of people with a uterus experience abnormal uterine bleeding during the perimenopause.[4] However, even when cycles are longer than 50 to 60 days, ovulation will occur in 25% of these cycles and therefore contraception is still needed if pregnancy is not desired.[5] Accordingly, contraception counseling remains a hallmark of care throughout the entire reproductive spectrum, including perimenopause. (See Chapter 4, Person-Centered Reproductive Health Conversations and Contraceptive Counseling.)

Other menopause-related symptoms include vaginal dryness, hot flushes, night sweats, sleep disturbances, reduced libido, mood swings, headaches, and bladder symptoms.[6-13] Other health issues to consider during this time include loss of bone mineral density, cardiovascular disease, mental health, and gynecologic cancers.[14] Changes of ovarian function have been linked to depression and increased cardiometabolic risk.[14-16] The timing of menopause is not affected by the use of contraception, but different contraceptive methods may delay symptoms indicative of perimenopause or the start of menopause.

Perimenopause and Menopause

What is the Probability of Pregnancy in Perimenopause?

The likelihood of pregnancy declines with age.[17] Women over the age of 40 have lower fecundity (chance of live birth per menstrual cycle) compared with their younger cohort.[18] Fertility at first gradually then rapidly declines with age due to diminishing oocyte quality and ovarian reserve with an associated increase in anovulatory cycles and luteal insufficiency.[1] The probability of becoming pregnant is dependent on ovulation, coital frequency, partner fertility, contraceptive efficacy, and consistency of contraceptive use. However, evidence of luteal phase activity (ovulation) is seen in 87.9% of cycles up to 5 years before menopause and is still seen in 22.8% of cycles within 1 year of the final menstrual period.[1] The absolute risk of pregnancy is lower due to decreased fertility and decreased coital frequency but it is still not zero.[19] During the perimenopause, the chance of naturally occurring pregnancy is approximately 30% per year at ages 40–44 and decreases to 10% per year from ages 45–49.[9]

Spontaneous pregnancy over the age of 50 is rare but people at this age are still potentially fertile during the perimenopause.[9] Thus if an individual is engaging in heterosexual intercourse and a pregnancy is not desired, an effective method of contraception should be used consistently. Perimenopausal women may use contraception less consistently than younger women,[20] possibly due to a lower perceived risk of pregnancy. In a survey of women aged 40–45, 75% were sexually active, and only 4% of those women were actively trying to conceive.[22] However, undesired pregnancies occur at ratios similar to or even higher than younger age groups, and almost half of these pregnancies will be terminated.[21] In the United States, roughly one-third of pregnancies occurring in the 40- to 45-year age cohort are unintended.[21] Cost, travel expenses, and restrictions in available modality of abortion are often insurmountable barriers[23] and it is impossible to predict the future of safe and equitable abortion access.

Clinicians should continue to offer pregnancy prevention counseling and services to patients until they reach natural menopause if pregnancy is not desired. (See Chapter 4, Person-Centered Reproductive Health Conversations and Contraceptive Counseling.)

What are the Reproductive Outcomes if Pregnancy Occurs During Perimenopause?

Compared with younger women, pregnancies in older reproductive age women result in poorer obstetrical and maternal outcomes. Age itself is an independent risk factor for poorer reproductive outcomes. Further increased risk may be seen with advanced maternal age due to additional medical comorbidities such as diabetes, hypertension, and obesity.[24,25] Compared to pregnant persons aged 25–29, risk of severe maternal mortality and morbidity increased 1.6 times at 40–44 years old, 2.0 times at 45–49 years old, and to 5.2 times at 50 years or more.[26]

The risk of spontaneous abortion and chromosomal abnormalities increases markedly after the age of 40.[27] More than 50% of pregnancies between the ages of 40 and 44 years end in miscarriage, increasing to more than 90% over age 45.[28-30] The predicted odds of delivering a child at term with Trisomy 21 increases from 1:85 at age 40 to 1:35 at age 45.[30] The risks are even higher when considering aneuploidy. Conception after age 40 is associated with both an increased risk of early pregnancy loss as well intrauterine fetal death.[31] The risk of ectopic pregnancy and perinatal death also increases with age.[28]

In an ongoing pregnancy, there is an increase in maternal complications including gestational diabetes, placenta previa, gestational hypertension, severe pre-eclampsia, and placental abruption.[24,27,32] The likelihood of cesarean section over the age of 40 years is two to three times higher than in those younger than age 25.[32] Neonatal complications include increased risks of preterm delivery, low birth weight, intrauterine growth restriction, and perinatal mortality.[24,25,27,32,33] In the postpartum period, readmissions after birth are increased.[34] Advances in maternal and fetal monitoring allow most pregnancies in people older than 35 to progress without significant complications. However, it is important to approach the following review of contraceptive options through the lens of the risks of conception, pregnancy, and childbirth. The actual risks of pregnancy should be addressed during any discussions about family planning and contraceptive options during the perimenopause. These risks must be balanced against the risks of continuing contraception, particularly risks of acute cardiovascular events, loss of bone mineral density, or breast cancer. In general, the risks of pregnancy outweigh the risks of contraception for most people.

Contraception During the Later Reproductive Years

Contraceptive needs change over the course of one's lifetime. The failure rates of any contraceptive method are lower over the age of 40 compared to younger individuals because overall fertility is lower in this age group. If there is a lower risk of pregnancy, methods with lower inherent efficacy may be suitable. Considerations include coital frequency, partner fertility, predictability of ovarian reserve, and the health risk posed by pregnancy.

No contraceptive method is contraindicated on the basis of age alone,[35] as there are no data to suggest that age itself is a risk factor for contraceptive-related complications. As such, contraceptives may be used up to age 55, the age at which 90% of women will have experienced the final menstrual period, so long as doing so is medically prudent.[36]

While the contraindications for contraceptive use in older persons mirror younger users, medical conditions may develop with age that may preclude the use of certain methods, in particular estrogen-containing methods. Conditions to consider include hypertension, obesity, smoking, diabetes, migraine with aura, and cardiovascular disease. Other important aspects of the medical history include history of venous thromboembolism (VTE), malignancy, and medications.

Discussion about contraceptive options should always be person-centered. (See Chapter 4, Person-Centered Reproductive Health Conversations and Contraceptive Counseling.) Individualized counseling should take into account baseline health risk for adverse clinical outcomes, menopause-related symptoms of the perimenopause, and individual life circumstances and goals. Contraceptive options that align with patient preferences and are not contraindicated should be presented so that health care providers can support individuals in deciding what contraceptive method (or methods) fits their individual needs ("user-method fit") while minimizing provider bias. The American College of Obstetricians and Gynecologists recognizes the importance of a patient-centered approach to contraceptive counseling. The first step unequivocally establishes whether or not the patient is interested in contraception. The clinician explores patient's contraceptive preferences in the context of their values and goals. Clinicians share relevant information with the patient so that they can come to an informed decision.[37]

Contraception can provide noncontraceptive benefits, or health benefits that go beyond pregnancy prevention. Contraception counseling is an opportunity to discuss and offer methods that could improve quality of life and provide primary prevention of certain conditions. Different contraceptive methods may also confer considerable noncontraceptive benefits that improve quality of life for those experiencing distressing perimenopausal symptoms and decrease the risk of other adverse health conditions.

For those who have decided that childbearing is complete, permanent contraception methods such as bilateral tubal ligation or salpingectomy (complete removal of the Fallopian tubes), or partner vasectomy may be options. Older women are less likely to express regret after the procedure.[38] Furthermore, tubal sterilization (either with partial tubal removal or complete salpingectomy) has been shown to reduce ovarian cancer risk at a RR of 0.61 (95% CI 0.46–0.85).[39] This may be explained by growing evidence that most ovarian cancers originate in the fallopian tube epithelium. (See Chapter 8, Permanent Contraception.) It is worth mentioning, however, that the benefit–risk ratio as a contraceptive choice decreases with age.

There are many contraceptive methods to choose from that may be suitable and provide additional health benefits. During the perimenopause, patients may choose to use a contraceptive method for its noncontraceptive benefits, even when there is no risk of pregnancy (i.e., not sexually active, prior permanent birth control procedure). Until menopause is confirmed, contraceptive use and choice of method should be regularly reviewed, keeping in mind benefits, risks, and potential comorbidities that may develop. (See Chapter 4, Person-Centered Reproductive Health Conversations and Contraceptive Counseling.)

Contraceptive Options During the Later Reproductive Years

Earlier chapters focused on individual methods provide detailed information about each of them. This chapter will summarize the features of each of the methods that are significant for individuals in the later reproductive years. The methods are outlined in order of efficacy.

Contraceptive Options During Perimenopause

The Contraceptive Implant

Contraceptive subdermal implants are the most effective contraceptive methods and offer several features that are particularly relevant during the later reproductive years. They do not contain estrogen and have very few contraindications to their use, so even those with serious medical comorbidities can usually safely use the implant.[35] The progestin component provides endometrial protection against the risks of unopposed estrogen associated with either anovulation or obesity, which are common in this age group. Extended use of implants for up to 5 years' total duration may be appropriate in this age group.[40]

Changes in bleeding patterns are common; 20% of implant users experience amenorrhea and more than 50% of users experience irregular bleeding (which may be infrequent). Bleeding disturbances are consistently the top reason for discontinuation.[41] It is not known how the implant impacts the abnormal bleeding patterns typically seen during the perimenopausal transition, although hormonal fluctuations may theoretically increase the likelihood of bleeding problems with this method. Changes in bleeding patterns in older implant users may raise concerns about the possibility of underlying pathology and the question of how to interpret abnormal bleeding, especially in users with risk factors for endometrial hyperplasia, such as obesity and anovulation. If bleeding changes that coincide with implant initiation are characteristic of implant use, and any previous concerns regarding abnormal uterine bleeding have been appropriately investigated, generally this would not raise concerns for endometrial pathology. However, if other changes develop during implant use, evaluation with endometrial sampling or ultrasonography of the uterus may be prudent since the implant does not provide complete protection against all endometrial disease, especially neoplasia that are not hormonally sensitive.

Although ovulation is inhibited in etonogestrel implant users, endogenous estradiol production continues, and serum estradiol levels remain above the threshold for maintaining normal bone mass. There is no apparent detrimental effect on bone density with the implant, an important consideration given the postmenopausal changes in bone health.[42] The implant should provide adequate endometrial protection when estrogen therapies are being used to treat perimenopausal symptoms associated with hormonal fluctuations (off-label use); thus, there is no need for additional progestin therapy in these settings. However, if abnormal bleeding patterns emerge, investigation with ultrasonography of the uterus and/or endometrial sampling is warranted.

(See Chapter 9, Contraceptive Implant; Chapter 2, Understanding the Physiology of the Menstrual Cycle; Chapter 3, Menstrual Disorders; and Chapter 4, Person-Centered Reproductive Health Conversations and Contraceptive Counseling.)

Levonorgestrel Intrauterine Devices (LNG-IUDs)

Levonorgestrel intrauterine devices (LNG-IUDs) are highly effective contraceptive methods that also induce endometrial changes that may address perimenopausal uterine concerns. The LNG 52 mg IUD (Mirena® and Liletta®) is the most effective medical treatment for heavy menstrual bleeding.[43] The progestin core of the IUD acts directly on the endometrial lining, causing endometrial thinning and glandular atrophy. Additionally, for patients with endometrial hyperplasia, the LNG 52 mg IUDs are effective treatment for patients who are poor surgical candidates or who wish to preserve their fertility.[44,45]

Amenorrhea is often a desirable side effect of the LNG-IUD.[46] Therefore, LNG-IUDs can be attractive options for those experiencing perimenopausal bleeding patterns of heavy, irregular, and anovulatory menstrual bleeding. Perimenopausal patients with abnormal uterine bleeding have similar improvements in bleeding when compared to endometrial ablation, precluding the need for surgery[47] and reducing the risk of hysterectomy.[48] Bleeding from leiomyoma can be reduced by the LNG 52 mg IUD if the fibroids are small (< 4 cm) intramural fibroids and they do not block successful placement of the device. However, expulsion rates are higher when fibroids are present.

Internationally, over 100 countries have currently approved the LNG 52 mg IUD as the progestin for those with an intact uterus using estrogen therapy for menopausal symptoms.[46] The LNG-IUD provides adequate endometrial suppression for endometrial proliferation for those on estrogen menopausal therapy.[49,50] It is used as an off-label option in the United States for progestin treatment in menopausal hormone therapy in those with a uterus. Using the LNG 52 mg IUD for contraception and as a segue into menopausal hormone therapy is an accepted strategy.[51]

Lower-dose LNG IUD devices (LNG 19.5 IUD Kyleena® and LNG 13.5 mg IUD-Skyla®) induce amenorrhea at lower rates then the LNG 52 mg IUD. Their impact on bleeding patterns in older users is not well documented. However, the narrower diameter of the device may make placement easier in perimenopausal patients.[52] There are little data on its effectiveness for endometrial protection as part of menopausal hormone therapy regimens.

The LNG 52 mg IUD is now approved by the US Food and Drug Administration (FDA) for contraceptive use up to 8 years. Continued amenorrhea is a good sign of ongoing IUD function. In the later reproductive years, the LNG 52 mg IUD provides effective contraception for 8 years and likely 10 years of endometrial protection. Use of a LNG-IUD allows for a smoother transition into menopause, helping to avoid the abnormal uterine bleeding patterns that affect many in this age group and can disrupt their quality of life. Once menopause is diagnosed and it is more than 8 years since since the LNG 52 mg IUD was inserted, the IUD may be removed. (See Chapter 10, Intrauterine Devices [IUDs] and Chapter 4, Person-Centered Reproductive Health Conversations and Contraceptive Counseling.)

Copper Intrauterine Devices (Cu-IUD)

A copper 380 mm^2 IUD (Cu-IUD) is a highly effective contraceptive method. Patients may experience an increase in menstrual blood loss, and therefore may not be as suitable in the setting of abnormal or heavy uterine bleeding, particularly in the perimenopause when anovulatory cycling often occurs and uterine fibroids may be more common. Uterine fibroids that markedly distort the endometrial cavity may prevent IUD use. Fibroids that do not prevent IUD use may contribute to higher rates of expulsion.

Cu-IUDs may be effective far beyond their approved duration of use, depending on the type.[53,55] This may be particularly important when a patient in their mid-to-late 40s presents after 10 years of Cu-IUD use asking for removal and replacement of the device. It has been proposed that the TCu380A IUD could be used until menopause if it was inserted when the IUD user was 35 years or older.[53] It is quite reasonable in those instances to extend the use of the existing device until menopause. Although leaving the Cu-IUD in situ once menopause is diagnosed may have no effect on one's health, it may result in bleeding, pain, or infection; thus, removal is advised once menopause is confirmed.

Copper IUD use is associated with a decreased risk of endometrial and possibly cervical cancer.[56,57] The Cu-IUD is also very effective as emergency contraception if used within 1 week of an act of unprotected intercourse (within 5 days of ovulation).[58] (See Chapter 4, Person-Centered Reproductive Health Conversations and Contraceptive Counseling; Chapter 10, Intrauterine Devices [IUDs]; and Chapter 18, Emergency Contraception.)

Injectable Progestins: Depot Medoxyprogesterone Acetate

Depot medroxyprogesterone acetate (DMPA; Depo-Provera®) is an effective method of contraception that is associated with high amenorrhea rates.[59] Successful treatment of heavy menstrual bleeding (HMB) is less likely with DMPA compared to the LNG-IUD.[60] Nevertheless, DMPA can still be very useful for treating HMB in some patients, including leiomyoma-related HMB. Use of DMPA has been associated with a decreased prevalence of leiomyomas.[61] Early transitional undesirable bleeding may discourage use of DMPA, but concurrent treatment with estradiol or combination oral contraceptives (where appropriate), GnRH agonists, nonsteroidal anti-inflammatory drugs, tranexamic acid, or other agents to establish amenorrhea may significantly reduce undesirable bleeding.[62]

The US FDA added a warning to DMPA labeling about the potential loss of bone mineral density (BMD) in 2004. Lingering concerns about the adverse impact DMPA may have on BMD have led some to recommend early perimenopausal cessation of DMPA to allow BMD to rebuild prior to menopause. This ignores the fact that patients entering menopause on DMPA have already lost the bone density they would lose during the early years of menopause when estradiol levels fall. They do not experience that accelerated loss in bone density in the first 5 years of menopause, although they do continue with age-related bone loss as do nonusers.[63,64] A systematic review of observational studies found that DMPA users may have an increased fracture risk, although postmenopausal fracture rates among those who used DMPA earlier compared to nonusers did not show any increased risk after excluding women with prior fractures.[65]

DMPA is associated with a reduced risk of endometrial hyperplasia and endometrial cancer,[66] which may be of benefit in the later reproductive years when anovulatory cycles become more common and body mass index is often increasing. DMPA use may be associated with hypoestrogenic symptoms due to the suppression of follicle-stimulating hormone (FSH)–regulated ovarian estradiol production. DMPA can be combined with menopausal estrogen therapy in appropriate candidates to control vasomotor symptoms as an off-label use. Perimenopausal patients using DMPA who experience abnormal uterine bleeding should have a transvaginal ultrasound to assess the endometrial thickness and the uterus. A thickened endometrial lining would warrant endometrial sampling. DMPA continuation beyond age 50 should be individualized and careful consideration should be given to other potential risk factors for osteoporosis. Of note, DMPA does not stop the menopausal rise in FSH levels.[67] In perimenopausal patients, if FSH is suppressed, the levels generally return to the normal baseline prior to the next injection. (See Chapter 11, Injectable Contraceptives and Chapter 4, Person-Centered Reproductive Health Conversations and Contraceptive Counseling.)

Combined Hormonal Contraception (CHC)

During perimenopause, combined hormonal contraceptives (CHCs; oral contraceptive pills, transdermal patches, and vaginal rings) offer pregnancy prevention as well as cyclic and predictable menstrual patterns (with the possibility of amenorrhea with continuous use), decreased blood loss, treatment of vasomotor symptoms, at least partial protection against bone loss, and reduced risk of several cancers. A large cohort study in the United Kingdom found that women who had ever used CHCs had a 12% risk reduction of any cancer and a 29% risk reduction of gynecologic cancers.[68] Endometrial cancer risk and ovarian cancer risk have both been demonstrated to be decreased in users of combined oral contraceptive pills in several meta-analyses, with greatest benefit correlated with duration and proximity of use.[69]

While breast cancer risk may prove concerning for some potential users, high-quality studies have demonstrated no prolonged increased risk of CHC use on breast cancer development, regardless of ethinyl estradiol dose, duration of use, or formulation.[70,71] Newer studies have demonstrated a modest increase in risk that matches that of nonusers after 5 years following discontinuation.[72] CHCs that contain newer estrogens, such as estetrol (E4), appear to have less of a proliferative effect on breast tissue. The risks of thrombotic stroke (TS) and myocardial infarction (MI) associated with combined hormonal contraceptives increases with age.[5] Those over 39 years of age had four times the risks compared to adolescents. In a Danish study, the risks of TS and MI increased by a factor of 20 and 10, respectively, in women age 45–49 compared to those age 15–19 after adjusting for CHC use. Higher estrogen dose formulations had higher risks.[73]

Careful monitoring for the development of category 4 conditions (i.e., conditions that pose an unacceptable health risk) or some combination of category 3 conditions (theoretical or proven risk outweighs advantages) is needed in this age group.[35] Given the prevalence of obesity and underdiagnosed hypertension, diabetes, and cardiovascular risks, a more thorough periodic analysis of the health status of users may be justified. Those found to be healthy can certainly continue to use combined hormonal methods until menopause in the United States, although recommendations in Canada and the United Kingdom suggest considering changing to a progestin-only method at the age of 50.[74]

In this age group, continuous use or extended cycle use of combined hormonal contraceptives may not only achieve amenorrhea but also avoid development of vasomotor symptoms by avoiding the hormone-free intervals. If the user wants scheduled bleeding, try to limit the number of hormone free days by using a 24/4 regimen. Two low-dose pill brands (Mircette®, Lolo®/Lo Loestrin®) have only two placebo pills. One pill with estradiol valerate (E2V, Natazia®) rather than ethinyl estradiol may be preferred in this age group because of its potential lower risk for VTE (not demonstrated in prospective observational studies), its high rate of amenorrhea, and its use of only two placebo pills per cycle. Combined oral contraceptives (COCs) containing 17-beta-estradiol appear to have less procoagulant effect than COCs containing ethinyl estradiol. Similarly, a COC E4 (NEXTSTELLIS®) may be preferred due to its 24/4 regimen, lower procoagulant effect, E4's lack of stimulatory effect on the breast, and its lack of metabolism by cytochrome P450. Of note, the vaginal contraceptive ring increases vaginal lubrication and may help relieve perimenopausal symptoms of vaginal dryness and dyspareunia. (See Chapter 12, Combined Hormonal Contraception and Chapter 4, Person-Centered Reproductive Health Conversations and Contraceptive Counseling.)

Progestin-Only Pills

Progestin-only pills (POPs) can be used by virtually everyone; only current breast cancer is listed as a category 4 condition by the US MEC.[35] They have not been shown to increase the risk of VTE, risk of arterial thromboembolism, or affect BMD. POPs are excellent options to use when a patient is transitioning from longer acting methods (DMPA, LNG-IUD) that commonly induce amenorrhea or from those that can schedule cyclic bleeding (pills, patches, rings). There are several different POPs (levonorgestrel-, norethindrone-, desogestrel-, and drosperinone-containing pills), with only the norethindrone and drosperinone options available in the United States as of April 2023. Unlike the norethindrone option, which relies on the cervical mucus changes it produces and requires users to use back-up for 2 days if they are more than 3 hours late in taking their daily pill, the drosperinone POP option has a better bleeding profile, more frequently achieving amenorrhea, and a longer "window of forgiveness" for missed pills.[75] (See Chapter 13, Progestin-Only Pills.)

While POPs reduce blood loss and can help reduce vasomotor symptoms, not all formulations will provide predictable scheduled bleeding. Notably, norethindrone-only pills may have increased episodes of unfavorable bleeding, while drosperinone-only pills may allow users to induce a scheduled bleed.[76] Amenorrhea and undesirable bleeding rates are generally higher than with CHCs, but this does not seem to increase POP discontinuation rates in older users. The POP does not suppress the menopausal rise in FSH levels.[67]

Barrier/Nonhormonal Methods

Fertility awareness–based methods (FABM) rely on knowledge of the timing of ovulation. During the perimenopause, changes in the hypothalamic-pituitary-ovarian axis cause unpredictable changes to menstrual cycle length and ovulation, making it difficult to predict cycle length and interpret markers of ovulation. FABMs are not usually reliable in the perimenopause. However, those techniques that monitor reproductive signs on a daily basis (symptothermal technique or 2-days method) may still have some degree of effectiveness during these years of transition, though studies examining this efficacy remain low to moderate in quality.[77] (See Chapter 15, Fertility Awareness-Based Methods.)

Patients with medical conditions or preferences that preclude use of other contraceptive options may still find FABMs desirable. While there is an increased rate of contraceptive failure with use of FABMs during perimenopause, this option may still be acceptable for patients who do not prioritize effectiveness and when considering the decreased fecundity in this age group. (See Chapter 4, Person-Centered Reproductive Health Conversations and Contraceptive Counseling.)

Barrier methods include external and internal condoms, diaphragms, and cervical caps. Barrier methods may be more effective during perimenopause compared to younger age groups; however, consistent use is still required to prevent pregnancy. Condoms have the additional advantage of protecting against sexually transmitted infections (STIs). Individuals in this age group may be entering into new relationships, and the need for STI prevention should be addressed. Condom use may be more problematic if the partner is older and/or has erectile dysfunction. In this case, internal condoms may be an option. Similarly, condom use in the setting of menopausal vaginal dryness may make penetrative intercourse painful or uncomfortable. Use of lubricants may help ameliorate these symptoms. (See Chapter 14, External [Male]Condoms and Chapter 16, On-Demand Internal Methods.) Decreased fecundity in the perimenopause may make less-effective methods like diaphragms and cervical caps an acceptable option for some patients. Correct use of the diaphragm or cervical cap may be difficult for patients with vaginal vault prolapse or significant urethral hypermobility. (See Chapter 16, On-Demand Internal Method.)

Patients using barrier or FABM methods should be offered counseling regarding the availability, efficacy, and safety of emergency contraception (EC) so that it can be used in the event of a method disruption/malfunction (e.g., condom slips or breaks, diaphragm is dislodged).

In 2020, the FDA approved a *vaginal gel contraceptive* containing lactic acid, citric acid, and potassium bitartrate (Phexxi®).[78] While there are no data specific to efficacy in the perimenopausal population, the vaginal contraceptive gel may be a favorable option for those who desire on-demand contraception and who are accepting of a lower efficacy rate. Its role as a lubricant may be a noncontraceptive benefit during the perimenopause. Condoms and other on-demand contraception such as the vaginal contraceptive gel could also complement FABMs to increase overall effectiveness. (See Chapter 16, On-Demand Internal Method.)

Emergency Contraception

If a reversible contraceptive method is chosen (with the exception of implants or intrauterine devices), offer counseling about the availability, efficacy, and safety of EC so that it can be used in the event of unprotected intercourse or a method disruption/malfunction. The choice of oral EC will depend upon body mass index and the ongoing contraceptive method to be used. (See Chapter 18, Emergency Contraception.) A copper IUD should also be considered at the time of EC counseling given its dual benefit as emergency contraception and as an ongoing contraceptive.[79]

When Can Contraception Be Reliably Stopped?

The precise time at which there is no longer a risk of pregnancy is unknown for any individual patient. However, as long as the potential to ovulate exists, the patient would need to use contraception if they want to avoid pregnancy. There are no reliable laboratory tests to confirm when there is definitive loss of fertility, and FSH levels may not be accurate in the perimenopausal period. Measurements of FSH in the face of the dramatic swings in hormone levels during the perimenopause can incorrectly diagnose menopause and put the patient at risk for pregnancy if contraception were to be discontinued. Patients who want to avoid pregnancy will need to continue their use of contraception until menopause is confirmed.

Amenorrhea alone cannot be used to diagnose menopause in users of hormonal contraception. Thus, recommendations for diagnosing menopause will vary depending on age, type of contraception used, clinical signs, and laboratory testing.

Menopause may be confirmed in the following instances:

- Amenorrhea for more than 1 year after age 50
- Amenorrhea for 2 or more years if less than 50 years of age
- Some authorities recommend an elevated FSH (FSH ≥ 30 IU/L) on two separate occasions 6 to 8 weeks apart.
    - FSH levels are not usually impacted by DMPA, In perimenopausal women, if FSH is suppressed, the levels generally return to baseline prior to the next injection. FSH can be checked on the day of injection and 13 weeks later at the next injection. If both FSH levels are > 30 IU/L, then contraception can be stopped.
    - FSH levels are not affected by POPs or the implant. If the FSH level is > 30 IU/L, contraception should be continued for one more year and then can be stopped. If it is < 30 IU/L, then contraception should be continued and FSH checked again in one year.
    - FSH levels may be affected by use of CHCs. Due to the potential for false negative results after only 7 hormone-free days, FSH levels should be drawn while off CHC for at least 2 weeks (preferably at least 6 weeks if the patient is able to use a reliable back-up method of contraception). If the FSH level is subsequently elevated on two occasions at least 6 to 8 weeks apart, contraception can be discontinued.

It is recommended that individuals continue their contraception until age 55 or at least 1 year after final menstrual period for individuals over 50, and for 2 years after final menstrual period for individuals under 50.[36] It is usually assumed that one is no longer fertile at age 55, when 95% of individuals have reached menopause. When CHC is discontinued, menopausal symptoms may start, including vasomotor symptoms, sleep disturbances, genitourinary symptoms, and changes in sexual function. It must be remembered that standard menopausal hormone therapy is NOT a method of contraception.

Transitioning to Menopausal Hormone Therapy

For patients who wish to avoid pregnancy before menopause can be confirmed, the recommendation is to continue contraception until the age of 55 if hormonal methods are being used. Nonhormonal methods, such as copper IUD, can be used safely until menopause is confirmed.[36,80] Understanding that with increasing age there is an increased incidence of medical conditions, providers should remain vigilant about making sure the patient's contraception is still safe for them to use.

The desire for menopausal hormone therapy (HT) is determined by patient preference and desire for symptom management. Exact formulations and dosages of HT are beyond the scope of this chapter. However, it is important to note that conventional menopausal HT is NOT an effective contraceptive option.[81] The LNG 52 mg IUD can provide effective contraception while also providing adequate endometrial protection for those who opt for estrogen menopausal therapy.[49,50]

Summary

- During the later reproductive years, one's contraceptive needs may change. New health problems or concerns may arise that require a method change or the use of a contraceptive method for its noncontraceptive benefits. Long-acting methods of reversible contraception are an alternative to permanent birth control methods and may offer important noncontraceptive benefits.
- The need for and safety of ongoing use of a contraceptive method should be reassessed at each health care provider visit. Noncontraceptive benefits of the method should be documented.
- Patients may want to consider changing methods during the later reproductive years, particularly as new situations arise. LNG-IUDs have additional benefits, including a decrease in menstrual bleeding and easing of the transition to HT. In the absence of contraindications, CHCs may also provide relief from many perimenopausal symptoms. However, during the later reproductive years, associated risks of CHC use may increase.
- External and internal condoms can be added for STI protection and providers should offer counseling about STI prevention when appropriate. Emergency contraception should be available in advance of need.
- Careful counseling should be provided regarding when to stop using contraception and how to transition to hormone therapy (HT) if desired.

Author Disclosures—Black: Consulting and Advisory Boards for Searchlight, Mithra, Organon, Pfizer, Bayer. Sherman: none. Miller: none.

References

1. Santoro N. Using antimullerian hormone to predict fertility. JAMA. 2017;318:1333-4.
2. Shifren JL, Gass ML, Group NRfCCoMWW. The North American Menopause Society recommendations for clinical care of midlife women. Menopause. 2014;21:1038-62.
3. Nichols HB, Trentham-Dietz A, Hampton JM, et al. From menarche to menopause: Trends among US women born from 1912 to 1969. Am J Epidemiol. 2006;164:1003-11.
4. Paramsothy P, Harlow SD, Greendale GA, et al. Bleeding patterns during the menopausal transition in the multi-ethnic Study of Women's Health Across the Nation (SWAN): a prospective cohort study. BJOG. 2014;121:1564-73.
5. Long ME, Faubion SS, MacLaughlin KL, Pruthi S, Casey PM. Contraception and hormonal management in the perimenopause. J Womens Health (Larchmt). 2015;24:3-10.
6. Hale GE, Shufelt CL. Hormone therapy in menopause: An update on cardiovascular disease considerations. Trends Cardiovasc Med. 2015;25:540-9.
7. Martin VT, Pavlovic J, Fanning KM, Buse DC, Reed ML, Lipton RB. Perimenopause and menopause are associated with high frequency headache in women with migraine: Results of the American Migraine Prevalence and Prevention Study. Headache. 2016;56:292-305.

8. Jones HJ, Huang AJ, Subak LL, Brown JS, Lee KA. Bladder symptoms in the early menopausal transition. J Womens Health (Larchmt). 2016;25:457-63.
9. Avis NE, Brockwell S, Randolph JF, Jr., et al. Longitudinal changes in sexual functioning as women transition through menopause: results from the Study of Women's Health Across the Nation. Menopause. 2009;16:442-52.
10. Santoro N. Perimenopause: From research to practice. J Womens Health (Larchmt). 2016; 25:332-9.
11. Jackson EA, El Khoudary SR, Crawford SL, et al. Hot flash frequency and blood pressure: Data from the Study of Women's Health Across the Nation. J Womens Health (Larchmt) 2016; 25:1204-9.
12. Kravitz HM, Joffe H. Sleep during the perimenopause: a SWAN story. Obstet Gynecol Clin North Am. 2011;38:567-86.
13. Avis NE, Crawford SL, Greendale G, et al. Duration of menopausal vasomotor symptoms over the menopause transition. JAMA Intern Med. 2015;175:531-9.
14. Chang PY, Gold EB, Cauley JA, et al. Triglyceride levels and fracture risk in midlife women: Study of Women's Health Across the Nation (SWAN). J Clin Endocrinol Metab. 2016;101:3297-305.
15. Bleil ME, Bromberger JT, Latham MD, et al. Disruptions in ovarian function are related to depression and cardiometabolic risk during premenopause. Menopause. 2013;20:631-9.
16. El Khoudary SR, Wang L, Brooks MM, Thurston RC, Derby CA, Matthews KA. Increase HDL-C level over the menopausal transition is associated with greater atherosclerotic progression. J Clin Lipidol. 2016;10:962-9.
17. Menken J, Trussell J, Larsen U. Age and infertility. Science. 1986;233:1389-94.
18. Chandra A, Copen CE, Stephen EH. Infertility and impaired fecundity in the United States, 1982-2010: data from the National Survey of Family Growth. Natl Health Stat Rep. 2013:1-18, 1 p. following 19.
19. Steiner AZ, Jukic AM. Impact of female age and nulligravidity on fecundity in an older reproductive age cohort. Fertil Steril. 2016;105:1584-8.e1.
20. Black A, Yang Q, Wu Wen S, Lalonde AB, Guilbert E, Fisher W. Contraceptive use among Canadian women of reproductive age: results of a national survey. J Obstet Gynaecol Can. 2009; 31:627-40.
21. Finer LB, Zolna MR. Declines in unintended pregnancy in the United States, 2008-2011. N Engl J Med. 2016;374:843-52.
22. Finer LB, Philbin JM. Trends in ages at key reproductive transitions in the United States, 1951-2010. Womens Health Iss. 2014;24:e271-9.
23. Higgins JA, Lands M, Valley TM, Carpenter E, Jacques L. Real-time effects of payer restrictions on reproductive healthcare: A qualitative analysis of cost-related barriers and their consequences among U.S. abortion seekers on Reddit. Int J Environ Res Public Health. 2021;18.
24. Jacobsson B, Ladfors L, Milsom I. Advanced maternal age and adverse perinatal outcome. Obstet Gynecol. 2004;104:727-33.
25. Klemetti R, Gissler M, Sainio S, Hemminki E. At what age does the risk for adverse maternal and infant outcomes increase? Nationwide register-based study on first births in Finland in 2005-2014. Acta Obstet Gynecol Scand. 2016;95:1368-75.
26. Lisonkova S, Potts J, Muraca GM, et al. Maternal age and severe maternal morbidity: A population-based retrospective cohort study. PLoS Med. 2017;14:e1002307.
27. Cleary-Goldman J, Malone FD, Vidaver J, et al. Impact of maternal age on obstetric outcome. Obstet Gynecol. 2005;105:983-90.
28. Nybo Andersen AM, Wohlfahrt J, Christens P, Olsen J, Melbye M. Maternal age and fetal loss: population based register linkage study. BMJ. 2000;320:1708-12.
29. Heffner LJ. Advanced maternal age--how old is too old? N Engl J Med. 2004;351:1927-9.
30. Morris JK, De Vigan C, Mutton DE, Alberman E. Risk of a Down syndrome live birth in women 45 years of age and older. Prenat Diagn. 2005;25:275-8.
31. Bouzaglou A, Aubenas I, Abbou H, et al. Pregnancy at 40 years old and above: obstetrical, fetal, and neonatal outcomes. Is age an independent risk factor for those complications? Front Med (Lausanne). 2020;7:208.
32. Joseph KS, Allen AC, Dodds L, Turner LA, Scott H, Liston R. The perinatal effects of delayed childbearing. Obstet Gynecol. 2005;105:1410-8.

33. Olapeju B, Hong X, Wang G, et al. Birth outcomes across the spectrum of maternal age: dissecting aging effect versus confounding by social and medical determinants. BMC Pregnancy Childbirth. 2021;21(1):594.
34. Wen T, Overton EE, Sheen JJ, et al. Risk for postpartum readmissions and associated complications based on maternal age. J Matern Fetal Neonatal Med. 2021 May;34(9):1375-81.
35. Curtis KM, Tepper NK, Jatlaoui TC, et al. U.S. medical eligibility criteria for contraceptive use, 2016. MMWR Recomm Rep. 2016;65:1-103.
36. ESHRE Capri Workshop Group. Female contraception over 40. Hum Reprod Update. 2009; 15:599-612.
37. American College of Obstetricians and Gynecologists' Committee on Health Care for Underserved Women, Contraceptive Equity Expert Work Group, and Committee on Ethics. Patient-centered contraceptive counseling: ACOG Committee Statement Number 1. Obstet Gynecol. 2022;139(2):350-3.
38. ACOG Practice bulletin no. 133: benefits and risks of sterilization. Obstet Gynecol 2013; 121:392-404.
39. Green A, Purdie D, Bain C, et al. Tubal sterilisation, hysterectomy and decreased risk of ovarian cancer. Survey of Women's Health Study Group. Int J Cancer. 1997;71:948-51.
40. Ali M, Akin A, Bahamondes L, et al. Extended use up to 5 years of the etonogestrel-releasing subdermal contraceptive implant: comparison to levonorgestrel-releasing subdermal implant. Hum Reprod. 2016;31:2491-8.
41. Moray KV, Chaurasia H, Sachin O, Joshi B. A systematic review on clinical effectiveness, side-effect profile and meta-analysis on continuation rate of etonogestrel contraceptive implant. Reprod Health. 2021;18:4.
42. Hadji P, Colli E, Regidor PA. Bone health in estrogen-free contraception. Osteoporos Int. 2019;30:2391-400.
43. Lethaby A, Hussain M, Rishworth JR, Rees MC. Progesterone or progestogen-releasing intrauterine systems for heavy menstrual bleeding. Cochrane Database Syst Rev. 2015:CD002126.
44. Pal N, Broaddus RR, Urbauer DL, et al. Treatment of low-risk endometrial cancer and complex atypical hyperplasia with the levonorgestrel-releasing intrauterine device. Obstet Gynecol. 2018;131:109-16.
45. Joo JK, Shin JH, Lee JR, Kim MR. Levonorgestrel-releasing intrauterine system use in perimenopausal women. J Menopausal Med. 2021;27:49-57.
46. Bednarek PH, Jensen JT. Safety, efficacy and patient acceptability of the contraceptive and non-contraceptive uses of the LNG-IUS. Int J Womens Health. 2010;1:45-58.
47. Kaunitz AM, Meredith S, Inki P, Kubba A, Sanchez-Ramos L. Levonorgestrel-releasing intrauterine system and endometrial ablation in heavy menstrual bleeding: a systematic review and meta-analysis. Obstet Gynecol .2009;113:1104-16.
48. Lahteenmaki P, Haukkamaa M, Puolakka J, et al. Open randomised study of use of levonorgestrel releasing intrauterine system as alternative to hysterectomy. BMJ. 1998;316:1122-6.
49. Sitruk-Ware R. The levonorgestrel intrauterine system for use in peri- and postmenopausal women. Contraception. 2007;75:S155-60.
50. Sturdee D. Levonorgestrel intrauterine system for endometrial protection. J Br Menopause Soc. 2006;12 Suppl 1:1-3.
51. Depypere HT, Hillard T, Erkkola R, et al. A 60-month non-comparative study on bleeding profiles with the levonorgestrel intrauterine system from the late transition period to estrogen supplemented menopause. Eur J Obstet Gynecol Reprod Biol. 2010;153:176-80.
52. Allen RH, Cwiak CA. Contraception for midlife women. Menopause. 2016;23:111-3.
53. Wu JP, Pickle S. Extended use of the intrauterine device: a literature review and recommendations for clinical practice. Contraception. 2014;89:495-503.
54. Ronnerdag M, Odlind V. Health effects of long-term use of the intrauterine levonorgestrel-releasing system. A follow-up study over 12 years of continuous use. Acta Obstet Gynecol Scand. 1999;78:716-21.
55. Sivin I, Stern J, Coutinho E, et al. Prolonged intrauterine contraception: a seven-year randomized study of the levonorgestrel 20 mcg/day (LNg 20) and the Copper T380 Ag IUDS. Contraception. 1991;44:473-80.

56. Felix AS, Gaudet MM, La Vecchia C, et al. Intrauterine devices and endometrial cancer risk: a pooled analysis of the Epidemiology of Endometrial Cancer Consortium. Int J Cancer. 2015; 136:E410-22.
57. Castellsague X, Diaz M, Vaccarella S, et al. Intrauterine device use, cervical infection with human papillomavirus, and risk of cervical cancer: a pooled analysis of 26 epidemiological studies. Lancet Oncol. 2011;12:1023-31.
58. Turok DK, Godfrey EM, Wojdyla D, Dermish A, Torres L, Wu SC. Copper T380 intrauterine device for emergency contraception: highly effective at any time in the menstrual cycle. Hum Reprod. 2013;28:2672-6.
59. Hubacher D, Lopez L, Steiner MJ, Dorflinger L. Menstrual pattern changes from levonorgestrel subdermal implants and DMPA: systematic review and evidence-based comparisons. Contraception. 2009;80:113-8.
60. Kucuk T, Ertan K. Continuous oral or intramuscular medroxyprogesterone acetate versus the levonorgestrel releasing intrauterine system in the treatment of perimenopausal menorrhagia: a randomized, prospective, controlled clinical trial in female smokers. Clin Exp Obstet Gynecol. 2008;35:57-60.
61. Harmon QE, Baird DD. Use of depot medroxyprogesterone acetate and prevalent leiomyoma in young African American women. Hum Reprod 2015;30:1499-504.
62. Abdel-Aleem H, d'Arcangues C, Vogelsong KM, Gaffield ML, Gulmezoglu AM. Treatment of vaginal bleeding irregularities induced by progestin only contraceptives. Cochrane Database Syst Rev. 2013:CD003449.
63. Cundy T, Cornish J, Roberts H, Reid IR. Menopausal bone loss in long-term users of depot medroxyprogesterone acetate contraception. Am J Obstet Gynecol. 2002;186:978-83.
64. Beksinska ME, Smit JA, Kleinschmidt I, Farley TM, Mbatha F. Bone mineral density in women aged 40-49 years using depot-medroxyprogesterone acetate, norethisterone enanthate or combined oral contraceptives for contraception. Contraception. 2005;71:170-5.
65. Lopez LM, Chen M, Mullins Long S, Curtis KM, Helmerhorst FM. Steroidal contraceptives and bone fractures in women: evidence from observational studies. Cochrane Database Syst Rev. 2015:CD009849.
66. Kaunitz AM. Depot medroxyprogesterone acetate contraception and the risk of breast and gynecologic cancer. J Reprod Med. 1996;41:419-27.
67. Beksinska ME, Smit JA, Kleinschmidt I, Farley TM. Assessing menopausal status in women aged 40 - 49 using depot-medroxyprogesterone acetate, norethisterone enanthate or combined oral contraception. S Afr Med J. 2011;101:131-5.
68. Hannaford PC, Selvaraj S, Elliott AM, Angus V, Iversen L, Lee AJ. Cancer risk among users of oral contraceptives: cohort data from the Royal College of General Practitioner's oral contraception study. BMJ. 2007;335:651.
69. Miller TA, Allen RH, Kaunitz AM, Cwiak CA. Contraception for midlife women: a review. Menopause. 2018;25:817-27.
70. Marchbanks PA, McDonald JA, Wilson HG, et al. Oral contraceptives and the risk of breast cancer. N Engl J Med. 2002;346:2025-32.
71. Marchbanks PA, Curtis KM, Mandel MG, et al. Oral contraceptive formulation and risk of breast cancer. Contraception. 2012;85:342-50.
72. Burchardt NA, Eliassen AH, Shafrir AL, et al. Oral contraceptive use by formulation and breast cancer risk by subtype in the Nurses' Health Study II: a prospective cohort study. Am J Obstet Gynecol. 2022;226(6):821.e1-26. https://doi.org/10.1016/j.ajog.2021.12.022
73. Lidegaard O, Lokkegaard E, Jensen A, Skovlund CW, Keiding N. Thrombotic stroke and myocardial infarction with hormonal contraception. N Engl J Med. 2012;366:2257-66.
74. Faculty of Sexual & Reproductive Healthcare. FSRH Guideline: Contraception for Women Aged Over 40 Years. 2017 (amended 2019):1-66. (https://www.fsrh.org/documents/fsrh-guidance-contraception-for-women-aged-over-40-years-2017/)
75. Chiara Del Savio M, De Fata R, Facchinetti F, Grandi G. Drospirenone 4 mg-only pill (DOP) in 24+4 regimen: a new option for oral contraception. Expert Rev Clin Pharmacol. 2020;13:685-94.
76. Prior JC. Progesterone for treatment of symptomatic menopausal women. Climacteric. 2018; 21:358-65.

77. Peragallo Urrutia R, Polis CB, Jensen ET, Greene ME, Kennedy E, Stanford JB. Effectiveness of fertility awareness-based methods for pregnancy prevention: A systematic review. Obstet Gynecol. 2018 Sep;132(3):591-604.
78. Evofem. Phexxi package insert. 2022. (https://22077562.fs1.hubspotusercontent-na1.net/hubfs/22077562/Hcp_phexxi_October2022/pdf/PhexxiUSPI.pdf)
79. Turok DK, Gero A, Simmons RG, et al. Levonorgestrel vs. copper intrauterine devices for emergency contraception. N Engl J Med. 2021;384:335-44.
80. Baldwin MK, Jensen JT. Contraception during the perimenopause. Maturitas. 2013;76:235-42.
81. The NAMS 2017 Hormone Therapy Position Statement Advisory Panel. The 2017 hormone therapy position statement of The North American Menopause Society. Menopause. 2017; 24:728-53.

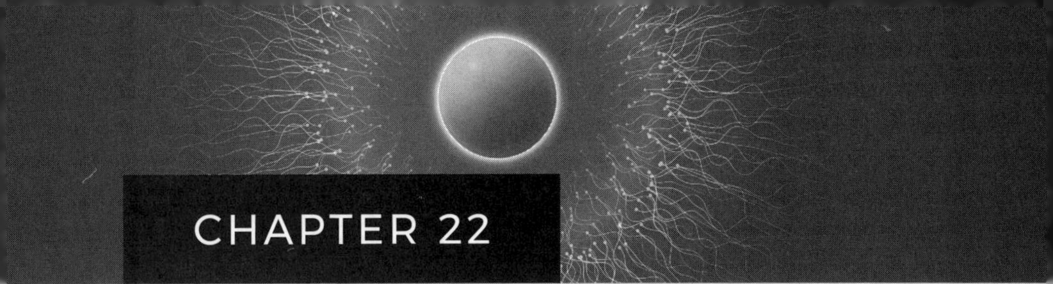

CHAPTER 22

Contraception for Lesbian, Gay, Bisexual, Transgender, Gender Diverse, Queer/Questioning, Intersex, and Asexual Individuals

Chance Krempasky, BSN, MSN, FNP-BC, WHNP-BC, AAHIVS
Lola Pellegrino, BSN, MSN, ANP-BE, WHNP-BC
Miles S. Harris, BSN, MSN, FNP-BC, AAHIVS
Frances Grimstad, MD, MS

KEY POINTS

- The contraceptive needs of lesbian, gay, bisexual, transgender, nonbinary, queer/questioning, intersex, and asexual (LGBTQIA) individuals may be overlooked by health care providers.
- Clinicians should use language that is accurate and affirming.
- LGBTQIA contraceptive care should not assume anatomy based on identity or sex assigned at birth.
- Gender-affirming hormone therapy should not be relied on as a contraceptive method.
- Some methods suppress menses or ovulation as a noncontraceptive benefit that many individuals may value as a means of gender affirmation.
- Clinicians should discuss reproductive desires and options for family building with LGBTQIA individuals.

KEY ACRONYMS

AFAB: Assigned female at birth
AMAB: Assigned male at birth
GAHT: Gender-affirming hormone therapy
LGBTQIA: lesbian, gay, bisexual, transgender, gender diverse, and queer/questioning, intersex, and asexual
LGBTQ: lesbian, gay, bisexual, transgender, gender diverse, and queer
LGBQ: lesbian, gay, bisexual, queer
TGD: Transgender and gender diverse

The contraceptive needs of LGBTQIA individuals are frequently overlooked by their health care providers. An individual's sexual orientation or gender identity does not limit the diverse range of desires regarding current or future childbearing and family building, and many LGBTQIA people engage in sexual activity that could result in pregnancy.[1–3] Yet, health care providers may assume that LGBTQIA people are not at risk for pregnancy or for getting a partner pregnant. Furthermore, sexuality education, and specifically information regarding contraception, is rarely inclusive of LGBTQIA people.[4,5] As a result, LGBTQIA people who may benefit from contraception have reduced access to culturally appropriate information about contraception and services.

Inclusive contraceptive counseling and care must be grounded in anatomically accurate discussions about pregnancy risk. For example, not all individuals with sex assigned female at birth are born with the same reproductive anatomy, and not all individuals maintain the same reproductive anatomy throughout their lives (e.g., hysterectomy, oophorectomy, salpingectomy). LGBTQIA contraceptive care should be anatomically inclusive, recognizing that some individuals are born with diverse sex traits (including those who identify as intersex), and not assume anatomy based on identity or sex assigned at birth.

Contraceptive methods also serve an important role in menstrual suppression for LGBTQIA people. While menstrual suppression may be utilized by people of any sexual orientation or gender identity, it has important significance for people for whom menstruation is associated with distress related to one's gender identity.[6]

Language and Terminology

LGBTQIA persons include those who have diverse sexual orientations and/or gender identities. Understanding the difference between sexual orientation and gender identity is necessary for understanding the identities and health care needs of LGBTQIA patients. Sexual orientation is not synonymous with sexual behavior. For example, a lesbian-identified person who identifies as a woman may have male-identified partners. It is important for providers to ask patients both about their sexual orientation as well as their behaviors and partners when taking a sexual history.[7]

Gender identity refers to a person's internal sense of being a girl/woman/female, a boy/man/male, something else, or having no gender. Gender identity is distinct from sex assigned at birth, which is the designation assigned to a newborn typically based on the appearance of the newborn's genitals, i.e. assigned male at birth (AMAB) or assigned female at birth (AFAB). Most states in the United States still require newborns to be AFAB or AMAB on their birth certificate. The term "sex assigned at birth" should be used in place of outdated terms such as "true sex," "original sex," or "biological sex." Similarly, AMAB and AFAB should be used instead of "biologically" or "originally" male or female.

While the sex assigned on birth certificates and other identity documents is most often binary, sex itself is not. Intersex traits, or differences in sex development, are variations in primary or secondary sex traits. As not all individuals who are assigned the same sex have the same anatomy at birth, it is important not to assume a patient or their partners' anatomy based on sex assigned at birth. As of 2017, several states are offering nongendered birth certificates, which signals a future sunsetting of the use of AFAB and AMAB as medically appropriate language.

People whose gender identity matches what is expected for their sex assigned at birth are described as *cisgender*, and those whose gender identity does not match their sex assigned at birth are *transgender*. Some people whose gender identity is different from their sex assigned at birth may describe themselves as being of transgender experience, but not as having a transgender identity. A person may also have an identity that falls outside the traditional gender binary structure of girl/woman and boy/man. The authors use "transgender and gender diverse" (TGD) to describe people with noncisgender identities throughout this chapter. This umbrella term includes many identities, such as transgender, two-spirit, gender fluid, agender, genderqueer, and nonbinary.

Gender expression is distinct from gender identity. Gender expression describes the way a person communicates their gender to the world through attributes including speech patterns, clothing, hair style, and mannerisms. What is considered masculine or feminine gender expression varies widely depending on culture, context, and historical period. Both TGD and cisgender people may alter their gender expression based on activity and circumstance. A person having a gender expression that does not conform to societal gender norms does not inherently confer a TGD identity. Additionally, TGD people may or may not have a gender expression consistent with others' expectations about how they should look or act based on their gender identity.

TGD people may engage in gender affirmation, which is the process of enacting social, legal, and/or medical changes to recognize, accept, and express one's gender identity. This may include gender-affirming hormone therapy (GAHT) and gender-affirming surgeries. Not all TGD people will desire hormones and/or surgery; *this does not make their TGD identity less valid*. Other examples of gender affirmation include using gendered facilities (such as public restrooms) that align with one's gender identity and changing one's name and gender marker on identity documents.

Gender dysphoria describes the distress TGD people may experience arising from difference between their gender identity and sex assigned at birth. Not all TGD people experience gender dysphoria; for many, an equal driver may be gender euphoria: the state of enjoyment, comfort, or joy when feeling aligned or affirmed in one's gender identity. Gender dysphoria refers to the specific diagnoses in the World Health Organization's International Classification of Diseases, version 10 (ICD-10) and the *Diagnostic and Statistical Manual of Mental Disorders*, Fifth Edition (DSM-5). Many TGD people find the categorization of gender dysphoria as a psychiatric diagnosis to be pathologizing. ICD-11, released globally January 1, 2022, removed gender dysphoria from "Mental and behavioral disorders" and instead recognized *gender incongruence* under "Conditions related to sexual health." The DSM-5 also underwent a text revision in 2022 (DSM-5-TR) that clarifies gender dysphoria in a similar manner.

Please see the following definitions of select common terms, modified from "LGBTQIA+ Glossary of Terms for Health Care Teams" by the National LGBTQIA+ Health Education Center, https://www.lgbtqiahealtheducation.org/wp-content/uploads/2020/02/Glossary-2022.02.22-1.pdf and Standards of Care for the Health of Transgender and Gender Diverse People, Version 8.[8]

Agender *(adjective)*: A gender-identity term used by a person who identifies as having no gender, or who does not experience gender as a primary identity component.

Asexual *(adjective)*: A sexual orientation term used by a person who experiences little or no sexual attraction to others. Asexual people may still engage in sexual activity.

Bisexual *(adjective)*: A sexual orientation term used by a person who is emotionally and physically attracted to women/females and men/males. Some people define bisexuality as attraction to their own gender and other genders.

Cisgender *(adjective)*: A person whose gender identity is consistent in a traditional sense with their sex assigned at birth; for example, a person assigned female sex at birth whose gender identity is woman/female.

Gay *(adjective)*: A sexual orientation term used by people who are primarily emotionally and physically attracted to people of the same sex and/or gender as themselves. Commonly used to describe men who are primarily attracted to men, but can also describe women attracted to women.

Gender affirmation *(noun)*: The process of making social, legal, and/or medical changes to recognize, accept, and express one's gender identity. Sometimes referred to as Transition.

Gender diverse *(adjective)*: Describes the community of people who fall outside of the gender binary structure (e.g., two-spirit, agender, nonbinary, genderqueer, gender fluid people).

Gender dysphoria *(noun)*: A state of distress or discomfort that may be experienced because a person's gender identity differs from that which is physically and/or socially attributed to their sex assigned at birth. Gender dysphoria is also a diagnostic term in the DSM-5-TR denoting an incongruence between the sex assigned at birth and experienced gender accompanied by distress. Not all transgender and gender diverse people experience gender dysphoria.

Gender euphoria *(noun)*: A distinct enjoyment or satisfaction caused by the correspondence between the person's gender identity and gendered features associated with a gender other than the one assigned at birth.[9]

Gender expression *(noun)*: The way a person communicates their gender to the world through mannerisms, clothing, speech, behavior, etc. Gender expression varies depending on culture, context, and historical period.

Gender fluid *(adjective)*: A gender identity term used by a person whose gender identity is not fixed. A person who is gender fluid may always feel like a mix of more than one gender, but may feel more aligned with a certain gender some of the time, another gender at other times, both genders sometimes, and sometimes no gender at all.

Gender identity *(noun)*: A person's inner sense of being a girl/woman/female, boy/man/male, something else, or having no gender.

Gender incongruence *(noun)*: Diagnostic term used in the ICD-11 that describes a person's marked and persistent experience of an incongruence between that person's gender identity and the gender expected of them based on their birth-assigned sex.

Genderqueer *(adjective)*: A gender identity term used by a person whose gender identity falls outside the traditional gender binary of male and female. Some people use the term gender expansive.

Gender nonbinary *(adjective)*: Describes a person whose gender identity falls outside of the traditional gender binary structure of female and male.

Intersex *(adjective)*: Describes a group of congenital conditions in which the reproductive organs, genitals, and/or other sexual anatomy do not develop according to traditional expectations for females or males. The medical community sometimes uses the term "differences (or disorders) of sex development" to describe intersex conditions.

Lesbian *(adjective, noun)*: A sexual orientation term used by a woman who is primarily emotionally and physically attracted to other women.

Pansexual *(adjective)*: A term used by someone to describe their sexual orientation, meaning emotionally and physically attracted to people of all gender identities, or that attractions are not related to other people's gender.

Polyamory *(noun)*: A sexual and/or romantic relationship structure that allows for more than one partner. A similar term is consensual nonmonogramy. Polyamorous also describes a person who romantically loves or has sex with more than one person consensually. Sometimes abbreviated as poly.

Pronouns *(noun)*: Pronouns are the words people should use when they are referring to you, but not using your name. Examples of pronouns are she/her/hers, he/him/his, and they/them/theirs. The appropriate phrasing is "What are your pronouns?" when seeking this information.

Queer *(adjective)*: An umbrella term used by people who think of their sexual orientation and/or gender identity as outside of societal norms. Some people view the term queer as more fluid and inclusive than traditional categories for sexual orientation and gender identity. Although queer was historically used as a slur, it has been reclaimed by many as a term of empowerment. Nonetheless, some still find the term offensive.

Sex assigned at birth *(noun)*: A person's status as male, female, or intersex based on physical characteristics. Sex is usually assigned at birth based on appearance of the external genitalia. AFAB is an abbreviation for "assigned female at birth." AMAB is an abbreviation for "assigned male at birth."

Sexual orientation *(noun)*: How a person characterizes their emotional and sexual attraction to others.

Transgender *(adjective)*: Gender identity term used by a person whose gender identity and sex assigned at birth do not correspond based on traditional expectations.

Trans man/transgender man/man of transgender experience *(noun)*: A transgender person whose gender identity is boy/man/male may use the terms trans man/transgender man to describe themselves. Some will simply use the term man.

Trans woman/transgender woman/woman of transgender experience *(noun)*: A transgender person whose gender identity is girl/woman/female may use the terms trans woman/transgender woman to describe themselves. Some will simply use the term woman.

It is important to use LGBTQIA-inclusive language with all people, not only those who clinicians know (or "suspect") to be LGBTQIA-identified. The landmark study, "When Health Care Isn't Caring: Lambda Legal's Survey on Discrimination Against LGBT People and People Living with HIV," documented high rates of mistreatment of LGBQ and TGD people in health care settings. Reported experiences of discrimination included being provided worse care, use of excessive precautions, and physical roughness.[10] As a result of personal and/or communal history of these negative experiences, many LGBQ and TGD people do not feel safe disclosing their sexual orientation or gender identity to a health care provider.[11,12]

In using LGBTQIA-inclusive language, providers can increase the likelihood that LGBTQIA patients will feel safe to disclose their sexual orientation and/or gender identity. Additionally, any cisgender and/or heterosexual patient may have LGBTQIA partners. Assuming that a partner is cisgender, for example, could result in failure to identify a patient who is at risk for pregnancy.

LGBTQIA-inclusive language affirms the patient's gender, gender(s) of their partner(s), and how the patient describes their body. Many electronic medical records now capture sexual orientation and gender identity (SOGI) data. SOGI sections typically include fields for sex assigned at birth and pronouns, as well as sexual orientation and gender identity. Many electronic medical records also include an "organ inventory" function. The organ inventory allows providers to note which reproductive organs a patient currently has, which organs were present or expected at birth, and if any of these organs have been changed via surgery or exogenous hormone use. As gender and sexuality are fluid and may change throughout a person's life, it is important to periodically reassess SOGI information.

Many TGD patients prefer nongendered, nonanatomical terms to refer to their body parts and functions. Asking patients which words they would like providers to use when speaking with them about their body provides an opportunity for patients to share this information. For example, a person AFAB may prefer the term "chest" instead of "breasts" (**Table 22-1**).

Gender-Affirming, Anatomy-, Identity-, and Activity-Inclusive Sexual History

Providers may desire guidance on how to formulate sexual history questions and address follow-up questions for LGBTQIA individuals. First, since LGBTQIA people are frequently asked intrusive and sometimes irrelevant questions about their bodies and sexual practices in health care settings, it is important to explain the reasoning for asking these questions. A clinician might frame the conversation by saying, "I talk to all of my patients about sex to help them get the health care they need," before asking about sexual partners and practices. In other settings, the relevance of sexual health related questions might be less clear; for example, a clinician might need to know if a patient could be pregnant before performing a colposcopy. In these circumstances, explaining why sensitive information is needed gives context that can help decrease an individual's discomfort.

Instead of attempting to specialize sexual health counseling for LGBTQIA individuals, clinicians should utilize a universal framework for sexual health assessment that encompasses all possible configurations of a person's, and their partners', anatomy (natal or current). This framework should be applied to patients of all sexual orientations and gender identities. The CDC's "Guide to Taking a Sexual History"

Table 22-1 Less Gendered Sexual and Reproductive Health Language

Use (less gendered language)[1]	Instead of (gendered language)
People who menstruate, people who are pregnant	Female, women; pregnant women
People who produce sperm	Male, men
Not trans, non-trans, cisgender	Biologically male/female
Assigned male at birth	Biologically male
Assigned female at birth	Biologically female
Sexual or genital ("GEN") health	Women's/gynecological health care
External genitals, external pelvic area	Vulva, clitoris
Outer parts	Penis, testicles
Genital opening, frontal opening, internal canal	Vagina
Outer folds	Labia, lips
Internal reproductive organs	Female reproductive organs
Internal organs	Uterus, ovaries
Internal gland	Prostate
Chest	Breasts[2]
Chest or breastfeeding[2]	Breastfeeding
Absorbent product	Pad/tampon
Internal condom	Female condom
Uterine bleeding	Period/menstruation
Parent or gestational parent	Mother
Hypothalamic-pituitary-gonadal – ovarian axis	Female gonadal steroid axis
Hypothalamic-pituitary-gonadal – testicular axis	Male gonadal steroid axis

[1] The terms in these columns are offered as suggestions, but we recommend asking patients which words they use for their own body parts and experiences.
[2] Transfeminine persons may prefer breasts.
Reproduced from Krempasky C, Harris M, Abern L, & Grimstad F. Contraception across the transmasculine spectrum. *Am J Obstet Gynecol* 2020 Feb;222(2):134-143. DOI:10.1016/j.ajog.2019.07.043

provides detailed information on this comprehensive and affirming approach to sexual history using five domains: Partners, Practices, Protection from STIs, Past History of STIs, and Pregnancy Intention.[14]

Another approach, the GOALS framework, seeks to address evidence showing that patients are more likely to obtain preventive health services when benefits are emphasized over risks. It features open-ended questions that focus on sexual health, not risk, with the goal of advancing motivation around sexual health behaviors. This framework incorporates a 6th "P," pleasure.[15] The National Coalition for Sexual Health has created a video series that clinicians may find useful, *The 6 Ps: A New Approach to Sexual History Taking*: https://nationalcoalitionforsexualhealth.org/tools/for-healthcare-providers/video-series.[7]

Examples of recommended sexual history questions include, "What are the genders and bodies of your partners?", "How do you have sex with them?", and "Which body parts do you use?" Suggested gender-inclusive sexual history scripts are available.[13] (Refer to Chapters 4, 6, and 23 for further discussion on sexual history-taking.)

Box 22-1 Trauma-Informed Care (TIC)

As with sexual history-taking, we recommend a "universal precautions" approach to pelvic exams: assume that everyone may have a trauma history and hold trauma-informed care as the standard of practice[16] *for people of all identities*. However, it is known that LGBTQIA people experience higher rates of sexual trauma.[17,18] In addition to the TIC recommendations below, clinicians should seek education on assessment and examination of the natal anus, prostate, and testes, as well as postoperative anatomy in those who have undergone gender-affirming genital surgeries (vaginoplasty, metoidioplasty, phalloplasty, scrotoplasty, etc.). The recommendations below are some suggestions. They are not comprehensive and should not replace a formal training. A foundational part of TIC is for providers to take every opportunity to keep the locus of control with the patient. When they are in control, people can take better care of themselves and can let providers know what they need. Take care with language. Avoid words or phrases that can have sexual connotations, such as "bed" versus "exam table," or phrases that an abuser might use, such as, "Relax and this will be less uncomfortable."

Prior to Exam

1. Position chairs and exam tables to face the door.
2. When possible, offer the patient a choice about the gender of the clinician performing the exam, as well as gender of chaperone, if desired.
3. Allow a support person during the exam.[19]
4. Offer to discuss the exam at the current visit and perform the exam at a separate visit.
5. Establish how much or little information/narration they want during the exam, then provide accordingly.

During Exam

1. Ask for consent to begin the exam and confirm consent as you proceed to examine other sensitive areas.
2. Notice any signs of distress. Offer examination positions other than lithotomy using footrests. Some use the pull-out extension at the end of the table; others use frog-leg position.
3. Never physically move a patient's legs during an exam. Ask patients to move their knees as far to the side as is comfortable, or to let their legs "fall towards the walls."

4. When possible, offer to replace provider collection of vaginal, cervical, and/or anorectal specimens with patient collection (self-swab).
5. Use of a smaller speculum may be more tolerable in TGD people on testosterone who have vaginal atrophy. Offer self-placement (done by positioning the speculum handle up). An anoscope may be used for both anal and vaginal exams in TGD people postvaginoplasty. Offering a hand mirror is appreciated by some, but use discretion based on patient behavior, as examining genitalia may be dysphoria-inducing.
6. Always use nongendered terms, but especially during exam narration; for example, "bring your lower half down towards me," "Is it okay if I examine the outside?" See Table 22-1 for a list of nongendered terms.
7. Provide opportunities for the patient to pause or stop the examination. If, at any point, the patient says to stop, stop the exam.

After Exam

1. Have tissues available to remove lubricant.
2. Leave the room to give the patient privacy to dress.
3. Once the patient is dressed, ask the patient how they are doing before ending the encounter.
4. Build skills and resources for supporting a distressed patient.

Data from Owens L, Terrell S, Low LK, et al. Universal precautions: the case for consistently trauma-informed reproductive healthcare. Am J Obstet Gynecol 2022;226(5):671–7; United States Department Of Health And Human Services, Centers For Disease Control And Prevention, National Center For Injury Prevention And Control. National Intimate Partner and Sexual Violence Survey (NISVS): General Population Survey Raw Data, 2010: Archival Version [Internet]. 2014 [cited 2022 Oct 23]. Available from: https://www.icpsr.umich.edu/web/NACJD/studies/34305; James S, Herman J, Rankin S, Keisling M, Mottet L, Anafi M. The Report of the 2015 U.S. Transgender Survey. 2016 [cited 2022 Aug 14]. Available from: https://ncvc.dspacedirect.org/handle/20.500.11990/1299; American Medical Association. Use of Chaperones [Internet]. Am. Med. Assoc. [cited 2022 Aug 14]. Available from: https://www.ama-assn.org/delivering-care/ethics/use-chaperones

Bodily Autonomy

Threats to contraceptive and abortion access for all people are integrally connected to the attacks on gender-affirming health care for TGD adolescents and adults, marriage equality, and the way people have sex.[20] At the same time that abortion bans take hold across the country, there is a growing flurry of legislation that prohibits TGD adolescents (and their parents), as well as TGD adults, from making decisions about their bodies and accessing life-saving health care services. So-called "conscience clauses" are enacted to limit both contraceptive and TGD care provision.[21-23] Citizens are being deputized to surveil their neighbors and criminalize people seeking abortions and adolescent TGD care, those who assist them, and the clinicians that provide them with these services.[24] The policing of TGD bodies in the forms of restricting bathroom access and sports participation further exemplify these trends outside of the medical sphere. These threats further add to the personal trauma histories of TGD persons. Trauma-informed care should be a standard of practice for these patients, as well as being a part of universal precautions for patients of all identities. See **Box 22-1**.

Reproductive justice and valuing the reproductive and family planning choices of all individuals are critical to honoring bodily autonomy.[25] Clinicians should avoid making assumptions about patient desires regarding pregnancy or parenting.[26] (See Chapter 4, Person-Centered Reproductive Health Conversations and Contraceptive Counseling.)

Furthermore, clinicians must be aware that no part of gender transition should require a TGD patient to undergo sterilization; this was historically the case and is still required in some areas of the world as well as in several states in the Unites States.[27]

Contraception for TGD Individuals Assigned Female at Birth

AFAB individuals may experience pregnancy, both planned and unintentionally. This includes those with current or previous testosterone use, as well as people who are amenorrheic secondary to testosterone use. Few studies address pregnancy rates and outcomes among TGD persons; a 2014 study by Light et al. found that 20% of TGD AFAB respondents were amenorrheic from testosterone when they became pregnant.[28]

Those who are amenorrheic at the time of conception may take longer to recognize an unintended pregnancy, especially if they incorrectly believe that testosterone is a contraceptive. The misconception that testosterone is a contraceptive is common among both patients and clinicians. Between 16.4% and 31% of TGD AFAB people incorrectly believe testosterone is a contraceptive; 5.5% to 9% report receiving this information from a health care provider.[29]

Physiology of Gender-Affirming Testosterone, Implications for Contraception, and Fertility

The effect of exogenous testosterone at gender-affirming care levels on the hypothalamic-pituitary-gonadal axis with ovaries is incompletely understood. Both gonadotropins and ovarian hormones must be adequately regulated to prevent pregnancy, which may not be achieved with gender-affirming testosterone use. While ovulation is impaired by increased androgen levels, it is not fully suppressed in all individuals on testosterone.[30] Breakthrough ovulation among TGD AFAB patients on testosterone is also supported by studies showing that elevated androgen levels alter gonadotropin production but do not suppress luteinizing hormone and follicle-stimulating hormone to prepubertal levels.[31-33] There are currently no data available regarding the effect of testosterone on cervical mucus thickness.

Inconsistent testosterone use may also contribute to breakthrough ovulation. Patients frequently experience barriers to GAHT access, which may result in missed, delayed, or incomplete dosing.[18,34] Patients may also desire to use low doses of testosterone ("microdosing"), which may increase likelihood of ongoing ovulation.

People with the capacity for pregnancy who use testosterone should be counseled on the potential teratogenic effect on a pregnancy; however, contraceptive use should never be mandated for a patient to access GAHT. An XX-chromosome fetus exposed to testosterone is at risk for labial fusion, variation in vaginal development, persistence of a urogenital sinus, and clitoromegaly. The effects of testosterone on a fetus mainly take place during the first trimester, when an pregnancy that was not expected is most likely to be unrecognized.[8] The World Professional Association for Transgender Health (WPATH) Standards of Care 8 state that testosterone use is contraindicated for any individual who is currently pregnant or attempting to become pregnant.[8]

Contraceptive Counseling for TGD Individuals Assigned Female at Birth

Given the potential for continued ovulation and teratogenic effects of testosterone, it is essential that providers educate TGD AFAB patients on pregnancy risk and contraception. Not all TGD AFAB people will be at risk for pregnancy based on current anatomy and sexual practices, as previously discussed. Accurate assessment of pregnancy risk is essential; as organs present, partners, and practices may change over time, periodic reassessment of these factors is important.

TGD AFAB individuals, including those on testosterone, may be offered the full range of available contraceptive options.[13] When working with TGD AFAB patients in selecting a contraceptive method, many considerations will be similar to the needs of cisgender women. Clinicians should consult the United States Medical Eligibility Criteria (US MEC) for contraceptive use for guidelines when determining if a given method is appropriate for a patient.[35] For example, a 40-year-old nonbinary AFAB patient who smokes one pack of cigarettes per day is recommended not to use an estrogen-containing contraceptive method. Reproductive desires should be discussed and taken into consideration. For example, a patient planning to become pregnant a year from now should be counseled on the potential for delayed return to fertility after discontinuing depot medroxyprogesterone acetate (DMPA).

No research currently exists on whether testosterone impacts the efficacy of any hormonal contraceptive methods; however, based on the mechanisms of action of combined estrogen/progestin and progestin-only methods, no decrease in efficacy is expected.[13] Testosterone-associated changes include increased body mass, increased low-density lipoprotein levels, and increased blood pressure.[36,37] While there is no evidence for increased risk of venous thromboembolism risk among TGD AFAB patients on testosterone,[38] there may be concern for increased risk of thrombosis in patients on testosterone taking estrogen-containing contraceptives.[39] Clinicians should consider monitoring lipid levels and be familiar with age-based screening recommendations for testosterone-dominant individuals, particularly for those using DMPA.

There are numerous factors unique to TGD patients. A primary concern is reducing potential exacerbation or worsening of gender dysphoria related to the contraceptive method, and alleviation of gender dysphoria in relation to menstruation. Use of both contraceptive and noncontraceptive methods for menstrual suppression are reviewed later in this chapter. Sources of gender dysphoria will be different for each TGD patient; it is important to discuss with every patient what their individual priorities are and offer anticipatory guidance regarding potential effects of each method.

While not medically contraindicated, TGD patients may associate use of estrogen- or progestin-containing contraceptive methods with cisgender women and thus desire to avoid the use of a hormonal method.[40] Methods with a need for frequent dosing, such as a daily combined oral contraceptives (COCs) or progestin-only pills (POPs), may worsen gender dysphoria due to repeated reminders of this association.[13]

Patients may also express concern that hormonal contraceptive methods will have feminizing effects.[41] While studies did not find elevated estradiol levels among

TGD AFAB patients on testosterone taking COCs,[42] COCs may affect androgen levels in two ways: (1) reduction in endogenous androgen production by the ovaries and (2) increasing sex hormone-binding globulin, which can bind testosterone, thus reducing bioavailable testosterone.[43] No data are available regarding whether a potential reduction in testosterone levels related to combined hormonal contraceptives use is clinically significant. TGD AFAB patients may benefit from monitoring of their testosterone level in the months following combined hormonal contraceptive start and dose adjustment of their testosterone, if appropriate. TGD individuals taking testosterone may want to avoid oral contraceptives containing drospirenone due to its antiandrogenic profile, and TGD AFAB patients may prefer COCs containing progestins with higher androgenic properties such as norethindrone, levonorgestrel, and gestodene.[44]

Chest or breast tenderness may result from use of hormonal contraceptives; TGD patients may experience this as a feminizing effect that exacerbates gender dysphoria. This effect is more common with use of estrogen-containing methods, typically occurring at initiation and resolving within 3–5 months of use.[45] Chest or breast tenderness is less common with use of progestin-only contraceptive methods; however, when it does occur, it is less likely to resolve spontaneously. Breast hypertrophy is a rare side effect of the etonogestrel implant, occurring in less than 1% of users.[26,46] Incidents of glandular breast tissue development have also been reported in TGD people using combined hormonal contraceptives.[26]

Ease of discontinuation of the contraceptive method is important to consider, especially for a patient concerned about potential side effects. Ease of discontinuation is affected by the need for a clinic visit to discontinue (i.e., implant and intrauterine device [IUD]), as well as by a lengthy washout period (i.e., DMPA). Patients may be more willing to try a method that is easily self-discontinued.[13]

Privacy, or ease of concealability, may have increased importance for a TGD patient who has concerns about another person finding their contractive supplies, which could also reveal their TGD identity. Methods that do not require storage of any supplies, such as DMPA, an IUD, and the implant, may afford more privacy compared with pills, patches, or rings.[13]

TGD patients, especially those who experience gender dysphoria related to their genitals or pelvic organs, may desire to avoid a contraceptive method that involves a pelvic procedure or vaginal placement.[13] Patients who select an IUD may benefit from interventions to reduce distress related to the IUD placement, including thorough preprocedure anticipatory guidance, preprocedure anxiolytic administration, and local analgesia (cervical block); sedation may be considered in some circumstances.[47] Use of smaller IUDs and a pediatric speculum may also be beneficial as difficulty tolerating a speculum exam may not only be due to atrophy but also to dysphoria in general.

Testosterone use may result in atrophic vaginitis similar to that experienced by postmenopausal cisgender women, making the IUD placement process more painful.[48] Patients with atrophic vaginitis may benefit from use of a vaginal estradiol preparation for 7–14 days prior to the IUD placement.[49]

Both progestin and copper IUDs may cause uterine bleeding and cramping immediately following placement, even in those amenorrheic prior to placement. In the case of progestin IUDs, bleeding and cramping is typically self-limited. Over time, progestin implants decrease dysmenorrhea and uterine bleeding; however, individuals may experience unpredictable bleeding and unfavorable bleeding that may or may not improve over the duration of use.[50] (See Chapter 9, Contraceptive Implant and Chapter 10, Intrauterine Devices [IUDs].) This bleeding pattern may be unacceptable to some TGD patients. Copper IUDs, in contrast, can make menses longer, heavier, or increase rates of dysmenorrhea and heavier menses among cisgender women.[51] No data are available on rates of dysmenorrhea and heavier menses among TGD patients using copper IUDs. Clinicians should use a low threshold for discontinuation of IUDs in TGD patients given the potential implications of uterine bleeding and cramping for gender dysphoria.[13]

Emergency Contraception

TGD patients should also receive counseling regarding emergency contraception (EC) options. Oral levonorgestrel, ulipristal acetate, copper IUDs, and levonorgestrel 52 mg IUDs may be used by TGD patients, regardless of testosterone use.[52] There are no studies regarding EC use among AFAB people using testosterone; however, expert opinion finds no expected loss of efficacy for any EC method when used together with testosterone.[13]

Anticipatory guidance prior to EC use as well as nonsteroidal anti-inflammatories may reduce distress associated with cramping and bleeding caused by IUDs and oral EC. All EC methods may change bleeding patterns, with pills causing a change in bleeding in the next cycle, and IUDs likely having longer-term effects. Even patients who are amenorrheic may experience bleeding, spotting or cramping following IUD placement or EC pill use.[53]

TGD people who are amenorrheic or have irregular menstrual cycles cannot rely on the arrival of their next menses to confirm they are not pregnant following EC use. In this circumstance, checking a urine pregnancy test 2–3 weeks after EC use is needed to confirm absence of a pregnancy.[53] Patients who do become pregnant despite oral EC use should receive counseling regarding the full range of pregnancy options. If a patient desires to terminate a pregnancy, they should be referred to an abortion provider, preferably one with experience working with TGD patients.[54]

Encounters at the Pharmacy

Pharmacy staff may question or reject a claim for a prescription for contraception or EC if an individual's insurance identifies them as male or if the patient's name differs from that on their insurance. Consider indicating on the prescription that the medication is intended for this patient, regardless of the gender marker on the patient's insurance or identification. Ensure that patients can contact the provider's office for assistance, especially in the case of EC, in which obtaining the medication promptly is vital for efficacy.[53]

Permanent Contraception and Hysterectomy

Vas and tubal procedures may also be considered by TGD patients. Hysterectomy may be desired for gender affirmation in addition to pregnancy prevention. For patients who desire permanent contraception but not a hysterectomy, tubal ligation or salpingectomy may be appropriate. Clinicians should not assume that all TGD patients desire a hysterectomy. Additionally, TGD patients should not be required to undergo procedures for permanent contraception at any point in their transition, or in order to change their gender marker on identity documents.[13] No recommendation for risk-reducing surgery is made for users of gender-affirming testosterone as data do not exist on increased risk for endometrial or ovarian cancer.[42,55]

Menstrual Suppression

LGBTQIA individuals may utilize contraceptive methods for menstrual suppression for reasons similar to non-LGBTQIA individuals,[13,56] such as for dysmenorrhea or heavy menstrual bleeding, or simply because they do not desire menses.[56,57] Additionally, some TGD individuals may suppress their bleeding and ovulation due to dysphoria experienced with these events, and may use it as a steppingstone prior to accessing gender-affirming androgen therapy.[13,58,59]All contraceptive methods that have a chance of producing menstrual suppression are options for LGBTQIA individuals, each of which has a different potential for achieving suppression.[60,61] No contraceptive method is universally successful. There are no comparative data available on the rates of menstrual suppression for individuals using a combination of testosterone and hormonal contraceptive methods.

There are also noncontraceptive medications that can be used to achieve menstrual suppression.[56] Norethindrone acetate is a progestin with estrogen-like activity that can be dosed 2.5–20 mg oral daily. Danazol is a synthetic androgen-progestin and is also effective for menstrual suppression (200–400 mg twice daily oral). It was previously used for endometriosis management but fell out of favor due to mild virilizing changes at higher doses. For this reason, it appeals to some TGD individuals who desire menstrual suppression and less virilization than would occur with testosterone use.[62] Finally, gonadotropin-releasing hormone (GnRH) analogs are another noncontraceptive menstrual suppression option. Due to the menopausal side effects, including hot flashes and bone mineral density loss, experts recommend against using GnRH analogs long term in isolation for this purpose; however, it is acceptable to use them concomitantly with testosterone or add-back estradiol.[56]

Some TGD individuals who take testosterone will experience breakthrough bleeding and desire concomitant menstrual suppression.[56,63] All of the above menstrual suppression methods are available alongside testosterone. No one method has been proven superior and as such all methods should be offered.[56] While progestins may be used as an adjunct at testosterone initiation to accelerate the onset of amenorrhea,[26,64] patients should be counseled that even this combination does not guarantee amenorrhea:, some will experience breakthrough bleeding on both.

Contraception for TGD Individuals Assigned Male at Birth

Although GAHT with estradiol and/or testosterone blockers for TGD people assigned male at birth has been shown to impair spermatogenesis, the use of feminizing GAHT does not guarantee lack of fertility.[65,66] The effects of feminizing GAHT on sperm production and semen quality are under-studied.[67] Some may experience permanent loss of fertility, and others may require assisted reproductive technologies. Sperm-producing patients may seek contraceptive options to prevent pregnancy in their sexual partners and are eligible for all anatomically appropriate options.

TGD people AMAB have markedly fewer options compared to people AFAB. Nonsurgical contraceptive options for individuals AMAB include withdrawal and condoms. Feminizing GAHT may alter an individual's experience of arousal, orgasm, and ejaculation/seminal release; for some, this may make use of the withdrawal method less reliable.[68] GAHT may cause a decrease in penile size and erectile function. Improperly sized condoms are less reliable for pregnancy prevention; thus, standard-size condoms may be less effective for some TGD patients. Smaller external condoms may provide a better fit; commercially available options include LifeStyles® Snugger Fit and Atlas® True Fit. Internal condoms, which are placed in the partner's vagina or rectum, do not require a fit to the AMAB person's external genitals. Internal condoms are also more likely than external condoms to remain correctly positioned with decreased erectile strength or consistency. Surgical contraceptive options include orchiectomy and vasectomy. Some TGD people will also choose to pursue orchiectomy as a standalone gender-affirming surgery or undergo it as part of vaginoplasty. Patients should be counseled that, unlike for an orchiectomy, a vasectomy does not decrease endogenous testosterone production.

Contraception for Lesbian, Gay, and Bisexual Cisgender Women

One in five cisgender women in the United States identifies as LGBQ,[69] and more than 20% of females in grades 9–12 in the United States describe their sexual identity as lesbian, gay, bisexual, or queer.[70] LGBQ cisgender women are as likely as heterosexual cisgender women to have had sex with cisgender men.[7] Many LGBQ cisgender women engage in sex that could lead to pregnancy (i.e., sex with partners who are capable of producing sperm, including transgender, nonbinary, and cisgender individuals assigned male at birth with natal anatomy).[72] Despite this, providers often assume that LGBQ cisgender women are not at risk for pregnancy and are less likely to offer them contraceptive counseling,[73,74] while in fact, both LGBQ adults and adolescents have higher rates of "unintended" pregnancy compared to heterosexual cisgender women, potentially due to use of less effective contraception.[75-77]

Additional obstacles to contraception exist for LGBQ cisgender women. Some may fear stigmatization by clinicians due to their sexual orientation and/or lack of community acceptance of sex with cisgender men, as well as feel that a regular contraceptive method isn't necessary due to infrequent sex with sperm-producing partners.[78]

One-third of cisgender women seeking contraception are LGBQ cisgender women.[79] Black, Latina, and White lesbian and bisexual cisgender women are less likely to receive contraceptive counseling than White heterosexual cisgender women.[80] Black and White bisexual cisgender women, and Black, Latina, and White lesbian cisgender women have lower rates of receiving contraception compared with White heterosexual cisgender women, with Black and Latina LGBQ cisgender women using contraception less than their White counterparts.[81] One study showed that LGBQ cisgender women preferred not to use an implant or IUD because they have intercourse with cisgender men infrequently.[73] Lesbian-identified cisgender women use contraceptive methods including condoms the least. Bisexual cisgender women have higher rates of contraception and condom use than heterosexual cisgender women and are twice as likely to use an implant or an IUD.[82,83]

It is imperative that providers address the reproductive desires of all cisgender women (and men) regardless of sexual orientation and offer relevant services including contraceptive counseling and prepregnancy care. (See Chapter 4, Person-Centered Reproductive Health Conversations and Contraceptive Counseling.)

Fertility Counseling

Certain GAHT may impact fertility, which is important to understand in the context of contraceptive counseling. GAHT includes pubertal suppression methods as well as testosterone and estrogen (with or without anti-androgens). It is important to remember that fertility is but one method of family building; foster care, adoption, using a gestational carrier, blended family, and chosen family are other common ways.

TGD adolescents who initiate pubertal suppression with GnRH analogs in early (Tanner II-III) puberty and then subsequently take gender-affirming hormones will arrest gonadal maturation, which impacts the use of gametes (both sperm and oocytes).[36] If pubertal suppression is discontinued, it is expected that oocyte maturation would proceed, and it appears that spermatogenesis does return in 3 or more months.[8,84] Fertility preservation at this stage is predominantly gonadal tissue preservation.[85] Despite this, GnRH analogs have not been researched as forms of contraception and patients should be advised that infertility is not guaranteed; therefore, contraceptive counseling is warranted. There are no literature describing the use of gonadal tissue preservation in TGD individuals, and there are no prospective studies available evaluating the effect of long-term hormone use or hormone use following GnRH analog treatment early in puberty.[8]

TGD people who have undergone natal puberty with ovaries and/or uteri who are on testosterone should be counseled that while testosterone mostly suppresses ovulation and induces amenorrhea, these appear to be at least somewhat reversible as patients who have discontinued testosterone have been able to retrieve eggs as well as carry a pregnancy.[28,86] Those who desire maximal fertility preservation are counseled to preserve eggs prior to initiation of testosterone,[36] as data are not available on the likelihood of return of fertility. Unlike testosterone, estrogen (with or without anti-androgens) is known to reduce fertility in sperm-producing individuals.[65] They are counseled to preserve sperm prior to initiation. For those who do not, there have been cases of patients successfully retrieving sperm after discontinuation of estrogen. The authors of this chapter have seen cases where partners of patients on feminizing GAHT became pregnant unexpectedly.[66] For those who desire pregnancy who have ovaries and a uterus and are on testosterone, the recommendation is to discontinue testosterone and allow the endogenous hormone levels to return. Testosterone can virilize an XX fetus, and as such is contraindicated in early pregnancy.[87]

While GAHT is not considered to cause infertility overall, some gender-affirming surgeries will remove the capacity for pregnancy. Gonadectomy (orchiectomy/oophorectomy) will render a patient infertile. Hysterectomy will render a patient unable to carry a pregnancy. Some patients will additionally desire removal of their ovaries at the time of hysterectomy.[34,88] This is not required for gender-affirming masculinizing genital surgeries but may be desired by some patients.[89] Those who retain ovaries after hysterectomy will be able to undergo oocyte retrieval and use their eggs in another individual for a future pregnancy if they desire.

For LGBTQIA individuals, physiologic fertility is the same as for heterosexual cisgender individuals; however, they may be more likely to be in relationships where assisted reproductive technologies are needed to achieve conception.[90] All assisted reproductive technology options (including intrauterine insemination and in vitro fertilization) available to heterosexual cisgender individuals are available to LGBTQIA people.[91] This also includes donor gametes and surrogacy. For partnerships where there are two individuals with ovaries and uteri, reciprocal in vitro fertilization, where the eggs of one partner are used with donor sperm to implant a pregnancy in another partner, is another option.[92] While all these options are medically available to LGBTQIA individuals, lack of insurance coverage for LGBTQIA individuals is often still a significant barrier to access.[93]

Summary

All clinicians should be prepared to assess the family-building desires and contraceptive needs of all patients, including those who identify as LGBTQIA. Many TGD and LGBQ people engage in sex that could result in pregnancy, yet report receiving limited and sometimes incorrect education from clinicians. Understanding and utilizing accurate and affirming language, eliciting a gender-inclusive sexual history, and practicing TIC techniques are skills that improve the quality of care and benefit all patients, including those who identify as LGBTQIA. Appropriate contraception and fertility counseling for TGD-identified patients should consider past, current, and planned gender-affirming surgeries and gender-affirming hormone therapy, if applicable. By offering comprehensive and accurate information, clinicians can support the diversity of reproductive choices made by TGD and LGBQ people.

Author Disclosures—Krempasky: none. Pellegrino: none. Harris: none. Grimstad: none.

References

1. Carpenter E, Niesen R. "It's just constantly having to make a ton of decisions that other people take for granted": Pregnancy and parenting desires for queer cisgender women and non-binary individuals assigned female at birth. J GLBT Fam Stud. 2021;17(2):87-101.
2. Goldberg AE. LGBTQ family building: A guide for prospective parents. Washington, DC: American Psychological Association; 2022.
3. Garborcauskas G, McCabe E, Boskey ER, Grimstad FW. Family building perspectives of assigned female at birth transgender and gender diverse adolescents seeking testosterone gender-affirming hormone therapy. LGBT Health. 2022;9(7):463-70.
4. Kosciw, J. G., Greytak, E. A., Palmer, N. A., & Boesen, M. J. The 2013 National School Climate Survey: The experiences of lesbian, gay, bisexual and transgender youth in our nation's schools. GLSEN; 2014. (https://www.glsen.org/research/2013-national-school-climate-survey.)
5. Let's Talk Poll. New York: Planned Parenthood Federation of America, Center for Latino Adolescent and Family Health; 2015. (https://www.nyu.edu/about/news-publications/news/2014/october/lets-talk-month-poll-shows-parents-need-to-be-more-direct-and-specific-with-teens-about-sexuality-and-relationships.html)
6. Chrisler JC, Gorman JA, Manion J, et al. Queer periods: attitudes toward and experiences with menstruation in the masculine of centre and transgender community. Cult Health Sex. 2016;18(11):1238–50.
7. National Coalition for Sexual Health. The 6 Ps: A new approach to sexual history taking. National Coalition for Sexual Health; 2021. (https://nationalcoalitionforsexualhealth.org/tools/for-healthcare-providers/video-series.)

8. Coleman E, Radix AE, Bouman WP, et al. Standards of care for the health of transgender and gender diverse people, version 8. Int J Transgender Health. 2022;23(sup1):S1-259.
9. Ashley F, Ells C. In favor of covering ethically important cosmetic surgeries: facial feminization surgery for transgender people. Am J Bioeth. 2018;18(12):23-5.
10. When Health care isn't caring. Lambda Legal; 2014. (https://www.lambdalegal.org/publications/when-health-care-isnt-caring)
11. Brooks H, Llewellyn CD, Nadarzynski T, et al. Sexual orientation disclosure in health care: a systematic review. Br J Gen Pract. 2018;68(668):e187-96.
12. Center for American Progress. Discrimination prevents LGBTQ People from accessing health care. (https://www.americanprogress.org/article/discrimination-prevents-lgbtq-people-accessing-health-care/.)
13. Krempasky C, Harris M, Abern L, Grimstad F. Contraception across the transmasculine spectrum. Am J Obstet Gynecol. 2020;222(2):134-43.
14. Centers for Disease Control and Prevention. A guide to taking a sexual history. (https://www.cdc.gov/std/treatment/sexualhistory.pdf.)
15. New York State Department of Health AIDS Institute. Clinical guidelines program: GOALS framework for sexual history taking in primary care. (https://www.hivguidelines.org/hiv-care/selected-resources/goals-framework/.)
16. Owens L, Terrell S, Low LK, et al. Universal precautions: the case for consistently trauma-informed reproductive healthcare. Am J Obstet Gynecol. 2022;226(5):671-7.
17. Centers for Disease Control and Prevention. National Center for Injury Prevention and Control. National Intimate Partner and Sexual Violence Survey (NISVS): General population survey raw data, 2010: Archival version. 2014. (https://www.icpsr.umich.edu/web/NACJD/studies/34305.)
18. James S, Herman J, Rankin S, Keisling M, Mottet L, Anafi M. The report of the 2015 U.S. transgender survey. 2016. (https://ncvc.dspacedirect.org/handle/20.500.11990/1299.)
19. American Medical Association. Use of chaperones. (https://www.ama-assn.org/delivering-care/ethics/use-chaperones.)
20. Savage C. Abortion ruling poses new questions about how far Supreme Court will go. The New York Times. August 8, 2022. (https://www.nytimes.com/2022/06/25/us/supreme-court-abortion-contraception-same-sex-marriage.html.)
21. Kidd KM, Sequeira GM, Paglisotti T, et al. "This could mean death for my child": Parent perspectives on laws banning gender-affirming care for transgender adolescents. J Adolesc Health. 2021;68(6):1082-8.
22. Hughes LD, Kidd KM, Gamarel KE, Operario D, Dowshen N. "These laws will be devastating": Provider perspectives on legislation banning gender-affirming care for transgender adolescents. J Adolesc Health. 2021;69(6):976-82.
23. Barbee H, Deal C, Gonzales G. Anti-transgender legislation—a public health concern for transgender youth. JAMA Pediatr. 2022;176(2):125-6.
24. Charo RA. Vigilante injustice — deputizing and weaponizing the public to stop abortions. N Engl J Med. 2021;385(16):1441-3.
25. Dehlendorf C, Akers AY, Borrero S, et al. Evolving the preconception health framework: A call for reproductive and sexual health equity. Obstet Gynecol. 2021;137(2):234-9. (https://journals.lww.com/greenjournal/fulltext/2021/02000/evolving_the_preconception_health_framework__a.6.aspx.)
26. Bonnington A, Dianat S, Kerns J, et al. Society of Family Planning clinical recommendations: Contraceptive counseling for transgender and gender diverse people who were female sex assigned at birth. Contraception. 2020;102(2):70-82.
27. Identity document laws and policies. Movement Advancement Project. (https://www.lgbtmap.org/equality-maps/identity_document_laws).
28. Light AD, Obedin-Maliver J, Sevelius JM, Kerns JL. Transgender men who experienced pregnancy after female-to-male gender transitioning. Obstet Gynecol. 2014;124(6):1120-7.
29. Abern L, Maguire K. Contraception knowledge in transgender individuals: Are we doing enough? Obstet Gynecol. 2018;131:65S.
30. Taub RL, Ellis SA, Neal-Perry G, Magaret AS, Prager SW, Micks EA. The effect of testosterone on ovulatory function in transmasculine individuals. Am J Obstet Gynecol. 2020;223(2):229.e1-8.

31. Haraldsen IR, Haug E, Falch J, Egeland T, Opjordsmoen S. Cross-sex pattern of bone mineral density in early onset gender identity disorder. Horm Behav. 2007;52(3):334-43.
32. Spinder T, Spijkstra JJ, van den Tweel JG, et al. The effects of long term testosterone administration on pulsatile luteinizing hormone secretion and on ovarian histology in eugonadal female to male transsexual subjects. J Clin Endocrinol Metab. 1989;69(1):151-7.
33. Van Caenegem E, T'Sjoen G. Bone in trans persons. Curr Opin Endocrinol Diabetes Obes. 2015;22(6):459–66.
34. Barrera EP, Grimstad FW, Boskey ER. Young adult patients with testosterone management concerns after gender-affirming hysterectomy and bilateral oophorectomy: A case series. J Pediatr Adolesc Gynecol. 2023;36(1):89-91.
35. Curtis KM. U.S. Medical eligibility criteria for contraceptive use, 2016. MMWR Recomm Rep. 2016;65(3):1-103. (https://www.cdc.gov/mmwr/volumes/65/rr/rr6503a1.htm.)
36. Hembree WC, Cohen-Kettenis PT, Gooren L, et al. Endocrine treatment of gender-dysphoric/gender-incongruent persons: An Endocrine Society clinical practice guideline. J Clin Endocrinol Metab. 2017;102(11):3869-903.
37. Maraka S, Singh Ospina N, Rodriguez-Gutierrez R, et al. Sex steroids and cardiovascular outcomes in transgender individuals: A systematic review and meta-analysis. J Clin Endocrinol Metab. 2017;102(11):3914-23.
38. Shatzel JJ, Connelly KJ, DeLoughery TG. Thrombotic issues in transgender medicine: A review. Am J Hematol. 2017;92(2):204-8.
39. Abou-Ismail MY, Sridhar DC, Nayak L. Estrogen and thrombosis: A bench to bedside review. Thromb Res. 2020;192:40-51.
40. Kanj RV, Conard LAE, Corathers SD, Trotman GE. Hormonal contraceptive choices in a clinic-based series of transgender adolescents and young adults. Int J Transgenderism. 2019;20(4):413-20.
41. Gomez A, Walters PC, Dao LT. "Testosterone in a way is birth control": contraceptive attitudes and experiences among transmasculine and genderqueer young adults. Contraception. 2016;94(4):422-3.
42. Grimstad FW, Fowler KG, New EP, et al. Uterine pathology in transmasculine persons on testosterone: a retrospective multicenter case series. Am J Obstet Gynecol. 2019;220(3): 257.e1-7.
43. Goodman NF, Cobin RH, Futterweit W, et al. American Association of Clinical Endocrinologists, American College of Endocrinology, and Androgen Excess and PCOS Society Disease State Clinical Review: Guide to the best practices in the evaluation and treatment of polycystic ovary syndrome--Part 1. Endocr Pract 2015;21(11):1291-300.
44. Hatcher RA, ed. Contraceptive technology. 21st ed. New York: Ayer Company Publishers, Inc.; 2018.
45. Fritz MA, Speroff LS (eds.) Clinical gynecologic endocrinology and infertility (8th ed.). Philadelphia, PA: Lippicott Williams & Wilkins; 2010.
46. Merck & Co, Inc. Etonogestrel implant prescribing information. Kenilworth, NJ: 2011.
47. Hillard PJA. Practical tips for intrauterine devices use in adolescents. J Adolesc Health Off Publ Soc Adolesc Med. 2013;52(4 Suppl):S40-6.
48. Baldassarre M, Giannone FA, Foschini MP, et al. Effects of long-term high dose testosterone administration on vaginal epithelium structure and estrogen receptor-α and -β expression of young women. Int J Impot Res. 2013;25(5):172-7.
49. Bachmann GA, Nevadunsky NS. Diagnosis and treatment of atrophic vaginitis. Am Fam Physician. 2000;61(10):3090-6.
50. Villavicencio J, Allen RH. Unscheduled bleeding and contraceptive choice: increasing satisfaction and continuation rates. Open Access J Contracept. 2016;7:43-52.
51. Milsom I, Andersson K, Jonasson K, Lindstedt G, Rybo G. The influence of the Gyne-T 380S IUD on menstrual blood loss and iron status. Contraception. 1995;52(3):175-9.
52. Turok DK, Gero A, Simmons RG, et al. Levonorgestrel vs. copper intrauterine devices for emergency contraception. N Engl J Med. 2021;384(4):335-44.
53. American Society for Emergency Contraception. (https://www.americansocietyforec.org.)
54. Moseson H, Fix L, Ragosta S, et al. Abortion experiences and preferences of transgender, nonbinary, and gender-expansive people in the United States. Am J Obstet Gynecol. 2021;224(4):376.e1-11.

55. Joint R, Chen ZE, Cameron S. Breast and reproductive cancers in the transgender population: a systematic review. BJOG Int J Obstet Gynaecol. 2018;125(12):1505-12.
56. Grimstad F, Kremen J, Shim J, Charlton BM, Boskey ER. Breakthrough bleeding in transgender and gender diverse adolescents and young adults on long-term testosterone. J Pediatr Adolesc Gynecol. 2021;34(5):706-16.
57. Pradhan S, Gomez-Lobo V. Hormonal contraceptives, intrauterine devices, gonadotropin-releasing hormone analogues and testosterone: Menstrual suppression in special adolescent populations. J Pediatr Adolesc Gynecol. 2019;32(5S):S23-9.
58. Carswell JM, Roberts SA. Induction and maintenance of amenorrhea in transmasculine and nonbinary adolescents. Transgender Health. 2017;2(1):195-201.
59. Schwartz BI, Effron A, Bear B, et al. Experiences with menses in transgender and gender non-binary adolescents. J Pediatr Adolesc Gynecol. 2022;35(4):450-6.
60. Hillard PA. Menstrual suppression: current perspectives. Int J Womens Health. 2014;6:631-7.
61. American College of Obstetricians and Gynecologists. General approaches to medical management of menstrual suppression. Clinical consensus No. 3. Obstet Gynecol. 2022;(140):528-41.
62. Barbieri RL, Evans S, Kistner RW. Danazol in the treatment of endometriosis: analysis of 100 cases with a 4-year follow-up. Fertil Steril. 1982;37(6):737-46.
63. Defreyne J, Vanwonterghem Y, Collet S, et al. Vaginal bleeding and spotting in transgender men after initiation of testosterone therapy: A prospective cohort study (ENIGI). Int J Transgender Health. 2020;21(2):163-75.
64. Murad MH, Elamin MB, Garcia MZ, et al. Hormonal therapy and sex reassignment: a systematic review and meta-analysis of quality of life and psychosocial outcomes. Clin Endocrinol (Oxf). 2010;72(2):214-31.
65. Cheng PJ, Pastuszak AW, Myers JB, Goodwin IA, Hotaling JM. Fertility concerns of the transgender patient. Transl Androl Urol. 2019;8(3):209-18.
66. Schneider F, Neuhaus N, Wistuba J, et al. Testicular functions and clinical characterization of patients with gender dysphoria (GD) undergoing sex reassignment surgery (SRS). J Sex Med. 2015;12(11):2190-200.
67. Sinha A, Mei L, Ferrando C. The effect of estrogen therapy on spermatogenesis in transgender women. FS Rep. 2021;2(3):347-51.
68. Garcia M, Zaliznyak M. MP45-20 effects of feminizing hormone therapy on sexual function of transgender women. J Urol 2020;203(Suppl 4):e672.
69. Centers for Disease Control and Prevention. Key statistics from the National Survey of Family Growth: sexual identity, attraction, and activity. 2018. (https://www.cdc.gov/nchs/nsfg/key_statistics/s.htm.)
70. Centers for Disease Control and Prevention. 2019 Number and percentage of students, by sexual identity 2021. (https://www.cdc.gov/healthyyouth/data/yrbs/2019_tables/students_by_sexual_identity.htm.)
71. Tornello SL, Riskind RG, Patterson CJ. Sexual orientation and sexual and reproductive health among adolescent young women in the United States. J Adolesc Health Off Publ Soc Adolesc Med. 2014;54(2):160-8.
72. Morrow KM, Allsworth JE. Original Research: Sexual risk in lesbians and bisexual women. J Gay Lesbian Med Assoc. 2000;4(4):159-65.
73. Porsch L, Zhang H, Paschen-Wolff M, Grosskopf N, Grov C. Contraceptive use by women across multiple components of sexual orientation: Findings from the 2011–2017 National Survey of Family Growth. LGBT Health. 2020;7(6):321-31.
74. Everett BG, Higgins JA, Haider S, Carpenter E. Do sexual minorities receive appropriate sexual and reproductive health care and counseling? J Womens Health. 2019;28(1):53-62.
75. Everett BG, McCabe KF, Hughes TL. Sexual orientation disparities in mistimed and unwanted pregnancy among adult women. Perspect Sex Reprod Health. 2017;49(3):157-65.
76. Everett BG, McCabe KF, Hughes TL. Unintended pregnancy, depression, and hazardous drinking in a community-based sample of sexual minority women. J Womens Health. 2002 2016;25(9):904-11.
77. Goldberg SK, Reese BM, Halpern CT. Teen pregnancy among sexual minority women: Results from the National Longitudinal Study of Adolescent to Adult Health. J Adolesc Health Off Publ Soc Adolesc Med. 2016;59(4):429-37.

78. Higgins JA, Carpenter E, Everett BG, Greene MZ, Haider S, Hendrick CE. Sexual minority women and contraceptive use: Complex pathways between sexual orientation and health outcomes. Am J Public Health. 2019;109(12):1680-6.
79. Everett BG, Sanders JN, Myers K, Geist C, Turok DK. One in three: challenging heteronormative assumptions in family planning health centers. Contraception. 2018;98(4):270-4.
80. Agénor M, Pérez AE, Wilhoit A, et al. Contraceptive care disparities among sexual orientation identity and racial/ethnic subgroups of U.S. women: A national probability sample study. J Womens Health. 2021;30(10):1406-15.
81. Kumnick A, Hanfling SN, Dowlut-McElroy T, Maher JY, Gomez-Lobo V. An intersectional analysis of contraceptive types chosen among sexual minority women: A nationally representative study. Contraception. 2022;110:42-7.
82. Charlton BM, Janiak E, Gaskins AJ, et al. Contraceptive use by women across different sexual orientation groups. Contraception. 2019;100(3):202-8.
83. Kerr DL, Ding K, Thompson AJ. A comparison of lesbian, bisexual, and heterosexual female college undergraduate students on selected reproductive health screenings and sexual behaviors. Womens Health Iss. 2013;23(6):e347-55.
84. Bertelloni S, Baroncelli GI, Ferdeghini M, Menchini-Fabris F, Saggese G. Final height, gonadal function and bone mineral density of adolescent males with central precocious puberty after therapy with gonadotropin-releasing hormone analogues. Eur J Pediatr. 2000;159(5):369-74.
85. Nahata L, Chen D, Moravek MB, et al. Understudied and under-reported: Fertility issues in transgender youth-a narrative review. J Pediatr. 2019;205:265-71.
86. Moravek MB, Kinnear HM, George J, et al. Impact of exogenous testosterone on reproduction in transgender men. Endocrinology. 2020;161(3):bqaa014.
87. Lee PA, Nordenström A, Houk CP, et al. Global disorders of sex development update since 2006: Perceptions, approach and care. Horm Res Paediatr. 2016;85(3):158-80.
88. Grimstad F, Boskey E. Empowering Transmasculine youth by enhancing reproductive health counseling in the primary care setting. J Adolesc Health. 2020;66(6):653-5.
89. Grimstad F, Boskey ER, Taghinia A, Ganor O. Gender-affirming surgeries in transgender and gender diverse adolescent and young adults: A pediatric and adolescent gynecology primer. J Pediatr Adolesc Gynecol 2021;34(4):442-8.
90. Wingo E, Ingraham N, Roberts SCM. Reproductive health care priorities and barriers to effective care for LGBTQ people assigned female at birth: A qualitative study. Womens Health Iss. 2018;28(4):350-7.
91. Ethics Committee of the American Society for Reproductive Medicine. Access to fertility treatment irrespective of marital status, sexual orientation, or gender identity: an Ethics Committee opinion. Fertil Steril. 2021;116(2):326-30.
92. Núñez A, García D, Giménez-Bonafé P, Vassena R, Rodríguez A. Reproductive outcomes in lesbian couples undergoing reception of oocytes from partner versus autologous in vitro fertilization/intracytoplasmic sperm injection. LGBT Health. 2021;8(5):367-71.
93. Montoya MN, Peipert BJ, Whicker D, Gray B. Reproductive considerations for the LGBTQ+ community. Prim Care. 2021;48(2):283-97.

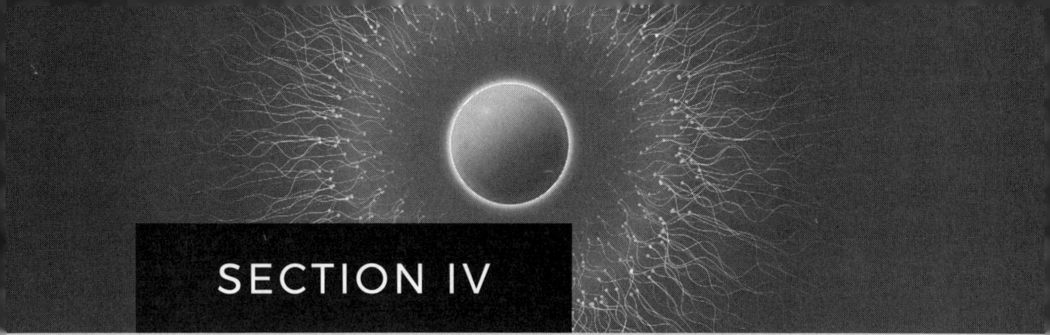

SECTION IV

Reproductive Tract Conditions

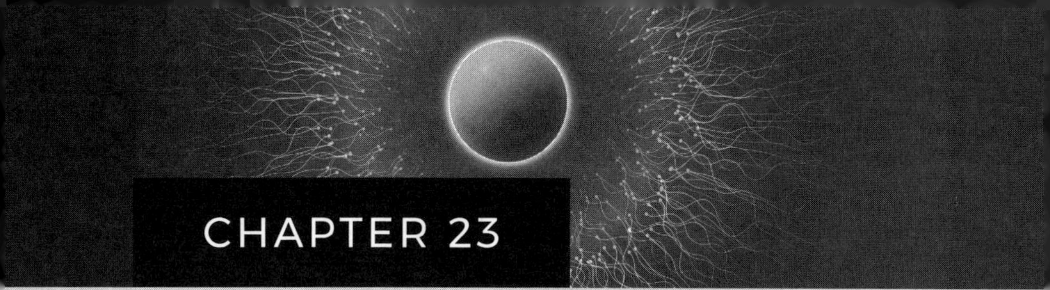

CHAPTER 23

Reproductive Tract Infections, Including HIV and Other Sexually Transmitted Infections

Jeanne M. Marrazzo, MD, MPH
Ina U. Park, MD, MS

KEY POINTS

- Reproductive tract infections (RTIs) are frequently encountered by reproductive health professionals.
- RTIs include both sexually transmitted infections (STIs) and other common infections of the genital tract, such as bacterial vaginosis (BV) and vulvovaginal candidiasis. Other infectious diseases with effects on perinatal health, such as Zika virus, also can be sexually transmitted.
- RTIs can have serious health consequences:
  - Tubal occlusion leading to infertility and ectopic pregnancy
  - Pregnancy loss and neonatal morbidity/mortality caused by transmission of the infection to the infant during pregnancy and childbirth
  - Anogenital cancers
  - Enhanced transmission and acquisition of human immunodeficiency virus (HIV)
- Assessing a patient's chances of exposure to RTIs can help them better select appropriate contraceptive methods and help the clinician provide better care. Ask each patient, "How do you protect yourself from infection with HIV and other STIs?"
- Adoption of safer sex behaviors and effective screening, diagnosis, and treatment of existing infections can help prevent RTIs and their consequences.
- Because reproductive-age patients constitute a major segment of the HIV epidemic in the United States, reproductive health care settings are a critical conduit to HIV testing and provision of preventive services, including HIV pre-exposure prophylaxis (PrEP). The United States Preventive Services Task Force (USPSTF) recommends counseling on PrEP be provided to persons at high risk of HIV acquisition, while the Centers for Disease Control and

Prevention (CDC) recommends all sexually active adults and adolescents be informed about PrEP. Offering all patients HIV prevention counseling (including a discussion of HIV PrEP) and voluntary HIV testing is a patient-centered approach that affords patients the opportunity to self-assess their risk. Subsequently, those interested in PrEP should be linked to services. A useful resource is the PrEP in Family Planning Tool Kit, available at www.hiveonline.org/prep4familyplanning/.

- Routine HIV testing for all pregnant patients is the standard of care for prenatal services. Ensure that HIV-positive pregnant patients have access to antiretroviral treatment to improve health status, suppress viral load, and eliminate the likelihood of perinatal transmission.

In *Contraceptive Technology*, the generic term reproductive tract infections (RTIs) covers three types of infections: (1) sexually transmitted infections (STIs), (2) vaginal infections including bacterial vaginosis (BV) and candidiasis, and (3) iatrogenic infections associated with placement of an intrauterine device (IUD) or induced abortion. Prevention of infection through safer sex practices and screening/treatment are the most effective ways to reduce the adverse consequences of RTI, while recognition and correct management of RTIs that do occur can prevent complications in the individual and interrupt transmission in the community. This chapter provides general background about RTI management in the reproductive health care setting.

Magnitude and Risks of RTI

The number of people infected with RTIs or affected by their consequences is a major problem for society.[1] For example, 2019 marked the highest number of sexually transmitted *Chlamydia trachomatis* cases (1,808,703 cases) ever reported to the Centers for Disease Control and Prevention (CDC).[2] Chlamydia is the most common bacterial infection reportable to the CDC, and STIs are the most common cause of pelvic inflammatory disease (PID). Infertility caused by PID accounts for billions of dollars in health care costs as well as major emotional costs. STIs such as syphilis can cause neurologic sequelae such as blindness and devastating consequences to the fetus in pregnancy, including stillbirth. Lifetime costs associated with the morbidity and mortality due to the eight most common STIs contracted in a single year is nearly 16 billion dollars.[3]

While the prevalence of RTIs by individual pathogen and across different geographic regions varies considerably, some general trends are notable. For example, individuals under 25 years of age account for a majority of RTI cases, with nearly two-thirds of chlamydia and 40% of gonorrhea reported in persons less than 25 years of age. Rates of chlamydia, gonorrhea, and PID are highest in adolescents and young adults and decline steadily with increasing age. RTIs are also concentrated in socio-geographic clusters that generally reflect sexual networks, regional variation in disease prevalence, disparities related to systemic racism, and access to sexual health care services.

Finally, most RTIs exhibit a "biological sexism." Compared with males, females suffer more severe long-term consequences, including PID, infertility, ectopic pregnancy, chronic pelvic pain, and cervical cancer. Females also may not seek health care for assessment of RTIs, because a higher proportion of their RTIs are asymptomatic or unrecognized as being serious. Females who have sex with males are more likely than their male partners to acquire RTI, due to the transmission dynamics during an act of vaginal intercourse. The risk of acquisition increases when trauma occurs to the genital mucosa, as may be the case in sexual assault. Mucosal trauma can also occur during receptive anal sex. RTI acquisition is less likely if friction during sexual activity is reduced with lubrication (either naturally occurring or exogenous) or involves activities that are less traumatic to the receptive epithelium, including oral sex, digital penetration, or sex acts other than vaginal or anal intercourse.

Transmission of RTI

The probability that condomless sexual intercourse will lead to RTIs or their consequences differs from the probability of pregnancy (see **Table 23-1**). The risk of pregnancy varies according to the menstrual cycle. In contrast, while numerous complex factors modulate susceptibility to RTIs, the risk of acquisition depends

Table 23-1 Comparative Risk of Adverse Consequences from Vaginal or Anal Intercourse: RTI and Unintended Pregnancy

Unintended pregnancy (per coital act)[14,15]	■ 17% to 30% midcycle ■ < 1% during menses
HIV transmission (per coital act)	■ 0.08% receptive vaginal sex ■ 0.04% insertive vaginal sex ■ 1.3% receptive anal sex ■ 0.11% insertive anal sex
Gonococcal transmission (per coital act)	■ 50% receptive vaginal sex[6] ■ 22% insertive vaginal sex[16]
PID per patient infected with cervical chlamydia	■ 22% if not treated[17] ■ 0% if promptly and adequately treated
Tubal infertility per PID episode[18]	■ 8% after first episode ■ 20% after second episode ■ 40% after third or more episodes

Data from Trussell J, Kost K. Contraceptive failure in the United States: a critical review of the literature. Stud Fam Plann 1987;18(5):237-83. http://www.ncbi.nlm.nih.gov/entrez/query.fcgi?cmd=Retrieve&db=PubMed&dopt=Citation&list_uids=3318006; Centers for Disease Control and Prevention. HIV Risk Behaviors. https://www.cdc.gov/hiv/risk/estimates/riskbehaviors.html; Holmes KK, Johnson DW, Trostle HJ. An estimate of the risk of men acquiring gonorrhea by sexual contact with infected females. Am J Epidemiol 1970;91(2):170-4. DOI: 10.1093/oxfordjournals.aje.a121125; Herzog SA, Heijne JC, Althaus CL, Low N. Describing the progression from Chlamydia trachomatis and Neisseria gonorrhoeae to pelvic inflammatory disease: systematic review of mathematical modeling studies. Sex Transm Dis 2012;39(8):628-37. DOI: 10.1097/OLQ.0b013e31825159ff; Westrom L, Joesoef R, Reynolds G, Hagdu A, Thompson SE. Pelvic inflammatory disease and fertility. A cohort study of 1,844 women with laparoscopically verified disease and 657 control women with normal laparoscopic results. Sex Transm Dis 1992;19(4):185-92. http://www.ncbi.nlm.nih.gov/entrez/query.fcgi?cmd=Retrieve&db=PubMed&dopt=Citation&list_uids=1411832; Platt R, Rice PA, McCormack WM. Risk of acquiring gonorrhea and prevalence of abnormal adnexal findings among women recently exposed to gonorrhea. JAMA 1983;250(23):3205-9. https://www.ncbi.nlm.nih.gov/pubmed/6417362

on (1) having sex with an infected person, (2) the genitalia of the infected partner, (3) transmissibility of the particular RTI, and (4) use of barriers or other protective measures.[4,5] For example, the risk of acquiring gonorrhea from a single act of penile-vaginal intercourse (where one partner is infectious) is approximately 20% to 30% for the person with the penis and 60% to 90% for the person with the vagina.[6,7] The probability of suffering consequences from an RTI depends on whether or not proper diagnosis and treatment are readily obtained.

In the case of human immunodeficiency virus (HIV), the quantity of serum (and presumably genital) HIV viral load directly influences the likelihood of transmitting HIV to vulnerable partners. HIV viral load is extremely high in the context of early infection (the first several months after a person acquires the virus). Because sexual transmission of HIV frequently occurs during this early infection interval,[8] persons who may be exposed to HIV need to consider HIV-prevention methods at all times.

There have been several breakthroughs related to preventing sexual transmission of HIV, including use of HIV antiretroviral medication for pre-exposure prophylaxis (PrEP).[9-12] Currently there are three medications approved by the US Food and Drug Administration (FDA) for HIV PrEP: (1) daily oral tenofovir-emtricitabine, (2) daily oral tenofovir alafenamide-emtricitabine (not studied for receptive vaginal intercourse, not FDA-approved for cisgender women), and (3) injectable cabotegravir given every 2 months. Studies in Africa have also demonstrated that circumcision of adult males can significantly reduce their risk of acquiring HIV and other RTIs from their female partners.[13]

RTI Risk Assessment, Prevention, and Risk Behaviors

Different individuals accept different levels of risk. Not everyone will follow every safer sex recommendation, but, with the proper knowledge, each person can make their own informed choices about reducing risk. Some prevention messages are universal and should be reinforced (for example, barrier methods when appropriate). Additionally, person-centered counseling (see Chapter 4, Person-Centered Reproductive Health Conversations and Contraceptive Counseling) highlights the need to individualize risk assessment and tailor risk-reduction plans. The latter may include a discussion on selecting sex partners and building skills for negotiating safer sex.

Preventive measures for avoiding RTI transmission generally are consistent with guidelines for reducing risk of HIV infection. Risk-free options include having a mutually monogamous relationship with an uninfected partner or completely abstaining from sexual activities that involve semen, blood or other body fluids, or skin-to-skin contact. Examining a partner for visible abnormalities of genital skin and discussing each new partner's previous history of STIs/HIV and most recent test results can augment other measures to prevent RTI transmission. Educating people about their bodies and teaching them to be active participants in their health care gives them more control over their sexual and reproductive health.

Contraceptive Choice

Choice of contraception directly affects the risk of RTIs (**Table 23-2**). Condoms reduce the risks of both bacterial and viral RTIs; the evidence is strongest for condom

Table 23-2 Effects of Contraceptives on Bacterial and Viral RTIs

Contraceptive Method	Bacterial RTI	Viral RTI
Condoms	Protective	Protective
Spermicides	Not protective	Not protective; elevates risk of HIV acquisition
Diaphragm	Protective against cervical infection	Protective against cervical neoplasia, not protective against HIV
Hormonal contraception	Somewhat protective against symptomatic PID but not silent endometritis Effect modified by estrogen vs. progestin components	Not protective against HIV
IUD	Not protective	Not protective

See chapters on specific contraceptive methods for details.

Data from Morrison CS, Turner AN, Jones LB. Highly effective contraception and acquisition of HIV and other sexually transmitted infections. Best Pract Res Clin Obstet Gynaecol 2009;23(2):263-84. DOI: 10.1016/j.bpobgyn.2008.11.004; Polis CB, Curtis KM. Use of hormonal contraceptives and HIV acquisition in women: a systematic review of the epidemiological evidence. Lancet Infect Dis 2013;13(9):797-808. DOI: 10.1016/S1473-3099(13)70155-5.

effectiveness against HIV, trichomoniasis, genital herpes, and gonorrhea.[19] No data support spermicides' ability to prevent bacterial or viral infections, and nonoxynol-9 has been associated with an increased risk of HIV acquisition.[4] Diaphragms provide a barrier against cervical infection but have not demonstrated protection against HIV and most other RTIs.[20,21] In addition, diaphragms have been associated with changes in vaginal flora and urinary tract infections. Although oral contraceptives usually are associated with an increase in chlamydia detected in the cervix, they decrease the risk of symptomatic PID but not asymptomatic endometritis.[22] Depot medroxyprogesterone acetate (DMPA) was associated with a modestly increased risk of HIV acquisition and of chlamydial infection in some observational studies,[21,23] but did not confer increased risk in a recent large, randomized trial designed to definitively answer the question.[24] Although older data suggested that copper IUD insertion was associated with a transient increased risk of PID in the first month after insertion, newer data indicate that RTI risk is both very low and not elevated after IUD insertion.[25] The overall risk of PID within 90 days of IUD insertion is less than 0.6%.[26,27] Routine antibiotic prophylaxis is not recommended before IUD placement. The IUD has a strong record of safety, even for patients with HIV.[28] At present, the data are insufficient to state whether the levonorgestrel IUD has a differential effect on RTI acquisition or natural history. Of note, the copper IUD was associated with incidence of BV in one large study[29]; the relevance of this at the individual level is not clear.

Microbicides, defined as substances used topically that interrupt the ability of infectious agents to establish infection, continue to hold promise for prevention of both HIV and other STIs. The search for a nonspecific microbicide that offers protection against a wide variety of STIs, including HIV, has yielded disappointing results, and no available microbicide offers broad protection against RTIs. Furthermore, frequent use of certain topical agents such as nonoxynol-9 gel was associated with an increased risk of HIV acquisition.[30] Vaginal delivery of drugs such as tenofovir, with specific antiretroviral activity against HIV and herpes simplex virus (HSV), appears more promising. Use of tenofovir gel applied vaginally before and after sexual intercourse significantly reduced the rate of HIV acquisition (by 39%) in a study of South African women and of HSV-2 acquisition by 50%.[31] Importantly, the dapivirine vaginal ring has been approved by the World Health Organization (WHO) for prevention of HIV infection (but is not available or FDA-approved in the United States).[32,33] Additional delivery systems in the form of subcutaneous implants and other vaginal rings are under study, and multipurpose prevention products that also include contraceptive agents are of particular interest. One such product is a vaginal contraceptive gel composed of lactic acid, citric acid, and potassium bitartrate (brand name Phexxi), which reduced risk of chlamydia by 50% and of gonorrhea by 78% in an initial trial; however, these protective effects were not confirmed in the follow-up EVOGUARD study, making future development of this product for STI protection uncertain.[34]

Other Behaviors Linked to RTIs

In addition to sexual behaviors, other practices have been linked to RTI risk. Routine douching for personal preference has been associated with an increased risk of PID and ectopic pregnancy. Douching also is a risk factor for BV because it eradicates commensal hydrogen peroxide–producing vaginal *Lactobacillus* species.[35] Genital washing has been poorly studied but appears to have little effect, if any, on reducing the risk of acquiring an RTI. In some studies, these practices have been associated with an increased risk of HIV acquisition.[36]

Substance use influences the transmission of RTI. While hepatitis C (often associated with drug use) is not typically considered an RTI, cases of sexual transmission have occurred, particularly among men who have sex with men.[37] Use of drugs such as methamphetamine and cocaine—through intravenous, intranasal, or other routes—has been associated with acquisition of RTIs. Outbreaks of syphilis, antibiotic-resistant gonorrhea, and chancroid have been linked to drug-related sexual behaviors and to sexual networks of drug users. Crystal methamphetamine has figured prominently in national outbreaks of syphilis in men who have sex with men and in reproductive-age women, and the drug is especially harmful for its disinhibitory effects on sexual behavior. Abuse of alcohol, particularly binge drinking, also has been associated with condomless sex.[38] Alcohol abuse is a notable concern for adolescents and young adults.

Assessment, Diagnosis, and Treatment of RTI

Comprehensive RTI-related care begins with routine risk assessment. Risk assessment should not be discarded due to common assumptions about either an individual patient (for example, a married patient) or "representative" types of patients (for example, patients who identify as lesbian).

At a minimum, ask about the following: (1) number of sex partners in the last 3 months; (2) anatomic sites exposed during sex (vagina, rectum, oropharynx); and (3) use of personal protective measures (e.g., condoms). (Refer to Chapters 4 and 6 for complete descriptions of sexual history taking). Risk assessment also helps clinicians to provide better contraceptive counseling and more cost-efficient RTI management. Balance the demographic, behavioral, and clinical information (other than laboratory test results) to assess the likelihood that someone is infected with an RTI or is at high risk of future infection. Include that information when counseling clients who are selecting contraceptive methods.

Laboratory diagnosis of most RTIs can be performed in nearly every reproductive health care setting. Over the past decade, routine screening for chlamydia has been associated with declines in PID and ectopic pregnancy.[39] In addition, some family planning clinics have extended their range of services to clients of all genders, including RTI diagnosis, treatment, and counseling. Many clinics provide *expedited partner treatment* (EPT), defined as provision of medications or a prescription for the partner of the index patient being treated, without a requirement for examination. (see Partner Management, p. 629).

Routine Screening for RTI

Because most RTIs are asymptomatic and do not cause clinical signs such as cervicitis or PID, routine screening can provide early detection and prompt treatment, thus interrupting the progression to the sequelae of untreated disease. Counsel patients about the asymptomatic nature of most RTIs and that transmission typically occurs in the absence of symptoms. Chlamydial infections are the prototype, because up to 90% of these infections cause neither symptoms nor clinical signs (namely, cervicitis). The United States Preventive Services Task Force (USPSTF) and the CDC recommend routine annual screening for target groups of patients, as delineated in **Table 23-3**. Screening can be considered on a case-by-case patients for individuals outside these groups who perceive themselves to be at risk.[40] Individuals between the ages of 15 and 64 in the United States should be screened for HIV at least once, and more frequently if at ongoing risk of acquisition.[41] In contrast, the USPSTF recommends against routine screening for asymptomatic HSV infection (genital herpes) using serology, citing the associated cost, issues with performance of available screening assays (which may lead to false positive diagnoses), and lack of evidence that routine screening effects significant health benefit at the individual or population level.[42,43]

Counseling Patients About RTI Diagnosis and Treatment

Patients who are being screened for, diagnosed with, and treated for RTIs deserve respectful care that is not stigmatizing. People who feel judged are less likely to trust their provider and to hear and fully understand the information given to them. Patients with RTIs need important information about their condition to understand about risk, prognosis, and treatment so they can make informed choices about their sexual behavior and adhere to treatment. These choices can either prevent or allow reinfection as well as spread of infection to partners or offspring. Therefore, a patient's understanding of the risk and consequences associated with specific behaviors is critical.

Table 23-3 Recommendations for Screening Patients for Infection with *Chlamydia trachomatis* (CT) and *Neisseria gonorrhoeae* (GC) in Reproductive Health Settings

Genital Infection

- All sexually active females and transgender/gender diverse patients with a cervix < 25 years old
- Men who have sex with women < 25 years old (consider)
- Men who have sex with men, or transgender persons who have sex with men (regardless of age)
- Patients of any age at risk for infection, defined as having any of the following risk factors since their last negative test:
    - A new sex partner
    - More than one sex partner (concurrent)
    - A sex partner with concurrent partners or a sex partner who has an STI
    - Inconsistent condom use when not in a mutually monogamous relationship
    - Previous or coexisting STI
    - Exchanging sex for money or drugs
    - A history of incarceration

Rectal Infection

- Men who have sex with men, or transgender/gender diverse persons who have sex with men
- Rectal screening can be considered for females based on sexual exposure (shared decision making)

Pharyngeal Infection

- Men who have sex with men, or transgender/gender diverse persons who have sex with men
- Pharyngeal screening can be considered for females based on sexual exposure (shared decision making)

Screening (genital, rectal, pharyngeal sites) should occur at least annually, or more frequently based on risk.
Note: The USPSTF recommends routine screening for genital CT/GC in females only. The CDC's 2021 STI Treatment Guidelines recommends screening in high-prevalence settings, such as reproductive health clinics for men.
Data from US Preventive Services Task Force. Screening for Chlamydia and Gonorrhea: US Preventive Services Task Force Recommendation Statement. JAMA 2021;326(10):949-56. DOI: 10.1001/jama.2021.14081; Workowski KA, Bachmann LH, Chan PA, et al. Sexually transmitted infections treatment guidelines, 2021. MMWR Recomm Rep 2021;70(4):1-187. DOI: 10.15585/mmwr.rr7004a1.

Trusted providers can help patients learn what they need to know about the importance of adherence to treatment and follow-up and can offer guidance about talking to partners about their RTI exposure. They also can help patients explore and potentially problem-solve when their life situation or relationship(s) present barriers to adherence or behavior change. (See Chapter 4, Person-Centered Reproductive Health Conversations and Contraceptive Counseling, particularly the section describing the *Affirm-Share-Ask Cycle*.) This facilitates listening on the part of the provider and helps providers individualize information and offer strong, clear recommendations that are specifically pertinent to the patient. Striving to ensure that patients feel respected and heard and that they fully understand the relevant information maximizes the possibility that they will recognize why they need to adhere to treatment and consider the risk attendant to specific sexual behaviors.

Education About Infection and Treatment

Ensure that patients understand what RTI they have, how it is transmitted, why it must be treated, and exactly when and how to take prescribed medication. Because unpleasant side effects from some medications may discourage patients from continuing treatment, discuss what to expect and ways to minimize side effects. For example, both azithromycin and doxycycline taken on an empty stomach may cause nausea that prompts the patient to stop taking the medication. Advise taking the medication with food unless directions specify otherwise.

Completion of Treatment. Underscore to patients that it is critically important they finish their entire supply of medication even though symptoms, if present, may diminish or disappear in a few days. Explain that discontinuing antibiotics before the infection is completely cured can lead to recurrent infection and increase the likelihood that hard-to-cure strains of the pathogen may flourish.

Abstinence During Treatment. Advise patients to avoid sex (oral, anal, or vaginal) until they complete the full course of therapy. For single-dose therapy like azithromycin, patients should abstain for the week following treatment.[40]

Partner Management

Failure to treat the partners of patients with RTIs is the most important factor influencing the high rates of chlamydia and gonorrhea recurrence in the months after initial treatment. An increasing number of family planning professionals are being trained in partner management skills. Confidentiality is crucial, just as it is in all aspects of family planning and RTI care. It is key to treat sex partner(s) to prevent both reinfection of the patient and spread of disease through the community. Assist patients in notifying their partners by coaching them in partner notification techniques (patient referral) and, if available, using trained public health program STI staff (provider referral) to help evaluate and treat partners. Another approach is asking patients to bring their partner with them for concurrent treatment (concurrent patient-partner therapy); this may be feasible for patients with one primary partner. EPT, in which the patient is given either drugs or a prescription to give to partners without requiring that the partner(s) be examined, is a highly effective way to increase the likelihood that partners are treated and to reduce the rate of recurrence in the index patient.[44-46] While legal regulations about the provision of EPT vary by state, EPT is now legally permissible in 46 states, and potentially allowable in the remaining four states (www.cdc.gov/std/ept).

Comfort and Support

Be attentive to patients' physical and psychosocial comfort. Treat nausea, pain, itching, or other physiologic discomforts symptomatically whenever possible. This is especially critical for patients who may be experiencing a first episode of symptomatic genital herpes, for example, or for patients with highly symptomatic vulvovaginal candidiasis. Overcoming the psychosocial component of genital discomfort is exceedingly important in RTI treatment. Patients may be afraid or ashamed to ask a partner to seek treatment, embarrassed to admit their sexual practices, or concerned about confidentiality. Reinforcing the messages that many RTIs are common and can often be transmitted when people are experiencing no symptoms can help to minimize the stigma associated with these infections.

Concurrent Infections

Managing an RTI requires that clinicians have a high index of suspicion for other infections. A patient can have two or more RTIs concurrently; therefore, patients with an RTI should be tested for other STIs and HIV. Be alert for symptoms that differ from those normally associated with the primary RTI.

STI Reporting

All states require that certain STIs, including chlamydia, gonorrhea, and syphilis, be reported by laboratories to public health officials. Reporting is not a breach of confidentiality; in fact, statutory protection of patients' names is a crucial part of control strategies. Accurate reporting helps identify trends in disease, gain resources for high-prevalence communities, and evaluate RTI control efforts. Laboratory reporting of STIs is not a substitute for the clinician reporting of certain conditions or pathogens, as required by your state. Questions about reporting should be directed to the individual state STD program. Email contacts for each state are listed on the National Coalition of STD Directors website at https://www.ncsddc.org/ncsd-full-members/.

RTIs During Pregnancy

Question pregnant patients and their sex partners about their risk of RTIs; counsel them about the possibility of transmitting an infection to their fetus and newborn. Because of the severe effects that RTIs may have on both the pregnancy and the developing fetus, all pregnant patients should be screened for infections with HIV, syphilis, and hepatitis B. Pregnant patients < 25 years of age also should be screened for chlamydia and gonorrhea (see **Tables 23-4** and **23-5**). Cervical cancer

Table 23-4 Risks of Sexually Transmitted *Bacteria* and Related Syndromes in Pregnancy and Childbirth

Organism/ Syndrome	Infant Effects	Transmission Risk from Infected Mother	Prevention	Treatment of Mother/ Neonate
Neisseria gonorrhoeae	Conjunctivitis, sepsis, meningitis	Approximately 30%	Screening: test mother; apply ocular prophylaxis	Ceftriaxone
Chlamydia trachomatis	Conjunctivitis, pneumonia, bronchiolitis, otitis media	25% to 50% conjunctivitis, 5% to 15% pneumonia	Screening in third trimester: test mother; apply ocular prophylaxis	Azithromycin Amoxicillin Erythromycin

Organism/ Syndrome	Infant Effects	Transmission Risk from Infected Mother	Prevention	Treatment of Mother/ Neonate
Treponema pallidum	Congenital syphilis, neonatal death	50%	Serologic screening in early and late pregnancy	Penicillin
Trichomonas vaginalis	Low birth weight, preterm delivery	N/A	Diagnostic testing	Metronidazole
Bacterial vaginosis	Low birth weight, preterm delivery	N/A	Diagnostic testing	Metronidazole Clindamycin

Data from Cates, W., Jr, & Alexander, E. R. (1988). Sexually transmitted diseases and the fetus. A continuing challenge. Annals of the New York Academy of Sciences, 549, 1–16. https://doi.org/10.1111/j.1749-6632.1988.tb23952.x; American College of Obstetricians and Gynecologists and the American Academy of Pediatrics. Guidelines for perinatal care, 7th edition; 2012

Table 23-5 **Risks of Sexually Transmitted *Viruses* and Related Syndromes in Pregnancy and Childbirth**

Organism/ Syndrome	Infant Effects	Transmission Risk from Infected Mother	Prevention	Treatment of Mother/ Neonate
Hepatitis B Virus (HBV)	Hepatitis, cirrhosis	10% to 90%	Active HBV immunization	Postexposure passive HBV immunization
Herpes Simplex Virus	Disseminated, central nervous system, localized lesions	Recurrent: 3% at delivery Primary: 30% at delivery	Cesarean delivery if lesions present at delivery	Acyclovir
Human Papillomavirus (HPV)	Laryngeal papillomatosis	Rare	HPV immunization	Surgical
Human Immunodeficiency Virus	Pediatric HIV infection	27% without ART; < 5% with ART	ART during pregnancy	Antivirals (ART)

Data from Cates, W., Jr, & Alexander, E. R. (1988). Sexually transmitted diseases and the fetus. A continuing challenge. Annals of the New York Academy of Sciences, 549, 1–16. https://doi.org/10.1111/j.1749-6632.1988.tb23952.x; American College of Obstetricians and Gynecologists and the American Academy of Pediatrics. Guidelines for perinatal care, 7th edition; 2012

screening should occur at the same intervals as for nonpregnant patients. (See Chapter 24, Screening for Cervical, Ovarian, and Breast Cancer.) Routine screening for HSV-2 infection is not recommended, although depending on the individual patient's concerns and sexual behavior, HSV serologic screening can be considered on a case-by-case basis. If serologic screening is ordered, it is critical to use a glycoprotein-G–based test, because this is the only type of assay that can distinguish between antibody formed in response to HSV-2 infection from that formed in response to HSV-1 infection (a common cause of oral cold sores). These assays can still produce false positive results, particularly at low positive index values (1.0–3.5).[47]

The management of some important RTI syndromes and related pathogens is discussed in more detail below. For more complete information, refer to the 2021 CDC STI Treatment Guidelines (www.cdc.gov/std/treatment)[48] and for RTIs in pregnant patients, refer to the *Guidelines for Perinatal Care*, jointly published by the American College of Obstetricians and Gynecologists and the American Academy of Pediatrics.[49]

RTIs and Sexual Assault

In cases of sexual assault and abuse, clinicians must attend not only to physical and psychological trauma, but also to the possibility of pregnancy or RTI. The following section describes the recommendations regarding evaluation and presumptive treatment for RTI, but does not discuss forensic examination or approaches to psychological care of sexual assault survivors. Based on the survivor's wishes, they should be offered referral to a local sexual assault response team (SART), sexual assault nurse examiner (SANE), or other clinician trained in provision of trauma-informed sexual assault services.

Any of the STIs, including HIV, can be acquired during a sexual assault. Some RTIs, such as gonorrhea or syphilis, are almost exclusively sexually transmitted and therefore are useful markers of assault in persons who have not previously been sexually active. To reduce the risk of pregnancy, offer emergency contraception (see Chapter 18, Emergency Contraception). To reduce risk of RTIs, the CDC recommends the following approach.[40]

Adult Evaluation

If possible, evaluate the survivor within 24 hours of the assault and take specimens for nucleic acid amplification testing (NAAT) for *N. gonorrhoeae* and *C. trachomatis* at all sites of penetration. NAAT for *T. vaginalis* also should be performed if vaginal penetration occurred. Examine vaginal fluid microscopically for trichomoniasis and BV. Perform a pregnancy test. If treatment is not administered, schedule a repeat evaluation for 2 weeks later.

Presumptive treatment is recommended for chlamydia and gonorrhea for all clients, and trichomonas treatment is recommended if vaginal penetration occurred. Advise clients to use condoms for vaginal or anal sex until the test results are reported. While no regimen provides coverage against all potential pathogens, the following should be effective against the most frequent RTIs:

- Ceftriaxone 500 mg intramuscularly (IM) PLUS
- Doxycycline 100 mg twice daily orally for 7 days PLUS
- Metronidazole 500 mg twice daily orally for 7 days (if vaginal penetration occurred)

- Hepatitis B vaccination, first dose (if survivor has not been vaccinated). If the assailant is known to be HBsAg positive, unvaccinated survivors should receive both hepatitis B vaccine and hepatitis B immunoglobulin (HBIG)
- HPV vaccination for all survivors between 9 and 26 years of age, who have not initiated or completed the vaccine series
- Postexposure prophylaxis against HIV, depending on risk assessment

Child Evaluation

In general, the presence of an RTI in a child beyond the neonatal period suggests sexual abuse. However, unlike gonorrhea, chlamydia, trichomonas, or syphilis, infections such as BV and genital warts are not conclusive evidence of sexual abuse. Evaluation is essentially the same as described for adult victims (see previous section), except both culture or NAAT may be used for diagnosis of chlamydia and gonorrhea. Specimens should be collected from the pharynx and rectum as well as from the vagina or urethra because the child's report of assault may not be complete. Presumptive treatment may be given at the family's request. For more complete information regarding laboratory procedures, diagnosis, and treatment for child sexual assault and abuse victims, refer to the CDC's 2021 Guidelines for Treatment of Sexually Transmitted Infections (see www.cdc.gov/std/treatment).

Special Considerations Regarding RTI Evaluation in the Reproductive Health Setting

For many young people, reproductive health care clinics may be the only source of health care. Each patient should be asked, "What do you do to protect yourself from infection with HIV and other sexually transmitted infections?" Providers may be able to determine readiness for behavior change by assessing this answer. The patient who answers, "I thought I would get some condoms while I'm here today," may be more receptive to behavioral change than the patient who answers, "Who, me?"

Although reproductive health providers are more likely than other primary care providers to ask about sex and drug use behavior, many are reluctant to risk offending patients. It may be helpful to begin with, "I'm going to ask you some questions about your sexual history I ask everyone, because I think it is important to your health. Is that all right with you?"

Other Key Points

Avoid making assumptions about a patient's sexual and other behaviors based on appearances. In particular, avoid assumptions based on age, gender identity, marital status, employment status, prior sexual history, educational status, or income.

Remember that terminology can sometimes get in the way of clarity with this type of risk assessment. For example, teens may not know the word "monogamous." Some may think "sexually active" means vigorous sex, or many partners. Some people who engage in same-sex behavior do not identify as gay or lesbian, particularly in settings or cultures where acknowledging same-sex behavior or gay identity is stigmatized. (See Chapter 4, Person-Centered Reproductive Health Conversations and Contraceptive Counseling and Chapter 6, Sexuality and Contraception.)

Counseling About Safer Sex

Offer information about safer sex skills, including correct use of condoms and other latex and plastic barriers, to all patients (**Table 23-6**). Advise all patients that a crucial time for diligent safer sex practices is the first few months of a new relationship. Delaying intercourse may allow the couple the opportunity to get screened for common STIs, including HIV, together. Oral sex also may transmit gonorrhea, syphilis, HSV-1, and (to a much lower extent) HIV, especially with activities that expose the mouth to semen or blood.

Customize teaching methods for individual patients. Use audiovisual, print, and electronic teaching aids appropriate to the patient's age, language, culture, and learning style. (See Chapter 4, Person-Centered Reproductive Health Conversations and Contraceptive Counseling.) Be sure to make your guidance specific to an individual's particular issues, rather than giving vague, global advice:

- "Starting today, you could put condoms on the nightstand beside the bed," rather than "always use condoms."
- "Tell me about the last time you used a condom. What has worked for you in the past?"

Table 23-6 Options for Sexual Intimacy and HIV and STI Prevention

No risk of STI/HIV transmission*	All unprotected sexual activities, when both partners are monogamous and known by testing to be free of HIV and other STIs; also mutual masturbation without contact with partner's semen, vaginal secretions, blood, or broken skin, as well as sexual fantasies, massage, hugging, body rubbing, dry kissing, erotic conversation, books, movies, videos, electronic images, showering/bathing together, nonpenetrative behaviors that eroticize body parts other than genitals, anus, or mouth, including feet, hands, hips, abdomen, ears
Low potential risk for STI/HIV transmission	All sexual activities, when both partners are monogamous but have not been tested; includes wet kissing with no broken skin, cracked lips, or damaged mouth tissue; hand-to-genital touching; vaginal or anal intercourse using latex or plastic condom correctly with adequate lubrication; oral sex to a penis covered by a latex or plastic condom; oral sex on a vulva covered by a latex or plastic barrier such as an internal condom, dental dam, or plastic wrap; hand-vaginal penetration with a glove
Higher risk for STI/HIV transmission	Blood contact of any kind, including menstrual blood; any vaginal or anal intercourse without a latex or plastic condom; oral sex without a latex or plastic barrier (especially if there is any oral contact with menstrual blood, infected vaginal secretions, or semen); oral-anal contact; shared sex toys or douching equipment; any sex that causes tissue damage or bleeding, such as rough vaginal or anal intercourse, fisting, or sexual assault

*HPV and HSV status may not be known by both partners and may be transmitted within monogamous partnerships despite negative testing for other STIs.

- "You can consider whether to date someone who is also dating other people," rather than "Have fewer, safer partners."
- "Next time you're out with friends and might have sex, you might want to avoid getting high on drugs or alcohol," rather than "Have safer sex."

Specific Concerns Related to HIV

Postexposure Prophylaxis, Sex, and Drugs

In cases of isolated high-risk exposures to HIV—unprotected vaginal or anal intercourse, sexual assault, receptive oral sex with ejaculation, or sharing injection equipment when the partner is known or suspected to be infected—consider offering postexposure prophylaxis for HIV (HIV-PEP).[49] Although data on efficacy are limited, health care providers often offer treatment to survivors of sexual assault as well. HIV-PEP should begin as soon as possible, and no later than 72 hours after the exposure. Treatment consists of a 28-day course of drugs combined from three antiretroviral drug groups, much like the combination therapy regimens used by persons with HIV. Discuss treatment protocol options with your local sexual assault service provider (call 1.800.656.HOPE [4673] to be routed to local resources), or call the Postexposure Prophylaxis Hotline operated by the National HIV/AIDS Clinicians' Consultation Center for guidance on individual cases. The hotline is based at the University of California at San Francisco and can be reached toll-free 24 hours a day, 7 days a week at 1.888.448.4911.

Treatment may be costly and may not be covered by health insurance. However, patient assistance programs from pharmaceutical companies can offset some or all of the costs (see https://nastad.org/sites/default/files/2021-11/PDF-PrEP-PEP-Pharma-Co-Patient-Assistance.pdf).

Thus, the decision to undertake HIV-PEP should be informed by a thorough discussion of all components of the risk-benefit assessment, including the risk associated with the exposure and the patient's individual concerns. Patients with ongoing risk for HIV exposure should be offered the opportunity to transition from HIV-PEP to HIV-PrEP once their course of HIV-PEP is completed. See updated 2021 CDC HIV-PrEP guidelines: https://www.cdc.gov/hiv/pdf/risk/prep/cdc-hiv-prep-guidelines-2021.pdf.

Factors Affecting Sexual Transmission of HIV

The likelihood of sexual HIV transmission is variable. The major determining factor is the HIV viral load in the infected partner's genital secretions (semen or vaginal fluid), which is directly proportional to the HIV viral load in their plasma.[50] Risk of sexual transmission may be increased under certain circumstances:

- During early HIV infection (the weeks after the infection is acquired), because HIV viral load, and thus infectivity, is very high
- During late or uncontrolled HIV infection, when viral replication is not suppressed by antiretroviral treatment
- When either partner, but especially the partner with HIV, has a concurrent STI including trichomoniasis, syphilis, gonorrhea, genital herpes, BV, or chlamydia, and their HIV is not virally suppressed
- When there is exposure to blood or bloody secretions, or when tears in the exposed mucous membranes are present
- With anal sex (especially for the receptive partner), relative to vaginal or oral sex

The risk of sexual transmission from a partner with HIV may be decreased or eliminated under the following circumstances:

- If the partner with HIV is being treated with antiretroviral medication and plasma HIV viral load is undetectable, the partner cannot transmit HIV sexually.
- If an HIV-negative partner's penis is circumcised, their risk of acquiring HIV from insertive sex is reduced by approximately half.

Advice for Patients Seeking Contraceptive Services

Note that when creating written materials, prioritize health literacy, language, and cultural considerations. Until further data are available, it is prudent to advise all patients as follows:

- For vaginal or anal intercourse, use latex or plastic condoms each time you suspect any risk of exposure to HIV. Consider use of HIV PrEP.
- For oral sex, use latex or plastic condoms for fellatio and latex or plastic vulvar barriers for cunnilingus any time you suspect any risk of HIV.
- Vaginal spermicides do not protect against HIV or other STIs.
- Any tissue damage to the vulva, vagina, anus, or penis could increase susceptibility to HIV. Avoid any intercourse until lesions are healed.

HIV Testing and Counseling

Reproductive health care providers represent the most important access point for patients to receive HIV testing. Thus, HIV testing should be a standard component of care.

When To Offer Testing

Routinely offer HIV testing to *all adolescents and adults* between the ages 15 to 64 if they have never been tested previously. Routine HIV testing for all pregnant patients already is the standard of care in the United States.[51] Certain situations outside the prenatal setting call for health care providers to (1) make strong recommendations in favor of testing and (2) undertake extra efforts to assure patients have reasonable access to counseling and testing services, and PEP, if needed:

- Patient's request
- Known sexual exposure to a person with HIV
- Shared injection equipment with a person with HIV
- Possible recent occupational exposure
- Clinical settings with a ≥ 1% HIV seroprevalence
- Settings serving "populations at increased behavioral or clinical HIV risk," such as STI clinics, teen clinics with high rates of RTIs, or correctional facilities, regardless of that setting's HIV seroprevalence
- Clinical signs or symptoms suggesting HIV infection (e.g., fever or illness of unknown origin, opportunistic infection without known reason for immune suppression)
- Diagnosis suggesting increased risk for HIV (such as another RTI or blood-borne infection)

Prenatal Testing

Many patients learn they have HIV when testing is done as part of routine prenatal care. Prospective studies have indicated that pregnancy itself also confers an increased risk of acquiring HIV infection.[52]

Counseling about pregnancy options is an especially important component of posttest counseling if the HIV diagnosis is made early in pregnancy; the patient may be overwhelmed by the news, and by the amount of information to absorb. Pregnant patients with HIV are faced with the same sorts of reproductive decisions as those without HIV, with similar percentages of terminated pregnancies and live births. For the patient with HIV who chooses to continue the pregnancy, refer to a specialist with expertise in managing HIV in pregnancy.

Test Counseling

Reproductive health care providers should be prepared to explain how the test is done, what the routine screening procedure will and will not reveal, implications of anonymous vs. confidential testing, and instructions on how to obtain test results. A guide (**Table 23-7**) for providing this information and for giving negative and positive test results may be helpful.

Table 23-7 Components of Counseling in the Setting of HIV Testing

Deciding whether to have the test

- Your right to decide whether to be tested
- Voluntary informed consent (some settings may offer opt-out testing)
- Who will see the results if test is done at clinic site; state law implications
- Anonymous sites for testing; home test options

Benefits of being tested

- Peace of mind, knowing one's status
- If results are positive:
  - Options for HIV therapy, managing related problems
  - Prevention of transmission to others
  - Make informed childbearing decisions
  - Diagnose illness or symptoms
  - Access assistance programs
  - Referral to an expert in clinical HIV care

Difficulties with being tested

- Learning you have a serious illness
- Disclosing results to sex or injection drug equipment–sharing partners (public health departments can provide help with this task)

What results mean

- If positive:
  - You have HIV in your body
  - You can pass the virus on to other people
  - You need to establish care with knowledgeable provider and undergo further assessment
- If negative or indeterminate:
  - You do not have HIV, or
  - You have HIV, but you are in a window period before testing becomes positive

Reducing risk for HIV

- Offer to develop a personalized risk-reduction plan
- Offer condoms and other safer sex supplies
- Referral for substance or alcohol use disorder treatment
- If testing is negative, consider using pre-exposure prophylaxis (PrEP)

Counseling and Testing Issues

Confidentiality. Confidential testing is name-linked, and information is protected to a degree determined by state law and, at the testing site, by formal policies and staff commitment to confidentiality.

Testing technology. Recommendations for laboratory-based HIV testing involve testing serum with a dual antigen/antibody immunoassay followed, if positive, by confirmation with an HIV-1/HIV-2 differentiation assay, or in uncertain cases, an HIV nucleic acid test (**Figure 23-1**). While the antigen/antibody and differentiation assays are both are very sensitive and specific, neither is perfect, so an HIV test is reported as positive only after obtaining positive results from both the screening and confirmatory tests. As with any test, prevalence of the infection within the client's population is the major factor in determining a test's predictive value; the higher the prevalence, the greater the likelihood that a positive test result means that the person truly has HIV. Always regard HIV test results in the context of the patient history and clinical picture and re-evaluate when they are not in agreement.

Clinic-based point-of-care tests and home-based rapid antibody testing are all FDA-approved and provide sensitivity and specificity comparable to those of traditional tests. Updated information on the types of tests available for rapid HIV testing

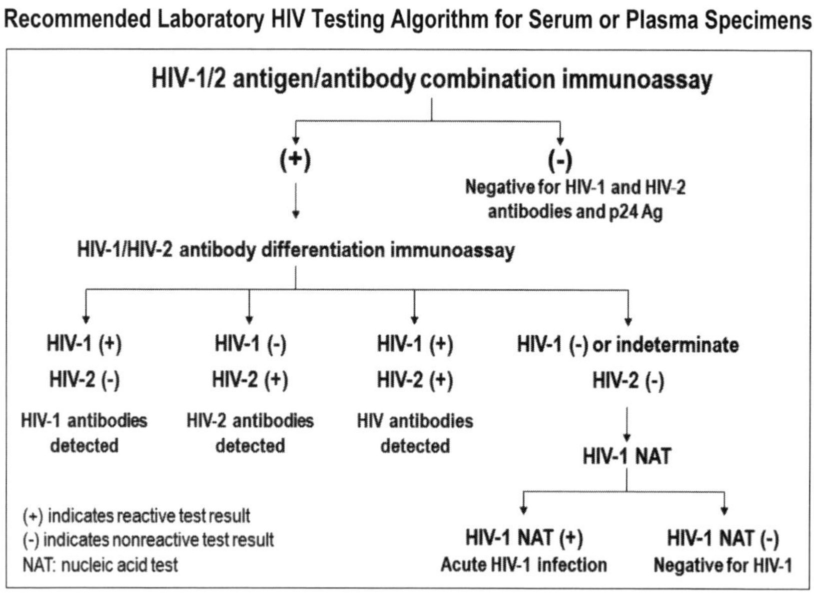

Figure 23-1 The 2018 Quick Reference Guide: Recommended laboratory HIV testing algorithm for serum or plasma specimens.

National Center for HIV/AIDS, Viral Hepatitis, and TB Prevention (US). Division of HIV/AIDS Prevention. Association of Public Health Laboratories. January 2018.

Note: This 2018 document is to be used in conjunction with the 2014 document Laboratory Testing for the Diagnosis for the Diagnosis of HIV Infection.

Reproduced from National Center for HIV/AIDS, Viral Hepatitis, and TB Prevention (U.S.). Division of HIV/AIDS Prevention.; Association of Public Health Laboratories. .2018 Quick reference guide: Recommended laboratory HIV testing algorithm for serum or plasma specimens; 2018. This 2018 document is to be used in conjunction with the 2014 document. Available free of charge from https://stacks.cdc.gov/view/cdc/50872. Reference to specific commercial products, manufacturers, companies, or trademarks does not constitute its endorsement or recommendation by the U.S. Government, Department of Health and Human Services, or Centers for Disease Control and Prevention.

can be found for clinic-based settings at https://www.cdc.gov/hiv/pdf/testing/rapid-hiv-tests-clinical-moderate-complexity.pdf

For rapid HIV testing outside of clinic settings, see https://www.cdc.gov/hiv/pdf/testing/rapid-hiv-tests-non-clinical.pdf

Documentation of HIV Test Results

Recording HIV test results is important for ongoing medical care, although minimizing any risk to confidentiality should be prioritized. State and local professional associations may offer guidance for appropriate, lawful charting that does not compromise the patient, provider, or health care delivery. However, many states require reporting when HIV is detected; specific information is available at https://www.cdc.gov/hiv/guidelines/reporting.html.

Clinical Characteristics of HIV Infection

The current standard of care for HIV is antiretroviral therapy (ART), a combination of antiretroviral agents that inhibit different targets of the virus. ART regimens can be composed of drugs from two, three, or more classes, including nucleoside analog reverse transcriptase inhibitors (NRTIs), non-nucleoside reverse transcriptase inhibitors (NNRTIs), protease inhibitors (PIs), and integrase strand transfer inhibitors; CCR-5 inhibitors and fusion inhibitors are used less commonly, largely in the setting of viral resistance.

ART should be initiated and managed by—or in close consultation with—an experienced HIV clinician in order to optimize care and achieve a high likelihood of adherence, which is the main determinant of future success. HIV mutation and resistance can occur if the patient is not adherent with the regimen. While single daily dosing regimens and formulations that combine agents from several classes are the standard of care and have greatly simplified the approach to treatment, side effects may still occur. Still, early initiation of therapy (e.g., on the day of diagnosis) is beneficial for patients, regardless of their CD4 count at the time of diagnosis.[53] Viral load testing uses DNA or RNA detection assays to measure the actual amount of HIV in plasma, permitting an accurate determination of real-time viral activity and a rapid assessment of antiretroviral drug efficacy. For complete information on recommended regimens, see www.aidsinfo.nih.gov/guidelines/.

Reproductive health care ideally would be managed in the primary care/HIV care setting also, but in some cases, these are two providers in two different sites, so careful attention to shared information, shared decision making, and collaboration is essential. Advice on medical management of patients with HIV is available from the National HIV/AIDS Clinicians' Consultation Center based at the University of California at San Francisco. This no-cost "warmline" is staffed Monday through Friday from 6:00 a.m. to 5:00 p.m. Pacific Time, and voicemail is available 24 hours a day, 7 days a week at 1.800.933.3413.

Gynecologic Management in HIV-Positive Patients

The keys to successful management of gynecologic infections among patients with HIV are a high index of suspicion, prompt diagnosis, aggressive treatment, and primary or secondary prophylaxis when appropriate. **Table 23-8** outlines general stages of HIV infection and related concerns; a discussion of some specific conditions follows.[58]

Table 23-8 Contraception for the HIV-Positive Patient

Method	Possible Benefits	Possible Drawbacks
Oral Contraceptives	■ Good effectiveness with consistent use ■ Less blood loss to avoid anemia	■ Unclear interaction of steroids and immune function ■ Possible interaction with certain antibiotics, antiretrovirals, other drugs ■ No RTI protection ■ No HIV protection for partner
Depo-Provera	Good low-maintenance effectiveness	■ Unclear interaction of steroids and immune function ■ No RTI function ■ No HIV protection for partner
IUD	Good low-maintenance effectiveness	■ Risk of infection during insertion interval ■ No RTI protection ■ No HIV protection for partner ■ Increased days of bleeding, possible anemia (copper IUD only)
Diaphragm	Some RTI protection for the cervix	■ Increases vulnerability to urinary tract infections for some users ■ Requires good technique
External, Internal Condom	Good RTI protection, HIV protection for partner	■ Male condom requires partner cooperation; partner cooperation helpful with female condom ■ Requires good technique
Permanent Contraception	Good low-maintenance efficacy for women who desire no more children	■ No RTI protection ■ No HIV protection for partner

Data from US Medical Eligibility Criteria for Contraceptive Use, 2016. https://www.cdc.gov/reproductivehealth/contraception/mmwr/mec/summary.html

Vulvovaginal Candidiasis (VVC). VVC is common in patients with HIV and may recur frequently if immune status deteriorates. Non–*Candida albicans* species may be involved and may be less responsive to topical imidazole or oral azole therapy. First-line treatment is a 7-day course of one of the topical imidazole antifungal agents, oral fluconazole (a single dose, 150 mg orally), or oral itraconazole.[54] Boric acid may be useful for infections with resistant *Candida* species.

Human Papillomavirus and Cervical Disease. Genital warts caused by certain types of HPV (types 6 and 11) may progress more rapidly with immune compromise. Patients with HIV have significantly higher rates of cytology-detected abnormalities, cervical intraepithelial neoplasia, and progression to cervical cancer relative to HIV-negative patients.

- Patients with HIV < 30 years of age: Patients 21–29 years old should have a cervical cytology test at the time of initial diagnosis with HIV. If the initial cytology result is negative, the next cytology test should be in 12 months. If the results of three consecutive cytology tests are negative, follow-up cytology tests should be every 3 years. Co-testing (cytology and an HPV test) is not recommended for HIV-infected patients < 30 years of age.
- Patients with HIV 30 years of age and older: can be screened with either cytology testing only or cytology testing and HPV co-testing. For screening with cytology tests alone, patients should have a cytology test at the time of HIV-diagnosis (baseline), then every 12 months. If the results of three consecutive cytology tests are normal, follow-up cytology tests should be completed every 3 years.
    - If co-testing with cytology and HPV is available, then co-testing can be done at the time of diagnosis or age 30. Co-test–negative patients (i.e., a negative cytology and HPV tests) should have their next cervical cancer screening in 3 years. Those who are cytology negative but positive for HPV should have repeat co-testing in 1 year (unless genotype testing for 16 or 16/18 is positive). If either of the co-tests at 1 year is abnormal (i.e., abnormal cytology or positive HPV), referral to colposcopy is recommended.
    - If the initial HPV results identify HPV16 or HPV16/18, then referral to colposcopy is recommended. If the HPV testing is positive, but the genotype specific testing for HPV16 or HPV16/18 is negative, then repeat co-testing in 1 year is recommended. If either of the co-tests at 1 year is abnormal (i.e., abnormal cytology or positive HPV), referral to colposcopy is recommended.

Cervical cancer screening should continue throughout the patient's lifetime, and not stop at age 65 as in the general population.

Recommendations for management of abnormal cytology in patients with HIV are available at https://clinicalinfo.hiv.gov/en/guidelines/adult-and-adolescent-opportunistic-infection/human-papillomavirus-disease?view=full

Finally, while the nonavalent HPV vaccine has not been extensively studied in patients with HIV, the vaccine is protein-based (no live virus) and currently is recommended for all persons with HIV between 9 and 26 years of age with shared decision making advised for individuals 27–45 years of age, according to ACIP guidelines.

See Chapter 24, Screening for Cervical, Ovarian, and Breast Cancer for more information on screening for cervical precancer.

Pelvic Inflammatory Disease (PID). In general, PID does not require more aggressive treatment for patients with HIV, but the approach should be individualized. Depending on the severity of PID and immune status, providers should consider parenteral therapy and hospitalization, based on similar factors and considerations for patients without HIV.

Genital Herpes. In the presence of immune dysfunction, herpes lesions may be more extensive, more painful, atypical in location or appearance, and slower to heal. In a large study in Africa, suppressive therapy with twice daily oral acyclovir was associated with a reduction in plasma HIV viral load relative to placebo.[59]

Benefits of suppressive therapy include reduction of symptomatic outbreaks, reduction in risk of HSV-2 transmission to sex partners (demonstrated in heterosexual couples), and possibly, a favorable effect on HIV itself due to direct activity against HIV. Symptomatic episodes of genital herpes should be treated in accordance with standard guidelines for people with HIV.

Psychological Care and Support for Patients with HIV

People with HIV often experience significant psychosocial stress. They will often need guidance, support, and referral to assist with concerns that may include stable housing, economic stability, childcare, and substance use.

Reproductive Health Care for Patients with HIV

For patients with HIV, the decision about whether to get pregnant is similar to that of HIV-negative patients, and their desire for a child often is profound. Counseling patients who are pregnant or contemplating pregnancy includes important medical issues:

- Impact of HIV on pregnancy
- Impact of pregnancy on HIV progression
- Effect of antiretroviral medication and other drugs on both the patient and developing fetus
- Risk of perinatal transmission and options for reducing risk
- Risk of breast/chest feeding for HIV transmission
- Course of HIV in perinatally infected infants
- Access to HIV-experienced obstetric and pediatric care
- Access to antiretroviral medications

Counseling for pregnancy optimally includes a full understanding of the patient's personal goals, support network, stressors in their life, and overall physical and emotional status. Once this groundwork is in place, guide the patient through specific questions to help them predict how they would feel, how others would feel, and what might happen. (See Chapter 4, Person-Centered Reproductive Health Conversations and Contraceptive Counseling.)

Patients with HIV who do not wish to become pregnant are more likely to succeed with a contraceptive method they have chosen for themselves and feel comfortable using (Table 23-8). (See Chapter 4, Person-Centered Reproductive Health Conversations and Contraceptive Counseling.) In addition to contraception, patients may also wish to lower risk of HIV transmission to partners (if applicable), and lower risk of STI acquisition. Adding either external or internal condoms will decrease risk of STI transmission/acquisition and increase effectiveness of other contraceptive methods.

Thousands of patients with HIV give birth each year in the United States. Generally, patients with HIV with competent immune systems have uneventful pregnancies with normal labor and delivery. Just as with any patient with a serious systemic illness, patients with HIV may have complicated pregnancies, including prematurity, low birth weight, and premature rupture of membranes. However, factors other than HIV may influence poor birth outcomes, including effects of poverty, lack of access to prenatal care, or substance use. Pregnancy itself does not appear to speed HIV progression.

Risks of HIV Transmission in the Perinatal Period

Without ART, each child born to someone with HIV in the United States faces approximately a 25% risk of being infected in utero, during birth, or while breast/chest feeding. With ART, the risk falls to 2% or less (see below).

Reducing Perinatal Transmission Risk. Strategies to reduce perinatal HIV transmission continue to evolve rapidly. ART is recommended for all pregnant patients with the goal of suppressing plasma HIV RNA to undetectable levels. ART also is recommended for HIV-exposed infants in their first weeks of life. ART initiation for this purpose may be delayed until the second trimester.

Labor and Delivery. In the absence of breast/chest feeding, an estimated 60% to 75% of perinatal HIV transmissions occur around the time of labor and delivery, and a number of strategies can reduce exposure of the neonate to blood and secretions. In addition to intrapartum ART, suggested approaches include ART treatment throughout pregnancy to lower viral shedding at term, avoidance of intrapartum invasive procedures, and cesarean delivery. Scheduled cesarean delivery before rupture of membranes is recommended for patients whose HIV viral load at 36 weeks or later is above 1,000 copies/mL. Avoid delays in delivery once membranes have ruptured. The risk of perinatal HIV transmission can double when fetal membranes rupture more than 4 hours before delivery.

Breast/Chest Feeding. Currently in the United States, bottle-feeding is recommended for infants to reduce the risk of postnatal HIV transmission via breast milk. The precise risk of HIV transmission via breast milk is difficult to quantify and is influenced by the stage of the HIV disease (with high viral loads during primary infection and late-stage disease), use of ART, breast/chest feeding patterns, and other factors. Approximately 10% to 15% of vertical transmissions are associated with breast/chest feeding. (See Chapter 19, Contraception After Pregnancy.) Little is known about the impact of breast/chest feeding on the birthing parent's nutritional status and overall health, or about the immunoprotective qualities of the breast milk produced by an immunocompromised patient.

SUMMARY OF MAJOR REPRODUCTIVE TRACT INFECTIONS (OTHER THAN HIV) BY SYNDROME

Vulvovaginal Syndromes

Vulvovaginal complaints may be the most common reasons for seeking medical attention from reproductive health care providers. These complaints range from changes in normal vaginal discharge (increased amount, abnormal odor or color) to vulvar pruritus or pain. While the number of conditions that may be responsible is broad, a solid knowledge of the conditions discussed here is essential in the reproductive health care setting.

Bacterial Vaginosis

BV is a clinical syndrome in which several species of vaginal bacteria (including *Gardnerella vaginalis* and other anaerobes) replace the normal hydrogen peroxide–producing *Lactobacillus* species. BV is a sexually associated condition, but it is not usually considered a specific STI; however, it probably results at least initially from transfer of the associated bacteria from a sex partner who harbors them. For example, BV occurs frequently in women who regularly have sex with women, and BV-associated bacteria have been consistently detected on the scrotum and penis, especially underneath the foreskin. While treatment of male partners has not been effective in improving cure rates or decreasing recurrence rates for BV, the concept continues to be studied. Because of the increased risk for postoperative infectious complications associated with BV, screening prior to pelvic surgery is recommended (for example, hysterectomy). Prior to surgical abortion, providers can consider screening and treating for BV in addition to providing routine antibiotic prophylaxis (with an anti-chlamydial regimen such as doxycycline). Guidelines for BV screening prior to medication abortion are lacking, but there are no data to support this practice.[61]

Symptoms and Diagnosis. Excessive or malodorous discharge is a common finding. Erythema, edema, and pruritus of the external genitalia may be observed. The clinical diagnosis of BV is made if three of the following four (Amsel) criteria are present:

1. Increased amounts of white or grey homogenous discharge
2. Elevated vaginal pH (greater than 4.5)
3. Fishy odor after addition of 10% KOH
4. Identification of clue cells (small coccobacillary organisms associated with epithelial cells) on saline wet mount (> 20% of vaginal epithelial cells)

Alternatively, rapid tests that detect high numbers of *G. vaginalis* bacteria, or byproducts of anaerobic metabolism such as sialidase, also are available. Primarily used in research, a Gram stain of the vaginal discharge reveals the relative absence of lactobacilli with replacement by other anaerobic organisms. Cultures and NAAT such as polymerase chain reaction (PCR) for individual bacteria are not useful and should not be performed, though detection of bacteria in specific combinations and quantities using this technology can be useful, as discussed below.

There are multiple NAATs that provide a result based on measuring the combination of bacteria present in vaginal fluid for symptomatic patients. Two tests are FDA cleared: BD Max Vaginal Panel (Becton Dickinson) and Aptima BV (Hologic). Three tests are laboratory-developed: NuSwab VG (LabCorp), OneSwab BV Panel PCR with Lactobacillus Profiling by qPCR (Medical Diagnostic Laboratories), and SureSwab BV (Quest Diagnostics).

Treatment. Patients with symptomatic disease should be offered treatment. The three recommended regimens are:

1. Metronidazole, 500 mg orally twice daily for 7 days, OR
2. Metronidazole gel, 0.75%, one full applicator (5 g) vaginally at bedtime for 5 days, OR
3. Clindamycin cream, 2%, one full applicator (5 g) vaginally at bedtime for 7 days.

Other alternatives are oral clindamycin 300 mg two times a day for 7 days; clindamycin ovules 100 mg vaginally at bedtime for 3 days; secnidazole 2 g oral granules in a single dose; tinidazole 2 g orally once daily for 2 days; or tinidazole 1 g orally once daily for 5 days. In pregnancy, oral regimens generally are preferred.

Nitroimidazoles and alcohol. Prior recommendations to avoid alcohol with nitroimidazoles (e.g., metronidazole) were due to concerns of a disulfiram-like reaction when taken together. The 2021 CDC STI Guidelines[48] included a review of *in vitro* data, animal studies, adverse event reporting, and clinical studies, and concluded that there is no evidence of an interaction between alcohol and metronidazole. Therefore, patients do not need to refrain from alcohol use during metronidazole or tinidazole therapy (note that symptoms of gastrointestinal distress, nausea, vomiting, and dizziness may occur independently with either metronidazole or alcohol use).

Potential complications. Recurrent infections are common. BV is associated with an increased risk of PID and also may cause cervicitis. BV is associated with an increased risk of adverse pregnancy outcomes, including preterm delivery and low birth weight. BV increases risk of acquiring chlamydia, gonorrhea, trichomoniasis, and HIV, and of transmitting HIV to male sex partners.

Behavioral messages to emphasize. The use of external condoms by male partners has been associated with a reduced risk of recurrence of BV and may be a useful adjunct to antibiotic treatment, especially for patients with recurrent episodes of BV. Avoid douching, as this promotes loss of vaginal lactobacilli and likely exacerbates the problem. Exchange of vaginal fluid between sex partners should be minimized during treatment to prevent recurrences.

Trichomoniasis

Trichomoniasis is caused by *Trichomonas vaginalis*, a motile protozoan with an undulating membrane and four flagella. Trichomoniasis is the most common nonviral STI in the United States and worldwide. Each year an estimated 6.9 million US women become infected.

Screening. Screening is routinely recommended for sexually active females with HIV upon entry to HIV care, and annually thereafter. Females aged ≤ 35 years in correctional facilities should be screened for trichomonas at intake; annual screening can be considered thereafter. Screening can also be considered for females attending STI clinics, or those at elevated risk of infection (e.g., multiple partners, transactional sex, substance use, history of other STIs or incarceration).

Symptoms. Excessive, frothy, diffuse, yellow-green vaginal discharge can occur, although clinical presentation varies from no signs or symptoms to erythema, edema, and pruritus of the external genitalia. Dysuria and dyspareunia also are frequent. The type of symptoms or signs alone does not distinguish the microbial etiology. Sex partners with a penis may develop urethritis, balanitis or prostatitis; however, the majority are asymptomatic. Sex partners with a vagina may be either symptomatic or asymptomatic.

Diagnosis. Trichomoniasis is diagnosed when a vaginal culture, nucleic acid amplification test, or antigen test is positive for *T. vaginalis* OR typical motile trichomonads are identified in a saline wet mount of vaginal discharge. Trichomonads visualized on liquid-based cervical cytology (Pap smear) is specific (unlikely to be false positive), but cervical cytology should not be used as a screening test for trichomoniasis.

Treatment. Recommended treatment is metronidazole 500 mg orally twice daily for 7 days for vaginal infections and metronidazole 2 g orally in a single dose for penile infections. The alternative regimen for patients of all genders is tinidazole 2 g orally in a single dose. Most treatment failures are due to failure to treat the index patient's sex partners; initial management should include retreatment of the patient and partners with the same therapy they received for initial treatment. Metronidazole-resistant *T. vaginalis*, although uncommon, can occur. Most treatment failures respond to higher doses of metronidazole therapy or to a single dose of tinidazole (2 g). Additional regimens for persistent trichomonas are available from the CDC at https://www.cdc.gov/std/treatment-guidelines/trichomoniasis.htm. Sex partners should be simultaneously treated at the same time as t client, with 7 days of abstinence from vaginal sex.

Potential complications. Secondary excoriation may occur. Recurrent infections are common. Trichomoniasis has been associated with an increased risk of salpingitis, low birthweight, prematurity, and acquisition of HIV.

Behavioral messages to emphasize. Make sure sex partner(s) are treated. Abstain from vaginal sex for 7 days (the last day of therapy for 7-day regimens, or 7 days after a single dose regimen). Use condoms to prevent future infections.

Candidiasis

Candidiasis (VVC) is caused by *Candida* species—usually *C. albicans*—that are dimorphic fungi that grow as oval, budding yeast cells and as chains of cells (hyphae). *Candida* are normal flora of the skin, mouth, and vagina. VVC is not considered an STI; however, sex partners do exchange orogenital strains of *Candida*. Risk factors for VVC are incompletely understood, but include immunosuppressed states, glucose intolerance, and (in some patients) antibiotic therapy.

Symptoms. Clinical presentation includes whitish vaginal discharge and erythema, edema, and pruritus of the external genitalia. Symptoms or signs alone do not distinguish the microbial etiology. Sex partners may develop balanitis or cutaneous lesions on the penis.

Diagnosis. The presumptive criteria are typical clinical symptoms of vulvovaginitis and microscopic identification of yeast forms (budding cells) or pseudohyphae in potassium hydroxide (KOH) wet-mount preparations of vaginal discharge. VVC is definitively diagnosed when a vaginal culture is positive for *C. albicans* or other *Candida* species in the presence of symptoms. Because up to 40% of patients are vaginally colonized with *Candida* species in the absence of VVC, cultures are not recommended unless chronic suppressive therapy is under consideration, in which case they are used to confirm the etiology and susceptibility to antifungal agents Several commercial laboratories offer PCR-based testing for *Candida* species, providers should be familiar with performance characteristics of these tests prior to use, as most are not FDA-approved.

Treatment. Single-dose oral fluconazole, 150 mg, is a convenient therapy. In addition, many topical formulations provide effective candidiasis treatment. Examples include miconazole vaginal suppositories, 200 mg intravaginally at bedtime for 3 days; OR miconazole, 2%, vaginal cream, one full applicator (5 g) intravaginally at bedtime for 3 days (and applied externally for vulvitis); OR clotrimazole vaginal tablets, 100 mg intravaginally, daily for 3 days; OR butoconazole cream, 2%, 5 g intravaginally for 3 days. A variety of other effective treatment regimens exist. In general, more severe infections may need treatment of longer duration. Over-the-counter preparations for intravaginal administration of miconazole, clotrimazole, and butaconazole are available. Resistant VVC may respond to treatment with boric acid, provided as 600 mg in a type O gelatin capsule administered vaginally once daily for 2 weeks (avoid in pregnancy).

Potential complications. Secondary excoriation may occur. Recurrent infections are common, particularly with antibiotic use, immunosuppression, or diabetes.

Behavioral messages to emphasize. Wear a sanitary pad to protect clothing if using topical treatment. Change pads frequently. To reduce moisture in the area, avoid panty hose, tight fitting clothing, and non-cotton underwear. Store suppositories in a refrigerator. Continue taking medicine even during menses.

Other Causes of Noninfectious Vaginitis that Reproductive Health Clinicians Might Encounter

Desquamative inflammatory vaginitis (DIV) is a relatively uncommon, but probably underdiagnosed, form of vaginitis characterized by copious, purulent (green or yellow) vaginal discharge, typically accompanied by vulvovaginal pain or burning and dyspareunia. DIV may be more common in older (peri- or postmenopausal) patients, though the epidemiology is poorly defined. Occasionally, frank vestibulitis or excoriations will occur. On examination of vaginal fluid, the characteristic findings are copious white blood cells, elevated vaginal pH (usually 5.5 to 7.4), few lactobacilli, and numerous gram-positive cocci. Group B *Streptococcus* may be involved in the pathogenesis of this condition; however, it is thought to be most likely an inflammatory or possibly autoimmune process, rather than a response to infection. Treatment uses antibiotics to reduce inflammation (not eradicate bacteria), and includes a prolonged course of clindamycin 2% cream administered vaginally at bedtime, usually given for at least 14 days OR 10% hydrocortisone cream 5 g administered nightly at bedtime for at least 14 days (often requires a compounding pharmacy). Longer courses of therapy are often required.

Irritant/chemical vaginitis occurs commonly, though few population-based data are available. Any substance that can elicit a mucosal inflammatory response, including douches, lubricants, spermicides, soaps or other cleansing agents, or other feminine-hygiene products, can be responsible if administered vaginally. This condition may result in vaginal discharge characterized by numerous white blood cells (WBCs). When evaluating a patient with vulvovaginal complaints, take a careful history of use of any vaginal products or of products applied directly to the vulva.

Discrete Genital Lesions: Genital Ulcer Diseases (GUD), Including Genital Herpes and Warts

Genital ulceration is often caused by STIs, especially herpes, which is the leading cause of this condition worldwide. The other main cause is syphilis. Chancroid is very uncommon in the United States but should be suspected if herpes has been ruled out and there is a painful, single ulcer with inguinal lymphadenopathy, particularly if the patient reports transactional sex. Two other STIs that may involve GUD are lymphogranuloma venereum (LGV), discussed in the section on chlamydia, and granuloma inguinale. Granuloma inguinale (also known as donavanosis) is caused by a bacteria called *Klebsiella granulomatis* and is rare in the United States. Initially, single or multiple subcutaneous nodules appear at the site of inoculation. Nodules erode to form granulomatous, heaped ulcers that are painless, bleed on contact, and enlarge slowly. It has been referred to as a "flesh-eating" STI because of the tissue destruction that can result from infection. The typical clinical presentation is sufficient to suggest the diagnosis.

Genital Herpes

Genital herpes is caused by HSV types 1 and 2, DNA viruses that cannot be distinguished clinically; however, initial infection with HSV-1 typically is less severe and causes less frequent recurrences (sometimes none) relative to HSV-2. HSV-2 is responsible for nearly all recurrent genital herpes.

Prevalence. Incident (or initial) HSV-2 infections affect an estimated 572,000 persons each year in the United States. An estimated 18.6 million Americans are currently infected with genital HSV-2, though most infections are asymptomatic.[58] Persons without symptoms transmit most HSV infections.

Symptoms. Some individuals will experience a prodrome prior to developing anogenital symptoms, including systemic symptoms such as headache, myalgias, and/or fatigue, as well as local symptoms such as itching, tingling, or skin hypersensitivity. During an outbreak, single or multiple vesicles, which are usually pruritic, can appear anywhere on the anogenital region. Vesicles spontaneously rupture to form shallow ulcers that may be very painful. Lesions resolve spontaneously with minimal scarring. The first clinical occurrence is termed the first episode infection (mean duration 12 days). Subsequent, usually milder, occurrences are termed recurrent infections (mean duration 4.5 days). The interval between clinical episodes is termed latency. Viral shedding from the cervix, vulva, or penile skin occurs intermittently without clinical symptoms during latency. HSV-2 genital infections are more likely to recur than are HSV-1 infections, thus identification of the type of infecting virus at initial infection has prognostic value.

Diagnosis. When typical genital lesions are present or a pattern of recurrence has developed, suspect herpes infection. HSV nucleic acid amplification tests can provide type-specific results from genital or other mucocutaneous lesions and are the most sensitive diagnostic tests. HSV viral culture has low sensitivity, particularly for recurrent lesions; sensitivity declines rapidly as lesions begin to heal. Tzanck preparation, which detects cellular changes associated with HSV, is insensitive and nonspecific and is not recommended for diagnosis. Type-specific HSV serologic assays may help in diagnosis for patients with a history of recurrent anogenital symptoms, and in management of sex partners of those with HSV.

Treatment. No cure for HSV exists; however, antiviral drugs are helpful in reducing or suppressing symptoms. Oral administration is effective both in treating clinically symptomatic episodes and in suppressing or reducing recurrent outbreaks.

Topical therapy is ineffective. Initial episodes can be treated with any of the following oral regimens, each given for 7–10 days, although treatment can be extended if healing is incomplete after 10 days of therapy:

- Acyclovir: 400 mg three times per day, OR
- Famciclovir: 250 mg three times per day, OR
- Valacyclovir: 1 g twice daily

  Recurrent infections can be treated with any of the following oral regimens:
- Acyclovir
  - 800 mg twice daily for 5 days, OR
  - 800 mg three times per day for 2 days
- Famciclovir
  - 125 mg twice daily for 5 days, OR
  - 1000 mg twice daily for 1 day, OR
  - 500 mg initial dose, then 250 mg twice daily for 2 days
- Valacyclovir
  - 500 mg twice daily for 3 days, OR
  - 1 g once a day for 5 days.

Daily prophylaxis with valacyclovir taken by HSV-infected persons reduces the risk of transmission to uninfected partners. Regimens given orally to prevent recurrences include the following (these regimens have been shown to be safe for long periods [years], so the duration of prophylaxis may be tailored to the individual patient's situation).

- Acyclovir 400 mg twice daily OR
- Famciclovir 250 mg twice daily OR
- Valacyclovir
  - 500 mg once a day OR
  - 1 g once a day.

(Valacylovir 500 mg once a day may be less effective than the higher-dose regimen or acyclovir regimen for patients with $\geq$ 10 recurrences per year)

Famciclovir and valacyclovir offer more convenient dosing but are not more effective clinically at treating symptomatic disease than acyclovir; however, famciclovir is less effective at suppressing subclinical shedding. For persons infected with HIV, increased dosages and/or extended duration of therapy is recommended.[59]

Potential complications. HSV infection can cause neuralgia, meningitis, ascending myelitis, urinary retention, urethral strictures, and lymphatic suppuration. These outcomes generally are more common in the female genital tract. Disseminated HSV also can cause severe hepatitis in pregnancy and may not be associated with genital or skin lesions. Pregnancy loss and preterm delivery have been associated with HSV infections, usually in primary infection occurring in the third trimester.

Neonates. During vaginal delivery, virus from an active genital infection can cause neonatal herpes. This condition ranges in severity from clinically inapparent infections to local infections of the eyes, skin, or mucous membranes or to severely disseminated infection that may involve the central nervous system. Full-blown neonatal herpes has a high fatality rate, and survivors often have ocular or neurologic sequelae.

Behavioral messages to emphasize. Because both the initial and recurrent HSV lesions shed high concentrations of the virus, abstain from sexual activity while ulcers are present and during the prodrome period prior to an outbreak. However, most genital HSV transmission occurs during asymptomatic intervals. Condoms offer protection from HSV acquisition during vaginal sex: a 65% reduction in transmission from females-to-males, and 96% reduction from males to females.[19] Prophylactic acyclovir and valacyclovir reduce HSV transmission. The risk of transmission to the neonate is highest with primary herpes infection (the first time they have been infected with either HSV-1 or HSV-2) during the third trimester, lower with nonprimary first episodes (first recognized outbreak, but patient with prior HSV antibodies) of the disease, and lowest with recurrent herpes. At the onset of labor, patients should be asked about symptoms and examined for lesions. If no symptoms or signs are present, the infant may be delivered vaginally. Infants delivered through an infected birth canal should be tested and followed carefully. Genital herpes (and other diseases causing genital ulcers) have been associated with an increased risk of acquiring HIV infections. Clinically evaluating asymptomatic partners has little value for preventing transmission of HSV.

Syphilis

Syphilis is caused by *Treponema pallidum*, a spirochete with 6 to 14 regular spirals and characteristic motility.

Prevalence. Primary and secondary syphilis, as well as congenital syphilis, are currently increasing dramatically across the United States. While the burden of syphilis is highest among men who have sex with men, rates of syphilis among reproductive-age women (15–44 years) nearly tripled between 2015 and 2019 (3.2 to 8.7 cases per 100,000 population).

In the United States, southeastern and western states have the highest rates of both syphilis and congenital syphilis. Early detection and treatment are key to avoid serious sequelae, particularly in pregnancy.

Symptoms

Primary. The classical chancre is a painless, indurated ulcer, located at the site of exposure (e.g., genitals, rectum, oral cavity). However, patients can present with multiple ulcers, and ulcers can be painful, especially if they are secondarily infected. Therefore, the differential diagnosis for all genital lesions should include syphilis.

Secondary. Patients may have a highly variable skin rash, mucous patches, condylomata lata (fleshy, moist tissue growths), lymphadenopathy, alopecia, or other signs.

Latent. Patients are without clinical signs of infection.

Diagnosis. The 2021 CDC STI Treatment Guidelines[50] discuss the types of serologic testing that are available. Serology is the mainstay of syphilis diagnosis and requires two types of reactive tests to confirm an initial diagnosis: nontreponemal tests (e.g., rapid plasma reagin test [RPR] and Venereal Disease Research Laboratory [VDRL]) and treponemal tests (e.g., *T. pallidum* particle agglutination, treponemal immunoassays). Refer to the 2021 CDC STI Treatment Guidelines[50] for more details about testing algorithms and interpretation of serology results.

The clinical presentation by stage is as follows:

Primary. Patients have lesion(s) (genital ulcers/chancres) and may have reactive treponemal serology (e.g., EIA and/or TP-PA) and reactive RPR (although RPR may be negative in early primary syphilis); or they have been exposed to syphilis within 90 days of lesion onset.

Primary and secondary syphilis can be definitively diagnosed by demonstrating *T. pallidum* with darkfield microscopy or fluorescent antibody technique in material from a chancre, lymph node, or other lesion, but access to these diagnostics is very limited.

Secondary. Patients have a typical clinical presentation (rash, mucocutaneous lesions, lymphadenopathy) and reactive serologic tests (RPR titers will often be high). If present, condyloma lata will be darkfield positive.

Latent. Patients have serologic evidence of syphilis (reactive treponemal and nontreponemal tests) without clinical signs.

Treatment

Primary, secondary, or early latent syphilis of less than 1 year duration. Benzathine penicillin G 2.4 million units IM in a single dose. Alternative regimens include ceftriaxone 1 g IV or IM daily for 10 days.

Syphilis of indeterminate length or of more than 1 year duration. Benzathine penicillin G 7.2 million units total; 2.4 million units IM, weekly, for 3 successive weeks.

Patients allergic to penicillin. Doxycycline 100 mg orally two times a day. [Note: Duration of therapy depends on the estimated duration of infection. If duration has been less than 1 year, treat the infection for 14 days; otherwise, treat for 28 days.] For penicillin-allergic pregnant patients or for doxycycline-intolerant individuals, consult the 2021 CDC STI Treatment Guidelines.[48]

Congenital syphilis. Refer to the 2021 CDC STI Treatment Guidelines.[48]

Potential complications. Late syphilis and congenital syphilis, both of which are complications of early syphilis, are preventable with prompt diagnosis and treatment. Sequelae of late syphilis include neurosyphilis (general paresis, tabes dorsalis, and focal neurologic signs), cardiovascular syphilis (thoracic aortic aneurism, aortic insufficiency), and localized gumma formation.

Behavioral messages to emphasize. Follow-up to monitor response to treatment is critical and involves periodic testing. Timing of repeat testing depends on stage of disease, pregnancy status, and HIV status. (Refer to the CDC STI Treatment Guidelines.[48] For early syphilis (primary, secondary, early latent), sex partner(s) from the prior 90 days should be evaluated and treated. Avoid sexual activity until treatment is completed, or at least 7 days if treated with benzathine penicillin injection.

Human Papillomavirus

Human papillomavirus (HPV) is a common DNA virus that includes over 200 types, with 40 types specific to the human genital tract, stratified as low- or high-risk depending on oncogenic potential. HPV can be transmitted sexually as well as through nonpenetrative skin-to-skin contact. Two major clinical syndromes arise from these infections: genital warts and epithelial (cervical, vulvar, vagina, anal) neoplasia. HPV vaccination should be a standard practice in reproductive health care. Genital warts are discussed below; cervical neoplasia is discussed in Chapter 24.

Genital Warts

Genital warts (condyloma accuminata) are caused by several low-risk types of human papillomavirus (HPV). Types 6 and 11 cause 90% of genital warts.

Prevalence. Nearly every sexually active person will be exposed to HPV, and the CDC estimates that there are currently 42.5 million people infected. Genital warts are a common RTI, but they can be prevented effectively with HPV vaccination. In the postvaccine era, condyloma diagnoses have decreased significantly by 31% to 67% (RR 0.33, 95% CI 0.24–0.46) among girls and women aged 15–29 years; among boys and men aged 15–24 years, diagnoses have decreased significantly by 32% to 48%. Risk for condyloma includes earlier onset of sexual activity, multiple sex partners, and a higher frequency of casual relationships.

Symptoms. Single or multiple soft, fleshy, papillary or sessile, painless keratinized growths appear around the vulvovaginal area, penis, anus, urethra, or perineum. Condyloma may manifest as typical growths on the walls of the vagina or cervix, and patients may be unaware of their existence. Regular genital self-examinations may be helpful in detecting such growths on the external genitalia.

Diagnosis. No evidence supports the use of HPV DNA tests in the routine diagnosis or management of visible genital warts. A diagnosis is made from the typical clinical signs on the external genitalia. Colposcopy may be valuable for diagnosing flat warts, which are difficult to see. Exclude the possible diagnosis of condylomata lata by obtaining a serologic test for syphilis. A biopsy usually is unnecessary but can be done if the diagnosis is in question. When neoplasia is a possibility, take a biopsy of any atypical lesions or persistent warts before initiating therapy.

Treatment. Several different treatment regimens can be used, depending on client preference, available resources, and the experience of the health care provider. None of the currently available treatments is superior to others or ideal for all patients. The currently available treatments for visible genital warts consist of two types: (1) patient-applied therapies and (2) provider-administered therapies.

Patient-applied therapies include:

- *Podofilox 0.5% solution or gel.* Patients apply podofilox solution with a cotton swab, or a podofilox gel with a finger, to visible genital warts twice daily for 3 days, followed by 4 days of no therapy. This process may be repeated up to a total of 4 times. Podofilox should not be used during pregnancy.
- *Imiquimod 3.75% or 5% cream.* Patients should apply imiquimod 3.75% cream with a finger, at bedtime nightly for up to 8 weeks. Imiquimod 5% cream is applied at bedtime, 3 times a week, for up to 16 weeks. For both formulations, patients should wash the area with mild soap and water after 6 to 10 hours. Imiquimod should not be used during pregnancy.
- *Sinecatechins 15% ointment.* Ointment should be applied to each wart 3 times daily, for up to 16 weeks. It should not be washed off after use.

Provider-administered therapies include:

- *Cryotherapy* with liquid nitrogen or cryoprobe. Repeat applications every 1 to 2 weeks.
- *Trichloroacetic acid (TCA) or bichloroacetic acid (BCA)* 80% to 90%. Apply a small amount to only the warts and allow to dry, at which time a white "frosting" develops. Repeat weekly as needed.

- *Surgical removal.* Scissor or shaving excision, curette, or electrosurgery is possible.
- *Alternative regimen:* Podophyllin resin, topical cidofovir, intralesional interferon, and photodynamic therapy may all be used as alternative regimens. More information on dosing schedules and treatment considerations can be found in the 2021 CDC STI Treatment Guidelines.[48]

HPV is infectious even when asymptomatic. For most people, it has a benign natural history; some individuals may not be infectious for long periods of time, and later have periods of time where HPV is redetected. Genital warts often regress on their own without treatment among people without HIV as well as those with HIV. The effect of genital wart treatment on HPV transmission and the natural history of HPV are unknown. Therefore, the goal of treatment is the temporary removal of visible genital warts and the amelioration of symptoms and signs, *not* the eradication of HPV.

Potential complications. Lesions may enlarge and destroy tissue. Giant condyloma, while histologically benign, may simulate carcinoma. In pregnancy, warts enlarge, are extremely vascular, and may obstruct the birth canal to necessitate a cesarean delivery. Neither routine HPV screening tests nor cesarean delivery is indicated for prevention of the transmission of HPV to the newborn. The perinatal transmission rate is unknown, although probably low. Juvenile onset respiratory papillomatosis can result from perinatal transmission. Persons with HIV disease can have rapidly growing genital warts. Patients infected with HIV have an increased risk of progressive HPV-related cervical disease.

Prevention. There is currently a nonavalent vaccine on the US market (Gardasil9®) to prevent genital HPV infection that protects against acquisition of types 6, 11, 16, 18, 31, 33, 45, 52, and 58. Large, multicenter studies in young women and men indicate that it is nearly 100% effective in preventing HPV infection and associated disease outcomes, including anogenital warts, cervical neoplasia, and anal neoplasia in men when given prior to HPV exposure. HPV vaccination should be routinely given to all 11- to 12-year-olds, prior to the onset of sexual activity. Catch-up vaccination is recommended for all patients through 26 years of age, with shared decision making for vaccination recommended through 45 years of age.[60] (See Chapter 24, Screening for Cervical, Ovarian, and Breast Cancer.)

Behavioral messages to emphasize

For external genital warts. Return for regular treatment until lesions have resolved. Once warts have responded to therapy, no special follow-up is necessary. Because most partners probably are already infected, examination of sex partners is not necessary. Most new HPV infections are acquired from sex partners who have no symptoms or signs of the infection.

For high-risk HPV. To reduce risks of sequelae from cervical cancer, regular cervical cancer screening is crucial, regardless of whether a patient has received HPV vaccine. See Chapter 24, Screening for Cervical, Ovarian, and Breast Cancer for further information. Additional resources may be found at:

- USPSTF Cervical Cancer Screening Recommendations [update pending]. https://www.uspreventiveservicestaskforce.org/uspstf/draft-update-summary/cervical-cancer-screening-adults-adolescents
- American Cancer Society Guidelines for the Prevention and Early Detection of Cervical Cancer. https://www.cancer.org/cancer/cervical-cancer/detection-diagnosis-staging/cervical-cancer-screening-guidelines.html.

Molluscum Contagiosum

Molluscum contagiosum is caused by the *Molluscum contagiosum* virus, the largest DNA virus of the poxvirus group. Transmission occurs via skin-to-skin contact. This infection manifests as lesions that are 1 to 5 mm, smooth, rounded, firm, shiny, flesh-colored to pearly-white papules with characteristically umbilicated centers. They are most commonly seen on the trunk and anogenital region and are generally asymptomatic. Exceptions occur in immunosuppressed patients (particularly those with HIV with low CD4 counts), in whom the lesions can be diffuse or become bulky.

Diagnosis. Infection is usually diagnosed on the basis of the typical clinical presentation. Microscopic examination of lesions or lesion material reveals the pathognomonic molluscum inclusion bodies.

Treatment. Lesions may resolve spontaneously without scarring. However, they may be removed by curettage after cryoanesthesia. Treatments with caustic chemicals (podophyllin, trichloroacetic acid, silver nitrate) and cryotherapy (liquid nitrogen) have been successful. If every lesion is not extirpated, the condition may recur.

Potential complications. Secondary infection, usually with *Staphylococcus*, may occur. Lesions rarely attain a size greater than 10 mm in diameter.

Behavioral messages to emphasize. Return for reexamination 1 month after treatment so any new lesions can be removed. Sex partner(s) should be examined.

Human Monkeypox

Human monkeypox (MPX) is caused by the monkeypox virus, a member of the orthopox genus and poxvirus family. Transmission occurs via skin-to-skin contact (including sexual contact), and can also occur via respiratory droplets. MPX causes a rash that progresses from macules, to papules, to vesicles, to pustules (often umbilicated similar to molluscum contagiosum), before developing crusts or scabs. Lesions are often painful and can be itchy as healing occurs.

Diagnosis. Clinical diagnosis can be made on the basis of typical lesions appearing after exposure to MPX. Definitive diagnosis can be made with PCR testing of lesions, which is offered by multiple commercial and public health laboratories. Testing may occur in two phases, first with PCR for orthopox viruses, and a second PCR to confirm monkeypox virus. (Some laboratories offer orthopox virus testing only, with presumption of monkeypox virus if initial testing is positive.)

Treatment. Lesions may resolve spontaneously without scarring; however, hypo- or hyperpigmentation may occur. Tecovirimat (TPOXX or ST-246) is FDA-approved for treatment of human smallpox disease and has been used off-label under an expanded access Investigational New Drug (EA-IND) protocol for MPX. Use of tecovirimat should be considered for patients with severe disease, those who are at high risk of severe disease, and those with involvement in anatomic areas where MPX might pose risk of complications (eyes, mouth, genitals, or anus, particularly periurethral or perianal regions). Guidance is updated regularly by the CDC and can be found here:

https://www.cdc.gov/poxvirus/monkeypox/clinicians/Tecovirimat.html

Potential complications. Lesions in the anogenital region may lead to procitis or urinary retention/dysuria. Secondary infection can also occur, including skin and soft-tissue infections, bronchopneumonia, sepsis, encephalitis, and corneal infection with vision loss. Death may occur due to secondary infection.

Behavioral messages to emphasize. Patients with MPX should abstain from skin-to-skin contact, including sexual activity, until all lesions are fully healed. Autoinnoculation can occur, and patients should use gloves or wash their hands after touching affected areas of their bodies. MPX can be transmitted via fomites including bedding and clothing, so these items should not be shared while a patient has lesions. Sex partner(s) should receive prophylactic vaccination, ideally within 4 days of exposure (up to 2 weeks after exposure).

Chlamydia- and Gonorrhea-Related Syndromes: Cervicitis, Urethritis, and Pelvic Inflammatory Disease

Chlamydia and Gonorrhea

These two infections often grouped are together because they are often asymptomatic (especially cervical infection), cause similar clinical syndromes, have similar adverse effects on reproductive health and risk of HIV transmission, and are targeted with national screening guidelines. They are discussed separately below.

Chlamydia. Chlamydia is the common name for infections caused by *Chlamydia trachomatis*. Genital chlamydial infection is the leading cause of preventable infertility and ectopic pregnancy. Chlamydia is the most commonly reported bacterial infectious disease in the United States. An estimated 4 million new cases occur annually. Because many chlamydial infections are asymptomatic and probably chronic, widespread screening is necessary to control this infection and its sequelae. The CDC recommends that all sexually active females age younger than 25 years of age be screened annually for *C. trachomatis* (Table 23-3). For further information about the syndromes caused by *C. Trachomatis*, see the sections on Cervicitis, Acute Urethral Syndrome, Nongonococcal Urethritis, and Pelvic Inflammatory Disease (PID) in this chapter.

The recommended regimen for all sites of uncomplicated chlamydial infection is doxycycline 100 mg orally twice daily for 7 days.

The alternatives are azithromycin 1 g orally in a single dose OR levofloxacin 500 mg orally for 7 days.

Test of cure is not necessary in nonpregnant patients after treatment with recommended or alternative regimens. Test of cure should be performed if therapeutic adherence is in question, symptoms persist, or reinfection is suspected. Test of cure with a NAAT should be performed 4 or more weeks after completion of therapy to avoid false positive results due to nonviable organisms.

During pregnancy, the recommended regimen is azithromycin 1 g orally in a single dose, and the alternative regimen is amoxicillin 500 mg orally three times daily for 7 days.

Test of cure with a NAAT should be performed approximately 4 weeks after completion of therapy for all pregnant patients with chlamydia.

Lymphogranuloma venereum (LGV) is caused by serovars L1, L2, or L3 of *C. trachomatis*. LGV infections are endemic in Asia and Africa and have occurred in the United States among men who report condomless receptive anal sex. LGV should be suspected in any men who have sex with men with proctitis that does not respond to routine treatment for chlamydia and gonorrhea or is especially severe. Such cases should be treated with 3 weeks of oral doxycycline and a specific diagnosis pursued, if possible.

Gonorrhea. Gonorrhea is caused by *Neisseria gonorrhoeae*, a gram-negative bacterium seen as a diplococcus on Gram stain. The CDC estimates that 1.6 million new cases of gonorrhea occur each year, making it the second most commonly reported STI in the United States.

Symptoms. Cervical infections are most commonly asymptomatic, but patients may also present with abnormal vaginal discharge, abnormal vaginal bleeding, or dysuria. Infections of the penile urethra often are associated with dysuria, increased frequency of urination, and purulent discharge; an estimated one-fourth of these infections can be asymptomatic. Pharyngeal gonorrhea can occasionally produce symptoms of pharyngitis, but most infections are asymptomatic.

Diagnosis. Definitive diagnosis requires recovery of bacteria either by culture or molecular testing (NAAT). NAATs can be performed on urine and vaginal, pharyngeal, or rectal swabs. Although the use of culture allows for antimicrobial susceptibility testing, greater use of NAATs has increased the number of patients tested and offers a noninvasive method for diagnosis. A definitive diagnosis by culture is required if important for medico-legal reasons (child abuse, sexual assault), or in cases of suspected treatment failure. Gram stain or methylene blue stain also can be used for presumptive diagnosis of gonorrhea but is not commonly performed outside of STI clinics.

Treatment. Gonococcal antibiotic resistance is a growing concern, and treatment options are limited. The recommended regimen for gonorrhea is ceftriaxone 500 mg IM in a single dose (or 1 g IM if weight $\geq$ 150 kg). See the CDC's website on this topic for updates (www.cdc.gov/std/treatment).

Potential complications. Up to 40% of untreated patients with cervical gonorrhea develop PID and are at risk for its sequelae (see the section on PID), including infertility and pelvic abscesses. Complications in males can include epididymitis, urethral stricture, and infertility. Newborns are at risk for ophthalmia neonatorum, scalp abscess at the site of fetal monitors, rhinitis, or anorectal infection. All infected untreated persons are at risk for disseminated gonococcal infection.

Behavioral messages to emphasize. Anyone the index patient had sex with in the 60 days prior to diagnosis should be treated (see section on Expedited Partner Treatment). Avoid sex until completion of the prescribed course of medication and/or for 1 week after treatment was started. Understand how to take prescribed oral medications. Use condoms to prevent future infections and understand potential consequences to future reproductive health if the infection is reacquired or not optimally treated.

Cervicitis. Cervicitis is a term used to refer to the syndrome of cervical inflammation that can accompany infection with some STIs, notably *C. trachomatis*, *N. gonorrhoeae*, and *Mycoplasma genitalium*, and occasionally trichomoniasis and genital herpes. It is defined as the presence of endocervical mucopurulent discharge, easily induced bleeding, and/or edematous ectopy. Cervicitis can have noninfectious causes, including chemical trauma, and also may be promoted by progestin-based hormonal therapy or BV.

Symptoms. Cervical mucopurulent discharge may be exuded from the cervix and may be perceived as abnormal vaginal discharge, and cervical bleeding may manifest as intermenstrual bleeding.

Diagnosis. Diagnosis is made by visualizing either mucopus on a swab of endocervical secretions or friability (bleeding) on gentle passage of a cotton-tipped swab. A definitive etiologic diagnosis is made when a specific organism is isolated. However, in many cases, a microbial organism cannot be identified. NAAT is the preferred method of detection for chlamydia, gonorrhea, *M. genitalium*, or trichomonas.

Treatment. Presumptive treatment should be provided based on the individual patient's risk for chlamydial and/or gonococcal infections (e.g., age < 25 years, new/multiple partners, sex partner with an STI). Evaluation for BV or trichomonas should also be performed. In patients at low risk for STIs, the results of NAATs for *C. trachomatis*, *N. gonorrhoeae*, or *T. vaginalis* should determine the need for treatment. If presumptive treatment is given, it should include coverage for chlamydia with doxycycline 100 mg orally twice daily for 7 days, or an alternative regimen of azithromycin 1 g orally in a single dose. If concurrent treatment for gonorrhea is administered, the recommended regimen is ceftriaxone 500 mg IM in a single dose. BV and/or trichomonas should be treated, if detected, with metronidazole 500 mg twice daily for 7 days.

If treatment for these infections is ineffective, testing for *M. genitalium* should be considered. If testing is positive, the recommended treatment is doxycycline 100 mg orally twice daily for 7 days, followed by moxifloxacin 400 mg orally once daily for 7 days.

Potential complications. PID (with subsequent infertility) may complicate infection. In addition, neonatal chlamydial infections, such as ophthalmia neonatorum or pneumonia, may be acquired during delivery if the cervix is infected. Postpartum endometritis also may occur.

Behavioral messages to emphasize. If infection involves *C. trachomatis*, *N. gonorrhoeae*, or *T. vaginalis*, sex partner(s) should be treated for these infections. Anyone the index patient had sex with in the 60 days prior to diagnosis should be treated (see section on Expedited Partner Treatment). Avoid sex (anal, vaginal, or oral) until completion of the prescribed course of medication and/or for 1 week after treatment was started. Understand how to take prescribed oral medications. Return early if symptoms persist or recur. Use condoms to prevent future infections and understand potential consequences to future reproductive health if the infection is reacquired or not optimally treated.

Pelvic Inflammatory Disease. PID can be caused by varying combinations of *N. gonorrhoeae*, *C. trachomatis*, anaerobic bacteria, facultative gram-negative rods (such as *Escherichia coli*), *Mycoplasma* (*genitalium* or *hominis*), and a variety of other microbial agents. Clinical PID is usually of polymicrobial etiology. *N. gonorrhoeae* and *C. trachomatis* may cause antecedent inflammation, which makes the tubes susceptible to invasion by anaerobic organisms.

Symptoms. Patients with PID can have atypical symptoms or be asymptomatic. Symptoms can include pain and tenderness involving the lower abdomen, cervix, uterus, or adnexae, occasionally with fever, chills, and elevated WBC count and erythrocyte sedimentation rate (ESR). The condition is more likely if the patient has multiple sex partners or a history of PID, or is in the first 5 to 10 days of a menstrual cycle.

Diagnosis. Patients with the typical clinical symptoms are presumed to have PID if other serious conditions, such as acute appendicitis or ectopic pregnancy, can be excluded. The diagnosis of PID often is based on imprecise clinical findings. Maintain a low threshold for diagnosing PID, because even mild or moderate PID has the potential for reproductive sequelae. Use objective criteria to monitor response to antibiotics, especially if ambulatory treatment is given. More specific criteria, such as endometrial biopsy, magnetic resonance imaging, or diagnostic laparoscopy, are warranted only in selected instances. Direct visualization of inflamed tube(s) (with edema, hyperemia, or tubal exudate) during laparoscopy or laparotomy confirms the diagnosis of PID. Cultures of tubal exudate may help establish the microbiologic etiology.

Treatment. Because the causative organism is usually unknown at the time of the initial therapy, use treatment regimens that are active against the broadest possible range of pathogens. Antimicrobial coverage should include *N. gonorrhoeae*, *C. trachomatis*, anaerobes, *T. vaginalis*, gram-negative facultative bacteria, and streptococci.

Hospitalization and inpatient care: Consider hospitalizing patients with acute PID when (1) surgical emergencies, such as appendicitis and ectopic pregnancy, are not definitely excluded; (2) severe illness precludes outpatient management; (3) the patient is unable to follow or tolerate an outpatient regimen; or (4) symptoms have not responded to outpatient therapy. Special consideration may be given to adolescents and those with social challenges (e.g., experiencing homelessness) to improve their adherence.

Combined drug therapy is recommended in all cases since the full bacterial etiology of PID is not clear and the infection generally is polymicrobial.

Parenteral treatment: Parenteral therapy may be transitioned to oral therapy within 24–48 hours of clinical improvement.

- Recommended:
  - Ceftriaxone 1 g IV every 24 hours, OR
  - Cefotetan 2 g IV every 12 hours, OR
  - Cefoxitin 2 g IV every 6 hours PLUS doxycycline 100 mg orally or IV every 12 hours PLUS metronidazole 500 mg orally or IV every 12 hours.
- *Alternative* A:
  - Clindamycin 900 mg, IV three times a day, PLUS gentamicin 2 mg per kilogram (kg) IV loading dose followed by maintenance 1.5 mg/kg IV every 8 hours.
- *Alternative B*: Ampicillin-sulbactam 3 g IV every 6 hours PLUS Doxycycline 100mg orally or IV every 12 hours PLUS

Continue doxycycline 100 mg orally twice daily after discharge to complete at least 14 days of therapy.

Intramuscular/oral treatment: Either of the following regimens is recommended:

- Ceftriaxone 500 mg IM in a single dose,* OR
- Cefoxitin 2 g IM along with probenecid 1 g orally in a single dose, OR
- Other parenteral third-generation cephalosporin (e.g., cefotaxime) PLUS doxycycline 100 mg taken orally twice daily for 14 days PLUS metronidazole 500 mg orally twice daily for 14 days.

*Persons weighing $>$ 150 kg with documented gonococcal infection should receive 1 g of ceftriaxone.

Potential complications. Potentially life-threatening complications include ectopic pregnancy and pelvic abscess. Other sequelae may include infertility, recurrent or chronic PID, chronic abdominal pain, pelvic adhesions, and premature hysterectomy.

Behavioral messages to emphasize. For outpatient therapy, return for evaluation 2 to 3 days after initiation of therapy. Return for further evaluation 4 days after completing therapy. Refer sex partner(s) for evaluation and treatment (even if they are asymptomatic). Avoid penile-vaginal sex throughout the course of treatment. Understand how to take prescribed oral medications.

Urethritis, Including Nongonococcal Urethritis (NGU)

Urinary Tract Infections and Acute Urethral Syndrome

Acute urethral syndrome (dysuria-pyuria syndrome) is a term reserved for the presentation of an acute urethral inflammation in patients that is distinct from bacterial cystitis and typically results from a direct urethral infection with the sexually transmitted pathogens *C. trachomatis* or *N. gonorrhoeae*. Bacterial cystitis itself is not sexually transmitted per se; however, it can be sexually associated. "Honeymoon" cystitis—that is, cystitis that occurs after frequent vaginal intercourse—is believed to be caused by friction against the urethra during sexual intercourse. In this case, the underlying etiology is mechanical, and coital movements help vaginal/fecal organisms ascend into the bladder. Use of the diaphragm with spermicides have been associated with a higher risk of acute urethral syndrome.

Prevalence. Urinary tract infections are second in incidence only to upper respiratory infections. Depending on the population studied, as many as 10% to 25% of reproductive-age women report dysuria during the previous year. Among women with genital chlamydial infections, approximately 10% are infected at the urethra only.

Symptoms. Painful, urgent, and frequent urination as well as dyspareunia characterize this syndrome. Occasionally, hematuria is the precipitating event for seeking clinical evaluation. Consider pyelonephritis in the presence of fever, or if costovertebral angle pain or tenderness are present.

Diagnosis. Patients with > 10 organisms (coliform bacteria or other uropathogens) per milliliter (ml) of urine have bacterial cystitis; however, a smaller number of organisms also may cause symptoms. In women with dysuria, frequency, pyuria (≥ 10 WBCs per 400× field on microscopic examination of urinary sediment), and lack of bacteriuria on standard urine culture, chlamydia should be strongly suspected. A definitive diagnosis of the etiologic organism requires cultures or nucleic acid amplification testing (for gonorrhea and chlamydia) of the urethra or urine. Dysuria also may be caused by vulvovaginitis or genital HSV infection.

Treatment. Bacterial cystitis can be treated with a variety of antibiotics that achieve a high concentration in urine. Initial episodes of bacterial cystitis can be treated with sulfamethoxazole 800 mg plus trimethoprim 160 mg (e.g., Bactrim

DS) orally twice daily for three days. Nitrofurantoin monohydrate/macrocrystals 100 mg twice daily for 5 days or fosfomycin 3 g (powder mixed in water) as a single dose also are first-line agents. Alternative regimens include fluoroquinolones such as ciprofloxacin 250 mg twice daily OR levofloxacin 250 mg daily for 3 days. If bacteriuria is absent in the presence of pyuria, consider presumptive treatment for chlamydial infection.

Potential complications. Left untreated, bacterial infections of the lower genitourinary tract can ascend to the upper tract, leading to pyelonephritis.

Behavioral messages to emphasize. Understand how to take any prescribed oral medications. Drink copious fluids to flush the genitourinary system. If *C. trachomatis* or *N. gonorrhoeae* organisms are isolated or strongly suspected, arrange for treatment of sex partner(s). (See the sections on these specific infections.)

Urethritis. Urethritis is caused by *C. trachomatis* or *N. gonorrhoeae* in less than half of cases. Other sexually transmissible agents, which may cause more than half of the cases, include *T. vaginalis, M. genitalium*, HSV, and *Ureaplasma urealyticum*. Among patients who engage in unprotected insertive anal sex, rectal coliform bacteria, such as *E. coli*, may contribute. The etiology of the remaining cases is unknown.

Symptoms. Dysuria, urinary frequency, and mucoid or mucopurulent urethral discharge are common.

Diagnosis. The syndrome of urethritis is defined by the sign of urethral discharge as noted above, and/or by the presence of at least two or more polymorphonuclear neutrophils (PMN) per high-power field (HPF) on Gram stain or methylene blue stain of urethral discharge. The latter test can also rule out gonorrhea if no gram-negative intracellular diplococci are seen. However, urine NAAT for chlamydia and gonorrhea can test for both pathogens.

Treatment. When the etiology is *C. trachomatis*, or unknown, the following treatment is recommended: doxycycline 100 mg orally twice daily for 7 days. The alternative regimen is azithromycin 1 g orally in a single dose OR azithromycin 500 mg orally in a single dose followed by 250 mg orally daily for 4 days.

For patients who fail their first trial of antibiotics and whose partners have been treated, the persistent urethritis should be documented (either by visual examination of discharge or microscopy to quantify WBCs). Patients initially treated with doxycycline who have insertive vaginal sex should be tested for *T. vaginalis* and presumptively treated with metronidazole 2 g or tinidazole 2 g orally in a single dose. If trichomonas is unlikely (MSM or patient has negative *T. vaginalis* NAAT), testing for *M. genitalium* with an NAAT should be performed. If *M. genitalium* is detected, the recommended treatment is doxycycline 100 mg twice daily for 7 days, followed by moxifloxacin 400 mg once daily for 7 days. For urethritis caused by genital herpes, see the relevant sections of this chapter.

Potential complications. Urethral strictures or epididymitis may occur. If *C. trachomatis* is transmitted to sex partners, the condition may result in mucopurulent cervicitis, PID, or proctitis. If *C. trachomatis* is acquired in pregnancy, complications may include neonatal infections such as conjunctivitis or pneumonia.

Behavioral messages to emphasize. If chlamydial infection or other STI is diagnosed, sex partner(s) with contact within the prior 60 days should be treated. Avoid anal or vaginal sex until treatment is completed. Use condoms to prevent future infections.

Viral Hepatitis

Hepatitis A, hepatitis B, and hepatitis C may be sexually transmitted. Infections are clinically indistinguishable and are often asymptomatic. When symptoms occur, they may include fatigue, anorexia, nausea, vomiting, headache, fever, dark urine, jaundice, and moderate liver enlargement with tenderness. In all cases, diagnosis is made by serologic testing, sometimes in combination with measurement of plasma viral load by PCR testing. Specific features of each infection are described below.

Hepatitis A

Hepatitis A is caused by hepatitis A virus (HAV), an RNA virus that is typically transmitted by the fecal-oral route. For this reason, HAV can be transmitted through oral-anal sexual contact.

Diagnosis. Serum IgM antiHAV almost always is detectable at the onset of symptoms, and IgG antiHAV levels rise soon thereafter. Measurement of serum IgM anti-HAV is the diagnostic test of choice for acute hepatitis A infection.

Treatment/Prevention. Therapy is supportive. Vaccination and postexposure prophylaxis strategies prevent the infection. Vaccinating all men who have sex with men, persons who use illicit drugs, persons experiencing homelessness, and travelers to endemic areas against hepatitis A currently is recommended.

Potential complications. Long-term sequelae are rare. Rarely, acute fulminant hepatitis can occur, resulting in hepatic failure and death.

Behavioral messages to emphasize. HAV vaccination is strongly encouraged for target groups. Consult public health authorities regarding recommendations for postexposure prophylaxis of household contacts and sex partners.

Hepatitis B

Hepatitis B is caused by hepatitis B virus (HBV), a DNA virus with multiple antigenic components. In the United States, about 4% of the general population show evidence of past HBV infections. Sexual transmission traditionally has been the predominant mode of HBV transmission in the United States, with men who have sex with men, heterosexual persons with multiple partners, or those who engage in transactional sex at increased risk. However, between 2006 and 2011, most new cases of acute HBV were associated with drug use.[61]

Diagnosis. Diagnosis involves interpretation of several serologic tests as well as HBV serum PCR in some cases.

- Hepatitis B surface antigen (HBsAg): May indicate acute HBV infection or a chronic active state (infectious in both)
- HBe antigen: Indicates active replication of the virus, and infectiousness
- AntiHBs (surface antibody): Indicates immunity conferred by past infection or successful immunization
- AntiHBc (core antibody): May indicate past or current infection; does not result from immunization

Guidance for interpretation of hepatitis B serology is available from the CDC at www.cdc.gov/hepatitis/hbv/pdfs/serologicchartv8.pdf.

Treatment. Chronic active HBV can be treated with a variety of agents, including tenofovir, entecavir, lamivudine, adefovir, and telbivudine, and should be initiated in consultation with a specialist. Guidelines can be found at https://www.aasld.org/publications/practice-guidelines.

Potential complications. Long-term sequelae include chronic, persistent, active hepatitis; cirrhosis; hepatocellular carcinoma; hepatic failure; and death. Rarely, the course may be fulminant with hepatic failure.

Behavioral messages to emphasize. HBV vaccination is strongly encouraged for all young, sexually active people. Specific vaccination and postexposure prophylaxis strategies are of proven efficacy in preventing hepatitis B. Vaccinating all newborn infants and adolescents against hepatitis B currently is recommended. In addition, the CDC Advisory Committee on Immunization Practices recommends HBV vaccination for all men who have sex with men, persons seeking evaluation or treatment for an STI, and those who have a history of sexual activity with more than one partner in the previous 6 months. Subsidized HBV vaccine programs are available in many states.

Hepatitis C

Hepatitis C is caused by hepatitis C virus (HCV), an RNA virus that is typically transmitted by the parenteral route (needle sharing or transfusion with contaminated blood). HCV has been detected in genital secretions, and sexual transmission has been documented, particularly in men who have sex with men. Transmission is more likely if sexual activity includes exchange of blood or bloody secretions, which may be more likely occur during anal sex (versus vaginal or oral sex).

Diagnosis. Serum IgM antiHCV almost always is detectable at the onset of symptoms, and IgG antiHCV levels rise soon thereafter. Measurement of serum IgM antiHCV, possibly combined with HCV PCR, is the diagnostic approach of choice in the setting of acute hepatitis.

Treatment/Prevention. Direct-acting oral agents capable of curing HCV infection have been approved for use in the United States since 2011. Numerous antiviral combinations may be utilized; selection of therapy depends on genotype and presence of cirrhosis, and typically lasts 8–12 weeks in duration. Existing guidelines for management can be found at www.hcvguidelines.org. No vaccine is available. Patients should be educated about ways to avoid transmission through contaminated needles or by sharing such items as razors with household or sexual contacts who are infected.

Potential complications. Long-term sequelae include chronic, persistent, active hepatitis; cirrhosis; hepatocellular carcinoma; hepatic failure; and death. Rarely, the course may be fulminant with hepatic failure.

Behavioral messages to emphasize. As risk of sexual transmission between male-female partners is low, persons in an established relationship do not need to change their sexual practices if in one partner is found to have HCV infection; the partner of unknown status should be screened. (Due to a lack of data, no recommendations exist for men who have sex with men or gender-diverse persons). If a person has HCV and is beginning a new sexual relationship, use safer sex precautions as applicable for routine STI protection and reduction of HCV transmission (e.g., condoms).

Zika Virus

Sexual transmission of Zika virus has been documented for male-female, female-male, and male-male sex. The virus may be shed in semen for prolonged periods (as late as 188 days following the onset of illness), though in most cases will clear by 3 months. The main risk is for those who are pregnant, in whom high rates of congenital infection occur and may be manifested by a wide range of disorders, including microcephaly, macular scarring, and arthrogryposis (congenital contractures). The CDC recommends that before having unprotected sex, men should wait at least 6 months after symptom onset or last possible Zika virus exposure (if asymptomatic); women (symptomatic or not) are advised to wait at least 8 weeks after symptom onset or, if asymptomatic, after the last possible Zika virus exposure. More detailed information is available at www.cdc.gov/zika/index.html.

Consultation for Complex RTI Cases

The National Network of Clinical STD Prevention Training Centers (NNPTC) has a national consultation service (STD Clinical Consultation Network) available for providers managing complex RTI cases who would like advice from a subject matter expert. Consults are answered in 1 to 5 business days depending on the urgency of the request. The STDCCN warm-line is staffed from Monday through Friday 8AM to 5PM, but consults can be entered anytime online at http://stdccn.org.

Author Disclosures—Marrazzo: none. Park: none.

References

1. Vermund SH, Geller AB, Crowley JS (eds.). Sexually transmitted infections: Adopting a sexual health paradigm. Washington DC: National Academies of Sciences, Engineering, and Medicine; Health and Medicine Division; Board on Population Health and Public Health Practice; Committee on Prevention and Control of Sexually Transmitted Infections in the United States; 2021. (https://nap.nationalacademies.org/catalog/25955/sexually-transmitted-infections-adopting-a-sexual-health-paradigm.)
2. Centers for Disease Control and Prevention. Sexually transmitted disease surveillance, 2020 [Internet]. Last Reviewed: August 22, 2022. (https://www.cdc.gov/std/statistics/2020/default.htm).
3. Chesson HW, Spicknall IH, Bingham A, et al. The estimated direct lifetime medical costs of sexually transmitted infections acquired in the United States in 2018. Sex Transm Dis. 2021;48(4):215-21. DOI: 10.1097/OLQ.0000000000001380.
4. Cates W, Jr. Review of non-hormonal contraception (condoms, intrauterine devices, nonoxynol-9 and combos) on HIV acquisition. J AIDS.2005;38 Suppl 1:S8-10. DOI: 10.1097/01.qai.0000167025.87783.31
5. Garnett G. The transmission dynamics of sexually transmitted infections. In: Holmes KK, Sparling PF, Stamm WE, et al. (eds.). Sexually transmitted diseases. 4th ed. New York: McGraw-Hill; 2008:27-39.
6. Platt R, Rice PA, McCormack WM. Risk of acquiring gonorrhea and prevalence of abnormal adnexal findings among women recently exposed to gonorrhea. JAMA. 1983;250(23):3205-9. DOI: 10.1001/jama.1983.03340230057031.
7. Hooper RR, Reynolds GH, Jones OG, et al. Cohort study of venereal disease. I: the risk of gonorrhea transmission from infected women to men. Am J Epidemiol. 1978;108(2):136-44. DOI: 10.1093/oxfordjournals.aje.a112597.

8. Pilcher CD, Tien HC, Eron JJ, Jr., et al. Brief but efficient: acute HIV infection and the sexual transmission of HIV. J Infect Dis. 2004;189(10):1785-92. (https://academic.oup.com/jid/article/189/10/1785/2191338).
9. Baeten JM, Donnell D, Ndase P, et al. Antiretroviral prophylaxis for HIV prevention in heterosexual men and women. N Engl J Med. 2012;367(5):399-410. DOI: 10.1056/NEJMoa1108524.
10. Landovitz RJ, Donnell D, Clement ME, et al. Cabotegravir for HIV prevention in cisgender men and transgender women. N Engl J Med. 2021;385(7):595-608. DOI: 10.1056/NEJMoa2101016.
11. Ogbuagu O, Ruane PJ, Podzamczer D, et al. Long-term safety and efficacy of emtricitabine and tenofovir alafenamide vs emtricitabine and tenofovir disoproxil fumarate for HIV-1 pre-exposure prophylaxis: week 96 results from a randomised, double-blind, placebo-controlled, phase 3 trial. Lancet HIV. 2021;8(7):e397-407. DOI: 10.1016/S2352-3018(21)00071-0.
12. Delany-Moretlwe S, Hughes JP, Bock P, et al. Cabotegravir for the prevention of HIV-1 in women: results from HPTN 084, a phase 3, randomised clinical trial. Lancet. 2022;399(10337):1779-89. DOI: 10.1016/S0140-6736(22)00538-4.
13. UNAIDS and WHO. New data on male circumcision and HIV prevention: policy and programme implications; WHO/UNAIDS technical consultation male circumcision and HIV prevention: research implications for policy and programming montreux. Geneva: Joint United Nations Programme on HIV/AIDS and World Health Organization, 2007. 2007.
14. Trussell J, Kost K. Contraceptive failure in the United States: a critical review of the literature. Stud Fam Plann. 1987;18(5):237-83.
15. Centers for Disease Control and Prevention. HIV risk behaviors. (https://www.cdc.gov/hiv/risk/estimates/riskbehaviors.html).
16. Holmes KK, Johnson DW, Trostle HJ. An estimate of the risk of men acquiring gonorrhea by sexual contact with infected females. Am J Epidemiol. 1970;91(2):170-4. DOI: 10.1093/oxfordjournals.aje.a121125.
17. Herzog SA, Heijne JC, Althaus CL, Low N. Describing the progression from *Chlamydia trachomatis* and *Neisseria gonorrhoeae* to pelvic inflammatory disease: systematic review of mathematical modeling studies. Sex Transmit Dis. 2012;39(8):628-37. DOI: 10.1097/OLQ.0b013e31825159ff.
18. Westrom L, Joesoef R, Reynolds G, Hagdu A, Thompson SE. Pelvic inflammatory disease and fertility. A cohort study of 1,844 women with laparoscopically verified disease and 657 control women with normal laparoscopic results. Sex Transmit Dis. 1992;19(4):185-92. (http://www.ncbi.nlm.nih.gov/entrez/query.fcgi?cmd=Retrieve&db=PubMed&dopt=Citation&list_uids=1411832).
19. Magaret AS, Mujugira A, Hughes JP, et al. Effect of condom use on per-act HSV-2 transmission risk in HIV-1, HSV-2-discordant couples. Clin Infect Dis. 2016;62(4):456-61. DOI: 10.1093/cid/civ908.
20. Padian NS, van der Straten A, Ramjee G, et al. Diaphragm and lubricant gel for prevention of HIV acquisition in southern African women: a randomised controlled trial. Lancet. 2007;370(9583):251-61. (https://www.ncbi.nlm.nih.gov/pmc/articles/PMC2442038/).
21. Polis CB, Phillips SJ, Curtis KM, et al. Hormonal contraceptive methods and risk of HIV acquisition in women: a systematic review of epidemiological evidence. Contraception. 2014;90(4):360-90. DOI: 10.1016/j.contraception.2014.07.009.
22. Ness RB, Keder LM, Soper DE, et al. Oral contraception and the recognition of endometritis. Am J Obstet Gynecol. 1997;176(3):580-5. (https://www.ajog.org/article/S0002-9378(97)70551-9/fulltext).
23. Morrison CS, Bright P, Wong EL, et al. Hormonal contraceptive use, cervical ectopy, and the acquisition of cervical infections. Sex Transmit Dis. 2004;31(9):561-7. (http://www.ncbi.nlm.nih.gov/entrez/query.fcgi?cmd=Retrieve&db=PubMed&dopt=Citation&list_uids=15480119).
24. HIV incidence among women using intramuscular depot medroxyprogesterone acetate, a copper intrauterine device, or a levonorgestrel implant for contraception: a randomised, multicentre, open-label trial. Lancet. 2019;394(10195):303-13. DOI: 10.1016/s0140-6736(19)31288-7.
25. Steenland MW, Zapata LB, Brahmi D, Marchbanks PA, Curtis KM. Appropriate follow up to detect potential adverse events after initiation of select contraceptive methods: a systematic review. Contraception. 2013;87(5):611-24. DOI: 10.1016/j.contraception.2012.09.017.

26. Sufrin CB, Postlethwaite D, Armstrong MA, Merchant M, Wendt JM, Steinauer JE. Neisseria gonorrhea and Chlamydia trachomatis screening at intrauterine device insertion and pelvic inflammatory disease. Obstet Gynecol. 2012;120(6):1314-21. DOI: http://10.1097/AOG.0b013e318273364c.
27. Turok DK, Eisenberg DL, Teal SB, Keder LM, Creinin MD. A prospective assessment of pelvic infection risk following same-day sexually transmitted infection testing and levonorgestrel intrauterine system placement. Am J Obstet Gynecol. 2016;215(5):599 e1-6. DOI: 10.1016/j.ajog.2016.05.017.
28. Tepper NK, Curtis KM, Nanda K, Jamieson DJ. Safety of intrauterine devices among women with HIV: a systematic review. Contraception. 2016;94(6):713-24. DOI: 10.1016/j.contraception.2016.06.011.
29. Peebles K, Kiweewa FM, Palanee-Phillips T, et al. Elevated risk of bacterial vaginosis among users of the copper intrauterine device: A prospective longitudinal cohort study. Clin Infect Dis. 2021;73(3):513-520. DOI: 10.1093/cid/ciaa703.
30. Van Damme L, Ramjee G, Alary M, et al. Effectiveness of COL-1492, a nonoxynol-9 vaginal gel, on HIV-1 transmission in female sex workers: a randomised controlled trial. Lancet. 2002;360(9338):971-7. (https://www.thelancet.com/journals/lancet/article/PIIS0140-6736(02)11079-8/fulltext).
31. Karim QA, Karim SS, Frohlich JA, et al. Effectiveness and safety of tenofovir gel, an antiretroviral microbicide, for the prevention of HIV infection in women. Science. 2010;10:1126.
32. Nel A, van Niekerk N, Kapiga S, et al. Safety and efficacy of a dapivirine vaginal ring for HIV prevention in women. N Engl J Med. 2016;375(22):2133-43. DOI: 10.1056/NEJMoa1602046.
33. Baeten JM, Palanee-Phillips T, Brown ER, et al. Use of a vaginal ring containing dapivirine for HIV-1 prevention in women. N Engl J Med. 2016;375(22):2121-32. DOI: 10.1056/NEJMoa1506110.
34. Chappell BT, Mena LA, Maximos B, Mollan S, Culwell K, Howard B. EVO100 prevents chlamydia and gonorrhea in women at high risk of infection. Am J Obstet Gynecol. 2021;225(2):162 e1-14. DOI: 10.1016/j.ajog.2021.03.005.
35. Klebanoff MA, Nansel TR, Brotman RM, et al. Personal hygienic behaviors and bacterial vaginosis. Sex Transmit Dis. 2010;37(2):94-9. DOI: 10.1097/OLQ.0b013e3181bc063c.
36. McClelland RS, Lavreys L, Hassan WM, Mandaliya K, Ndinya-Achola JO, Baeten JM. Vaginal washing and increased risk of HIV-1 acquisition among African women: a 10-year prospective study. AIDS 2006;20(2):269-73. DOI: 10.1097/01.aids.0000196165.48518.7b.
37. Jin F, Matthews GV, Grulich AE. Sexual transmission of hepatitis C virus among gay and bisexual men: a systematic review. Sex Health. 2017;14(1):28-41. DOI: 10.1071/SH16141.
38. Leigh BC. Alcohol and condom use: a meta-analysis of event-level studies. Sex Transmit Dis. 2002;29(8):476-82. DOI: 10.1097/00007435-200208000-00008.
39. US Preventive Services Task Force, Davidson KW, Barry MJ, et al. Screening for chlamydia and gonorrhea: US Preventive Services Task Force Recommendation statement. JAMA. 2021;326(10):949-56. DOI: 10.1001/jama.2021.14081.
40. Workowski KA, Bachmann LH, Chan PA, et al. Sexually transmitted infections treatment guidelines, 2021. MMWR Recomm Rep. 2021;70(4):1-187. DOI: 10.15585/mmwr.rr7004a1.
41. US Preventive Services Task Force. Screening for gonorrhea: recommendation statement. Ann Fam Med. 2005;3(3):263-7. (https://www.ncbi.nlm.nih.gov/pmc/articles/PMC1466867/).
42. Feltner C, Grodensky C, Ebel C, et al. Serologic screening for genital herpes: An updated evidence report and systematic review for the US Preventive Services Task Force. JAMA. 2016;316(23):2531-43. DOI: 10.1001/jama.2016.17138.
43. US Preventive Services Task Force, Bibbins-Domingo K, Grossman DC, et al. Serologic screening for genital herpes infection: US Preventive Services Task Force recommendation statement. JAMA. 2016;316(23):2525-30. DOI: 10.1001/jama.2016.16776.
44. Golden MR, Whittington WL, Handsfield HH, et al. Effect of expedited treatment of sex partners on recurrent or persistent gonorrhea or chlamydial infection. N Engl J Med. 2005;352(7):676-85. DOI: 10.1056/NEJMoa041681.
45. Kissinger P, Mohammed H, Richardson-Alston G, et al. Patient-delivered partner treatment for male urethritis: a randomized, controlled trial. Clin Infect Dis. 2005;41(5):623-9. DOI: 10.1086/432476.

46. Yu YY, Frasure-Williams JA, Dunne EF, Bolan G, Markowitz L, Bauer HM. Chlamydia partner services for females in California family planning clinics. Sex Transmit Dis. 2011;38(10):913-8. DOI: 10.1097/OLQ.0b013e3182240366.
47. Agyemang E, Le QA, Warren T, et al. Performance of commercial enzyme-linked immunoassays for diagnosis of herpes simplex virus-1 and herpes simplex virus-2 infection in a clinical setting. Sex Transm Dis. 2017;44(12):763-67. DOI: 10.1097/OLQ.0000000000000689.
48. Centers for Disease Control and Prevention. STI treatment guidelines, 2021 [Internet]. 2021. (https://www.cdc.gov/std/treatment-guidelines/default.htm).
49. American Academy of Pediatrics Committee on Fetus and Newborn; American College of Obstetricians and Gynecologists Committee on Obstetric Practice. Guidelines for perinatal care (8th ed.). 2017.
50. Dominguez KL, Smith DK, Vasavi T, et al. Updated guidelines for antiretroviral postexposure prophylaxis after sexual, injection-drug use, or other nonoccupational exposure to HIV-- United States, 2016. Atlanta, GA: Centers for Disease Control and Prevention; 2016. (https://stacks.cdc.gov/view/cdc/38856).
51. Gray RH, Wawer MJ, Brookmeyer R, et al. Probability of HIV-1 transmission per coital act in monogamous, heterosexual, HIV-1-discordant couples in Rakai, Uganda. Lancet. 2001; 357(9263):1149-53. (https://www.thelancet.com/journals/lancet/article/PIIS0140-6736(00)04331-2/fulltext).
52. Centers for Disease Control and Prevention. Revised recommendations for HIV testing for adults, adolescents, and pregnant women in healthcare settings. MMWR 2006;55 (RR-14).
53. Thomson KA, Hughes J, Baeten JM, et al. Increased risk of HIV acquisition among women throughout pregnancy and during the postpartum period: A prospective per-coital-act analysis among women with HIV-infected partners. J Infect Dis. 2018;218(1):16-25. DOI: 10.1093/infdis/jiy113.
54. INSIGHT START Study Group, Lundgren JD, Babiker AG, et al. Initiation of antiretroviral therapy in early asymptomatic HIV infection. N Engl J Med. 2015;373(9):795-807. DOI: 10.1056/NEJMoa1506816.
55. Clinicalinfo.HIV.gov. Guidelines for the prevention and treatment of opportunistic infections in HIV-infected adults and adolescents: Recommendations from the Centers for Disease Control and Prevention, the National Institutes of Health, and the HIV Medicine Association of the Infectious Diseases Society of America. (https://clinicalinfo.hiv.gov/en/guidelines/adult-and-adolescent-opportunistic-infection/whats-new-guidelines).
56. Lingappa JR, Baeten JM, Wald A, et al. Daily aciclovir for HIV-1 disease progression in people dually infected with HIV-1 and herpes simplex virus type 2: a randomised placebo-controlled trial. Lancet. 2010;375(9717):824-33. DOI: 10.1016/S0140-6736(09)62038-9.
57. Centers for Disease Control and Prevention. US medical eligibility criteria (US MEC) for contraceptive use, 2016. [Last reviewed May 18, 2022]. (https://www.cdc.gov/reproductivehealth/contraception/mmwr/mec/summary.html).
58. Muzny CA, Schwebke JR. Asymptomatic bacterial vaginosis: To treat or not to treat? Curr Infect Dis Rep. 2020;22(12):32. DOI: 10.1007/s11908-020-00740-z.
59. Kreisel KM, Spicknall IH, Gargano JW, et al. Sexually transmitted infections among US women and men: Prevalence and incidence estimates, 2018. Sex Transm Dis. 2021;48(4):208-214. DOI: 10.1097/OLQ.0000000000001355.
60. Centers for Disease Control and Prevention. Human papillomavirus (HPV) ACIP vaccine recommendations. 2014. (https://www.cdc.gov/vaccines/hcp/acip-recs/vacc-specific/hpv.html).
61. Iqbal K, Klevens RM, Kainer MA, Baumgartner J, Gerard K, Poissant T, Sweet K, Vonderwahl C, Knickerbocker T, Khudyakov Y, Xia GL, Roberts H, Teshale E. Epidemiology of Acute Hepatitis B in the United States From Population-Based Surveillance, 2006-2011. Clin Infect Dis. 2015 Aug;61(4):584-92. Epub 2015 Apr 22.

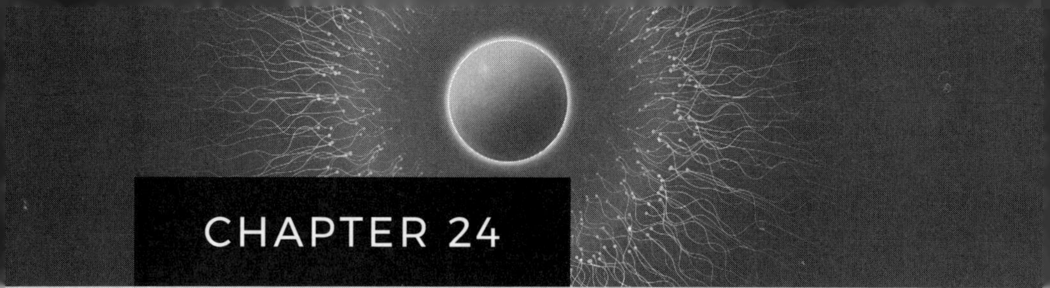

CHAPTER 24

Screening for Cervical, Ovarian, and Breast Cancer

Michael S. Policar, MD, MPH
George F. Sawaya, MD
Patty Cason, MS, FNP-BC

KEY POINTS

- Evidence-based cervical and breast cancer screening guidelines are put out by the United States Preventive Services Task Force (USPSTF) and the American Cancer Society (ACS). These guidelines apply to all asymptomatic people in the United States. These guidelines, as well as the breast cancer screening guidelines from the American College of Obstetricians and Gynecologists (ACOG), differ from one another regarding the ages at which to start and stop.
- Those aged younger than 21 years should not be screened for cervical cancer regardless of the age of sexual debut or behavior-related risk factors.
- After hysterectomy with removal of the cervix, individuals who do not have a history of a high-grade cervical precancer or cancer should discontinue screening.
- The *ASCCP Risk-Based Consensus Management Guidelines* were published by the ASCCP (also known as American Society for Colposcopy and Cervical Pathology) in 2019, emphasizing a personalized approach to management of those with abnormal cervical cancer screening test results or biopsies. An app is available to recommend management strategies.
- Screening for ovarian cancer in people who are at higher than average risk is individualized.
- Screening for ovarian cancer with current modalities has no benefit for those at average risk and has substantial false-positive results that can lead to complications during diagnostic evaluations.
- For most asymptomatic individuals, a screening pelvic exam and screening breast exam may not be necessary. If indicated, a person can collect a self-administered vaginal swab or urine sample for nucleic acid amplification testing (NAAT) to screen for chlamydia and gonorrhea.

A reproductive health care visit represents an ideal opportunity to offer periodic health screening services, including screening for genital tract and breast cancers. As early as the 1920s, the prevalent philosophy of the American medical community was that individuals of all ages should receive an annual physical examination and a battery of routine screening tests to detect early, asymptomatic disease.[1] However, the wisdom of this practice has been challenged. Research studies and health policy discussions have focused on the optimal content of periodic health screening: which tests should or should not be performed, how often each screening test should be done, and whether each test should be performed routinely or limited to persons with certain risk factors. While many approaches to periodic health screening have been proposed, the recommendations of the United States Preventive Services Task Force (USPSTF) are considered the blueprint for the screening guidelines developed by professional specialty societies and health plans. Using an evidence-based methodology, the USPSTF guidelines gauge the strength of each recommendation with a letter grade, which is assigned using a combination of the balance of net benefits and harms of the intervention and the level of certainty regarding net benefit, based upon the quality of the research studies used to develop the recommendation. In 2007, the USPSTF updated the definitions of the grades it assigns to recommendations and now includes "suggestions for practice" for each grade. In 2012, it further updated the definition of, and suggestions for practice, for the grade C statement.[2] (See **Table 24-1**.)

Another helpful preventive health screening guideline is the Women's Preventive Services Initiative (WPSI), a federally supported collaborative program led by the American College of Obstetricians and Gynecologists (ACOG) to review and recommend updates to the current Health Resources and Services Administration (HRSA) *Women's Preventive Services Guidelines* (https://www.womenspreventivehealth.org/). The recommendations, if adopted by HRSA, help ensure that patients receive a comprehensive set of preventive services without having to pay a health insurance copayment, coinsurance, or deductible.

In the past, the concept of the "annual well-woman visit" included a screening breast exam, cervical cytology screening, and a screening pelvic exam in persons who had initiated sexual activity. Owing in part to the changes in cancer screening recommendations, however, most people will no longer require yearly visits to receive preventive health screening tests, irrespective of their choice of contraceptive method. The USPSTF recommends that people undergo a health screening visit once every 1–3 years, depending upon their underlying health status, sexual behaviors, the intervals of the recommended screening tests, and their own personal preferences. If the person chooses not to receive this service, offer "opportunistic prevention" by discussing prevention guidance and screening tests at the time of problem-oriented visits.

Another issue that may arise at a health-screening visit is whether to provide comprehensive preventive health services or only those related to sexual and reproductive health. One original intention of the 2010 Patient Protection and Affordable Care Act (ACA)'s individual mandate clause was that a majority of people would be insured and have an established relationship with a primary care provider (PCP) from whom they will receive some or all preventive health services. While this provision was repealed in 2019, in the years that it was in force, many formerly uninsured persons did initiate a PCP relationship.[3] For patients who have this relationship with a PCP, it is important for the sexual and

Table 24-1 Recommendation Grades Used By the USPSTF, 2023

Grade	Definition	Suggestions for Practice
A	The USPSTF recommends the service. There is high certainty that the net benefit is substantial.	Offer or provide this service.
B	The USPSTF recommends the service. There is high certainty that the net benefit is moderate or there is moderate certainty that the net benefit is moderate to substantial.	Offer or provide this service.
C	The USPSTF recommends selectively offering or providing this service to individual patients based on professional judgment and patient preferences. There is at least moderate certainty that the net benefit is small.	Offer or provide this service for selected patients depending on individual circumstances.
D	The USPSTF recommends against the service. There is moderate or high certainty that the service has no net benefit or that the harms outweigh the benefits.	Discourage the use of this service.
I	The USPSTF concludes that the current evidence is insufficient to assess the balance of benefits and harms of the service. Evidence is lacking, of poor quality, or conflicting, and the balance of benefits and harms cannot be determined.	Read the clinical considerations section of USPSTF Recommendation Statement. If the service is offered, patients should understand the uncertainty about the balance of benefits and harms.

Reproduced from U.S. Preventive Services Task Force. Grade definitions; 2012. https://www.uspreventiveservicestaskforce.org/uspstf/about-uspstf/methods-and-processes/grade-definitions

reproductive health care provider to avoid duplicating tests already completed, and ideally, with the permission of the individual, to transmit the record of their health care visits to the PCP and vice-versa. In some cases, the only opportunity available to receive preventive health care services is during a person's sexual and reproductive health care visit, so if you are adequately equipped in your practice, it is appropriate to offer the full range of recommended preventive interventions. The USPSTF has a free app, the Prevention Task Force application (formerly ePSS), that facilitates point-of-care decisions about appropriate preventive services (https://www.uspreventiveservicestaskforce.org/apps/). The WPSI website has interactive tables as well (https://www.womenspreventivehealth.org/wellwomanchart/#interactive).

(See Chapter 27 on digital resources.)

Many years ago, a health screening visit was linked with the provision of prescription hormonal contraceptives, so that a person could receive a prescription for combined hormonal contraceptives only if they underwent a well-person visit. This attitude is outdated, and only those medical conditions that could influence contraceptive choice, safety, or usage should be the subject of screening before prescribing hormonal contraception. For example, the 2016 Selected Practice Recommendations (SPR) for contraceptive use published by the Centers for Disease Control and Prevention (CDC) do not recommend breast or genital tract examination, cervical cancer screening, sexually transmitted infection assessment, hemoglobin determination, or other routine lab tests as "contributing substantially to safe and effective use of a contraceptive method."[4] No published domestic or international guidelines require screening for genital tract cancer or sexually transmitted infections prior to prescribing contraceptives, based on the attitude that doing so is unnecessary for safe contraceptive use and that any unnecessary barriers to contraceptive services should be removed.[5] Furthermore, hormonal methods need not be withheld from a person solely because of an abnormal cervical cytology or positive high-risk human papillomavirus (hrHPV) test. There is no reason to believe that the use of any contraceptive method will hasten the progression of an existing preinvasive lesion to cervical cancer. All too often, the unfortunate result of withholding contraceptives from a person with an abnormal cytology or cervical biopsy result is undesired pregnancy, which makes assessment of the abnormal cervical test more difficult and often delays treatment.

Cervical Cancer

The Natural History of Cervical Cancer

The cause of preinvasive cervical lesions and invasive cancer is an accumulation of DNA mutations in immature metaplastic cells in the cervix as a consequence of persistent hrHPV infection, in concert with other carcinogenic cofactors.

Infection With High-Risk HPV

Genital HPV infections are transmitted by skin-to-skin contact during sex. Although more than 100 DNA types of HPV have been identified, only a limited number are associated with premalignant and malignant epithelial lesions of the lower genital tract: HPV types 16 and 18 account for about 70% of high-grade squamous intraepithelial lesions (HSIL; also referred to as cervical intraepithelial neoplasia [CIN] 2 and 3 lesions) and cervical cancers. The remaining 30% are due to HPV types 31, 33, 35, 39, 45, 51, 52, 56, 58, 59, 66, and 68.[6] The high-risk HPV types exert their cancer-causing effects through a series of events leading to the degradation of the p53 tumor suppressor protein in infected cells, reducing the host's ability to reject cells with random DNA mutations. Infections due to HPV types 6 and 11, the cause of genital warts and low-grade cervical lesions, exhibit no malignant potential.

HPV infections are widespread among sexually active adults and cannot be eradicated with antiviral drugs. HPV infections are transient in the large majority of infected individuals, while persistent infection with hrHPV types is necessary for the development of high-grade lesions and cancer. (See Chapter 23, Reproductive Tract Infections, Including HIV and Other Sexually Transmitted Infections.)

Squamous Metaplasia Within the Transformation Zone

The cervix consists of two types of epithelium:

- *Squamous epithelium*, covering the vagina and the vaginal portion of the cervix
- *Columnar epithelium*, covering the endocervical canal, and in some individuals, the area around the external cervical os

Prior to menarche, columnar epithelial cells cover much of the face of the cervix. At menarche, the vaginal pH drops into an acidic range and causes the fragile columnar epithelial cells around the cervical os to be replaced by squamous epithelium, a process referred to as squamous metaplasia. As this process proceeds over decades, the advancing edge of the squamous epithelium (referred to as the squamocolumnar junction or SCJ) migrates centrally toward the cervical os and ultimately into the endocervical canal. The immature metaplastic cells found in younger people are particularly vulnerable to infection with HPV. Because squamous cell cancers and their precursors virtually always develop within the field of metaplasia (also called the transformation zone), both cytological and colposcopic evaluation focus upon this area.

An Oncogenic Cofactor

Since not all people who have persistent hrHPV infection of their cervix develop a preinvasive cervical lesion, it seems that persistent hrHPV infection alone is insufficient to initiate the development of a preinvasive cervical lesion. A facilitating agent, or oncogenic cofactor, appears to be necessary to act in concert with hrHPV to initiate these premalignant changes. For example, cigarette smoking has been identified as a powerful cofactor,[7] doubling the risk of cervical cancer.

Risk Factors for Cervical Cancer

Epidemiologic observations are consistent with the biological mechanism of cervical cancer. Anything that increases the possibility of acquiring an HPV infection increases risk for cervical cancer: a sex partner whose previous partner had cervical cancer; more than five lifetime sexual partners; and sexual debut before 20 years old. Metaplasia is most active during adolescence, making a young person more vulnerable to cell changes that result from hrHPV infection. Clinical history of condyloma acuminata, which is caused by an infection with a low-risk type of HPV, is a risk marker for coinfection with a high-risk type.[8] Infection with the human immunodeficiency virus (HIV) and other medical conditions associated with immunodeficiency decrease the ability of the immune system to recognize and reject abnormal cells. People who use immunosuppressive drugs, especially after a major organ transplant, also are at increased risk of cervical cancer.

Behavioral protective factors include no history of partnered sexual activity, lifelong mutual monogamy, and long-term use of condoms. Factors that appear to have no effect on cervical cancer risk include a history of herpes simplex virus infection or the circumcision status of the partner.

Rather than to rely on a behavioral strategy that focuses on the sexual transmissibility of HPV, it makes more sense from a public health viewpoint, as well as from the perspective of minimizing harm to patients, to prevent cervical cancer and its precursors with primary prevention via HPV immunization before sexual debut and secondary prevention through screening programs that will detect and lead to treatment of high-grade preinvasive lesions before life-threatening invasive cervical cancers have a chance to develop.

Disparities in Incidence and Mortality from Cervical Cancer

Studies show higher rates of cervical cancer and higher rates of death from cervical cancer among Black and Hispanic/Latinx patients.[9,10] Rates of cancer deaths are higher for Black patients (3.4 per 100,000 people) and Hispanic/Latinx patients (2.6 per 100,000 people), respectively, than White patients (2.1 per 100,000).[11,12] Racial and ethnic differences persist despite HPV vaccination,[13,14] a variety of screening modalities,[15,16] and programs for under- and uninsured patients such as State Plan Amendments to Medicaid and the National Breast and Cervical Cancer Early Detection Program. Among the many ways racism leads to these higher rates is through lack of appropriate follow-up; inequities in management and treatment; differences in cancer type (adenocarcinoma); differences in predominant hrHPV types; and barriers to accessing medical care for cervical cancer screening, management, and treatment. A Black patient's risk of dying from cervical cancer is even higher than previously thought. An earlier risk estimate based on population-based mortality statistics had not been corrected for prior hysterectomy; the corrected cervical cancer mortality rate for African American patients is 10.1 per 100,000, whereas the uncorrected rate is 5.7 per 100,000. The corrected rate for White patients is 4.7 per 100,000, whereas the uncorrected rate is 3.2 per 100,000. Without the correction, the disparity in mortality was underestimated by 44%.[17,18]

Primary Prevention of Cervical Cancer with HPV Vaccination

Vaccination against hrHPV infection has been shown to be successful for primary prevention of cancer precursors and cancers caused by certain hrHPV subtypes. Almost 100% of cervical cancers are caused by hrHPV, and many other cancers can be hrHPV-related, including vaginal, vulvar, penile, anal, and head and neck cancers. The only product currently available in the United States is the nonavalent HPV (9vHPV) vaccine, Gardasil9®. The earlier quadrivalent and bivalent HPV vaccines had been available since 2006 and 2009, respectively, but are no longer sold in the United States.

The vaccine consists of genetically manufactured viral envelope proteins, rather than live or attenuated virus, to stimulate the production of anti-HPV antibodies. When given to uninfected individuals, the vaccine has very high efficacy in preventing HSIL and cancers attributable to HPV types 16, 18, 31, 33, 45, 52, and 58. The 9vHPV vaccine also has high efficacy in protecting against genital warts, which are induced by HPV types 6 and 11. The vaccine does not appear to cause any serious long-term adverse effects, but pain at the injection site can trigger a vasovagal fainting episode.

Current guidelines recommend that individuals who have been vaccinated receive routine cervical screening. Ten percent of HSIL lesions contain hrHPV types not included in the vaccine, and there are data showing that some non-Hispanic Black and Latinx/Hispanic people have predominant hrHPV types not covered by the available nonavalent HPV vaccine.[23-25] These types are, however, included in

Preventing Vasovagal Syncope

If a patient feels dizzy, nauseated, ringing in their ears, vision changes, or like they may faint, have them isometrically contract the muscles in their arms, hands, feet, and legs to push blood back to the center of their body.[19-22] This can immediately stop the reflex and prevent syncope. Consider offering anticipatory guidance to the patient prior to giving the immunization by telling them that it is not uncommon for people getting an injection to get dizzy or even faint. You can go over some of the more common prodromal symptoms with them and then have them practice tensing their muscles so they know how to stop the reaction if it starts. In addition, individuals receiving the vaccine should be monitored for at least a few minutes after the injection to prevent an injury from an unwitnessed fall, and clinicians should be familiar with the recognition and treatment of vasovagal episodes.

hrHPV tests, so routine hrHPV-based screening (either primary or as part of co-testing) would be able to detect the hrHPV and precancer. The information about hrHPV genotype patterns among Black and Hispanic women in the United States should have implications for future cervical cancer prevention strategies.

The 2016 CDC Advisory Committee on Immunization Practices (ACIP) has published guidelines regarding the use of HPV vaccine in individuals of any gender.[26]

Important points:

- It is ideal to immunize before an individual has potential exposure to HPV through sexual skin-to-skin contact.
- Routine vaccination at age 9–12 years is recommended. The immune response in 9- and 10-year-olds in particular is excellent and enduring, and there may be less resistance from parents who accept the vaccine as "cancer prevention" at an age distant from sexual activity.
- Vaccination is recommended for everyone through age 26. If a person reaches age 26 before the vaccination series is complete, remaining doses should be administered.
- Discuss HPV vaccination with unvaccinated adults aged 27–45 years. Vaccination of people in this age range may provide less benefit than being vaccinated at a younger age, for several reasons, including that more people in this age range have already been exposed to one or more types of HPV. People with few lifetime sexual partners, those who may have a new partner in the future, patients who have had preinvasive lower genital tract lesions, and cigarette smokers may have the most to benefit from vaccination. In this age group, the CDC recommends a shared-decision-making discussion, not on an opt-out or opt-in basis.
- Initially, the HPV vaccination was a three-dose schedule for those of any age: first dose, second dose 1 to 2 months later, and third dose 6 months after the first. In 2016, the CDC added a two-dose schedule for 9- to 14-year-olds (first dose, then second dose after a minimum of 6 to 12 months), based on studies that showed seroconversion and antibody titers after two doses were not inferior to three doses in this age group.
- The 9vHPV vaccine can be given at the same time as other vaccines, including TDaP, TD, and MCV4 vaccines. Lactating people can receive the HPV vaccine.

- People should be advised that vaccination has no therapeutic (treatment) effect on a patient's HPV infection, genital warts, or abnormal cytology. However, it is recommended that they get immunized to prevent future acquisition of HPV.
- Prevaccination assessments (e.g., cervical cytology, screening for hrHPV DNA, type-specific HPV tests, or HPV antibody) to establish the appropriateness of HPV vaccination are not recommended at any age.
- Routine pregnancy testing is not indicated before vaccination. HPV vaccination is not recommended during pregnancy; however, if a vaccine dose is administered during pregnancy, no intervention is needed. If a person is found to be pregnant after initiating the vaccination series, the remainder of the series should be delayed until the patient is no longer pregnant. Pregnancy registries for 4vHPV and 2vHPV vaccines have been closed because reports of problems in pregnant people or their newborns were no greater than in nonvaccinated persons. The U.S. Food and Drug Administration (FDA) has established a registry for people immunized with the 9vHPV vaccine to track the rate of adverse effects.
- HPV vaccines are not live vaccines and can be administered to those who are immunosuppressed from disease or medications. However, the immune response and vaccine efficacy may be less than that in immunocompetent persons. The ACS 2020 guideline[27] adds the caveat that late vaccination should be completed as soon as possible and that individuals should be informed that vaccination may not be effective at older ages.

In the United States, providers follow recommendations from CDC; however, it is interesting to note that the World Health Organization[28] published guidance in December 2022 recommending a two-dose schedule for people of all ages. They also present an alternative single-dose schedule for those aged 9–20 years old based on data showing that a single dose has duration of protection and efficacy comparable to a two-dose schedule.

Secondary Prevention of Cervical Cancer with Cervical Cancer Screening

Based upon current screening patterns in the United States, early detection and treatment of preinvasive cervical lesions prevents at least 70% of potential cervical cancers. ACS estimates that in 2022, of the 14,100 Americans[29] who develop new cases of cervical cancer:

- One-half had not had a cervical cytology in the past 5 years.[30]
- Among those who had been screened, tests results were either falsely negative, the patient was not managed correctly, or there was inadequate follow-up.

False-negative results occur in about 25% of cervical cytology tests and occur either because the lesion exfoliated too few cells to be detected, there was a sampling error by the clinician, or there was an interpretive error in the cytopathology lab. In 1996, the FDA approved liquid-based cytology (LBC) with thin-layer preparation technique (for example, Thin Prep and BD SurePath), which removes blood, mucus, and debris from the background of the sample. Early studies suggested that LBC improved screening accuracy over conventional slides[31,32]; however, a large, randomized clinical trial (RCT) from the Netherlands[33] and a meta-analysis of eight studies[34] concluded that LBC is neither more sensitive nor more specific for detection of HSIL compared with the conventional cervical cytology test. Virtually all cytopathology labs in the United States use this technology because it improves the efficiency of cytotechnicians, facilitates computerized screening or rescreening, and serves as a platform for evaluation of other pathogens in the cytology sample, specifically hrHPV, gonorrhea, and chlamydia.

Technical Aspects of Cytological Screening

High accuracy in cytological screening depends on a good-quality cervical sample, appropriately performed preparation, and competent cytopathologic interpretation.

- Cytological screening may be performed at any time of the cycle because the presence of menstrual blood is not problematic in the interpretation of LBC. It is still prudent to avoid high-flow days.
- Moisten the speculum with warm water or a small amount of lubricating gel applied at the introitus and away from the tip of the speculum. Samples most easily contaminated by blood should be taken early in the sampling sequence: NAATs for chlamydia and gonorrhea should be performed before the cervical cytology sample.
- LBC sampling:
    - It is important to obtain sufficient cellular material for interpretation.
    - The material covering the cervix should not be wiped away, as this practice can remove a significant amount of cellular material, resulting in a scanty sample. If necessary, the vagina may be very gently dabbed with a swab to wipe away heavy mucus or discharge prior to collecting an LBC sample.
    - Use the specific sampling devices that have been provided by the cytopathology lab used by your practice; avoid using other sampling instruments.
    - The optimal collection is with a spatula plus endocervical brush or a broom plus brush. Adequate sampling of the endocervical canal is essential.
    - When using the spatula, place it gently against the cervical tissue with the contoured end resting in the dimple of the os. With even pressure, turn the spatula 360 degrees.
    - When using the brush, insert the brush into the cervix until only the bottom fibers are visible. Slowly rotate one-quarter to one-half turn in one direction. Do not over-rotate or use pressure when moving the brush, as this may cause bleeding and loss of endocervical cells.
    - For ThinPrep, vigorously twirl the brush and spatula in the liquid at least 10 times. Push the brush against the side of the vial to remove any mucus. Use the spatula to mechanically remove mucus and cells from the brush. For SurePath, the spatula/brush tips are snapped off into the vial.

HPV Testing Used Alone or As an Adjunct to Cytological Screening

hrHPV DNA testing for 13 or 14 high-risk HPV types is used in one of four ways:

1. **Primary hrHPV screening**, using an FDA-approved hrHPV test *alone*, and then triaging to cytology if positive. USPSTF recommends not switching to primary hrHPV screening until age 30, whereas the ACS recommends starting screening with primary hrHPV screening at age 25.

2. **Screening with cytology and hrHPV (cotesting)**, in which a hrHPV test and cervical cytology are performed simultaneously, in those 30 years old and older.
3. **Triage** of a cervical cytology result of atypical squamous cells of undetermined significance (ASC-US) in patients aged 25 and older. With this strategy, once the laboratory determines an ASC-US result, a "reflex" hrHPV test is performed on the same sample. This may also be useful for low-grade squamous intraepithelial lesion results.
4. **HPV-based follow-up testing.** Use of either cotesting or an approved hrHPV alone as follow-up after colposcopy showing no high-grade lesion and for post-treatment surveillance.

Primary hrHPV screening should be done with a test that is FDA-approved specifically for primary hrHPV screening such as Cobas or Onclarity; both test for 14 hrHPV types, including HPV type 16/18. If HPV testing is positive, it is recommended that a "reflex" cervical cytology test be performed on the same sample that was sent to the lab. If the genotype test is positive for HPV 16/18, colposcopy is recommended. If negative for HPV 16/18, the cytology result is used to triage the person to colposcopy (if ASC-US or worse) or repeat screening in 1 year if negative. Rescreening after a negative primary hrHPV screen should occur no sooner than 5 years.

Cervical cancer screening with cotesting improves the sensitivity of screening for HSIL or cancer to at least 92% when compared with a sensitivity of about 75% for cytology alone.[35,36] Of importance is the higher negative predictive value; people with negative results on both cytology and HPV tests have a less than 1% likelihood of developing HSIL or cancer within the next 10 years. Cotesting is not recommended for screening people under 30 years old due to the high prevalence of transient hrHPV infections in younger individuals. People who cotest negative (hrHPV negative and normal cervical cytology) should not be rescreened before 5 years, in part because even if the person were to acquire a new hrHPV infection during these 5 years, they are highly likely to clear the infection without negative sequelae, and the risk of a significant new lesion developing in that time frame is negligible. However, while it is highly unlikely that a new hrHPV infection detected soon after a negative cotest will persist, the likelihood of a new positive hrHPV test result causing distress and unnecessary follow-up is substantial.

Recommended Routine Cervical Cancer Screening Intervals

The national recommendations for cervical cancer screening intervals have changed over time, which often resulted in inconsistent, or even incorrect, practices among providers.[37] Between the 1940s and 2002, women in the United States were advised to have cervical cytology screening performed annually at the time of their well-woman visit. Currently, two major national organizations, the USPSTF and the ACS, have issued recommendations regarding the periodicity of cervical cancer screening in the general, asymptomatic population. ASCCP and ACOG endorse the USPSTF guidelines and support the ACS guidelines.[38-40]

Those who are "under surveillance" for prior abnormal results or who have undergone treatment for a preinvasive cervical lesion are followed under the 2019 ASCCP management guidelines.[35] Once a patient has completed the recommended follow up, if the ASCCP management guideline recommends they return to routine screening, they should go back to being screened according to the screening guidelines. However, if there is a history of treatment for cervical intraepithelial neoplasia

(CIN) 2 or worse, rather than a return to hrHPV-based testing every 5 years, the 2019 ASCCP management guidelines[35] recommend that after a patient exits from management, HPV-based testing continue every 3 years for at least 25 years.

There are minor differences between the USPSTF and ACS guidance, but overall, they constitute a single "national standard" regarding screening periodicity. Consequently, clinicians should be careful to explain the rationale in the medical record if a decision is made to deviate from the guideline used in your practice.

The USPSTF[39] cervical cancer screening guidelines recommend the following:

- Age under 21: do not screen
- Age 21–29: screen every 3 years with cervical cytology alone
- Age 30–65: perform hrHPV alone or cotesting every 5 years; or cervical cytology every 3 years
- Discontinue at age 65 after three consecutive negative cytology screening tests or two negative cotests or hrHPV tests in the prior 10 years, with the last test performed within the prior 3 years (if cytology) and 5 years (if a hrHPV test).*
- Discontinue routine screening after hysterectomy with removal of the cervix (total hysterectomy) if no prior CIN2+, not immunocompromised, and no diethylstilbestrol exposure in utero. Once discontinued, routine cytology screening and hrHPV testing should not be restarted.

The 2020 ACS[40] cervical cancer screening guidelines recommend:

- Age under 25: do not screen
- Age 25–65: screening with hrHPV alone every 5 years is preferred
- Discontinue all cervical cancer screening for individuals aged > 65 years who have no history of CIN 2 or more severe disease within the past 25 years, and who have documented adequate negative screening in the prior 10 years.*
- If primary hrHPV testing is not available, it is acceptable to screen individuals aged 25–65 years with cotesting every 5 years or cytology alone every 3 years.

* The current national guidelines recommend exiting screening over age 65 for those without a history of CIN2+ who have been adequately screened. This is considered a weak recommendation by ACS/ASCCP/ACP, and reviews of the available data suggest that it is based on expert opinion and limited evidence. In part, this recommendation stems from the potential for distress that screening may cause for the person getting screened, tipping the perceived balance of harms and benefits. However, approximately 20% of new cervical cancers are in those over age 65 and there are large racial disparities. People over age 65 and Black-identified people are more often diagnosed at a later stage and have worse outcomes and higher mortality rates. The characteristics and demographics of people in the United States over age 65 are changing in many ways including life expectancy, sexual behaviors, and hysterectomy rates. The data on disparities and changes in the population over age 65 are not reflected in the current guidelines.[41,42]

The USPSTF guideline allows for more options and recommends screening 21- to 24-year-olds. The ACS guideline is similar to screening guidelines in countries like Australia and England that have robust, coordinated screening programs and a well-vaccinated population. To some extent, the ACS guidance can be considered aspirational. Providers and patients are often slow to incorporate changes in screening and management protocols, and it will take time for laboratories to adapt workflows and for adequate coordination between payers, laboratories, health care systems, and health centers to implement primary hrHPV screening. For these and other reasons, we are in a transition period with a choice of acceptable screening methods. FDA clearance of additional hrHPV testing platforms for use in primary HPV screening will facilitate the transition.

Clarification for screening in individuals in specific circumstances:

- Individuals 21 years of age and older who have never had genital sexual contact with another person should be advised that their risk of cervical cancer is extremely low, but not zero. Once counseled, they may choose to postpone cervical cancer screening until sexually active or opt to be screened.
- Pregnant persons should be screened at the same intervals as those who are not pregnant. Unless the patient is due for screening at the time they enter antepartum care, no additional "routine screening" is needed if prior results are available and negative.
- People having an intrauterine device (IUD) placed or starting contraception do not need cervical cancer screening unless they are due for their routine screening.
- People with a new sexual partner or multiple partners should have the same cervical cancer screening as the general population.
- People with a cervix who are not cisgender women should be screened according to national guidelines. (See Chapter 22 for specific recommendations about sensitive exams.)
- Recommend screening to patients who are LGBTQIA+-identified and screen according to national guidelines.

The 2021 National Institutes of Health (NIH) Guidelines for the Prevention and Treatment of Opportunistic Infections in Adults and Adolescents with HIV[43] recommends that women with HIV (WWH) have age-based cervical cancer screening:

- **WWH ages 21–29 years** should have annual cytology testing. If the results of three consecutive cytology tests are normal, follow-up cytology tests should be every 3 years. Cotesting (cytology and hrHPV) is not recommended for WWH $<$ 30 years of age.
- **WWH aged $\geq$ 30 years**
  - Either cytology alone or cotesting are acceptable for screening.
  - If screening with cytology alone, WWH should have a cytology test at the time of HIV diagnosis (baseline), then every 12 months. If the results of three consecutive cytology tests are normal, follow-up cytology tests should be every 3 years.
  - If cotesting is available, it can be done at the time of diagnosis or at age 30 years. Patients who cotest negative can have their next cervical cancer screening in 3 years.
  - Cervical cancer screening should not stop at 65 years of age.
- The ASCCP management guidelines[35] recommend screening people with non-HIV immunocompromise (for example, a major organ transplant or use of immunosuppressive medications) in the same way as HIV-positive individuals, starting at 21 years of age.

A problem for clinicians is that there has been no national consumer education campaign regarding the rationale for increased screening intervals, and many patients reject them as being financially motivated and not in the best interest of their health.[44] Some clinicians are reluctant to change their screening practices as well; in one study, physicians felt that patients were uncomfortable with extended screening intervals and were concerned that people would not come for health screening visits without the need for concurrent cytology screening. Providers are fearful of encountering a person with an interval cancer and being sued for a missed diagnosis.[45]

Despite these obstacles, clinicians should discuss the particular screening interval that applies to the individual patient. It is helpful to frame the idea of longer intervals by pointing out that screening with hrHPV tests every 5 years will miss fewer precancerous and cancerous lesions than screening more often, every 3 years, with cytology tests. Screening every 3 years with cytology has lower positive predictive value than screening every 5 years with hrHPV-based testing and the longer screening interval minimizes false-positive test results. It is logical with cotesting, for example, that one would need less frequent screening because they are having two tests rather than just one. Some clinicians counsel that being screened too often can be harmful to their health. (See Chapter 4, Person-Centered Reproductive Health Conversations and Contraceptive Counseling.)

Overscreening minimally improves lesion detection rates, but it results in an excess risk of false-positive tests, which can lead to unnecessary colposcopy and biopsies, with attendant distress, anxiety, and inconvenience, as well as unnecessary financial costs to the patient[46] and the health delivery system. Health plans now recognize this as a patient safety issue. Going forward, expect quality metrics for cervical cancer screening to evaluate your practice, not only on the percentage of eligible patients who are screened for cervical cancer, but also for the average interval between tests in those who should be routinely screened every 3–5 years, which is intended to detect overutilization of resources.

Management of Abnormal Screening Test Results

Epithelial Cell and Glandular Abnormalities

The goal of screening and management is to discover premalignant cervical lesions and to treat them before invasion occurs. This is done by screening for cytologic abnormalities and/or the presence of hrHPV, followed by a histologic diagnosis (biopsy) of HSIL (CIN 2 or 3). Additionally, glandular cancer precursor lesions can be detected (cytologically, as atypical glandular cells [AGC] and histologically, as adenocarcinoma in situ [AIS]) and treated before invasion to adenocarcinoma occurs. Consequently, the clinical endpoint that screening and evaluation seeks to identify is CIN 2+ (which includes CIN 2, CIN 2/3, CIN3, AIS, and cancer). Low-grade lesions are highly likely to regress (or at least, not to progress to CIN 3+), and therefore, should not be treated in almost all circumstances.

The management of abnormal test results is detailed in the 2019 ASCCP updated consensus guidelines for the management of abnormal cervical cancer screening tests and cancer precursors.[34] These guidelines are available online (https://www.asccp.org/guidelines) and a convenient app for iPad, iPhone, and Android phones is available (https://www.asccp.org/mobile-app). Both the mobile device app and the website allow you to incorporate both current and past test results (including no prior testing or unknown past testing) when determining personalized risk assessment and next steps in management. This improvement results in management decisions that are more tailored to the individual, rather than relying on the "generic" algorithms that were used in the earlier consensus management guidelines. For many clinicians, this will be the biggest change in how the guidelines are used.

Management of abnormal screening results in persons with HIV is according to ASCCP Management Guidelines.[43]

Other Abnormal Results Not Reflecting Epithelial Cell and Glandular Abnormalities

The classification system recommended by the third Bethesda workshop (2014 Bethesda System for Reporting Cervical Cytology) contained a number of modifications to include new screening technologies, as well as to remedy points of confusion between pathologists and clinicians.[47]

Negative, But Endocervical/Transformation Zone Component Absent or Insufficient. The Bethesda System has eliminated the category of "satisfactory, but limited by . . .", but comments regarding suboptimal specimen quality still may be made. The finding that most often limits interpretation is a paucity of endocervical cells. Their presence confirms that in the process of sampling the transformation zone, the active squamocolumnar junction was included. Endocervical cells are absent in 10% to 20% of cervical cytology samples obtained from premenopausal patients and as many as 50% from those who are postmenopausal.[48] For normal cytology results with no endocervical cells or transformation zone elements, the 2019 ASCCP guidelines recommend the following:[37,27]

- Age 21–29: Routine screening
- Age 30 or older:
    - If HPV is negative, routine screening.
    - If HPV is unknown, HPV testing is preferred, but repeat cytology in 3 years is acceptable.
    - If the HPV test is positive, HPV-based testing should be done in 1 year.

Unsatisfactory for Evaluation. Inadequate sampling, too much lubricant, or obscuring inflammation, blood, or cellular debris from necrosis makes interpretation impossible. Because unsatisfactory smears have a greater likelihood of being abnormal[49]:

- Repeat screening in 2–4 months (sooner is acceptable), preferably at mid-cycle and at least 24 hours after the most recent intercourse or use of vaginal products.
- If the original test was HPV negative or no HPV test was done, repeat screening in 2–4 months.
- If repeat cytology is negative, return to routine screening.
- If the repeat cytology again is unsatisfactory, refer for colposcopy.

If the proportion of unsatisfactory cytology tests within a practice is greater than 5%, remedial action in consultation with the cytopathologist is recommended.

Negative for Intraepithelial Lesion or Malignancy (NILM): Organisms

Trichomonas vaginalis. While cervical cytology is a relatively insensitive test for the detection of *T. vaginalis* (it detects trichomonads in only about half of infected patients), its specificity is as high as 98%.[50] Because the prevalence of *T. vaginalis* vaginal colonization in reproductive-aged people is about 5%, the positive predictive value of a cytological report of *T. vaginalis* is about 72%. When the report indicates the presence of *T. vaginalis*, review the patient's medical record to determine whether the infection was recently treated. If it has been, no further action is required. If not, offer treatment to avoid horizontal transmission to a new sexual partner and to prevent conversion of asymptomatic *T. vaginalis* colonization into an uncomfortable case of symptomatic vaginal trichomoniasis. The practice of requiring microscopic saline suspension to confirm vaginal trichomonads is illogical because the sensitivity of this test is only 60%. Instead, if the saline suspension is negative and confirmation is desired, use a molecular *Trichomonas* test (NAAT or PCR) with high sensitivity and specificity. Repeat the cytology test after the next routine screening interval, unless the narrative report mentions obscuring inflammation and indicates the need to repeat the cytology test after treatment.

Fungus morphologically consistent with *Candida* spp. In most cases, *Candida* detected on cervical cytology is due to normal vaginal colonization with low levels of *Candida* rather than frank vaginal candidiasis. While *Candida* colonization is not dangerous to the patient or to sexual partner(s), it is reasonable to let the patient know so they can decide if they would like to treat it. Repeat the cytology test only if the inflammation due to the candidiasis is of sufficient severity that the cytopathologist recommends that the test be repeated after treatment is complete.

Shift in flora suggestive of bacterial vaginosis. This result refers to changes detected in the bacterial flora of the vagina in which the normal *Lactobacillus* are not abundant, but coccobacilli are seen in numbers greater than normal. While this description was devised to suggest the possibility of bacterial vaginosis (BV), it is both an insensitive and nonspecific indicator of BV. Neither vaginal culture nor cervical cytology findings have any role in the diagnosis of BV. (See Chapter 23, Reproductive Tract Infections, Including HIV and Other Sexually Transmitted Infections.) Subsequent cervical cancer screening should be performed at the routine interval.

Bacteria morphologically consistent with *Actinomyces* spp. *Actinomyces israelii* is an anaerobic bacterium capable of causing a rare, but severe, pelvic infection called pelvic actinomycosis, especially in long-term IUD users over 35 years of age. The vast majority of IUD users with "*Actinomyces*-like organisms (ALO)" on cytology have an asymptomatic cervical colonization (not infection) that does not require either antibiotic therapy or removal of the IUD. However, IUD users with *Actinomyces* on their cytology report should have a bimanual pelvic examination to determine whether they have evidence of pelvic infection. If symptoms or physical findings suggest pelvic actinomycosis, remove the IUD and initiate intensive antibiotic therapy (see Chapter 10, Intrauterine Devices [IUDs]).

Cellular changes consistent with herpes simplex virus (HSV). Although an insensitive test of cervical herpes simplex shedding, cytology is a specific indicator. If the patient requests confirmation, a positive HSV-2 type-specific serology will confirm prior infection, but an HSV culture or PCR should be avoided, because viral shedding is intermittent and unpredictable. Unless inflammation interferes with the interpretation of the cytology sample, the next test should be performed at the routine interval.

NILM: Other Non-Neoplastic Findings

Reactive cellular changes associated with inflammation. Nonspecific reactive inflammatory changes may be associated with benign metaplasia, mechanical or chemical irritation, posttraumatic repair, chlamydial or gonococcal endocervicitis, trichomoniasis, mycoplasmas or ureaplasmas, viral infection, invasive cervical cancer with necrosis, or other unknown factors. Of these possibilities, the only infectious conditions amenable to antibiotic therapy are gonococcal and chlamydial endocervicitis, *Mycoplasma genitalium* infections, and vaginal trichomoniasis. Evaluate those who have not been screened recently by performing gonorrhea and chlamydia tests and treating patients who test positive. Rarely, the only cytological finding in a patient with an invasive cervical carcinoma is the persistent finding of inflammation. Some experts recommend that for those who have had consecutive cytology results with unexplained inflammation be evaluated by colposcopy, although the recommendation is not evidence-based.

Atrophy. Thinned epithelium in the lower genital tract is most common in postmenopausal patients or those with estrogen-deficiency states. Treatment is indicated only if the patient has symptomatic genitourinary syndrome of menopause (GSM). Cervical cytology screening intervals do not need to be modified, and the patient does not need to be notified. However, if there is concern that adequate sampling is hindered, or the result is unsatisfactory, or when patients are going to have colposcopy, it can be helpful if they use intravaginal estrogen for 4–6 weeks before repeat cytology or colposcopy.

Endometrial cells, cytologically benign, in someone 40 years of age or older. Endometrial cells found on cervical cytology are an insignificant finding in those who are premenopausal with normal ovulatory cycling. However, because the endometrium of postmenopausal people normally is atrophic, the finding of endometrial cells may be the result of exfoliation from a focus of endometrial hyperplasia or adenocarcinoma. For this reason, consider the finding of endometrial cells in someone postmenopausal as a danger sign and evaluate the endometrium with either endometrial biopsy or pelvic ultrasound to measure endometrial stripe thickness. Someone who is premenopausal with factors that put them at increased risk for endometrial hyperplasia, such as obesity or chronic anovulation, should have the finding of endometrial cells followed up by endometrial biopsy.

Ovarian Cancer

In the United States in 2022, the ACS estimated that 19,880 patients would be diagnosed with ovarian cancer, making this cancer the 10th most common among American women.[51] However, because of the low 5-year survival rates with this disease, especially in the later stages when it is more commonly diagnosed, it is the leading cause (53%) of gynecologic cancer deaths, accounting for 12,810 deaths in the United States in 2022. The average age at diagnosis is 63 years. It is more common in White patients than in African American patients. The lifetime risk of ovarian cancer is about 1 in 78, and the lifetime risk of dying of ovarian cancer is about 1 in 108.

Although some risk factors for ovarian cancer are well known, a majority of people diagnosed with this condition have none.[52] Geographic differences are marked; rates in Sweden and the United States are 13 to 15 cases per 100,000 women per year, while the rate in Japan is 3 cases per 100,000 women per year. This difference in part may be related to dietary fat intake, which is higher in the United States and Scandinavia and lower in Japan. A long interval of ovulatory cycles also is associated with ovarian cancer; low parity, delayed childbearing, body mass index of 30 kg/m^2 or higher, and infertility are weak risk factors.[52]

Familial predisposition accounts for 5% to 10% of cases, and the risk of ovarian cancer is 5% if one first-degree relative had ovarian cancer and 7% if two or more first-degree relatives had the condition. A site-specific familial ovarian cancer syndrome has been described, which is mediated through a highly penetrant autosomal dominant gene; in these cases, the risk to a first-degree relative is up to 50%. In addition, persons with ovaries who have *BRCA* mutations are at greater risk of ovarian cancer, about 35% to 70% for *BRCA-1* and 10% to 30% for *BRCA-2* by age 70.[52,53] Another genetic syndrome called hereditary non-polyposis colon cancer (Lynch syndrome) also is associated with increased risk of both ovarian and endometrial cancer. There is no accurate method to detect early ovarian cancer in these high-risk patients, and expert consensus guidelines recommend discussing prophylactic oophorectomy with patients who have completed childbearing and have either tested positive for one of the genetic syndromes or have two or more first-degree relatives with ovarian cancer.[54]

Other factors are known to protect against ovarian cancer. People who have had a term pregnancy before age 26 have a lower risk of ovarian cancer than those who have not, and risk goes down with each full-term pregnancy.[53] Oral contraceptive use reduces the risk of ovarian cancer by as much as 80% in people aged 40 to 59 years. Not only does longer duration of use provide more protection, but the effect lasts for as long as 15 years after oral contraceptives are discontinued.[55] Oral contraceptives are also effective in reducing the risk of ovarian cancer in those with *BRCA-1* and *BRCA-2* mutations, both of which increase the risk of ovarian cancer.[56,57] The same effect is seen with depot medroxyprogesterone acetate (DMPA); a case-control study in Thailand[58] showed an 83% risk reduction for epithelial ovarian cancer when the duration of DMPA use was longer than 3 years. Patients who have chronic anovulation (i.e., polycystic ovarian syndrome) have a decreased risk of ovarian cancer; protection also is seen with greater duration of lactation. Tubal surgery for permanent contraception is associated with a 40% to 50% reduction in the risk of ovarian cancer, and hysterectomy (without oophorectomy) with a 35% reduction. This may be explained by growing evidence that most ovarian cancers originate in the fallopian tube epithelium, both in those that are at high-risk and in the general population.[59] As a result, prophylactic salpingectomy with conservation of the ovaries until menopause has become a more common practice for premenopausal patients undergoing risk-reducing surgery,[60,61] as well as offering bilateral salpingectomy as an option for those having tubal surgery for permanent contraception instead of a tubal occlusion procedure.[62] (See Chapter 8, Permanent Contraception.) Additional recommendations have emerged for offering bilateral salpingectomy to any person who no longer desires pregnancy and is undergoing a gynecologic surgery.[63]

Ovarian Cancer Screening

Ovarian cancer usually is diagnosed during an evaluation of someone who is symptomatic, but it may be detected as a mass found incidentally during pelvic examination or ultrasound. While early ovarian cancer has been long considered a "silent cancer," over 70% of patients recall having symptoms for 3 months or longer before their diagnosis.[64] In a recent study by Chan et al.[65] of 419 patients with ovarian cancer evaluated for symptoms, 301 (72%) presented with one or more symptoms, and 118 (28%) were asymptomatic but had a mass found on examination. Ovarian cancer can be associated with pelvic pain, abdominal discomfort and distention, bloating after meals, feeling full quickly, constipation, nausea, urinary frequency, and rarely, irregular vaginal bleeding. In advanced stages, ovarian cancer is often accompanied by fatigue, nonspecific gastrointestinal symptoms, poor appetite and weight loss, increased abdominal girth, or shortness of breath due to pleural effusion. Patients who experience such symptoms daily for more than a few weeks should be evaluated. The best way to promptly diagnose ovarian cancer is for both the patient and their clinician to have a high index of suspicion when characteristic symptoms occur.[66]

Three techniques have been suggested to screen for the early stages of asymptomatic ovarian cancer: periodic bimanual pelvic examination, serum CA-125 measurement, and transvaginal ultrasound. The USPSTF recommends against routine screening for ovarian cancer with any of these modalities (D Statement), because the potential harms outweigh the potential benefits.[67] However, guidelines from the NIH state that these tests should be offered annually to women who have familial risk factors for ovarian cancer, starting at 25–30 years of age.[54]

For decades, clinicians conducting a screening pelvic exam (SPE) as part of a well-woman visit has as a way to screen for ovarian cancer and other abnormalities, but it is insensitive and has poor specificity. Recent national guidelines contain inconsistent recommendations.

- The USPSTF issued a statement in March 2017 that "current evidence is insufficient to assess the balance of benefits and harms of performing SPE in asymptomatic, non-pregnant adult women...", an [I] statement.[67-69]
- ACOG recommends an annual screening pelvic exam in those 21 years of age and older, despite acknowledging that no evidence supports or refutes the benefits of routine exam in low-risk individuals (also an [I] statement). However, they qualify this recommendation by stating that the inclusion of speculum exam, bimanual exam, or both, in an otherwise healthy woman should be a shared, informed decision between patient and provider.[70]
- The American College of Physicians (ACP) recommends against routine screening bimanual pelvic examination.[71] Their rationale is that the accuracy of SPE for detecting ovarian cancer is low and that no studies have assessed the benefit of SPE for other conditions, such as PID, benign conditions, or other gynecologic cancers. They emphasize that SPE rarely detects noncervical cancer or other treatable conditions, and of note, that outcomes are not improved. However, the harms of SPE include false-positive findings that lead to unnecessary laparoscopies or laparotomies; fear, anxiety, embarrassment, pain, and discomfort for the patient; and unnecessary costs to the health care system.

Given the differences in guidelines, clinicians will need to decide for themselves which guideline to follow and what to advise asymptomatic people about the need for a screening pelvic exam at the time of a well visit.

Screening with the serum tumor marker CA-125 will detect up to 80% of advanced nonmucinous ovarian cancers, but the test is only 50% to 70% sensitive for early-stage cancers and has poor specificity (many false-positive results), which may lead to unnecessary invasive and costly workups.[66] Screening those at average risk with this test is not recommended because of the low prevalence of ovarian cancer and the test's moderate sensitivity and poor specificity. Vaginal-probe pelvic ultrasound also has been suggested as a screening test because of its high sensitivity (98%), but it has poor specificity and the highest cost of any of the screening modalities.

The utility of screening asymptomatic average-risk people for ovarian cancer was evaluated in the Prostate, Lung, Colorectal and Ovarian (PLCO) Cancer Screening RCT.[72] This clinical trial was conducted between 1993 and 2001 and enrolled 78,216 women who were 55–74 years of age. Each was assigned to annual screening or usual care; the screened participants had a CA-125 for 6 years and transvaginal ultrasound for 4 years. The cohorts were followed on average for 12.4 years [range, 10.9–13.0 years] with a cancer diagnosis and death as primary outcomes. Simultaneous screening with CA-125 and transvaginal ultrasound compared with usual care did not reduce ovarian cancer mortality. However, diagnostic evaluation following a false-positive screening test result was associated with complications.[73] Of 3,285 women with false-positive results, 1,080 underwent surgery as part of the diagnostic workup. Of these women, 15% experienced distinct major complications, resulting in a rate of 20.6 complications per 100 surgical procedures. This large RCT is consistent with others in showing that screening for ovarian cancer, at least with these modalities, has no benefit for those at average risk, but it does have substantial risk of false-positive results that can lead to complications during diagnostic evaluation.

Breast Cancer

It is estimated there were 288,000 new cases of breast cancer in the United States in 2022. Breast cancer is the second leading cause of female cancer deaths in the United States (following lung cancer), accounting for 28% of all cancer cases and 15% of cancer deaths in women (about 43,250 deaths in 2022).[74] Incidence rates of breast cancer increased 1% per year since the 1970s, but from 1999 to 2006 the rates decreased by 2% per year. Mortality also has been falling since 1990 as a result of earlier diagnosis and improved treatments. A woman's lifetime risk of breast cancer, assuming she lives to old age, is 13% (about 1 in 8). The likelihood that a woman will die from breast cancer is about 1 in 39 (about 2.6%).[66]

Risk factors are helpful indicators of risk but do not predict the development of breast cancer in the majority of cases. Of patients with breast cancer, 21% of those age 30–54 years have risk factor(s), as do 29% of those between 55 and 84 years old.[75] (See **Table 24-2**.)

Given the multiplicity of breast cancer risk factors, and their relative contribution to breast cancer risk, it is challenging for a clinician to forecast an individual patient's likelihood of acquiring breast cancer. Three free internet-based programs are available to quickly calculate a person's breast cancer risk:

- *The Breast Cancer Risk Assessment Tool*, sponsored by the National Cancer Institute, projects a person's individualized of risk for invasive breast cancer over a 5-year period and over a lifetime. It can be found at http://www.cancer.gov/bcrisktool.
- *Breast Cancer Surveillance Consortium Risk Calculator*. This tool integrates mammographic breast density: https://tools.bcsc-scc.org/bc5yearrisk/calculator.htm.
- *The Detailed Breast Cancer Risk Calculator* produces estimates using each of the Gail Model 1 and NSABP model-2. It is located at http://www.halls.md/breast/risk.htm.

Breast Density

Recent studies have focused on the role of breast density as a risk factor for breast cancer. Breast density normally decreases with advancing age, menopause, heavier body weight, and earlier childbearing, while in general there is increased breast density in those using hormone therapies. Patients with dense breasts have a modestly increased

Table 24-2 **Risk Characteristics of Breast Cancer**

Factor	High-Risk Group	Low-Risk Group
Relative risk >4.0		
Age	Old	Young
Country of origin	North America, Northern Europe	Asia, Africa
Two first-degree relatives with breast cancer diagnosed at an early age	Yes	No
History of cancer in one breast	Yes	No
Relative risk = 2.1–4.0		
Nodular densities on mammogram (postmenopausal)	Densities occupy > 75% of breast volume	Parenchyma composed entirely of fat
One first-degree relative with breast cancer	Yes	No
Biopsy-confirmed atypical hyperplasia	Yes	No
High-dose radiation to chest	Yes	No
Oophorectomy before age 35	No	Yes
Relative risk = 1.1–2.0		
Socioeconomic status	High	Low
Place of residence	Urban	Rural
Race/ethnicity		
—Breast cancer at ≥ 40 years	White (European ancestry)	Asian
—Breast cancer at < 40 years	Black (African-American/ Afro-Caribbean ancestry)	Asian
Religion	Jewish	Adventist, Mormon
Age at first full-term pregnancy	≥ 30 years	< 20 years
Age at menarche	< 12 years	> 14 years
Age at menopause	> 55 years	< 45 years
Obesity (postmenopausal)	Obese	Slender

Factor	High-Risk Group	Low-Risk Group
Breastfeeding	None	Several years
Hormone replacement therapy > 10 years	Yes	No
Height	Tall	Short
History of primary cancer in endometrium, ovary, or colon	Yes	No
Alcohol consumption	Yes	No

Source: Adapted from Hulka et al.,[75] with updates.
Modified from Hulka BS, Stark AT. Breast cancer: cause and prevention. Lancet 1995;346(8979):883-7. DOI: 10.1016/s0140-6736(95)92713-1.

Table 24-3 **BI-RADS Breast Density Categories, Demographics, Sensitivity of Cancer Detection, and Breast Cancer Risk[77]**

Category	Description	Percentage of Population*	Sensitivity (%)	Relative Risk of Breast Cancer‡
1	Almost entirely fat	10	88	---
2	Scattered fibroglandular densities	43	82	---
3	Heterogeneously dense	39	69	1.2 (compared with average breast density)
4	Extremely dense	8	62	2.1 (compared with average breast density)

Chan et al.[63]
Data from Spak DA, Plaxco JS, Santiago L, Dryden MJ, & Dogan BE. ACR BI-RADS® fifth edition: A summary of changes. Diagn Interv Imaging 2017;98(3):179–190. https://doi.org/10.1016/j.diii.2017.01.001

risk of breast cancer and experience a 10% to 20% reduction in the sensitivity of mammography to detect breast cancer. In postmenopausal patients, an increase in mammographic breast density score over time (when it should be stable or decreasing) is an important risk factor for breast cancer.[76] A four-category scoring system for mammographic breast density is now used with all screening mammograms.[77] (See **Table 24-3**.) Numerous states have passed legislation that requires health care providers to inform patients with dense breasts of the modest increased risk of breast cancer and reduced sensitivity of mammography, and several states require practitioners to discuss supplemental tests to screening mammography. This is despite a lack of evidence about which additional tests should be done and the degree to which they improve screening outcomes, as well as the fact that health insurance often does not cover these additional tests. In their 2015 guidance, ACOG[78] does not recommend routine use of alternative or adjunctive tests to screening mammography for those with dense breasts who are asymptomatic and have no additional risk factors, based on the fact that published evidence does not demonstrate meaningful outcome benefits with supplemental tests, such as ultrasonography, magnetic resonance imaging (MRI), breast tomosynthesis, or thermography. The recommendations for screening mammography intervals are the same for individuals with dense breasts as for others.

Disparities

As with cervical cancer, there are significant racial and ethnic disparities evident in breast cancer incidence and outcomes. In response to these inequities, USPSTF changed their screening mammogram recommendations to begin screening at age 40. USPSTF makes this comment:

"Black women are 40 percent more likely to die from breast cancer than White women and too often get aggressive cancers at young ages. Ensuring Black women start screening at 40 is an important first step, yet it is not enough to improve these inequities. It's important that health care professionals involve patients in a conversation on how best to support them to ensure equitable follow-up after screening and timely and effective treatment of breast cancer."

Breast Cancer Screening

Breast Self-Examination (BSE)

The longstanding recommendation that clinicians should advise all adult women to practice monthly BSE has been abandoned. Although BSE may provide those who perform them with a sense of agency and may, at times, result in earlier detection of a breast mass than might be found by coincidence, two very large RCTs have shown that breast cancer mortality and survival are no greater in those who are taught BSE than in those who are not. The larger study, involving 266,000 women in Shanghai, China, concluded that BSE actually might cause more hazard than benefit, owing to the many false positives that result from BSE.[79] From a public health standpoint, these studies suggest that financial and educational resources should not be used to implement population-based BSE programs. For individuals, the message in these studies is that a formal, timed regimen of BSE is no more effective in preventing death from breast cancer than the incidental discovery of unusual breast changes. Nonetheless, patients still should be supported in efforts to be very familiar with their breasts and to take note of changes, and if they feel something different or concerning, bring the finding to the attention of their clinician. ACOG refers to this as "breast awareness."[80]

For people choosing to examine their own breasts, the optimal time is 1 to 7 days after the end of the menses. Performing the exam in a shower while the skin wet or with body cream may improve accuracy. It is helpful to inspect the breasts while sitting or standing in front of a mirror and palpate each breast in turn, with the hand on the side of the breast being examined placed behind the head. The objective is to detect a significant change in the breasts from one month to the next, not necessarily the finding of a dominant nodule.

Screening Clinical Breast Examination (CBE)

CBE is not a highly accurate screening test, having a sensitivity of only 54% and a false-positive rate of 6%. However, 2% to 6% of breast cancers missed on mammography can be palpated on CBE. As with screening pelvic exams, three national guidelines differ regarding the benefits and harms of screening CBE.

- The USPSTF has concluded that the current evidence is insufficient (I statement) to assess the additional benefits and harms of screening CBE beyond screening mammography in women 40 years or older.[81]
- ACOG recommends that screening CBE may be offered to asymptomatic, average-risk women in the context of an informed, shared decision-making approach that recognizes the uncertainty of additional benefits and the possibility of adverse consequences of CBE beyond mammography. Screening intervals of every 1–3 years for women aged 25–39 and annually for women 40 and older are reasonable.[80]
- The ACS does not recommend CBE for breast cancer screening for those of average risk at any age, because there is no evidence of any benefit of a CBE alone or in conjunction with screening mammography.[40] However, moderate-quality evidence suggests that adding CBE to mammography increases the false-positive rate, resulting in harms that are not balanced by improved outcomes.

For people who are not screened with mammography, there are data showing a mortality benefit from CBE, so it is reasonable to offer CBE to those individuals.[82] When performing CBE for screening or diagnostic purposes, having good technique is important for optimal detection of abnormalities.[83] Examine the breasts while the patient is sitting with hands on hips or behind the head. Ask the patient to flex their chest muscles and watch for changes or dimpling. Repeat the exam while the patient is lying down. Examine each breast in either overlapping vertical stripes or in overlapping circles. Take care to examine the entire breast, including the axillary tail. Palpate with the flat portion of your fingers rather than your fingertips. If a patient has very pendulous breasts, place your hand between the breast and chest wall, then palpate the tissue between your hands. Palpation of the supraclavicular and axillary nodes is an integral component of the examination. Draw a diagram in the medical record indicating the position and size of abnormalities, noting that dominant nodules have measurable dimensions, while fibrocystic changes do not.

Mammography

When used as a screening test, the purpose of mammography is to detect preclinical breast cancer before a mass can be palpated clinically. Large-scale studies show that in those who receive at least biennial mammograms over a 10-year period, breast cancer mortality is reduced by an average of 24%, with the largest reduction in those 50–69 years old. The accuracy of mammography as a screening test has improved over the last two decades, resulting in a false-negative rate of 5% to 15% and a false-positive rate of 3% to 6%.

Digital screening mammography has almost completely replaced film mammography in the United States. A newer version of digital breast imaging called digital breast tomosynthesis (DBT), also known as 3D mammography, uses a computer algorithm to reconstruct multiple low-dose digital images of the breast into thin "slices" to include the entire breast. Tomosynthesis is typically performed as a supplement to standard two-view digital screening mammography, which more than doubles the total radiation exposure compared to a standard digital mammography screening examination alone. DBT reduces follow-up for additional imaging or testing (lower recall rates) and increases cancer detection rates compared with conventional digital mammography alone.[84] However, these studies did not evaluate whether an incremental clinical benefit exists to detecting these cancers earlier than with conventional digital mammography. In addition, no studies of DBT looked at clinical outcomes, such as breast cancer morbidity or mortality or quality of life.

The three national guidelines differ regarding the benefits and harms of screening mammograms, as reflected in the age ranges for when to start and stop screening mammograms, as well as how often they should be performed.

- The USPSTF 2023 guidelines for breast cancer screening recommend[81]:
    - The USPSTF recommends biennial screening mammography for women ages 40 to 74 years. (B statement).
    - Current evidence is insufficient to assess the benefits and harms of DBT as a primary screening method for breast cancer (I statement).
    - For women identified as having dense breasts on an otherwise negative screening mammogram, evidence is insufficient to recommend breast ultrasonography, MRI, or other methods as additional screening modalities (I statement).
- For those at average risk of breast cancer, ACOG guidelines recommend[80]:
    - Beginning at age 40, offer screening mammography.
    - Begin screening with mammography by no later than age 50.
    - Use shared decision making and include information about the potential benefits and harms when patients are deciding at what age they will begin mammography screening.
    - Once an individual begins screening mammography, continue to screen every 1 or 2 years.
    - Use shared decision making to discuss the option of screening every 2 years. Discuss the potential for biennial screening mammogram to reduce the likelihood of harm, as well as the fact that with decreased screening comes some reduction in benefits.
- The ACS guidelines[40]:
    - Made a qualified recommendation that women should have the opportunity to begin screening at age 40 years.
    - Made a strong recommendation that women should undergo regular screening mammography starting at age 45 years.
    - Women aged 45 to 54 should be screened every year and biennially starting at 55 years of age.

People with an increased risk of breast cancer should initiate mammographic screening before age 40. According to the guidelines of the American College of Radiology,[85] younger people should start mammograms at the following times:

- 10 years before the age of diagnosis of a first-degree relative with breast cancer, but not before the age of 30
- After the diagnosis of breast cancer
- Age 25–30 years if known or suspected carrier of the *BRCA*-2 breast cancer gene

- Age 20–25 years if known or suspected carrier of *BRCA-1* breast cancer gene
- 6 to 12 months after radiation therapy if breast tissue is conserved, then every 6 to 12 months for 1 to 2 years, then annually
- A breast biopsy result of lobular carcinoma in situ (LCIS) or atypical ductal hyperplasia
- Eight years after radiation therapy to the chest or mediastinum, or by age 25, whichever occurs last

An international reporting system for mammogram results, developed by the American College of Radiologists and adopted internationally, is entitled BI-RADS (Breast Imaging Reporting and Data System).[77,86] The seven categories of assessment and management of each are contained in **Table 24-4**. Patients with assessments of BI-RADS 4 or 5 should be referred immediately for breast biopsy. Pay special attention to patients with category "zero" results, as they will need to receive additional imaging studies. Also pay special attention to those with category 3 results, because they will need further follow-up imaging studies at an interval specified by the radiologist. Patients with BI-RADS category 3 results who are at increased risk of breast cancer should be referred to a breast specialist.

When used as a diagnostic test in someone with a breast abnormality, diagnostic mammography paired with ultrasound can suggest malignancy at the location of the finding and exclude malignancy elsewhere in the same or opposite breast. In

Table 24-4 BI-RADS Mammogram, Breast Ultrasound, and Breast MRI Reporting System[77]

Category	Assessment	Cancer risk	Recommendation
0	Incomplete		Further studies needed until a final category can be assigned
1	Negative	0	Routine screening interval
2	Benign finding	0	Routine screening interval
3	Probably benign	$> 0\%$ to $< 2\%$	Short-interval (6 month) follow-up
4	Suspicious	50%	Biopsy
4A	Low suspicion	2% to $< 10\%$	Biopsy
4B	Moderate suspicion	$> 10\%$ to $\leq 50\%$	Biopsy
4C	High suspicion	$> 50\%$ to $< 95\%$	Biopsy
5	Highly suspicious	$> 95\%$	Biopsy
6	Known biopsy-proven malignancy	N/A	Surgical excision

Reproduced from American College of Radiology. ACR BI-RADS® ATLAS – MAMMOGRAPHY; 2013. https://www.acr.org/-/media/ACR/Files/RADS/BI-RADS/Mammography-Reporting.pdf

the presence of a dominant breast nodule, a negative diagnostic mammogram does not exclude the diagnosis of breast cancer. In this case, tissue sampling, either by core needle biopsy, fine-needle aspiration cytology, or excisional biopsy, is the only definitive procedure to exclude cancer.

Author Disclosures—Policar: none; Sawaya: none; Cason: Board of Directors for ASCCP, Organon, Merck, Sebela Women's Health.

References

1. American Medical Association. Periodic health examination: a manual for physicians. Chicago: American Medical Association; 1940.
2. U.S. Preventative Services Task Force. Grade Definitions. 2018.
3. Zhu B, Glied SA. More is more: Expanding access to primary care while maintaining quality. The Commonwealth Fund. 2021. (https://www.commonwealthfund.org/publications/issue-briefs/2021/jul/more-is-more-expanding-access-primary-care-maintaining-quality)
4. Curtis KM, Jatlaoui TC, Tepper NK, et al. U.S. Selected Practice Recommendations for Contraceptive Use, 2016. MMWR Recomm Rep. 2016;65:1-66.
5. Stewart FH, Harper CC, Ellertson CE, Grimes DA, Sawaya GF, Trussell J. Clinical breast and pelvic examination requirements for hormonal contraception: Current practice vs evidence. JAMA. 2001;285:2232-9.
6. Munoz N, Bosch FX, de Sanjose S, et al. Epidemiologic classification of human papillomavirus types associated with cervical cancer. N Engl J Med. 2003;348:518-27.
7. Winkelstein W, Jr. Smoking and cervical cancer--current status: a review. Am J Epidemiol. 1990;131:945-57; discussion 58-60.
8. Bennetts LE, Wagner M, Giuliano AR, Palefsky JM, Steben M, Weiss TW. Associations of anogenital low-risk human papillomavirus infection with cancer and acquisition of HIV. Sex Transm Dis. 2015;42:541-4.
9. Centers for Disease Control. Black-white differences in cervical cancer mortality--United States, 1980-1987. MMWR Morb Mortal Wkly Rep. 1990;39:245-8.
10. Musselwhite LW, Oliveira CM, Kwaramba T, et al. Racial/ethnic disparities in cervical cancer screening and outcomes. Acta Cytol. 2016;60:518-26.
11. U.S. Cancer Statistics Data Visualizations Tool, based on 2019 submission data (1999–2017): U.S. Department of Health and Human Services, Centers for Disease Control and Prevention and National Cancer Institute. 2020. (www.cdc.gov/cancer/dataviz)
12. Singh GK, Williams SD, Siahpush M, Mulhollen A. Socioeconomic, rural-urban, and racial inequalities in US cancer mortality: Part I-all cancers and lung cancer and Part II-colorectal, prostate, breast, and cervical cancers. J Cancer Epidemiol. 2011;2011:107497.
13. Abdalla E, Troy R, Fall S, Elhussin I, Egiebor-Aiwan O, Nganwa D. Racial differences in 5-year relative survival rates of cervical cancer by stage at diagnosis, between African American (black) and white women, living in the state of Alabama, USA. BMC Cancer. 2020;20:830.
14. Burger EA, Lee K, Saraiya M, et al. Racial and ethnic disparities in human papillomavirus-associated cancer burden with first-generation and second-generation human papillomavirus vaccines. Cancer. 2016;122:2057-66.
15. Karuri AR, Kashyap VK, Yallapu MM, et al. Disparity in rates of HPV infection and cervical cancer in underserved US populations. Front Biosci (Schol Ed). 2017;9:254-69.
16. Benard VB, Thomas CC, King J, et al. Vital signs: cervical cancer incidence, mortality, and screening - United States, 2007-2012. MMWR Morb Mortal Wkly Rep. 2014;63:1004-9.
17. McDaniel CC, Hallam HH, Cadwallader T, Lee HY, Chou C. Persistent racial disparities in cervical cancer screening with Pap test. Prev Med Rep. 2021;24:101652.
18. Rositch AF, Nowak RG, Gravitt PE. Increased age and race-specific incidence of cervical cancer after correction for hysterectomy prevalence in the United States from 2000 to 2009. Cancer. 2014;120:2032-8.
19. Grubb BP. Clinical practice. Neurocardiogenic syncope. N Engl J Med. 2005;352:1004-10.

20. Krediet CT, van Dijk N, Linzer M, van Lieshout JJ, Wieling W. Management of vasovagal syncope: controlling or aborting faints by leg crossing and muscle tensing. Circulation. 2002;106:1684-9.
21. Brignole M, Croci F, Menozzi C, et al. Isometric arm counter-pressure maneuvers to abort impending vasovagal syncope. J Am Coll Cardiol. 2002;40:2053-9.
22. Romme JJ, Reitsma JB, Go-Schon IK, et al. Prospective evaluation of non-pharmacological treatment in vasovagal syncope. Europace. 2010;12:567-73.
23. Montealegre JR, Varier I, Bracamontes CG, et al. Racial/ethnic variation in the prevalence of vaccine-related human papillomavirus genotypes. Ethn Health. 2019;24:804-15.
24. Vidal AC, Smith JS, Valea F, et al. HPV genotypes and cervical intraepithelial neoplasia in a multiethnic cohort in the southeastern USA. Cancer Causes Control. 2014;25:1055-62.
25. Shokar NK, Doan A, Calderon-Mora J, et al. The prevalence of genital human papillomavirus subtypes in a cohort of hispanic women presenting for cervical cancer screening along the US-Mexico border. Cancer Control. 2020;27:1073274820951780.
26. Meites E, Szilagyi PG, Chesson HW, Unger ER, Romero JR, Markowitz LE. Human papillomavirus vaccination for adults: Updated recommendations of the Advisory Committee on Immunization Practices. MMWR Morb Mortal Wkly Rep. 2019;68:698-702.
27. Saslow D, Andrews KS, Manassaram-Baptiste D, Smith RA, Fontham ETH, American Cancer Society Guideline Development G. Human papillomavirus vaccination 2020 guideline update: American Cancer Society guideline adaptation. CA Cancer J Clin. 2020;70:274-80.
28. Human papillomavirus vaccines: WHO position paper, December 2022. World Health Organization [Organisation Mondiale de la Santé]. Human papillomavirus vaccines: WHO position paper (2022 update). Wkly Epidemiol Record. 2022;97:64-72.
29. American Cancer Society. Key statistics for cervical cancer. 2022. (https://www.cancer.org/cancer/cervical-cancer/about/key-statistics.html)
30. Benard VB, Jackson JE, Greek A, et al. A population study of screening history and diagnostic outcomes of women with invasive cervical cancer. Cancer Med. 2021;10:4127-37.
31. Hessling JJ, Raso DS, Schiffer B, Callicott J, Jr., Husain M, Taylor D. Effectiveness of thin-layer preparations vs. conventional Pap smears in a blinded, split-sample study. Extended cytologic evaluation. J Reprod Med. 2001;46:880-6.
32. Wertlake P. Results of AutoPap system-assisted and manual cytologic screening. A comparison. J Reprod Med. 1999;44:11-7.
33. Siebers AG, Klinkhamer PJ, Grefte JM, et al. Comparison of liquid-based cytology with conventional cytology for detection of cervical cancer precursors: a randomized controlled trial. JAMA. 2009;302:1757-64.
34. Arbyn M, Bergeron C, Klinkhamer P, Martin-Hirsch P, Siebers AG, Bulten J. Liquid compared with conventional cervical cytology: a systematic review and meta-analysis. Obstet Gynecol. 2008;111:167-77.
35. Perkins RB, Guido RS, Castle PE, et al. 2019 ASCCP Risk-Based Management Consensus Guidelines for Abnormal Cervical Cancer Screening Tests and Cancer Precursors. J Low Genit Tract Dis. 2020;24:102-31.
36. Egemen D, Cheung LC, Chen X, et al. Risk estimates supporting the 2019 ASCCP Risk-Based Management Consensus Guidelines. J Low Genit Tract Dis. 2020;24:132-43.
37. Yabroff KR, Saraiya M, Meissner HI, et al. Specialty differences in primary care physician reports of papanicolaou test screening practices: a national survey, 2006 to 2007. Ann Intern Med. 2009;151:602-11.
38. Marcus JZ, Cason P, Downs LS Jr, Einstein MH, Flowers L. The ASCCP Cervical Cancer Screening Task Force Endorsement and Opinion on the American Cancer Society Updated Cervical Cancer Screening Guidelines. J Low Genit Tract Dis. 2021 Jul 1;25(3):187-191. DOI: 10.1097/LGT.0000000000000614. PMID: 34138787
39. U.S. Preventive Services Task Force, Curry SJ, Krist AH, et al. Screening for cervical cancer: US Preventive Services Task Force Recommendation Statement. JAMA. 2018;320:674-86.
40. Fontham ETH, Wolf AMD, Church TR, et al. Cervical cancer screening for individuals at average risk: 2020 guideline update from the American Cancer Society. CA Cancer J Clin. 2020;70:321-46.
41. Dilley S, Huh W, Blechter B, Rositch AF. It's time to re-evaluate cervical cancer screening after age 65. Gynecol Oncol. 2021;162:200-2.

42. Grabinski E, Dunsmoor-Su R. Pap smear recommendations in older women, does the data support stopping? Curr Opin Obstet Gynecol. 2023;35:160-3.
43. National Institutes of Health, the Centers for Disease Control and Prevention, and the HIV Medicine Association of the Infectious Diseases Society of America Panel on Guidelines for the Prevention and Treatment of Opportunistic Infections in Adults and Adolescents with HIV. 2021. Guidelines for the prevention and treatment of opportunistic infections in adults and adolescents with HIV. https://clinicalinfo.hiv.gov/en/guidelines/hiv-clinical-guidelines-adult-and-adolescent-opportunistic-infections/human-0?view=full
44. Meissner HI, Tiro JA, Yabroff KR, Haggstrom DA, Coughlin SS. Too much of a good thing? Physician practices and patient willingness for less frequent pap test screening intervals. Med Care. 2010;48:249-59.
45. Perkins RB, Anderson BL, Gorin SS, Schulkin JA. Challenges in cervical cancer prevention: a survey of U.S. obstetrician-gynecologists. Am J Prev Med. 2013;45:175-81.
46. Bettigole C. The thousand-dollar Pap smear. N Engl J Med. 2013;369:1486-7.
47. Nayar R, Wilbur DC. The Bethesda System for reporting cervical cytology: A historical perspective. Acta Cytol. 2017;61:359-72.
48. Kivlahan C, Ingram E. Papanicolaou smears without endocervical cells. Are they inadequate? Acta Cytol. 1986;30:258-60.
49. Ransdell JS, Davey DD, Zaleski S. Clinicopathologic correlation of the unsatisfactory Papanicolaou smear. Cancer. 1997;81:139-43.
50. Hobbs MM, Sena AC. Modern diagnosis of Trichomonas vaginalis infection. Sex Transm Infect. 2013;89:434-8.
51. American Cancer Society. Key statistics for ovarian cancer. 2022. (https://www.cancer.org/cancer/ovarian-cancer/about/key-statistics.html)
52. Whittemore AS, Harris R, Itnyre J. Characteristics relating to ovarian cancer risk: collaborative analysis of 12 US case-control studies. II. Invasive epithelial ovarian cancers in white women. Collaborative Ovarian Cancer Group. Am J Epidemiol. 1992;136:1184-203.
53. American Cancer Society. Ovarian cancer risk factors. 2021. (https://www.cancer.org/cancer/ovarian-cancer/causes-risks-prevention/risk-factors.html)
54. NIH Consensus Development Panel on Ovarian Cancer. Ovarian cancer: Screening, treatment, and follow-up. JAMA. 1995;273:491-7.
55. Rosenberg L, Palmer JR, Zauber AG, et al. A case-control study of oral contraceptive use and invasive epithelial ovarian cancer. Am J Epidemiol. 1994;139:654-61.
56. Schrijver LH, Antoniou AC, Olsson H, et al. Oral contraceptive use and ovarian cancer risk for BRCA1/2 mutation carriers: an international cohort study. Am J Obstet Gynecol. 2021;225:51.e1-.e17.
57. Huber D, Seitz S, Kast K, Emons G, Ortmann O. Use of oral contraceptives in BRCA mutation carriers and risk for ovarian and breast cancer: a systematic review. Arch Gynecol Obstet. 2020;301:875-84.
58. Wilailak S, Vipupinyo C, Suraseranivong V, et al. Depot medroxyprogesterone acetate and epithelial ovarian cancer: a multicentre case-control study. BJOG. 2012;119:672-7.
59. Corzo C, Iniesta MD, Patrono MG, Lu KH, Ramirez PT. Role of fallopian tubes in the development of ovarian cancer. J Minim Invasive Gynecol. 2017;24:230-4.
60. Hartmann LC, Lindor NM. The role of risk-reducing surgery in hereditary breast and ovarian cancer. N Engl J Med. 2016;374:454-68.
61. Long Roche KC, Abu-Rustum NR, Nourmoussavi M, Zivanovic O. Risk-reducing salpingectomy: Let us be opportunistic. Cancer. 2017;123:1714-20.
62. ACOG Committee Opinion No. 774. Opportunistic salpingectomy as a strategy for epithelial ovarian cancer prevention. Obstet Gynecol. 2019;133:e279-e84.
63. Ovarian Cancer Research Alliance. Ovarian cancer screening and symptom awareness consensus statement. 2023. (https://ocrahope.org/news/ovarian-cancer-screening-and-symptom-awareness-consensus-statement/)
64. Creinin MD, Zite N. Female tubal sterilization: the time has come to routinely consider removal. Obstet Gynecol. 2014;124:596-9.
65. Chan JK, Tian C, Kesterson JP, et al. Symptoms of women with high-risk early-stage ovarian cancer. Obstet Gynecol. 2022;139:157-62.

66. ACOG Committee Opinion No. 477. The role of the obstetrician-gynecologist in the early detection of epithelial ovarian cancer. Obstet Gynecol. 2011;117:742-6.
67. Grossman DC, Curry SJ, Owens DK, et al. Screening for ovarian cancer: US Preventive Services Task Force Recommendation Statement. JAMA. 2018;319:588-94.
68. Bibbins-Domingo K, Grossman DC, Curry SJ, et al. Screening for gynecologic conditions with pelvic examination: US Preventive Services Task Force Recommendation Statement. JAMA. 2017;317:947-53.
69. Guirguis-Blake JM, Henderson JT, Perdue LA. Periodic screening pelvic examination: Evidence report and systematic review for the US Preventive Services Task Force. JAMA. 2017;317:954-66.
70. ACOG Committee Opinion No. 755. Well-woman visit. Obstet Gynecol. 2018;132:e181-e6.
71. Qaseem A, Humphrey LL, Harris R, Starkey M, Denberg TD, Clinical Guidelines Committee of the American College of Physicians. Screening pelvic examination in adult women: a clinical practice guideline from the American College of Physicians. Ann Intern Med. 2014;161:67-72.
72. Buys SS, Partridge E, Black A, et al. Effect of screening on ovarian cancer mortality: the Prostate, Lung, Colorectal and Ovarian (PLCO) Cancer Screening Randomized Controlled Trial. JAMA. 2011;305:2295-303.
73. Doroudi M, Kramer BS, Pinsky PF. The bimanual ovarian palpation examination in the Prostate, Lung, Colorectal and Ovarian cancer screening trial: Performance and complications. J Med Screen. 2017;24:220-2.
74. Giaquinto AN, Sung H, Miller KD, et al. Breast cancer statistics, 2022. Cancer J Clinicians. 2022;72:524-41.
75. Hulka BS, Stark AT. Breast cancer: cause and prevention. Lancet. 1995;346:883-7.
76. Kerlikowske K, Ichikawa L, Miglioretti DL, et al. Longitudinal measurement of clinical mammographic breast density to improve estimation of breast cancer risk. J Natl Cancer Inst. 2007;99:386-95.
77. Spak DA, Plaxco JS, Santiago L, Dryden MJ, Dogan BE. BI-RADS((R)) fifth edition: A summary of changes. Diagn Interv Imaging. 2017;98:179-90.
78. ACOG Committee Opinion No. 625. Management of women with dense breasts diagnosed by mammography: Correction. Obstet Gynecol. 2016;127:166.
79. Thomas DB, Gao DL, Ray RM, et al. Randomized trial of breast self-examination in Shanghai: final results. J Natl Cancer Inst 2002;94:1445-57.
80. ACOG Practice Bulletin No. 179. Breast cancer risk assessment and screening in average-risk women. Obstet Gynecol. 2017;130:e1-e16.
81. https://www.uspreventiveservicestaskforce.org/uspstf/draft-recommendation/breast-cancer-screening-adults#bcei-recommendation-title-area
82. Ngan TT, Nguyen NTQ, Van Minh H, Donnelly M, O'Neill C. Effectiveness of clinical breast examination as a 'stand-alone' screening modality: an overview of systematic reviews. BMC Cancer. 2020;20:1070.
83. Oeffinger KC, Fontham ET, Etzioni R, et al. Breast cancer screening for women at average risk: 2015 Guideline Update From the American Cancer Society. JAMA. 2015;314:1599-614.
84. Lowry KP, Coley RY, Miglioretti DL, et al. Screening performance of digital breast tomosynthesis vs digital mammography in community practice by patient age, screening round, and breast density. JAMA Netw Open. 2020;3:e2011792.
85. Monticciolo DL, Newell MS, Moy L, Niell B, Monsees B, Sickles EA. Breast Cancer screening in women at higher-than-average risk: Recommendations from the ACR. J Am Coll Radiol. 2018;15:408-14.
86. Liberman L, Abramson AF, Squires FB, Glassman JR, Morris EA, Dershaw DD. The breast imaging reporting and data system: positive predictive value of mammographic features and final assessment categories. AJR Am J Roentgenol. 1998;171:35-40.

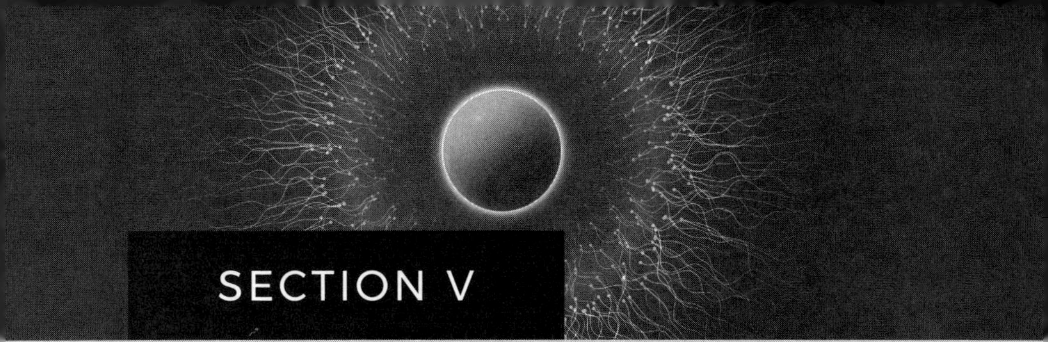

SECTION V

Pregnancy Testing and Termination

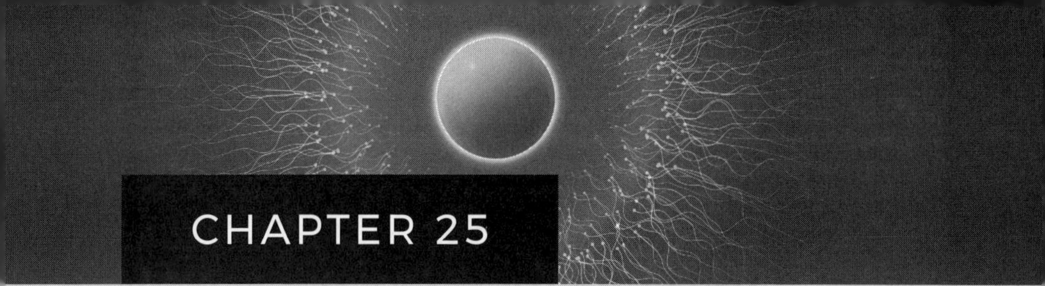

CHAPTER 25

Pregnancy Testing

Maureen K. Baldwin, MD, MPH
Beatrice A. Chen, MD, MPH

KEY POINTS

- Contraception can be initiated without pregnancy testing if it is reasonably certain that the patient is not pregnant based on history.
- Early pregnancy diagnosis allows consideration of all options for pregnancy care: parenthood, adoption, and abortion.
- A positive pregnancy test after contraceptive failure requires additional counseling.
- A negative pregnancy test permits rapid initiation of preferred contraception and preconception counseling.

Pregnancy Testing Opportuntities

Many types of clinical visits provide key opportunities to educate people regarding person-centered reproductive desires.[1] For example, clinician visits to screen for sexually transmitted infection (STI) are a common and underutilized opportunity to offer contraception counseling. As many as one-quarter of all adolescents with a positive pregnancy test have previously had one or more visits for pregnancy screening, representing an opportunity for education and counseling.[2]

Since a person's reproductive goals and health care needs may vary based on their life circumstances, and people may not always have a binary intention about whether they want to become pregnant or avoid pregnancy, using these opportunities to discuss their reproductive desires can help tailor counseling, including both preconception health counseling and contraceptive counseling as needed.[3] Encounters for pregnancy test visits allow for opportunities to review medical history and medications; timely completion of recommended screening tests and immunizations; and planning and preparing for pregnancy, including initiation of folic acid, in order to optimize health prior to conception (**Box 25-1**).[1,4]

Family planning is a complex issue influenced by social, familial, biological, and psychological factors. Many people experience pregnancies that they do not want,"[5] suggesting there is unmet need for effective discussions of how to meet

Box 25-1 Pregnancy Test Visit Goals

1. Determine if patient is pregnant.
2. Assess patient preferences.
3. Educate the patient about relevant options and implement a plan if and when they are ready.
4. Identify other issues that might require further evaluation or urgent intervention.
5. Review use of medications (over-the-counter, prescription), herbs/vitamins, nicotine, and recreational substances.
6. Assess gestational dating.
7. Screen for sexually transmitted infections.
8. Document Rh status and obtain relevant laboratory tests.

Data from ACOG Committee Opinion No. 762: Prepregnancy counseling. Obstet Gynecol 2019;133(1):e78-e89. (In eng). DOI: 10.1097/aog.0000000000003013; Wilkes J. AAFP Releases Position Paper on Preconception care. Am Fam Physician 2016;94(6):508-10. https://www.ncbi.nlm.nih.gov/pubmed/27637129

reproductive goals. A pregnancy test visit with a negative test result can be an important time to offer this conversation. (See Chapter 4, Person-Centered Reproductive Health Conversations and Contraceptive Counseling.)

Disclosing a Pregnancy Test Result

Before conducting the pregnancy test, find out how the patient feels about the possibility of pregnancy. Realize that it is common for feelings about the acceptability of pregnancy to be nuanced and complex. When presenting the test result, allow time for them to express feelings. If it is not already clear, consider asking if the patient has already considered their options or made a decision. If they have decided, offer to tell them about options that are consistent with their decision. If they are undecided, offer to tell them about all available options. Assess the patient's support system. Provide referrals if a patient feels counseling would be helpful, or if the patient is unsupported or alone with this decision. Emphasize that a decision regarding the outcome of this pregnancy does not need to be made that day, but do provide any relevant timelines regarding when access to options might change. Encourage the patient to talk with a partner, family, or friends. Some topics to include based on the outcome of the pregnancy test and the patient's decision or goals might include the following:

- **Pregnant and planning to continue the pregnancy:**
  - Provide education about healthy antenatal practices and resources for prenatal care.
  - Review the pregnancy warning signs (severe pain, bleeding, faint or dizzy, fever).
- **Pregnant and planning to continue the pregnancy, but does not want to parent:**
  - In addition to the above initial prenatal care education and resources, provide resources for adoption services.
  - Provide resources for an unbiased counselor.

- **Pregnant and does not plan to continue the pregnancy:**
    - Review preferences for type of abortion.
    - Provide abortion or a referral for abortion services or, at a minimum, provide contact information for abortion resources such as abortionfinder.org.
    - Provide a general overview of what can be expected with the process to obtain an abortion based on state laws, access to services, and gestational dating. (See Chapter 26, Abortion.)
- **Not pregnant but wants to be pregnant:**
    - Provide age-based fertility counseling (such as from www.reproductive-facts.org).
    - If appropriate, provide a referral for fertility evaluation.
    - Provide preconception education, including advice to take a daily vitamin that includes folic acid (400 mcg daily) before and during the first trimester of pregnancy.[1,6]
    - Provide assessment to optimize medical conditions and medications.
    - Review if up to date on vaccinations (especially vaccines that cannot be given when pregnant and common respiratory illnesses with worse outcomes in pregnancy, like COVID-19 and pertussis).
    - Update travel warnings (Zika exposure, see www.cdc.gov/zika/).
- **Not pregnant and does not want or unsure about pregnancy:**
    - Offer to discuss contraceptive options. (See Chapter 4, Person-Centered Reproductive Health Conversations and Contraceptive Counseling.)
    - If interested, provide relevant information about method attributes, such as relative effectiveness and side effects. (See Chapter 5, Effectiveness, Safety, and Comparative Side Effects.)
    - If appropriate, initiate preferred contraceptive method.
    - Provide risk-based STI screening.
    - Provide age-based fertility counseling.

Pregnancy Care Referral

If the patient is pregnant and plans to continue the pregnancy, encourage early entry into pregnancy care so gestational dating can be confirmed and baseline vital signs can be documented. If the patient selects to continue the pregnancy, perform screening tests in the first trimester, which can also include prenatal diagnosis for genetic abnormalities (if desired).

If the patient is pregnant and selects pregnancy termination, expedient care is important as earlier access to abortion is associated with less morbidity.[7,8] While placing a referral might not be required for abortion care, it might facilitate easier transfer of records or insurance coverage, especially in the setting of medical conditions. Providing information about abortion resources such as abortionfinder.org and National Abortion Federation's National Abortion Hotline may also help expedite care.

If prenatal or abortion care is not provided on-site, then facilitate the patient's access to care. In making a referral, consider factors such as the patient's insurance coverage, primary language, indications for high-risk perinatal care, accessibility of the clinic/hospital logistically and financially, and any special delivery needs (e.g., need for cesarean section) or desires (e.g., epidural or water-birth delivery, access to permanent contraception, availability of immediate postpartum or postabortion contraception).

There is often a delay of several weeks until the patient will have a first pregnancy care appointment, so review the signs and symptoms (i.e., severe pain or bleeding, faint or dizzy, fever) that may signal problems during early pregnancy such as miscarriage or ectopic pregnancy. Consider referral for a first trimester ultrasound to confirm pregnancy dating and location, if there is an expected delay. Provide instructions to the patient, including whom to contact if a problem or emergency arises in the interim. Patients who have medical conditions such as diabetes, heart disease, or hypertension may need an urgent referral to a high-risk obstetrician.

Pregnancy Tests and Contraception

Pregnancy Tests Prior to Contraception

A pregnancy test is not required prior to initiating contraception as long as the health care provider and patient can reasonably rule out pregnancy based on absence of signs and symptoms of pregnancy and use of contraception, timing of menses, intercourse, or recent completed pregnancy (see **Box 25-2**).[9] Standard of care and manufacturer labeling often dictate obtaining a pregnancy test prior to initiation of injectable or long-acting contraception (implant or intrauterine device [IUD]) regardless of being able to rule out pregnancy based on history. This is typically done with a urine pregnancy test in the same clinical environment as the injection or procedure. If an unexpected positive result is obtained, consider repeating the same test or confirming with a serum human chorionic gonadotropin (hCG) test.

Contraception Initiation During Luteal Phase

Pregnancy cannot be reliably excluded if recent intercourse occurred without contraception or with inconsistent contraception, particularly during mid-cycle.

Box 25-2 How to be Reasonably Certain that a Person is Not Pregnant

A health care provider can be reasonably certain that a person is not pregnant if there are no symptoms or signs of pregnancy and they meet any one of the following criteria:

The patient

- Is ≤ 7 days after the start of normal menses
- Has not had sexual intercourse since the start of last normal menses
- Has been correctly and consistently using a reliable method of contraception
- Is ≤ 7 days after spontaneous or induced abortion
- Is within 4 weeks postpartum
- Is fully or nearly fully breastfeeding/chest feeding (exclusively or the vast majority [> 85%] of feeds), amenorrheic, and < 6 months postpartum

Reproduced from Curtis KM, Jatlaoui TC, Tepper NK, et al. U.S. Selected practice recommendations for contraceptive use, 2016. MMWR Recomm Rep 2016;65(4):1-66. Available free of charge from https://www.cdc.gov/mmwr/volumes/65/rr/pdfs/rr6504.pdf. Reference to specific commercial products, manufacturers, companies, or trademarks does not constitute its endorsement or recommendation by the U.S. Government, Department of Health and Human Services, or Centers for Disease Control and Prevention.

Pregnancy tests may not detect pregnancy for up to 2 weeks after intercourse between the time that a conception might have already occurred and the next expected menses. When there is a chance of undetectable pregnancy during this time, this is considered a possible *luteal phase pregnancy* (See Chapter 2, Understanding the Physiology of the Menstrual Cycle.) Initiation of contraception during this time period does not interrupt an established pregnancy, though it is possible that a method such as the copper IUD may prevent embryo implantation. (See Chapter 18, Emergency Contraception.) Contraception can be initiated during this phase after discussion with the patient about the possible chance of pregnancy, the implications of using the specific method during early pregnancy, and the next steps should a pregnancy be detected. A follow-up plan should be developed to be able to exclude pregnancy. This is particularly important with use of methods that might induce amenorrhea, since the absence of bleeding due to pregnancy would not raise concern.

Positive Pregnancy Test with Contraceptive Use

The finding of a positive pregnancy test may be an unexpected shock for someone who has been using a contraceptive method consistently and correctly. For others, a pregnancy that occurs while using contraception, often called a "contraceptive failure," may bring about a wide variety of feelings ranging from delight to shame. Regardless of decisions about continuation or termination of the pregnancy, respect that the patient will primarily need to process an unexpected pregnancy and could be negatively affected by any implication of culpability brought on by a discussion about imperfect use. Future contraceptive discussions may be appropriate for determining whether the pregnancy might have been a result of medication interaction, misunderstanding about correct use, inconsistent use due to dissatisfaction with side effects, partner coercion, acceptability of pregnancy, or incidental failure. Chapter 4 presents in-depth recommendations for person-centered, nondirective pregnancy options counseling.

Pregnancy After Exposure to Hormonal Contraception

If a pregnancy is detected while using hormonal contraception, counseling about the safety of exposure to the method may be helpful to the patient in making their decision about the course of the pregnancy. While there have been many claims that hormonal contraceptives are teratogenic, evidence does not support these concerns.[10] Information about exposures during pregnancy can be accessed by patients with support from teratogenic specialists at www.mothertobaby.org.

Pregnancy Test Positive With an IUD

Rarely, a pregnancy may occur with an IUD in place. A pregnancy may also be the reason that an IUD malposition or extrauterine location (perforation or expulsion) is identified. Perform an exam to determine whether the IUD strings are visible. After obtaining informed consent, if the strings are present, any available provider should remove the IUD immediately, regardless of whether the patient plans to continue the pregnancy or intends to have an abortion. Patients considering an abortion may ultimately decide to continue the pregnancy, or they may choose an abortion (medical or procedural) — but in all instances, it is important to remove the IUD. The passage of time (even a couple of days) may lead to retraction of the strings as the uterus increases in size. An IUD left in place increases the risk of septic abortion and other complications such as late miscarriage, preterm delivery, and placental abruption.[11] Counsel the patient that the risk of miscarriage with immediate removal is less than the risk with keeping it in place. Beyond the risk associated with removing the IUD or leaving it in place, miscarriage is a risk for *all* pregnancies.[12] If the IUD strings are not visualized, they may have retracted, there might have been an unrecognized expulsion, or the IUD could be intraperitoneal. Further management is necessary to confirm IUD location. (See Chapter 10, Intrauterine Devices [IUDs].)

If the strings are not visible with an IUD correctly positioned within the uterus and the patient desires to continue the pregnancy, then provide urgent referral to a specialized family planning service. The patient could potentially be offered ultrasound-guided or hysteroscopic removal. Always, earlier is better. For a patient who chooses to have an abortion, an IUD without visualized strings can be removed simultaneously during a vacuum aspiration. While the number of pregnancies that occur with an IUD in place is extremely low, the proportion of these pregnancies that are ectopic is higher than for patients not using an IUD. Therefore, localize the site of the pregnancy by ultrasound as soon as possible or follow the hCG trend to assess for possible ectopic pregnancy.

Pregnancy Test Positive With an Implant

If a patient presents with symptoms of pregnancy with a contraceptive implant in place, the first step is to repeat the pregnancy test, as contraceptive failures of the implant are extremely rare. Most contraceptive failures occur due to implant placement during the luteal phase, prior to the ability to detect an early pregnancy. Luteal phase placement frequently includes a recommendation for the patient to perform a pregnancy test at a 2- to 4-week interval after placement. Ask the patient about timing and location for implant placement and about their recent menstrual pattern. Perform an abdominal exam to assess for a gravid uterus, since it may be possible for patients with implant contraceptive failure to be unaware they are pregnant until the second trimester.[13] Ask about medications, in case there might have been a medication interaction that could have impacted implant effectiveness. Once pregnancy is confirmed, perform an exam to assess the implant. Confirm whether it is palpable subdermally in the expected position in the upper arm. If not palpable, check both arms, inspecting for a placement scar. (See Chapter 9, Contraceptive Implant.) If you are unable to palpate the implant, do not attempt to remove it. Nonpalpable implants should be referred to a regional specialty center with expertise in removal of nonpalpable implants where imaging and laboratory analysis can confirm that the implant is present and aid with complex removal. Contact the manufacturer (Organon, 1-844-674-3200) if needed to obtain a referral. Implant removal is recommended by the manufacturer regardless of decisions about the pregnancy. However, if the pregnancy occurred after implant placement during the luteal phase rather than a medication interaction that affected contraceptive effectiveness, and the patient plans to terminate the pregnancy, the patient may choose to leave the implant in place for continuing contraception postabortion with appropriate counseling.

Pregnancy Tests for Human Chorionic Gonadotropin (hCG)

Pregnancy tests are now readily available and even automated in some cases. It is important to understand the timing of events that would result in a positive hCG test either following conception or following pregnancy completion.

Introduction to hCG Tests

Pregnancy tests are useful for many scenarios to diagnose or rule out pregnancy. In most cases, urine tests are adequate. Serum hCG may be necessary in symptomatic patients at risk for abnormal pregnancy or those undergoing serial trend analysis.

Urine hCG tests are used:

- To rule out pregnancy prior to initiation of contraception
- To screen for pregnancy prior to surgery or medical treatments
- To test for pregnancy after a missed menstrual cycle

Serum hCG tests are used:

- To provide hCG trend prior to the time when a pregnancy is expected to be visualized on ultrasound examination
- To confirm hCG decline after abortion to rule out an ongoing pregnancy

Timing of Early Pregnancy Events

Following ovulation, fertilization of the ovum by sperm occurs within the ampulla of the fallopian tube and the fertilized ovum remains in the tube until it is a ball of cells (the *morula*), when it then enters the uterine cavity. By 6 days after ovulation, the morula has developed into a *blastocyst*, which implants into the *decidua*, which is the modified endometrium specialized for implantation and support of a pregnancy. The blastocyst typically begins to secrete hCG by 7–8 days after fertilization,[14] though hCG has been detectable in urine as early as 6 days after ovulation.[15] hCG is then secreted by placental cells in order to maintain the corpus luteum of the ovary, which continues to secrete progesterone until the placental tissue produces increasing quantities of progesterone by 6 to 7 weeks after fertilization. The hCG is the molecule that is detected by a pregnancy test.[16]

hCG Detection in Pregnancy

Pregnancy tests detect the hCG in a pregnant person's urine or the component of blood called serum. Serum or urine pregnancy tests today detect four independent molecules[17]:

- Intact hCG
- Hyperglycosylated hCG (H-hCG)
- Free β-subunit
- Pituitary hCG

hCG is the term used in this text to denote the types of hCG tested in pregnancy and replaces the formerly used term β-hCG.

The First Pregnancy Tests

Early pregnancy tests in the 1920s and 1930s were based on injecting urinary extracts from pregnant people into animals such as mice and rabbits to identify ovarian stimulation.[18,19] These early tests were only available to clinicians and hospitals, and typically required mailing urine samples to a laboratory for testing.[18] An immunoassay method based on passive agglutination to detect urinary hCG was developed in 1960 and could detect pregnancy at about 21–23 days after ovulation. It was later marketed by Organon as a commercial pregnancy test under the name Pregnosticon in 1962 and as a home pregnancy test under the name Predictor.[20] Radio-immunosorbent assays were later developed, including specific assays that could detect the β-subunit at levels as low as 5 IU/L in serum, or as early as 7.5 days after fertilization.[19] Modern pregnancy tests use two-antibody immunometric assays to bind and label hCG for detection.[17]

Highly Sensitive Urine Pregnancy Tests

The over-the-counter (OTC) pregnancy tests sold for home use and those used in clinics are essentially the same. Cross-reactions with other hormones are not a problem for highly sensitive urine pregnancy tests.

Home Pregnancy Tests

Home pregnancy test kits offer the advantages of privacy, anonymity, and convenience. Because home pregnancy tests are easily accessible, patients may identify pregnancies early and thus be more able to be active managers of their own health care. Most have a stated sensitivity of 20–25 mIU/mL.[22] However, the diagnostic accuracies of the tests can vary,[21-23] and one study found consistently positive results only at an hCG level of 100 mIU/mL.[22] This may be due in part to differences in detection of hCG variants in the urine.[24]

Test accuracy can be affected by the technique and experience of the user, and by the user's ability to follow the test instructions precisely.[22] The most common error with home pregnancy tests is a negative result because the test was performed too early in pregnancy. In addition, a person using a home pregnancy test may have difficulty understanding the directions packaged in the test kit. In an evaluation of instructions from 13 OTC urine pregnancy tests, the reading level required to understand the instructions ranged from a seventh-grade to college-level reading level.[25] A false-positive test can occur if the test is not read within the designated number of minutes. This phenomenon occurs because a negative test appears faintly positive due to evaporation of the urine sample, which gives rise to an evaporation line.

Sensitivity and Specificity

Highly sensitive urine pregnancy tests, including home pregnancy tests, are intended to provide accurate qualitative (positive/negative) results with hCG levels as low as 5 to 100 mIU/mL. Tests can be positive as early as the day of the first missed menses, depending on the sensitivity of the test. One study reported that 98% of women have a positive pregnancy test within 28 days after their last menstrual period (LMP).[26] On the other hand, another study reported that, even using an extremely sensitive test (0.13 mIU/mL), among 142 women with self-reported onset of LMP, 10% of clinical pregnancies were undetectable on the first day of missed menses. This is due to the variable timing of implantation, which can even occur after the first day of the next expected menses.[27]

Early pregnancies produce quite a variable range of hCG levels, and the time at which a pregnancy is detected accurately by different pregnancy tests varies widely. Moreover, few clinic pregnancy tests or home tests have been calibrated against the three critical forms of hCG: intact hCG, H-hCG, and free β-subunit.[16]

Accuracy

A study investigated the validity of 18 different OTC home urine pregnancy tests in well-dated pregnancies 28–30 days from LMP demonstrating hCG levels ranging from 23 to 2,438 mIU/mL.[22] In order to detect 95% of pregnancies at the time of missed menses, a test would need to consistently detect hCG of at least 12.4 mIU/mL. This study found that most tests were consistently accurate at a urine hCG of 100 mIU/mL and that some brands had technical or design problems.[22] Manufacturers' claims that a pregnancy test can detect pregnancy "as early as the day of the missed menstrual period" are based on data that are almost 30 years old that assumed that urine hCG concentrations were the same as serum hCG concentrations. In fact, the average urine hCG concentration is generally less than half of the corresponding serum hCG concentration, depending on the duration of pregnancy and specificity of the test.[16]

Low-Sensitivity Urine Pregnancy Tests

Low-sensitivity urine pregnancy tests can detect hCG from 200 to 2,000 mIU/mL. These tests are not currently available in the United States. They have a narrow range of use. They are not appropriate to "rule out" pregnancy, because early pregnancy, ectopic pregnancy, impending spontaneous abortion, and, in rare cases, even later pregnancies (16 to 20 weeks) may be missed due to their low hCG levels. Low-sensitivity tests can be used to confirm pregnancy at ≥ 6 weeks after LMP or to document the decline of hCG after abortion. However, even for this use, a low-sensitivity test (sensitivity 1,500 to 2,000 mIU/mL) had sensitivities ranging from 67% to 100% for detecting ongoing pregnancy 2 weeks after successful medication abortion.[28] A negative low-sensitivity pregnancy test after medication abortion is reassuring, but a positive test may not mean much.

Semi-quantitative Urine Pregnancy Tests

Semi-quantitative, or multilevel, pregnancy tests are designed to provide both high- and low-sensitivity urine pregnancy test readings at various ranges.[29] They have mostly been evaluated in the research setting for follow-up after medication abortion,[29-31] but have also been studied for follow-up after assisted reproductive technology.[32] Semi-quantitative pregnancy tests have also been hypothesized as an alternative for follow-up after molar pregnancy.[33] Since hCG levels should decline rapidly after completion of a medication abortion, a stable or higher hCG result would raise concern for an ongoing pregnancy. A meta-analysis of seven studies evaluating semi-quantitative pregnancy tests after medication abortion at ≤ 63 days' gestation found that they were a reliable and efficient method to exclude ongoing pregnancy.[31]

Quantitative Serum hCG Tests

A quantitative serum hCG test is designed to provide a *level* or number of hCG mIU/mL; thus, the rise or fall of the hCG level may provide important information about the status of the pregnancy. Use of a serum *quantitative* hCG test only to confirm early pregnancy does not have any advantages over *qualitative* (yes/no) highly sensitive urine tests. Highly sensitive urine pregnancy kits are equally specific for hCG and provide immediate results at much lower cost. Only certain clinical situations justify the additional expense of serum hCG testing.

Accuracy and Reliability

Serum quantitative hCG tests provide accurate results with levels as low as 5 mIU/mL. Thus, they reliably detect pregnancy sooner after implantation, around 21 days LMP. Tests are usually "batched" because of expense; test processing requires 1 to 2 hours. Be sure to specify *quantitative* hCG when ordering this test. In addition, it is optimal but not essential to use the same laboratory for serial hCG tests to limit inter-assay variation between laboratories.[34] Given that some patients often have to travel significant distances for repeat hCG tests, it may be difficult to have all samples sent to the same laboratory.

Uses for Serum hCG Trend

Repetitive or serial testing of serum hCG can be used to check the increasing or decreasing trend of hCG levels. A single serum hCG result alone is rarely meaningful[35] and, as mentioned earlier, if you just need a yes/no answer (pregnant or not pregnant), then a qualitative highly sensitive urine test works just as well. The hCG trend in conjunction with other diagnostic tests, such as ultrasound examination, clinical evaluation of the patient, and consideration of risk factors, can help to differentiate between a normal or abnormal intrauterine pregnancy or ectopic pregnancy.[35] Very high levels of hCG (> 100,000 prior to 10 weeks) can be associated with molar pregnancy or multiple pregnancies, such as twins.

Pitfalls of Pregnancy Tests

Any test result can be wrong. Laboratory errors do occur, including specimen mix-up, decimal point errors, and incorrectly performed test procedures. Consider repeating the test when an unexpected result occurs.

Incorrectly Performed Home Pregnancy Tests

A urine pregnancy test result should be read only at the indicated timing, usually 3–5 minutes after administration. A common scenario occurs when the negative test is viewed again much later and found to have a faintly positive test line. The faint line is often referred to as an "evaporation line" and does not represent a positive result. Digital tests avoid this issue.

False-Negative Pregnancy Tests

False-negative results can occur either when the test is performed too early or when there are extremely high hCG levels. Urine that is too diluted can also be responsible for false-negative results. It is rare but known in the literature that urine and serum pregnancy tests may yield false-negative results when hCG is present at extreme concentrations. Known as the *high-dose hook effect*, the *secondary* antibody binding sites become saturated with free hCG so that the *primary* antibody complex is unable to bind, preventing detection of the antigen.[36] In one case of molar pregnancy, only after multiple dilutions of the serum was hCG of 1.5 million mIU/mL detected.[37] In complete molar pregnancy, hCG levels as high as 3,704,085 mIU/mL have been reported.[38] If you suspect a molar pregnancy, but hCG is much lower than expected (in the hundreds), notify the laboratory so that they can perform dilutions. The important thing to remember is that laboratory test results should be questioned if they are discordant with clinical findings.

False-Positive Pregnancy Tests

In very rare cases, urine pregnancy test results are positive even when the patient is not pregnant or has not recently been pregnant. This occurs when hCG is present and originating from a source other than pregnancy. A false-positive result could occur if the person has had treatment involving an hCG injection within the preceding 14 days. hCG injections are used in fertility treatments to stimulate ovulation. Faint false-positive results have also been reported with urine samples contaminated by blood or recent use of Chinese herbal medication and with the fad hCG diet.[39] If you suspect a false-positive result, repeat the test and/or obtain a serum quantitative hCG.

A serum or urine pregnancy test may also be positive if hCG is present due to incomplete resolution of a previous pregnancy, including gestational trophoblastic disease, or due to an hCG-secreting tumor. Low levels of hCG (5 to 30 mIU/mL) may be associated with tumors of the pancreas, ovaries, breast, and many other sites.[40] Some normal postmenopausal patients also have low levels of circulating hCG-like substance of pituitary origin.[41-43] In addition, patients with end-stage renal disease may produce hCG, which registers as a false-positive pregnancy test, due to decreased urinary clearance.[44]

Phantom hCG or heterophilic antibodies can cause a *serum* hCG to be positive (typically at low levels) but urine tests to be negative. These antibodies are present only in the blood and at high enough levels to interfere with serum hCG radioimmunoassay in a small number of women (1 in 3,300).[38,45,46] In these cases, hCG is falsely detected due to interfering antibodies found in human serum. While uncommon, false-positive or phantom hCG tests have led to the misdiagnosis of ectopic pregnancy, or to the erroneous assumption of postgestational choriocarcinoma. Since these interfering antibodies are present only in blood, perform a urine pregnancy test as a confirmatory hCG measurement when clinically indicated to rule out the false-positive serum hCG results due to heterophilic antibodies.[16] For confirmation, the laboratory should be notified to perform serial dilutions, since the hCG results will not decrease in parallel with increasing dilutions.

Biochemical Pregnancy

Very early pregnancy loss, or a *biochemical pregnancy*, refers to a pregnancy that initially establishes implantation but fails to grow successfully. Serum hCG levels appear approximately 1 week after conception, peak at approximately 10 to 100 mIU/mL, then drop. A normal or heavier-than-usual menstrual period follows, which may or may not be delayed. A positive pregnancy test may be detected in the last week of the menstrual cycle, but if the test is repeated later, the test is negative; transient hCG may extend to 5 days after the time of the missed menses.[22]

Serum hCG Levels in Early Pregnancy

Normal hCG Levels and Trends

Elevated hCG can be detected in serum at low levels as early as 21 days from LMP, very soon after implantation occurs.[48] In general, serum levels of hCG reach 50 to 250 mIU/mL by the time of the first missed menstrual period; hCG reaches a peak of >100,000 mIU/mL at approximately 10–12 weeks LMP and then declines to a plateau that is maintained until delivery (**Figure 25-1**).[47,49] Low levels of hCG may simply indicate that a normal pregnancy is earlier in gestation than menstrual dates suggest. These values can also vary significantly between individuals. During the first 10 weeks of pregnancy, an hCG rise of 66% over 2 days or 48 hours had generally been considered acceptable evidence of a viable intrauterine pregnancy.[50] However, hCG increase over 48 hours can be as high as 228% and as low as 33% for a viable pregnancy, though trends are dependent on initial hCG levels.[51,52] With an hCG trend that is less than expected, consider obtaining a third value for confirmation.[53] Elevated levels of hCG are seen with a multiple gestation, reflecting the increased placental mass, as well as in the setting of gestational trophoblastic disease.[49]

A single hCG value tells you if a person is pregnant, but it does not determine the pregnancy's location or whether it is growing normally.[54] An hCG level of 2,000 to 3,000 mIU/mL or higher generally correlates with the ability to visualize a pregnancy via transvaginal ultrasound, also called the "discriminatory zone,"[55-57] although there have been reported cases of intrauterine pregnancies being diagnosed

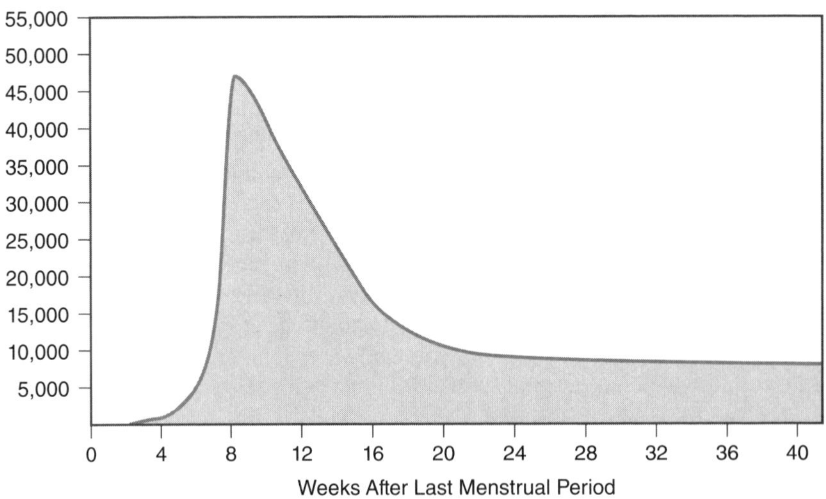

Figure 25-1 hCG levels during normal pregnancy.

Reproduced from Braunstein GD, Rasor J, Danzer H, Adler D, Wade ME. Serum human chorionic gonadotropin levels throughout normal pregnancy. Am J Obstet Gynecol 1976;126(6):678-81. https://www.ncbi.nlm.nih.gov/pubmed/984142

only after initial hCG levels as high as 6,567 mIU/mL.[58] In practice, an hCG level of 3,500 may have a 99% probability of detecting an intrauterine pregnancy.[59] In a hemodynamically stable patient with a pregnancy of unknown location, serial assessments of hCG change over time, usually over 48 hours, can provide more information for diagnosis.[54,57] If an intrauterine pregnancy can be visualized on ultrasound examination, the appearance of anatomic landmarks and growth of the embryo over time on ultrasound should be the primary method of assessing viability. If there is a question about viability of an intrauterine pregnancy, the ultrasound is generally repeated in 7–10 days.[60]

hCG Trends in Abnormal Pregnancy

A pregnancy that is ultimately found to be abnormal could initially have already stopped growing, or could have continued growth with a normal or abnormal trend. Similarly, in abnormal pregnancies, hCG levels often increase abnormally, plateau, or decrease, but can also have a normal trend initially. One study demonstrated that almost 30% of women with ectopic pregnancies had initial patterns of hCG change that mimicked either an intrauterine pregnancy or a complete miscarriage.[61] The rate of rise of hCG in ectopic pregnancy generally is lower than for intrauterine pregnancies, but the curves overlap.[62]

Extremely high hCG production, with hCG levels as high as 2 million mIU/mL, can occur with a molar pregnancy, such as hydatidiform mole or gestational trophoblastic disease, though some molar gestations have normal hCG levels.[49] Abnormally low hCG levels often occur with an abnormal pregnancy, such as before a spontaneous abortion or with an ectopic pregnancy, but they can also represent a normal pregnancy that is earlier than expected.

If an abnormal hCG trend occurs but the pregnancy is desired, obtain an ultrasound as soon as the hCG level reaches the discriminatory zone. Consider following an abnormally low rise of serum hCG with a third serial hCG value for confirmation since a third value can help to reduce misclassification of an intrauterine pregnancy.[53]

Typically, the pattern of hCG rise, fall, or plateau, in combination with the clinical picture, ultrasound examination (if performed), and risk factors for ectopic pregnancy is more important than a single hCG value in determining the location and status of the pregnancy (See **Box 25-3**).

hCG Trends After Pregnancy

After a pregnancy ends and the placenta has separated from the uterus, hCG levels decrease, first quickly and then more slowly. **Figure 25-2** represents the hCG

Box 25-3 Risk Factors for Ectopic Pregnancy

- Previous ectopic pregnancy[63]
- History of tubal surgery (female sterilization or tubal reconstruction)
- Intrauterine contraceptive in place[62]
- Pelvic inflammatory disease[64]

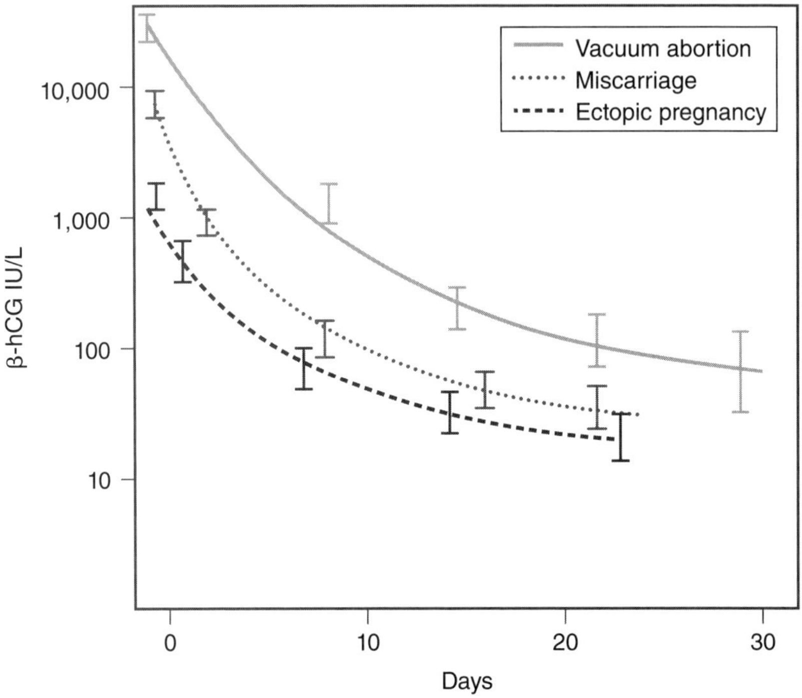

Figure 25-2 Disappearance curve of hCG after abortion, miscarriage, and surgical treatment of ectopic pregnancy. Disappearance curves of serum hCG in three groups of women. Semilogarithmic scale. Upper curve represents women (*n* = 36) who had elective vacuum aspiration abortion at 7–13 weeks LMP. Middle curve represents women (*n* =35) with spontaneous abortion at 6–15 weeks LMP treated with uterine aspiration. Lower curve represents women (*n* =35) with ectopic pregnancies diagnosed 2.5–11.0 weeks after LMP and removed surgically.

disappearance curve following uterine aspiration abortion at 7–13 weeks (upper curve), miscarriage at 6 to 15 weeks (middle curve), and surgical treatment of ectopic pregnancy (bottom curve).[65] Following complete evacuation of a pregnancy of any gestation, hCG becomes undetectable by 3–4 weeks in most patients.

If a medication abortion or a first-trimester vacuum aspiration successfully ended the pregnancy, the hCG level initially declines steadily, halving by 48 hours.[66-69]

The outcome of medication abortion can be followed by quantitative hCG instead of ultrasound, making a return to the clinic for an in-person examination unnecessary. This is especially helpful for those who must travel a great distance to obtain mifepristone and misoprostol and for those who have received the medication by mail for self-administration. For patients undergoing a medication abortion, hCG may continue to increase following mifepristone but then declines precipitously after expulsion of the pregnancy.[70] By day 3 and day 5 after mifepristone, hCG levels can decrease by 57% and 86%, respectively.[71,72] By 6 to 18 days after taking mifepristone, the hCG level is expected to drop by at least 80% from the initial value (measured on the day of mifepristone) in 98.5% of successful medication abortions.[71-73]

When an hCG level is used to confirm completed vacuum aspiration abortion, a 50% decline in hCG by 48 hours is considered successful uterine evacuation based on trends after medication abortion.[69] Often, hCG will drop 50% in 24 hours, allowing for a faster confirmation. Likewise, if hCG is used to confirm complete uterine evacuation in the setting of pregnancy of unknown location or uterine aspiration without identification of gestational tissue, a 50% decline is considered to confirm completed pregnancy and is suggestive of intrauterine location.[54] (See Chapter 16, Abortion.)

Follow-up After Spontaneous Abortion

Serum hCG is not recommended following a spontaneous abortion if a prior ultrasound documented an intrauterine pregnancy or if the gestational sac and placental tissue were confirmed by direct visualization after uterine evacuation.[60] Ultrasound examination can be used to identify whether the gestational sac has completely expelled. If intrauterine pregnancy has not been confirmed by one of these methods, then serial hCG testing should demonstrate a rapid decline if complete expulsion has occurred. Without prior evidence of intrauterine pregnancy, these cases should be treated as pregnancy of unknown location with appropriate documentation of adequate hCG decline to rule out ectopic pregnancy. hCG measurements typically decrease as a quadratic curve with a steeper rate of decline at higher initial hCG concentrations when a spontaneous abortion resolves without intervention.[74] In some cases, weekly serial hCG followed to nonpregnant levels might be necessary to ensure completion of the pregnancy.

Author Disclosures—Baldwin: none; Chen: receives funding for contraceptive research from Medicines360, Sebela, and Mylan, all of which are managed by Magee-Womens Research Institute.

References

1. ACOG Committee Opinion No. 762: Prepregnancy counseling. Obstet Gynecol. 2019;133(1): e78-89. DOI: 10.1097/aog.0000000000003013.
2. Zabin LS, Emerson MR, Ringers PA, Sedivy V. Adolescents with negative pregnancy test results. An accessible at-risk group. JAMA. 1996;275(2):113-7. (https://www.ncbi.nlm.nih.gov/pubmed/8531305).
3. Callegari LS, Aiken AR, Dehlendorf C, Cason P, Borrero S. Addressing potential pitfalls of reproductive life planning with patient-centered counseling. Am J Obstet Gynecol. 2017;216(2):129-34. DOI: 10.1016/j.ajog.2016.10.004.
4. Wilkes J. AAFP releases position paper on preconception care. Am Fam Physician. 2016;94(6):508-10. (https://www.ncbi.nlm.nih.gov/pubmed/27637129).
5. Finer LB, Zolna MR. Declines in unintended pregnancy in the United States, 2008-2011. N Engl J Med. 2016;374(9):843-52. DOI: 10.1056/NEJMsa1506575.
6. Erickson JD. Folic acid and prevention of spina bifida and anencephaly. 10 years after the U.S. Public Health Service recommendation. MMWR Recomm Rep. 2002;51(RR-13):1-3. (https://www.ncbi.nlm.nih.gov/pubmed/12353506).
7. Kapp N, Whyte P, Tang J, Jackson E, Brahmi D. A review of evidence for safe abortion care. Contraception. 2013;88(3):350-63. DOI: 10.1016/j.contraception.2012.10.027.

8. National Academies of Sciences, Engineering, Medicine, et al. The safety and quality of abortion care in the United States. Washington DC: National Academies Press; 2018.
9. Curtis KM, Tepper NK, Jamieson DJ, Marchbanks PA. Adaptation of the World Health Organization's Selected Practice Recommendations for Contraceptive Use for the United States. Contraception. 2013;87(5):513-6. DOI: 10.1016/j.contraception.2012.08.024.
10. Phillips O, Simpson J. Contraception and congenital malformations. Glob Lib Womens Med. [Internet]. 2008. DOI 10.3843/GLOWM.10398
11. Kim SK, Romero R, Kusanovic JP, et al. The prognosis of pregnancy conceived despite the presence of an intrauterine device (IUD). J Perinat Med. 2010;38(1):45-53. DOI: 10.1515/JPM.2009.133.
12. Rai R, Regan L. Recurrent miscarriage. Lancet. 2006;368(9535):601-11. DOI: 10.1016/S0140-6736(06)69204-0.
13. Lazorwitz A, Coleman-Minahan K, Teal SB, Guiahi M. Ongoing etonogestrel contraceptive implant use throughout pregnancy. J Adolesc Health. 2018;63(3):363-4. DOI: 10.1016/j.jadohealth.2018.03.021.
14. Taylor HS, Pal L, Seli E. Speroff's clinical gynecologic endocrinology and infertility. Philadelphia, PA: Wolters Kluwer; 2019.
15. Wilcox AJ, Baird DD, Weinberg CR. Time of implantation of the conceptus and loss of pregnancy. N Engl J Med. 1999;340(23):1796-9. DOI: 10.1056/nejm199906103402304.
16. Davies S, Byrn F, Cole LA. Human chorionic gonadotropin testing for early pregnancy viability and complications. Clin Lab Med. 2003;23(2):257-64, vii. (https://www.ncbi.nlm.nih.gov/pubmed/12848444).
17. Cole LA. Human chorionic gonadotropin and associated molecules. Expert Rev Mol Diagn. 2009;9(1):51-73. DOI: 10.1586/14737159.9.1.51.
18. Olszynko-Gryn J. The demand for pregnancy testing: the Aschheim-Zondek reaction, diagnostic versatility, and laboratory services in 1930s Britain. Stud Hist Philos Biol Biomed Sci. 2014;47 Pt B:233-47. DOI: 10.1016/j.shpsc.2013.12.002.
19. Braunstein GD. The long gestation of the modern home pregnancy test. Clin Chem. 2014;60(1):18-21. DOI: 10.1373/clinchem.2013.202655.
20. Wide L. Inventions leading to the development of the diagnostic test kit industry--from the modern pregnancy test to the sandwich assays. Ups J Med Sci. 2005;110(3):193-216. DOI: 10.3109/2000-1967-066.
21. Butler SA, Khanlian SA, Cole LA. Detection of early pregnancy forms of human chorionic gonadotropin by home pregnancy test devices. Clin Chem. 2001;47(12):2131-6.
22. Cole LA, Khanlian SA, Sutton JM, Davies S, Rayburn WF. Accuracy of home pregnancy tests at the time of missed menses. Am J Obstet Gynecol. 2004;190(1):100-5. DOI: 10.1016/j.ajog.2003.08.043.
23. Cole LA. The utility of six over-the-counter (home) pregnancy tests. Clin Chem Lab Med. 2011;49(8):1317-22. DOI: 10.1515/cclm.2011.211.
24. Cervinski MA, Lockwood CM, Ferguson AM, et al. Qualitative point-of-care and over-the-counter urine hCG devices differentially detect the hCG variants of early pregnancy. Clin Chim Acta. 2009;406(1-2):81-5. DOI: 10.1016/j.cca.2009.05.018.
25. Wallace LS, Zite NB, Homewood VJ. Making sense of home pregnancy test instructions. J Womens Health (Larchmt). 2009;18(3):363-8. DOI: 10.1089/jwh.2008.0985.
26. Chard T. Pregnancy tests: a review. Hum Reprod. 1992;7(5):701-10. (https://www.ncbi.nlm.nih.gov/pubmed/1639991).
27. Wilcox AJ, Baird DD, Dunson D, McChesney R, Weinberg CR. Natural limits of pregnancy testing in relation to the expected menstrual period. JAMA. 2001;286(14):1759-61. (https://www.ncbi.nlm.nih.gov/pubmed/11594902).
28. Raymond EG, Shochet T, Bracken H. Low-sensitivity urine pregnancy testing to assess medical abortion outcome: A systematic review. Contraception. 2018;98(1):30-5. DOI: 10.1016/j.contraception.2018.03.013.
29. Lynd K, Blum J, Ngoc NT, Shochet T, Blumenthal PD, Winikoff B. Simplified medical abortion using a semi-quantitative pregnancy test for home-based follow-up. Int J Gynaecol Obstet. 2013;121(2):144-8. DOI: 10.1016/j.ijgo.2012.11.022.

30. Grossman D, Berdichevsky K, Larrea F, Beltran J. Accuracy of a semi-quantitative urine pregnancy test compared to serum beta-hCG measurement: a possible screening tool for ongoing pregnancy after medication abortion. Contraception. 2007;76(2):101-4. DOI: 10.1016/j.contraception.2007.04.008.
31. Raymond EG, Shochet T, Blum J, et al. Serial multilevel urine pregnancy testing to assess medical abortion outcome: a meta-analysis. Contraception. 2017;95(5):442-8. DOI: 10.1016/j.contraception.2016.12.004.
32. Shochet T, Comstock IA, Ngoc NTN, et al. Results of a pilot study in the U.S. and Vietnam to assess the utility and acceptability of a multi-level pregnancy test (MLPT) for home monitoring of hCG trends after assisted reproduction. BMC Womens Health. 2017;17(1):67. DOI: 10.1186/s12905-017-0422-y.
33. Hoppenot C, Zimmerman L, Arlandson M, Lurain JR, Patel A. Follow-up after molar pregnancy evacuation: Feasibility of using semi-quantitative urine pregnancy tests. The J Reprod Med. 2016;61(5-6):192-6.
34. Desai D, Lu J, Wyness SP, et al. Human chorionic gonadotropin discriminatory zone in ectopic pregnancy: does assay harmonization matter? Fertil Steril. 2014;101(6):1671-4. DOI: 10.1016/j.fertnstert.2014.02.023.
35. Doubilet PM, Benson CB, Bourne T, Blaivas M. Diagnostic criteria for nonviable pregnancy early in the first trimester. N Engl J Med. 2013;369(15):1443-51. DOI: 10.1056/NEJMra1302417.
36. Kazemi MR, Vargas JE, Lo JC. Hyperthyroidism and a negative urine hCG test in molar pregnancy. Am J Med. 2004;117(11):889-90. DOI: 10.1016/j.amjmed.2004.09.007.
37. Tabas JA, Strehlow M, Isaacs E. A false negative pregnancy test in a patient with a hydatidiform molar pregnancy. N Engl J Med. 2003;349(22):2172-3. DOI: 10.1056/NEJM200311273492221.
38. Cole LA. Human chorionic gonadotropin tests. Expert Rev Mol Diagn. 2009;9(7):721-47. DOI: 10.1586/erm.09.51.
39. Butler SA, Cole LA. Evidence for, and associated risks with, the human chorionic gonadotropin supplemented diet. J Diet Suppl. 2016;13(6):694-9. DOI: 10.3109/19390211.2016.1156208.
40. Bandi ZL, Schoen I, Waters M. An algorithm for testing and reporting serum choriogonadotropin at clinically significant decision levels with use of "pregnancy test" reagents. Clin Chem. 1989;35(4):545-51. (https://www.ncbi.nlm.nih.gov/pubmed/2649272).
41. Cole LA, Khanlian SA, Muller CY. Normal production of human chorionic gonadotropin in perimenopausal and menopausal women and after oophorectomy. Int J Gynecol Cancer. 2009;19(9):1556-9. (https://www.ncbi.nlm.nih.gov/pubmed/19994471).
42. Cole LA, Khanlian SA, Muller CY. Detection of perimenopause or postmenopause human chorionic gonadotropin: an unnecessary source of alarm. Am J Obstet Gynecol. 2008;198(3):275 e1-7. DOI: 10.1016/j.ajog.2007.09.034.
43. Cole LA, Ladner DG. Background hCG in non-pregnant individuals: need for more sensitive point-of-care and over-the-counter pregnancy tests. Clin Biochem. 2009;42(3):168-75. DOI: 10.1016/j.clinbiochem.2008.09.107.
44. Fahy BG, Gouzd VA, Atallah JN. Pregnancy tests with end-stage renal disease. J Clin Anesth. 2008;20(8):609-13. DOI: 10.1016/j.jclinane.2008.05.025.
45. Knight AK, Bingemann T, Cole L, Cunningham-Rundles C. Frequent false positive beta human chorionic gonadotropin tests in immunoglobulin A deficiency. Clin Exp Immunol. 2005;141(2):333-7. DOI: 10.1111/j.1365-2249.2005.02837.x.
46. Rotmensch S, Cole LA. False diagnosis and needless therapy of presumed malignant disease in women with false-positive human chorionic gonadotropin concentrations. Lancet. 2000;355(9205):712-5. DOI: 10.1016/S0140-6736(00)01324-6.
47. Braunstein GD, Rasor J, Danzer H, Adler D, Wade ME. Serum human chorionic gonadotropin levels throughout normal pregnancy. Am J Obstet Gynecol. 1976;126(6):678-81. (https://www.ncbi.nlm.nih.gov/pubmed/984142).
48. Lohstroh PN, Overstreet JW, Stewart DR, et al. Hourly human chorionic gonadotropin secretion profiles during the peri-implantation period of successful pregnancies. Fertil Steril. 2007;87(6):1413-8. DOI: 10.1016/j.fertnstert.2006.11.053.
49. Cole LA, Laidler LL, Muller CY. USA hCG reference service, 10-year report. Clin Biochem. 2010;43(12):1013-22. DOI: 10.1016/j.clinbiochem.2010.05.006.

50. Kadar N, Caldwell BV, Romero R. A method of screening for ectopic pregnancy and its indications. Obstet Gynecol. 1981;58(2):162-6. (https://www.ncbi.nlm.nih.gov/pubmed/6454867).
51. Barnhart KT, Sammel MD, Rinaudo PF, Zhou L, Hummel AC, Guo W. Symptomatic patients with an early viable intrauterine pregnancy: HCG curves redefined. Obstet Gynecol. 2004;104(1):50-5. DOI: 10.1097/01.AOG.0000128174.48843.12.
52. Barnhart KT, Guo W, Cary MS, et al. Differences in Serum human chorionic gonadotropin rise in early pregnancy by race and value at presentation. Obstet Gynecol. 2016;128(3):504-11. DOI: 10.1097/AOG.0000000000001568.
53. Morse CB, Sammel MD, Shaunik A, et al. Performance of human chorionic gonadotropin curves in women at risk for ectopic pregnancy: exceptions to the rules. Fertil Steril. 2012;97(1):101-6 e2. DOI: 10.1016/j.fertnstert.2011.10.037.
54. Committee on Practice Bulletins—Gynecology. ACOG Practice Bulletin No. 191: Tubal ectopic pregnancy. Obstet Gynecol. 2018;131(2):e65-77. DOI: 10.1097/AOG.0000000000002464.
55. Timor-Tritsch IE, Rottem S. Transvaginal sonography. 2nd ed. New York: Elsevier; 1991.
56. Doubilet PM. Ultrasound evaluation of the first trimester. Radiol Clin North Am. 2014; 52(6):1191-9. DOI: 10.1016/j.rcl.2014.07.004.
57. Doubilet PM, Benson CB, Bourne T, Blaivas M, Society of Radiologists in Ultrasound Multispecialty Panel on Early First Trimester Diagnosis of Miscarriage and Exclusion of a Viable Intrauterine Pregnancy. Diagnostic criteria for nonviable pregnancy early in the first trimester. Ultrasound Q. 2014;30(1):3-9. DOI: 10.1097/RUQ.0000000000000060.
58. Doubilet PM, Benson CB. Further evidence against the reliability of the human chorionic gonadotropin discriminatory level. J Ultrasound Med. 2011;30(12):1637-42. DOI: 10.7863/jum.2011.30.12.1637.
59. Connolly A, Ryan DH, Stuebe AM, Wolfe HM. Reevaluation of discriminatory and threshold levels for serum beta-hCG in early pregnancy. Obstet Gynecol. 2013;121(1):65-70. DOI: http://10.1097/AOG.0b013e318278f421
60. American College of Obstetricians and Gynecologists' Committee on Practice Bulletins—Gynecology. ACOG Practice Bulletin No. 200: Early pregnancy loss. Obstet Gynecol. 2018;132(5):e197-207. DOI: 10.1097/AOG.0000000000002899.
61. Dart RG, Mitterando J, Dart LM. Rate of change of serial beta-human chorionic gonadotropin values as a predictor of ectopic pregnancy in patients with indeterminate transvaginal ultrasound findings. Ann Emerg Med. 1999;34(6):703-10. (https://www.ncbi.nlm.nih.gov/pubmed/10577398).
62. Barnhart KT. Clinical practice. Ectopic pregnancy. N Engl J Med. 2009;361(4):379-87. DOI: 10.1056/NEJMcp0810384.
63. Ankum WM, Mol BW, Van der Veen F, Bossuyt PM. Risk factors for ectopic pregnancy: a meta-analysis. Fertil Steril. 1996;65(6):1093-9. (https://www.ncbi.nlm.nih.gov/pubmed/8641479).
64. Hillis SD, Owens LM, Marchbanks PA, Amsterdam LF, Mac Kenzie WR. Recurrent chlamydial infections increase the risks of hospitalization for ectopic pregnancy and pelvic inflammatory disease. Am J Obstet Gynecol. 1997;176(1 Pt 1):103-7. (https://www.ncbi.nlm.nih.gov/pubmed/9024098).
65. Steier JA, Bergsjo P, Myking OL. Human chorionic gonadotropin in maternal plasma after induced abortion, spontaneous abortion, and removed ectopic pregnancy. Obstet Gynecol 1984;64(3):391-4. (https://www.ncbi.nlm.nih.gov/pubmed/6462569).
66. Aral K, Gurkan Zorlu C, Gokmen O. Plasma human chorionic gonadotropin levels after induced abortion. Adv Contracept. 1996;12(1):11-4. (https://www.ncbi.nlm.nih.gov/pubmed/8739512).
67. Schaff EA, Fielding SL, Eisinger S, Stadalius L. Mifepristone and misoprostol for early abortion when no gestational sac is present. Contraception. 2001;63(5):251-4. (https://www.ncbi.nlm.nih.gov/pubmed/11448464).
68. Walker K, Schaff E, Fielding S, Fuller L. Monitoring serum chorionic gonadotropin levels after mifepristone abortion. Contraception. 2001;64(5):271-3. (https://www.ncbi.nlm.nih.gov/pubmed/11777484).
69. Baldwin MK, Bednarek PH, Russo J. Serum human chorionic gonadotropin decline following aspiration abortion in early pregnancy less than 42 days gestation. Contraception. 2021;103(2):113-5. DOI: 10.1016/j.contraception.2020.11.010.

70. Rorbye C, Norgaard M, Nilas L. Prediction of late failure after medical abortion from serial beta-hCG measurements and ultrasonography. Hum Reprod. 2004;19(1):85-9. (https://www.ncbi.nlm.nih.gov/pubmed/14688162).

71. Pocius KD, Bartz D, Maurer R, Stenquist A, Fortin J, Goldberg AB. Serum human chorionic gonadotropin (hCG) trend within the first few days after medical abortion: a prospective study. Contraception. 2017;95(3):263-8. DOI: 10.1016/j.contraception.2016.09.007.

72. Pocius KD, Maurer R, Fortin J, Goldberg AB, Bartz D. Early serum human chorionic gonadotropin (hCG) trends after medication abortion. Contraception. 2015;91(6):503-6. DOI: 10.1016/j.contraception.2015.03.004.

73. Fiala C, Safar P, Bygdeman M, Gemzell-Danielsson K. Verifying the effectiveness of medical abortion; ultrasound versus hCG testing. Eur J Obstet Gynecol Reprod Biol. 2003;109(2):190-5. (http://www.ncbi.nlm.nih.gov/pubmed/12860340).

74. Barnhart K, Sammel MD, Chung K, Zhou L, Hummel AC, Guo W. Decline of serum human chorionic gonadotropin and spontaneous complete abortion: defining the normal curve. Obstet Gynecol. 2004;104(5 Pt 1):975-81. DOI: 10.1097/01.AOG.0000142712.80407.fd.

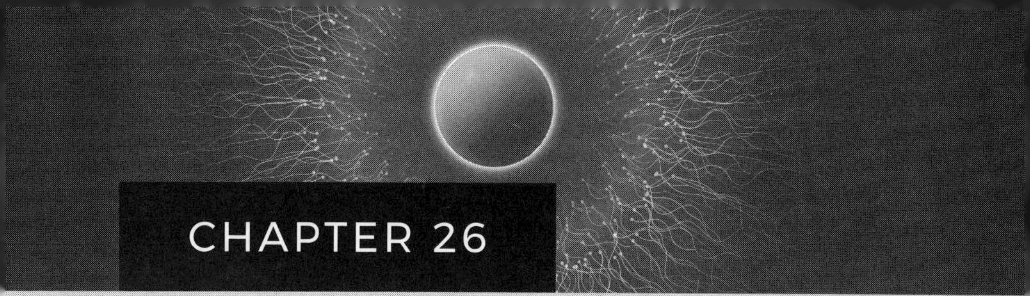

CHAPTER 26

Abortion

Siripanth Nippita, MD, MS
Maureen Paul, MD, MPH

KEY POINTS

- Access to high-quality, safe abortion is a critical part of primary health care.
- Restrictions on abortion disproportionately affect access for people living on low incomes, adolescents, people of color, people living in rural communities, immigrants, and incarcerated individuals.
- Over 90% of all abortions in the United States occur early in pregnancy; three-quarters take place at or before 9 weeks following the onset of the person's last normal menstrual period.
- Medication methods (most commonly mifepristone followed by misoprostol) are effective and safe options for people seeking abortion up to 11 weeks' gestation.
- Clinicians should confirm pregnancy as soon as possible and provide information about all options, with referrals and services for abortion as appropriate. (See Chapter 4, Person-Centered Reproductive Health Conversations and Contraceptive Counseling)
- Resources are available for facilitating abortion referrals, and for providing financial and logistical assistance to those in need of these services.
- Where allowed by law, medication abortion using telehealth for eligible patients is a safe and convenient option.

Autonomy is a critical ethical tenet in the provision of medical care. This principle is fundamental to the Reproductive Justice framework, a theory based in human rights that Black women in the United States coined following the 1994 International Conference of Population and Development in Cairo, Egypt.[1] The Reproductive Justice framework recognizes that people of color and other oppressed communities experience many factors, such as systemic racism, gender discrimination, inadequate financial resources, environmental injustice, incarceration, and employment and housing inequities, that may affect their reproductive decisions and aspirations. The Reproductive Justice framework asserts that all persons have the right to bodily autonomy; to decide whether and when to parent; and to raise families in safe, healthy, and sustainable communities. As such, it moves the right to abortion from simply an individual choice to one inextricably linked to social justice and unfettered health care access.

People have abortions for many reasons. The decision to terminate a pregnancy is based on an individual's unique situation and often involves complex considerations regarding responsibilities to self and others. Individuals often cite financial concerns, family obligations, continuing school or work, or relationship problems as reasons for having an abortion.[2] Other common reasons include wanting to delay or space childbearing and risk to the individual's own health or to that of the embryo/fetus. Those seeking abortions later in pregnancy may have a delayed diagnosis or encounter logistical difficulties in accessing services, such as finding a provider, paying for an abortion, or arranging transportation.[3-5] Patients who decide to have an abortion are typically sure of their decision and deserve to feel respected and supported. In studies that follow people long after abortion, those who end a pregnancy feel that it was the right decision for them over 95% of the time.[6,7]

This chapter provides an overview for clinicians who evaluate and refer patients for abortion services, as well as those who offer early medication or aspiration abortion in their practices. Several excellent reviews describe the various clinical abortion techniques in more detail.[8-10]

Safety of Abortion

Modern methods of abortion are remarkably safe. Following the nationwide legalization of abortion in the United States in 1973, abortion-related mortality decreased by 90%, with most of the decline occurring from 1973 to 1976. The risk of dying from a modern legal abortion is less than 1 in 100,000 procedures, which represents the lowest mortality risk of all pregnancy outcomes. Pregnancy-related death rates are twice as high for spontaneous abortion and eight times higher for continuing pregnancy and childbirth.[11]

Abortion-related complications are rare. Major adverse events occur in less than 0.25% of early abortions and 0.4% of procedures after the first trimester. The single greatest factor influencing the safety of abortion is gestational duration. Abortions are safer when performed early in pregnancy, which emphasizes the importance of access for people seeking abortion.

The availability of safe abortion also has broader health implications. Research has documented associations between restrictive state abortion policies and increased rates of maternal and infant mortality.[12-14] Another study demonstrated an inverse relationship between the number of state abortion restrictions and the likelihood of policies that support the health and well-being of women and children, such as expanded Medicaid provisions, childhood educational programs, maternal mortality review boards, and liberal family/medical leave laws.[15]

Abortion and Public Health

Incidence

According to the Guttmacher Institute, the annual number of legal induced abortions rose dramatically following the *Roe v. Wade* decision to reach 1.5 million in 1980. The number remained stable throughout the 1980s, peaking at 1.6 million in 1990 and falling to a historic low of 862,320 in 2017.[16,17] Increased contraceptive access and use of highly effective contraception, facilitated by the Affordable Care Act, likely contributed to this decline. Data from 2020 showed an 8% increase in the number of reported abortions in the United States, compared with 2017 (**Figure 26-1**).[18] Trends varied across and within states, with such factors as expanded state funding for abortion in some areas and clinic closures forcing individuals to travel for care in others contributing to these changes.

About 92% of abortions take place before 14 weeks' gestation, a figure that has remained fairly stable over time (**Figure 26-2**).[19] Abortions at 6 weeks' gestation or less have become more common, accounting for nearly 40% of abortions performed at ≤ 13 weeks' gestation in 2019.[19] In 2020, medication abortion accounted for more than half of abortions in the United States.[20] In contrast, the small percentage of abortions (about 5%) performed at or after 16 weeks' gestation has remained largely unchanged.[19]

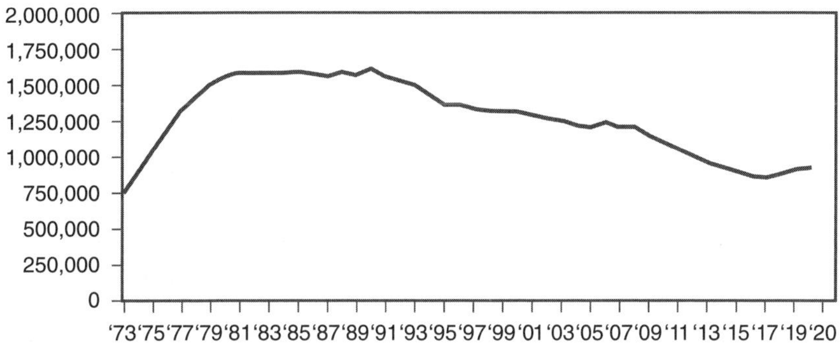

Figure 26-1 Abortion rates in the United States, 1973-2020.

Reproduced from Jones RK, Philbin J, Kirstein M, Nash E, Lufkin K. Long-term decline in US abortions reverses, showing rising need for abortion as Supreme Court is poised to overturn Roe v. Wade. Guttmacher Institute; 2022. https://www.guttmacher.org/article/2022/06/long-term-decline-us-abortions-reverses-showing-rising-need-abortion-supreme-court

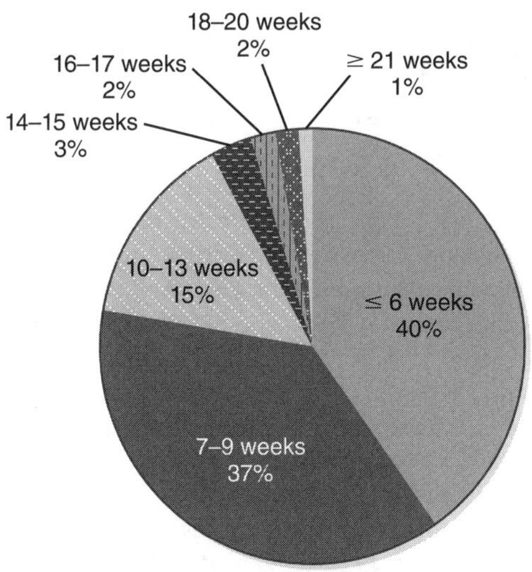

Figure 26-2 Gestational duration at the time of abortion in the United States, 2019.

Data from Kortsmit K, Mandel MG, Reeves JA, et al. Abortion surveillance - United States, 2019. MMWR Surveill Summ. 2021;70(9):1-29. DOI:10.15585/MMWR.SS7009A1

Characteristics of Individuals Who Obtain Abortions

Reflecting health disparities, people living on lower incomes bear a disproportionate share of the burden of unintended pregnancy and its consequences. In 2014, three-quarters of abortion patients were living below 200% of the federal poverty line.[21] Paying for an abortion can pose an extreme financial hardship, especially for people living in states where public insurance does not cover this care.[22-24]

Most people who have abortions are in their 20s, unmarried, or already have a child. Non-Hispanic White women and non-Hispanic Black women comprised 33.4% and 38.4%, respectively, of individuals who had an abortion in 2019, with the former having the lowest abortion rate (6.6 abortions per 1,000 women) and the latter the highest rate (23.8 abortions per 1,000 women).[19] The reasons for this disparity are complex and not well studied. Being marginalized from health systems or experiencing systemic racism in health care affects health outcomes.

Based on Guttmacher Institute data, nonhospital abortion facilities in the United States provided several hundred (452–530) abortions to transgender and gender nonbinary individuals in 2017.[25] Most of the abortions occurred in facilities that did not offer transgender-specific health services. These numbers may be underestimates, since some facilities do not document patients' gender identities, and stigma or confidentiality concerns may affect disclosure.

Although 51% of individuals obtaining abortions report that they used contraception during the month that they became pregnant, they may rely on less-effective methods or use methods inconsistently or incorrectly.[26] Providers of abortion care can offer person-centered contraceptive counseling while respecting autonomy and should be aware that some individuals do not want contraception at the time of abortion.[27-29] (See Chapter 4, Person-Centered Reproductive Health Conversations and Contraceptive Counseling.)

Public Health Benefits

The 1973 *Roe v. Wade* decision ushered in a new era in reproductive health, producing numerous public health benefits. In addition to improving the safety of abortion, legalization allowed people to obtain abortions earlier in pregnancy and closer to home. Abortion provision moved largely from hospitals to outpatient settings, which increased accessibility and reduced health care costs.[30]

Historically, the availability of contraception and abortion services bolstered women's agency, educational attainment, participation in the workforce, and earning potential. It facilitated decisions about if and when to have children. Increased economic stability benefited the well-being of women and their families and improved educational and economic outcomes for children.[31,32]

In the landmark Turnaway Study, researchers examined the benefits of obtaining wanted abortions by comparing outcomes among individuals who received abortions and those who were denied because they exceeded the facility's gestational age limit.[33] The study included nearly 1,000 participants seeking abortion care at 30 facilities in the United States who were each followed for 5 years. Compared with individuals made to continue an unwanted pregnancy, those who obtained abortions were significantly less likely to live in poverty, remain in relationships with abusive partners, and experience serious health problems. They were more likely to achieve aspirational life plans (e.g., education, employment) within the first year, and their existing children were more likely to achieve developmental milestones.

Recognizing the public health benefits of safe, legal abortion, in 2015 the American Public Health Association issued a policy upholding access to the full range of reproductive health services, including abortion, as a fundamental human right.[34] The policy calls for a public health strategy to advance health, equity, and Reproductive Justice, in part by demanding public funding of abortion, reversing all policies that restrict abortion access, and asserting support for the conscientious provision of abortion as an extension of clinicians' responsibility to center patients' needs in the provision of care.

Access to Legal Abortion: Brief History

In its *Roe v. Wade* ruling [410 U.S. 113 (1973)], the Supreme Court recognized the decision to continue or end a pregnancy as part of a fundamental constitutional right to privacy, thereby affording it high protection. Holding that the government could not interfere with a person's decision to have an abortion unless it had a "compelling" reason to do so, the justices sought to balance the interests involved by establishing a "trimester framework"[35,36]:

1. Up to the end of the first trimester, the abortion decision and procedure must be left to the judgment of the pregnant individual and their physician, largely unimpeded by governmental regulations.
2. After the first trimester, each state may choose to regulate abortion procedures in ways that are reasonably related to the pregnant person's health.
3. Subsequent to viability, the state may elect to promote its interest in potential human life by prohibiting abortion, as long as it provides an exception for abortions necessary to protect the pregnant person's life or health.

Following the *Roe v. Wade* decision, abortion opponents introduced legislation at the local, state, and national levels to reduce access to services. Passage of the Hyde Amendment in 1976 restricted federal funding for abortion, thereby curtailing access for people insured through Medicaid,[37,38] and numerous states regulated minors' access to abortion through provisions for parental involvement. The Supreme Court upheld these limitations, which disproportionately affected access to abortion for young people and people living on low incomes.[35]

The Supreme Court's 1992 landmark decision in *Planned Parenthood of Southeastern Pennsylvania v. Casey* [505 U.S. 833 (1992)] affirmed the fundamental right to abortion but abandoned *Roe's* trimester framework in favor of one based on fetal viability, thereby allowing states to impose restrictions early in pregnancy.[35] The Court also lowered the standard for determining the constitutionality of abortion restrictions, asserting that restrictions must not impose an "undue burden" on a person's ability to seek abortion. Under this less protective standard, the Supreme Court has upheld provisions such as mandatory waiting periods and biased counseling requirements. However, in its 2016 *Whole Woman's Health v. Hellerstedt* ruling, the Court found that a Texas law requiring abortion providers to maintain local hospital admitting privileges and imposing unnecessary design requirements for abortion facilities posed an undue burden to obtaining an abortion without any apparent benefit.[39]

Even though these Supreme Court rulings upheld the fundamental right to abortion, many states continued to accelerate efforts to limit abortion access and provision. In fact, nearly half of the abortion restrictions passed by states since *Roe* were enacted in the past decade alone. In addition to sheer volume, these laws increasingly shifted toward unconstitutional abortion bans and those designed to shutter abortion-providing facilities altogether.[40,41] Examples of such legislation included abortion bans as early as 6 weeks' gestation, limiting provision of medication abortion, bans on dilation and evacuation (D&E), and laws imposing onerous requirements on facilities and staff that provide abortion care. These restrictions are not based on sound scientific evidence.[42]

The long-standing erosion of reproductive rights culminated in the overturning of *Roe* in the 2022 *Dobbs v. Jackson Women's Health Organization* decision. *Dobbs* leaves abortion access subject to regulation by states, which already has had sweeping effects. The Guttmacher Institute reported that at least 43 clinics across 11 states stopped offering care in the month following the *Dobbs* decision, and they estimate that half the states are certain or likely to ban abortion with *Roe*'s demise.[43] Curtailment of abortion services and facility closures also limit training opportunities, exacerbating the long-standing shortage of abortion providers.[44,45] These changes affect pregnant people from marginalized communities most acutely. In many areas of the country, individuals must travel ever farther to obtain an abortion.[46-48] This travel burden not only adds to the time a person will be away from their work and family, but also compounds the costs of abortion to include transportation, lodging, and often childcare. These hurdles will prove insurmountable to some people, forcing them to continue undesired pregnancies.

To maintain the important public health benefits brought by the *Roe v. Wade* decision, abortions must remain not only safe and legal, but available to those who need them.[33] Advocates for reproductive rights and justice have worked diligently to challenge abortion restrictions and advance proactive legislation to protect abortion access. As of March 2023, 17 states and the District of Columbia had passed laws to protect and fund abortion access; 14 in anticipation of the *Dobbs* decision, 3 more in its aftermath.[49] Federal initiatives to repeal the Hyde Amendment and advance the Women's Health Protection Act, which would curtail many state abortion restrictions, are ongoing.[50] As health professionals, clinicians play a critical role in supporting efforts to protect abortion rights and advance the health and well-being of their patients.

Evaluation and Preparation of Patients for Abortion

Providers have advocated for and successfully used telehealth to improve access to abortion, where allowed by law.[51,52] The COVID-19 pandemic accelerated its adoption as patients and providers coped with stay-at-home orders and distancing measures to minimize contact.[53,54] Whether clinicians provide services on site or remotely, the basic components of abortion care are similar.

Deciding Whether to Continue a Pregnancy

The process of deciding whether to continue a pregnancy commonly begins as soon as an individual suspects pregnancy. Most people are certain of their decision, while some experience ambivalence or find the decision complicated.[55] Basic factual information and discussion will meet the needs of most individuals, and those who need more support can receive more extensive counseling and education. Clinicians can help explore feelings in a supportive and nonjudgmental way. (See Chapter 4, Person-Centered Reproductive Health Conversations and Contraceptive Counseling.)

Table 26-1 **Resources for Abortion Services and Funding**

Resource	Contact Information	Services
Abortion Finder	www.abortionfinder.org	Provides comprehensive directory of abortion services in the United States
I need an a	https://www.ineedana.com/	Provides information on clinics, funding, and telemedicine for individuals seeking abortion
National Abortion Federation	https://prochoice.org/find-a-provider/ Abortion referrals: 1-877-257-0012 Funding support: 1-800-772-9100	Multilingual hotline for abortion referrals and financial assistance in the United States and Canada
Planned Parenthood	http://plannedparenthood.org/abortion-access? 1-800-230-PLAN	Directs to Planned Parenthood clinics that provide abortion care
National Network of Abortion Funds	https://abortionfunds.org/	Connects patients with organizations providing logistical and financial support for abortion services
Brigid Alliance	https://brigidalliance.org/need-support/	Arranges and funds long-distance travel support for people seeking abortions at 15 weeks' gestation or more

Depending on the scope of services that your practice provides, you may need to refer patients for financial assistance, further counseling, abortion, prenatal care, adoption services, or other necessary care. Some helpful resources for abortion referrals and funding assistance are listed in **Table 26-1**.

Pre-abortion Evaluation

Because most individuals who request abortion are young and healthy, the pre-abortion medical evaluation is usually straightforward. The main goals of the evaluation include the following:

- Confirm and estimate duration of pregnancy
- Identify possible problems that require further evaluation or intervention, such as ectopic pregnancy
- Identify medical or gynecologic conditions that might influence the selection of abortion methods or necessitate a referral.

Some freestanding clinics are not able to accommodate patients with certain medical conditions. Referring providers should be aware of any such restrictions when coordinating care.

Much of the preabortion evaluation can be completed over the phone, which can shorten or even eliminate face-to-face time for patients. People who are eligible for abortion without further testing and desire medication abortion may be able to obtain mifepristone and misoprostol with minimal to no in-person contact (**Table 26-2**).[56]

Table 26-2 Sample Protocol for Medication Abortion With No or Limited Testing

Screening to Estimate Pregnancy Duration

Purpose: To confirm that the patient is within the gestational duration limit for medication abortion.

Screening questions:

- What was the first day of your last menstrual period (LMP)?
- Are you certain about that date?
- Did you have or perform a pregnancy test? If YES, document date and result.
- Did you have an ultrasound during this pregnancy? If YES, document date and result, including location of the pregnancy and gestational duration at the time of the ultrasound.

Eligible for no testing if:

- Pregnancy test positive
- Ultrasound, if done, confirms intrauterine pregnancy
- Based on ultrasound result or certain LMP, the gestational duration is 77 days or less on the anticipated day of mifepristone administration

Medical Screening

Purpose: To ensure the patient has no contraindications or conditions that would preclude safe medication abortion.

Screening questions:

- Do you have any of the following conditions
  - Chronic adrenal failure*
  - Currently using long-term systemic corticosteroids (does not include use of inhaled or topical steroids)*
  - Inherited porphyria*
  - Allergy to mifepristone*
  - Allergy to prostaglandins
  - Currently using anticoagulants
  - Hemorrhagic disorder
  - History of ectopic pregnancy
  - History of surgery or procedures on the fallopian tubes (including permanent contraception procedures)
  - Any serious medical condition such as chronic high blood pressure, heart disease, seizure disorder, or diabetes that is not well controlled?

*If using mifepristone. Individuals answering YES to these questions may be eligible for medication abortion with misoprostol only

- In the past several days, have you experienced vaginal spotting, bleeding, or pelvic pain (especially pain on one side of the pelvis)?
- Have you had an intrauterine device (IUD) in place at any time during this pregnancy? If YES, is the device still in place?

Eligible for mifepristone and misoprostol without further testing if patient answers NO to all medical questions.

If the patient has risk factors or symptoms suspicious for ectopic pregnancy or an uncontrolled medical condition, further evaluation is warranted.

An IUD must be removed before initiation of medication abortion.

Screening for Rh Status

Purpose: To determine if the patient requires administration of Rh_0(D)-immune globulin at the time of medication abortion, in accordance with your facility's Rh policy. The Society of Family Planning, National Abortion Federation, and World Health Organization do not recommend Rh testing and anti-D immunoglobulin prior to 12 weeks' gestation.[57-59]

Questions:

- Do you know whether your blood type is Rh positive or Rh negative?

Eligible for no testing if patient reports Rh positive blood type or does not require testing according to your facility's Rh policy.

Treatment

- Review the medication abortion protocol and what to expect.
- Complete any informed consent forms. Follow your facility's policy pertaining to verbal or signed consent.
- Explain the process for follow-up, including offering a phone call approximately 1 week post-mifepristone and self-administered home pregnancy testing 5 weeks post-misoprostol.[60] Verify the appropriate telephone number.
- Offer to discuss contraceptive methods if the patient desires.
- Make a plan for the patient to obtain the medications (mifepristone, misoprostol, analgesics, antiemetics), a high-sensitivity pregnancy test (HSPT), and written instructions (including 24-hour emergency contact information).
  - If the medications and supplies will be mailed to the patient, confirm mailing address.
  - If prescriptions will be sent, collect pharmacy information.
  - If the patient will pick up the medications and supplies, advise how to receive the medications at the health center.
- Answer any questions the patient may have.

Follow-Up

1 week post-mifepristone

Assess for continuing pregnancy or any symptoms or signs of ectopic pregnancy.

- If the patient had the expected amount of bleeding and cramping and thinks the pregnancy has passed, remind the patient to perform the HSPT 5 weeks after taking misoprostol and contact the provider if the test is positive.
- If the patient had no to little bleeding, still feels pregnant, or has pelvic pain suspicious for ectopic pregnancy, initiate prompt evaluation.

5 weeks post-misoprostol

- The patient performs a HSPT. If positive, initiate prompt evaluation.

Data from Raymond EG, Grossman D, Mark A, et al. Commentary: No-test medication abortion: A sample protocol for increasing access during a pandemic and beyond. Contraception. 2020;101(6):361-366. DOI:10.1016/J.CONTRACEPTION.2020.04.005

Clinicians should screen for anemia and perform other laboratory evaluation as indicated by history and symptoms.[57] At times, patients may request testing that is not medically necessary. Clinicians should elicit the reasons for such requests and validate their responses, explain why testing would or would not be indicated, and document the shared decision making that the discussion entailed.

History-Taking

The patient's history may affect the provider's recommendations for abortion method, preabortion testing, pain management, or follow-up. It may be appropriate to refer patients who are medically complex to a setting where staff and resources are readily available to manage any serious problems that may arise (**Table 26-3**).[61]

Ask the patient about their recent menstrual history, including cycle regularity and the onset of their LMP. Recording recent use of hormonal contraceptive methods helps to establish the accuracy of gestational dating based on LMP.

Clinical Examination

When indicated, perform a targeted physical assessment. A pelvic examination determines uterine size and position before aspiration abortion and helps to confirm gestational duration if the patient has not had an ultrasound or is unsure of their LMP.

If a pregnant patient has an intrauterine contraceptive device in place, remove it before proceeding with a medication abortion or during the aspiration abortion procedure.

Ultrasonography

Although many abortion providers in the United States use ultrasound routinely for gestational dating,[62] guidelines from the American College of Obstetricians and Gynecologists, Society of Family Planning, and National Abortion Federation do not require it before early abortion.[57,63] In many instances, clinical assessment of gestational duration by a certain or estimated LMP, combined with a protocol for ultrasound as needed, suffices for provision of safe early abortion.[64-66] Consider ultrasound evaluation if the patient has an uncertain LMP, if you suspect pregnancy beyond 77 days, if you detect an adnexal mass or suspect ectopic pregnancy, or to evaluate other pelvic examination findings. Ultrasound dating is the standard of care for second-trimester abortion in the United States.[57]

Laboratory Tests

For first-trimester abortion, routine hemoglobin or hematocrit evaluation is not required but may be indicated by clinical history.[57] Rh typing may be waived for people who report a positive Rh type, do not desire children in the future, decline anti-D immunoglobulin, or are having an early abortion, given the negligible risk of Rh-sensitization early in pregnancy,[67-71] but clinicians should follow their facility's protocol. The Society of Family Planning, National Abortion Federation, and World Health Organization do not recommend Rh testing and administration of anti-D immunoglobulin in patients having abortions at less than 12 weeks' gestation.[58-60,69]

Table 26-3 Considerations for Selected Conditions

Condition	Comment
Moderate to severe anemia	■ Consider aspiration with resources to manage and treat bleeding
Asthma	■ If mild or well controlled, may proceed with abortion ■ May need to delay care for a person with an acute asthma attack or poorly controlled asthma ■ Misoprostol is safe to use
Bleeding disorders	■ Early aspiration abortion is safe ■ Consider referral to higher-level facility as appropriate
Diabetes	■ May proceed with aspiration and local anesthesia without changes to diet or medication ■ May require insulin adjustment if fasting is required before IV sedation ■ High blood glucose levels are preferable to low levels at the time of aspiration
Hypertension	■ Avoid methylergonovine if hemorrhage occurs
Pregnancy of unknown location or suspected ectopic pregnancy	■ Evaluate and treat or refer according to local protocol ■ Aspiration with tissue examination may assist in diagnosis
Seizure disorder	■ If well controlled, may take antiseizure medications and proceed with aspiration or medication abortion ■ May use benzodiazepines for sedation or analgesia during aspiration
Substance use disorder	■ Individuals may require higher doses for analgesia or sedation due to tolerance
Uterine abnormalities, cervical stenosis	■ For aspiration, consider cervical preparation and/or ultrasound guidance ■ Consider medication abortion

Data from Turner KL, Huber A (Eds). Woman-centered, comprehensive abortion care: Reference manual. 2nd ed. Chapel Hill, NC: Ipas; 2013.

Infection Prevention

Infection associated with medication abortion is rare, as no uterine instrumentation occurs.[72] Current guidelines from the National Abortion Federation, Society of Family Planning, American College of Obstetricians and Gynecologists, and World Health Organization do not recommend routine antibiotic administration during medication abortion.[57,59,63,73]

In contrast, universal antibiotic prophylaxis at the time of aspiration or D&E abortion reduces the risk of postabortion infection, even in patients without risk factors.[74] The clinician should initiate the antibiotic shortly before the procedure, and a single dose or short-course regimen on the day of the abortion suffices. Many providers use doxycycline or azithromycin, and nitroimidazoles (metronidazole or tinidazole) are appropriate alternatives.[73] Although some providers use additional antibiotic prophylaxis for patients who may be at increased risk for subacute bacterial endocarditis, the American Heart Association does not recommend prophylaxis for genitourinary procedures.[75]

Clinicians also should offer testing or referral for reproductive tract infections and may opt to treat empirically for chlamydia based on history, signs, or symptoms.[57] Depending on their patient population, clinicians may universally screen for reproductive tract infection or follow US Preventive Services Task Force recommendations. Clinicians can initiate treatment for gonorrhea or chlamydia on the same day as the abortion.[57]

Patient Education and Informed Consent

An individual seeking abortion will need information about available methods; how they are done; their safety, success rates, risks, costs, and time required; and follow-up care. Although the patient may want their partner or other supportive persons involved in the information session, provide the opportunity to talk privately in case there are any confidential concerns, as well as to screen for intimate partner violence or coercion. Providers must follow any state regulations regarding the information given to patients, as well as those governing parental notification or consent for minors seeking abortion.[76] Once the patient has the information they need to make a decision and has all their questions answered, ask them to sign the appropriate consent forms before the abortion. Facilities offering medication abortion with telehealth may have secure mechanisms for sending required consent forms and educational materials electronically or they may permit verbal consent with appropriate documentation.

More than any other factor, gestational duration determines which abortion method the person may select (**Figure 26-3**). A patient may opt for an aspiration abortion during the first 14 to 15 weeks of pregnancy or an early medication

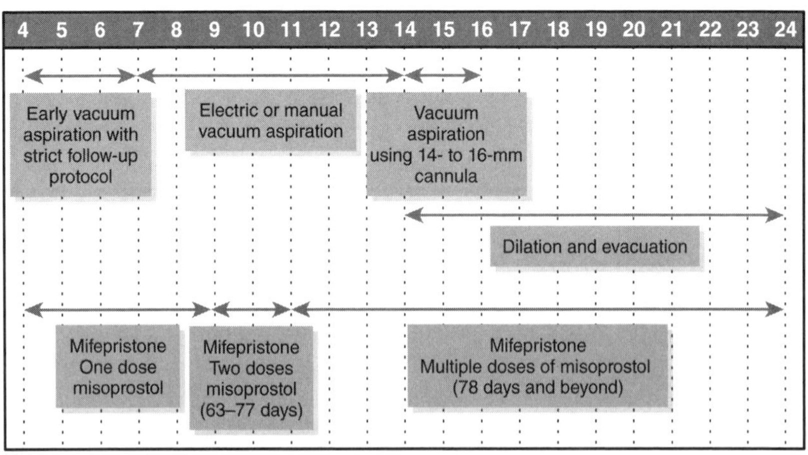

Figure 26-3 Options for terminating pregnancy, by duration of pregnancy.

Modified from Royal College of Obstetricians and Gynaecologists. The care of women requesting induced abortion. RCOG evidence-based clinical guideline No. 7. London: RCOG; 2011, with the permission of the Royal College of Obstetricians and Gynaecologists.

Table 26-4 Characteristics of Early Abortion Methods

Uterine Aspiration	Medication Abortion
Highly effective	Highly effective
Brief procedure time	Abortion process usually takes several hours or longer
Requires instrumentation	Avoids procedure (aspiration) if successful
Usually done with cervical anesthesia; allows option of oral analgesia/anxiolytics, sedation, or general anesthesia	Avoids anesthesia
Usually requires a single visit	May access via telehealth depending on eligibility without in-person provider contact, or may require one or more visits
Lighter perceived bleeding	Heavier perceived bleeding
Requires clinical setting	May occur in privacy of home

abortion during the first 77 days (11 weeks) of pregnancy.[77] For most people, the choice of method depends on their preferences. In helping the patient decide, explain the important features of each method (**Table 26-4**), emphasizing that both are highly effective. Most individuals will express a clear preference and be highly satisfied with the method they choose.[78]

After 14 to 15 weeks, abortion methods include dilation and evacuation (D&E) or induction with medications. A patient's options may be limited by other factors such as cost, availability of later medication abortion, or lack of skilled D&E providers in the community. In addition, some medical conditions or problems, such as severe anemia or abnormal uterine anatomy, may affect which abortion method or clinical setting would be safest.

Uterine aspiration is fast (usually around 5–10 minutes), highly effective, and reliably ends a pregnancy. Several options are available for pain management. The drawback is that aspiration is a procedure that takes place in an office or clinic, and it requires a pelvic exam and instrumentation. There is a small risk of complications from the procedure, including uterine perforation.

The advantage of medication abortion is that people can complete the process at home, in the setting and with the support people they prefer. Reasons commonly cited for choosing medication abortion include that it is noninvasive and that it affords individuals greater privacy and control over the abortion process.[79,80] In addition, medication abortion by telehealth expands access to abortion, particularly for people who face barriers to obtaining in person health care. Some individuals may consider a medication abortion similar to a miscarriage, and for them the experience may be more acceptable. Disadvantages include that it takes longer, and some people may still need an aspiration procedure for incomplete abortion or continuing pregnancy.

Many options are available for pain control during abortion, and often depend upon the clinical setting. Local anesthesia and oral pain control options are widely used, whereas intravenous sedation and general anesthesia require specialized equipment and trained providers. In one qualitative study, many participants felt that pain control decisions should be individualized.[81] Clinicians should discuss available options for pain control when obtaining informed consent for an abortion, as part of supporting patient autonomy.

Provision of Abortion Methods

Early Medication Abortion

Since the introduction of mifepristone in Europe more than two decades ago, its use for abortion has risen worldwide. The US Food and Drug Administration (FDA) approved mifepristone for abortion in September 2000, and Health Canada approved it in 2015. Planned Parenthood affiliates and most members of the National Abortion Federation currently offer early medication abortion services, and many private doctors, including obstetrician-gynecologists, pediatricians, and family practice physicians, provide abortion care within their primary care offices. In several states, advanced practice clinicians (nurse practitioners, certified nurse midwives, and physician assistants/associates) provide some or all aspects of early medication abortion care in accordance with state laws.[82]

Research supports the effectiveness of medication abortion up to 77 days' gestation. Use of mifepristone-misoprostol predominates as the most effective regimen, but misoprostol alone is a critical alternative where mifepristone is unaffordable or unavailable. In the United States a legal challenge to the FDA's approval of mifepristone is ongoing, but as of this writing, mifepristone is still available for use in the US market.

Medications Used in Early Abortion

Mifepristone. Mifepristone is a 19-norsteroid with a high affinity for progesterone receptors; it also binds to glucocorticoid receptors and, to a lesser extent, androgen receptors. The drug blocks the action of progesterone, which is necessary to establish and maintain placental attachment. Mifepristone also softens the cervix and stimulates synthesis of prostaglandins by cells of the early decidua.[63]

Millions of people worldwide have used the combination of mifepristone and misoprostol for early abortion with an impressive safety record. However, some limitations apply. The FDA drug label for mifepristone-misoprostol abortion advises against its use in the following circumstances:

- Intrauterine device in place (must be removed before treatment)
- Chronic adrenal failure
- Current long-term systemic corticosteroid therapy
- History of allergy to mifepristone, misoprostol, or other prostaglandin
- Hemorrhagic disorders or concurrent anticoagulant therapy
- Inherited porphyrias

Mifepristone does not appear to be teratogenic.[83] It is not as effective in ending pregnancy when used without misoprostol, and no evidence-based way exists to "reverse" its effects.[84,85]

Misoprostol. Misoprostol is a prostaglandin E1 analogue that softens the cervix and stimulates uterine contractions, thereby facilitating expulsion of the pregnancy. It is widely available and inexpensive, marketed for prevention of gastrointestinal ulcer disease. Although misoprostol alone induces abortion, protocols that combine it with mifepristone are more effective.[86]

Misoprostol can cause mild, short-term systemic prostaglandin effects, including nausea, vomiting, diarrhea, and temporary elevation of body temperature—side effects that patients commonly report with all medication abortion regimens. It can be administered vaginally, buccally (tucked between cheek and gum), or sublingually (placed under the tongue) for abortion. The pharmacokinetics of the drug differ by route of administration. Sublingual administration of misoprostol results in rapid peak blood levels that decrease in 1–3 hours, while vaginal or buccal dosing produces serum levels that rise more slowly but remain elevated longer.[87,88] Prenatal exposure to misoprostol has been associated with major congenital anomalies, primarily of the skull and limbs, but the absolute risk is low (less than 1%).[89,90]

Facility and Staffing Considerations

Medication abortion is well-suited to the scope of practice of primary care providers, including nurse practitioners, nurse midwives, and physician assistants/associates. For in-office visits, a typical medical office with space for private consultation, physical examination if indicated, and arrangements for a urine pregnancy test and lab services suffices. In addition, the practice must have a protocol for backup or referral, 24-hour emergency telephone service, and trained staff.

Provision of medication abortion by telehealth requires secure information and communications technologies as well as trained staff. However, some states have laws that explicitly prohibit telehealth for medication abortion.[91] Several others limit its implementation by requiring in-person counseling or prescribing by the clinician. Facilities wishing to offer telehealth medication abortion should be thoroughly familiar with state and local regulations governing its use.

To provide mifepristone, the FDA requires a risk evaluation and mitigation strategy (REMS).[92] Under this REMS, mifepristone prescribers must register directly with the drug distributor and meet certain qualifications. They must be able to determine gestational duration and diagnose ectopic pregnancy, as well as provide or refer for uterine aspiration or emergency treatment when necessary (e.g., hemorrhage or signs of sepsis). Personal expertise in ultrasound or aspiration is not required. These capabilities do not differ from those needed by any clinician caring for reproductive-aged patients who seek care for diagnosis or evaluation of early pregnancy. Although mifepristone prescribers are permitted to authorize practitioners under their supervision to provide the medication, laws in many states restrict the extent to which clinicians other than physicians can practice medication abortion.[93] Practitioners should verify state-specific requirements before initiating the service.

Before ordering or receiving mifepristone from the drug company, prescribers must attest to the above qualifications by signing a Prescribers Agreement.[92] They also must agree to provide a copy of a Medication Guide to each patient and secure a signed Patient Agreement. These materials are available at http://earlyoptionpill.com or https://genbiopro.com. The REMS initially mandated that patients receive mifepristone in person at a medical office, clinic, or hospital. In December 2021, the FDA permanently repealed this in-person requirement, allowing individuals to receive mifepristone by mail or delivery.[94,95]

Accumulated research confirms the safety and efficacy of medication abortion delivered by telehealth, including studies that involved delivery of the medications by mail.[53,66,96-99] Existing evidence does not support the assertion that the REMS program renders medication abortion with mifepristone safer.[100,101]

Mifepristone-Misoprostol Regimens

The combination of mifepristone and misoprostol is very effective. In 2016, the FDA revised labeling to reflect an evidence-based regimen of mifepristone 200 mg oral, followed by misoprostol 800 mcg buccal 24–48 hours later, up to 70 days' gestation.[102-105] Subsequent research confirmed acceptable efficacy up to 77 days, particularly with additional misoprostol doses (**Table 26-5**).[77,103,106,107,112]

Table 26-5 Efficacy of Mifepristone 200 mg Oral and Misoprostol 800 mcg Buccal Regimens by Gestational Duration

	Efficacy	Ongoing Pregnancy
≤ 49 days		
Misoprostol × 1 dose	98.1%	0.4%
50–56 days		
Misoprostol × 1 dose	96.7%	0.8%
57–63 days		
Misoprostol × 1 dose	93.5%	3.1%
64–70 days		
Misoprostol × 1 dose	92.3%	3.6%
Misoprostol × 2 doses, 4 hours apart	99.6%	0.4%
71–77 days		
Misoprostol × 1 dose	86.7%	8.7%
Misoprostol × 2 doses, 4 hours apart	97.6%	1.6%

Modified from National Abortion Federation. Clinical policy guidelines for abortion care; 2022. https://prochoice.org/providers/quality-standards/; Dzuba IG, Chong E, Hannum C, et al. A non-inferiority study of outpatient mifepristone-misoprostol medical abortion at 64–70 days and 71–77 days of gestation. Contraception. 2020;101(5):302-308; Dzuba IG, Castillo PW, Bousiéguez M, Lugo Hernández EM, Castañeda Vivar JJ, Sanhueza Smith P. A repeat dose of misoprostol 800 mcg following mifepristone for outpatient medical abortion at 64–70 and 71–77 days of gestation: A retrospective chart review. Contraception 2020;102(2):104-108. DOI:10.1016/j.contraception.2020.05.012; Hsia JK, Lohr PA, Taylor J, Creinin MD. Medical abortion with mifepristone and vaginal misoprostol between 64 and 70 days' gestation. Contraception. 2019;100(3):178-181. DOI:10.1016/j.contraception.2019.05.006; Chen MJ, Creinin MD. Mifepristone with buccal misoprostol for medical abortion. Obstetrics & Gynecology. 2015;126(1):12-21. DOI:10.1097/AOG.0000000000000897

Researchers have studied other doses, routes of administration, and timing of misoprostol following mifepristone ingestion:

- Shorter dosing intervals between mifepristone and misoprostol (24 hours for buccal and 6–24 hours for vaginal administration) do not decrease efficacy significantly.[108–110]
- Simultaneous administration of mifepristone and vaginal misoprostol also has acceptable efficacy through 63 days LMP.[111]

Misoprostol-only Regimens

Although misoprostol alone is not as effective as combined mifepristone regimens,[86,113] it remains an important alternative in settings where mifepristone is not available or abortion is illegal or inaccessible. Researchers have studied a variety of early-abortion regimens using misoprostol alone; most involve multiple doses and therefore higher rates of side effects than occur with mifepristone regimens (**Table 26-6**).[113-115] In a study involving more than 2,000 participants, success rates of 83% to 85% were achieved with use of misoprostol 800 mcg vaginally every 3 or 12 hours or sublingually every 3 hours; sublingual doses taken at 12-hour intervals were less effective. Side effects (primarily fever) are increased with sublingual administration compared with the vaginal route.[116] A randomized trial comparing misoprostol 800 mcg administered sublingually or buccally every 3 hours for three doses found similar rates of complete abortion (87% and 85%, respectively) but lower rates of ongoing pregnancy in the sublingual group (1.1% vs. 5.5%).[117] Providing additional misoprostol at the 7- to 14-day follow-up visit increased complete abortion rates to 94% in the sublingual group and 93% in the buccal group.

Table 26-6 Selected Clinical Protocols for Early Medication Abortion

Mifepristone and misoprostol (up to 77 days*)	Misoprostol only (≤ 13 weeks)[†]
Day 1 Give 200 mg mifepristone orally Up to **63 days**, provide four 200-mcg misoprostol tablets (800 mcg total) to take home, with instructions for: ■ Vaginal administration in 0–48 hours,[‡] OR ■ Buccal in 24–48 hours; swallow tablets after 30 minutes[§] At **64–70 days**, consider providing a second dose of misoprostol 800 mcg to use 4 hours following the first dose. At **71–77 days**, provide two doses of misoprostol 800 mcg to use 4 hours apart.	*Day 1* Provide 12 200-mcg misoprostol tablets to use as follows: ■ Four tablets (800 mcg) sublingually every 3 hours for 2–3 doses, OR ■ Four tablets (800 mcg) vaginally or buccally every 3–12 hours for 2–3 doses ■ Swallow buccal or sublingual tablets after 30 minutes.
Follow your facility's policy regarding Rh testing and administration of Rh_0(D)-immune globulin for Rh-negative individuals.[‖] Provide nonsteroidal anti-inflammatory medications (NSAIDs), such as ibuprofen, with instructions for use. Avoid narcotics. Antibiotic prophylaxis is not indicated for medication abortion.	

(continues)

Table 26-6 **Selected Clinical Protocols for Early Medication Abortion** *(continued)*

Mifepristone and misoprostol (up to 77 days*)	Misoprostol only (≤ 13 weeks)[†]
Day 3–14 (at least 24 hours after misoprostol) Assess outcome: ■ If ongoing pregnancy and ≤ 77 days gestation, repeat the regimen unless aspiration is desired; follow up in about 1 week. ■ If nonviable pregnancy, follow up in about 4 weeks unless aspiration is desired.	*Day 4–9 (at least 24 hours after misoprostol)* Assess outcome: ■ If abortion has not occurred, provide repeat doses of misoprostol (800 mcg) unless patient prefers aspiration. ■ If ongoing pregnancy, follow up at about day 14. ■ If nonviable pregnancy, follow up in about 4 weeks.
Day 14–21 (if ongoing pregnancy on previous visit) Schedule aspiration abortion if ongoing pregnancy persists.	*Day 14 (if ongoing pregnancy on previous visit)* Schedule aspiration abortion if ongoing pregnancy persists.
Follow up 4–5 weeks after initiation of treatment for patients who are awaiting resolution of a nonviable pregnancy. Offer aspiration if nonviable pregnancy persists.	

*In one study, treatment success was 87% at 71–77 days gestation, which was noninferior compared to 92% success rate at 64–70 days.[77] The National Abortion Federation recommends two doses of misoprostol 4 hours apart from 71–77 days and consideration of two doses at 64–70 days.[57]

[†]Regimen based on guidelines from the International Federation of Gynecology and Obstetrics (FIGO).[114]

[‡]Vaginal administration has fewer side effects compared with buccal and allows for a shorter dosing interval. Simultaneous administration of mifepristone and vaginal misoprostol has been found to have acceptable efficacy through 63 days LMP.[111]

[§]The FDA-approved regimen specifies buccal administration.

[||] Society of Family Planning, National Abortion Federation, and World Health Organization guidelines do not recommend Rh testing and Rh_0(D)-immune globulin for patients undergoing abortion before 12 weeks' gestation.[57-59]

Data from National Abortion Federation. Clinical policy guidelines for abortion care; 2022. https://prochoice.org/providers/quality-standards/; Horvath S, Goyal V, Traxler S, Prager S. Society of Family Planning committee consensus on Rh testing in early pregnancy. Contraception. 2022;114:1-5. DOI:10.1016/j.contraception.2022.07.002; World Health Organization. Abortion care guideline; 2022. http://www.who.int/publications/i/item/9789240039483; Dzuba IG, Chong E, Hannum C, et al. A non-inferiority study of outpatient mifepristone-misoprostol medical abortion at 64–70 days and 71–77 days of gestation. Contraception. 2020;101(5):302-308; Creinin MD, Schreiber CA, Bednarek P, et al. Mifepristone and misoprostol administered simultaneously versus 24 hours apart for abortion: a randomized controlled trial. Obstet Gynecol 2007;109(4):885-894. DOI:10.1097/01.AOG.0000258298.35143.d2; Morris JL, Winikoff B, Dabash R, et al. FIGO's updated recommendations for misoprostol used alone in gynecology and obstetrics. Int J Gynecol & Obstet 2017;138(3):363-366. DOI:10.1002/IJGO.12181

Providing Information to Patients

An individual undergoing medication abortion needs detailed information about the medications, when and how to take them, what to expect during the process, possible side effects and problems, and what to do if questions or concerns arise (**Table 26-7**).

Table 26-7 Patient Education for Early Medication Abortion

When creating patient education materials, prioritize health literacy, language, and cultural considerations.

1. Confirm that the decision to have an abortion is voluntary and the patient feels comfortable with their decision.
2. Discuss the treatment alternatives (medication abortion or aspiration abortion) and explain the benefits and risks of each method.
3. Describe the medication regimen the patient will use.
4. Explain what to expect regarding bleeding and cramping. These symptoms typically intensify during expulsion of the pregnancy (usually 2–4 hours) and then gradually subside. Passage of clots is common during expulsion. Lighter bleeding or spotting typically can last for up to 2 weeks but may last longer.
5. Explain that the patient is unlikely to see products of conception unless the pregnancy is close to 9 weeks' gestation or more, in which case the embryo will be very small and often obscured by blood clots.
6. Discuss known side effects of the medication abortion regimen, including mild gastrointestinal symptoms, short-term fever, warmth, or chills.
7. Explain that misoprostol may increase the risk of birth defects if the pregnancy were to continue. **Emphasize that aspiration abortion is advised if medication abortion fails.**
8. Discuss possible morbidity, including failed abortion (continuing pregnancy), incomplete abortion, hemorrhage, or infection.
9. Provide instructions about how to administer the misoprostol. Depending on the regimen used, routes of administration can include buccal (tucked between cheek and gum), sublingual (under the tongue), or vaginal (inserted deep into the vagina after washing hands). It may be helpful to reference a drawing of buccal placement, which can be found in patient medication guides offered by manufacturers Danco or GenBioPro. Advise the patient to swallow tablets used buccally or sublingually after 30 minutes.
10. Explain how to use pain medications.
11. Explain the time commitment and follow-up plan.
12. Provide 24-hour emergency contact information and emphasize warning signs that may require evaluation, including the following:
    a. Prolonged or heavy bleeding (≥ 2 soaked maxi-pads for 2 consecutive hours)
    b. Fever (≥ 100.4° F) lasting more than 4 hours or beginning in the days after misoprostol administration
    c. Abdominal pain or discomfort or "feeling sick" (including weakness, nausea, vomiting or diarrhea, with or without fever) more than 24 hours after using misoprostol
13. Offer person-centered contraception counseling and, if desired, information about and arrangements for initiating the chosen method (if any). (See Chapter 4, Person-Centered Reproductive Health Conversations and Contraceptive Counseling.)
14. Address any concerns about confidentiality.
15. Review all required consent forms, which must be executed before administration of the medication regimen.

Pain Control During Medication Abortion. No matter which drug combination or regimen they use, individuals undergoing medication abortion will experience cramping. In most cases, pain can be managed with NSAIDs, such as ibuprofen. NSAIDs do not interfere with the effectiveness of misoprostol.[118] Patients taking mifepristone and misoprostol have similar duration and intensity of pain whether NSAIDs are taken at regular intervals or as needed, and they tend to ingest more pills with the former approach.[119] Opioids at dosing regimens studied in clinical trials do not appear to decrease pain scores compared with NSAIDs alone.[120,121]

Bleeding During Medication Abortion. Bleeding is expected with medication abortion, and failure to bleed may indicate unsuccessful abortion. Although bleeding may seem abundant to those experiencing it, the amount of bleeding is rarely clinically significant. One study that used mifepristone with oral or vaginal misoprostol through 63 days' gestation found median blood losses ranging from 83 mL to 89 mL,[122] compared with the 50 mL typically lost during menses or the nearly 500 mL typically given in a blood donation. Although the range of bleeding varies widely among individuals, meaningful changes in hemoglobin seldom occur.[122] Bleeding is usually heaviest during expulsion of the pregnancy; lighter flow or spotting lasts about 2 weeks on average, but may last longer.[123] Use of combined oral contraceptives does not alter bleeding patterns after medication abortion.[123,124]

Providing parameters for excessive bleeding enhances safety. Advise the patient to call if they soak two or more large pads per hour for 2 consecutive hours. If they feel otherwise well, monitoring periodically by telephone for another 2 hours is acceptable. Those whose bleeding does not slow after this interval warrant prompt in-person evaluation. Some providers treat excessive bleeding with another dose of misoprostol or an ergot alkaloid such as methylergonovine maleate before resorting to aspiration. Bleeding heavy enough to require aspiration occurs in less than 1% of patients, and less than 1 in 1,000 patients will need a blood transfusion for excessive bleeding.[63,125,126]

Side Effects of Medications. Side effects common with all medication abortion regimens include nausea, headache, vomiting, diarrhea, dizziness, fever, and chills. These side effects typically subside within a few hours and seldom require treatment. Temperature elevation (100.4° F or more) that lasts more than 4 hours or that begins in the days after misoprostol administration, however, warrants clinical assessment.

Follow-up After Medication Abortion

During a follow-up encounter, the patient and clinician assess whether the pregnancy has ended. They may also discuss contraception, in accordance with the patient's desires. The evaluation may occur remotely or in-person, according to the patient's preferences or as medically indicated.[127,128]

History should include whether cramping, bleeding, and passage of tissue occurred, including amount and duration. Ask if the patient still feels pregnant or if they think the pregnancy has passed. Patients and clinicians are very often accurate in assessing whether the medication abortion was successful.[129,130]

Remote Assessment. Most patients do not need in-person follow-up for medication abortion. They can be followed at home with either a self-assessment of symptoms, a phone call, and/or a urine pregnancy test.

High-sensitivity home pregnancy tests are widely available. Although a negative test is reassuring, about 20% of patients will have a positive test 4 weeks after treatment.[60] To reduce the risk of false-positive tests, clinicians may consider having patients check a high-sensitivity test 5 weeks after treatment. (See Chapter 25, Pregnancy Testing.)

Clinical/In-Person Assessment

Ultrasound follow-up. Although most medication abortion researchers in the United States relied on ultrasonography to assess gestational duration and clinical outcomes, many providers offer safe medication abortion services without routine use of ultrasound.[129,131,132] If a patient has a gestational sac on initial ultrasound examination and no sac on follow-up, then the abortion is complete. Aspiration for a thickened endometrial stripe or "debris" in the uterus is not indicated unless the patient is bleeding heavily or has symptoms or signs of infection.[133]

Serum hCG follow-up. Patients may opt to have a baseline serum quantitative hCG level drawn at the initial visit (on Day 1, the day of mifepristone administration). They can either return for a second serum hCG or have the test done at a more convenient laboratory or facility. At gestational duration ≤ 63 days, hCG levels drop predictably by day 5 after mifepristone administration (with average decline of 70% by day 3 and 91% by day 5).[134]

For patients with a documented intrauterine pregnancy, clinicians can repeat the hCG 3–14 days after mifepristone (at least 24 hours after using misoprostol). For gestations of 63 days or less, the hCG level must drop by at least 50% to confirm complete abortion. Because serum hCG levels begin to decline naturally after 9–10 weeks' gestation, clinicians should use a decrease of at least 80% at 64–77 days' gestation.[135]

Serum hCG follow-up is particularly useful when an ultrasound does not demonstrate a gestational sac or yolk sac in a patient who is not eligible for a no- or limited-testing protocol (for example, a person who has a history of ectopic pregnancy or tubal surgery, or with an uncertain LMP). In these circumstances, the clinician should ensure that the patient has no symptoms or signs suspicious for ectopic pregnancy, provide ectopic precautions, and schedule the follow-up hCG 2–3 days after misoprostol. Prompt evaluation is warranted if the baseline hCG is 2,000 mIU/mL or more or if the follow-up hCG fails to decline by at least 50%. These findings are concerning for an ectopic or other abnormal pregnancy. Aspiration may assist in the diagnosis; failure to identify gestational sac material or villi on postprocedure tissue examination supports the diagnosis of ectopic pregnancy.

Incomplete Medication Abortion (Persistent Gestational Sac). If the pregnancy has stopped growing but has not completely passed out of the uterus, the patient may choose to have another course of misoprostol, an aspiration procedure, or simply wait for expulsion to occur.

Continuing Pregnancy. If a growing pregnancy persists for 2 to 3 weeks after treatment, aspiration abortion is strongly recommended because of the potential risk of birth defects following exposure to misoprostol. If the gestational duration is still less than 77 days when the patient returns, however, then clinicians may offer another course of mifepristone and misoprostol with close follow-up.

Self-Managed Medication Abortion

Throughout the world, many people use mifepristone-misoprostol or misoprostol alone to terminate their pregnancies outside of the formal health care system. Some reasons for doing so include individual preference, privacy or financial concerns, restricted access to care, or mistrust of health care institutions.[136-141] When people have access to appropriate medications and accurate information, self-managed abortion is a safe and important option.[142]

The COVID-19 pandemic laid bare racial and socioeconomic inequalities in the United States, as stay-at-home orders created disproportionate hardships among low-income communities and communities of color. The pandemic catalyzed the adoption of straightforward, de-medicalized access to medication abortion, which many stakeholders favor given its potential to improve equity and reduce stigma.[59,137,138]

Although the prevalence of self-managed abortion is not known, surveys of people seeking care in abortion clinics likely underestimate this value.[139] Studies of self-managed medication abortion from Ireland, Peru, and other countries have shown high efficacy and low rates of adverse events.[143,144] Self-managed abortion will become more common in the United States as access to abortion decreases. Some online resources that offer information about self-managed medication abortion include Aid Access (https://aidaccess.org), Self-managed Abortion Safe & Supported (https://abortionpillinfo.org), and Plan C (https://plancpills.org).

Individuals occasionally may present for follow-up or management of problems. Although some states have laws that criminalize self-managed abortion, no states legally mandate health care providers to report suspected or confirmed cases.[140] The clinical presentation of people who have self-managed their medication abortion is similar to those who have had medically supervised medication abortions or who are having a spontaneous abortion. Clinicians can provide appropriate care without knowing if the abortion is medication-induced or spontaneous.[140] For many individuals, confirming successful expulsion may suffice. Others may need evaluation for heavy bleeding, incomplete abortion, or infection. Providers can follow guidelines for management and referral discussed in this chapter.

Uterine Aspiration Abortion

Introduced in the United States in 1967, uterine aspiration is used for virtually all procedural abortions through 13 weeks in the United States,[19] and some providers use it up to 16 weeks. Aspiration is a safe and simple way to empty the uterus completely and quickly using modest cervical dilation and a hand-held syringe (manual vacuum aspiration [MVA]) or an electric vacuum pump. Most states limit abortion provision to physicians; however, in a few states without such restrictions, advanced practice clinicians have provided aspiration abortions for years with an impressive safety record.[145]

Vacuum aspiration using local cervical anesthesia with or without oral NSAIDs and/or anxiolytics or, alternatively, intravenous moderate sedation can be provided safely and appropriately in a medical office setting. The office should be equipped with the same emergency back-up equipment and supplies needed to provide injectable medications (drugs and resuscitation equipment to manage an allergic reaction, seizure, respiratory depression, or cardiac arrest). In addition, clinicians should have available the medications needed to treat uterine bleeding and a plan in place for transferring a patient to a surgical facility in the rare event that uterine perforation or severe hemorrhage occurs. The availability of portable and inexpensive manual vacuum aspirators has facilitated abortion provision in primary care settings that do not have electric pumps, as well as resource-poor settings worldwide. Research indicates that MVA is as effective and safe as electric vacuum aspiration (EVA);[146,147] although pain is comparable,[148,149] patients prefer the quietness of the MVA device.[149] The ability of providers to identify products of conception in the tissue aspirate after very early abortion (less than 6 weeks) does not differ significantly with use of MVA or EVA.[150]

Pain Management

Pain management options for aspiration abortion include cervical anesthesia used alone or in combination with oral or IV medications for analgesia or sedation. Practice patterns vary, and researchers have studied different approaches.

Local cervical anesthesia reduces pain associated with aspiration abortion regardless of gestational duration. A common technique uses 1% lidocaine 20 mL injected paracervically or intracervically at two or four injection sites. Adding sodium bicarbonate (8.4% solution 1 mL for each 10 mL of anesthetic solution) decreases the pain of injection, and injecting to a depth of about 3 cm is more effective than superficial injections.[151] Two- and four-site blocks have similar effects, and a 3-minute wait time prior to dilation does not affect pain scores in a clinically significant way.[152]

NSAIDs such as ibuprofen 600–800 mg administered orally 30–90 minutes prior to the abortion procedure help to reduce pain.[153,154] Studies have not shown a benefit to intramuscular or intracervical administration of NSAIDs over the oral route.[154,155] No evidence supports using oral opioids prior to abortion.[156,157] Oral anxiolytics can help reduce anxiety, but they do not affect pain associated with aspiration abortion.[158-160] Nonpharmacologic techniques such as verbal support and music may facilitate coping, but they do not necessarily reduce pain.[152] It is often helpful to ask the patient what, if anything, has worked for them in the past to help them cope with situations that are stressful, painful, or anxiety-provoking.

Research confirms the efficacy of moderate sedation for pain control during procedural abortions. Appropriately trained advanced practice clinicians administer moderate sedation in many facilities that provide abortions. A common regimen is midazolam 1–3 mg combined with fentanyl 50–100 mcg administered by slow IV push, with the amount titrated to achieve the desired level of sedation and anesthesia. Recommended monitoring during moderate sedation includes periodic vital signs and measurement of oxygen saturation using pulse oximetry.[161]

Steps of the Procedure

As the first step in an aspiration procedure, perform a bimanual examination to determine the size and position of the uterus. Place a short-bladed speculum, such as a Moore Graves design, which allows the cervix to remain close to the perineum for adequate visualization. Swabbing the cervix with an antiseptic solution is common practice but does not reduce the incidence of postprocedure infection.[162] To facilitate asepsis, many clinicians use a *no-touch technique*, i.e., not touching the parts of instruments, including the tips of dilators or cannulas, that will enter the sterile uterine cavity.[163] (See **Figure 26-4**.)

Next, administer cervical anesthesia. Inject 2–3 mL of the anesthetic into the lip of the cervix before placing a tenaculum to keep the cervix stabilized, and then administer the remaining solution at two (4 and 8 o'clock) to four sites (2, 4, 8, and 10 o'clock) either directly into the cervical stroma near the cervical os or paracervically. Using a 1.5-inch needle accomplishes deep injections, which are more effective than superficial injections.[151] Be sure to aspirate before injecting the anesthetic solution to avoid an intravenous bolus of the medication, which can cause toxicity. Occasionally, a patient will experience mild toxicity, such as numbing of the lips or tinnitus, but these symptoms dissipate quickly without intervention.

Using tapered, graduated metal or plastic dilators, stretch the cervix gently and incrementally as needed to accommodate an aspiration cannula of appropriate size for the gestation. Typically, the diameter of the cannula in millimeters corresponds to the duration of the pregnancy in weeks. For example, a clinician may select a 7-mm cannula to evacuate a pregnancy at 7 weeks. On occasion, smaller cannulas may be necessary due to cervical scarring, or may simply be equally effective. Insert a cannula connected to either a manual vacuum syringe or an electric vacuum pump through the dilated cervix and remove the products of conception by a combination of rotary and back-and-forth motions. Detection of a "gritty" sensation as the cannula moves across the endometrial surface typically indicates that the uterus is empty.

Examining the removed tissue helps to confirm complete evacuation. If the products of conception are not readily apparent, suspending the tissue in water, saline, or white vinegar and checking with backlighting may facilitate the evaluation.[163] If pregnancy tissue still is not identified, a postprocedure ultrasound may confirm retained products or assist in the diagnosis of uncommon events such as

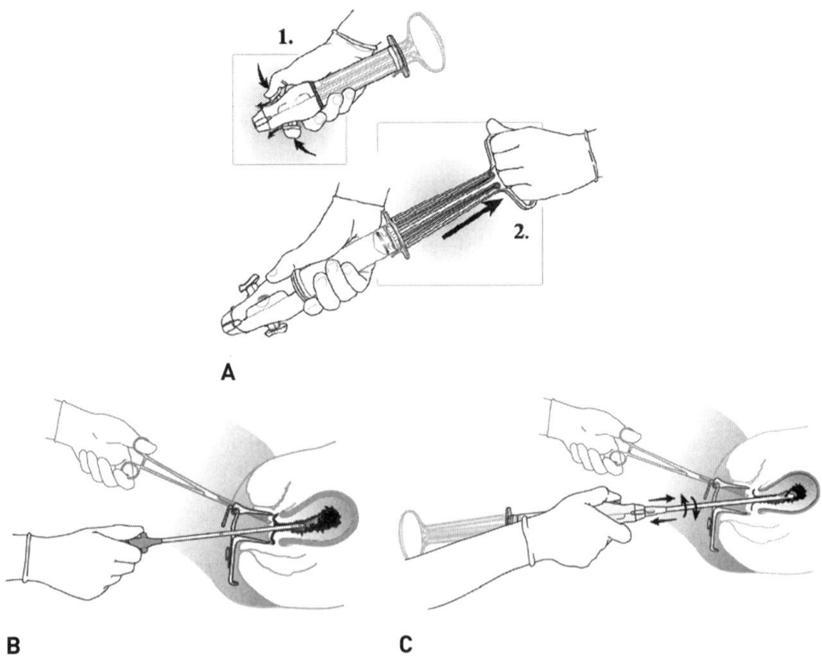

Figure 26-4 A-C: Performing an early abortion using a manual vacuum aspirator.

a missed ectopic pregnancy. If ectopic pregnancy is suspected in an asymptomatic patient, the clinician should provide ectopic precautions, obtain a serum quantitative hCG test, and repeat the test in 24–72 hours. The patient requires further evaluation if the hCG level does not decrease by 50% or more.

Dilation and Evacuation

After 13–15 weeks, the most common method for abortion in the United States is dilation and evacuation (D&E), a procedure that typically combines aspiration with the use of extracting forceps.[19] Complications are infrequent, especially with adequate cervical preparation and trained providers.

For patients undergoing D&E, cervical anesthesia reduces pain associated with osmotic dilator placement[164] as well as pain associated with the abortion procedure. Adding vasopressin to the anesthetic solution helps to reduce blood loss.[165] Moderate IV sedation is the most common pain control modality used for D&E in the United States and is safe and effective.[166] A few studies have examined the safety of deep IV sedation without tracheal intubation for patients undergoing first- and second-trimester procedural abortion, and found that anesthesia-related complications, such as intubation and hypoxemia, are extremely rare.[166-168]

Ultrasound dating is standard of care before D&E in the United States, and ultrasound guidance may be helpful during challenging procedures or in a teaching setting. The cervix requires more dilation for D&E to permit evacuation of the pregnancy. Thus, preoperative cervical preparation using osmotic dilators, mifepristone, misoprostol, or a combination is recommended (see Cervical Preparation, following below).

Medication Abortion Later in Pregnancy

Later medication abortion involves administration of medications that cause the uterus to contract and eventually expel the fetus and placenta. Although this method is used commonly in many European countries, it accounts for only a small proportion of abortions after 14 weeks in the United States.[19]

Most patients undergoing later medication abortion require analgesia. Options include oral medications (NSAIDs or opiates)[169] or patient-controlled IV or epidural analgesia,[170] all of which are effective and acceptable to patients. Paracervical anesthesia has no effect on pain intensity, amount of morphine used, or duration of induction.[171]

Clinicians may use mifepristone and misoprostol, or misoprostol alone, for later medication abortion. Based on current evidence, the most effective approach is mifepristone followed in 24–48 hours by repeated doses of misoprostol.[172] A commonly used regimen at $\geq$ 12 weeks is mifepristone 200 mg orally, followed in 24–48 hours by repeat doses of misoprostol 400 mcg vaginally every 4 hours.[59] Side effects are specific to the medications used.

The skills, support, and complications management for later medication abortion are identical to labor support and may be within the scope of practice for an advanced practice clinician with experience in labor and delivery care.

Cervical Preparation

Clinicians can use pharmacologic cervical preparation agents or osmotic dilators to facilitate abortion procedures. Placing osmotic dilators decreases the risk of cervical laceration or perforation, although the minimal risk of uterine injury in early abortion may not justify routine use. The Society of Family Planning recommends cervical preparation before D&E abortion and advises earlier consideration for some individuals (e.g., adolescents, those with pregnancies at 12–14 weeks, or those in whom the clinician anticipates difficulty dilating the cervix).[173-175]

Misoprostol

Treatment with misoprostol prior to D&E causes cervical softening, effacement, and dilation that can reduce the need for additional mechanical dilation or make it easier. Numerous studies suggest that an optimal regimen for first-trimester cervical preparation is 400 mcg administered vaginally 3 hours prior to the procedure.[175,176] Buccal misoprostol has pharmacokinetics similar to vaginal misoprostol[88] and represents an effective alternative route of administration.[175,177]

Experienced providers may use misoprostol safely in lieu of osmotic dilators before early D&E abortions or as an adjunct to osmotic dilators for later procedures.[174] Optimal regimens for these uses are not well defined.[173] Misoprostol may also induce contractions and can cause unscheduled expulsion of the pregnancy when used over an extended time period, as with overnight cervical preparation. Side effects include nausea, vomiting, diarrhea, cramping, and fever or shivering. Although uterine rupture has been reported following misoprostol use during later medication abortion, primarily in people who had a scar from prior uterine surgery, these cases are rare and do not contraindicate its use, as demonstrated by several large case series.[173]

Mifepristone

Mifepristone also is an excellent cervical ripening agent, and longer preparation times (24–48 hours) result in better effects. As such, it is well suited to multi-day rather than same-day procedures and is often used off-label for this purpose.

Cervical preparation with mifepristone as a single ripening agent given 24 hours prior to D&E at 14–16 weeks' gestation did not increase procedure time when compared with osmotic dilators.[178] In another study, researchers randomized patients undergoing D&E from 16 weeks' through 23 weeks' gestation to cervical preparation with osmotic dilators alone, or in conjunction with mifepristone or misoprostol.[179] They found no difference in procedure time among the groups. Providers found the procedure subjectively easier with mifepristone plus osmotic dilators compared with osmotic dilators alone, and mifepristone was better tolerated than misoprostol.[179] Mifepristone also may allow for fewer visits for cervical preparation and fewer osmotic dilators when used for D&E procedures between 19 weeks and 23 weeks and 6 days.[180]

Osmotic Dilators

Two types of osmotic dilators currently are available in the United States: laminaria dilators consist of sterile stalks of dried seaweed (*Laminaria japonica* or *L. digitata*), and Dilapan-S® is a synthetic polyacrylonitrile (plastic) rod. The clinician places osmotic dilators so they extend through the endocervical canal and dilate both the internal and external os. The devices absorb fluid and expand. The major effect of laminaria is mechanical (exerting radial pressure on the cervix), while the predominant effect of Dilapan-S is likely chemical (inducing prostaglandin release). Thus, using a combination of these two types of osmotic dilators is reasonable. Laminaria reach maximum dilation in 12–24 hours, so they are most commonly inserted the day before the D&E procedure. In contrast, Dilapan-S devices dilate quickly, achieving most of their effect within 4–6 hours, so their use often allows clinicians to complete D&E abortions in a shorter time frame. Many clinicians use a combination of osmotic dilators, and serial insertions may be necessary for procedures later in pregnancy.[174]

Managing Postabortion Adverse Events and Morbidity

Take seriously any complaint or problem after an abortion procedure and listen carefully to the patient's concerns. Advise all abortion patients to watch for warning signs (Table 26-7) and tell them how to contact you in case they have questions or problems. Prompt recognition and management can be critical in preventing the rare serious outcome. Adverse events can be emotionally difficult as well as physically complicated for the patient. Provide time for the patient to process the situation and react emotionally. Invite questions by asking, "What questions do you have about ____?" Acknowledge their experience and offer counseling or referral for counseling as appropriate. Adverse events and morbidity following abortion, while not common,[181,182] include the following immediate and short-term problems.

Excessive Bleeding

Excessive bleeding during or after abortion is rare. After a medication abortion, less than 1 in 100 patients require aspiration to stop bleeding, and less than 1 in 1,000 require transfusion.[125] Bleeding that requires treatment is often not due to immediate hemorrhage but rather persistent or delayed bleeding that occurs 3–5 weeks following mifepristone administration.[183] Therefore, medication abortion patients and providers need to remain vigilant for bleeding even if findings appear normal on initial follow-up. Clinicians can treat heavy bleeding with uterotonics, such as methylergonovine or misoprostol, or aspiration to remove retained tissue.

For aspiration or D&E abortion, the most common causes of hemorrhage are uterine atony and retained placental or fetal tissue. Atony, which typically occurs immediately after the procedure, almost always responds to uterotonic agents and uterine massage. Individuals with retained tissue may present with heavy bleeding several days to a few weeks following the abortion (see following section on Incomplete Abortion). Infrequent causes of hemorrhage include uterine injury, abnormal placental attachment, or bleeding disorders.

A systematic approach to hemorrhage management includes the following steps:

1. Evaluate the cause of bleeding. Perform a bimanual exam to evaluate uterine tone and perform uterine massage if the uterus feels boggy.
2. Perform a speculum exam to identify cervical lacerations. Superficial cervical lacerations can be treated with application of ferric subsulfate solution, but more extensive lacerations may require suturing.
3. Use ultrasound, if available, to identify retained intrauterine tissue and aspirate as indicated.
4. Administer one or more uterotonic agents such as methylergonovine maleate 0.2 mg intramuscular (IM), dilute vasopressin 4–6 units intracervical, misoprostol

600–800 mcg sublingual (rectal administration has slower onset of action), and/or oxytocin 10–40 units in IV solution or 10 units IM.
5. If bleeding persists, administer IV fluids and initiate transfer. If persistent uterine atony or cervical/uterine injury, consider placing a 30 mL intrauterine Foley catheter and inflate with 30–60 mL sterile saline while awaiting arrival of emergency medical services.

Some clinicians use tranexamic acid, an antifibrinolytic, for management of hemorrhage during procedural abortion. Although not specifically studied in the abortion setting, tranexamic acid is approved by the FDA for treatment of heavy menstrual bleeding and used off label for treatment of postpartum hemorrhage, where large studies have shown a reduction in maternal mortality when the drug is administered within 3 hours of birth.[184] Currently, ACOG does not support prophylactic use of the drug outside of research settings.[184]

Incomplete Abortion

When pregnancy tissue remains in the uterus, the abortion procedure is *incomplete*. Medication abortion regimens take a longer time to empty the uterus than aspiration, and an ultrasound examination may show residual tissue after the pregnancy sac has passed. This normal finding does not require intervention unless the patient is bleeding excessively or has symptoms or signs of an infection.[133]

Incomplete abortion occurs in less than 3% of aspiration procedures.[181,182] Retained pregnancy tissue is likely to cause continued bleeding and cramping that prompt an individual to seek care. Treatment with misoprostol, oral methylergonovine maleate, or uterine aspiration is appropriate.

Continuing Pregnancy

In less than 1% of cases, an attempt to terminate pregnancy fails altogether.[63,185] A patient with a continuing pregnancy may have ongoing symptoms of pregnancy and a soft or enlarged uterus. Ultrasound or hCG testing may help to identify this problem. Providing or referring the patient for an effective means to terminate the pregnancy is appropriate treatment. Continued pregnancy after an abortion can be particularly emotionally triggering for some people. Provide an opportunity for them to respond emotionally and to ask questions. Acknowledge their experience and offer counseling or referral for counseling as appropriate.

Ongoing pregnancy due to failed medication abortion potentially involves an increased risk for fetal malformation due to misoprostol exposure; available evidence indicates that mifepristone does not appear to be teratogenic.[83,186-189] Rarely, individuals change their minds about proceeding with medication abortion after they have already ingested mifepristone. No available evidence indicates that progesterone therapy is effective to “reverse” mifepristone’s effects.[84] Taking mifepristone without misoprostol within the usual timeframe for medication abortion may put the pregnant person at risk for hemorrhage.[85]

Meticulous tissue examination after an aspiration abortion minimizes the risk of a continuing pregnancy. Failure to visualize products of conception (gestational sac plus placental tissue/chorionic villi) in the aspirate warrants further investigation for a continuing intrauterine or ectopic pregnancy. Failed aspiration abortion occurs more often in people with uterine abnormalities, such as a bicornuate uterus or a cavity distorted by fibroids. Treatment options include medication abortion (if the patient is still within an eligible gestational duration) or re-aspiration using ultrasound guidance as needed.

Intrauterine Blood Clots (Hematometra)

Intrauterine blood clots can occur immediately or as long as a few days after an aspiration abortion; their presence may cause severe cramping and pain. This problem occurs after approximately 0.14% of first-trimester uterine aspiration abortion procedures.[185] Typical findings on pelvic examination include a large, tense, and tender uterus with little or no bleeding from the cervix. Uterine aspiration remedies the problem; pain and cramping resolve within a few minutes.

Perforation/Laceration

Uterine rupture has been reported with use of misoprostol for induction of labor at term and rarely in conjunction with mifepristone or other uterotonic agents in later medication abortion. Most cases occur in individuals with a previous uterine scar.[190]

External cervical tears can occur if the tenaculum detaches from the cervix. Management options include applying pressure and observing, applying ferric subsulfate solution, or rarely, placing suture. A small midline uterine perforation in the first trimester can be managed safely with careful observation for 2–4 hours, and hospitalization is not necessary unless evidence arises of internal bleeding, abdominal pain, or rebound tenderness. More severe cervical or uterine injury, including perforation with damage to nearby abdominal organs or vessels, is rare.[185] Depending on their severity, these adverse events may require exploratory surgery to identify and repair the uterus or abdominal organ injury, or even hysterectomy. To decrease the risk of such injuries, providers typically prepare the cervix with osmotic dilators or pharmacologic agents before D&E.[173,174,191]

Infection

Most US studies report an infection rate of < 2% following early aspiration abortion[182]; rates are 0.8% to 1.6% following D&E.[73] Infection rates are low following medication-induced abortion.[72]

In the decade following FDA approval of mifepristone, rare cases of clostridial infection occurred in patients who had medication abortions, and the clinical presentation differed from typical endometritis.[192-195] Health authorities never established a causal relationship, and the last reported case of clostridial infection associated with induced abortion occurred in 2009.[192] Nonetheless, clinicians should remain aware of signs and symptoms that may signal atypical infection in the days following misoprostol use for medication abortion:

- Nausea, vomiting, diarrhea, weakness with or without abdominal pain
- Tachycardia or hypotension
- Lack of fever with little tenderness on pelvic examination
- High hemoglobin or hematocrit value
- Marked leukocytosis (unusually high white blood cell count)

Any patient presenting with these findings after medication abortion requires immediate evaluation and referral.

Measures to minimize the risk of infection after aspiration abortion or D&E include:

- Screening for preexisting reproductive tract infections, with treatment before or at the time of the abortion
- Administering prophylactic antibiotics at the time of the procedure
- Using a no-touch technique
- Emptying the uterus completely

Common symptoms of postprocedure endometritis include some combination of persistent cramping, abdominal pain, fever, discharge, and malaise. Treatment of uncomplicated pelvic infection includes broad-spectrum antibiotics and aspiration of retained tissue, if present. The availability of parenteral cephalosporins and oral doxycycline and metronidazole permit the option of outpatient treatment in appropriately selected patients. Hospitalization for intravenous antibiotic therapy is warranted in patients with severe illness or suspected pelvic abscess and in those who are immunocompromised, are unable to tolerate oral medications, or who fail to respond to outpatient therapy.

Long-Term Health Outcomes

Individuals who seek abortion services may ask about possible long-term health effects. Public debate about long-term effects has been used inappropriately as a rationale for limiting people's access to abortion services. Reassuring expert reviews of this topic have been published.[196] The study of long-term health outcomes is methodologically challenging; as new research findings are published, pay attention to the quality of study design and the criteria for determining causality. Conclusions in three key areas are briefly summarized below.

Future Reproductive Health and Fertility

Research to date has found no association between mifepristone-misoprostol abortion and the risk of subsequent ectopic pregnancy, preterm birth, or low birthweight infants.[197,198] Some registry-based observational studies and systematic reviews have suggested a slight increase in the risk of preterm birth after aspiration abortion.[199-203] Increased risks for spontaneous abortion or preterm delivery and low birthweight infants have been reported after D&E abortion, but adequate preparation of the cervix before the procedure may mitigate these risks.[204-206]

Psychological Health

The contention that induced abortion causes lasting psychological harm is misleading and unsubstantiated. No causal association is evident between induced abortion and mental health problems.[207,208] If abortion caused incapacitating emotional responses frequently, this association would be evident because abortion is such a common procedure. Temporary feelings of loss or sadness may follow what is sometimes a difficult decision to terminate a pregnancy, but these normal reactions do not constitute mental health problems. Psychiatric problems following abortion are rare,[209] and they are more likely to occur among people with preexisting mental health conditions.[210] Individuals who are denied an abortion experience higher levels of stress and anxiety in the months after seeking this care.[211] Relief is a predominant emotion after abortion, and long-term follow-up studies confirm that most people remain satisfied with their decision to have had an abortion.[212]

Breast Cancer

The question of whether induced abortion has any effect on the risk of subsequent breast cancer has received intense scrutiny. Epidemiologic research on this topic is complex, as study design methods can lead to spurious association. For example, recall bias may explain some of the positive associations found in case-control studies that compare abortion histories of healthy individuals with those of people who have breast cancer, because healthy individuals are less likely than people with cancer to report sensitive events such as prior abortion. Prospective studies have found no association between induced abortion and breast cancer.[213-215] Numerous authoritative organizations, including the National Cancer Institute and the American College of Obstetricians and Gynecologists (ACOG), have concluded that no evidence supports a true association between induced abortion and subsequent breast cancer risk.[216,217]

Postabortion Contraception

Fertility returns quickly following abortion. Ovulation, and with it the possibility of another pregnancy, may occur as soon as 8 days after abortion.[218] Should an individual desire contraception on the same day as the abortion, clinicians can help address any personal, situational, or method-related factors that may contribute to satisfaction and success with their chosen method. (See Chapter 4, Person-Centered Reproductive Health Conversations and Contraceptive Counseling.) Lack of insurance coverage and availability, for example, may prevent a person from choosing or obtaining the method they desire.[219-224]

However, individuals may not be interested in contraceptive counseling at the time of a visit for an abortion.[27,28] Discussing different ways to avoid pregnancy may not be appropriate for a person who has already selected a method, plans to obtain contraception from someone other than the abortion provider, or does not want it at the time of an abortion. Clinicians must be cognizant of the legacy of coercive family planning policies, institutionalized racism, and any biased motivations we may hold[27,29] if discussing contraception. We must extend the same regard for bodily autonomy as it relates to contraceptive provision, as we do for abortion care.

Individuals can initiate most methods on the day of procedural abortion or at the time of mifepristone ingestion, with some exceptions (**Table 26-8**). If patients would like counseling about emergency contraception, the clinician may also discuss its availability and mechanism of action and, if possible, provide or prescribe a supply to have on hand.

Intrauterine Devices

Providers may place intrauterine devices safely at the time pregnancy expulsion is confirmed following medication abortion.[225] Studies have demonstrated expulsion rates of 4% to 12% for copper IUDs and the levonorgestrel devices when placed 1–4 weeks after early medication abortion.[226-230] These rates are higher compared with IUD placement remote from pregnancy. However, expulsion rates are similar when placement occurs within a week after medication abortion, compared to 3–6 weeks afterward.[230]

Table 26-8 Initiating Contraception After Abortion

Method	Initiation*	Special Considerations
Progestin-only methods		
Etonogestrel implant	On the day of procedural abortion or mifepristone ingestion	Does not affect success of medication abortion if placed on day of mifepristone; may initiate at follow-up visit with backup method for 7 days
DMPA		Rate of continuing pregnancy may be higher when initiated on the day of mifepristone; may initiate at follow-up visit with backup method for 7 days
Norethindrone-only pill		Use a backup method for 48 hours if initiated more than 7 days from abortion
Drospirenone-only pill		Use a backup method for 1 week if initiated more than 7 days from abortion
Intrauterine device		
	On the day of procedural abortion, or at follow-up visit after medication abortion	Not recommended in setting of septic abortion, or if uterine perforation or hemorrhage occurs during procedural abortion
Combined hormonal methods		
Pills, patch	On the day of procedural abortion or mifepristone ingestion	Use a backup method for 1 week if initiated more than 7 days from abortion
Etonogestrel ring	Within 1 week of medication or procedural abortion†	
Barrier methods		
Condoms Single-size diaphragm	With sexual intercourse	
Sized diaphragm		Ensure that pregnancy-related changes to the cervix have resolved‡

Method	Initiation*	Special Considerations
Permanent contraception		
Tubal surgery	When medication abortion is confirmed complete	May be restricted by federal or state regulations at the time of abortion
Vasectomy		Confirm azoospermia or wait 3 months prior to discontinuing other contraceptive methods

DMPA, depot medroxyprogesterone acetate

*Unless otherwise specified, individuals can initiate a method on the day of procedural abortion, or on the day of mifepristone or ingestion.[239,240,246]

†No lower or upper genital tract infections occurred within 3 months when placed within 5 days of procedural abortion.[238]

‡No evidence exists to support avoiding vaginal intercourse or tampons as a means to decrease risk of infection. The recommendation does not appear in the 2022 National Abortion Federation guidelines or the World Health Organization's Abortion Care Guidelines.[57,59]

Data from National Abortion Federation. Clinical policy guidelines for abortion care; 2022. https://prochoice.org/providers/quality-standards/; World Health Organization. Abortion care guideline; 2022. http://www.who.int/publications/i/item/9789240039483; Fine PM, Tryggestad J, Meyers NJ, Sangi-Haghpeykar H. Safety and acceptability with the use of a contraceptive vaginal ring after surgical or medical abortion. Contraception. 2007;75(5):367-371. DOI:10.1016/j.contraception.2007.01.009; Gemzell-Danielsson K, Kallner HK. Post abortion contraception. Women's Health. 2015;11(6):779-784. DOI:10.2217/whe.15.72; Curtis KM, Tepper NK, Jatlaoui TC, et al. U.S. Medical eligibility criteria for contraceptive use, 2016. MMWR Recomm Rep 2016;65(3):1-104. DOI:10.15585/mmwr.rr6503a1; Roe AH, Bartz D. Society of Family Planning clinical recommendations: contraception after surgical abortion. Contraception. 2019;99(1):2-9. DOI:10.1016/J.Contraception.2018.08.016

When individuals receive intrauterine contraception immediately after uterine aspiration or D&E, continuation is more common at 6 months postprocedure compared with later placement, but expulsion rates may be higher.[231,232] Reported expulsion rates when devices are placed immediately following procedural abortion range from 3.1% to 6.8%, versus 0% to 5% when placement occurs at 2–6 weeks. However, the proportion of participants in the later placement groups who did not return for IUD placement ranged from 45% to 71%; hence when assessed at 6 months or later, many more of the immediate insertion group are protected by IUDs.[233-235] Intrauterine device placement is not recommended at the time of abortion if uterine perforation or postprocedure hemorrhage occur.[236]

Combined Hormonal Methods

The patient may start a combined estrogen/progestin method of contraception on the day of mifepristone ingestion, or immediately after an aspiration or D&E.[237] If initiated within 7 days, a back-up contraceptive method is not needed.[238-240]

Progestin-only Methods

Progestin-only methods such as the etonogestrel subdermal contraceptive implant and depot medroxyprogesterone acetate (DMPA) may be initiated on the same day that a patient takes mifepristone for a medication abortion.[239,241,242] Available evidence demonstrates that the implant does not affect mifepristone's efficacy.[243,244] One study found that participants who received DMPA on the same day as mifepristone had a higher frequency of ongoing pregnancies compared with those who received it after the abortion (3.6% vs. 0.9%).[245] Although patients in the same-day mifepristone and DMPA group reported greater satisfaction with their assignment, clinicians should thoroughly counsel individuals considering this approach about the risk of ongoing pregnancy and need for close monitoring and possible further treatment.

Author Disclosures—Nippita: session physician, Planned Parenthood Greater NY; Paul: session physician, Planned Parenthood League of Massachusetts.

References

1. Ross LJ, Solinger R. Reproductive justice: A new vision for the 21st century. Oakland, CA: University of California Press; 2017.
2. Chae S, Desai S, Crowell M, Sedgh G. Reasons why women have induced abortions: a synthesis of findings from 14 countries. Contraception. 2017;96(4):233-41. DOI: 10.1016/j.contraception.2017.06.014.
3. Janiak E, Kawachi I, Goldberg A, Gottlieb B. Abortion barriers and perceptions of gestational age among women seeking abortion care in the latter half of the second trimester. Contraception. 2014;89(4):322-7. DOI: 10.1016/j.contraception.2013.11.009.
4. Drey EA, Foster DG, Jackson RA, Lee SJ, Cardenas LH, Darney PD. Risk factors associated with presenting for abortion in the second trimester. Obstet Gynecol. 2006;107(1):128-35. DOI: 10.1097/01.AOG.0000189095.32382.d0.
5. Kiley JW, Yee LM, Niemi CM, Feinglass JM, Simon MA. Delays in request for pregnancy termination: comparison of patients in the first and second trimesters. Contraception. 2010;81(5):446-51. DOI: 10.1016/j.contraception.2009.12.021.
6. Ralph LJ, Foster DG, Kimport K, Turok D, Roberts SCM. Measuring decisional certainty among women seeking abortion. Contraception. 2017;95(3):269-78. DOI: 10.1016/j.contraception.2016.09.008.
7. Rocca CH, Samari G, Foster DG, Gould H, Kimport K. Emotions and decision rightness over five years following an abortion: An examination of decision difficulty and abortion stigma. Soc Sci Med. 2020;248. DOI: 10.1016/J.SOCSCIMED.2019.112704.
8. ACOG Practice Bulletin No. 135: Second-trimester abortion. Obstet Gynecol. 2013;121(6):1394-406. DOI: 10.1097/01.aog.0000431056.79334.cc.
9. Costescu D, Guilbert É. No. 360-Induced abortion: surgical abortion and second trimester medical methods. J Obstet Gynaecol Can. 2018;40(6):750-83. DOI: 10.1016/J.JOGC.2017.12.010.
10. Royal College of Obstetricians and Gynaecologists. The care of women requesting induced abortion (evidence-based Clinical Guideline No. 7). (https://www.rcog.org.uk/guidance/browse-all-guidance/other-guidelines-and-reports/the-care-of-women-requesting-induced-abortion-evidence-based-clinical-guideline-no-7/)
11. Raymond EG, Grimes DA. The comparative safety of legal induced abortion and childbirth in the United States. Obstet Gynecol. 2012;119(2, Part 1):215-9. DOI: 10.1097/AOG.0b013e31823fe923.
12. Vilda D, Wallace ME, Daniel C, Evans MG, Stoecker C, Theall KP. State abortion policies and maternal death in the United States, 2015-2018. Am J Public Health. 2021;111(9):1696-704. DOI: 10.2105/AJPH.2021.306396.
13. Blackwell S, Louis JM, Norton ME, et al. Reproductive services for women at high risk for maternal mortality: a report of the workshop of the Society for Maternal-Fetal Medicine, the American College of Obstetricians and Gynecologists, the Fellowship in Family Planning, and the Society of Family Planning. Am J Obstet Gynecol. 2020;222(4):B2-18. DOI: 10.1016/J.AJOG.2019.12.008.
14. Karletsos D, Stoecker C, Vilda D, Theall KP, Wallace ME. Association of state gestational age limit abortion laws with infant mortality. Am J Prev Med. 2021;61(6):787-94. DOI: 10.1016/J.AMEPRE.2021.05.022.
15. Burns B, Dennis A, Douglas-Durham E. Evaluating priorities: Measuring women's and children's health and well-being against abortion restrictions in the states. Cambridge, MA: Ibis

Reproductive Health; 2014. (https://www.ibisreproductivehealth.org/publications/evaluating-priorities-measuring-womens-and-childrens-health-and-well-being-against-0).

16. Jones RK, Witwer E, Jerman J. Abortion incidence and service availability in the United States, 2017. New York, NY: Guttmacher Institute; 2019. DOI: 10.1363/2019.30760.
17. Finer LB, Zolna MR. Declines in unintended pregnancy in the United States, 2008–2011. N Engl J Med. 2016;374(9):843-52. DOI: 10.1056/NEJMsa1506575.
18. Jones RK, Philbin J, Kirstein M, Nash E, Lufkin K. Long-term decline in US abortions reverses, showing rising need for abortion as supreme court is poised to overturn Roe v. Wade. New York, NY: Guttmacher Institute; 2022. (https://www.guttmacher.org/article/2022/06/long-term-decline-us-abortions-reverses-showing-rising-need-abortion-supreme-court).
19. Kortsmit K, Mandel MG, Reeves JA, et al. Abortion surveillance - United States, 2019. MMWR Surveill Summ. 2021;70(9):1-41. DOI: 10.15585/MMWR.SS7009A1
20. Jones RK, Nash E, Cross L, Philbin J, Kirstein M. Medication abortion now accounts for more than half of all US abortions. New York, NY: Guttmacher Institute; 2022. (https://www.guttmacher.org/article/2022/02/medication-abortion-now-accounts-more-half-all-us-abortions).
21. Jerman J, Jones RK, Onda T. Characteristics of U.S. abortion patients in 2014 and Changes Since 2008. New York, NY: Guttmacher Institute; 2016. (https://www.guttmacher.org/report/characteristics-us-abortion-patients-2014).
22. Guttmacher Institute. State funding of abortion under Medicaid [as of March 1, 2023]. New York, NY: Guttmacher Institute; 2023. (https://www.guttmacher.org/state-policy/explore/state-funding-abortion-under-medicaid).
23. Zuniga C, Thompson TA, Blanchard K. Abortion as a catastrophic health expenditure in the United States. Womens Health Iss. 2020;30(6):416-25. DOI: 10.1016/j.whi.2020.07.001.
24. Coast E, Lattof SR, Rodgers YVDM, Moore B, Poss C. The microeconomics of abortion: A scoping review and analysis of the economic consequences for abortion care-seekers. PLoS One. 2021;16(6 June). DOI: 10.1371/journal.pone.0252005.
25. Jones RK, Witwer E, Jerman J. Transgender abortion patients and the provision of transgender-specific care at non-hospital facilities that provide abortions. Contracept X. 2020;2. DOI: 10.1016/J.CONX.2020.100019.
26. Jones RK, Frohwirth L, Moore AM. More than poverty: disruptive events among women having abortions in the USA. J Fam Plann Reprod Health Care. 2013;39(1):36-43. DOI: 10.1136/jfprhc-2012-100311.
27. Brandi K, Woodhams E, White KO, Mehta PK. An exploration of perceived contraceptive coercion at the time of abortion. Contraception. 2018;97(4):329-34. DOI: 10.1016/j.contraception.2017.12.009.
28. Cansino C, Lichtenberg ES, Perriera LK, Hou MY, Melo J, Creinin MD. Do women want to talk about birth control at the time of a first-trimester abortion? Contraception. 2018;98(6):535-40. DOI: 10.1016/j.contraception.2018.08.005.
29. Cannon R, White K, Seifert B, Woodhams E, Brandi K, Yinusa-Nyahkoon L. Exploring the physician's role in contraceptive counseling at the time of abortion in the US. Contraception. 2021;103(5):316-321. DOI: 10.1016/j.contraception.2021.01.014.
30. Cates W, Grimes DA, Schulz KF. The public health impact of legal abortion: 30 years later. Perspect Sex Reprod Health. 2003;35(1):25-8. DOI: 10.1111/j.1931-2393.2003.tb00081.x.
31. Sonfield A, Hasstedt K, Kavanaugh ML, Anderson R. The social and economic benefits of women's ability to determine whether and when to have children. New York, NY: Guttmacher Institute; 2013. (https://www.guttmacher.org/report/social-and-economic-benefits-womens-ability-determine-whether-and-when-have-children).
32. Bernstein A, Jones KM. The economic effects of abortion access: A review of the evidence. Washington DC: Institute for Women's Policy Research; 2019. (https://iwpr.org/iwpr-issues/reproductive-health/the-economic-effects-of-abortion-access-a-review-of-the-evidence/).
33. University of California San Francisco. ANSIRH: The Turnaway Study. (https://www.ansirh.org/research/ongoing/turnaway-study).
34. American Public Health Association. Restricted access to abortion violates human rights, precludes reproductive justice, and demands public health intervention. Published online 2015. https://www.apha.org/policies-and-advocacy/public-health-policy-statements/policy-database/2016/01/04/11/24/restricted-access-to-abortion-violates-human-rights.

35. Jones B, Dalven J. Abortion law and policy in the USA. In: Paul Maureen, Lichtenberg ES, Borgatta L, Grimes DA, Stubblefield PG, Creinin MD, eds. Management of unintended and abnormal pregnancy: Comprehensive abortion care. Blackwell-Wiley; 2009:36-47.
36. Library of Congress. U.S. Reports: *Roe v. Wade*, 410 U.S. 113 (1973). (https://www.loc.gov/item/usrep410113/).
37. Fried MG. The economics of abortion access in the US: restrictions on government funding for abortion is the post-Roe battleground. Conscience. 26(4):11-5.
38. Henshaw SK, Joyce TJ, Dennis A, Finer LB, Blanchard K. Restrictions on Medicaid funding for abortions: A literature review. New York, NY: Guttmacher Institute; 2009. (https://www.guttmacher.org/report/restrictions-medicaid-funding-abortions-literature-review).
39. Grossman D. The use of public health evidence in *Whole Woman's Health v Hellerstedt*. JAMA Intern Med. 2017;177(2):155-6. DOI: 10.1001/jamainternmed.2016.6839.
40. Nash E, Naide S. State policy trends at midyear 2021: Already the worst legislative year ever for U.S. abortion rights. New York, NY: Guttmacher Institute; 2021. (https://www.guttmacher.org/article/2021/07/state-policy-trends-midyear-2021-already-worst-legislative-year-ever-us-abortion#).
41. Nash E. For the first time ever, US states enacted more than 100 abortion restrictions in a single year. New York, NY: Guttmacher Institute; 2021. (https://www.guttmacher.org/article/2021/10/first-time-ever-us-states-enacted-more-100-abortion-restrictions-single-year/).
42. Benson Gold R, Nash E. Flouting the facts: State abortion restrictions flying in the face of science. Guttmacher Policy Rev. 2017;20:53-9. (https://www.guttmacher.org/gpr/2017/05/flouting-facts-state-abortion-restrictions-flying-face-science).
43. Kirstein M, Jones RK, Philbin J. One month post-Roe: At least 43 abortion clinics across 11 states have stopped offering abortion care. New York, NY: Guttmacher Institute; 2022. (https://www.guttmacher.org/article/2022/07/one-month-post-roe-least-43-abortion-clinics-across-11-states-have-stopped-offering).
44. American College of Obstetricians and Gynecologists. Abortion training and education. 2014;(612):1055-9. DOI: 10.1097/01.AOG.0000456327.96480.18.
45. American College of Obstetricians and Gynecologists' Committee on Health Care for Underserved Women AC of O and GAA and TEWG. Increasing access to abortion: ACOG Committee Opinion, Number 815. Obstet Gynecol. 2020;136(6):e107-15. DOI: 10.1097/AOG.0000000000004176.
46. Jerman J, Frohwirth L, Kavanaugh ML, Blades N. Barriers to abortion care and their consequences for patients traveling for services: Qualitative findings from two states. Perspect Sex Reprod Health. 2017;49(2):95-102. DOI: 10.1363/psrh.12024.
47. Johns NE, Foster DG, Upadhyay UD. Distance traveled for Medicaid-covered abortion care in California. BMC Health Serv Res. 2017;17(1):287. DOI: 10.1186/s12913-017-2241-0.
48. White K, Turan JM, Grossman D. Travel for abortion services in Alabama and delays obtaining care. Women's Health Iss. 2017;27(5):523-9. DOI: 10.1016/j.whi.2017.04.002.
49. Guttmacher Institute. State laws and policies: Abortion policy in the absence of Roe. New York, NY: Guttmacher Institute; 2023. (https://www.guttmacher.org/state-policy/explore/abortion-policy-absence-roe).
50. Guttmacher Institute. Roe v. Wade overturned: Our latest resources. (https://www.guttmacher.org/abortion-rights-supreme-court).
51. Gomperts RJ, Jelinska K, Davies S, Gemzell-Danielsson K, Kleiverda G. Using telemedicine for termination of pregnancy with mifepristone and misoprostol in settings where there is no access to safe services. BJOG. 2008;115(9):1171-8. DOI: 10.1111/j.1471-0528.2008.01787.x.
52. Raymond EG, Chong E, Hyland P. Increasing access to abortion with telemedicine. JAMA Intern Med. 2016;176(5):585. DOI: 10.1001/jamainternmed.2016.0573.
53. Upadhyay UD, Schroeder R, Roberts SCM. Adoption of no-test and telehealth medication abortion care among independent abortion providers in response to COVID-19. Contracept X. 2020;2:100049. DOI: 10.1016/j.conx.2020.100049.
54. Kaller S, Muñoz MGI, Sharma S, et al. Abortion service availability during the COVID-19 pandemic: Results from a national census of abortion facilities in the U.S. Contracept X. 2021;3:100067. DOI: 10.1016/j.conx.2021.100067.
55. Perrucci AC. Decision assessment and counseling in abortion care: Philosophy and practice. Lanham, MD: Rowman & Littlefield; 2012.

56. Raymond EG, Grossman D, Mark A, et al. Commentary: No-test medication abortion: A sample protocol for increasing access during a pandemic and beyond. Contraception. 2020;101(6):361-6. DOI: 10.1016/j.contraception.2020.04.005.
57. National Abortion Federation. Clinical policy guidelines for abortion care. Washington DC: NAF; 2022. (https://prochoice.org/providers/quality-standards/).
58. Horvath S, Goyal V, Traxler S, Prager S. Society of Family Planning committee consensus on Rh testing in early pregnancy. Contraception. 2022;114:1-5. DOI: 10.1016/j.contraception.2022.07.002.
59. World Health Organization. Abortion care guideline. Geneva, Switzerland: WHO; 2022. (http://www.who.int/publications/i/item/9789240039483).
60. Raymond EG, Anger HA, Chong E, et al. "False positive" urine pregnancy test results after successful medication abortion. Contraception. 2021;103(6):400-3. DOI: 10.1016/j.contraception.2021.02.004.
61. Turner KL, Huber A (Eds). Woman-centered, comprehensive abortion care: Reference manual. Chapel Hill, NC: Ipas, 2013.
62. White KO, Jones HE, Lavelanet A, et al. First-trimester aspiration abortion practices: a survey of United States abortion providers. Contraception. 2019;99(1):10-15. DOI: 10.1016/j.contraception.2018.08.011.
63. Creinin MD, Grossman DA. Medication abortion up to 70 days of gestation: ACOG Practice Bulletin, Number 225. Obstet Gynecol. 2020;136(4):e31-47. DOI: 10.1097/AOG.0000000000004082.
64. Chong E, Shochet T, Raymond E, et al. Expansion of a direct-to-patient telemedicine abortion service in the United States and experience during the COVID-19 pandemic. Contraception. 2021;104(1):43-8. DOI: 10.1016/j.contraception.2021.03.019.
65. Raymond E, Chong E, Winikoff B, et al. TelAbortion: evaluation of a direct to patient telemedicine abortion service in the United States. Contraception. 2019;100(3):173-7. DOI: 10.1016/j.contraception.2019.05.013.
66. Aiken ARA, Lohr PA, Lord J, Ghosh N, Starling J. Effectiveness, safety and acceptability of no-test medical abortion (termination of pregnancy) provided via telemedicine: a national cohort study. BJOG. 2021;128(9):1464-74. DOI: 10.1111/1471-0528.16668.
67. Hollenbach SJ, Cochran M, Harrington A. "Provoked" feto-maternal hemorrhage may represent insensible cell exchange in pregnancies from 6 to 22 weeks gestational age. Contraception. 2019;100(2):142-6. DOI: 10.1016/j.contraception.2019.03.051.
68. Wiebe ER, Campbell M, Aiken ARA, Albert A. Can we safely stop testing for Rh status and immunizing Rh-negative women having early abortions? A comparison of Rh alloimmunization in Canada and the Netherlands. Contracept X. 2019;1:100001. DOI: 10.1016/J.CONX.2018.100001.
69. Mark A, Foster AM, Grossman D, et al. Foregoing Rh testing and anti-D immunoglobulin for women presenting for early abortion: a recommendation from the National Abortion Federation's Clinical Policies Committee. Contraception. 2019;99(5):265-266. DOI: 10.1016/j.contraception.2019.02.008.
70. Horvath S, Tsao P, Huang ZY, et al. The concentration of fetal red blood cells in first-trimester pregnant women undergoing uterine aspiration is below the calculated threshold for Rh sensitization. Contraception. 2020;102(1):1-6. DOI: 10.1016/j.contraception.2020.02.011.
71. Chan MC, Gill RK, Kim CR. Rhesus isoimmunisation in unsensitised RhD-negative individuals seeking abortion at less than 12 weeks' gestation: a systematic review. BMJ Sex Reprod Health. 2022;48(3):163-8. DOI: 10.1136/bmjsrh-2021-201225.
72. Shannon C, Brothers LP, Philip NM, Winikoff B. Infection after medical abortion: A review of the literature. Contraception. 2004;70(3):183-90. DOI: 10.1016/j.contraception.2004.04.009.
73. Achilles SL, Reeves MF, Society of Family Planning. Prevention of infection after induced abortion. Contraception. 2011;83(4):295-309. DOI: 10.1016/j.contraception.2010.11.006.
74. Low N, Mueller M, Vliet HA Van, Kapp N. Perioperative antibiotics to prevent infection after first-trimester abortion. Cochrane Database Syst Rev. 2012;2012(3). DOI: 10.1002/14651858.CD005217.PUB2.
75. Wilson W, Taubert KA, Gewitz M, et al. Prevention of infective endocarditis: guidelines from the American Heart Association: a guideline from the American Heart Association Rheumatic Fever, Endocarditis, and Kawasaki Disease Committee, Council on Cardiovascular Disease in

the Young, and the Council on Clinical Cardiology, Council on Cardiovascular Surgery and Anesthesia, and the Quality of Care and Outcomes Research Interdisciplinary Working Group. Circulation. 2007;116(15):1736-54. DOI: 10.1161/CIRCULATIONAHA.106.183095.

76. Guttmacher Institute. An overview of abortion laws. (https://www.guttmacher.org/state-policy/explore/overview-abortion-laws).
77. Dzuba IG, Chong E, Hannum C, et al. A non-inferiority study of outpatient mifepristone-misoprostol medical abortion at 64–70 days and 71–77 days of gestation. Contraception. 2020;101(5):302-8.
78. Howie FL, Henshaw RC, Naji SA, Russell IT, Templeton AA. Medical abortion or vacuum aspiration? Two year follow up of a patient preference trial. Br J Obstet Gynaecol. 1997;104(7):829-33. DOI: 10.1111/J.1471-0528.1997.TB12028.X.
79. Winikoff B. Acceptability of medical abortion in early pregnancy. Fam Plann Perspect. 2013;27(4):142-8, 185. DOI: 10.2307/2136257.
80. Moseson H, Fix L, Ragosta S, et al. Abortion experiences and preferences of transgender, nonbinary, and gender-expansive people in the United States. Am J Obstet Gynecol. 2021;224(4):376.e1-11. DOI: 10.1016/J.AJOG.2020.09.035.
81. Allen RH, Fortin J, Bartz D, Goldberg AB, Clark MA. Women's preferences for pain control during first-trimester surgical abortion: a qualitative study. Contraception. 2012;85(4):413-8. DOI: 10.1016/j.contraception.2011.08.019.
82. Barnard S, Kim C, Park MH, Ngo TD. Doctors or mid-level providers for abortion. Cochrane Database Syst Rev. 2015;2015(7). DOI: 10.1002/14651858.CD011242.pub2.
83. Bernard N, Elefant E, Carlier P, et al. Continuation of pregnancy after first-trimester exposure to mifepristone: an observational prospective study. 2013;120(5):568-75. DOI: 10.1111/1471-0528.12147.
84. Grossman D, White K, Harris L, et al. Continuing pregnancy after mifepristone and "reversal" of first-trimester medical abortion: a systematic review. Contraception. 2015;92(3):206-11. DOI: 10.1016/j.contraception.2015.06.001.
85. Creinin MD, Hou MY, Dalton L, Steward R, Chen MJ. Mifepristone antagonization with progesterone to prevent medical abortion: a randomized controlled trial. Obstet Gynecol. 2020;135(1):158-65. DOI: 10.1097/AOG.0000000000003620.
86. Jain JK, Dutton C, Harwood B, Meckstroth KR, Mishell DR. A prospective randomized, double-blinded, placebo-controlled trial comparing mifepristone and vaginal misoprostol to vaginal misoprostol alone for elective termination of early pregnancy. Hum Reprod. 2002;17(6):1477-82. DOI: 10.1093/humrep/17.6.1477.
87. Schaff EA, DiCenzo R, Fielding SL. Comparison of misoprostol plasma concentrations following buccal and sublingual administration. Contraception. 2005;71(1):22-5. DOI: 10.1016/j.contraception.2004.06.014.
88. Meckstroth KR, Whitaker AK, Bertisch S, Goldberg AB, Darney PD. Misoprostol Administered by Epithelial Routes. Obstet Gynecol. 2006;108(3, Part 1):582-90. DOI: 10.1097/01.AOG.0000230398.32794.9d.
89. Tang OS, Gemzell-Danielsson K, Ho PC. Misoprostol: pharmacokinetic profiles, effects on the uterus and side-effects. Int J Gynaecol Obstet. 2007;99 Suppl 2:S160-7. DOI: 10.1016/j.ijgo.2007.09.004.
90. da Silva Dal Pizzol T, Knop FP, Mengue SS. Prenatal exposure to misoprostol and congenital anomalies: Systematic review and meta-analysis. Reprod Toxicol. 2006;22(4):666-71. DOI: 10.1016/j.reprotox.2006.03.015.
91. Donovan MK. Improving access to abortion via telehealth. Guttmacher Policy Rev. 2019;22:23-7.
92. US Food and Drug Administration. Risk Evaluation and Mitigation Strategies | REMS. https://www.fda.gov/drugs/drug-safety-and-availability/risk-evaluation-and-mitigation-strategies-rems.
93. Guttmacher Institute. Medication abortion. (https://www.guttmacher.org/state-policy/explore/medication-abortion).
94. American Civil Liberties Union. FDA response to ACOG April 2021. (https://www.aclu.org/letter/fda-response-acog-april-2021).
95. US Food and Drug Administration. Questions and answers on mifepristone for medical termination of pregnancy through ten weeks gestation. (https://www.fda.gov/drugs/postmarket-drug-safety-information-patients-and-providers/questions-and-answers-mifeprex).

96. Godfrey EM, Fiastro AE, Jacob-Files EA, et al. Factors associated with successful implementation of telehealth abortion in 4 United States clinical practice settings. Contraception. 2021;104(1):82-91. DOI: 10.1016/j.contraception.2021.04.021.
97. Tschann M, Ly ES, Hilliard S, Lange HLHH. Changes to medication abortion clinical practices in response to the COVID-19 pandemic. Contraception. 2021;104(1):77-81. DOI: 10.1016/j.contraception.2021.04.010.
98. Chong E, Shochet T, Raymond E, et al. Expansion of a direct-to-patient telemedicine abortion service in the United States and experience during the COVID-19 pandemic. Contraception. 2021;104(1):43-8. DOI: 10.1016/j.contraception.2021.03.019.
99. Kerestes C, Murayama S, Tyson J, et al. Provision of medication abortion in Hawai'i during COVID-19: Practical experience with multiple care delivery models. Contraception. 2021;104(1):49-53. DOI: 10.1016/j.contraception.2021.03.025.
100. Kaye J, Reeves R, Chaiten L. The mifepristone REMS: A needless and unlawful barrier to care. Contraception. 2021;104(1):12-5. DOI: 10.1016/j.contraception.2021.04.025.
101. Serpico JJ. Abortion exceptionalism and the mifepristone REMS. Contraception. 2021;104(1):8-11. DOI: 10.1016/j.contraception.2021.03.031.
102. Raymond EG, Shannon C, Weaver MA, Winikoff B. First-trimester medical abortion with mifepristone 200 mg and misoprostol: a systematic review. Contraception. 2013;87(1):26-37. DOI: 10.1016/j.contraception.2012.06.011.
103. Winikoff B, Dzuba IG, Chong E, et al. Extending outpatient medical abortion services through 70 days of gestational age. Obstet Gynecol. 2012;120(5):1070-6. DOI: http://10.1097/AOG.0b013e31826c315f.
104. Abbas D, Chong E, Raymond EG. Outpatient medical abortion is safe and effective through 70 days gestation. Contraception. 2015;92(3):197-9. DOI: 10.1016/j.contraception.2015.06.018.
105. US Food and Drug Administration. Information about mifepristone for medical termination of pregnancy through ten weeks gestation. (https://www.fda.gov/drugs/postmarket-drug-safety-information-patients-and-providers/information-about-mifepristone-medical-termination-pregnancy-through-ten-weeks-gestation).
106. Dzuba IG, Castillo PW, Bousiéguez M, Lugo Hernández EM, Castañeda Vivar JJ, Sanhueza Smith P. A repeat dose of misoprostol 800 mcg following mifepristone for outpatient medical abortion at 64–70 and 71–77 days of gestation: A retrospective chart review. Contraception. 2020;102(2):104-8. DOI: 10.1016/j.contraception.2020.05.012.
107. Hsia JK, Lohr PA, Taylor J, Creinin MD. Medical abortion with mifepristone and vaginal misoprostol between 64 and 70 days' gestation. Contraception. 2019;100(3):178-81. DOI: 10.1016/j.contraception.2019.05.006.
108. Winikoff B, Dzuba IG, Creinin MD, et al. Two distinct oral routes of misoprostol in mifepristone medical abortion. Obstet Gynecol. 2008;112(6):1303-10. DOI: 10.1097/AOG.0b013e31818d8eb4
109. Creinin MD, Fox MC, Teal S, et al. A randomized comparison of misoprostol 6 to 8 hours versus 24 hours after mifepristone for abortion. Obstet Gynecol. 2004;103(5 Pt 1):851-9. DOI: 10.1097/01.AOG.0000124271.23499.84.
110. Young D, Fitzgerald K, Laursen L, Whitaker AK. Comparison of vaginal and buccal misoprostol after mifepristone for medication abortion through 70 days of gestation: A retrospective chart review. Contraception. 2022;115:62-6. DOI: 10.1016/j.contraception.2022.06.012.
111. Creinin MD, Schreiber CA, Bednarek P, et al. Mifepristone and misoprostol administered simultaneously versus 24 hours apart for abortion: a randomized controlled trial. Obstet Gynecol. 2007;109(4):885-94. DOI: 10.1097/01.AOG.0000258298.35143.d2.
112. Chen MJ, Creinin MD. Mifepristone with buccal misoprostol for medical abortion. Obstet Gynecol. 2015;126(1):12-21. DOI: 10.1097/AOG.0000000000000897.
113. Blum J, Raghavan S, Dabash R, et al. Comparison of misoprostol-only and combined mifepristone-misoprostol regimens for home-based early medical abortion in Tunisia and Vietnam. Int J Gynaecol Obstet. 2012;118(2):166-71. DOI: 10.1016/j.ijgo.2012.03.039.
114. Morris JL, Winikoff B, Dabash R, et al. FIGO's updated recommendations for misoprostol used alone in gynecology and obstetrics. International Journal of Gynecology & Obstetrics. 2017;138(3):363-366. DOI: 10.1002/IJGO.12181.
115. Ngoc NTN, Blum J, Raghavan S, et al. Comparing two early medical abortion regimens: mifepristone+misoprostol vs. misoprostol alone. Contraception. 2011;83(5):410-7. DOI: 10.1016/j.contraception.2010.09.002.

116. von Hertzen H, Piaggio G, Huong NTM, et al. Efficacy of two intervals and two routes of administration of misoprostol for termination of early pregnancy: a randomised controlled equivalence trial. Lancet. 2007;369(9577):1938-46. DOI: 10.1016/S0140-6736(07)60914-3.
117. Sheldon WR, Durocher J, Dzuba IG, et al. Early abortion with buccal versus sublingual misoprostol alone: a multicenter, randomized trial. Contraception. 2019;99(5):272-7. DOI: 10.1016/j.contraception.2019.02.002.
118. Creinin MD, Shulman T. Effect of nonsteroidal anti-inflammatory drugs on the action of misoprostol in a regimen for early abortion. Contraception. 1997;56(3):165-8. DOI: 10.1016/S0010-7824(97)00120-0.
119. Raymond EG, Weaver MA, Louie KS, et al. Prophylactic compared with therapeutic ibuprofen analgesia in first-trimester medical abortion: a randomized controlled trial. Obstet Gynecol. 2013;122(3):558-64. DOI: 10.1097/AOG.0b013e31829d5a33.
120. Colwill AC, Bayer LL, Bednarek P, Garg B, Jensen JT, Edelman AB. Opioid analgesia for medical abortion: A randomized controlled trial. Obstet Gynecol. 2019;134(6):1163-1170. DOI: 10.1097/AOG.0000000000003576.
121. Jackson E, Kapp N. Pain control in first-trimester and second-trimester medical termination of pregnancy: a systematic review. Contraception. 2011;83(2):116-26. DOI: 10.1016/j.contraception.2010.07.014.
122. Tang OS, Lee SWH, Ho PC. A prospective randomized study on the measured blood loss in medical termination of early pregnancy by three different misoprostol regimens after pretreatment with mifepristone. Hum Reprod. 2002;17(11):2865-8. DOI: 10.1093/humrep/17.11.2865.
123. Davis A, Westhoff C, De Nonno L. Bleeding patterns after early abortion with mifepristone and misoprostol or manual vacuum aspiration. J Am Med Womens Assoc. 2000;55(3 Suppl): 141-4.
124. Tang OS, Gao PP, Cheng L, Lee SW, Ho PC. A randomized double-blind placebo-controlled study to assess the effect of oral contraceptive pills on the outcome of medical abortion with mifepristone and misoprostol. Hum Reprod. 1999;14(3):722-5.
125. Cleland K, Creinin MD, Nucatola D, Nshom M, Trussell J. Significant adverse events and outcomes after medical abortion. Obstet Gynecol. 2013;121(1):166-71. DOI: 10.1097/AOG.0b013e3182755763.
126. Grossman D, Grindlay K. Safety of medical abortion provided through telemedicine compared with in person. Obstet Gynecol. 2017;130(4):778-82. DOI: 10.1097/AOG.0000000000002212.
127. Baiju N, Acharya G, D'Antonio F, Berg RC. Effectiveness, safety and acceptability of self-assessment of the outcome of first-trimester medical abortion: a systematic review and meta-analysis. BJOG. 2019;126(13):1536-44. DOI: 10.1111/1471-0528.15922.
128. Schmidt-Hansen M, Cameron S, Lohr PA, Hasler E. Follow-up strategies to confirm the success of medical abortion of pregnancies up to 10 weeks' gestation: a systematic review with meta-analyses. Am J Obstet Gynecol. 2020;222(6):551-63.e13. DOI: 10.1016/j.ajog.2019.11.1244.
129. Rossi B, Creinin MD, Meyn LA. Ability of the clinician and patient to predict the outcome of mifepristone and misoprostol medical abortion. Contraception. 2004;70(4):313-7. DOI: 10.1016/j.contraception.2004.04.005.
130. Jackson A V., Dayananda I, Fortin JM, Fitzmaurice G, Goldberg AB. Can women accurately assess the outcome of medical abortion based on symptoms alone? Contraception. 2012;85(2):192-7. DOI: 10.1016/j.contraception.2011.05.019.
131. Clark W, Panton T, Hann L, Gold M. Medication abortion employing routine sequential measurements of serum hCG and sonography only when indicated. Contraception. 2007;75(2):131-135. DOI: 10.1016/j.contraception.2006.08.001.
132. Clark W, Bracken H, Tanenhaus J, Schweikert S, Lichtenberg ES, Winikoff B. Alternatives to a routine follow-up visit for early medical abortion. Obstet Gynecol. 2010;115(2, Part 1): 264-72. DOI: 10.1097/AOG.0b013e3181c996f3.
133. Cowett AA, Cohen LS, Lichtenberg ES, Stika CS. Ultrasound evaluation of the endometrium after medical termination of pregnancy. Obstet Gynecol. 2004;103(5, Part 1):871-5. DOI: 10.1097/01.AOG.0000124782.69622.48.

134. Pocius KD, Bartz D, Maurer R, Stenquist A, Fortin J, Goldberg AB. Serum human chorionic gonadotropin (hCG) trend within the first few days after medical abortion: a prospective study. Contraception. 2017;95(3):263-8. DOI: 10.1016/j.contraception.2016.09.007.
135. Korevaar TIM, Steegers EAP, de Rijke YB, et al. Reference ranges and determinants of total hCG levels during pregnancy: the Generation R Study. Eur J Epidemiol. 2015;30(9):1057-66. DOI: 10.1007/S10654-015-0039-0.
136. Aiken ARA, Starling JE, Gomperts R. factors associated with use of an online telemedicine service to access self-managed medical abortion in the US. JAMA Netw Open. 2021;4(5). DOI: 10.1001/jamanetworkopen.2021.11852.
137. Mark A, Foster AM, Perritt J. The future of abortion is now: Mifepristone by mail and in-clinic abortion access in the United States. Contraception. 2021;104(1):38-42. DOI: 10.1016/j.contraception.2021.03.033.
138. Yanow S, Pizzarossa LB, Jelinska K. Self-managed abortion: Exploring synergies between institutional medical systems and autonomous health movements. Contraception. 2021;104(3): 219-21. DOI: 10.1016/j.contraception.2021.06.006.
139. Ralph L, Foster DG, Raifman S, et al. Prevalence of self-managed abortion among women of reproductive age in the United States. JAMA Netw Open. 2020;3(12):e2029245. (https://jamanetwork.com/journals/jamanetworkopen/fullarticle/2774320).
140. Harris LH, Grossman D. Complications of unsafe and self-managed abortion. N Engl J Med. 2020;382(11):1029-40. DOI: 10.1056/nejmra1908412.
141. Upadhyay UD, Cartwright AF, Grossman D. Barriers to abortion care and incidence of attempted self-managed abortion among individuals searching Google for abortion care: A national prospective study. Contraception. 2022;106:49-56. DOI: 10.1016/j.contraception.2021.09.009.
142. World Health Organization. WHO consolidated guideline on self-care interventions for health sexual and reproductive health and rights. Geneva, Switzerland: WHO; 2019. (https://pubmed.ncbi.nlm.nih.gov/31334932/).
143. Aiken ARA, Digol I, Trussell J, Gomperts R. Self reported outcomes and adverse events after medical abortion through online telemedicine: population based study in the Republic of Ireland and Northern Ireland. BMJ. 2017;357:j2011. DOI: 10.1136/bmj.j2011.
144. Grossman D, Baum SE, Andjelic D, et al. A harm-reduction model of abortion counseling about misoprostol use in Peru with telephone and in-person follow-up: A cohort study. PLoS One. 2018;13(1). DOI: 10.1371/JOURNAL.PONE.0189195.
145. Weitz T, Anderson P, Taylor D. Advancing scope of practice for advanced practice clinicians: more than a matter of access. Contraception. 2009;80(2):105-7. DOI: 10.1016/j.contraception.2009.04.013.
146. Goldberg AB, Dean G, Kang MS, Youssof S, Darney PD. Manual versus electric vacuum aspiration for early first-trimester abortion: a controlled study of complication rates. Obstet Gynecol. 2004;103(1):101-7. DOI: 10.1097/01.AOG.0000109147.23082.25.
147. Wen J, Cai QY, Deng F, Li YP. Manual versus electric vacuum aspiration for first-trimester abortion: A systematic review. BJOG. 2008;115(1):5-13. DOI: 10.1111/j.1471-0528.2007.01572.x.
148. Bird ST, Harvey SM, Beckman LJ, Nichols MD, Rogers K, Blumenthal PD. Similarities in women's perceptions and acceptability of manual vacuum aspiration and electric vacuum aspiration for first trimester abortion. Contraception. 2003;67(3):207-12. DOI: 10.1016/S0010-7824(02)00484-5.
149. Dean G, Cardenas L, Darney P, Goldberg A. Acceptability of manual versus electric aspiration for first trimester abortion: A randomized trial. Contraception. 2003;67(3):201-6. DOI: 10.1016/S0010-7824(02)00485-7.
150. Dean G, Colarossi L, Porsch L, Betancourt G, Jacobs A, Paul ME. Manual compared with electric vacuum aspiration for abortion at less than 6 weeks of gestation: a randomized controlled trial. Obstet Gynecol. 2015;125(5):1121-9. DOI: 10.1097/aog.0000000000000787.
151. Renner RM, Jensen JT, Nichols MD, Edelman AB. Pain control in first-trimester surgical abortion: a systematic review of randomized controlled trials. Contraception. 2010;81(5):372-88. DOI: 10.1016/j.contraception.2009.12.008.
152. Allen RH, Singh R. Society of Family Planning clinical guidelines pain control in surgical abortion part 1 — local anesthesia and minimal sedation. Contraception. 2018;97(6):471-7. DOI: 10.1016/j.contraception.2018.01.014.

153. Wiebe ER, Rawling M. Pain control in abortion. Int J Gynecol Obstet. 1995;50(1):41-6. DOI: 10.1016/0020-7292(95)02416-A.
154. Braaten KP, Hurwitz S, Fortin J, Goldberg AB. Intramuscular ketorolac versus oral ibuprofen for pain relief in first-trimester surgical abortion: a randomized clinical trial. Contraception. 2014;89(2):116-21. DOI: 10.1016/j.contraception.2013.10.009.
155. Cansino C, Edelman A, Burke A, Jamshidi R. Paracervical block with combined ketorolac and lidocaine in first-trimester surgical abortion: a randomized controlled trial. Obstet Gynecol. 2009;114(6):1220-6. DOI: 10.1097/AOG.0b013e3181c1a55b.
156. Micks EA, Edelman AB, Renner RM, et al. Hydrocodone-acetaminophen for pain control in first-trimester surgical abortion: a randomized controlled trial. Obstet Gynecol. 2012;120(5):1060-9. DOI: http://10.1097/AOG.0b013e31826c32f0.
157. Allen RH, Fitzmaurice G, Lifford KL, Lasic M, Goldberg AB. Oral compared with intravenous sedation for first-trimester surgical abortion. Obstet Gynecol. 2009;113(2, Part 1):276-83. DOI: 10.1097/AOG.0b013e3181938758.
158. Wiebe E, Podhradsky L, Dijak V. The effect of lorazepam on pain and anxiety in abortion. Contraception. 2003;67(3):219-21. DOI: 10.1016/S0010-7824(02)00516-4.
159. Allen RH, Kumar D, Fitzmaurice G, Lifford KL, Goldberg AB. Pain management of first-trimester surgical abortion: effects of selection of local anesthesia with and without lorazepam or intravenous sedation. Contraception. 2006;74(5):407-13. DOI: 10.1016/j.contraception.2006.06.002.
160. Bayer LL, Edelman AB, Fu R, et al. An evaluation of oral midazolam for anxiety and pain in first-trimester surgical abortion. Obstet Gynecol. 2015;126(1):37-46. DOI: 10.1097/AOG.0000000000000913.
161. Cansino C, Denny C, Carlisle AS, Stubblefield P. Society of Family Planning clinical recommendations: Pain control in surgical abortion part 2 – Moderate sedation, deep sedation, and general anesthesia. Contraception. 2021;104(6):583-92. DOI: 10.1016/j.contraception.2021.08.007.
162. Varli IH, Lindelius A, Bergström M. Is preoperative vaginal cleansing necessary for control of infection after first trimester vacuum curettage? Acta Obstet Gynecol Scand. 2005;84(7):650-3. DOI: 10.1111/j.0001-6349.2005.00689.x.
163. Meckstroth KR, Paul ME. First trimester aspiration abortion. In: Paul ME, Lichtenberg ES, Borgatta L, Grimes DA, Stubblefield PG, Creinin MD, eds. Management of unintended and abnormal pregnancy: Comprehensive abortion care. Wiley-Blackwell; 2009:135-56.
164. Soon R, Tschann M, Salcedo J, Stevens K, Ahn HJ, Kaneshiro B. Paracervical block for laminaria insertion before second-trimester abortion. Obstet Gynecol. 2017;130(2):387-92. DOI: 10.1097/AOG.0000000000002149.
165. Schulz KF, Grimes DA, Christensen DD. Vasopressin reduces blood loss from second-trimester dilatation and evacuation abortion. Lancet. 1985;326(8451):353-6. DOI: 10.1016/S0140-6736(85)92496-1.
166. Wilson LC, Chen BA, Creinin MD. Low-dose fentanyl and midazolam in outpatient surgical abortion up to 18 weeks of gestation. Contraception. 2009;79(2):122-8. DOI: 10.1016/j.contraception.2008.08.005.
167. Mancuso AC, Lee K, Zhang R, Hoover EA, Stockdale C, Hardy-Fairbanks AJ. Deep sedation without intubation during second trimester surgical termination in an inpatient hospital setting. Contraception. 2017;95(3):288-91. DOI: 10.1016/j.contraception.2016.09.012.
168. Dean G, Jacobs AR, Goldstein RC, Gevirtz CM, Paul ME. The safety of deep sedation without intubation for abortion in the outpatient setting. J Clin Anesth. 2011;23(6):437-42. DOI: 10.1016/j.jclinane.2011.05.001.
169. Hamoda H, Ashok PW, Flett GMM, Templeton A. Analgesia requirements and predictors of analgesia use for women undergoing medical abortion up to 22 weeks of gestation. BJOG. 2004;111(9):996-1000. DOI: 10.1111/j.1471-0528.2004.00235.x.
170. Smith RL, Siddiqui N, Henderson T, Teresi J, Downey K, Carvalho JCA. Analgesia for medically induced second trimester termination of pregnancy: A randomized trial. J Obstet Gynaecol Can.. 2016;38(2):147-53. DOI: 10.1016/j.jogc.2015.12.015.
171. Andersson IM, Benson L, Christensson K, Gemzell-Danielsson K. Paracervical block as pain treatment during second-trimester medical termination of pregnancy: an RCT with bupivacaine versus sodium chloride. Human Reproduction. 2016;31(1):67-74. DOI: 10.1093/humrep/dev286.

172. Borgatta L, Kapp N, Society of Family Planning. Labor induction abortion in the second trimester: Release date February 2011 - SFP Guideline 20111. Contraception. 2011;84(1):4-18. DOI: 10.1016/j.contraception.2011.02.005.
173. Fox MC, Krajewski CM. Cervical preparation for second-trimester surgical abortion prior to 20 weeks' gestation: SFP Guideline #2013-4. Contraception. 2014;89(2):75-84. DOI: 10.1016/j.contraception.2013.11.001.
174. Diedrich JT, Drey EA, Newmann SJ. Society of Family Planning clinical recommendations: Cervical preparation for dilation and evacuation at 20–24 weeks' gestation. Contraception. 2020;101(5):286-92. DOI: 10.1016/j.contraception.2020.01.002.
175. Allen RH, Goldberg AB. Cervical dilation before first-trimester surgical abortion (< 14 weeks' gestation). Contraception. 2016;93(4):277-91. DOI: 10.1016/j.contraception.2015.12.001.
176. Kapp N, Lohr PA, Ngo TD, Hayes JL. Cervical preparation for first trimester surgical abortion. Cochrane Database Syst Rev. 2010;(2):CD007207. DOI: 10.1002/14651858.CD007207.pub2.
177. Panchal HB, Godfrey EM, Patel A. Buccal misoprostol for cervical ripening prior to first trimester abortion. Contraception. 2010;81(2):161-4. DOI: 10.1016/j.contraception.2009.10.002.
178. Borgatta L, Roncari D, Sonalkar S, et al. Mifepristone vs. osmotic dilator insertion for cervical preparation prior to surgical abortion at 14-16 weeks: A randomized trial. Contraception. 2012;86(5):567-71. DOI: 10.1016/j.contraception.2012.05.002.
179. Goldberg AB, Fortin JA, Drey EA, et al. Cervical preparation before dilation and evacuation using adjunctive misoprostol or mifepristone compared with overnight osmotic dilators alone. Obstet Gynecol. 2015;126(3):599-609. DOI: 10.1097/AOG.0000000000000977.
180. Shaw KA, Shaw JG, Hugin M, Velasquez G, Hopkins FW, Blumenthal PD. Adjunct mifepristone for cervical preparation prior to dilation and evacuation: a randomized trial. Contraception. 2015;91(4):313-9. DOI: 10.1016/j.contraception.2014.11.014.
181. Upadhyay UD, Desai S, Zlidar V, et al. Incidence of emergency department visits and complications after abortion. Obstet Gynecol. 2015;125(1):175-83. DOI: 10.1097/AOG.0000000000000603.
182. White K, Carroll E, Grossman D. Complications from first-trimester aspiration abortion: a systematic review of the literature. Contraception. 2015;92(5):422-38. DOI: 10.1016/j.contraception.2015.07.013.
183. Allen RH, Westhoff C, De Nonno L, Fielding SL, Schaff EA. Curettage after mifepristone-induced abortion: Frequency, timing, and indications. Obstet Gynecol. 2001;98(1):101-6. DOI: 10.1016/S0029-7844(01)01375-8.
184. Shields LE, Goffman D, Caughey AB. Postpartum Hemorrhage. Obstet Gynecol. 2017; 130(4):e168-86. DOI: 10.1097/AOG.0000000000002351.
185. Taylor D, Upadhyay UD, Fjerstad M, Battistelli MF, Weitz TA, Paul ME. Standardizing the classification of abortion incidents: the Procedural Abortion Incident Reporting and Surveillance (PAIRS) Framework. Contraception. 2017;96(1):1-13. DOI: 10.1016/j.contraception.2017.05.004.
186. Vauzelle C, Beghin D, Cournot MP, Elefant E. Birth defects after exposure to misoprostol in the first trimester of pregnancy: prospective follow-up study. Reprod Toxicol. 2013;36:98-103. DOI: 10.1016/j.reprotox.2012.11.009.
187. Schüler L, Pastuszak A, Sanseverino MT V., et al. Pregnancy outcome after exposure to misoprostol in Brazil: a prospective, controlled study. Reprod Toxicol. 1999;13(2):147-51. DOI: 10.1016/S0890-6238(98)00072-0.
188. Auffret M, Bernard-Phalippon N, Dekemp J, et al. Misoprostol exposure during the first trimester of pregnancy: Is the malformation risk varying depending on the indication? Eur J Obstet Gynecol Reprod Biol. 2016;207:188-92. DOI: 10.1016/j.ejogrb.2016.11.007.
189. Gonzalez CH, Marques-Dias MJ, Kim CA, et al. Congenital abnormalities in Brazilian children associated with misoprostol misuse in first trimester of pregnancy. Lancet. 1998;351(9116):1624-7. DOI: 10.1016/S0140-6736(97)12363-7.
190. Goyal V. Uterine rupture in second-trimester misoprostol-induced abortion after cesarean delivery. Obstet Gynecol. 2009;113(5):1117-23. DOI: 10.1097/AOG.0b013e31819dbfe2.
191. Grimes DA, Schulz KF, Cates WJ. Prevention of uterine perforation during curettage abortion. JAMA. 1984;251(16):2108-11.
192. Meites E, Zane S, Gould C. Fatal *Clostridium sordellii* infections after medical abortions. N Engl J Med. 2010;363(14):1382-3. DOI: 10.1056/NEJMc1001014.

193. Sinave C, Le Templier G, Blouin D, Léveillé F, Deland E. Toxic shock syndrome due to *Clostridium sordellii*: a dramatic postpartum and postabortion disease. Clin Infect Dis. 2002;35(11):1441-3. DOI: 10.1086/344464.
194. Cohen AL, Bhatnagar J, Reagan S, et al. Toxic shock associated with *Clostridium sordellii* and *Clostridium perfringens* after medical and spontaneous abortion. Obstet Gynecol. 2007;110(5):1027-33. DOI: 10.1097/01.AOG.0000287291.19230.ba.
195. Ho CS, Bhatnagar J, Cohen AL, et al. Undiagnosed cases of fatal *Clostridium*-associated toxic shock in Californian women of childbearing age. Am J Obstet Gynecol. 2009;201(5):459.e1-7. DOI: 10.1016/j.ajog.2009.05.023.
196. Hogue C, Boardman L. Answering questions about long-term outcomes. In: Paul ME, Lichtenberg ES, Borgatta L, Grimes DA, Stubblefield PG, Creinin MD, eds. Management of unintended and abnormal pregnancy: Comprehensive abortion care. Blackwell-Wiley; 2009:252-263.
197. Virk J, Zhang J, Olsen J. Medical abortion and the risk of subsequent adverse pregnancy outcomes. N Engl J Med. 2007;357(7):648-53. DOI: 10.1056/NEJMoa070445.
198. Liao H, Wei Q, Duan L, Ge J, Zhou Y, Zeng W. Repeated medical abortions and the risk of preterm birth in the subsequent pregnancy. Arch Gynecol Obstet. 2011;284(3):579-86. DOI: 10.1007/s00404-010-1723-7.
199. Klemetti R, Gissler M, Niinimaki M, Hemminki E. Birth outcomes after induced abortion: a nationwide register-based study of first births in Finland. Hum Reprod. 2012;27(11):3315-20. DOI: 10.1093/humrep/des294.
200. Bhattacharya S, Lowit A, Bhattacharya S, et al. Reproductive outcomes following induced abortion: a national register-based cohort study in Scotland. BMJ Open. 2012;2(4):e000911. DOI: 10.1136/bmjopen-2012-000911.
201. Saccone G, Perriera L, Berghella V. Prior uterine evacuation of pregnancy as independent risk factor for preterm birth: a systematic review and metaanalysis. Am J Obstet Gynecol. 2016;214(5):572-91. DOI: 10.1016/j.ajog.2015.12.044.
202. Scholten BL, Page-Christiaens GCML, Franx A, Hukkelhoven CWPM, Koster MPH. The influence of pregnancy termination on the outcome of subsequent pregnancies: a retrospective cohort study. BMJ Open. 2013;3(5):e002803. DOI: 10.1136/bmjopen-2013-002803.
203. Situ KC, Hemminki E, Gissler M, Virtanen SM, Klemetti R. Perinatal outcomes after induced termination of pregnancy by methods: A nationwide register-based study of first births in Finland 1996-2013. PLoS One. 2017;12(9). DOI: 10.1371/journal.pone.0184078.
204. Kalish RB, Chasen ST, Rosenzweig LB, Rashbaum WK, Chervenak FA. Impact of midtrimester dilation and evacuation on subsequent pregnancy outcome. Am J Obstet Gynecol. 2002;187(4):882-5. DOI: 10.1067/mob.2002.127139.
205. Chasen ST, Kalish RB, Gupta M, Kaufman J, Chervenak FA. Obstetric outcomes after surgical abortion at ≥20 weeks' gestation. Am J Obstet Gynecol. 2005;193(3):1161-4. DOI: 10.1016/j.ajog.2005.05.078.
206. Oliver-Williams C, Fleming M, Monteath K, Wood AM, Smith GCS. Changes in association between previous therapeutic abortion and preterm birth in Scotland, 1980 to 2008: A historical cohort study. Gulmezoglu M, ed. PLoS Med. 2013;10(7):e1001481. DOI: 10.1371/journal.pmed.1001481.
207. Herd P, Higgins J, Sicinski K, Merkurieva I. The implications of unintended pregnancies for mental health in later life. Am J Public Health. 2016;106(3):421-9. DOI: 10.2105/AJPH.2015.302973.
208. Steinberg JR, Rubin LR. Psychological aspects of contraception, unintended pregnancy, and abortion. Policy Insights Behav Brain Sci. 2014;1(1):239-47. DOI: 10.1177/2372732214549328.
209. Munk-Olsen T, Laursen TM, Pedersen CB, Lidegaard Ø, Mortensen PB. Induced first-trimester abortion and risk of mental disorder. N Engl J Med. 2011;364(4):332-9. DOI: 10.1056/NEJMoa0905882.
210. Steinberg JR, McCulloch CE, Adler NE. Abortion and mental health. Obstet Gynecol. 2014;123(2, Part 1):263-70. DOI: 10.1097/AOG.0000000000000092.
211. Foster DG, Steinberg JR, Roberts SCM, Neuhaus J, Biggs MA. A comparison of depression and anxiety symptom trajectories between women who had an abortion and women denied one. Psychol Med. 2015;45(10):2073-2082. DOI: 10.1017/S0033291714003213.

212. Rocca CH, Kimport K, Roberts SCM, Gould H, Neuhaus J, Foster DG. Decision rightness and emotional responses to abortion in the United States: a longitudinal study. PLoS One. 2015;10(7):e0128832. DOI: 10.1371/journal.pone.0128832.
213. Guo J, Huang Y, Yang L, et al. Association between abortion and breast cancer: an updated systematic review and meta-analysis based on prospective studies. Cancer Causes Control. 2015;26(6):811-9. DOI: 10.1007/s10552-015-0536-1.
214. Braüner CM, Overvad K, Tjønneland A, Attermann J. Induced abortion and breast cancer among parous women: A Danish cohort study. Acta Obstet Gynecol Scand. 2013;92(6):700-5. DOI: 10.1111/aogs.12107.
215. Melbye M, Wohlfahrt J, Olsen JH, et al. Induced abortion and the risk of breast cancer. N Engl J Med. 1997;336(2):81-5. DOI: 10.1056/NEJM199701093360201.
216. National Cancer Institute. Abortion, miscarriage, and breast cancer risk: 2003 Workshop. (https://www.cancer.gov/types/breast/abortion-miscarriage-risk).
217. Committee on Gynecologic Practice. ACOG Committee Opinion No. 434: Induced abortion and breast cancer risk. Obstet Gynecol. 2009;113(6):1417-8. DOI: 10.1097/AOG.0b013e3181ac067d.
218. Schreiber CA, Sober S, Ratcliffe S, Creinin MD. Ovulation resumption after medical abortion with mifepristone and misoprostol. Contraception. 2011;84(3):230-3. DOI: 10.1016/j.contraception.2011.01.013.
219. Krashin JW, Stuart GS, Garrett J, et al. Contraception insurance coverage and receipt of long-acting reversible contraception or depot medroxyprogesterone acetate on the day of abortion. Obstet Gynecol. 2017;130(1):109-17. DOI: 10.1097/AOG.0000000000002070.
220. Goyal V, Canfield C, Aiken ARA, Dermish A, Potter JE. Postabortion contraceptive use and continuation when long-acting reversible contraception is free. Obstet Gynecol. 2017;129(4): 655-62. DOI: 10.1097/AOG.0000000000001926.
221. Bell KN, Meyn LA, Chen BA. Long-acting reversible contraceptive uptake before and after the affordable care act contraceptive mandate in women undergoing first trimester surgical abortion. Womens Health Iss. 2018;28(4):301-5. DOI: 10.1016/j.whi.2018.04.007.
222. Jerman J, Berry A, Kavanaugh ML. Challenges and strategies for contraceptive care in independent abortion clinics in the United States, 2017. Sex Reprod Healthc. 2019;21:102-7. DOI: 10.1016/j.srhc.2019.07.001.
223. White K, Portz KJ, Whitfield S, Nathan S. Women's postabortion contraceptive preferences and access to family planning services in Mississippi. Womens Health Iss. 2020;30(3):176-83. DOI: 10.1016/j.whi.2020.01.004.
224. Goyal V, Madison AM, Powers DA, Potter JE. Impact of contraceptive counseling on Texans who can and cannot receive no-cost post-abortion contraception. Contraception. 2021;104(5): 512-7. DOI: 10.1016/j.contraception.2021.05.017.
225. Schmidt-Hansen M, Hawkins JE, Lord J, et al. Long-acting reversible contraception immediately after medical abortion: Systematic review with meta-analyses. Hum Reprod Update. 2020;26(2):141-60. DOI: 10.1093/humupd/dmz040.
226. Shimoni N, Davis A, Ramos ME, Rosario L, Westhoff C. Timing of copper intrauterine device insertion after medical abortion. Obstet Gynecol. 2011;118(3):623-8. DOI: 10.1097/AOG.0b013e31822ade67.
227. Betstadt SJ, Turok DK, Kapp N, Feng KT, Borgatta L. Intrauterine device insertion after medical abortion. Contraception. 2011;83(6):517-21. DOI: 10.1016/j.contraception.2010.10.006.
228. Pohjoranta E, Suhonen S, Mentula M, Heikinheimo O. Intrauterine contraception after medical abortion: factors affecting success of early insertion. Contraception. 2017;95(3):257-62. DOI: 10.1016/j.contraception.2016.10.012.
229. Korjamo R, Mentula M, Heikinheimo O. Fast-track vs. delayed insertion of the levonorgestrel-releasing intrauterine system after early medical abortion — a randomized trial. Contraception. 2017;96(5):344-51. DOI: 10.1016/j.contraception.2017.07.008.
230. Sääv I, Stephansson O, Gemzell-Danielsson K. Early versus delayed insertion of intrauterine contraception after medical abortion - a randomized controlled trial. PLoS One. 2012;7(11). DOI: 10.1371/journal.pone.0048948.
231. Okusanya BO, Oduwole O, Effa EE. Immediate postabortal insertion of intrauterine devices. Cochrane Database Syst Rev. 2014;2014(7):CD001777. DOI: 10.1002/14651858.CD001777.pub4.

232. Steenland MW, Tepper NK, Curtis KM, Kapp N. Intrauterine contraceptive insertion postabortion: a systematic review. Contraception. 2011;84(5):447-64. DOI: 10.1016/j.contraception.2011.03.007.
233. Cremer M, Bullard KA, Mosley RM, et al. Immediate vs. delayed post-abortal copper T 380A IUD insertion in cases over 12 weeks of gestation. Contraception. 2011;83(6):522-7. DOI: 10.1016/j.contraception.2010.10.005.
234. Bednarek PH, Creinin MD, Reeves MF, et al. Immediate versus delayed IUD insertion after uterine aspiration. N Engl J Med. 2011;364(23):2208-17. DOI: 10.1056/NEJMoa1011600.
235. Hohmann HL, Reeves MF, Chen BA, Perriera LK, Hayes JL, Creinin MD. Immediate versus delayed insertion of the levonorgestrel-releasing intrauterine device following dilation and evacuation: a randomized controlled trial. Contraception. 2012;85(3):240-5. DOI: 10.1016/j.contraception.2011.08.002.
236. Patil E, Bednarek PH. Immediate intrauterine device insertion following surgical abortion. Obstet Gynecol Clin North Am. 2015;42(4):583-91. DOI: 10.1016/j.ogc.2015.08.002.
237. Kim C, Nguyen AT, Berry-Bibee E, Ermias Y, Gaffield ME, Kapp N. Systemic hormonal contraception initiation after abortion: A systematic review and meta-analysis. Contraception. 2021;103(5):291-304. DOI: 10.1016/j.contraception.2021.01.017.
238. Fine PM, Tryggestad J, Meyers NJ, Sangi-Haghpeykar H. Safety and acceptability with the use of a contraceptive vaginal ring after surgical or medical abortion. Contraception. 2007;75(5):367-71. DOI: 10.1016/j.contraception.2007.01.009.
239. Gemzell-Danielsson K, Kallner HK. Post abortion contraception. Womens Health. 2015;11(6):779-784. DOI: 10.2217/whe.15.72.
240. Curtis KM, Tepper NK, Jatlaoui TC, et al. U.S. medical eligibility criteria for contraceptive use, 2016. MMWR Recomm Rep. 2016;65(3):1-103. DOI: 10.15585/mmwr.rr6503a1.
241. Barros Pereira I, Carvalho RM, Graça LM. Intra-abortion contraception with etonogestrel subdermal implant. Eur J Obstet Gynecol Reprod Biol. 2015;185:33-5. DOI: 10.1016/j.ejogrb.2014.11.025.
242. Douthwaite M, Candelas JA, Reichwein B, Eckhardt C, Ngo TD, Domínguez A. Efficacy of early induced medical abortion with mifepristone when beginning progestin-only contraception on the same day. Int J Gynecol Obstet. 2016;133(3):329-33. DOI: 10.1016/j.ijgo.2015.11.009.
243. Hognert H, Kopp Kallner H, Cameron S, et al. Immediate versus delayed insertion of an etonogestrel releasing implant at medical abortion—a randomized controlled equivalence trial. Hum Reprod. 2016;31(11):2484-90. DOI: 10.1093/humrep/dew238.
244. Raymond EG, Weaver MA, Tan YL, et al. Effect of immediate compared with delayed insertion of etonogestrel implants on medical abortion efficacy and repeat pregnancy. Obstet Gynecol. 2016;127(2):306-12. DOI: 10.1097/AOG.0000000000001274.
245. Raymond EG, Weaver MA, Louie KS, et al. Effects of depot medroxyprogesterone acetate injection timing on medical abortion efficacy and repeat pregnancy. Obstet Gynecol. 2016;128(4):739-45. DOI: 10.1097/AOG.0000000000001627.
246. Roe AH, Bartz D. Society of Family Planning clinical recommendations: contraception after surgical abortion. Contraception. 2019;99(1):2-9. DOI: 10.1016/j.contraception.2018.08.016.

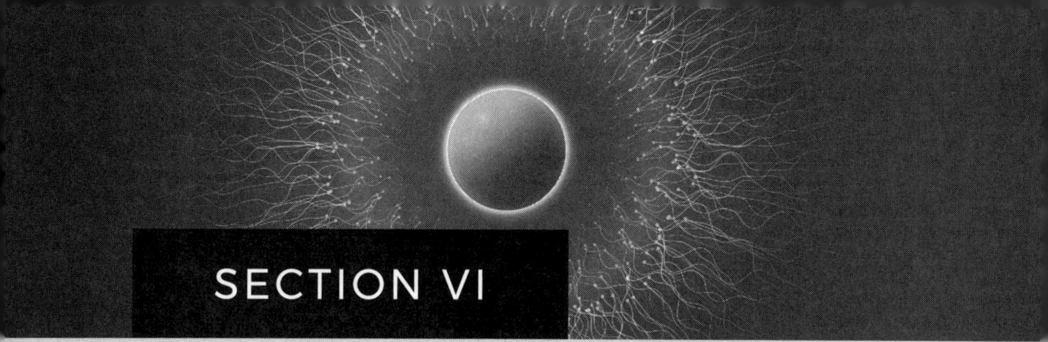

SECTION VI

Resources

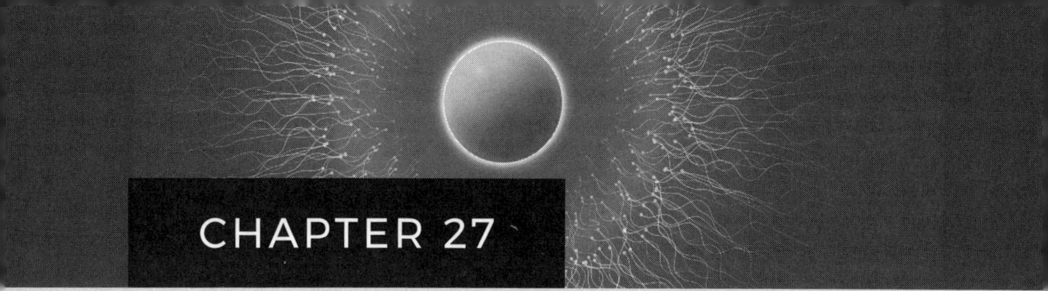

CHAPTER 27

Digital Resources for Health and Medical Information

Brian T. Nguyen, MD, MSc
Leo Han, MD, MPH

KEY POINTS

- Advances in information and communication technology have produced a vast universe of digital health and medical resources for both health care providers and individuals.
- While digital resources are easily accessible and constantly being updated, their quality can be variable and/or their sources not reputable. Consumers of reproductive health information may be more vulnerable to misinformation given the lack of consistent sex education in the United States and the young age at which this information becomes relevant.
- The Centers for Disease Control and Prevention's Medical Eligibility Criteria and Selective Practice Recommendations website and mobile app are key resources for *Contraceptive Technology* readers. These digital resources will have answers to most contraceptive questions that a health care provider might have when initiating contraceptives with their clients. These resources also are maintained regularly.

- **Top three family planning websites:**

The Centers for Disease Control and Prevention: https://www.cdc.gov/	Essential resource for health care providers. Reliable and regularly updated home to the US Medical Eligibility Criteria and Selective Practice Recommendations (MEC/SPR), sexually transmitted infection (STI) treatment guidelines, and updates on infectious disease outbreaks
Bedsider: https://www.bedsider.org/	One of the best person-centered contraceptive resources on the web, Bedsider now has tools to help individuals find family planning clinics, links to telehealth and birth control-by-mail services, a separate provider resource site, and now its very own contraceptive reminder app.

Innovating Education in Reproductive Health: https://innovating-education.org/	A free directory of curricula and downloadable multimedia learning tools about sexual and reproductive health, inclusive of contraception and abortion, for health professionals and health educators. This resource is unique in its inclusion of contraceptive guidance from a reproductive health equity lens.

- **Top three "must-have" family planning apps (*available on Apple* and *Android* (G) *platforms*):**

Contraceptive Guidance for Health Care Providers from the CDC	Easy-to-use, easily searchable mobile app version of the US Medical Eligibility Criteria and Selected Practice Recommendations (MEC/SPR).
STI Treatment Guidelines from the CDC (Updated August 2022)	A reference guide for health care professionals for quickly finding the most evidence-based screening and treatment regimens for STIs. There is also an online STI Tx Quick Guide on the CDC website (https://www.cdc.gov/stiapp/index.html).
The Prevention Task Force App (previously known as the AHRQ ePSS)	Interactive, patient characteristic-specific mobile app that compiles and simplifies preventative health recommendations from the US Preventative Services Task Force (USPSTF) for clinicians.

This section provides general background information regarding the rise and importance of digital health resources as well as a curated guide to digital resources, relevant to family planning, in the form of websites, mobile applications, and social media.

The Rise of Digital Resources

Prior to the rise of the internet, the volume of digital resources was limited to digital transcriptions of written media and audio and visual recordings from large academic institutions and publishers. Access to digital resources with the most up-to-date information was limited to affiliated parties, libraries, and individuals who could afford to purchase them. Consequently, access to digital health and medical information was limited primarily to health care providers (HCP). Prior to the internet, individuals were reliant on their HCPs to be their primary source of guidance for health and medical information and decision-making. However, rapid developments in the internet and communication technology in the last two decades have made information freely accessible and transformed the provider-client relationship such that today, HCPs are not only responsible for providing information, but also supporting their clients' search for and use of digital information.

Estimates from the United Nations and World Bank as of 2016 indicate that approximately half of the world population is using the internet, constituting nearly

3.5 billion users. As fewer than 5% of the world's population was using the internet two decades ago, this development represents unprecedented growth.[1] As both a freely accessible repository for information and a forum for the continuous discussion and development of new information in the form of websites and apps, the internet is a vast universe of digital resources. In the United States, more than 80% adults use the internet, nearly 75% of whom have used it to find health information in the past year; women are more likely than men to do so (79% vs. 65%).[2] With recent developments in mobile technology, the availability of digital health and medical information has never been greater. According to US survey data from 2021, 97% of US adults own a mobile phone,[3] and over half of users have some kind of health-related app downloaded on their phone.[4] Today, the majority of US internet use is accessed via mobile technology, most of which occurs in self-contained apps.[5] These are transforming the landscape of digital resources to include not only a wider breadth of available information, but also user-specific tools that directly impact health and/or help people access health care.

The Impact of Digital Resources

The availability of these digital resources has the potential to empower people by increasing individual awareness of and access to both health-related knowledge and services. These resources can support and contribute to patient autonomy, which forms the basis of person-centered care.[6] Given the quantity of information found on the internet and the individual's ability to access this information both conveniently and anonymously (particularly with respect to sensitive topics, such as reproductive and sexual health), people commonly resort to digital resources first, prior to meeting with HCPs, so that they are better able to have effective exchanges and make informed decisions.[7] Digital resources have effectively transformed how person-centered health care is provided, moving towards a model of improved quality through informed choices and shared decision making.[8,9] Additionally, digital resources serve as an important tool for people to continue to expand their knowledge after time-limited clinical encounters.

The amount of clinical research being published continues to grow at an increasing rate.[10] Health care providers are thus responsible for more information than ever and expected to constantly maintain up-to-date knowledge of medical evidence, health care policy, and professional guidelines. Fortunately, digital resources help HCPs to maintain their expertise. Online digital resources provide clinicians with mobile, easily accessible, up-to-date, immediate answers to their clients' clinical questions. Globally, the expansion of access to digital resources to academic physicians in developing countries has enabled them to train other HCPs, ultimately addressing the global shortage of medical personnel and protecting the human right to health.

The Perils of Digital Resources

While the expansion of information technology has created a digital universe of medical resources, finding the most reliable resource with the right information can be a challenge. Increases in the volume of digital information may decrease the user's chances of finding the most appropriate source of information in the least amount of time.[11] As there is no restriction on the content that can be uploaded to the internet or on the types of apps that are developed for mobile phones, digital resources do not necessarily receive oversight from experts and can vary widely in their quality.[12] Unlike traditional print sources, which have publishers and editors to ensure the quality of content, digital resources do not have the same controls. In a systematic review of 79 studies that examined the accuracy and utility of digital health resources found on the internet, nearly 75% expressed concerns regarding the quality of digital content.[13] While there are many high-quality digital resources available to consumers, there are arguably many more "resources" that represent anecdotal evidence, specific opinion, or commercial interest.

Furthermore, in a study examining how lay users searched for answers to specific health-related queries on the internet, users endorsed the importance of the credibility of their sources of information; however, in observations of their browsing practices, these users never examined the "About Us" sections of websites to verify credibility, and when interviewed, could not recall the sources from which they derived their health information.[14] Inexperienced or unguided users of digital resources likely will be met with frustration, misinformation, incomplete information, or even disinformation. Finally, social media platforms also increase the passage of person-to-person information. The interconnectedness of people through the internet creates even more ways health information can be found, amplified, and distorted.[15]

While digital resources for health and medical information can be more comprehensive than that which can be provided by a HCP during a clinical encounter, these resources do not always relay how the information should be used or how it may fit into the context of a patient's condition or concern. For this reason, helping clients navigate the digital landscape plays a new but increasingly important role in the overall counseling that HCPs provide. (See Chapter 4, Person-Centered Reproductive Health Conversations and Contraceptive Counseling.)

The Range of Digital Resources

The distinctions between websites and mobile apps are becoming increasingly blurred. Many professional organizations now offer the user the ability to subscribe and receive content updates via e-mail, as well as view content that is tailored to their specific interests. Additionally, several organizations have optimized their websites to be viewed on mobile phones, with others even developing their own mobile health apps. Consequently, rather than divide the following resource guide by website and mobile health app, we will provide a directory of relevant resources linked to a professional organization, followed by a general description of the types of commercial resources currently available. The goal of including commercial resources is not to endorse any particular one, but rather to ensure that readers are aware of the landscape of resources being utilized by their clients.

Digital Resources Within Contraceptive Technology

As the content in *Contraceptive Technology* remains static until the next edition, this section is meant to the direct the reader to additional, credible digital resources (websites and mobile apps) and consensus guidelines from organizations that are well-accepted by health care professionals.

In this section, we also provide a list with guidance specific to the HCP audience of *Contraceptive Technology* and their patients in how to better navigate and utilize the expanse of digital health and medical resources. As more than 75% of individuals will begin their search for health information by using popular search engines such as Google, they may face difficulty in parsing out the most appropriate sources for their queries. HCPs thus should have a repository of useful digital resources. HCPs can then direct clients to these trusted sites or applications for further information.

Our list is not exhaustive, nor does it guarantee that listed sites will be regularly maintained or updated. While we strive to choose digital resources without commercial interests or undertones, some of these still may contain endorsement of specific branded products or services. This list does not intend to make any endorsements of anything other than the digital resources themselves. The information in this section is only accurate up to the time of this edition's publication.

Digital Resources from Professional Groups and Societies[a]

1. **Contraceptive Guidance for Health Care Providers from the CDC (G) (C)** (https://www.cdc.gov/reproductivehealth/contraception/contraception_guidance.htm) The Centers for Disease Control and Prevention (CDC) is an essential resource for issues related to reproductive, maternal, and infant health. True to its name, it is also the first resource for clinical concerns regarding outbreaks, such as with COVID-19 (https://www.cdc.gov/vaccines/covid-19/clinical-considerations/interim-considerations-us.html#contraindications), as well as changes to clinical recommendations based upon changes in disease prevalence and antibiotic resistance, particularly in the case of sexually transmitted infections (https://www.cdc.gov/std/default.htm). Most pertinent to contraception, the CDC website has made digitally available in many formats their indispensable 2016 US Medical Eligibility Criteria for Contraceptive Use (US MEC) and 2016 US Selected Practice Recommendations for Contraceptive Use (US SPR). Full versions of the MEC and SPR, complete with clarification, comments, and evidence, are available from this portal. In addition, the popular color-coded MEC charts and visual patient-centered effectiveness charts are also available on the website. Additionally, the CDC has released a user-friendly phone app (CDC Contraception) that is available for both iPhone and Android platforms (see **Figure 27-1**). The MEC can be searched by multiple conditions or methods with the app while the SPR is organized by topic. This app is free to download and use.
2. **STI Treatment Guidelines from the CDC (C) (G)**
CDC's app for the 2021 CDC STI Treatment Guidelines is available at https://www.cdc.gov/std/treatment-guidelines/provider-resources.htm. Prior to its release in August 2022, providers could only access the 2015 version, which was outdated (and not recommended), illustrating one of the pitfalls of digital

a Digital resources listed with indication of intended audience as follows: **(C)** clinicians, **(I)** individuals, and **(C, I)** for both clinicians and individuals without a medical background. Mobile app available on the following platforms: **(G)** Android Apple

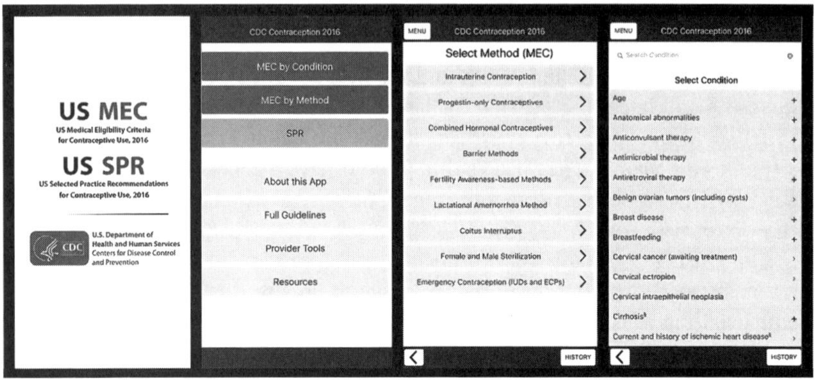

Figure 27-1 US MEC/SPR app screen.

Reproduced from Contraceptive Guidance for Health Care Providers from the CDC located https://www.cdc.gov/reproductivehealth/contraception/contraception_guidance.htm .

resources. Providers are also able to access a mobile-friendly version of the most up-to-date guidelines, called the "STI Tx Quick Guide," which can be found at https://www.cdc.gov/stiapp/index.html. The app and website are the go-to resources for HCPs looking for the most up-to-date STI treatment guidelines. The site is well-organized and easy to use in comparison to searching the full website for the appropriate treatment algorithm; the new app is organized similarly to its excellent predecessor.

3. **Bedsider** (https://www.bedsider.org/) **(G)** ** (C, I)**
   If you have a client who wants information about contraception, https://www.bedsider.org is a visually engaging, patient-centered website full of interactive, informative features that provide simplified yet comprehensive answers. For each contraceptive method, Bedsider provides people with information on efficacy, cost, side effects, use, and commonly encountered problems. Bedsider has a function that allows users to compare methods side-by-side, stratifying for multiple characteristics that may be important to a potential user. Beyond information about contraceptives, Bedsider also includes a large repository of content about sexuality and sexual health, called "Frisky Fridays," and about contraceptive behavior, pertinent to all genders. The site includes multimedia video "stories" from real users of the method, describing their experiences, as well as blog posts, reviews, web content–styled articles, and humorous, informational videos. In addition to contraceptive resources and sexual health/wellness content, Bedsider now has important links related to obtaining contraceptives. Individuals can input their zip code into the site and obtain an updated list of clinics in the area and online services that can prescribe and deliver contraception to the client. They also provide separate searches for reproductive health centers and abortion providers by zip code. Bedsider also offers a mobile app that provides clients with reminders for contraceptive use and administration, applicable to the pill, patch, ring, and injection. Bedsider also has a site designed for providers that contains, among other things, research summaries, educational materials, charts and posters, training opportunities, and links.

4. **The Agency for Healthcare Research & Quality** (https://www.ahrq.gov/) (G) (C)
   As family planning is considered to be an essential component of preventive health care, its provision often is paired with other preventive health services. The most up-to-date guidelines are located on the Agency for Healthcare Research and Quality's (AHRQ) website. The AHRQ is a component of the US Department of Health and Human Services. As such, the site links to the US Preventive Services Task Force (USPSTF) guidelines. Additionally, the site also is connected to the National Guidelines Clearinghouse, a centralized repository of guidelines from national and international health organizations. While the website is a comprehensive repository, users may find it difficult to find a streamlined set of practice guidelines. In such an event, users may want to use the revamped app now called the Prevention TaskForce app (**Figure 27-2**). This app allows HCPs to search and browse recommendations multiple ways. Additionally, the guidelines can be accessed offline once downloaded, making it a valuable resource for rural primary care providers.
5. **Innovating Education in Reproductive Health** (https://innovating-education.org/) **(C)**
   A project of the Bixby Center for Global Reproductive Health at UCSF, Innovating Education in Reproductive Health (Innovating Education) generates, curates, and disseminates free curricula and multimedia learning tools about sexual and reproductive health, inclusive of contraception and abortion, for health professionals and health educators. This resource emphasizes contraceptive guidance from a reproductive health equity lens. The site is notable for its video series that is aimed at helping medical educators improve their teaching on these topics.
6. **American Society for Colposcopy and Cervical Pathology (G) (C)**
   (http://www.asccp.org/) The American Society for Colposcopy and Cervical Pathology (ASCCP) is a nonprofit professional society for health care providers who care for patients with human papillomavirus (HPV)-related lower genital

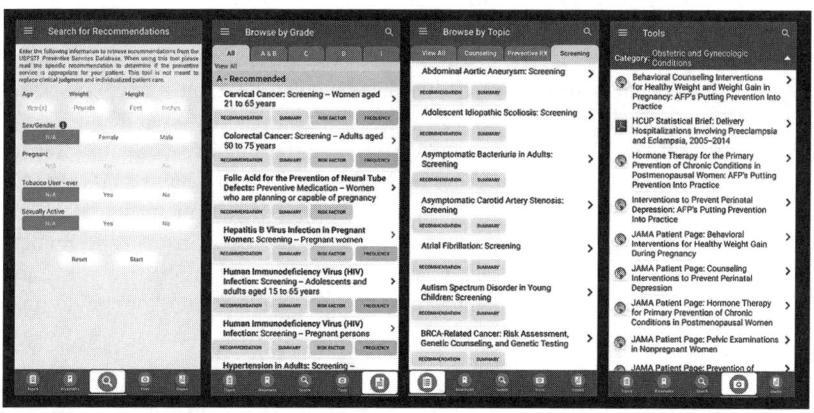

Figure 27-2 AHRQ app screen.

Courtesy of The Agency for Healthcare Research & Quality.

tract disease. ASCCP provides a forum for education and dissemination of knowledge about the lower genital tract. The ASCCP created the guidelines for management of abnormal screening results and cervical pathology. The ASCCP website offers invaluable practice guidelines that reflect the rapidly changing advances in data about HPV-related disease applied to prevention, and management of lower genital tract disease . The website also is a portal for one of the largest sources of training in colposcopy. There are additional resources available only to members, such as a digital image library for use in teaching.

The most widely used resource, however, is the mobile app developed by the ASCCP, which is available for both Apple and Android platforms. Although it is not available for free, the app is inexpensive and indispensable to any health care provider who performs cervical cancer screening. The app is the best digital resource for distilling the unwieldy guidelines into a specific management plan based upon the patient's age and results of their past screening and diagnostic testing. (See Chapter 24, Screening for Cervical, Ovarian, and Breast Cancer for additional guidelines and use of this app.)

7. **The American Congress of Obstetricians and Gynecologists (ACOG) website** (https://www.acog.org) **(G) (C)**
The American Congress of Obstetricians and Gynecologists is known for developing and distributing guidelines that serve as the standard of care for general obstetrician-gynecologists. In addition to the well-known, periodically released, and updated *Practice Guidelines* and *Committee Opinions*, ACOG offers a number of Patient Education FAQs on topics including postpartum permanent contraception, emergency contraception, implants, intrauterine devices (IUDs), and many others. A caveat to this is many of the patient education documents are written at an education level higher than sixth grade, which is the standard for optimizing health literacy. Extensive advice regarding Current Procedural Terminology and International Classification of Diseases, 11th Revision (ICD-11) coding can be found there as well. Many of the materials do not require membership, but some sections of the ACOG website require membership login for access, such as the practice bulletins that guide the practice of many obstetrician-gynecologists. ACOG provides a free app on both Android and Apple mobile platforms. The app allows members to receive up-to-date information valuable for clinical practice, as well as information on national and local meetings. The app also includes an estimated due date calculator for pregnancy, based on guidance from ACOG.
8. **The World Health Organization (WHO): Programme in Sexual and Reproductive Health** (https://www.who.int/health-topics/contraception) **(G) (C)**
For those who have more internationally focused practice questions, the WHO has its own version of the MEC and SPR available in both Spanish and French. Additionally, the WHO has launched its own app version of their MEC and SPR. The latest WHO statements and guidelines are still found online, in multiple languages and updated frequently.
9. **Planned Parenthood Federation of America (G) (I)**
(http://www.plannedparenthood.org/)
Planned Parenthood is one of the nation's leading providers of family planning services to women, men, and young people. Planned Parenthood health centers now offer family planning services in-person and by telemedicine, all of which can be scheduled through their website. Planned Parenthood also offers

a mobile app on both Apple and Android platforms, going beyond providing information to allowing users to order birth control from their phone. While the app is free to download, actual medical services obtained via the app are paid for upon linkage and verification of the user's health insurance plan.
(http://www.plannedparenthood.org/teens)
Providing up-to-date, clear, and medically accurate information, the Planned Parenthood for Teens website helps young people better understand their sexual health. It has nice, crisp webpage and delves into adolescent topics such as sexting, bullying, and LGBTQIA+ issues.
(https://www.plannedparenthood.org/learn/birth-control/birth-control-pill)
Given concerns about misinformation or the complexity of information found online surrounding the correct use of oral contraceptives, Planned Parenthood has developed a website with video instruction and answers to frequently asked questions about correct use and concerns regarding oral contraceptives.

10. **Reproductive Health National Training Center** (www.fpntc.org/ & www.ctcfp.org/) **(C)**
The Reproductive Health National Training Center (formerly the Family Planning National Training Center) and National Clinical Training Center for Family Planning (NCTCFP) are separate websites that have similar, but not identical, resources. They are clinical training resources in family planning supported by the Office of Population Affairs (OPA) for Title X service providers. The sites are a treasure trove of resources for HCPs and clinic administrators regarding provision of high quality, efficient, family planning services. In particular, the NCTCFP offers resources to connect providers with training opportunities for providing long-acting reversible contraceptive methods (https://www.ctcfp.org/larc-link/).
11. **The Office of Population Affairs (C)**
(https://www.hhs.gov/opa/)
The Office of Population Affairs (OPA) administers the Title X program, which is the federal program dedicated to the provision of family planning and other reproductive health services. While the site has basic information and links to information on family planning, it also has a search bar for finding the closest Title X clinic, which may be useful for HCPs looking for a practice where their clients may obtain contraception, particularly long-acting reversible methods if the HCP is not trained to provide them at their institution or office.
12. **American Sexual Health Association (C, I)**
(http://www.ashasexualhealth.org/)
This association provides a wealth of resources on sexual health for all genders and sexual orientations, and specific resources directed at adolescents and young adults. This is a relatively basic site with static content.
13. **The Pleasure Project (C, I)**
(http://thepleasureproject.org/)
The Pleasure Project is an international advocacy organization that seeks to provide sexual education and promote sexual health through a sex-positive, pleasure-based lens. Available resources online include a downloadable tool-kit with exercises that trainers can implement with learners to promote sexual awareness, openness, and more satisfying sexual practices.
14. **Center for Young Women's Health and Young Men's Health (Boston Children's Hospital)** (http://youngwomenshealth.org and http://youngmenshealthsite.org) **(I)**

These websites provide information targeted at adolescents, including guides on a variety of sexual health topics such as contraception, STIs, LGBTQIA+ health, and puberty.

15. **Go Ask Alice!** (http://www.goaskalice.columbia.edu) **(I)**
Geared to young adults, this question-and-answer website contains a large database of questions about a variety of reproductive and sexual health concerns.
16. **The Guttmacher Institute Website (C)**
(https://www.guttmacher.org/united-states/contraception)
For those seeking health policy-focused information on contraception and abortion, the Guttmacher Institute produces continuously updated fact sheets and articles on contraceptive usage, contraceptive coverage, and regulations surrounding contraceptive and abortion provision in the United States.

Conclusion and Future Directions

The amount of digital information available to HCPs and consumers today is unprecedented and is expected to continue to grow. Nevertheless, continued increases in the number of available resources may not translate into effective knowledge if the sources do not control for quality. Most of the resources listed in *Contraceptive Technology* represent sources that we believe will continue to be maintained by professional organizations and thus be updated to reflect the most current knowledge. However, the turnover speed of the internet cannot be overemphasized. Between this edition of *Contraceptive Technology* and the previous one, numerous apps and websites became defunct, and many new ones were introduced. Consequently, it is our additional hope that this chapter becomes a springboard for HCPs to collaborate in the digital space.

Author Disclosures—Nguyen: research advisory board for Myovant Sciences and Sebela Pharmaceuticals, neither of which have projects related to the submitted chapter; Han: none.

References

1. Internet Live Stats. Number of internet users (2016). Vol. 2017. The International Telecommunication Union (ITU), World Bank, and United Nations Population Division; 2016. (http://www.internetlivestats.com/internet-users/).
2. Fox S, Duggan M. Health online 2013. Washington, DC: Pew Internet & American Life Project; 2013. (https://www.pewinternet.org/wp-content/uploads/sites/9/media/Files/Reports/PIP_HealthOnline.pdf).
3. Pew Research Center. Internet/broadband fact sheet. Washington, DC: Pew Research Center; 2021. (https://www.pewresearch.org/internet/fact-sheet/internet-broadband/).
4. Krebs P, Duncan DT. Health app use among us mobile phone owners: A national survey. JMIR Mhealth Uhealth. 2015;3(4):e4924. DOI: 10.2196/mhealth.4924.
5. Wurmser Y. The majority of Americans' mobile time spent takes place in apps. Insider Intelligence; July 9, 2020. (https://www.emarketer.com/content/the-majority-of-americans-mobile-time-spent-takes-place-in-apps).
6. Clarke MA, Moore JL, Steege LM, et al. Health information needs, sources, and barriers of primary care patients to achieve patient-centered care: A literature review. Health Informatics J. 2016;22(4):992-1016. DOI: 10.1177/1460458215602939.
7. Rupert DJ, Gard Read J, Amoozegar JB, et al. Peer-generated health information: The role of online communities in patient and caregiver health decisions. J Health Commun. 2016;21(11):1187-97. DOI: 10.1080/10810730.2016.1237592.

8. Ziebland S, Powell J, Briggs P, et al. Examining the role of patients' experiences as a resource for choice and decision-making in health care: a creative, interdisciplinary mixed-method study in digital health. Program Grants Appl Res. 2016;4(17):1-214. DOI: 10.3310/pgfar04170.
9. McMullan M. Patients using the Internet to obtain health information: how this affects the patient–health professional relationship. Patient Educ Couns. 2006;63(1):24-8. DOI: 10.1016/j.pec.2005.10.006.
10. Larsen PO, Von Ins M. The rate of growth in scientific publication and the decline in coverage provided by Science Citation Index. Scientometrics. 2010;84(3):575-603. DOI: 10.1007/s11192-010-0202-z.
11. Damman OC, Hendriks M, Rademakers J, Delnoij DMJ, Groenewegen PP. How do healthcare consumers process and evaluate comparative healthcare information? A qualitative study using cognitive interviews. BMC Public Health. 2009;9(1):423. DOI: 10.1186/1471-2458-9-423.
12. Hirsch M, Aggarwal S, Barker C, Davis CJ, Duffy JMN. Googling endometriosis: a systematic review of information available on the Internet. Am J Obstet Gynecol. 2016;216(5):451-8.e1. DOI: 10.1016/j.ajog.2016.11.1007.
13. Eysenbach G, Powell J, Kuss O, Sa ER. Empirical studies assessing the quality of health information for consumers on the world wide web: a systematic review. JAMA. 2002;287(20): 2691-700. DOI: 10.1001/jama.287.20.2691.
14. Eysenbach G, Kohler C. How do consumers search for and appraise health information on the world wide web? Qualitative study using focus groups, usability tests, and in-depth interviews. BMJ. 2002;324(7337):573-7. DOI: 10.1136/bmj.324.7337.573.
15. Wilson K, Keelan J. Social media and the empowering of opponents of medical technologies: the case of anti-vaccinationism. J Med Internet Res. 2013;15(5):e103. DOI: 10.2196/jmir.2409.

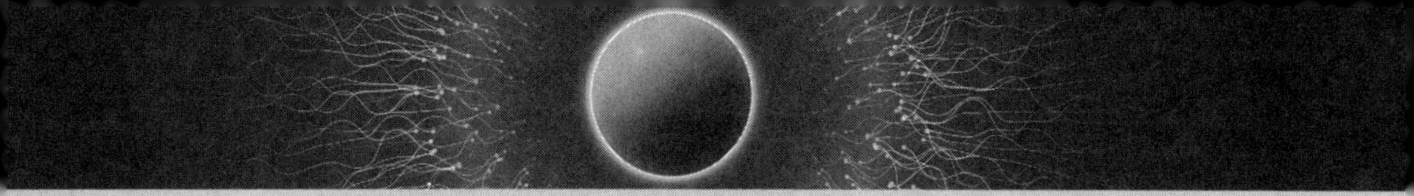

Appendix A

Summary Chart of United States Medical Eligibility Criteria for Contraceptive Use

A color version of this chart is available in the eBook.

Condition	Sub-Condition	Cu-IUD	LNG-IUD	Implant	DMPA	POP	CHC
		I / C	I / C	I / C	I / C	I / C	I / C
Age		Menarche to <20 yrs:**2** ≥20 yrs:**1**	Menarche to <20 yrs:**2** ≥20 yrs:**1**	Menarche to <18 yrs:**1** 18-45 yrs:**1** >45 yrs:**1**	Menarche to <18 yrs:**2** 18-45 yrs:**1** >45 yrs:**2**	Menarche to <18 yrs:**1** 18-45 yrs:**1** >45 yrs:**1**	Menarche to <40 yrs:**1** ≥40 yrs:**2**
Anatomical abnormalities	a) Distorted uterine cavity	4	4				
	b) Other abnormalities	2	2				
Anemias	a) Thalassemia	2	1	1	1	1	1
	b) Sickle cell disease‡	2	1	1	1	1	2
	c) Iron-deficiency anemia	2	1	1	1	1	1
Benign ovarian tumors	*(including cysts)*	1	1	1	1	1	1
Breast disease	a) Undiagnosed mass	1	2	2*	2*	2*	2*
	b) Benign breast disease	1	1	1	1	1	1
	c) Family history of cancer	1	1	1	1	1	1
	d) Breast cancer‡						
	i) Current	1	4	4	4	4	4
	ii) Past and no evidence of current disease for 5 years	1	3	3	3	3	3
Breastfeeding	a) <21 days postpartum			2*	2*	2*	4*
	b) 21 to <30 days postpartum						
	i) With other risk factors for VTE			2*	2*	2*	3*
	ii) Without other risk factors for VTE			2*	2*	2*	3*
	c) 30-42 days postpartum						
	i) With other risk factors for VTE			1*	1*	1*	3*
	ii) Without other risk factors for VTE			1*	1*	1*	2*
	d) >42 days postpartum			1*	1*	1*	2*
Cervical cancer	Awaiting treatment	4 / 2	4 / 2	2	2	1	2
Cervical ectropion		1	1	1	1	1	1
Cervical intraepithelial neoplasia		1	2	2	2	1	2
Cirrhosis	a) Mild (*compensated*)	1	1	1	1	1	1
	b) Severe‡ (*decompensated*)	1	3	3	3	3	4
Cystic fibrosis‡		1*	1*	1*	2*	1*	1*
Deep venous thrombosis (DVT)/Pulmonary embolism (PE)	a) History of DVT/PE, not receiving anticoagulant therapy						
	i) Higher risk for recurrent DVT/PE	1	2	2	2	2	4
	ii) Lower risk for recurrent DVT/PE	1	2	2	2	2	3
	b) Acute DVT/PE	2	2	2	2	2	4
	c) DVT/PE and established anticoagulant therapy for at least 3 months						
	i) Higher risk for recurrent DVT/PE	2	2	2	2	2	4*
	ii) Lower risk for recurrent DVT/PE	2	2	2	2	2	3*
	d) Family history (*first-degree relatives*)	1	1	1	1	1	2
	e) Major surgery						
	i) With prolonged immobilization	1	2	2	2	2	4
	ii) Without prolonged immobilization	1	1	1	1	1	2
	f) Minor surgery without immobilization	1	1	1	1	1	1
Depressive disorders		1*	1*	1*	1*	1*	1*

Key:	
1 No restriction (method can be used)	3 Theoretical or proven risks usually outweigh the advantages
2 Advantages generally outweigh theoretical or proven risks	4 Unacceptable health risk (method not to be used)

Condition	Sub-Condition	Cu-IUD I	Cu-IUD C	LNG-IUD I	LNG-IUD C	Implant I	Implant C	DMPA I	DMPA C	POP I	POP C	CHC I	CHC C
Diabetes	a) History of gestational disease	1		1		1		1		1		1	
	b) Nonvascular disease												
	i) Non-insulin dependent	1		2		2		2		2		2	
	ii) Insulin dependent	1		2		2		2		2		2	
	c) Nephropathy/retinopathy/neuropathy‡	1		2		2		3		2		3/4*	
	d) Other vascular disease or diabetes of >20 years' duration‡	1		2		2		3		2		3/4*	
Dysmenorrhea	Severe	2		1		1		1		1		1	
Endometrial cancer‡		4	2	4	2	1		1		1		1	
Endometrial hyperplasia		1		1		1		1		1		1	
Endometriosis		2		1		1		1		1		1	
Epilepsy‡	(*see also Drug Interactions*)	1		1		1*		1*		1*		1*	
Gallbladder disease	a) Symptomatic												
	i) Treated by cholecystectomy	1		2		2		2		2		2	
	ii) Medically treated	1		2		2		2		2		3	
	iii) Current	1		2		2		2		2		3	
	b) Asymptomatic	1		2		2		2		2		2	
Gestational trophoblastic disease‡	a) Suspected GTD (immediate postevacuation)												
	i) Uterine size first trimester	1*		1*		1*		1*		1*		1*	
	ii) Uterine size second trimester	2*		2*		1*		1*		1*		1*	
	b) Confirmed GTD												
	i) Undetectable/non-pregnant ß-hCG levels	1*	1*	1*	1*	1*		1*		1*		1*	
	ii) Decreasing ß-hCG levels	2*	1*	2*	1*	1*		1*		1*		1*	
	iii) Persistently elevated ß-hCG levels or malignant disease, with no evidence or suspicion of intrauterine disease	2*	1*	2*	1*	1*		1*		1*		1*	
	iv) Persistently elevated ß-hCG levels or malignant disease, with evidence or suspicion of intrauterine disease	4*	2*	4*	2*	1*		1*		1*		1*	
Headaches	a) Nonmigraine (mild or severe)	1		1		1		1		1		1*	
	b) Migraine												
	i) Without aura (includes menstrual migraine)	1		1		1		1		1		2*	
	ii) With aura	1		1		1		1		1		4*	
History of bariatric surgery‡	a) Restrictive procedures	1		1		1		1		1		1	
	b) Malabsorptive procedures	1		1		1		1		3		COCs: **3** P/R: **1**	
History of cholestasis	a) Pregnancy related	1		1		1		1		1		2	
	b) Past COC related	1		2		2		2		2		3	
History of high blood pressure during pregnancy		1		1		1		1		1		2	
History of Pelvic surgery		1		1		1		1		1		1	
HIV	a) High risk for HIV	1*	1*	1*	1*	1		1		1		1	
	b) HIV infection					1*		1*		1*		1*	
	i) Clinically well receiving ARV therapy	1	1	1	1	If on treatment, see Drug Interactions							
	ii) Not clinically well or not receiving ARV therapy‡	2	1	2	1	If on treatment, see Drug Interactions							

Abbreviations: ARV = antiretroviral; C=continuation of contraceptive method; CHC=combined hormonal contraception (pill, patch, and, ring); COC=combined oral contraceptive; Cu-IUD=copper-containing intrauterine device; DMPA = depot medroxyprogesterone acetate; I=initiation of contraceptive method; LNG-IUD=levonorgestrel-releasing intrauterine device; NA=not applicable; POP=progestin-only pill; P/R=patch/ring; SSRI=selective serotonin reuptake inhibitor; ‡ Condition that exposes a woman to increased risk as a result of pregnancy. *Please see the complete guidance for a clarification to this classification: https://www.cdc.gov/reproductivehealth/contraception/contraception_guidance.htm.

Condition	Sub-Condition	Cu-IUD (I / C)	LNG-IUD (I / C)	Implant (I / C)	DMPA (I / C)	POP (I / C)	CHC (I / C)
Hypertension	a) Adequately controlled hypertension	1*	1*	1*	2*	1*	3*
	b) Elevated blood pressure levels (*properly taken measurements*)						
	i) Systolic 140-159 or diastolic 90-99	1*	1*	1*	2*	1*	3*
	ii) Systolic ≥160 or diastolic ≥100‡	1*	2*	2*	3*	2*	4*
	c) Vascular disease	1*	2*	2*	3*	2*	4*
Inflammatory bowel disease	(*Ulcerative colitis, Crohn's disease*)	1	1	1	2	2	2/3*
Ischemic heart disease‡	Current and history of	1	2 / 3	2 / 3	3	2 / 3	4
Known thrombogenic mutations‡		1*	2*	2*	2*	2*	4*
Liver tumors	a) Benign						
	i) Focal nodular hyperplasia	1	2	2	2	2	2
	ii) Hepatocellular adenoma‡	1	3	3	3	3	4
	b) Malignant‡ (hepatoma)	1	3	3	3	3	4
Malaria		1	1	1	1	1	1
Multiple risk factors for atherosclerotic cardiovascular disease	(e.g., older age, smoking, diabetes, hypertension, low HDL, high LDL, or high triglyceride levels)	1	2	2*	3*	2*	3/4*
Multiple sclerosis	a) With prolonged immobility	1	1	1	2	1	3
	b) Without prolonged immobility	1	1	1	2	1	1
Obesity	a) Body mass index (BMI) ≥30 kg/m²	1	1	1	1	1	2
	b) Menarche to <18 years and BMI ≥ 30 kg/m²	1	1	1	2	1	2
Ovarian cancer‡		1	1	1	1	1	1
Parity	a) Nulliparous	2	2	1	1	1	1
	b) Parous	1	1	1	1	1	1
Past ectopic pregnancy		1	1	1	1	2	1
Pelvic inflammatory disease	a) Past						
	i) With subsequent pregnancy	1 / 1	1 / 1	1	1	1	1
	ii) Without subsequent pregnancy	2 / 2	2 / 2	1	1	1	1
	b) Current	4 / 2*	4 / 2*	1	1	1	1
Peripartum cardiomyopathy‡	a) Normal or mildly impaired cardiac function						
	i) <6 months	2	2	1	1	1	4
	ii) ≥6 months	2	2	1	1	1	3
	b) Moderately or severely impaired cardiac function	2	2	2	2	2	4
Postabortion	a) First trimester	1*	1*	1*	1*	1*	1*
	b) Second trimester	2*	2*	1*	1*	1*	1*
	c) Immediate postseptic abortion	4	4	1*	1*	1*	1*
Postpartum (*nonbreastfeeding women*)	a) <21 days			1	1	1	4
	b) 21 days to 42 days						
	i) With other risk factors for VTE			1	1	1	3*
	ii) Without other risk factors for VTE			1	1	1	2
	c) >42 days			1	1	1	1
Postpartum (*in breastfeeding or non-breastfeeding women, including cesarean delivery*)	a) <10 minutes after delivery of the placenta						
	i) Breastfeeding	1*	2*				
	ii) Nonbreastfeeding	1*	1*				
	b) 10 minutes after delivery of the placenta to <4 weeks	2*	2*				
	c) ≥4 weeks	1*	1*				
	d) Postpartum sepsis	4	4				

Condition	Sub-Condition	Cu-IUD I	Cu-IUD C	LNG-IUD I	LNG-IUD C	Implant I	Implant C	DMPA I	DMPA C	POP I	POP C	CHC I	CHC C
regnancy		4*		4*		NA*		NA*		NA*		NA*	
heumatoid rthritis	a) On immunosuppressive therapy	2	1	2	1	1		2/3*		1		2	
	b) Not on immunosuppressive therapy	1		1		1		2		1		2	
chistosomiasis	a) Uncomplicated	1		1		1		1		1		1	
	b) Fibrosis of the liver‡	1		1		1		1		1		1	
exually transmitted iseases (STDs)	a) Current purulent cervicitis or chlamydial infection or gonococcal infection	4	2*	4	2*	1		1		1		1	
	b) Vaginitis (*including trichomonas vaginalis and bacterial vaginosis*)	2	2	2	2	1		1		1		1	
	c) Other factors relating to STDs	2*	2	2*	2	1		1		1		1	
moking	a) Age <35	1		1		1		1		1		2	
	b) Age ≥35, <15 cigarettes/day	1		1		1		1		1		3	
	c) Age ≥35, ≥15 cigarettes/day	1		1		1		1		1		4	
olid organ ransplantation‡	a) Complicated	3	2	3	2	2		2		2		4	
	b) Uncomplicated	2		2		2		2		2		2*	
troke‡	History of cerebrovascular accident	1		2		2	3	3		2	3	4	
uperficial venous isorders	a) Varicose veins	1		1		1		1		1		1	
	b) Superficial venous thrombosis (acute or history)	1		1		1		1		1		3*	
ystemic lupus rythematosus‡	a) Positive (or unknown) antiphospholipid antibodies	1*	1*	3*		3*		3*	3*	3*		4*	
	b) Severe thrombocytopenia	3*	2*	2*		2*		3*	2*	2*		2*	
	c) Immunosuppressive therapy	2*	1*	2*		2*		2*	2*	2*		2*	
	d) None of the above	1*	1*	2*		2*		2*	2*	2*		2*	
hyroid disorders	Simple goiter/ hyperthyroid/hypothyroid	1		1		1		1		1		1	
uberculosis‡ (*ee also Drug Interactions*)	a) Nonpelvic	1	1	1	1	1*		1*		1*		1*	
	b) Pelvic	4	3	4	3	1*		1*		1*		1*	
nexplained vaginal leeding	(suspicious for serious condition) before evaluation	4*	2*	4*	2*	3*		3*		2*		2*	
terine fibroids		2		2		1		1		1		1	
alvular heart sease	a) Uncomplicated	1		1		1		1		1		2	
	b) Complicated‡	1		1		1		1		1		4	
aginal bleeding patterns	a) Irregular pattern without heavy bleeding	1		1	1	2		2		2		1	
	b) Heavy or prolonged bleeding	2*		1*	2*	2*		2*		2*		1*	
ral hepatitis	a) Acute or flare	1		1		1		1		1		3/4*	2
	b) Carrier/Chronic	1		1		1		1		1		1	1
rug Interactions													
ntiretrovirals used for revention (PrEP) or eatment of HIV	Fosamprenavir (FPV) All other ARVs are 1 or 2 for all methods.	1/2*	1*	1/2*	1*	2*		2*		2*		3*	
nticonvulsant therapy	a) Certain anticonvulsants (phenytoin, carbamazepine, barbiturates, primidone, topiramate, oxcarbazepine)	1		1		2*		1*		3*		3*	
	b) Lamotrigine	1		1		1		1		1		3*	
ntimicrobial erapy	a) Broad spectrum antibiotics	1		1		1		1		1		1	
	b) Antifungals	1		1		1		1		1		1	
	c) Antiparasitics	1		1		1		1		1		1	
	d) Rifampin or rifabutin therapy	1		1		2*		1*		3*		3*	
RIs		1		1		1		1		1		1	
John's wort		1		1		2		1		2		2	

pdated in 2020. This summary sheet only contains a subset of the recommendations from the U.S. MEC. For complete guidance, see: https://www.cdc.gov/reproductivehealth/ ntraception/contraception_guidance.htm. Most contraceptive methods do not protect against sexually transmitted diseases (STDs). Consistent and correct use of the male latex ndomreduces the risk of STDs and HIV.

CS314239-A

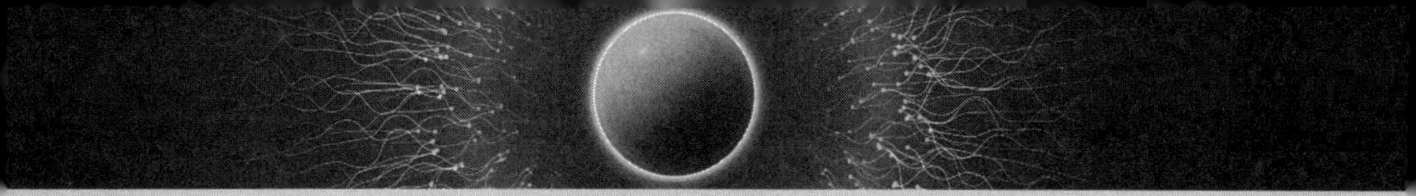

Index

Note: Page numbers followed by *b* denote boxes, *f* denote figures and *t* denote tables.

A

B

C

G

J

K

L

M

N

O

Q

R

S

T

X

Y

Z